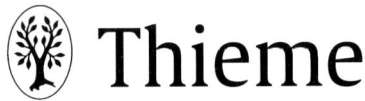

Cranial Neuroimaging and Clinical Neuroanatomy

Atlas of MR Imaging and Computed Tomography

Hans-Joachim Kretschmann, M.D.
Professor and Former Director, Department of Neuroanatomy
Hannover Medical School
Hannover, Germany

Wolfgang Weinrich, M.D.
Professor and Former Head, Neurological Clinic
Krankenhaus Nordstadt, Klinikum Hannover
Hannover, Germany

Foreword by Ruth G. Ramsey, M.D.

Third edition, revised and expanded

664 illustrations
Drawings by Ingeborg Heike and Rudolf Mutschall, D.D.S

Thieme
Stuttgart · New York

Library of Congress Cataloging-in-Publication Data is available from the publisher.

1st English edition 1986
(published under *Neuroanatomy and Cranial Computed Tomography*
2nd (published under Cranial Neuroimaging and Clinical Neuroanatomy) English edition 1992

1st German edition 1984
2nd German edition 1991
(has been merited as one of the most beautiful German books 1991)
3rd German edition 2003

1st Italian edition 1989

1st Japanese edition 1986
2nd Japanese edition 1995

1st Spanish edition 1988

Prof. Hans-Joachim Kretschmann, M.D.
Former Director of Department Neuroanatomy
Hannover Medical School
Carl-Neuberg-Straße 1
30625 Hannover
Germany

Prof. Wolfgang Weinrich, M.D.
Former Head of Neurological Clinic
Krankenhaus Nordstadt, Klinikum Hannover
Haltenhoffstr. 41
30169 Hannover
Germany

Illustrated by:
Ingeborg Heike, Department of Neuroanatomy, Hannover Medical School, Germany
Rudolf Mutschall, D.D.S, Hatten/Sandkrug, Germany

Important note: Medicine is an ever-changing science undergoing continual development. Research and clinical experience are continually expanding our knowledge, in particular our knowledge of proper treatment and drug therapy. Insofar as this book mentions any dosage or application, readers may rest assured that the authors, editors, and publishers have made every effort to ensure that such references are in accordance with **the state of knowledge at the time of production of the book.**
Nevertheless, this does not involve, imply, or express any guarantee or responsibility on the part of the publishers in respect to any dosage instructions and forms of applications stated in the book. **Every user is requested to examine carefully** the manufacturers' leaflets accompanying each drug and to check, if necessary in consultation with a physician or specialist, whether the dosage schedules mentioned therein or the contraindications stated by the manufacturers differ from the statements made in the present book. Such examination is particularly important with drugs that are either rarely used or have been newly released on the market. Every dosage schedule or every form of application used is entirely at the user's own risk and responsibility. The authors and publishers request every user to report to the publishers any discrepancies or inaccuracies noticed.

© 2004 Georg Thieme Verlag,
Rüdigerstrasse 14, 70469 Stuttgart, Germany
http://www.thieme.de
Thieme New York, 333 Seventh Avenue,
New York, NY 10001 USA
http://www.thieme.com

Cover drawing: Renate Stockinger, Stuttgart
Typesetting by primustype R. Hurler GmbH, Notzingen
Printed in Germany by Grammlich, Pliezhausen

ISBN 3-13-672603-0 (GTV)
ISBN 1-58890-145-9 (TNY)   1 2 3 4 5

Some of the product names, patents, and registered designs referred to in this book are in fact registered trademarks or proprietary names even though specific reference to this fact is not always made in the text. Therefore, the appearance of a name without designation as proprietary is not to be construed as a representation by the publisher that it is in the public domain.

This book, including all parts thereof, is legally protected by copyright. Any use, exploitation, or commercialization outside the narrow limits set by copyright legislation, without the publisher's consent, is illegal and liable to prosecution. This applies in particular to photostat reproduction, copying, mimeographing, preparation of microfilms, and electronic data processing and storage.

Foreword to the Third Edition

This is the third edition of the book *Cranial Neuroimaging and Clinical Neuroanatomy*. There have been changes and improvements in all chapters. It is a useful addition to any library as it provides accurate anatomic correlation with easy to read and understand vascular and neurofiber track illustrations, which are of the highest quality. The over-sized pages and well-designed layout allow for easy reading of the text. Furthermore, the use of standard terminology aids understanding.

The introduction includes an expanded discussion of the variety of neuroimaging tests that are presently available as well as the indications for each of these tests. This guidance is particularly helpful to those practicing clinicians who are faced with the dilemma of which neuroimaging studies to request and in what order they should be performed. The advantages and disadvantages of each are highlighted.

This new edition contains additional images that include the vascular supply to the posterior fossa. The rapid development of MRI and neurofunctional imaging has made this type of anatomic correlation even more valuable and welcome.

Dr. Kretschmann is a senior neuroanatomist at the Hannover School of Medicine and Dr. Weinrich a neurologist and neuroradiologist; they work with a dedicated team of young enthusiastic neuroscientists. Together they have used the thin gross anatomic slices of the brain that are then traced and outlined for the various images included in their text. The line drawings in three planes—axial, coronal and sagittal—identify the slice positions that are used and their relationship to the normal anatomic structures. These line drawings, taken from anatomic specimens, provide a clearer picture of the anatomy than the actual MR images and allow ready correlation with the MR images. Each of these slices is then outlined and highlighted to identify the various anatomic structures that are then also annotated in great detail.

The present third edition adds to the excellence of the previous two editions by including actual MR images of volunteers that correlate with the enhanced and annotated line drawings. The excellent quality of the images allows for easy identification on the anatomic structures on the MR images obtained in clinical practice. MR images and annotated line drawings are available in the axial, coronal and sagittal planes. This greatly aids in the three-dimensional localization of various anatomic structures.

As in the previous additions, there are also illustrations of the ventricles and cisterns and a discussion of CSF flow dynamics.

The clear, color-coded, identification of the vascular supply to various areas of the brain on individual slices is very instructive and especially helpful in today's practice where early stroke detection and localization of the areas of involvement are vital prior to interventional procedures.

The color-highlighted illustrations of the fiber tracts for the various neurological pathways are excellent. These can be used by the radiologist to understand the clinical setting and by neuroscientist to aid in the diagnosis and treatment. Many of the cranial nerve pathways and interconnections are complicated, and these illustrations greatly aid understanding of the anatomic locations and relationships. Those involved in functional imaging will find this chapter particularly helpful.

Every effort has been made to update and enliven the text. Consequently studying and learning is more fun and enjoyable. The images have been upgraded and improved throughout. There is also an up-to-date list of references for the reader who is interested in more in-depth reading.

Finally, the book is an excellent reference for day-to-day teaching on a wide variety of issues relating to neuroimaging, including vascular supply and neurofunctional studies. It is a plesure to recommend this excellent text to students at any level who are interested in neuroimaging of the cranium.

Ruth G. Ramsey, M.D., F.A.C.R.
President, Illinois Radiological Society
Councilor, American College of Radiology
Medical Director
Premier Health Sercvices
Clinical Professor of Radiology
University of Illinois Medical School, Chicago

Preface

Our book *Neuroanatomy and Cranial Computed Tomography* first appeared in 1984. At that time computed tomography revolutionized the field of medicine, particularly neurology and neurosurgery. The purpose of the illustrations and text of our book was to provide necessary neuroanatomic information using images of anatomic slices. Our aim was to enable the reader to identify the complex structure of the brain on the monitor for diagnostic purposes to correlate the loss of function with the localization of the cerebral lesion.

The technique of magnetic resonance imaging permitted multiplanar presentations in all desired planes. The second edition, published in 1992 under a new title *Cranial Neuroimaging and Clinical Neuroanatomy*, presented graphic illustrations of anatomic slices in three standard planes.

For this third edition the old MR and CT images of the atlas have been completely replaced with large-sized illustrations, and the number of images has almost doubled. Therefore, the amount of cerebral structures described has increased considerably. In addition, friends of the former editions encouraged us to introduce the arterial territories of the infratentorial space. Nevertheless, this book is intended as a tool for everyday practice. It aids the physician to correlate the patient's symptoms with the neuroimaging findings. This information considerably facilitates diagnosis and can be of great importance for the choice of therapy. The target readership includes neurologists, neurosurgeons, neuropediatricians, neurophysiologists, anatomists, physicians, traumatologists, oncologists, as well as students interested in the neurooriented specialities and especially physicians undergoing further training in clinical neurology.

Acknowledgments

We would like to thank all colleagues engaged in the closely associated departments at the Hannover Medical School. Our grateful thanks especially to Prof. H. Becker, Department of Neuroradiology, Dr. G. Berding, Department of Nuclear Medicine, Prof. K. Gärtner, Central Laboratory for Animal Experimentation, Prof. Claudia Grothe, Department of Neuroanatomy, Prof. H. Lippert, Prof. R. Pabst, and Dr. U. Thorns (†), Department of Functional and Applied Anatomy.

Prof. M. Samii gave us the opportunity to work in the recently opened International Neuroscience Institute (INI) in Hannover. The MR and CT images appearing in the third edition would not have been possible without the help of Prof. U. Piepgras, Dr. T. Liebig, Dr. C. Dalle Feste (INI), Mrs. B. Gehrmann, Mrs. M. Houbolt, and Mrs. A. Hohensee.

Prof. A. Schwartz and P. Brunotte of the Neurological Clinic, Nordstadt Krankenhaus, Klinikum Hannover were kind enough to give critical proposals and valuable clinical suggestions for improvements to the text. Prof. Jean A. Büttner-Ennever from the Institute of Anatomy, Ludwig-Maximilians-University, Munich was most helpful in her comments relating to the vestibular and oculomotor systems.

We would also like to express our thanks to the former co-workers of the Department of Neuroanatomy, Hannover Medical School, who presented excellent dissertations on three-dimensional reconstructions of the functional systems and cerebral arteries: Dr. C. Buhmann, Dr. Andrea Gloger, Dr. S. Gloger, Dr. Anja Schmidt, Dr. Britta Vogt, Dr. H. Vogt, and Dr. D. Weirich. The results of these papers have been mentioned in the text. The technical aspects of our work were supported by Mrs. Nicola van Dornick, Mrs. Ingeborg Heike, and Mr. K. Rust. Dr. Anja Schmidt and Dr. C. Schrader provided invaluable help in correcting the drafts of the manuscripts. Mrs. Claudia Loock, Mrs. Riem Hawi, and Mrs. Züleyha Demir dedicated many hours to reading through the completed manuscripts for final corrections.

Expertise and clinical advice were imparted by Prof. B. Terwey, Institute for Magnet Resonance Diagnostics, Zentralklinikum Bremen, Dr. W. Ruempler, Radiological, Oncological and Nuclear Practice, Stade, and by Dr. A. Majewski and R.-H. Prawitz, MRT-Practice, Nordstadt Hannover.

We appreciate the constructive ideas and advice regarding fMRI given by Prof. J. Frahm, Max Planck Institute, Göttingen. J. Graessner, Siemens Hamburg introduced to us newly specialized technical concepts in the presentation of MR atlas images and was of tremendous support in our work. We dedicate our thanks as well to H. Mahramzadeh, Regionales Rechenzentrum Niedersachsen, Hannover University for his practical assistance in the computergraphic processing of printed copies.

Dr. Gabriele Engelcke, Department of Radiology, Kinderkrankenhaus auf der Bult, Hannover and Dr. G. Glinzer together with Dr. R. Metz, Department of Neurology, Agnes-Karl-Krankenhaus, Laatzen/Hannover were kind enough to assist us with recommended omissions and additions to the texts.

Translation of new chapters and amendments to the third edition were undertaken by Mrs. Nicola van Dornick. Dr. Angela Krönauer kindly checked the complete text for any further changes required. For additional improvements we dedicate thanks to Mrs. Susanne Kretschmann and Dr. Anja Schmidt. The responsibility for the translation rests with the author (K) only.

Following completion of the English manuscript we were grateful for the improvements recommended by M. J. T. FitzGerald, M. D., Professor Emeritus of Anatomy, University of Galway, Ireland (author of the informative and awarded book Clinical Neuroanatomy and Related Neuroscience, Saunders 2002). For further improvements we thank Dr. V. Beckmann, Röttenbach, Dr. Louise McKenna, Siemens AG Erlangen, Prof. Ruth G. Ramsey, M. D., Medical Director Premier Health Services, Chicago, Ill., Dr. H. Requardt, Siemens AG Erlangen, and Prof. G. Vossius, Institute of Biomedical Technics, University of Karlsruhe.

A big thank-you is directed to our respective families for all their patience and understanding during the compilation of the book, especially to Dr. Britta Kretschmann and Mrs. Frauke Weinrich.

Mr. G. Krüger, Production Director of Thieme Publishers has been a supervisory figure behind our book since 1984 and is responsible for the excellent didactic compilation and the make-up of our work. Last but not least, we would like to express our thanks to Dr. C. Bergman, Dr. T. Pilgrim, and Dr. O Schneider at Thieme Publishers for their loyal cooperation in the presentation of the text and illustrations of our book.

Hannover, Autumn 2003
Hans-Joachim Kretschmann   Wolfgang Weinrich

Contents

1	**Introduction**	1

1.1	Background and Objectives	1
1.2	Three-dimensional Coordinate Systems for the Localization of Brain Structures	4
1.3	Intravital and Postmortem Neuroanatomy	10
1.4	Terminology	11
1.5	Abbreviations and Notes for the Reader	11

2	**Neuroimaging and Guideline Structures**	14

2.1	Computed Tomography	14
2.2	Magnetic Resonance Imaging	15
2.3	Emission Computed Tomography	16
2.4	Ultrasound Techniques	17
2.5	Guideline Structures in Imaging Procedures	18
2.5.1	Facial Skeleton	18
2.5.2	Head and Neck Region	19
2.5.3	Neurocranium	19
2.5.4	Cisterns and the Ventricular System	19
2.5.5	Blood Vessels	20
2.5.6	Dural Structures	20
2.6	Clinical Value of the New Imaging Techniques	21

3	**Topography of the Facial Skeleton and its Cavities in Multiplanar Parallel Slices**	210

3.1	Facial Skeleton	210
3.2	Nasal Cavity and Paranasal Sinuses	211
3.3	Orbit	218
3.4	Oral Cavity	227
3.5	Masticatory Apparatus	228
3.6	Lateral Facial Region	228

4	**Topography of the Pharynx and Craniocervical Junction in Multiplanar Parallel Slices**	230

4.1	Pharynx and Parapharyngeal Space	230
4.2	Craniocervical Junction	231
4.3	Blood Vessels in the Head and Neck	234

5	**Topography of the Neurocranium and its Intracranial Spaces and Structures in Multiplanar Parallel Slices**	236

5.1	Neurocranium	236
5.2	Cranial Cavity	238
5.3	Cerebrospinal-Fluid-Containing Spaces	239
5.4	Arteries of the Brain and their Vascular Territories	253
5.5	Veins of the Brain	283

5.6	Cranial Nerves 286	5.7.3	Cerebellum 303
5.7	Subdivisions of the Brain 288	5.7.4	Diencephalon and Pituitary Gland 305
5.7.1	Medulla Oblongata and Pons 288	5.7.5	Telencephalon 307
5.7.2	Midbrain 298		

6 Neurofunctional Systems 325

6.1	General Sensory Systems 326	6.7	Olfactory System 372
6.1.1	Anterolateral System 326	6.8	Motor Systems 375
6.1.2	Medial Lemniscus System 331	6.8.1	Pyramidal System 375
6.1.3	Trigeminal System 338	6.8.2	Motor Systems of the Basal Ganglia 383
6.1.4	Topography of Sensory Disorders 342	6.8.3	Oculomotor Systems 388
6.2	Gustatory System 345	6.9	Cerebellar Systems 394
6.3	Ascending Reticular System 348	6.10	Language Areas 400
6.4	Vestibular System 348	6.11	Limbic System 404
6.5	Auditory System 354	6.12	Autonomic Nervous System 412
6.6	Visual System 361		

7 Neurotransmitters and Neuromodulators 415

7.1	Catecholaminergic Neurons 416	7.6	Glutamatergic and Aspartatergic
7.1.1	Dopaminergic Neurons 416		Neurons 419
7.1.2	Noradrenergic Neurons 417	7.7	Peptidergic Neurons 419
7.1.3	Adrenergic Neurons 417	7.7.1	SP-Containing Neurons 419
7.2	Serotoninergic Neurons 417	7.7.2	VIP-Containing Neurons 420
7.3	Histaminergic Neurons 418	7.7.3	β-Endorphin-Containing Neurons 420
7.4	Cholinergic Neurons 418	7.7.4	Enkephalinergic Neurons 420
7.5	GABAergic Neurons 419		

8 Material and Methods 421

9 References 425

10 Index 435

1 Introduction

1.1 Background and Objectives

Medical and technical **advances in neuroradiology** over the last three decades have led to new diagnostic and therapeutic approaches in medicine. Due to the highly invasive nature of the classical neuroradiologic procedures (pneumoencephalography, ventriculography, cerebral and spinal angiography and myelography), they were diagnostic methods of last resort. Specific clinical neurologic indications and precautions were necessary before administration of such procedures. Today, pneumoencephalography, ventriculography, cerebral and spinal angiography and myelography have been replaced by neuroimaging or reserved for special questions.

Modern **neuroimaging** (computed tomography [CT], magnetic resonance imaging [MRI], emission computed tomography, and ultrasound scanning) for the main part is noninvasive. Therefore neuroimaging is frequently performed as an introduction to technical diagnostics and in many cases prior to laboratory tests. The risk of overlooking or belatedly detecting a critical intracranial space-occupying process, impairment of circulation of the cerebrospinal fluid (CSF), or compression of the spinal cord is thus considerably reduced. This holds true for many of the industrial nations that are able to provide the appropriate equipment in sufficient numbers and offer a well-balanced medical infrastructure.

MRI and CT of the central nervous system (CNS) are predominantly used as the **primary technical diagnostic tools**. Modern neuroimaging through the availability of immediate and short-term radiologic follow-up has replaced the long clinical observation of progress, e.g. for the observation of spontaneous regression of subdural hematoma or hygroma or the need for surgical intervention. MRI as **therapy control monitor** for multiple sclerosis has led to the development of new therapeutic concepts and made their evaluation possible. The high degree of sensitivity of MRI enables detection of millimeter-sized tumors (e.g. microadenoma of the pituitary gland, intracanalicular acoustic schwannoma), so that microsurgical operative removal may in individual cases take place without any functional loss.

Today, diagnostic neuroradiology has advanced to the extent that it accompanies and determines the methods of therapy. In addition, **interventional neuroradiology** has been introduced. Often, vascular impairments (especially vascular malformations) and stenosing vascular processes are able to be treated, or even cured, less aggressively using interventional neuroradiology as opposed to open surgical interventions.

The "ready availability" of the wide range of diagnostic possibilities of modern neuroimaging for all physicians may also result in a number of **disadvantages** and even risks for the patients. It must be emphasized that not all intracranial diseases can be detected or excluded at all times with either MRI or CT. Unilateral symptoms do not always stem from the cerebral region. The "image pathology" recognized at first glance may not in fact be responsible for the clinical findings. The correlation of image pathology and clinical findings requires functional and topical anatomic knowledge. The presentation of this neurofunctional correlation is one aim of our book.

Image pathology is neither described in the text nor depicted in the illustrations in this book. Relevant references have been made to neuroradiologic textbooks (17, 66a, 101, 198, 344, 375, 403, 404, 440, 467). Every physician and radiologist should not only be aware of the many positive aspects of the various neuroradiologic procedures but also of the associated limitations and drawbacks. In this way, incorrect investigations at the wrong anatomic location can be avoided. The referring physician must acquaint the radiologist with all relevant clinical data.

The **expectations of neuroscience** in regard to neuroradiology and its further development remain exceptionally high. This applies to magnetic resonance spectroscopy, the development of multidetector and multislice spiral CT, and especially to functional MRI. For this reason, **MR or CT images** and the large anatomic atlas illustrations are of equal size and have been printed side by side in this up-to-date version of our book. Newly introduced to this edition are the T2-weighted MR images corresponding to the T1-weighted MR images (Chap. 8). A number of atlas illustrations have undergone changes, for example where more exact information has appeared in the literature or as a result of our experience.

With **neuroimaging** of the living human body, slices with a thickness of 1–10 mm are usually scanned. These slices consist of small cuboids (**Voxel** = **Vo**lume **x El**ement). Their height corresponds to the thickness of the slice, and the length of their sides corresponds to the image matrix (Chap. 2.1). For each voxel the X-ray absorption is determined in CT, the intensity of the signal in MRI, and the radioactivity in positron emission tomography (PET). Each value determined from a voxel is represented on a monitor or a film carrier at the corresponding point of the image (**Pixel** = **Pi**cture **x El**ement) with a gray scale value or a specific color.

Using **CT** and PET, axial slices are usually taken (i.e. perpendicular to the long axis of the body) because of the necessary rotation of the scanner. Coronal images can be obtained by tilting of the gantry as well as by retroflexion of the head in the prone or supine position. Sagittal imaging of the head is limited when using a CT or PET scanner. Applying **MRI** the plane of the section can be selected freely, which is one of the advantages of this technique. For **ultrasound diagnosis**, the sectioning plane also can be freely chosen, depending on the object of examination. In infants the intracranial cavity can be investigated through the anterior fontanelle, the "acoustic window," in fan-shaped sections.

Nowadays, **computed tomographs with spiral technique** (helical CT) do not scan in a disciform manner, that is, the measured data are obtained disk for disk and then processed further. Here, a highly efficient X-ray tube rotates continuously around the patient who is continuously moved forward during this process. Serial images are processed from a greater measured volume (volume scan). Any desired slice and slice thickness may be generated from the measured volume. Scanning times significantly below one minute can be achieved with the so-called multi-slice technique with spiral CT (Chap. 2.1). Three-dimensional reconstructions of structures of interest can be made with a corresponding software and an efficient workstation. This way, cerebral vessels may be demonstrated following i. v. bolus injection of X-ray contrast medium (CT angiography [CTA]).

The development of digital imaging procedures required a **new orientation of the cerebral anatomy** and led to an altered topical alignment for clinical application. With the introduction of CT, sections were made which appear unconventional to the "classical" anatomist. During the course of evolution of the human brain, the forebrain moved from its original in-line horizontal relationship to the brainstem and became bent into an obtuse angle. This relocation was caused by the development of the upright posture and the enormous increase in size of the neocortex. In many textbooks of neuroanatomy the human brain is illustrated by using at least two series of cross-sections: one series (so-called coronal series) is oriented perpendicular to the longitudinal axis of the forebrain (Forel's axis), and the other perpendicular to the longitudinal axis of the brainstem (Meynert's axis) (219). This procedure is particularly useful in comparative anatomy as it facilitates the extrapolation to the human brain of neuroanatomic results originally derived from animals. In most mammals the axes of the forebrain and the brainstem approach a straight line. In the human brain the two axes form an obtuse angle of about 110°–120°. Therefore, no "ideal" imaging plane exists in the human with which simultaneously axial sections of the forebrain and of the brainstem can be obtained, so that they would correspond to the conventional neuroanatomic sections.

Ambrose (9) chose the **canthomeatal plane** as the most appropriate imaging plane for CT scans. It runs from the lateral corner of the eyelid (canthus) to the external acoustic meatus. Ambrose called this the orbitomeatal plane. The features and advantages of this and other axial sectional planes will be discussed in Chapter 1.2.

Brain images in the living, using coronal and canthomeatally oriented parallel slices, differ substantially from the conventional, postmortem neuroanatomic images (Chap. 1.3). The advantage of these new CT images can only be fully utilized if adequate knowledge of the three-dimensional structures is available to the investigator. As a result, a wide range of books has appeared in the last decades, demonstrating the macroscopic anatomy of the head in axial and **multiplanar sections** (41, 160, 168, 264, 422, 467). Neurofunctional systems, however, cannot be described by gross anatomy alone as they can only be inferred from a synthesis of macroscopic and microscopic findings, and above all from hodological results, hodology being the study of neuronal pathways and cross-linkages in the central nervous system (CNS) (Chap. 6). Graphic illustrations are superior to photographs for the depiction of these synaptic pathways of the neurofunctional systems.

The goals of this book are as follows:

1. **Representation of the anatomy of the brain in three common planes for digital tomographic diagnostics** (atlas section of the book), the illustrations are based on anatomic slices.

A **new illustration technique** has been developed for quick and accurate orientation in the scans. The anatomic structures are shown in the various shades of gray corresponding to those in the CT scans. The gray scale of the T1-weighted MR images only partly corresponds to the illustrations (Chap. 2). The wide spectrum of the MR signal gained from biologic structures, which is dependent on the chosen investigation sequence, could not be taken into consideration in the illustrations. By means of corresponding, large-sized (new) CT and MR images in the atlas section (colored lines at the edge of the page), the reader is given the opportunity to compare the images. All graphic illustrations are based on original anatomic sections (Chap. 8). Macrophotography can only show the surface of the slices. The CT, MRI, single photon emission computed tomography (SPECT), and PET techniques, however, represent the contents of a slice, as they transform voxels into pixels as described above. The advantage of graphic illustrations is that they can show, by means of dotted lines or hatched areas, important anatomic structures such as tracts or nuclear areas that lie within the slice and are not visible on its surface. In our illustrations, microscopically recognizable structures such as certain cortical areas that cannot be shown by macrophotography are also included.

The **illustrations in the atlas portion of this book** (Figs. 4–17, 32–37, 47–60, 69a–78a) are reproduced to scale and **in a defined coordinate system,** according to principles used in stereotactic atlases (4, 11, 44, 337a, 337b, 406, 453, 454), in order to be able to transfer anatomic details of the "model brain" to the patient's brain by means of a particular coordinate system. A detailed explanation is given in Chapter 1.2.

2. Graphic reproduction of the most important arterial territories in the supratentorial and infratentorial space.

The blood vessels and their territories in the coronal, sagittal, and axial brain slices are depicted. The territories of the brainstem and cerebellum within the infratentorial space are included in this edition. In addition, these slices are compared with angiographic images. In this manner, evaluation of the angio CT images, angio MR images (MRA), and the relationship of CT and MR findings to the angiographic findings (DSA) will be made much easier for the clinician.

3. Description and illustration of the most important neurofunctional systems in multiplanar parallel sections.

The main tracts of the **neurofunctional systems** are graphically displayed in axial sections, the most important ones also in coronal and/or sagittal sections. We used serial slices of equal thickness in a rectangular coordinate system. The distance between the slices in the coronal, sagittal, and canthomeatal series is 1 cm, in the brainstem series it is 5 mm. The slices are drawn to scale on a gray background; those in the canthomeatal plane appear as seen from above, the coronal ones as seen from the front, and the sagittal ones as seen from the left. Because of the accurate, to-scale reproduction and the precise positioning of the individual slices in a three-dimensional coordinate system, it is possible for the reader to mentally reconstruct individual structures (Figs. 79–108) or neurofunctional systems (Figs. 109–151).

A computergraphic representation of the neurofunctional systems and the cerebral arteries has been published as a book and also CD-ROM (243, 244). In these publications the above-mentioned systems are portrayed in a pseudo-three-dimensional and in three-dimensional form. True three-dimensional reconstructions in a number of different projections and combinations may be achieved on the computer with the aid of red–blue spectacles.

4. Explanation of the topography of the neurofunctional systems including the location of a lesion and the associated clinical symptoms.

A display of the topography of the neurofunctional systems should assist in the elucidation of monosymptomatic or polysymptomatic conditions from the site of the lesion. The neurofunctional systems and their presenting symptoms will, therefore, be described. Thus, topographic knowledge should help to improve diagnostic accuracy. An agreement between the clinical syndrome and the lesion detected in the corresponding neurofunctional system confirms the topical diagnosis. Any discrepancy between the clinical findings and the neuroimaging may call for reevaluation and for further diagnostic procedures. In addition, the relationship of the lesion to neurofunctional systems can be of prognostic value.

5. Magnified illustrations of the brainstem including T1- and T2-weighted MR images.

In the brainstem the nuclei and the fiber tracts are particularly crowded and they require magnification for their graphic display. The bony artifacts of CT examinations prevent satisfactory imaging of these fine structures. Only with MRI has an almost artifact-free display of the brainstem become possible. Furthermore, the signal difference between the white and the gray matter is greater in MR scans than in CT scans. For this reason a series of 5-mm slices through the brainstem using the coordinate system based on the Meynert plane is incorporated here (Chap. 1.2). Anatomic structures with their variants relevant to clinical practice are described in the text. On the other hand systematic, embryologic, comparative, and descriptive microscopic details of the anatomy of the head are only briefly dealt with. As regards the neurofunctional systems, we have limited ourselves to definite results already published. Speculative statements and research not yet generally accepted were not included. References are given in parentheses (Chap. 9).

The main emphasis of the atlas, its additional illustrations, and text is the reproduction and description of the **brain and its neurofunctional systems**. The normal topography of the head and craniocervical junction are also discussed and illustrated, as diseases of these regions can affect the brain and vice versa. The **normal** tomographic anatomy achievable today with CT and MR imaging will always be the main objective. We did not use any special imaging planes, magnifications, or contrast medium for better MR and CT imaging of a region of interest (pituitary gland, blood vessels etc.) Emission computed tomography and ultrasound will only be mentioned in passing.

The graphic representation and reproduction of pathologic MR and CT images have been deliberately omitted. However, information on pathologic changes and their clinical significance have been included in the text. This gives the physician an indication of the best methods of investigation and imaging to increase the information content. With the knowledge of the clinical findings including the neurophysiologic data, the appropriate imaging procedure can be selected. With precise questions the diagnostic process can be simplified and the therapy optimized.

Neuroradiologists should be familiar with the complex, functionally oriented neuroanatomic knowledge in order to interpret the clinical questions. Neurologists, neurosurgeons, radiotherapists, physicians, pediatricians etc. should be acquainted with the advantages as well as diagnostic drawbacks of modern neuroimaging so as to be able to profit from the beneficial aspects of the procedure. One aim of this book is to bring together all these disciplines, giving them common knowledge and terminology.

1.2 Three-dimensional Coordinate Systems for the Localization of Brain Structures

In 1637 the philosopher and mathematician Descartes (Latinized: Cartesius) published the analytic-geometric basis for **three-dimensional coordinate systems**. A coordinate system is the intermediary between points and numbers. Points in space are determined by means of a right-angled or Cartesian coordinate system. It consists of three coordinate axes at right angles to each other, which meet at the origin or zero point.

In 1906 Clarke and Horseley introduced the Cartesian coordinates for the localization of brain structures into experimental animal research. Based on Clarke's idea, an apparatus was constructed from brass. Its coordinate system was oriented along the median plane of the head and the plane through the external acoustic meatus and the upper margin of the orbit. This orientation served as the basis for the localization and investigation of individual brain structures in experimental research (44). It was not until 40 years later that this stereotactic principle was used in humans. In 1947 Spiegel and Wycis undertook the first human stereotactic operation. In the meantime, extracerebral or intracerebral coordinate systems have been used.

Sagittal Planes

A basic plane of orientation for coordinate systems on the human head is the median plane, which divides the "bilaterally symmetrical" head into two almost equal parts. Clarke and Horseley found that the asymmetry of the head in humans was greater than in cats and in Rhesus monkeys. The median plane can be defined as the y,z-plane of the coordinate system. In comparison with other reference planes, the median plane is easily established, since the bilaterality aids orientation. The planes parallel to the median plane are the sagittal planes.

Axial Planes

The horizontal plane in the erect human is called the transverse plane. In clinical usage a slight tilt of the horizontal plane is also termed an axial plane. An axial plane that uses bony reference points is the German horizontal ("Deutsche Horizontale" [DH], Frankfurt line). This line connects the lower border of the orbit with the upper border of the external acoustic meatus (Fig. 1). **Reid's base line** has as its points of reference the lower border of the orbit and the center of the external acoustic meatus. The difference between Reid's base line and the German horizontal is negligible. Reid's base line is an approximation for the German horizontal.

The **canthomeatal plane** joins the external canthi (lateral angles of the eyelids) with the centers of the external acoustic meatus. Ambrose (9) called this plane the orbitomeatal plane. However this term is also used for the German horizontal plane. In order to avoid confusion, the term canthomeatal plane should be used in preference to orbitomeatal plane.

In cranial CT and PET the brain is generally examined in planes parallel to the canthomeatal plane. With this setting, using slices of uniform thickness, fewer slices are required for a complete examination of the brain than in horizontal planes. This is due to the flattened external form of the forebrain, the long axis of which is not perpendicular to the long axis of the body, but runs almost parallel to the canthomeatal plane. In practice, use of the canthomeatal plane shortens the examination time and reduces the patient's total radiation dose. However, the radiosensitive lens of the eye lies in the field of investigation (see below, supraorbitomeatal plane). Furthermore, medical personnel can easily identify the canthomeatal plane, ensuring reproducible results. From the theoretic point of view, the canthomeatal plane is favored because of the parallel location of the bicommissural line (on a statistical average). This line is an important landmark in stereotactic procedures (see below).

The **bicommissural line**, according to **Talairach** (453, 454), joins the upper border of the anterior commissure with the lower border of the posterior commissure. In a sample of 50 brains a mean difference of less than 2° in the angle between the canthomeatal plane and the bicommissural line was found. In individual cases the differences lay between +9° and −5° (standard deviation s = 1.4).

The retrievable digital image available with **CT investigations** (scoutview, topogram) has led some investigators to choose slices parallel to the orbital roof as a routine procedure for the head. With the help of a scoutview the plane tangential to the orbital roof can easily be adjusted, while the external canthus is not visible in this scoutview. The **plane of the orbital roof**, according to our measurements, varies between 5° and 23° (on average about 14° in 200 individuals) from the canthomeatal plane and approaches the supraorbitomeatal plane. The advantages of the orbital roof plane are: rapid adjustment by tilting of the gantry, the high level of intraindividual consistency in repeated examinations, and in most examinations the lens of the eye being outside the field of radiation. It is also of value in investigations of the posterior cranial fossa (see below). The interindividual variations are, however, greater than with the canthomeatal views (see above).

The slices parallel to the **supraorbitomeatal plane** are particularly suitable for CT examination of the contents of the posterior cranial fossa. In the supraventricular slices the central sulcus appears more ventral in comparison with the slices parallel to the canthomeatal plane. This becomes obvious if the reader adjusts the position of the supraorbitomeatal plane in Figure 46 by tilting the frontal end of the canthomeatally oriented planes upward.

For **MRI** of the brain the patient must be made as comfortable as possible in order to avoid movement artifacts. For anatomic orientation a midsagittal image should be visualized first. For the next views axial slices should usually be chosen. Depending on the particular problem, additional coronal or sagittal views, or both, may follow.

For standard investigations a uniform angle setting is desirable to avoid additional variability in the topographic relations through varying angles. For the axial series we selected slices parallel to the canthomeatal plane (Figs. 44–66, canthomeatal series), and for the brainstem slices vertical to Meynert's axis (Figs. 67, 69–78, brainstem series).

Coronal Planes

For the coronal slices in this book planes of the section vertical to Reid's base line were chosen (Figs. 1–28, coronal series). On the teleradiograph Reid's base line was determined for the head S 63/86 and transferred to the skin of the head. With the help of a set-square and a special locking mechanism, coronal slices perpendicular to Reid's base line were obtained (Chap. 8). A plane constructed through the zig-zag course of the coronal suture does not cut Reid's base line at an angle of 90° as does the "coronal" plane, but at an angle of about 65°. Due to the bilateral symmetry, coronal and axial slices allow a comparison of the two sides, so that one-sided pathology like space-occupying lesions and circumscribed areas of atrophy, differing density and signal intensity can be easily recognized. In the isolated, nonbisected brain there are no landmarks for the determination of the coronal plane. Therefore, pictures of coronal sections of the brain in conventional atlases often differ significantly because of different angles of sectioning (85, 99, 182, 350, 370). The topographic relations of the brain structures appear to change, giving a variable picture.

Intracerebral Coordinates

The experiences in stereotactic interventions showed that the bony and extracerebral reference planes show a greater variability in relation to the brain structures than the intracerebral landmarks (44). The intracerebral landmark most frequently used by neurosurgeons in the **supratentorial space** is the bicommissural line. The aforementioned definition of the bicommissural line according to Talairach uses the upper border of the anterior commissure and the lower border of the posterior commissure, because in the days of ventriculography these were most easily recognizable. With MR technique both commissures can be accurately recognized in the median plane. The diameter of the anterior commissure varies between 2 mm and more than 5 mm. In comparison with a line which running through the midpoint of both commissures, the bicommissural line of Talairach can lead to a deviation of 7°. With an average distance of 17 cm between the frontal and occipital poles of the brain this can lead to a deviation of more than 1 cm on the outside of the brain. Therefore, the use of the **bicommissural line**, which is defined **by the midpoints** of the anterior commissure and the posterior commissure, can reduce potential mistakes in the localization of brain structures. Furthermore, as a result of the partial volume effect, the centers of the two commissures can be more accurately determined than their borders. Consequently, the definition of the bicommissural line, which runs through the central point of both commissures, should be internationally accepted. The central point of the line between the anterior and posterior commissures can be used as the origin (zero point) of the bicommissural coordinate system.

Sagittal slices do not allow any direct comparison between the two sides. The sagittal parallel slices have as their sole reference plane the median (midline) plane. The particular advantage of sagittal slices is that they enable identification and assessment of the midline structures of the brain, particularly the brainstem and some sulci and gyri on the medial surface of the cerebral hemisphere. This applies especially to the calcarine sulcus that runs almost parallel to the axial plane and is often cut tangentially in these sections. In contrast, in sagittal sections this sulcus has a more vertical course within the section and is imaged more clearly because it is affected less by the partial volume effect. The sagittal images are also used to evaluate the presence or absence of the Chiari malformation.

The reference points necessary for the intracerebral coordinate system (bicommissural plane and Meynert's plane) are easy to recognize in the midline section. In the atlas pictures of the sagittal series, in addition to Reid's base line (DH), the bicommissural line (B) will also be given (Figs. 32–37). The **bicommissural line** chosen by us joins the midpoints of the anterior and posterior commissures and runs in the bicommis-

1 Introduction

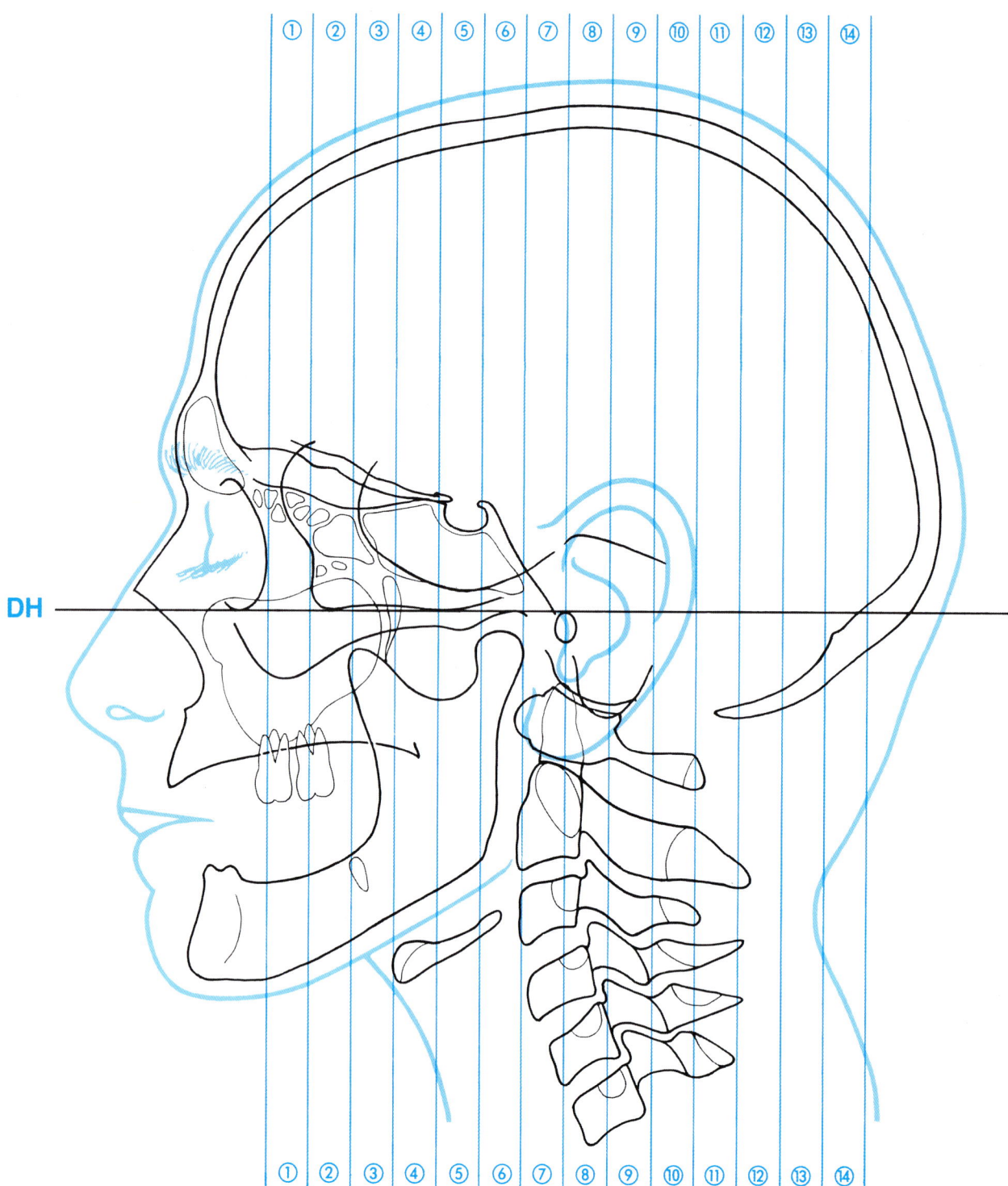

Fig. 1 Position of the coronal slices in lateral view. The 14 slices are described in an anterior to posterior order in the atlas of this book (Figs. 4a–17a and 4c–17c). The encircled numbers indicate the number of the 1-cm-thick slices that are illustrated as viewed from the front. The illustrated surface of each section, therefore, represents the line to the left of the encircled number of the corresponding slice (Chap. 8 Material).
DH Reid's base line

1.2 Three-dimensional Coordinate Systems for the Localization of Brain Structures

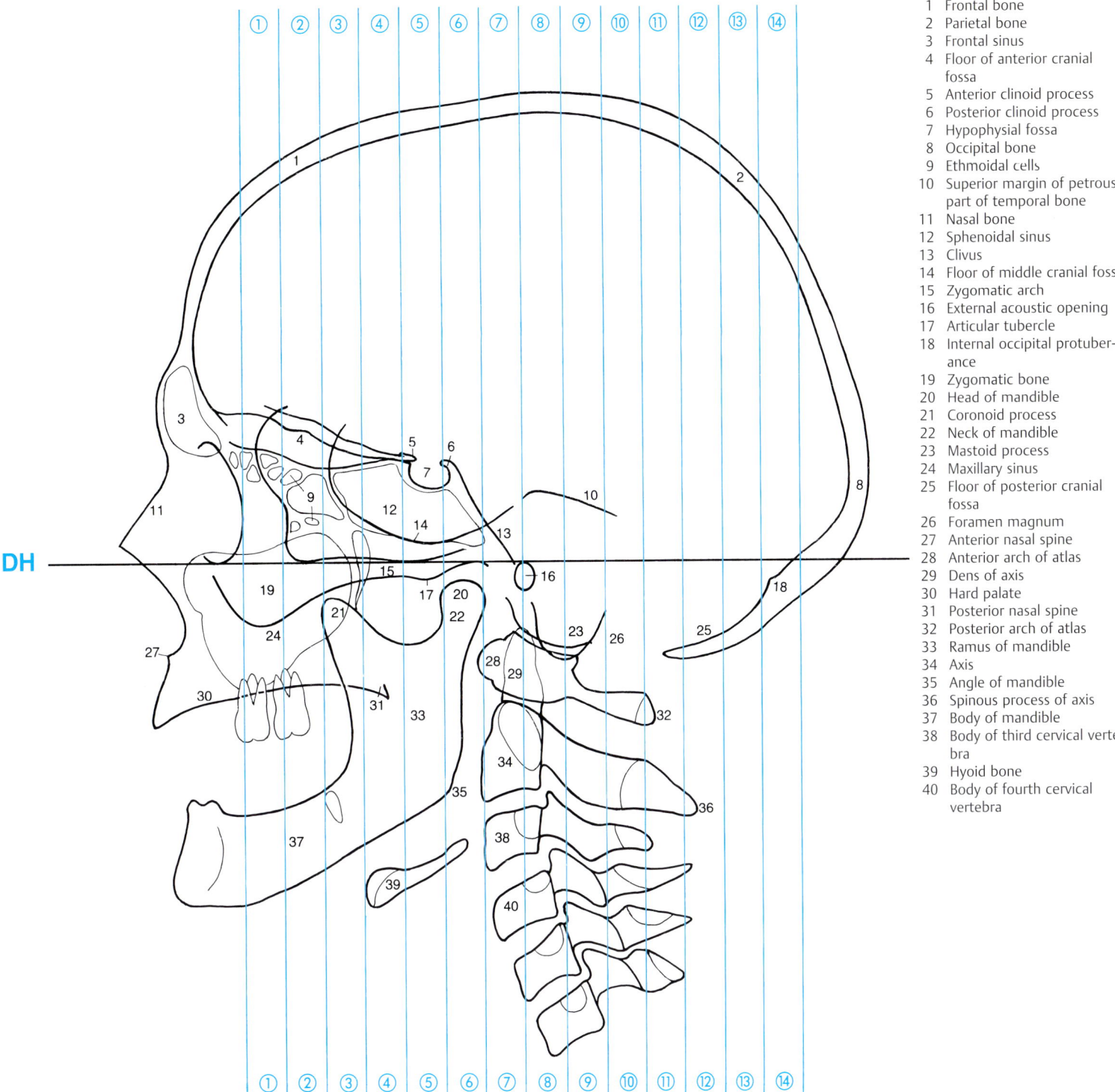

Fig. **2a** Tracing of lateral teleradiograph of the head (Chap. 8). The 14 coronal slices were assembled in their original anatomic form and numbered in anteroposterior sequence. The encircled number indicates the number of the slice.
DH Reid's base line

1. Frontal bone
2. Parietal bone
3. Frontal sinus
4. Floor of anterior cranial fossa
5. Anterior clinoid process
6. Posterior clinoid process
7. Hypophysial fossa
8. Occipital bone
9. Ethmoidal cells
10. Superior margin of petrous part of temporal bone
11. Nasal bone
12. Sphenoidal sinus
13. Clivus
14. Floor of middle cranial fossa
15. Zygomatic arch
16. External acoustic opening
17. Articular tubercle
18. Internal occipital protuberance
19. Zygomatic bone
20. Head of mandible
21. Coronoid process
22. Neck of mandible
23. Mastoid process
24. Maxillary sinus
25. Floor of posterior cranial fossa
26. Foramen magnum
27. Anterior nasal spine
28. Anterior arch of atlas
29. Dens of axis
30. Hard palate
31. Posterior nasal spine
32. Posterior arch of atlas
33. Ramus of mandible
34. Axis
35. Angle of mandible
36. Spinous process of axis
37. Body of mandible
38. Body of third cervical vertebra
39. Hyoid bone
40. Body of fourth cervical vertebra

1 Paracentral lobule
2 Cingulate sulcus
3 Cingulate gyrus
4 Precuneus
5 Trunk (body) of corpus callosum
6 Parieto-occipital sulcus
7 Septum pellucidum
8 Frontal pole
9 Genu of corpus callosum
10 Fornix
11 Interventricular foramen (of Monro)
12 Splenium of corpus callosum
13 Interthalamic adhesion
14 Anterior commissure
15 Third ventricle
16 Cuneus
17 Lamina terminalis
18 Posterior commissure
19 Pineal gland
20 Optic chiasm
21 Superior colliculus
22 Mammillary body
23 Calcarine sulcus
24 Olfactory bulb
25 Olfactory tract
26 Optic nerve
27 Pituitary gland
28 Infundibulum
29 Oculomotor nerve
30 Aqueduct of midbrain
31 Inferior colliculus
32 Culmen (IV, V)
33 Primary fissure of cerebellum
34 Occipital pole
35 Declive (VI)
36 Temporal lobe
37 Pons
38 Fourth ventricle
39 Nodule of vermis (X)
40 Folium of vermis (VII A)
41 Uvula of vermis (IX)
42 Tuber of vermis (VII B)
43 Pyramis of vermis (VIII)
44 Medulla oblongata
45 Tonsil of cerebellum (H IX)
46 Spinal cord

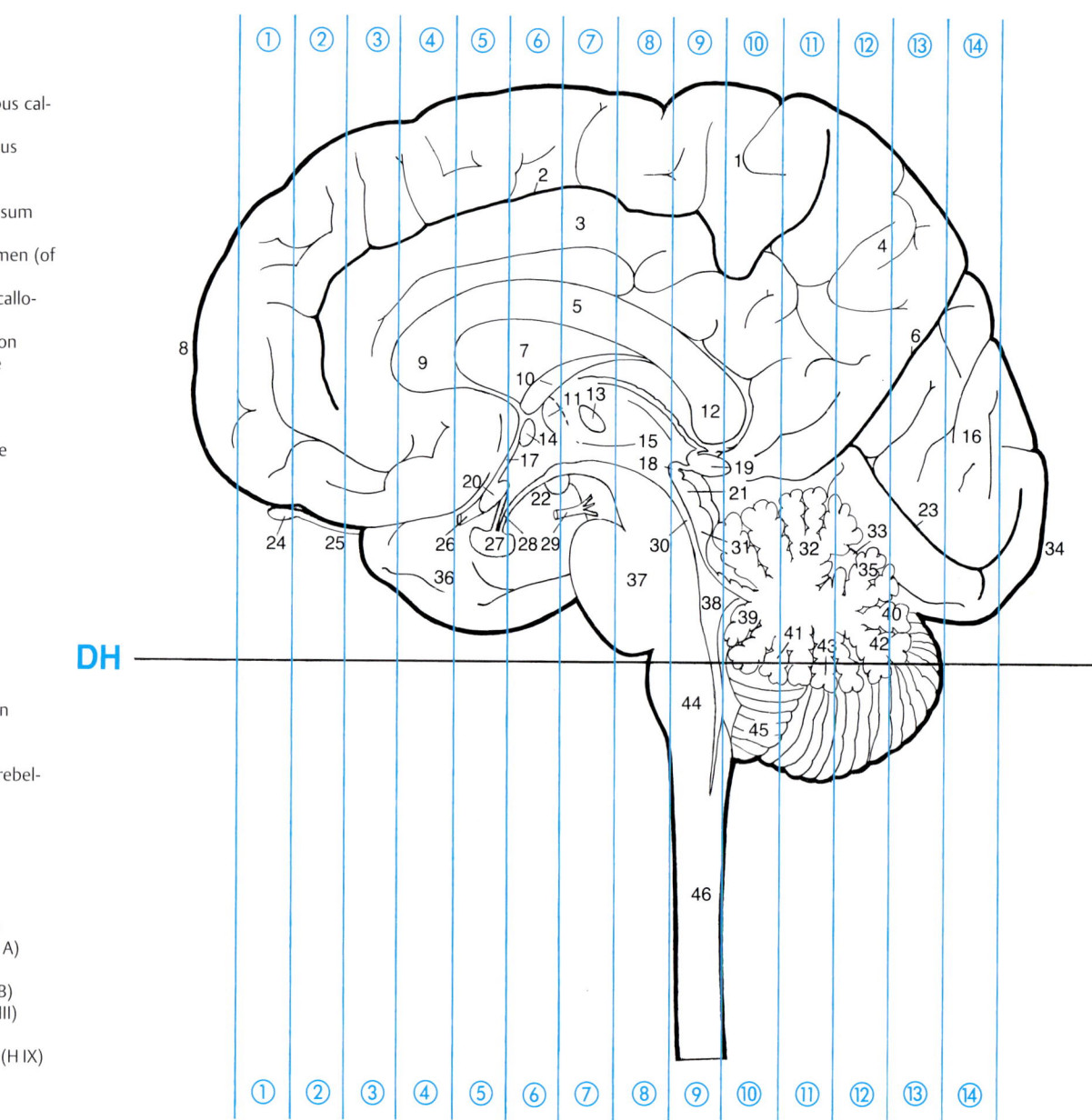

Fig. **2b** Median view of the brain and the cranial part of the spinal cord taken from the same head as in Figs. 1 and 2a. The coronal slices were assembled and numbered as shown in Fig. 2a (Chap. 8).
DH Reid's base line

1.2 Three-dimensional Coordinate Systems for the Localization of Brain Structures

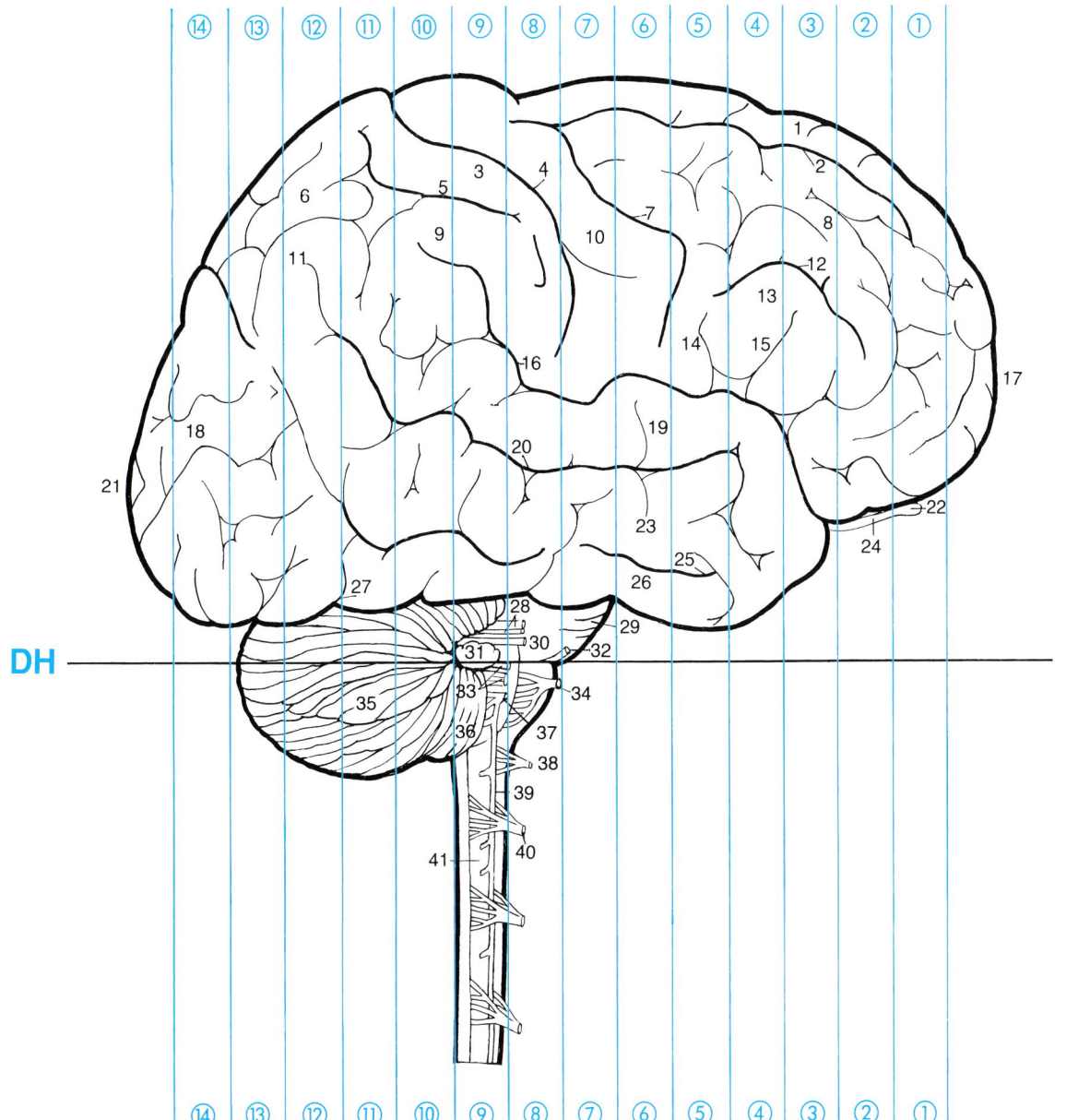

Fig. 3 Lateral view of the brain and the cranial part of the spinal cord taken from the same head as in Figs. 1, 2a, and 2b (Chap. 8). The coronal slices were assembled and numbered as shown in Fig. 2b.
DH Reid's base line

1 Superior frontal gyrus
2 Superior frontal sulcus
3 Postcentral gyrus
4 Central sulcus
5 Postcentral sulcus
6 Superior parietal lobule
7 Precentral sulcus
8 Middle frontal gyrus
9 Supramarginal gyrus
10 Precentral gyrus
11 Angular gyrus
12 Inferior frontal sulcus
13 Inferior frontal gyrus
14 Ascending ramus of lateral sulcus (Sylvian fissure)
15 Anterior ramus of lateral sulcus (Sylvian fissure)
16 Posterior ramus of lateral sulcus (Sylvian fissure)
17 Frontal pole
18 Occipital gyri
19 Superior temporal gyrus
20 Superior temporal sulcus
21 Occipital pole
22 Olfactory bulb
23 Middle temporal gyrus
24 Olfactory tract
25 Inferior temporal sulcus
26 Inferior temporal gyrus
27 Preoccipital notch
28 Facial nerve and intermediate nerve
29 Pons
30 Vestibulocochlear nerve
31 Flocculus (H X)
32 Abducens nerve
33 Glossopharyngeal nerve and vagus nerve
34 Hypoglossal nerve
35 Cerebellum
36 Tonsil of cerebellum (H IX)
37 Accessory nerve
38 Anterior (ventral) root of first cervical spinal nerve
39 Spinal root of accessory nerve
40 Second cervical spinal nerve
41 Spinal cord

sural plane, which is vertical to the median plane (Figs. 32a.8, 32a.11, 32b.12, 32b.15). The bicommissural plane allows a comparison with the stereotactic atlases (11, 406, 453, 454) and facilitates the three-dimensional orientation of extracerebral structures such as the cranial nerves, blood vessels, bones, and soft parts, which are not mentioned in the atlases referred to. The large variability of cortical gyri and sulci of the cerebrum restricts application of the standardized localization systems (441), such as the stereotactic system used by Talairach (453, 454). Therefore, neuroradiologic guideline structures were developed for clinical practice for the purpose of identifying the gyri and sulci that are of clinical importance and significance for orientation (508).

For the **infratentorial space** a Cartesian coordinate system is used; this system is defined by the midline plane, the plane through the floor of the fourth ventricle (Meynert's plane) and through the plane of the fastigium (4). The **plane of the fastigium** is vertical to the midline plane and to the floor of the fourth ventricle and runs through the fastigium (Fig. 67.28). The straight line that runs in the midline plane tangential to the floor of the fourth ventricle is called **Meynert's axis**. It determines Meynert's plane, which is vertical to the median plane. The origin (zero point) of this coordinate system is the point of intersection of these three chosen planes. The brainstem series of the atlas (Figs. 69–78) is depicted in this coordinate system. Due to the clinical importance of this area and to the great number of nuclei and tracts in this small region, a magnified reproduction of the brainstem (Figs. 69b–78b) was chosen. It should illustrate those structures that are of significance in microsurgery of the brainstem.

These geometric–analytic principles on the localization of anatomic structures have been incorporated by the manufacturers of CT, MR, and PET apparatus so that the CT, MR, and PET images are oriented in a coordinate system. A scale or the letters L (left) or R (right) always reproduced at the same place of the coordinate frames serve as orientation guides in this coordinate system.

Coordinate crosses or frames are used in stereotactic atlases (11, 44, 406, 453, 454). Their advantage in comparison with conventional atlases is that they provide the opportunity to reconstruct "in the mind" brain structures such as the caudate nucleus, internal capsule, or central sulcus, using coordinate frames for orientation from one to the following section. In this way one can follow their course in the series of slices and hence locate pathologic lesions in relation to anatomic structures and neurofunctional systems. For this reason the four series of sections in this book have been oriented, cut, and reproduced in well-defined coordinate systems. In the atlas pictures of the coronal, sagittal, and brainstem series, the corresponding 10-mm coordinate frame has been accurately reproduced around the head slices.

The idea of using the **coordinate systems** for the localization of bony structures is also valid for the "mental" reconstruction of complicated bony cavities such as the canal for the facial nerve or the inner ear in the petrous part of the temporal bone. The bony reference planes such as Reid's base line, infraorbital and supraorbital planes retain their localizing significance for surgeons who, when planning an operation, must orient themselves to the skull so that during the procedure they are able to protect the venous channels and the arteries.

With the help of Reid's base line and the meatovertical plane (MV) the inconstancy of the relationship between the skull bones and the brain can be shown. The MV lying perpendicular to Reid's base line is the coronal plane that runs through the center of the external acoustic meatus. In a sample of 25 heads the larger group (14 heads) could be classified as of **frontopetal type** and the smaller group (11 heads) as **occipitopetal type** (136). In the frontopetal type the cerebrum in the lateral view appears to be displaced forward and the central sulcus runs more steeply upward than in the occipitopetal type. The occipital lobes lie far above Reid's base line. In the lateral view the occipital bone is shorter than in the occipitopetal type. With the occipitopetal type in the lateral view the cerebrum is shifted backward and the central sulcus runs less steeply upward and reaches further posteriorly in comparison with the frontopetal type. The base of the occipital lobe lies immediately above Reid's base line or actually touches it. The relationship of the cerebrum in the coronal series (Fig. 3) to Reid's base line is that of the occipitopetal type. The topography of the brain portrayed in the canthomeatal series (Fig. 46) corresponds with a frontopetal type.

1.3 Intravital and Postmortem Neuroanatomy

The new imaging techniques have clearly demonstrated the differences between living and postmortem brain morphology. After death gases collect in the subarachnoid space. The borders between gray and white matter become less sharp postmortem, particularly in CT scans. In MR images there are of course no signals from blood circulation. Postmortem MR images of brains fixed intracranially show so many artifacts that intravital MR images are more suitable for a comparison with the atlas pictures of an anatomic series than MR images in the postmortem state. Although MR images from the heads depicted in the atlas exist, we preferred comparable intravital MR images of other individuals.

Attention must be paid to changes occuring postmortem and changes caused by histologic techniques if findings derived from anatomic preparations are transferred to the living. The volumes of the intracranial compartments, blood, **CSF**, and brain tissue are very difficult to determine exactly, either antemortem or postmortem. There are reasons, however, for assuming that the CSF is partially absorbed by the brain tissue after death. Measurements of the CSF (424) show that after death its volume decreases. In 159 investigated cases the average volume of CSF was 100 ml three hours postmortem and only 49 ml after 21 hours (424). The difference between the volumes of the cranial cavity and of the brain substance becomes smaller after death (348). After death the brain volume increases as CSF is absorbed, the degree of absorption depending on the time interval between death and autopsy. Assuming an average of 100–150 ml of CSF and 1200–1400 ml brain volume in living adults, an error of 5% can be expected after half of the CSF has steadily diffused into the brain tissue after death. This diffusion is likely to be nonlinear in nature, and the postmortem volume increase in more heavily affected brain areas will be correspondingly higher. Any correlation of the size of the cisterns found at autopsy with intravital conditions should be made with caution.

A change in the topographic relation of the brainstem and the forebrain usually develops in brains fixed outside the cranial cavity (extracranial fixation). In most cases the brain is suspended by the basilar artery during fixation. Because the specific gravity of the brain is slightly higher than that of the formalin mixture used for fixation, the forebrain, which hangs downward in the fixation solution, sinks. As the occipital pole generally sinks first, the forebrain alters its proportion and position relative to the brainstem. As a result, sections of brains that have been fixed outside the skull can differ markedly from their anatomy in vivo. Consequently, for anatomic comparisons with CT and MR images, brains fixed inside the skull (**intracranial fixation**) rather than outside should be used. All atlas illustrations in this book are taken from intracranially fixed brains (Chap. 8).

When embedded in paraffin or celloidin for **histologic preparation**, the brain loses 40–50% of its volume (177, 240). In the paraffin process the brain does not shrink evenly. The gray matter, which has a higher water content, shrinks more than the white matter. The frontal cortex contains about 84% water and shrinks on average 51%, while the white matter contains 71% water and loses about 42% of its volume (241). Findings concerning the size and shape of brain structures taken from histologic preparations can be correlated only approximately with in vivo conditions.

1.4 Terminology

The international anatomic nomenclature offers a better supranational understanding of the terminology. The International Federation of Associations of Anatomists established a new nomenclature commission (Federative Committee on Anatomical Terminology) for which delegates were appointed by the national anatomical associations. All anatomists were called up to discuss their draft of the nomenclature in 1997. The final version was agreed on and published as the **Terminologia Anatomica** in 1998 (122). For the first time each Latinized anatomic name was coupled with the equivalent english term, thus enabling scientists and physicians worldwide to use the same names for any anatomic structure. This is an essential prerequisite for international medical communication. Therefore, we too decided to use the Terminologia Anatomica.

In the Terminologia Anatomica the anatomic terms of the head regarding the direction have been replaced e.g. cranialis-caudalis with superior-inferior and ventralis-dorsalis with anterior-posterior. Therefore, the topographic relations regarding the head are described as superior or inferior and anterior or posterior. Eponyms are given in nonlatinized and nondeclined form.

In the case of individual arterial branches, the Terminologia Anatomica distinguishes between artery and branch. Frequently the diameter of the so-called branch is greater than that of the artery (e.g. parietooccipitalis branch and anterolateral central arteries). The term "branch" is customary also for branches of veins, nerves, bones, and bronchi. We, therefore, decided in accordance with clinical usage to use the unambiguous term "artery" for all arteries (238, 474, 501).

Numbers in parentheses refer to publications that appear in the references (Chap. 9).

1.5 Abbreviations and Notes for the Reader

The following abbreviations are used:
ACTH   Adrenocorticotropic hormone
ADH   Antidiuretic hormone
AEP   Auditory evoked potentials
AICA   Anterior inferior cerebellar artery
ASP   Aspartate
B   Bicommissural line
BERA   Brainstem electric response audiometry
Ch   Cholinergic
CNS   Central nervous system
CSF   Cerebrospinal fluid
CT   Computed tomography
CTA   Computed tomography angiography, CT-Angio
DH   Reid's base line (Deutsche Horizontale)
DSA   Digital subtraction angiography
EEG   Electroencephalogram
EP   Evoked potentials
FISP   Fast imaging with steady precession
FLASH   Fast low angle shot

fMRI	functional magnetic resonance imaging
FSH	Follicular stimulating hormone
GABA	gamma- (γ-) aminobutyric acid
GH	Growth hormone
GLU	Glutamate
HU	Hounsfield unit
IF	Inhibiting factor
i.v.	intravenous
LH	Luteinizing hormone
M	Median plane
MA	Meynert's axis
ME	Meynert's plane
MEG	Magnetencephalogram
MEP	Motor evoked potentials
MR	Magnetic resonance
MRA	Magnetic resonance angiography
MRI	Magnetic resonance imaging
MV	Meatovertical line
PET	Positron emission tomography
PICA	Posterior inferior cerebellar artery
PPRF	Paramedian pontine reticular formation
PRL	Prolactin
RF	Releasing factor
SEP	Somatosensory evoked potentials
SPECT	Single photon emission computed tomography
SP	Substance P
STH	Somatotropic hormone
TE	Time of echo
TR	Time of repetition
TSH	Thyrotropic hormone
(Var.)	Variant
VEP	Visual evoked potentials
VIP	Vasoactive intestinal polypeptide

The **atlas pictures and serial illustrations** in this book are described in the following order: the coronal slices (Figs. 4–17) are shown in a sequence from front to back (anterior-posterior), the sagittal slices of the right side of the head (Figs. 32–37) from medial to lateral, and the axial slices (Figs. 47–60, 69–78) from inferior to superior. The axial slices are shown as viewed from above. The left side of the body is therefore always represented on the left side of the axial illustrations. This corresponds to the usual view of the brain in neurosurgery or in autopsies of the head. Accordingly, this orientation was used for the first CT scans of the head.

With the introduction of whole-body CT the images were reproduced as though viewed from below. Consequently the left side of the body appeared on the right side of the image. This portrayal of the images has also gained acceptance for CT of the head. For the evaluation of a CT scan in which voxels are transformed into pixels it does not make a difference whether it is viewed from below or from above; only the indications of the side—right or left—must be considered. MRI and CT are analyses of volume of the slices and not surface observations of the slices. For a "mental" reconstruction of the contents of an anatomic slice it is, on the other hand, important to know if the picture comes from the upper or the under side of the slice.

In the MR technique the axial slices are viewed from below. The sagittal slices are viewed from the lateral side to the midline and then from the midline to the other side. Coronal MR images are mostly arranged in a series from front to back.

For **allocating the level** of the individual parallel slice the numbers of the slices are given:
- For the 14 coronal slices in Figures 1–3
- For the 6 sagittal slices in Figures 29–31
- For the 14 slices of the canthomeatal series in the Figures. 44–46
- For the 10 slices of the brainstem series in Figure 67.

The different planes of the atlas pictures are color-coded at the outer border of the pages:
- The coronal series **blue**
- The sagittal series **green**
- The canthomeatal series **red**
- The brainstem series **yellow**
- Spaces of CSF, arteries with their vascular territories and veins **violet**.

In the corresponding serial illustrations (Figs. 79–151) the numbers of the slices are placed in circles. This **circled number** of the slices can be found for the respective series in the above-mentioned figures for better orientation.

In the pictures the various **anatomic structures** are labeled **with numbers**. As far as possible these numbers are placed in the optical center of the structure. Where this is graphically impossible, an indicating line has been added. In the illustrations the numbers are arranged continuously from left to right and from top to bottom. This corresponds to the normal reading sequence for the Western reader. In regions with a high density of numbers, as an exception to this rule, neighboring structures are numbered consecutively without regard to their arrangement from left to right or from top to bottom. Paired structures that appear symmetrically in the pictures are numbered once only. Paired structures that appear in different positions in the two hemispheres of the brain are labeled twice with the same number. If a structure is cut more than once in the same plane of section, e.g. the superior sagittal sinus, (Fig. 59b.2, 59c.2) then it retains its number throughout the illustration (e.g. 2). In the serial illustrations the same structure may have two different numbers according to its position on the surface or within the slice; for example, in one part of the drawing the head of the caudate nucleus is not seen on the surface of the slice (it lies in the posterior part of the slice) (Fig. 136.1.) and in another part it is seen on the surface (Fig. 136.2). **Each picture in the atlas is numbered**

independently. In the index, for example, the insula appears as F8a.10, F8b.11, F8d.11, F9a.18, etc. In the diagrams of the blood vessels (Figs. 88–97b) the numbering takes into account the area of distribution of the vessels and the direction of flow. In the case of the neurofunctional systems the individual structures are labeled throughout the sequence of the sections.

References to anatomic structures in different figures are often numerous in the text. These may disturb the flow of the text for the reader, but they facilitate the finding of the corresponding pictures. In this way the reader can combine the verbal and graphic-visual information. If many references exist for one anatomic structure, a selection is given. The reader will find all numbers of the figures corresponding to the structures listed in the index (Chap. 10). In the case of the T1- and T2-weighted MR images, often the text refers to one illustration only. Nevertheless, it is recommended to compare both illustrations.

Special notes in the atlas section (Figs. 1–78):
The graphic atlas illustrations have been taken from **four individuals** (Figs. 4a,c–17a,c; 32a,c–37a,c; 47a, 48a,c–60a,c; 69a,b–78a,b).

The coronal, sagittal, and brainstem series were complemented by MR images in T1- and T2-weighted images from a **fifth individual** (Figs. 4b,d–17b,d; 32b,d–37b,d; 48b–60b, 69c,d–78c,d). The T1-weighted MR images of the canthomeatal series were also taken from this individual.

Instead of the T2-weighted MR images, we chose a CT series for the canthomeatal series from a **sixth individual** (Figs. 47b, 48d–60d). For details, see Chapter 8.

References to chapters in parenthesis indicate the decimal classification of the heading of the chapter. Their pages are found in the contents. The decimal classification is also given in the column headings on the right-hand pages.

2 Neuroimaging and Guideline Structures

With the development of computed tomography (CT), magnetic resonance imaging (MRI), single photon emission computed tomography (SPECT), positron emission tomography (PET), and ultrasound B-scans new imaging techniques were introduced into medicine. These techniques are based on different physical principles and, accordingly, different measuring techniques. Some of them are based on common mathematical methods of image generation via electronic data processing (403, 425, 440, 462, 515). When applied to the examination of the nervous system, these five techniques can be clustered under the heading **neuroimaging**. These techniques were developed in the second half of the 20th century and within a few decades replaced the traditional invasive X-ray contrast media procedures, pneumoencephalography, and ventriculography in neuroradiology. Indications for angiography (also digital subtraction angiography [DSA]) and myelography were considerably restricted.

The first digital tomographic technique using X-rays was called computed tomography. After the introduction of further computer-assisted techniques for image generation, computed tomography should have been called X-ray computed tomography or transmission computed tomography. However, the term computed tomography (CT) has been generally accepted and will also be used here on account of its brevity (Chap. 2.1). MRI (Chap. 2.2) and emission computed tomography (Chap. 2.3, SPECT and PET) are physically quite different, but similar in their calculation of images. With these methods three-dimensional slices of a selected thickness are measured. Following data processing, two-dimensional digital images are generated. The B-image sonography uses ultrasound echos for imaging. It is now possible to combine color-coded Doppler information with this technique. In contrast to the aforementioned techniques, layers or the layer thickness cannot be adjusted. Spatial resolution is then achieved by manual positioning of the transducer and the choice of transmitting frequency (1–20 MHz).

2.1 Computed Tomography

In CT a slice of the body is visualized using X-ray transmission. Finely collimated X-ray beams scan the object to be examined in a circular or helical fashion. The differences in the intensity of the transmitted radiation are measured by a highly sensitive detector that is opposite the source of the X-rays. Today, the scanning of the object is almost exclusively carried out with a fan-beam source-detector system that rotates around the subject. This is known as a **transverse X-ray tomographic procedure**. The measurements from the detectors are transmitted to a computer which divides the scanned slice into a selected number of single volume elements (voxels) of specified size and calculates the absorption coefficient for each volume element. The size of the voxel varies according to the individual scanner and can be selected within a certain range. The base area is approximately 1 mm^2 or less depending on the size of the scanning field and the image matrix. The total volume depends on slice thickness, which can be selected between 0.5 mm and 10 mm in defined steps according to the particular equipment being used. The volume elements of the region to be examined (slices or spirals from the human body) are displayed in a matrix format in a gray scale on the monitor with the help of a television technique (198, 275). Each picture element (pixel) corresponds to a voxel of the object being measured. A brighter gray value for a pixel signifies stronger absorption of the radiation by the tissue present in the voxel. With modern equipment these computed individual layers with a slice thickness of 0.5–10 mm are obtained through continuous measurements applying a **helical technique**. Layers in every desired three-dimensional orientation and thickness can be reconstructed from the data obtained from the helical scanning (126, 198, 220, 275, 337, 403).

Images are generated after measurement of X-ray absorption of the voxels in the examined volume. The X-ray density of every voxel is expressed in **Hounsfield units (HU)**. The Hounsfield scale is arranged according to specific standard values. The limited **gray scale** of the monitor does not allow satisfactory visual differentiation of the clinically interesting structures when the entire Hounsfield scale is used (broad window). For this reason, electronic manipulation of the monitor image is necessary for viewing and evaluating the structures examined. By selecting the "window level" and the "window width" the gray scale of the monitor is adjusted to the radiodensity of special interest. With a broad window width the bony structures appear "spatial." A narrow window improves visualization of structures with only small differences in density, such as brain tissue. With large differences in densities (e.g. between bone and brain tissue or air), disproportionate beam hardening and distorted measurements lead to image computation errors.

CT technique is limited by the accuracy of measurement, and anatomic inaccuracies may be produced. The **partial volume effect** is of particular significance: The gray value of each pixel of the monitor image represents the average of all measured compartmental densities in the corresponding volume unit. Large differences in the densities of adjacent structures in one volume unit lead to misinterpretation of these component densities and hence to misrepresentation of the structural borders, masking of fissures, as well as coarser illustration and distortion of these structures especially if thick slices are scanned. The partial volume effect can be reduced by using high-resolution matrices and examining thinner sections. The partial volume effect, artifacts, and varying conditions of each examination (use of contrast medium, movement during examination, position of the patient) result in specific features that have to be taken into account when evaluating the images (198, 310, 403, 462). Artifacts can be reduced by using thin slices and avoiding beam hardening or by the addition of several thin layers to form one layer of desired thickness (198).

Intravenous (i.v.) administration of iodine-containing **contrast media** increases image quality by increasing the density of physiologic blood vessels as well as of pathologic structures (many tumors and inflammation, for example) (101). Use of faster CT scanners (shorter scanning times with continuous helical measurement) resulting in shorter examination times, together with the bolus injection of i.v. contrast media has made **computed tomography angiography** (CTA, dynamic CT) possible. Acquisition of data using the spiral technique allows smaller cerebral vessels to be visualized either as a so-called three-dimensional surface reconstruction by maximum intensity projection (MIP) or by the volume rendering technique (101, 198, 391, 403).

2.2 Magnetic Resonance Imaging

In MRI no ionizing radiation is used. For image generation the magnetic effect of the spin (angular momentum) of atomic nuclei with an odd nucleon number (number of protons plus neutrons) is used. The hydrogen nucleus has a relatively large magnetic moment and is abundant in living organisms. Consequently, tissues containing much water, lipids and proteins, can be demonstrated particularly well with MRI, due to their high content of hydrogen atoms (17, 101, 275, 344, 403, 440).

In a MRI exam the patient lies in a strong, homogeneous **magnetic field**, which in most systems is produced by superconductive coils. By superimposing a so-called gradient magnetic field with three additional coil pairs during slice selection, phase encoding and read-out of the signal, the homogeneous main magnetic field is changed linearly for a short period. This creates a unique assignment of every volume element of interest to a unique frequency- and angle-(phase) coding after slice selective excitation, a precondition for spatial encoding of cross-sectional images. The excitation of the protons occurs temporally parallel to the slice selection (by means of the gradient coils) with a transmitting body resonator, which delivers a high frequency, alternating electromagnetic field (irradiation of radiowaves). Once they have been stimulated they return to their previous, lower level of energy, emitting electromagnetic energy in the form of radiofrequency (RF). These spatially coded **nuclear resonance signals** are received by an antenna. Special head and surface coils improve the signal-to-noise ratio and hence the spatial resolution without prolongation of the examination time.

For a given strength of the magnetic field the MR signal is determined by the proton density, the relaxation times T1 (longitudinal or spin-lattice relaxation time) and T2 (transverse or spin-spin relaxation time), and the proton movements in the volume measured. The signal intensity in the respective volume unit (voxel) determines the gray scale values in a point of the picture element (pixel) on the monitor.

The protons can be stimulated by various **measuring sequences** that influence the image contrast and consequently the diagnostic value. The spin-echo (SE) technique is widely used. This technique involves the sequential generation of a 90° pulse (excitation pulse) and a 180° pulse (echo pulse). A short repetition time (time between two excitation pulses [TR]) in combination with a short echo-time (TE) leads to the so-called T1-weighted image. A long repetition time TR in combination with a long echo time TE leads to a T2-weighted image. T1-weighted images and sequences, which mainly measure the proton density, demonstrate the anatomy best due to the very favourable signal-to-noise ratio. The cerebrospinal fluid (CSF) produces a low signal and hence appears dark. In T2-weighted images the CSF produces a high signal and so appears white. Edema and many other pathologic changes can be easily visualized.

Using a rapid gradient-echo sequence (FLASH = Fast Low Angle Shot, FISP = Fast Imaging with Steady Precession) examination time can be shortened, movement artifacts can be reduced, liquid and blood flow can be demonstrated with a high resolution in time, and even isolated vessels can be displayed **Magnetic Resonance Angiography (MRA)**.

The gradient-echo sequences are based on an excitation of a total volume segment and parallel layered signal read-out corresponding to the increase of gradients in the transverse plane. The quick gradient-echo sequences enable volume-selective 3D measurements, the advantage of which, are the thin layers without intermediate gaps and the secondary reconstruction of other scanning planes (101, 440, 468). The disadvantage, however, is the hybrid character and a low T2 contrast, respectively.

The clinical questions to be answered determine the measuring conditions of an MRI investigation. Choices include the volume to be examined, the slice positions and the measuring parameters (e.g. the slice thickness and gaps), the matrix and the measuring sequence. The respective critical pixels must be clearly represented and free from artifacts (so-called quality criteria). Investigation of the skull should be carried out in T1- and T2-weighted images with high-contrast representation of gray and white matter. Certain clinical questions require additional T2*-weighted sequences, for example in the case of cerebrovascular impairments (101, 344, 403). Due to the large number of variable measuring parameters dependent on one another, the **chance of errors** occurring through artifacts and inadequate conduction of investigation is considerably higher than with other imaging procedures. Therefore, it is not only the quality control plays a significant role, but also the medical qualification for choice of indication, conduction of investigation, evaluation and interpretation of the MR image (101, 344, 375, 440, 445).

MRI uses several parameters (e.g., proton density, relaxation times) to be examined for image acquisition (117, 212b, 375, 440). In MRI the image processing and reconstruction are similar to that in CT with the choice of appropriate window center and window width by the investigator who determines the outcome of the investigation. Quality of outcome is highly dependent upon the clinical assumptions made when choosing the exam parameters.

Paramagnetic substances (Gadolinium-DTPA, Gadolinium-Diamid, manganese) used as **contrast media** can improve the diagnostic value. They shorten the T1 relaxation time in the area of distribution. This leads to a higher signal of the lesion compared with the total surroundings in the T1-weighted image (205, 440). Prior to administration of contrast medium injection, a T1-weighted imaging examination should be performed with the same parameters.

In general, the following features will influence the decision to use contrast media:
- to reveal the presence or lack of contrast enhancement in a lesion
- to characterize the size of contrast-enhanced region
- to evaluate the pattern of enhancement of this region (101).

The structures at the base of the brain, in the infratentorial space, and in the vertebral canal can be much better visualized using MRI than using CT due to the higher contrast of soft tissues and the absence of bony artifacts.

The **high sensitivity** for pathologic cerebral and spinal lesions resulting from the exceptionally good contrast resolution justified the rapid acceptance of MRI (440). Even without contrast media, MRI allows a more sensitive registration of proton flow, and therefore of the cerebral blood vessels, than CT. Spatial resolution is equal for both procedures (13, 403).

In infants, MRI can be used to depict myelinization of the central nervous system (CNS) and is, therefore, able to demonstrate myelinization impairment and delay of myelinization as well as diffuse or localized demyelinization in adults (232, 344, 403, 468).

Similar to CT and CTA, MRI in combination with morphologic and functional methods can be used for diagnosing acute infarcts in the case of hemorrhage and is more effective in the exclusion of tumors. By means of a diffusion-weighted sequence, infarcts and the size of the affected region can be accurately detected within minutes following vascular occlusion.

Magnetic resonance spectroscopy (MRS) in vivo has not yet been introduced as a routine procedure due to the complex technique involved (372, 374a, 509), despite the numerous promising observations (93, 101, 259). In vivo MRS has a high specificity for tissue in the imaging volume based on the detection of the so-called "chemical shifts" of molecules in the magnetic field. MRS is not only suitable for identification of abnormal tissue (e.g., tumors, inflammation, necrosis) in the central nervous system (CNS) but may also offer an alternative to emission computed tomography in the differentiation of various tumors (509).

Functional MRI (fMRI)

has been an interesting method for mapping of brain functions (96, 162, 229, 248, 311, 334, 374a). Local changes in the cerebral blood flow can be registered by means of vasoneuronal coupling after specific motor, visual, or sensory stimulation and then used under defined paradigms for localization of short-term altered cerebral functions (403, 445). This technique is time-consuming and the signal output is low, thus limiting the practical value to a number of stable paradigms (motor, visual, auditory, tactile). fMRI can aid in the decision for or against cochlear implants and for or against the left or right side (417).

2.3 Emission Computed Tomography

Emission computed tomography is a computed tomographic variant of classic **scintigraphy** (66). Usually radioactive tracer substances are injected intravenously and serve as the radiation source. In emission computed tomography the technical difficulties of the measurement are due to the spatial position and the distribution of intensity of the radioactive tracer within a medium of variable absorption. Furthermore, the number of recorded photons (which determine the flow of information) is much smaller than with X-ray CT. The local resolution of emission computed tomography is considerably lower than that of MRI and CT.

In **single photon emission tomography (SPECT)**, radionuclides are used that emit γ- and X-rays during their decay. SPECT images are mainly produced by a rotating γ-camera system. Using this technique, disturbances of the blood–brain barrier can be detected and regional cerebral blood flow can be measured (66, 97a, 221, 374a). The main advantages of SPECT are the relatively uncomplicated technical measuring equipment and the ready availability of γ-emitting radionuclides.

For **positron emission tomography (PET)** a β+-emitting nuclide is necessary (206, 221, 374a). With this technique the distribution of a radioactive tracer is shown by means of axial tomography. Thus, metabolic processes and perfusion of organs and their subdivisions as well as of tumors can be measured (66, 489). PET enlarges our understanding of functional processes of the brain beyond the structural changes seen through CT and MRI (76, 209). PET can also be used for investigations of functional neuroanatomy (Chaps. 6 and 7). The glucose metabolism of the brain, including regional changes during various activities, has been examined most extensively so far. For a number of years several radiopharmaceuticals have been available for imaging of transmitter receptors and neurotransmitters with SPECT and PET (32a, 32b, 57a, 66, 471a).

PET represents, from the physiologic and technical point of view, the best method of emission computed tomography. Nevertheless, the elements carbon, nitrogen, and oxygen, which are directly involved in metabolic processes, are available in a suitable radioactive form only with a very short half-life period of a few minutes to a few hours. Consequently, a generator system, a cyclotron and a radiochemical laboratory are most commonly needed for PET (206).

2.4 Ultrasound Techniques

Ultrasound techniques initially produced only the one-dimensional **A-image** (A-Amplitude, A-mode) for the identification of structure and organ boundaries. With this method an exact intravital measurement of distance was achieved by calculation of the echo depth (451). The A-imaging was discontinued due to its low anatomic information content and replaced with the **B-image** (B = brightness, B-mode) and CT (272, 374a). Today ultrasound waves are mainly used for generating sectional images (sonography) and to visualize morphologic tissue properties. Piezoelectric elements are used for ultrasound generation and for detection of echo-ultrasonic pulses. The advantages of the B-scan technique for sonographic diagnosis are the relatively free choice of sectioning plane and the good demonstration of borders between different tissues (451). The amplitudes of the reflected pulses from the borderline structures between different tissues influence the brightness on the monitor and a brightness-modulated image is created.

Because of the high absorption of sound waves by the intact skull, **ultrasound examination of the adult brain** did not prove effective in the past. The steadily advancing development of equipment and the use of echo-contrast-enhancing substances have made visualization of an increasing number of intracranial structures possible (231). Midline shifts, ventricular width, or extent of hemorrhage can be detected and used for follow up. In the examination of neonates and infants, however, ultrasound imaging has gained great practical significance (167, 377). The examination can be best performed while the anterior fontanelle (physiologic acoustic window) is still open in neonates. Modern equipment with automatic three-dimensional scanning and an image store enable the display of sectional images in three planes. The absence of ionizing radiation and the **mobility of the equipment** with real-time technique are significant advantages for its use in pediatrics, particularly in premature infant units. In dealing with certain clinical problems this technique can either replace or supplement CT and MRI (98, 165), even in adults (27a, 27b). During surgery the opened cranial cavity allows sonography from the access angle of the surgeon to demonstrate the boundaries between the anatomic and pathologic structures (403, 422).

Sonography is of great clinical importance as a technique for investigating the eyeball and the retrobulbar structures, as well as for examining the soft tissues of the neck, particularly the thyroid gland. The paranasal sinuses, especially the frontal and maxillary sinuses, can also be assessed well sonographically. Fine-needle biopsy controlled by ultrasound allows accurate removal of tissue from various regions with minimal risk (451).

Doppler sonography is a noninvasive ultrasound technique for measuring the speed of flow in vessels using the Doppler effect. Ultrasound waves reflected from moving objects undergo a shift in frequency that is proportional to the speed of the reflecting particles. Thus the speed of flow in the vessel can be calculated (98, 374a). Doppler sonography is used for the examination of blood vessels located close to the body surface and increasingly recent years for measurement of flow in larger, intracranial arteries (63, 374a, 488). In infants with an open fontanelle all larger arteries can be examined easily by Doppler sonography. Characteristic changes in flow profiles and speed of flow can be found in localized vascular stenoses, vascular wall processes, vasospasms, and increased intracranial pressure. From these changes clinically relevant information about the cerebral blood flow can be deduced.

The combination of a B-scan and Doppler sonography is called a **duplex scan**. This method is used to obtain a good anatomic and hemodynamic-functional imaging of the common carotid artery, its bifurcation and the subsequent intracranial arteries. Stenoses and plaques attached to the wall, and thromboses can be recognized (183a). Doppler sonography with color coding and the sonospectrogram will be used increasingly in the future. Doppler sonography is frequently used at the start of apparative-technical diagnosis because it offers the possibility of examining the patient at bedside location and can be repeated as often as required (15, 231, 451, 488, 498).

2.5 Guideline Structures in Imaging Procedures

The term **guideline structures** refers to the anatomic structures that can reliably and constantly be displayed using imaging techniques and used as landmarks in topographic orientation of the images created.

With **conventional neuroradiologic procedures** (pneumoencephalography, angiography, and myelography), the guideline structures are predominantly the topographic relationships of the bony structures to the CSF spaces and the blood vessels. Lesions in the cranial and spinal cavities are recognized by deformation of the contrast-enhanced CSF spaces, as well as by displacement and changes of cerebral vessels. Only one system, the contrast-enhanced CSF space or the contrast-enhanced vascular system, can be used for the image generation. Outside the cranial cavity topical orientation is aided by the air-filled cavities, such as the nasal cavity, the paranasal sinuses, the pharynx, and the trachea. These guideline structures are important landmarks for spatial orientation. They also serve as controls for the accuracy of alignment in imaging.

CT, MRI, and sonography have the advantage of simultaneously displaying numerous anatomic structures in the region examined. This is due to the very high-resolution of soft tissues based on various physical, and also to some extent chemical, parameters. They allow a far better and more **detailed recognition of the anatomic structures** and a significantly improved demonstration of lesions. Constant visualization of various anatomic landmarks and cavities greatly enhances the interpretation of the images. At the same time, topical orientation becomes more difficult as a result of the sectioning technique. A prerequisite for a correct interpretation and topographic arrangement is the synoptic or general study of all slices and also, as far as possible, the use of different sectioning planes. For **spatial orientation of an image**, especially in the vertebral column, digital images in sagittal and coronal planes (scoutview, pilot, scanogram, radiogram, topogram) are necessary and generally used in CT and MRI. This has led us to add a sketch of the sequence of slices (signet) to the ana-tomic drawings and to the MR and CT images. It is meant to aid in the topographic localization of each individual slice.

In **CT** the two-dimensional image of the picture elements (pixels) in its gray values is determined by the absorption coefficients of the corresponding volume elements (voxels). The scale of absorption coefficients is related in its extreme values to biologically important structures. Thus air (which appears black) has the lowest absorption coefficient −1000 **Hounsfield Units (HU)**, water 0 HU, and dense bone +1000 HU (198, 375). A scan of the head allows the following categories to be distinguished (198, 375):

Air		−1000 HU
Fatty tissue	−100 to	−30 HU
CSF spaces	+5 to	+10 HU
Brain, gray and white matter	+20 to	+40 HU
Blood vessels with contrast medium	+50 to	+200 HU
Calcification	+30 to	+1000 HU
Skull		to +1000 HU and above

In contrast to emission computed tomography and most sequences of MRI, the bony structures of the skull and the vertebral column are good landmarks, as are the CSF spaces and the air-filled cavities (nose, paranasal sinuses, pharynx, and trachea).

In **MRI** the imaging is influenced by complex physical and chemical processes. Different pulse sequences and various imaging selection procedures lead to changing gray values of the same anatomic structures. The particular clinical problem and the part of the body or the organ being examined determine the choice of the examination sequences (T1-weighted, T2-weighted, proton density). For detailed information one should consult the specialized literature (286, 344, 403, 468).

In **emission computed tomography** the imaging takes place through measuring the radioactivity of the respective volume elements. For a better recognition of image and function, color coding is frequently used. In the intracranial cavity the internal CSF space aids orientation.

2.5.1 Facial Skeleton

In **CT** the bony structures and the **air-filled cavities** (nasal cavity, paranasal sinuses [Figs. 79, 47–51], oral cavity) allow anatomic orientation in the coronal and axial slices. This is greatly enhanced by the numerous bilateral symmetrical structures in this region. Thus correct positioning of the head in the scan field can be controlled.

For the examination of the orbit in axial planes, an angle inclined at about 10° to the canthomeatal plane is preferred (198). This plane approximates the infraorbital plane (Chap. 1.2). In this way the optic nerve and rectus muscles can be clearly visualized. The optic nerve, which in normal forward gaze runs a slightly tortuous course, can be straightened by means of a slight upward gaze (198). The **mass of orbital fat** provides a good contrast for the remaining contents of the orbit. The examination can be supplemented by additional coronal slices (198, 203, 403).

MRI must, to a large extent, dispense with any bony orientation in the images. At the same time bony artifacts are not found at the skull base, which impair CT images. The possibility of multiplanar scans with a free choice of sectioning plane, and the greater soft-tissue contrast, are definite advantages particularly in the facial skeleton. Teeth artifacts remain localized and do not disturb the image. The **bicommissural line** (connection of anterior with posterior commissure) is used for anatomic orientation in MRI. In the orbit the retrobulbar fat gives a high MR signal in T1-weighted images. The extraocular muscles can be clearly visualized. In the diagnosis of orbital diseases various superficial coils or special pulse sequences for suppression of the MR signals of retrobulbar fat are used for improvement of the images (344, 404, 440). For optimal visualization of the optic nerve (Figs. 6b.10, 6d.10, 7b.14, 7d.14, 50b.5, 77c.1, 77d.1) as far as the optic chiasm (Figs. 8b.15, 8d.15, 32b.18, 32d.18, 77c.4, 77d.4), examination in paraxial (oblique sagittal) planes is suitable (203). For imaging the paranasal cavities and the retromaxillary space the head coil is preferred. The nasal conchae (Figs. 4d.8, 5d.10, 6d.17, 33d.25, 33d.26, 69d.2) and the muscles aid the anatomic orientation. In the nasopharynx in axial slices, one can frequently distinguish a superficial mucosal compartment from the deeper tissue layers, which can be of clinical significance (17, 440).

2.5.2 Head and Neck Region

Using **CT** an optimal assessment of the width of the vertebral canal can be obtained. For orientation regarding the correct height, survey radiographs (scoutviews, topograms) are necessary. The air-filled cavities (nasopharynx, Fig. 47b.6), are easily recognizable, as well as the dens of the axis (Fig. 47b.11), the atlas (Fig. 47b.8), the squamous part of the occipital bone (Fig. 48d.6, 50d.25), and the spinal cord (Fig. 47b.13).

The bony parts of the **skull base and its foramina** are important guideline structures. For demonstrating the detailed structures special sectioning planes are required (198). In canthomeatal views the internal acoustic meatus are always identifiable and, therefore, are important landmarks. In the radiograph of the fourth slice of the canthomeatal series (comparable to the bony "window" of the CT image), the internal acoustic meatus is shown (Fig. 64.12). Information about the clinically useful views for optimal demonstration of fine bony structures in the skull base can be found in the following references (198, 237, 450).

In **MRI** other landmarks, apart from the cervical vertebrae, include the spinal cord and the medulla oblongata (Figs. 12b.27, 32b.34, 48b.11, 69c.8), as well as the spinal subarachnoid space and the basal CSF cisterns. The great vessels in the neck (the internal and external carotid arteries and internal jugular vein) are clearly identifiable. The air-filled spaces (oral cavity, pharynx; Figs. 8d.20, 69c.3, 69d.3, 70c.3, 70d.3) are recognizable in all MR sequences used. Concerning the soft tissues in the neck the anatomy is best demonstrated in the proton-density or T1-weighted images and pathologic lesions in the T2-weighted images. For technical details see special references (16, 344, 440).

Dopplersonography and **duplexsonography**-can be used to examine the large arteries supplying the brain both from the thorax to the skull and, with restriction, the intracranial space. Duplexsonography is superior to Dopplersonography for these types of exam.

2.5.3 Neurocranium

With **CT** the bony parts of the base of the skull and its foramina are the guideline structures. They give information about the sectioning plane chosen and its position. Orientation is provided by the occipital bone (Figs. 48d.6, 49d.23, 50d.25), petrous part of temporal bone (Figs. 49d.10, 50d.19), mastoid cells (Figs. 48d.12, 49d.20), sphenoidal sinus (Figs. 49d.4, 50d.7), sella turcica, ethmoidal cells (Figs. 49d.2, 50d.2), zygomatic arch (Fig. 48d.3), and orbital margin. The hypoglossal canal, jugular foramen, external acoustic meatus (Figs. 48d.9, 49d.16), tympanic cavity, foramen lacerum, carotid canal, foramen spinosum, and foramen ovale are small structures in the base of the skull not regularly identifiable. If they are demonstrated they can serve as anatomic landmarks for other intracranial structures. Thinner slices and variations from the canthomeatal plane, as well as an additional coronal series, are necessary for imaging individual structures of the base of the skull.

Examination of bony structures should be carried out using the **high-resolution technique** (HR-CT) (403). Conventional radiographs of anatomic slices of the bony structures of the base of the skull illustrate accurately the small bony structures. For this reason, we have preferred such radiographs for displaying the anatomy of the skull base (Figs. 18–28, 38–43, 61–66).

2.5.4 Cisterns and the Ventricular System

In **CT** the CSF-filled spaces are crucial **guideline structures** (141). Narrow spaces might not be displayed due to the partial volume effect or be obscured by denser structures. The unpaired cisterna magna (cerebellomedullary cistern) (Fig. 48d.16), the pontine cistern, and the paired cerebellopontine cisterns (Fig. 50d.13) at the level of the petrous part of temporal bone are visible in slices roughly parallel to the supraorbitomeatal plane (Chap. 1.2). Immediately above this plane the anterior basal cistern, the interpeduncular cistern (Fig. 52d.11), and the superior cerebellar cistern can be seen. The anterior basal cistern including the interpeduncular cistern are referred to as the suprasellar cistern, which generally appears five-sided in CT scans. It surrounds the stalk of the pituitary gland, the optic nerves, and the optic chiasm. Anteriorly the suprasellar cistern borders on the gyri recti, laterally on the uncus and parahippocampal gyrus, and posteriorly on the pons. Other important CSF-containing guideline structures are the ambient cistern and the quadrigeminal cistern (Figs. 52d.20, 53d.21). The interhemispheric cistern and the cistern of the Sylvian fissure (of lateral sulcus, insular cistern) are very small in young patients. They are particularly well-marked in older patients and in those with cerebral atrophy. A better imaging of the cisterns can be achieved by **enhancing the contrast** with the lumbar intrathecal injection of a suitable iodine-containing water-soluble contrast medium, such as Iopamidol or Iotrolan.

Due to the considerable physiologic variation in the size of the ventricular system and its deformation by space-occupying lesions, no uniform images can be given for the different parts of the ventricles. Images with wide bilateral temporal horns indicate hydrocephalus. The volume of the ventricles can be calculated by measurement of the ventricular pixels in serial CT images (305, 394, 510).

In **MRI** the CSF spaces are guideline structures in the cranial cavity. The images of the CSF spaces appear to be free from bony artifacts. This can be of clinical importance in the basal regions and also at the craniocervical junction (440). The cisterna magna (Figs. 13b.22, 13d.22, 32b.36, 32d.36, 48b.16, 69c.12, 69d.12), cerebellopontine cistern (Figs. 73c.9, 73d.9), pontine cistern (Figs. 74c.5, 74 d.5), interpeduncular cistern (Figs. 11b.17, 11d.17, 52b.11, 77c.9, 77d.9), ambient cistern (Figs. 52b.18, 77c.13, 77d.13, 78c.11, 78d.11), quadrigeminal cistern (Figs. 52b.20, 53b.21), and the cistern of vallecula cerebri (Figs. 78c.3, 78d.3) give a low signal in T1-weighted images but a high signal in T2-weighted images. The cistern of the lateral cerebral fossa (Figs. 11b.11, 36b.9, 53b.16) is useful for the localization of the frontal and parietal opercula in comparison with the temporal operculum.

With **sonography** a reliable assessment of the shape and size of the ventricles and of cerebral structures is possible through the open fontanelle during the first months of life, or intraoperatively after craniotomy regardless of age (451). It can be difficult to visualize smaller extraaxial hematoma (403). CT should be performed if such a lesion is suspected.

2.5.5 Blood Vessels

With **CT** sections of the larger vessels can be demonstrated, such as the basilar artery (Figs. 50d.12, 51d.12) and the internal carotid arteries (Figs. 49d.8, 51d.6). If contrast medium is used, these arteries can be seen particulary well. With special techniques, further blood vessels can be visualized even in noncontrast views as in the orbit for example. If contrast medium is used, the middle cerebral artery in the lateral sulcus and parts of the circle of Willis can usually be seen. Of the venous channels the great cerebral vein (of Galen), the inferior sagittal sinus, the straight sinus (Fig. 55d.20), as well as the superior sagittal sinus (Figs. 54d.29, 57d.2) and less constantly the transverse sinus, are guideline structures.

In **MRI** the large blood vessels are easily seen, though usually with reduced signal intensity in conventional sequences (flow void). For this reason the blood vessels are important guideline structures for the assessment of MR images. Use of contrast medium is not necessary. Using special techniques MR angiograms can be obtained. Cerebral vascular malformations are significantly better visualized with MRI than with CT (17). MRA without contrast media has generally replaced conventional and digital subtraction angiography (DSA). Angiography is often a necessary supplement for the visualization of small arteries and veins, and for the assessment of hemodynamics and small vascular abnormalities (101, 183a, 440).

Transcranial **Doppler sonography** allows the non-invasive assessment of blood flow in the larger cerebral arteries, gives evidence of vasospasm, and frequently suggests arterial stenoses (104, 183a, 488).

2.5.6 Dural Structures

In **CT** the dura mater over the convexity of the brain is not (or only rarely) outlined as a separate structure. The falx cerebri is always demonstrated (Figs. 53d.3, 54d.2, 55d.3, 56d.7, 57d.4, 58d.3, 59d.3) with an increase in density after administration of contrast medium. In the venous phase the superior and inferior sagittal sinuses, the straight sinus, and also the bridging veins are contrasted and hence outline the boundaries of the falx cerebri. The tentorium cerebelli borders below and laterally on the confluence of sinuses (the transverse sinus, superior petrosal sinus, and parts of the straight sinus). The free borders of the tentorium cannot be demonstrated consistently and often are visible only after administration of contrast medium (344, 345). The position of the tentorial notch in relation to the midbrain varies considerably. Sections through the tentorium and falx cerebri may be Y-shaped (Fig. 54a.40, 54a.3), V-shaped, or M-shaped. The **tentorial notch** (incisura) is indicated in contrast CT scans by the ventromedial segments of the diverging bands (329). When the tentorium is not visualized in axial CT, the position of the diverging bands can be constructed using an auxillary line. This line extends from the lateral portion of the ambient cistern in an occipital–lateral direction toward the skull, and forms a 45° angle with the sagittal plane. Structures lateral to this auxiliary line are located supratentorially and those medial infratentorially (329). In coronal sections the tentorium cerebelli is usually clearly visible.

In **MRI** the dura mater is demonstrated only after administration of contrast medium. The dura is related to the interhemispheric cistern (Figs. 4d.2, 5d.2, 7d.2, 16d.4, 17d.3, 76d.11, 78c.1, 78d.1) and to the transverse cerebral fissure, which is the space between the occipital lobe and the cerebellum (Fig. 16d.11). These spaces are both easily discerned and hence are important guideline structures. Calcifications of the dura mater usually give no MR signal but ossifications may produce a low or, rarely, a high signal.

2.6 Clinical Value of the New Imaging Techniques

The new imaging techniques (CT, CTA, MRI, MRA, PET, SPECT, and ultrasound) have changed our way of thinking and our method of practicing clinical medicine. This holds particularly true for diagnostic procedures of the cranial and spinal cavities. The classical X-ray examinations such as pneumoencephalography and myelography were used less frequently due to their invasive nature. Therefore, they were performed at the end of the diagnostic process and were not suitable for follow-up examinations. Their minimal invasiveness, their use in facilitating lower-cost outpatient exams (as compared with inpatient examinations) make these new procedures ideal for **follow-up examinations**. In special clinical situations myelography and angiography are still in use.

In recent years the new imaging techniques have assured themselves an important place among other diagnostic procedures. Depending on the particular speciality, the clinical problem, and the organ being examined, each new technique has its individual indications. For good clinical practice, choosing the correct technique, and describing and evaluating the results of neuroimaging, functional neuroanatomic knowledge is essential. This book aims to provide the reader with this neccessary information.

Atlas

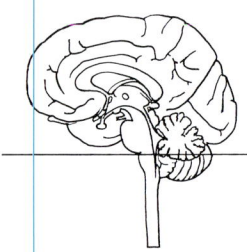

1 Longitudinal cerebral (interhemispheric) fissure
2 Superior frontal gyrus
3 Falx cerebri
4 Middle frontal gyrus
5 Dura mater
6 Supraorbital nerve
7 Ethmoidal cells
8 Optic disc
9 Fovea centralis of retina
10 Ethmoidal bulla
11 Eyeball
12 Semilunar hiatus
13 Middle nasal meatus
14 Middle nasal concha
15 Infraorbital nerve
16 Nasal cavity
17 Nasal septum
18 Inferior nasal meatus
19 Maxillary sinus
20 Inferior nasal concha
21 Oral cavity
22 Tongue
23 Hypoglossal nerve
24 Inferior alveolar nerve

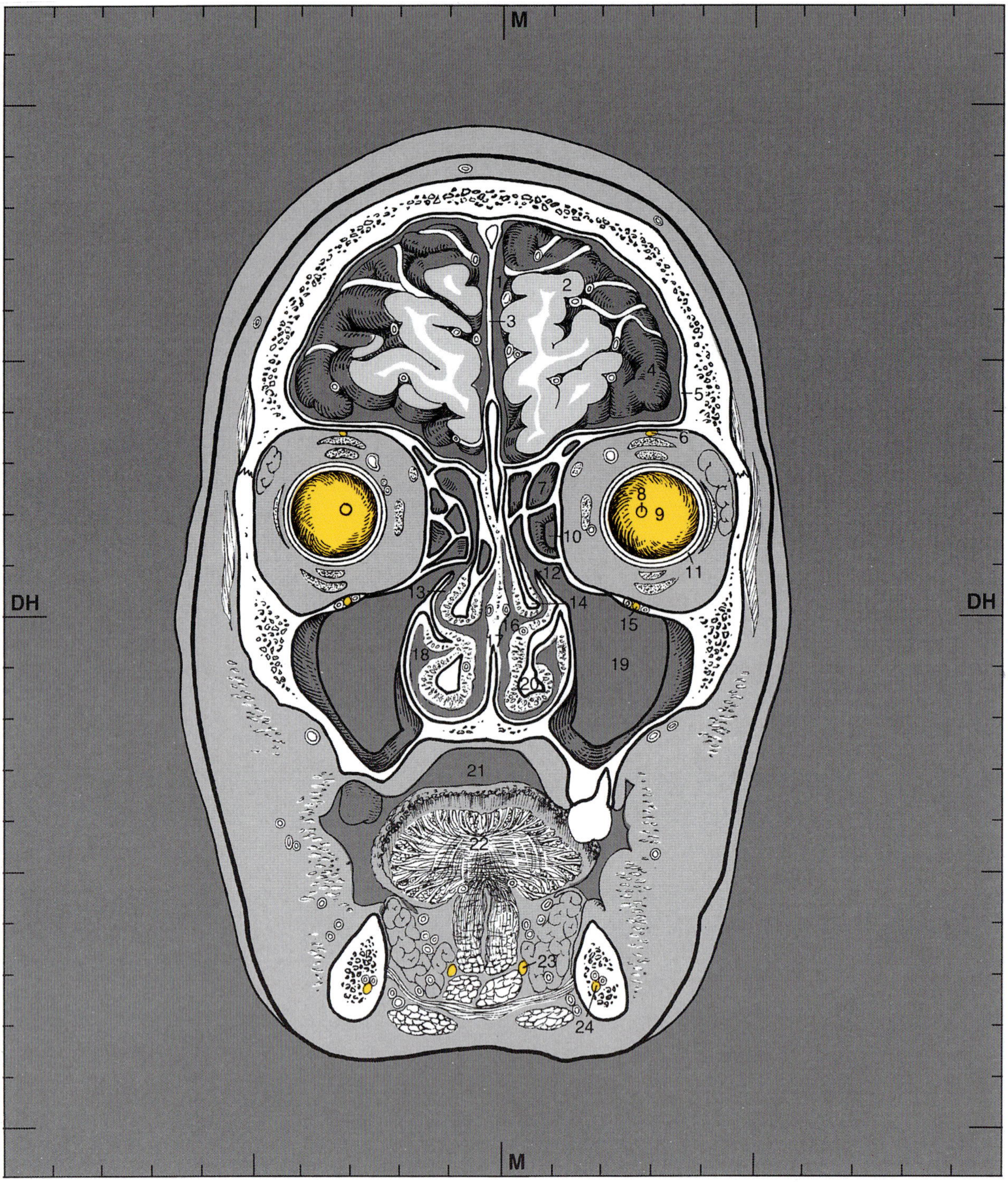

Fig. **4a** Anterior section surface of the first coronal slice showing nasal cavity, nasal sinuses, oral cavity, brain structures, retina, and cranial nerves. In the upper left corner of the page, the blue line through the median view of the brain indicates the location of the sectional plane through the frontal lobe (Fig. 2b).

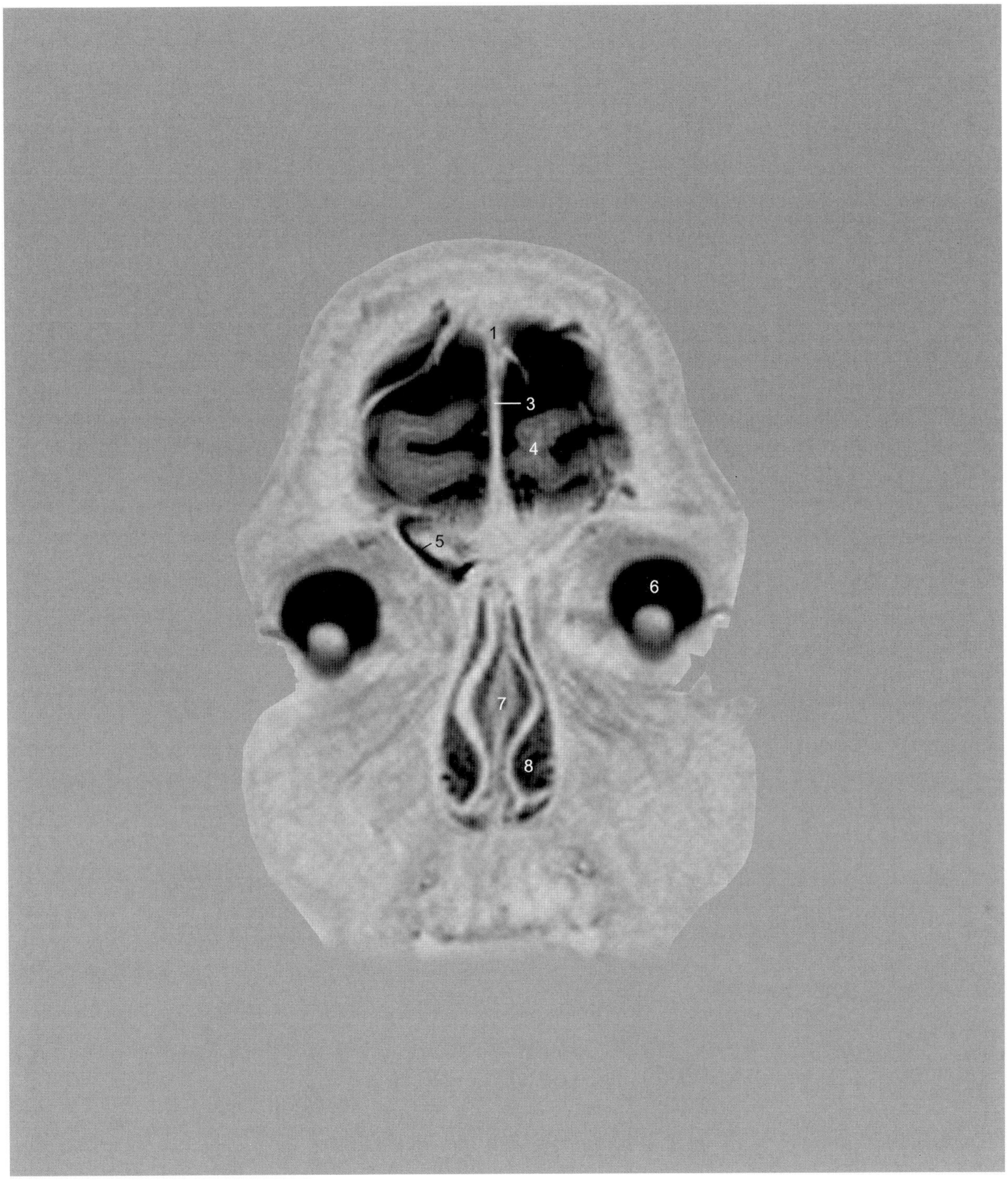

Coronal Slices

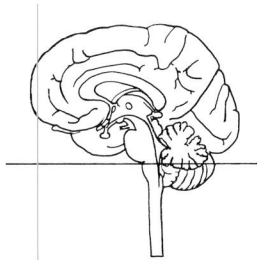

1 Superior sagittal sinus
3 Falx cerebri
4 Superior frontal gyrus
5 Frontal sinus
6 Eyeball with lens
7 Nasal septum
8 Inferior nasal concha

Fig. **4b** Coronal, T1-weighted MR image (Turbo-Inversion-Recovery-Sequence) corresponding approximately to the sectional plane of Figs. 4a and 4c. The selected sequence emphasizes the brain structures and suppresses the surrounding soft tissues. The two coronal MR series (Figs. 4b–17b and 4d–17d) were obtained from a 38-year-old female. A missing number with its label indicates here and in the following legends of MR images that this number can be found in the other corresponding T2-weighted MR image. See following page (Fig. 4d). Technical data (Chap. 8).

24 Atlas

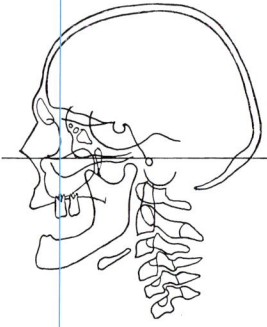

1 Superior sagittal sinus
2 Intermediomedial frontal artery
3 Anteromedial frontal artery
4 Frontal bone
5 Polar frontal artery
6 Temporalis
7 Crista galli
8 Medial frontobasal artery
9 Roof of orbit
10 Levator palpebrae superioris
11 Superior ophthalmic vein
12 Superior oblique
13 Superior rectus
14 Lacrimal gland
15 Medial rectus
16 Orbital plate
17 Zygomatic bone
18 Tendon of lateral rectus
19 Orbicularis oculi
20 Inferior rectus
21 Inferior oblique
22 Floor of orbit
23 Infraorbital artery and vein
24 Maxilla
25 Hard palate
26 Second molar tooth
27 First molar tooth (cut)
28 Submandibular duct
29 Buccinator
30 Genioglossus
31 Sublingual artery and vein
32 Sublingual gland
33 Body of mandible
34 Geniohyoid
35 Inferior alveolar artery and vein
36 Submental artery and vein
37 Mylohyoid
38 Anterior belly of digastric

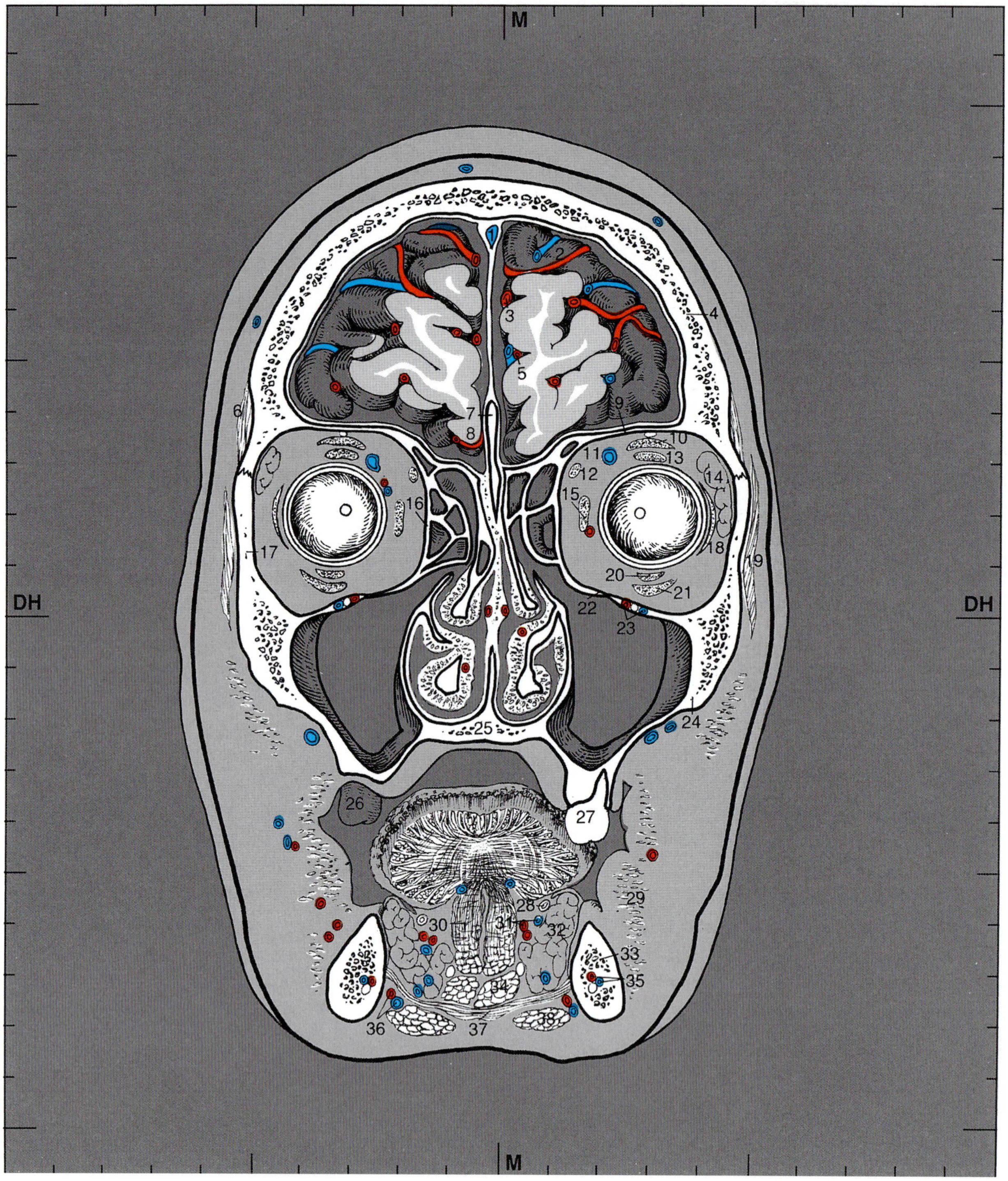

Fig. 4c Anterior section surface of the first coronal slice showing bony structures, muscles, and blood vessels. In the upper left corner of the page, the blue line through the skull indicates the position of the sectional plane through the crista galli, orbit, and the anterior molar teeth (Fig. 2a).
DH Reid's base line
M Median plane

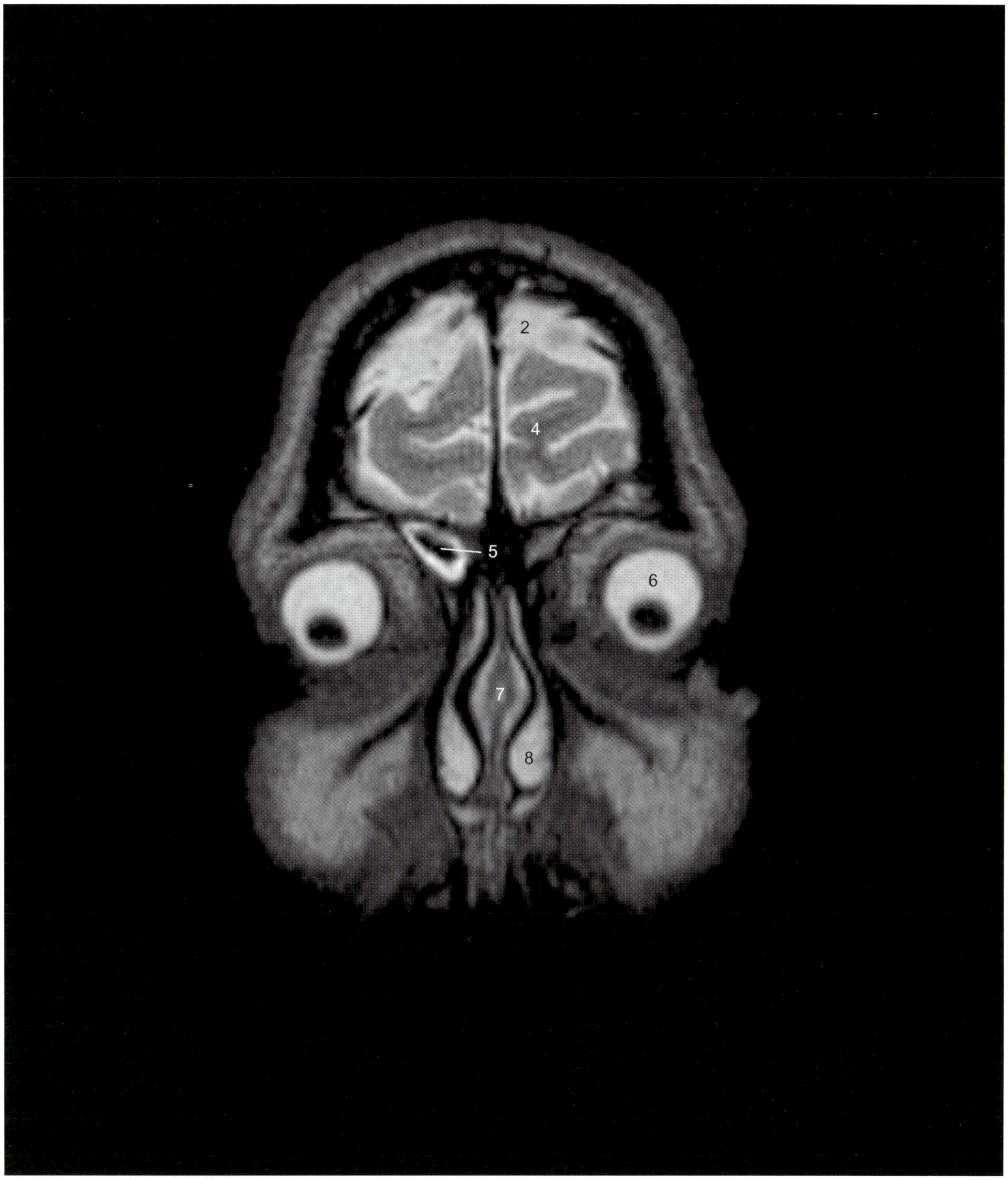

Coronal Slices

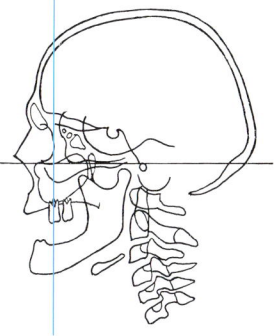

2	Interhemispheric cistern
4	Superior frontal gyrus
5	Frontal sinus (swelling of mucous membrane)
6	Eyeball with lens
7	Nasal septum
8	Inferior nasal concha

Fig. **4d** Coronal, T2-weighted MR image corresponding approximately to the sectional plane of Figs. 4a and 4c. The T2-weighted MR image is positioned approximately 3 mm posterior to Fig. 4b. A missing number with its label indicates here and in the following legends of MR images that this number can be found in the other corresponding T1-weighted MR image. See previous page (Fig. 4b). The two coronal MR series (Figs. 4b–17b and 4d–17d) were obtained from a 38-year-old female. Technical data (Chap. 8).

26 Atlas

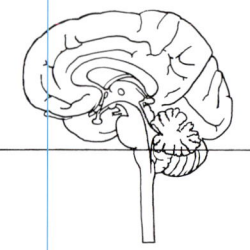

1 Superior frontal gyrus
2 Falx cerebri
3 Middle frontal gyrus
4 Dura mater
5 Orbital gyri
6 Inferior frontal gyrus
7 Straight gyrus
8 Supraorbital nerve
9 Nasociliary nerve
10 Olfactory bulb
11 Optic nerve
12 Ethmoidal cells
13 Semilunar hiatus
14 Infraorbital nerve
15 Middle nasal meatus
16 Middle nasal concha
17 Nasal septum
18 Nasal cavity
19 Maxillary sinus
20 Inferior nasal concha
21 Inferior nasal meatus
22 Greater palatine nerve
23 Oral cavity
24 Tongue
25 Lingual nerve
26 Hypoglossal nerve
27 Inferior alveolar nerve

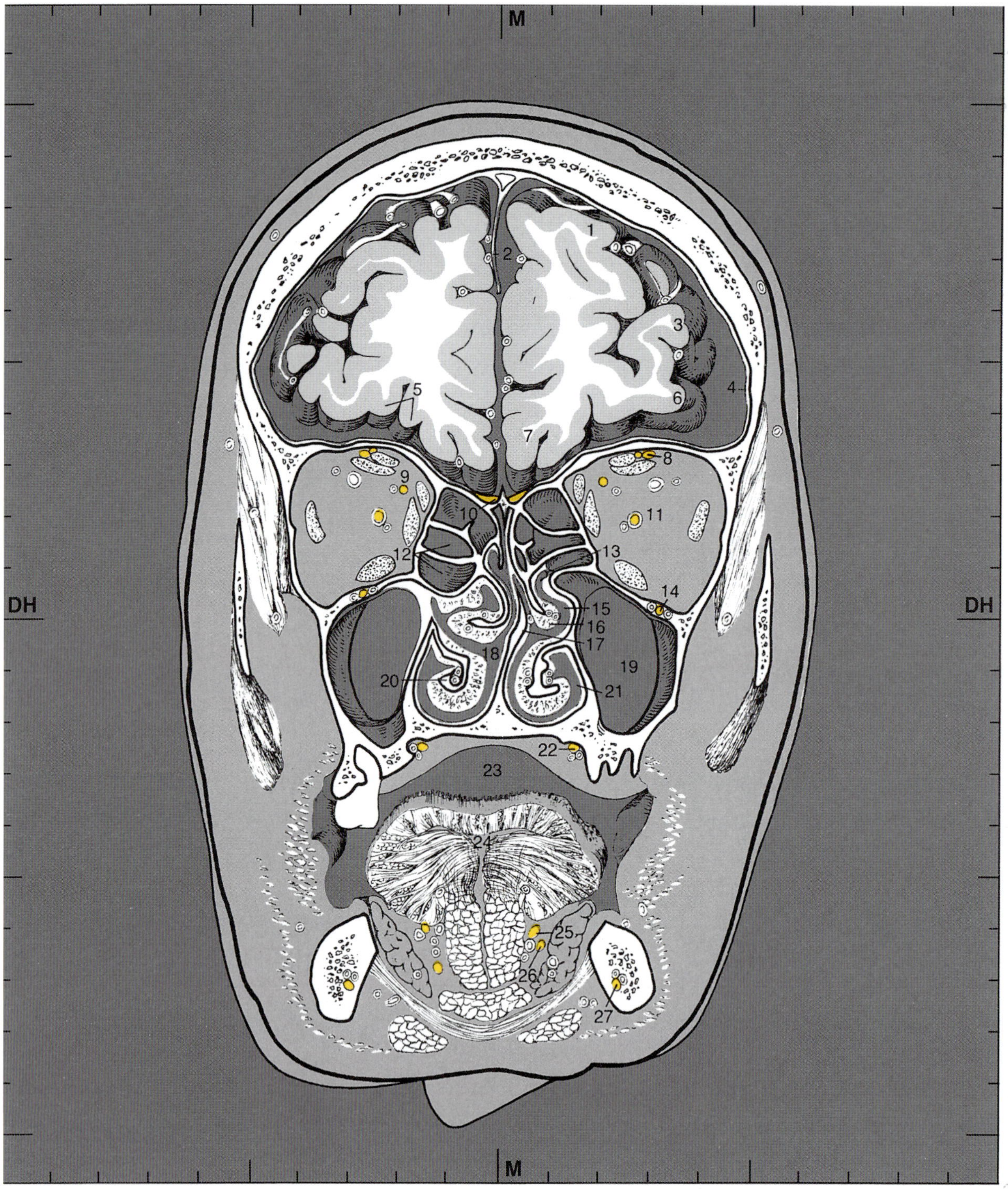

Fig. 5a Anterior section surface of the second coronal slice showing nasal cavity, nasal sinuses, brain structures, and cranial nerves. The frontal lobes are cut at the site of the olfactory bulb.

Coronal Slices

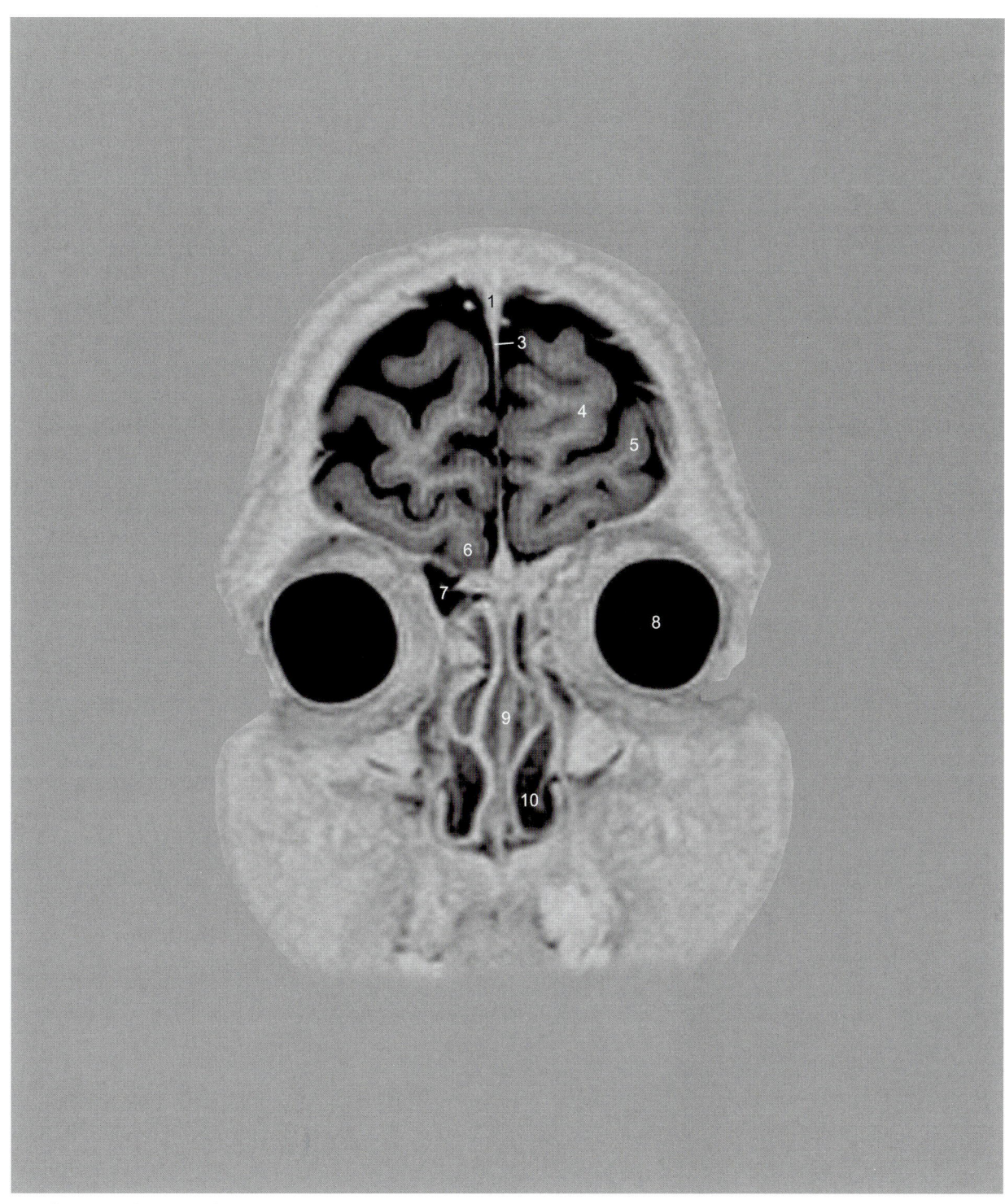

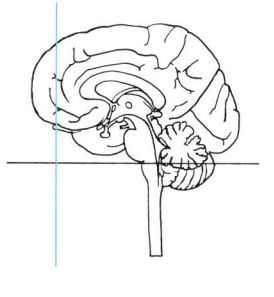

1 Superior sagittal sinus
3 Falx cerebri
4 Superior frontal gyrus
5 Middle frontal gyrus
6 Straight gyrus
7 Frontal sinus
8 Eyeball
9 Nasal septum
10 Inferior nasal concha

Fig. **5b** Coronal, T1-weighted MR image corresponding approximately to the sectional plane of Figs. 5a and 5c. The MR image shows the facial skeleton to be situated more posteriorly than is shown in Figs. 5a and 5c, thus the olfactory bulb can be seen in this MR image.

28   Atlas

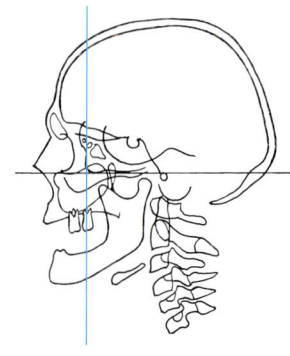

1 Superior sagittal sinus
2 Anteromedial frontal artery
3 Frontal bone
4 Intermediomedial frontal artery
5 Polar frontal artery
6 Roof of orbit
7 Medial frontobasal artery
8 Levator palpebrae superioris
9 Superior oblique
10 Superior rectus
11 Superior ophthalmic vein
12 Ophthalmic artery
13 Ethmoid, cribriform plate
14 Medial rectus
15 Lateral rectus
16 Temporalis
17 Orbital plate
18 Inferior rectus
19 Infraorbital artery and vein
20 Floor of orbit
21 Zygomatic bone
22 Buccal fat pad (of Bichat)
23 Alveolar process of maxilla
24 Hard palate
25 Masseter
26 Greater palatine artery and vein
27 Second molar tooth (cut)
28 Buccinator
29 Sublingual gland
30 Submandibular duct
31 Body of mandible
32 Genioglossus
33 Sublingual artery
34 Inferior alveolar artery and vein
35 Submental artery and vein
36 Platysma
37 Geniohyoid
38 Mylohyoid
39 Anterior belly of digastric

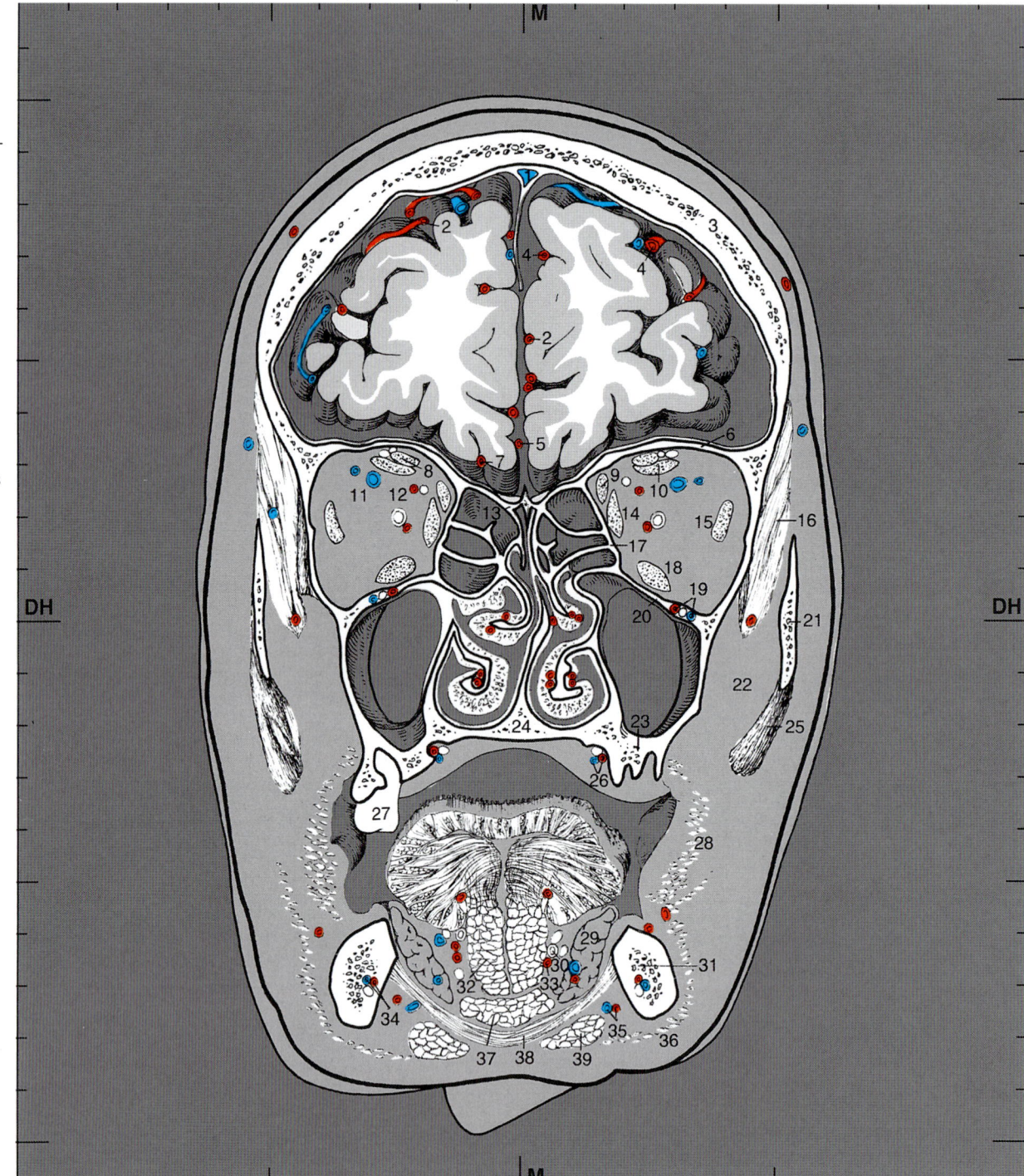

Fig. 5c Anterior section surface of the second coronal slice showing bony structures, muscles, and blood vessels. The sectional plane is positioned approximately 6 mm posterior to the eyeball and in the middle of the body of mandible.

Coronal Slices

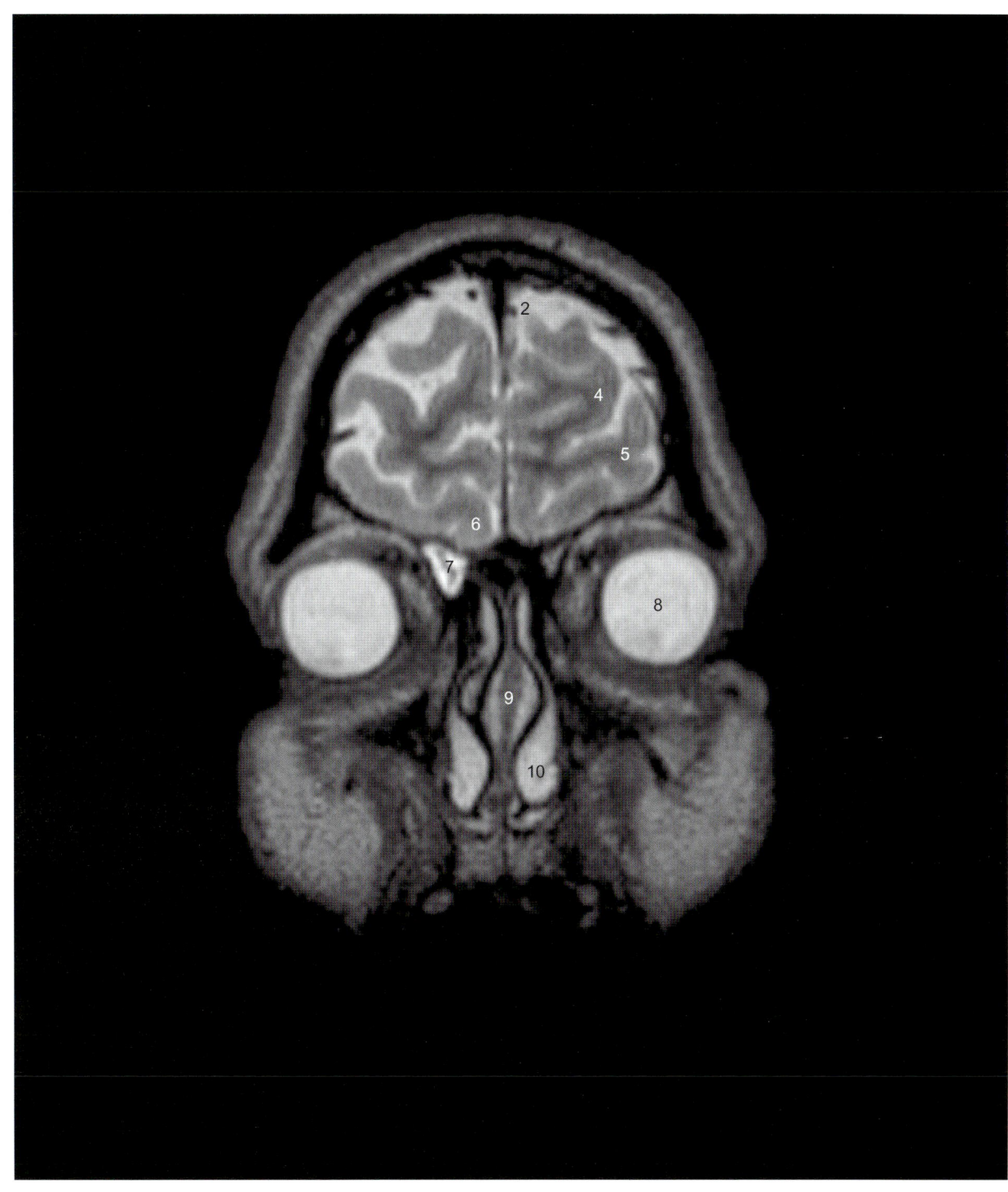

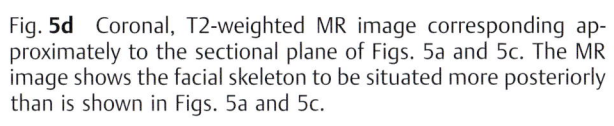

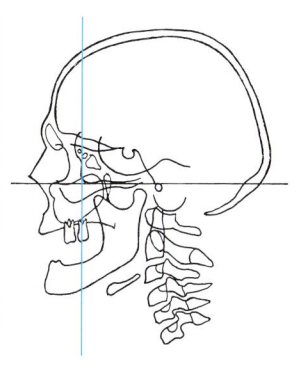

2 Interhemispheric cistern
4 Superior frontal gyrus
5 Middle frontal gyrus
6 Straight gyrus
7 Frontal sinus (swelling of mucous membrane)
8 Eyeball
9 Nasal septum
10 Inferior nasal concha

Fig. **5d** Coronal, T2-weighted MR image corresponding approximately to the sectional plane of Figs. 5a and 5c. The MR image shows the facial skeleton to be situated more posteriorly than is shown in Figs. 5a and 5c.

30 Atlas

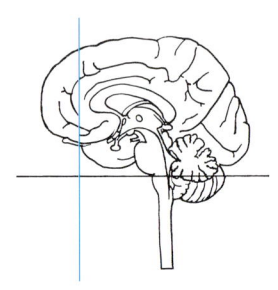

1 Falx cerebri
2 Superior frontal gyrus
3 Middle frontal gyrus
4 Cingulate sulcus
5 Cingulate gyrus
6 Dura mater
7 Inferior frontal gyrus
8 Orbital gyri
9 Straight gyrus
10 Trochlear nerve
11 Olfactory tract
12 Frontal nerve
13 Nasociliary nerve
14 Ethmoidal cells
15 Abducens nerve
16 Optic nerve
17 Inferior branch of oculomotor nerve
18 Middle nasal concha
19 Middle nasal meatus
20 Infraorbital nerve
21 Nasal septum
22 Maxillary sinus
23 Inferior nasal concha
24 Nasal cavity
25 Inferior nasal meatus
26 Palatine nerves
27 Oral cavity
28 Tongue
29 Lingual nerve
30 Inferior alveolar nerve
31 Hypoglossal nerve

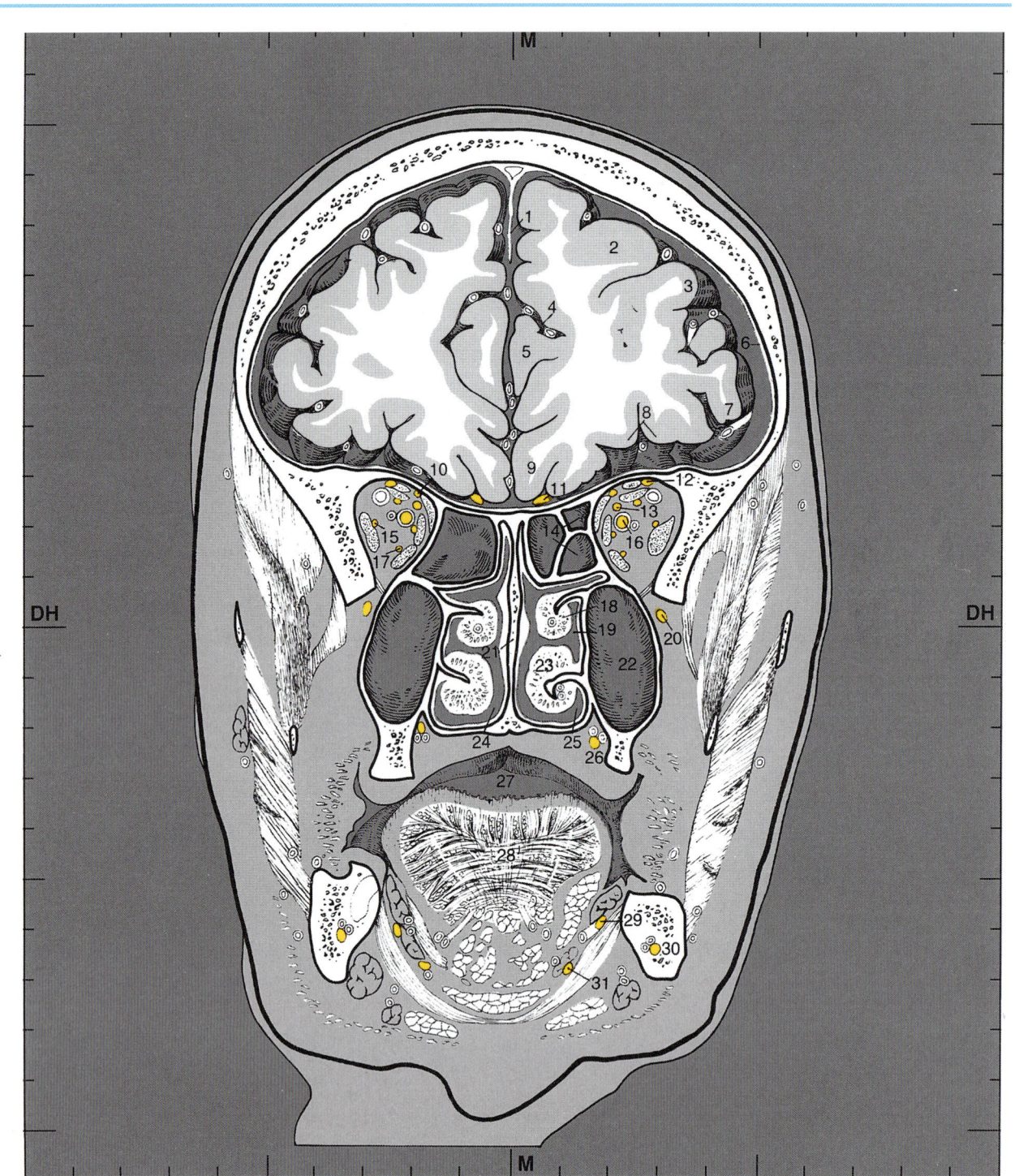

Fig. **6a** Anterior section surface of the third coronal slice showing nasal cavity, nasal sinuses, oral cavity, brain structures, and cranial nerves. The sectional plane is located in the frontal lobe approximately 8 mm anterior to the genu of the corpus callosum (Fig. 2b). The optic nerve, the branches of the trigeminal nerve, and the hypoglossal nerve are also demonstrated in the facial skeleton.

Coronal Slices

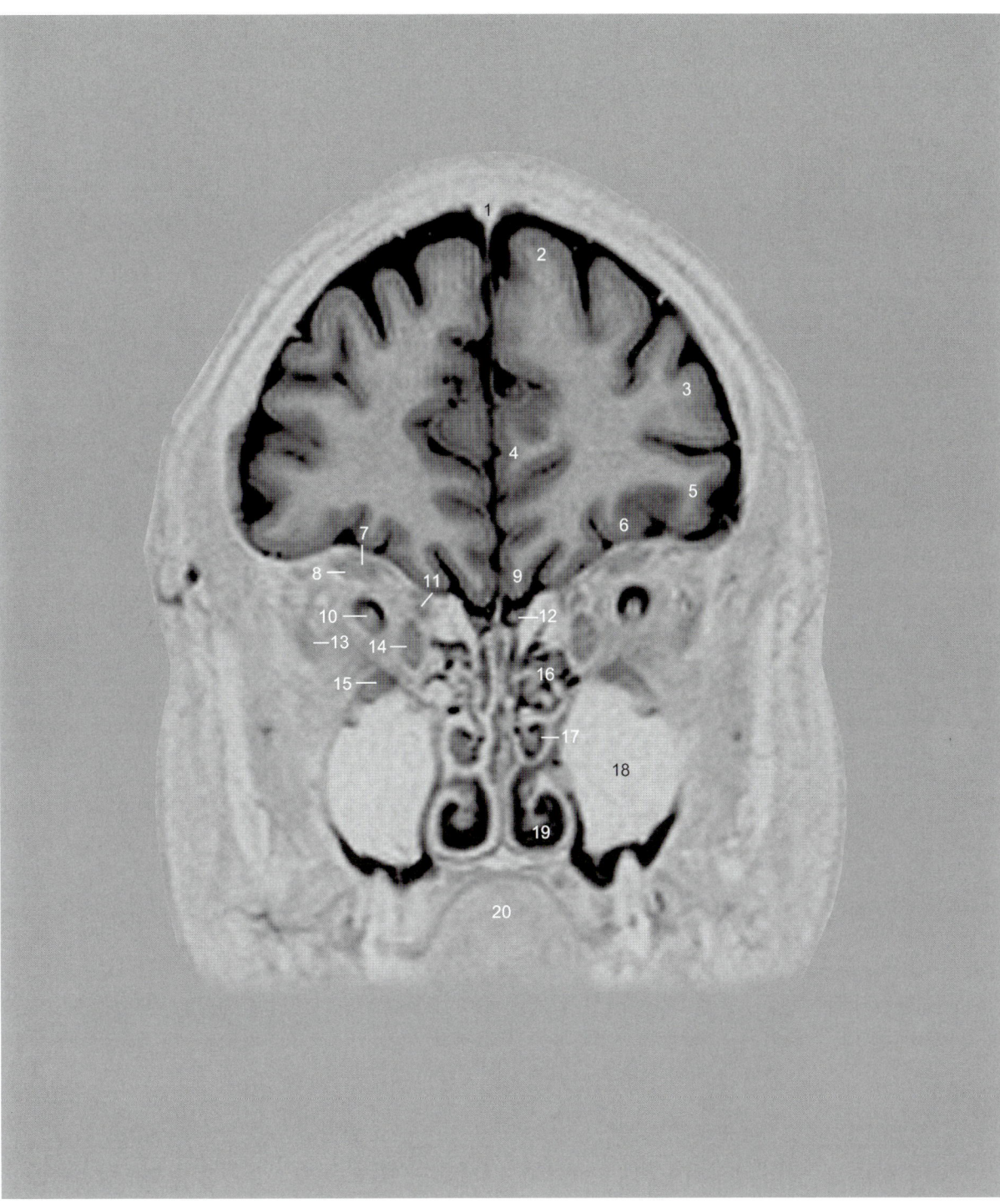

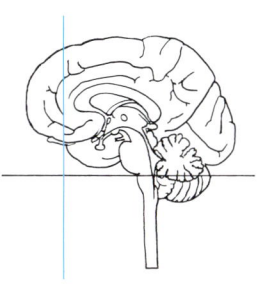

1 Superior sagittal sinus
2 Superior frontal gyrus
3 Middle frontal gyrus
4 Cingulate gyrus
5 Inferior frontal gyrus
6 Orbital gyrus
7 Levator palpebrae superioris
8 Superior rectus
9 Straight gyrus
10 Optic nerve
11 Superior oblique
12 Olfactory bulb
13 Lateral rectus
14 Medial rectus
15 Inferior rectus
16 Ethmoidal cells
17 Middle nasal concha
18 Maxillary sinus
19 Inferior nasal concha
20 Tongue

Fig. **6b** Coronal, T1-weighted MR image corresponding approximately to the sectional plane of Figs. 6a and 6c.

32 Atlas

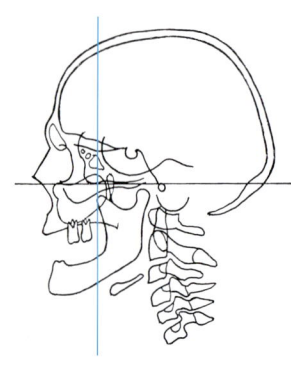

1 Superior sagittal sinus
2 Frontal bone
3 Intermediomedial frontal artery
4 Prefrontal artery
5 Anteromedial frontal artery
6 Lateral frontobasal artery
7 Polar frontal artery
8 Medial frontobasal artery
9 Superior ophthalmic vein
10 Levator palpebrae superioris
11 Superior rectus
12 Superior oblique
13 Superficial temporal artery, frontal branch
14 Greater wing of sphenoid
15 Medial rectus
16 Ophthalmic artery
17 Lateral rectus
18 Temporalis
19 Inferior rectus
20 Orbitalis
21 Zygomatic arch
22 Maxilla
23 Hard palate
24 Descending palatine artery and vein
25 Coronoid process
26 Parotid duct
27 Masseter
28 Buccinator
29 Body of mandible
30 Facial artery and vein
31 Inferior alveolar artery and vein
32 Submandibular duct
33 Genioglossus
34 Sublingual artery
35 Submental artery and vein
36 Submandibular gland
37 Anterior belly of digastric
38 Geniohyoid
39 Mylohyoid
40 Platysma

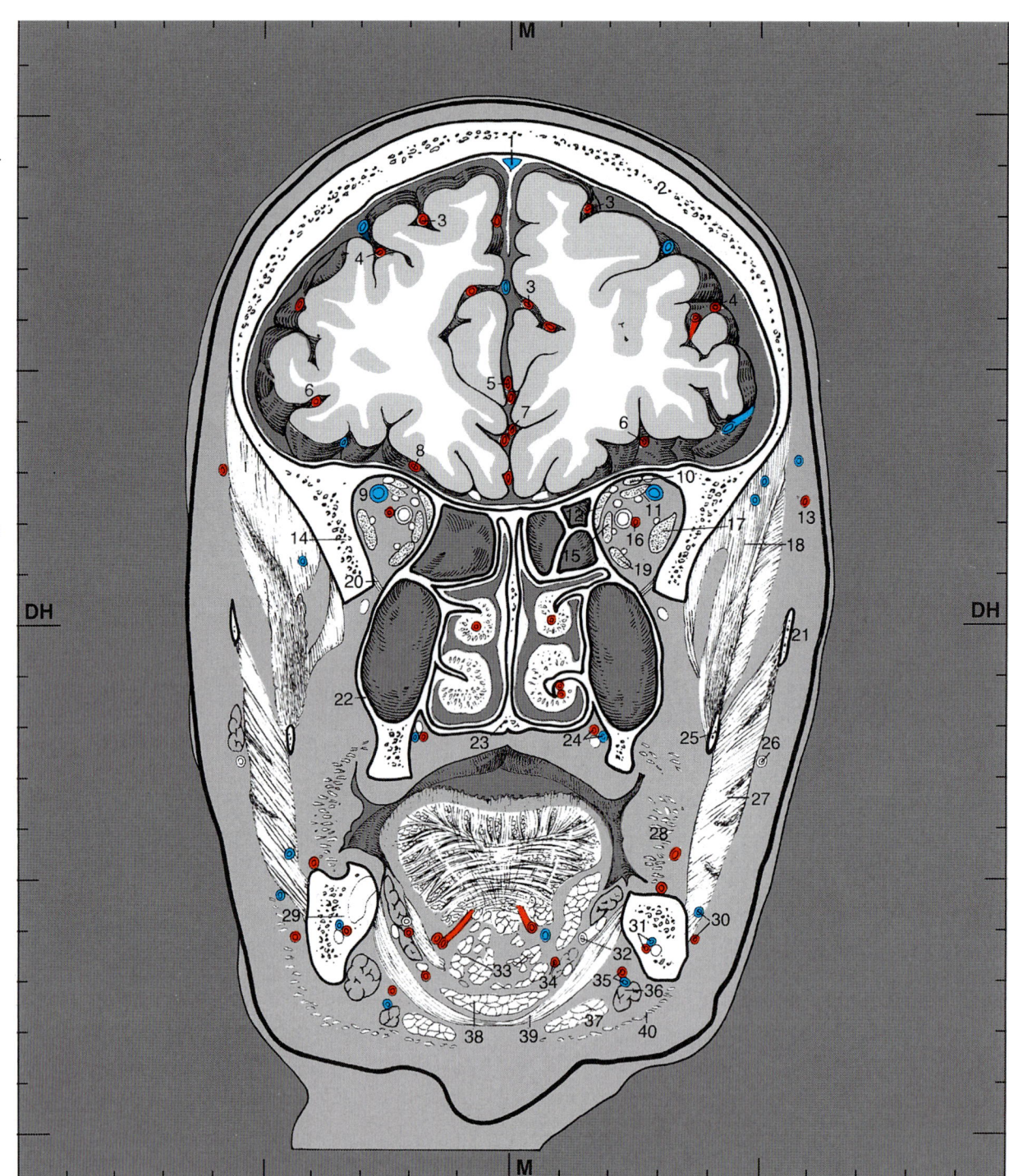

Fig. **6c** Anterior section surface of the third coronal slice showing bony structures, muscles, and blood vessels. The sectional plane runs posteriorly to the middle of the anterior cranial fossa, through the posterior third of the orbit and through the coronoid process of the mandible.

Coronal Slices

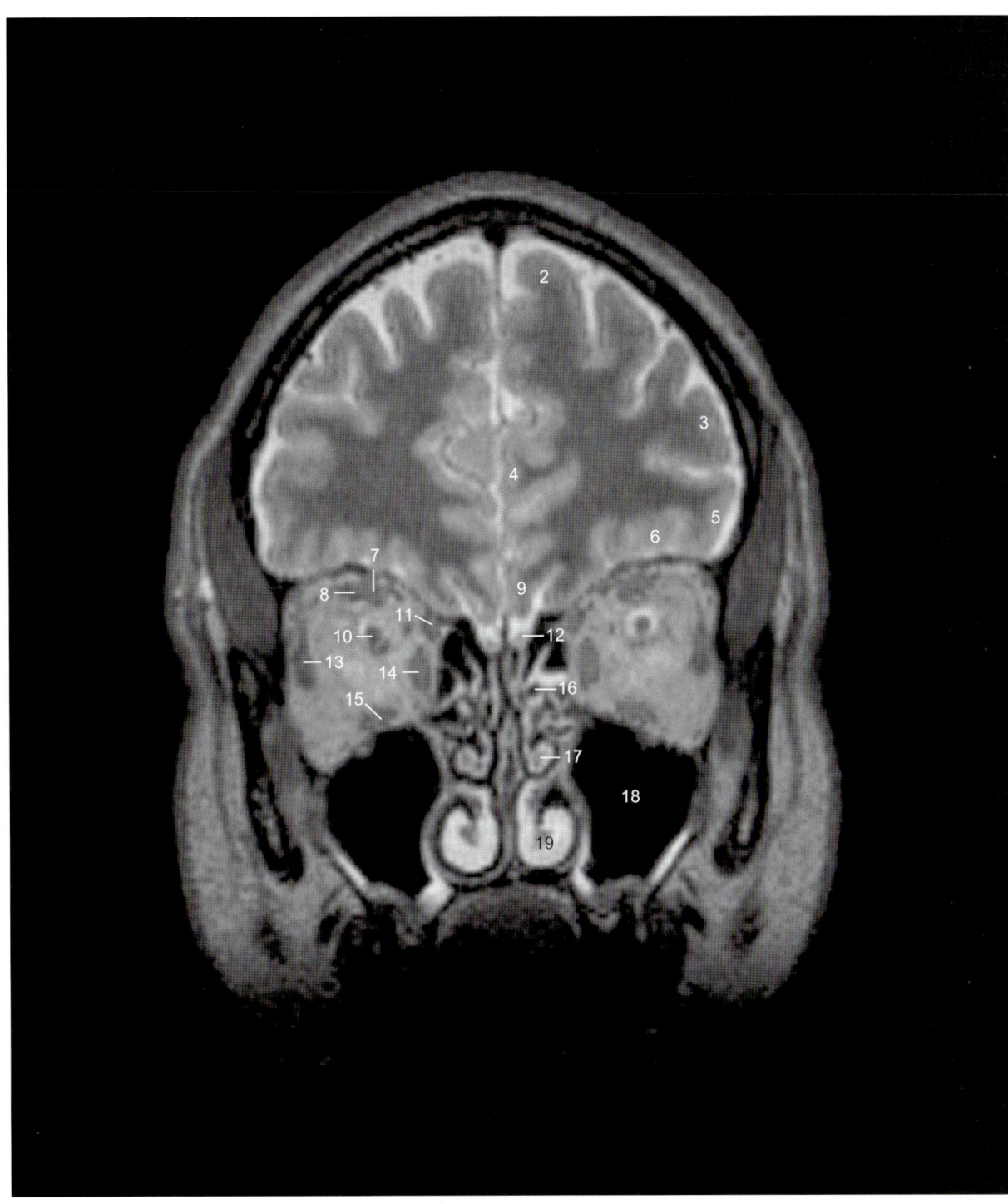

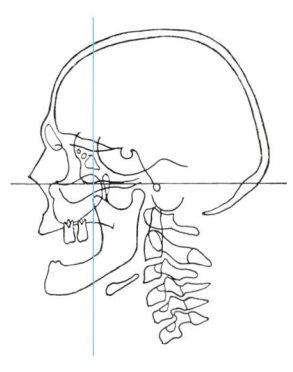

2 Superior frontal gyrus
3 Middle frontal gyrus
4 Cingulate gyrus
5 Inferior frontal gyrus
6 Orbital gyrus
7 Levator palpebrae superioris
8 Superior rectus
9 Straight gyrus
10 Optic nerve
11 Superior oblique
12 Olfactory bulb
13 Lateral rectus
14 Medial rectus
15 Inferior rectus
16 Ethmoidal cells
17 Middle nasal concha
18 Maxillary sinus
19 Inferior nasal concha

Fig. **6d** Coronal, T2-weighted MR image corresponding approximately to the sectional plane of Figs. 6a and 6c.

34 Atlas

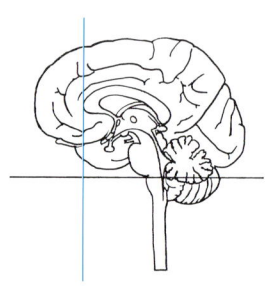

1 Falx cerebri
2 Superior frontal gyrus
3 Cingulate sulcus
4 Middle frontal gyrus
5 Cingulate gyrus
6 Genu of corpus callosum
7 Inferior frontal gyrus
8 Dura mater
9 Longitudinal cerebral (inter-hemispheric) fissure
10 Straight gyrus
11 Orbital gyrus
12 Olfactory tract
13 Optic nerve
14 Trochlear nerve
15 Oculomotor nerve
16 Pole of temporal lobe
17 Ophthalmic nerve
18 Abducens nerve
19 Sphenoidal sinus
20 Maxillary nerve
21 Nasal septum
22 Middle nasal concha
23 Nasal cavity
24 Inferior nasal concha
25 Oral cavity
26 Tongue
27 Lingual nerve
28 Inferior alveolar nerve
29 Hypoglossal nerve

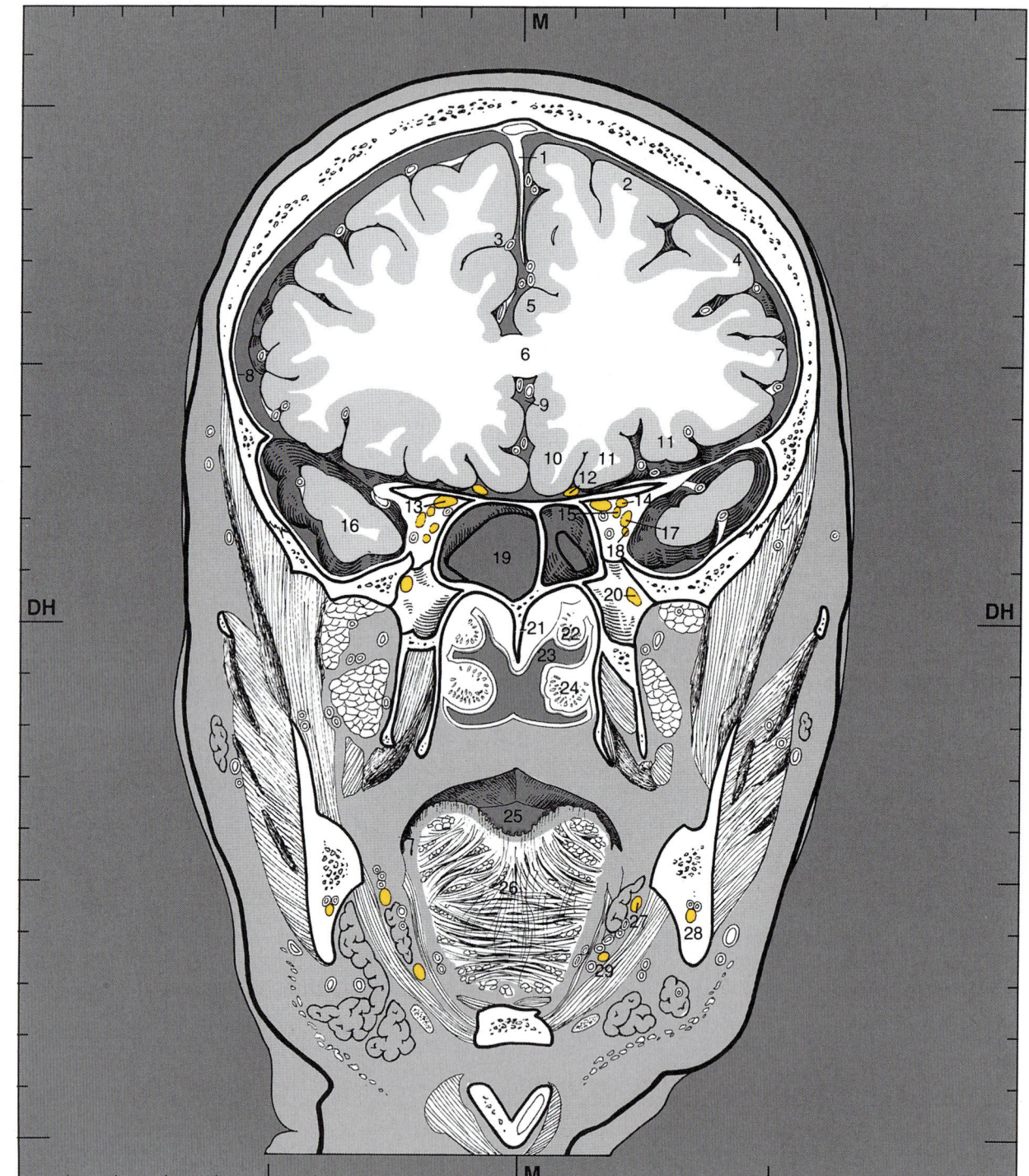

Fig. **7a** Anterior section surface of the fourth coronal slice showing nasal cavity, nasal sinuses, brain structures, and cranial nerves. The frontal lobe is cut at the level of the genu of the corpus callosum. The optic nerve and the third, fourth, and sixth cranial nerves are positioned in close proximity in the orbital apex. The hypoglossal nerve and the branches of the mandibular nerve are found on the floor of the oral cavity.

Coronal Slices

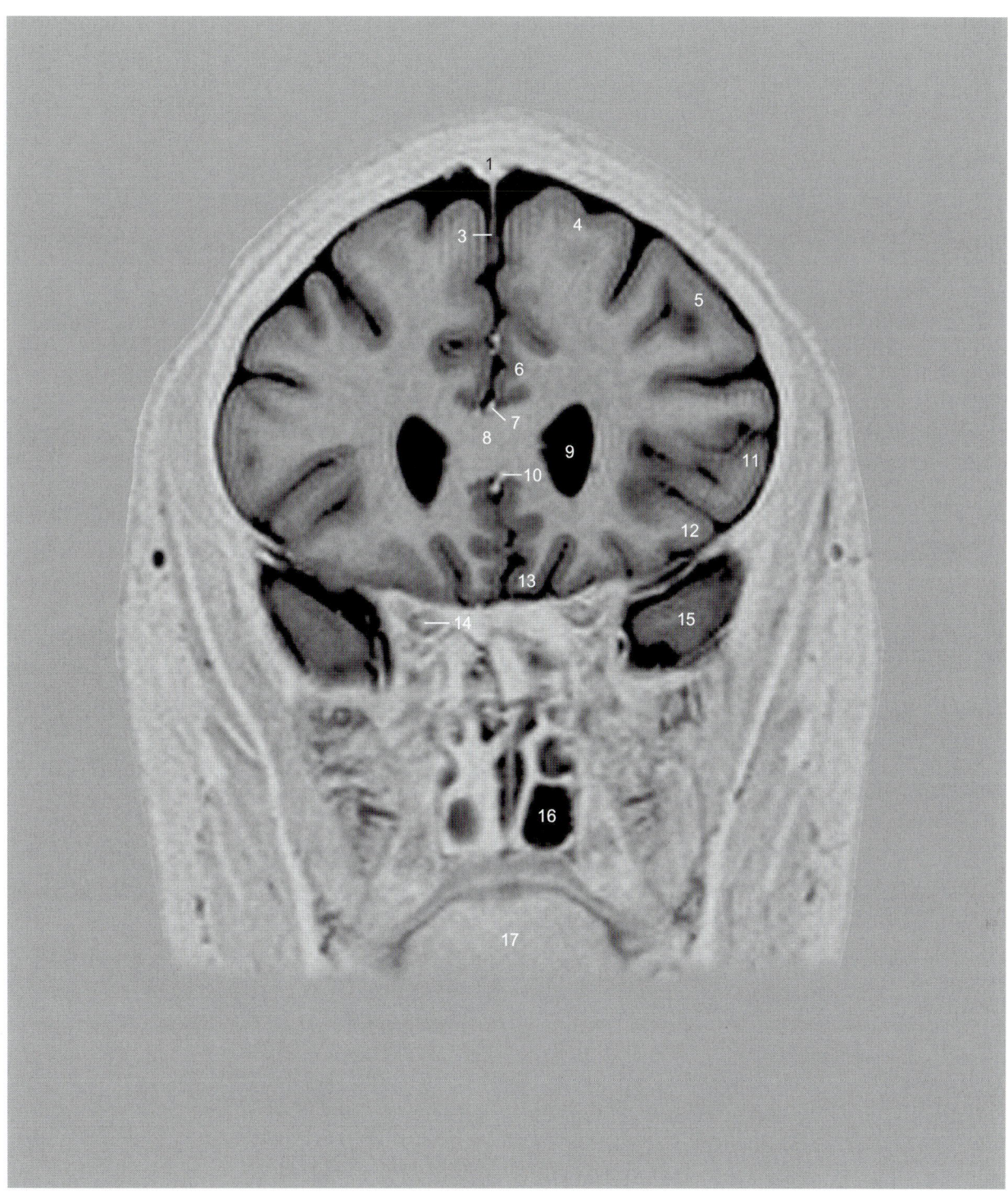

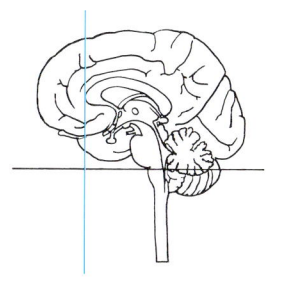

1 Superior sagittal sinus
3 Falx cerebri
4 Superior frontal gyrus
5 Middle frontal gyrus
6 Cingulate gyrus
7 Pericallosal artery
8 Genu of corpus callosum
9 Frontal (anterior) horn of lateral ventricle
10 Anterior cerebral artery
11 Inferior frontal gyrus
12 Orbital gyrus
13 Straight gyrus
14 Optic nerve
15 Pole of temporal lobe
16 Inferior nasal concha
17 Tongue

Fig. **7b** Coronal, T1-weighted MR image. Nonconformity with the sectional plane of Figs. 7a and 7c is shown by the frontal (anterior) horns of the lateral ventricles and the sphenoidal sinus.

Atlas

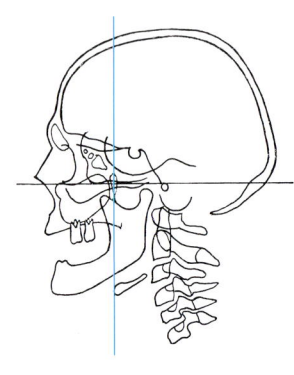

1 Superior sagittal sinus
2 Intermediomedial frontal artery
3 Prefrontal artery
4 Pericallosal artery
5 Anterior cerebral artery
6 Lateral frontobasal artery
7 Polar temporal artery of middle cerebral artery
8 Lesser wing of sphenoid
9 Ophthalmic artery
10 Superior ophthalmic vein
11 Inferior orbital fissure
12 Superficial temporal artery, frontal branch
13 Pterygopalatine fossa
14 Zygomatic arch
15 Temporalis
16 Maxillary artery
17 Lateral pterygoid plate
18 Lateral pterygoid
19 Medial pterygoid
20 Medial pterygoid plate
21 Soft palate
22 Tensor veli palatini
23 Coronoid process
24 Parotid duct
25 Pterygoid hamulus
26 Masseter
27 Ramus of mandible
28 Inferior alveolar artery and vein in mandibular canal
29 Sublingual artery
30 Mylohyoid
31 Submental artery and vein
32 Submandibular gland
33 Platysma
34 Digastric tendon
35 Hyoid bone
36 Thyroid cartilage

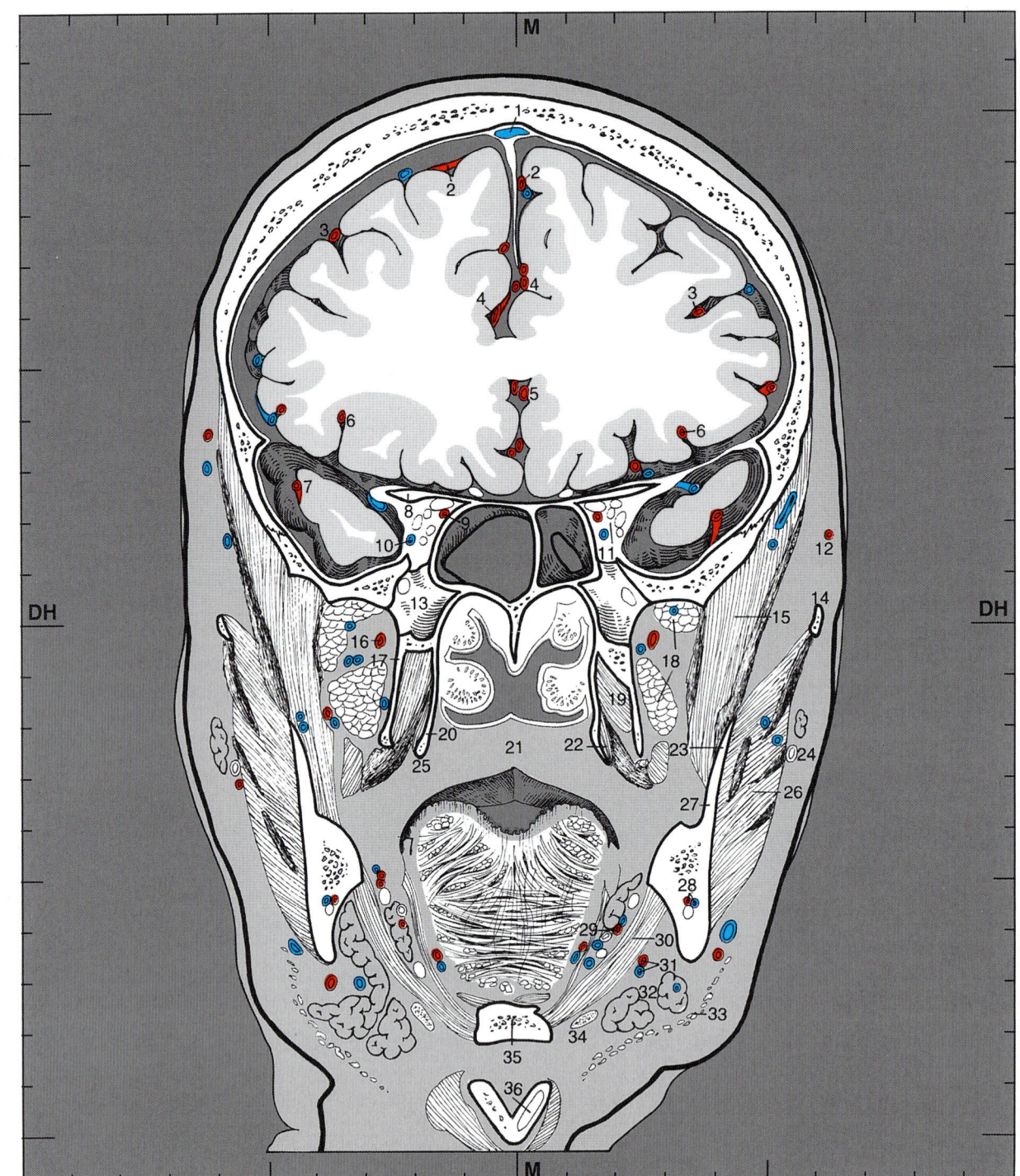

Fig. **7c** Anterior section surface of the fourth coronal slice showing bony structures, muscles, and blood vessels. The anterior poles of the middle cranial fossae are positioned lateral and inferior to the lesser wing of the sphenoid. The optic canal and the superior orbital fissure are also shown. The tongue is cut at the level of the hyoid bone.

Coronal Slices

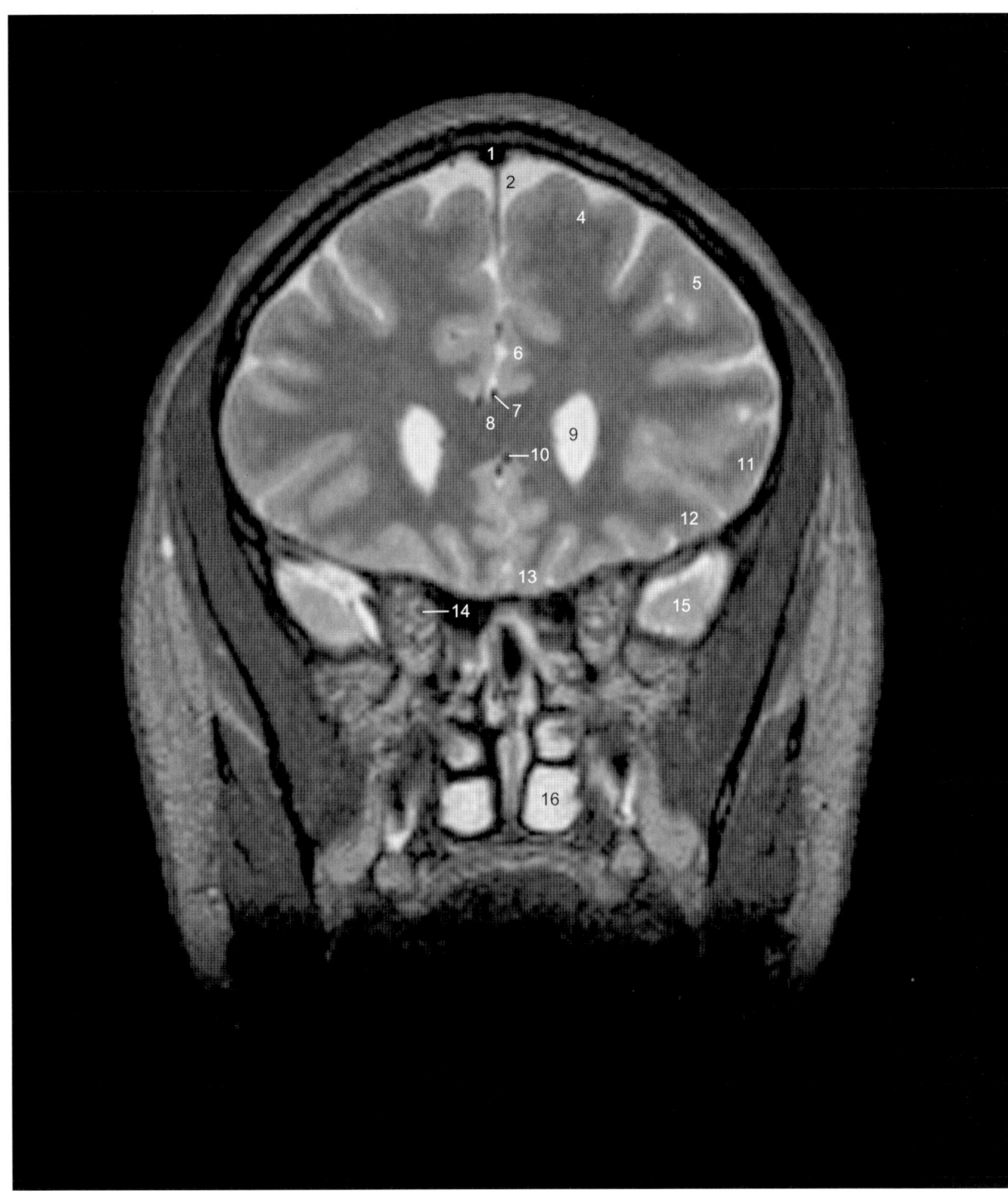

Fig. **7d** Coronal, T2-weighted MR image. Nonconformity with the sectional plane of Figs. 7a and 7c is shown by the frontal (anterior) horns of the lateral ventricles and the sphenoidal sinus.

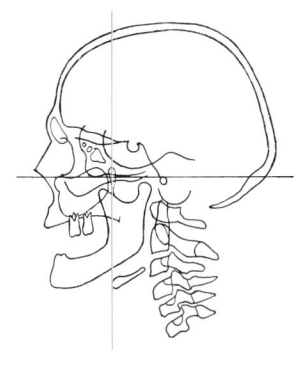

1 Superior sagittal sinus
2 Interhemispheric cistern
4 Superior frontal gyrus
5 Middle frontal gyrus
6 Cingulate gyrus
7 Pericallosal artery
8 Genu of corpus callosum
9 Frontal (anterior) horn of lateral ventricle
10 Anterior cerebral artery
11 Inferior frontal gyrus
12 Orbital gyrus
13 Straight gyrus
14 Optic nerve
15 Pole of temporal lobe
16 Inferior nasal concha

38 Atlas

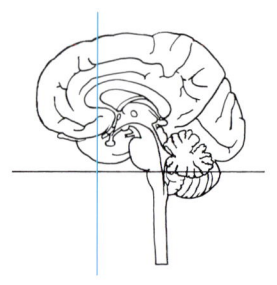

1 Superior frontal gyrus
2 Falx cerebri
3 Middle frontal gyrus
4 Cingulate sulcus
5 Cingulate gyrus
6 Inferior frontal gyrus
7 Genu of corpus callosum
8 Frontal (anterior) horn of lateral ventricle
9 Head of caudate nucleus
10 Insula
11 Lateral sulcus (Sylvian fissure)
12 Putamen
13 Superior temporal gyrus
14 Straight gyrus
15 Olfactory tract
16 Optic chiasm
17 Optic nerve
18 Oculomotor nerve
19 Trochlear nerve
20 Middle temporal gyrus
21 Ophthalmic nerve
22 Abducens nerve
23 Sphenoidal sinus
24 Maxillary nerve
25 Nasopharynx
26 Uvula
27 Inferior alveolar nerve
28 Palatine tonsil
29 Lingual nerve
30 Isthmus of fauces
31 Hypoglossal nerve

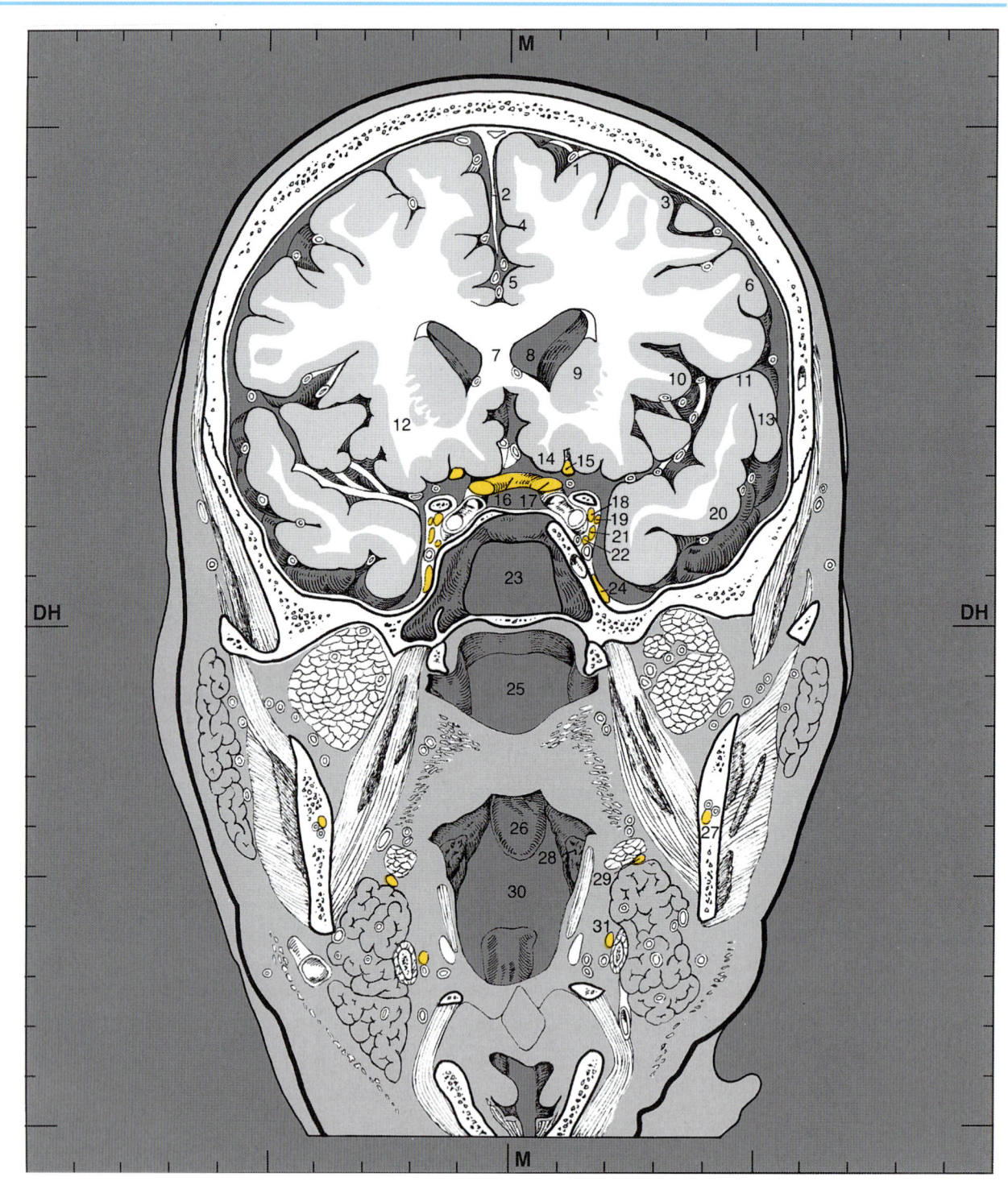

Fig. 8a Anterior section surface of the fifth coronal slice showing brain structures and cranial nerves. The frontal (anterior) horns of the lateral ventricles are cut at this level. The section shows the optic chiasm. The lingual nerve and the hypoglossal nerve are positioned lateral to the isthmus of fauces.

Coronal Slices 39

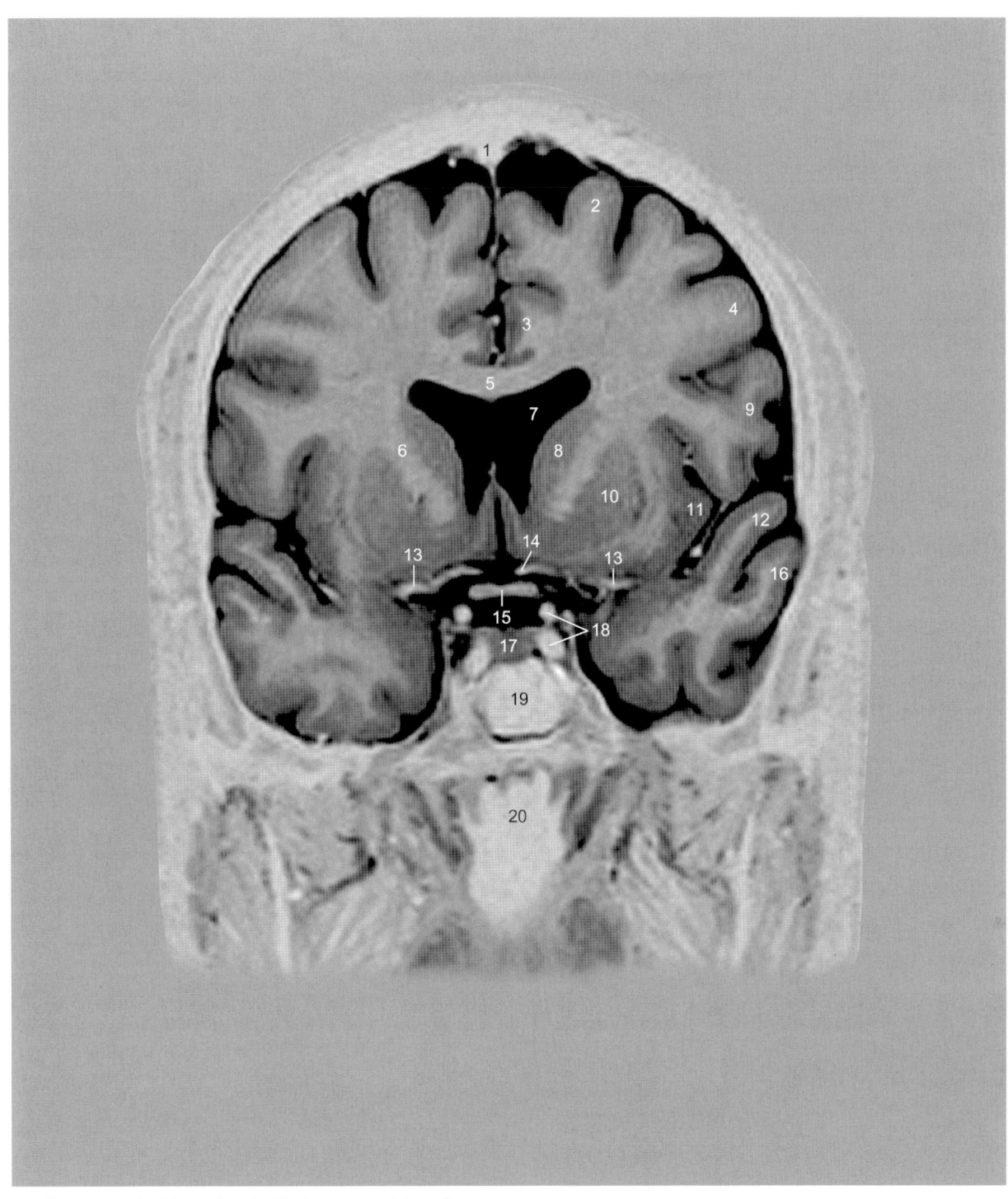

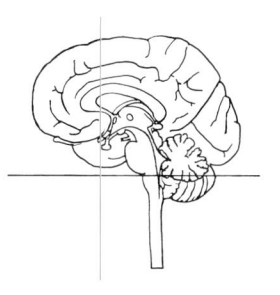

1 Superior sagittal sinus
2 Superior frontal gyrus
3 Cingulate gyrus
4 Middle frontal gyrus
5 Corpus callosum
6 Internal capsule
7 Frontal (anterior) horn of lateral ventricle
8 Head of caudate nucleus
9 Inferior frontal gyrus
10 Putamen
11 Insula
12 Superior temporal gyrus
13 Middle cerebral artery
14 Anterior cerebral artery
15 Optic chiasm
16 Middle temporal gyrus
17 Pituitary gland
18 Internal carotid artery
19 Sphenoidal sinus
20 Nasopharynx

Fig. **8b** Coronal, T1-weighted MR image positioned more posteriorly than the sectional plane of Figs. 8a and 8c.

40 Atlas

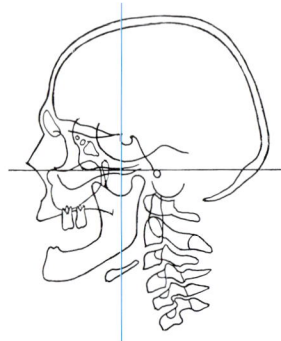

1 Superior sagittal sinus
2 Parietal bone
3 Posteromedial frontal artery
4 Bridging vein
5 Intermediomedial frontal artery
6 Prefrontal artery
7 Paracentral artery
8 Pericallosal artery
9 Insular arteries
10 Anterior cerebral artery
11 Basal vein (of Rosenthal)
12 Anterior clinoid process
13 Internal carotid artery
14 Temporal artery of middle cerebral artery
15 Cavernous sinus
16 Temporal bone
17 Superficial temporal artery, frontal branch
18 Temporalis
19 Sphenoid
20 Zygomatic arch
21 Maxillary artery
22 Lateral pterygoid
23 Nasopharynx
24 Parotid gland
25 Soft palate
26 Medial pterygoid
27 Inferior alveolar artery and vein
28 Masseter
29 Uvula
30 Styloglossus
31 Ramus of mandible
32 Submandibular gland
33 Facial artery
34 Epiglottis
35 Stylohyoid ligament
36 Lingual artery
37 Digastric tendon and stylohyoid
38 Greater cornu of hyoid bone
39 Platysma
40 Vestibular fold
41 Thyroid cartilage
42 Vocal fold

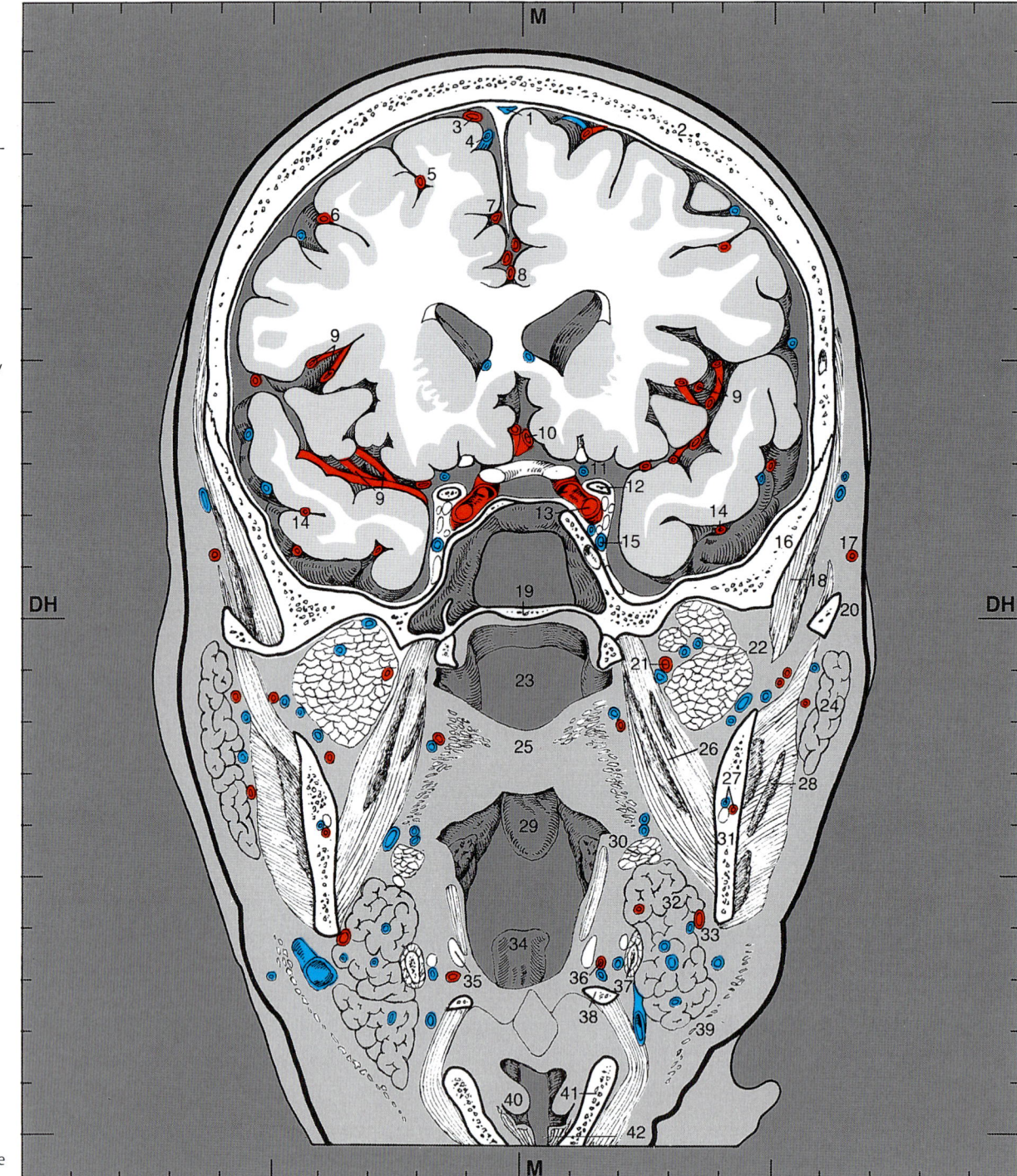

Fig. **8c** Anterior section surface of the fifth coronal slice showing bony structures, muscles, and blood vessels. The sectional plane lies close to the middle of the sphenoid at the level of the anterior clinoid processes and the middle of the zygomatic arch. Demonstrated in this section are the nasopharynx, the soft palate, and the uvula.

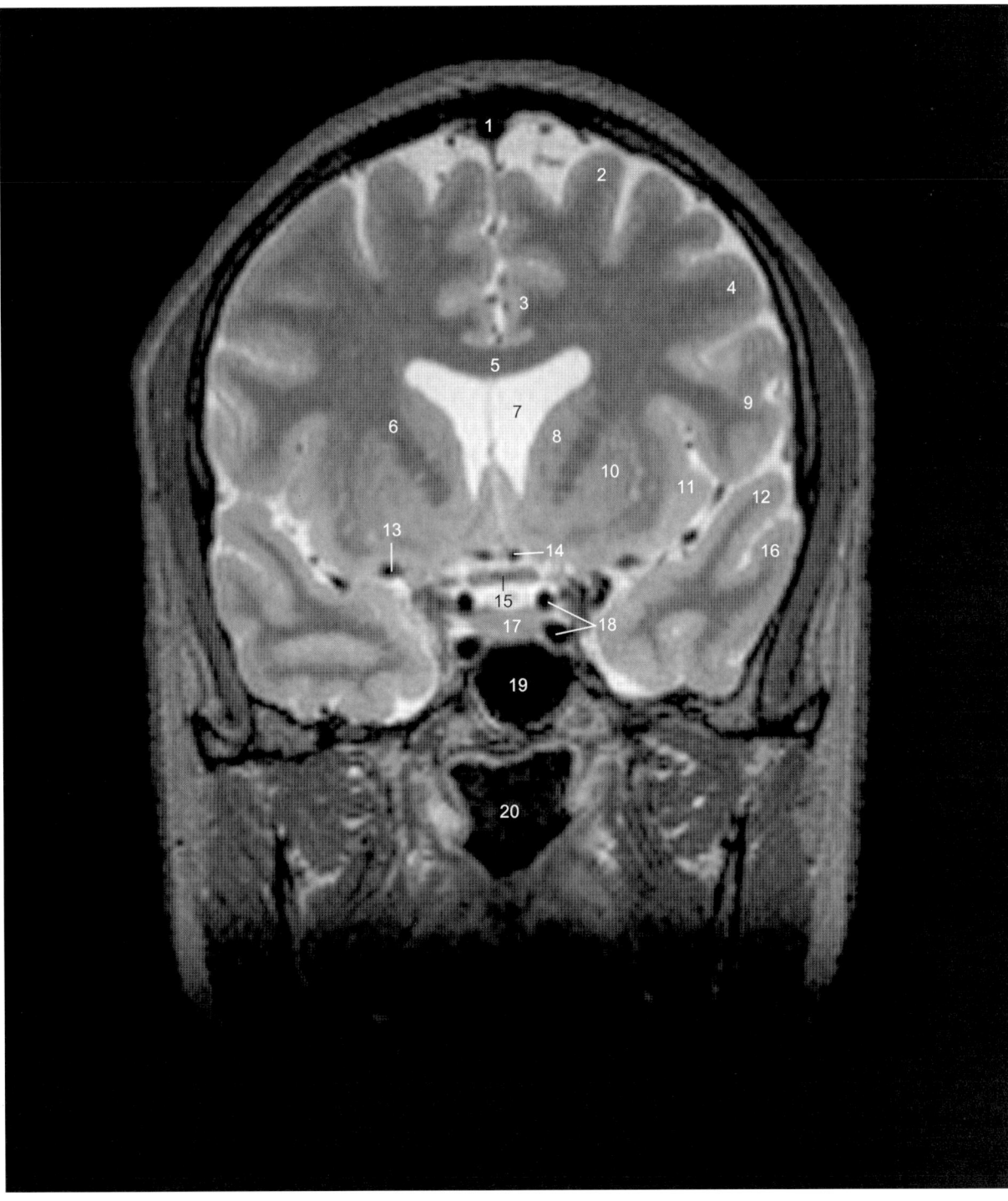

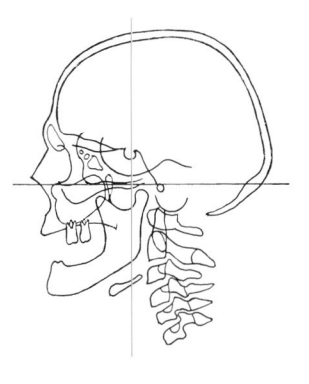

Coronal Slices

1 Superior sagittal sinus
2 Superior frontal gyrus
3 Cingulate gyrus
4 Middle frontal gyrus
5 Corpus callosum
6 Internal capsule
7 Frontal (anterior) horn of lateral ventricle
8 Head of caudate nucleus
9 Inferior frontal gyrus
10 Putamen
11 Insula
12 Superior temporal gyrus
13 Middle cerebral artery
14 Anterior cerebral artery
15 Optic chiasm
16 Middle temporal gyrus
17 Pituitary gland
18 Internal carotid artery
19 Sphenoidal sinus
20 Nasopharynx

Fig. **8d** Coronal T2-weighted MR image positioned more posteriorly than the sectional plane of Figs. 8a and 8c.

42 Atlas

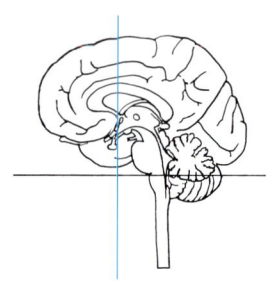

1 Superior frontal gyrus
2 Falx cerebri
3 Middle frontal gyrus
4 Cingulate sulcus
5 Cingulate gyrus
6 Stratum subependymale
7 Trunk (body) of corpus callosum
8 Inferior frontal gyrus
9 Frontal (anterior) horn of lateral ventricle
10 Head of caudate nucleus
11 Septum pellucidum
12 Anterior limb of internal capsule
13 Lateral sulcus (Sylvian fissure)
14 Putamen
15 External capsule
16 Claustrum
17 Extreme capsule
18 Insula
19 Superior temporal gyrus
20 Anterior commissure (within the slice)
21 Anterior commissure
22 Superior temporal sulcus
23 Third ventricle
24 Optic tract
25 Middle temporal gyrus
26 Infundibular recess
27 Oculomotor nerve
28 Trochlear nerve
29 Parahippocampal gyrus
30 Abducens nerve
31 Trigeminal ganglion
32 Inferior temporal gyrus
33 Inferior temporal sulcus
34 Sphenoidal sinus
35 Lateral occipitotemporal gyrus
36 Mandibular nerve
37 Glossopharyngeal nerve
38 Hypoglossal nerve

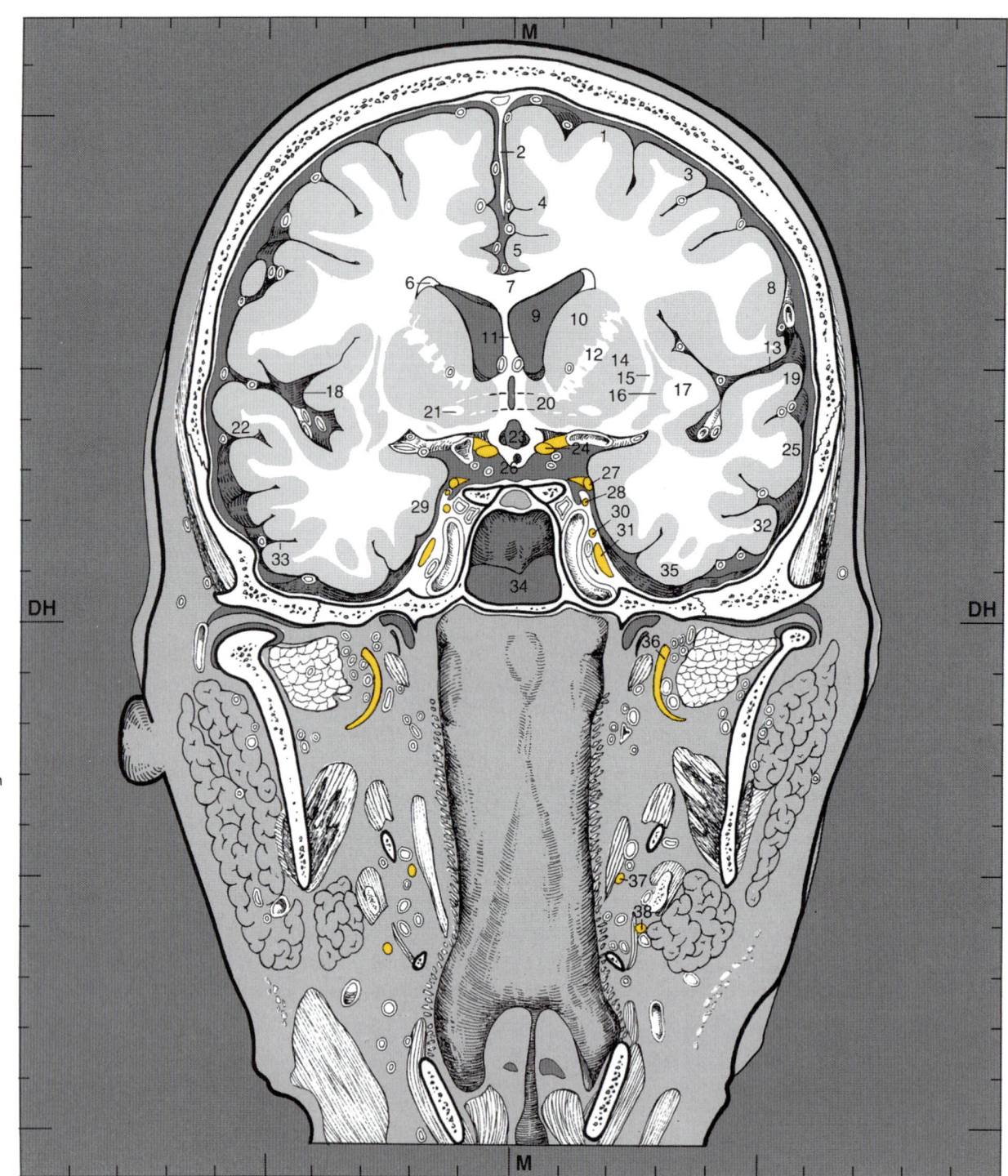

Fig. **9a** Anterior section surface of the sixth coronal slice showing brain structures and cranial nerves. The sectional plane lies in the median region 2 mm anterior to the anterior commissure (dashed line within the slice). The anterior branches of the anterior commissure are located laterally in the basal ganglia. The third, fourth, and sixth cranial nerves lie in a lateral aspect to the pituitary gland.

Coronal Slices

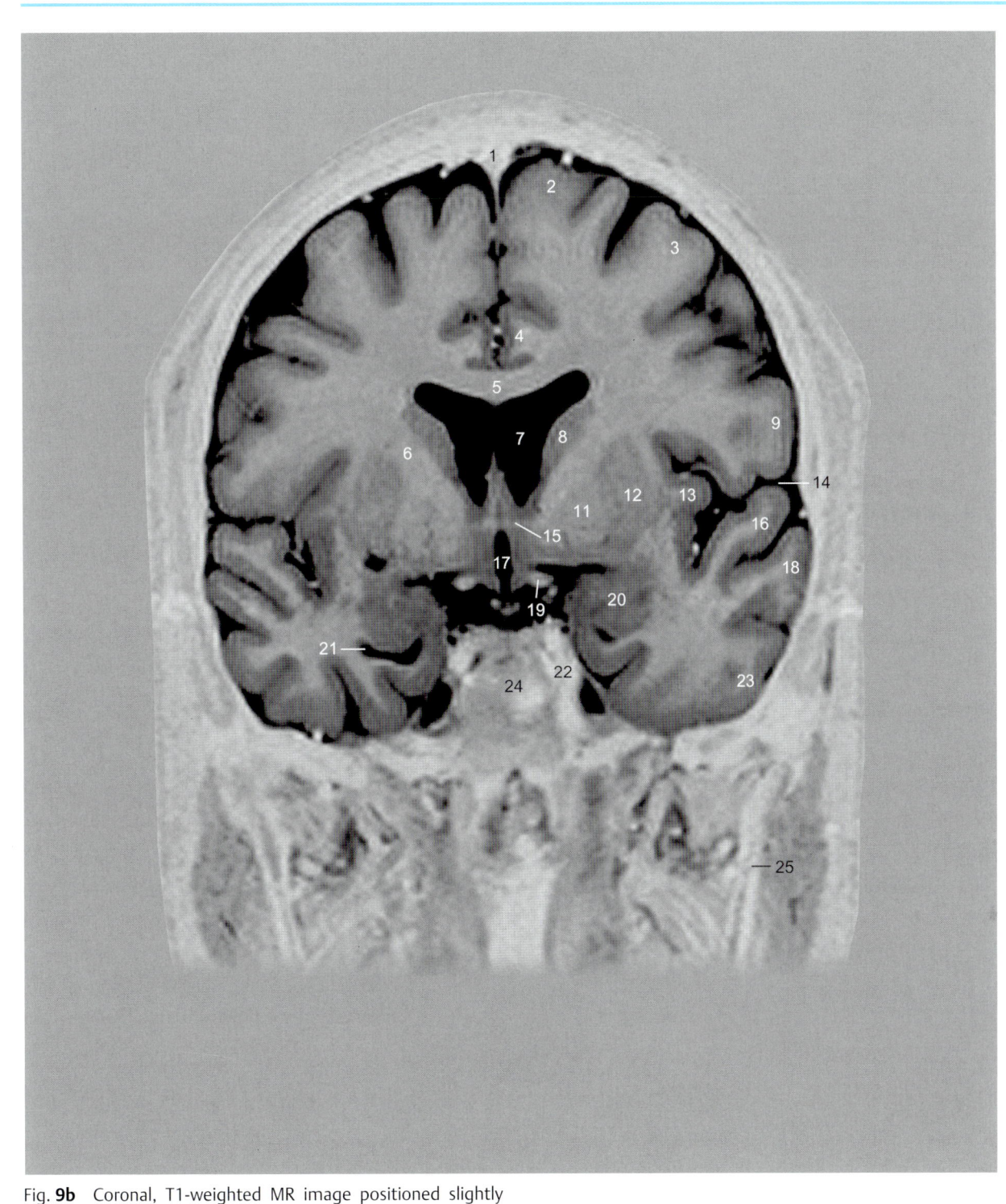

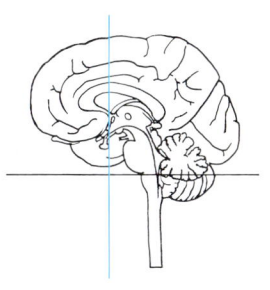

1 Superior sagittal sinus
2 Superior frontal gyrus
3 Middle frontal gyrus
4 Cingulate gyrus
5 Corpus callosum
6 Anterior limb of internal capsule
7 Frontal (anterior) horn of lateral ventricle
8 Caudate nucleus
9 Inferior frontal gyrus
11 Globus pallidus
12 Putamen
13 Insula
14 Lateral sulcus
15 Anterior commissure
16 Superior temporal gyrus
17 Third ventricle
18 Middle temporal gyrus
19 Optic tract
20 Amygdaloid body
21 Temporal (inferior) horn of lateral ventricle
22 Internal carotid artery
23 Inferior temporal gyrus
24 Sphenoidal sinus
25 Ramus of mandible

Fig. **9b** Coronal, T1-weighted MR image positioned slightly more posteriorly than the sectional plane of Figs. 9a and 9c.

44   Atlas

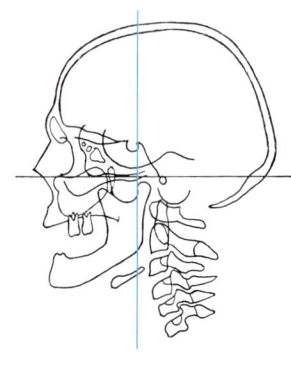

1 Superior sagittal sinus
2 Posteromedial frontal artery
3 Parietal bone
4 Paracentral artery
5 Pericallosal artery
6 Artery of precentral sulcus
7 Superior thalamostriate (terminal) vein
8 Insular arteries
9 Middle cerebral artery
10 Anterior choroidal artery
11 Basal vein (of Rosenthal)
12 Posterior clinoid process
13 Cavernous sinus
14 Pituitary gland
15 Temporalis
16 Temporal artery of middle cerebral artery
17 Internal carotid artery
18 Sphenoid
19 Temporal bone
20 Superficial temporal artery
21 Mandibular fossa
22 Articular disc of temporomandibular joint
23 Head of mandible
24 Cartilage of pharyngotympanic tube
25 Pterygoid venous plexus
26 Levator veli palatini
27 Lateral pterygoid
28 Maxillary artery
29 Posterior pharyngeal wall of nasopharynx
30 Ramus of mandible
31 Medial pterygoid
32 Styloglossus
33 Constrictor of pharynx
34 Parotid gland
35 Posterior pharyngeal wall of oropharynx
36 Facial artery
37 Masseter
38 Stylohyoid ligament (ossified)
39 Posterior belly of digastric
40 Stylopharyngeus
41 Lingual artery
42 Greater cornu of hyoid bone
43 Platysma
44 Superior thyroid artery
45 Sternocleidomastoid
46 Thyroid cartilage

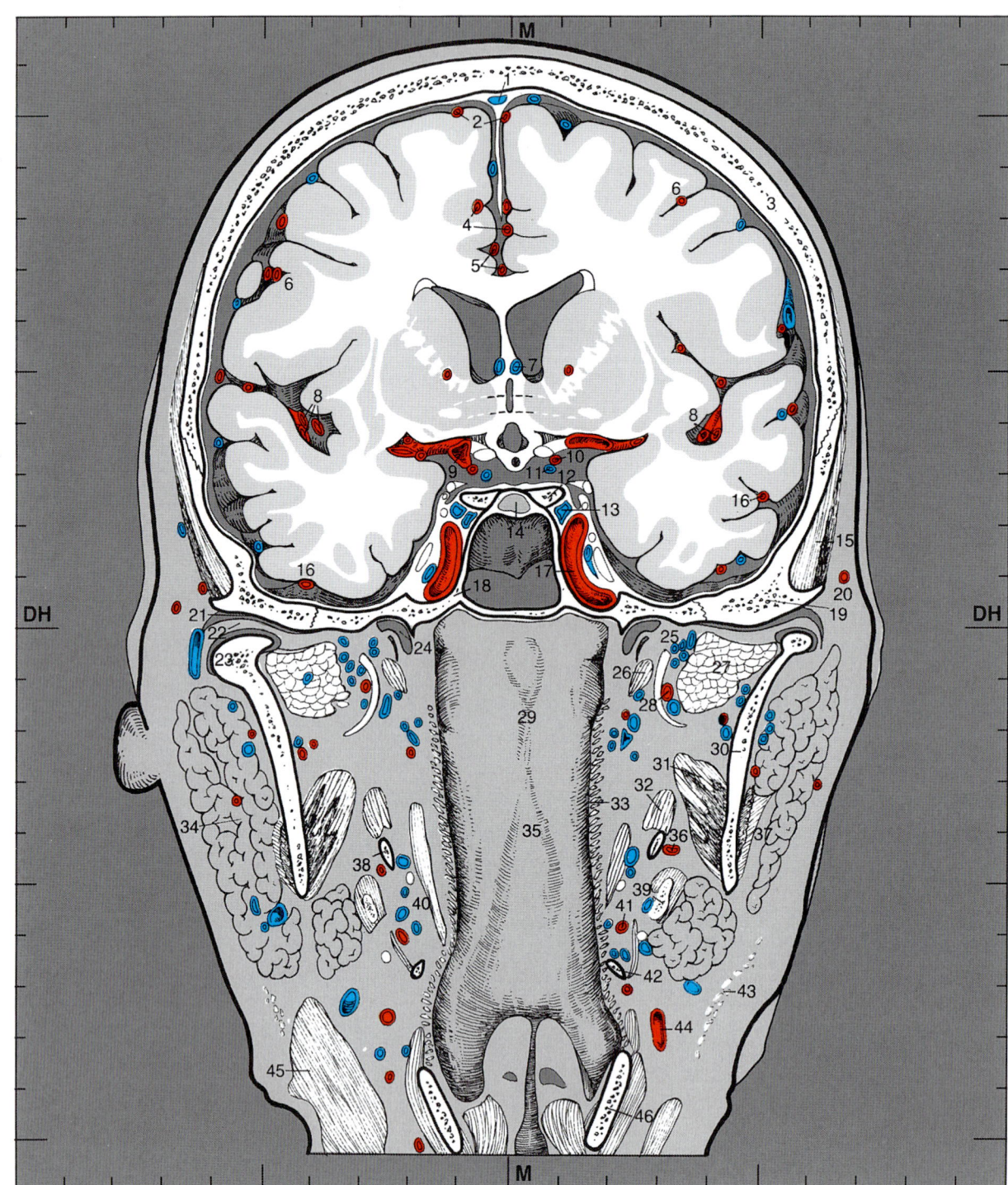

Fig. **9c** Anterior section surface of the sixth coronal slice showing bony structures, muscles, and blood vessels. The sectional plane runs through the hypophysial fossa at the level of the posterior clinoid processes and through both temporomandibular joints. The posterior wall of the pharynx is positioned in the anterior half of the 1-cm-thick slice.

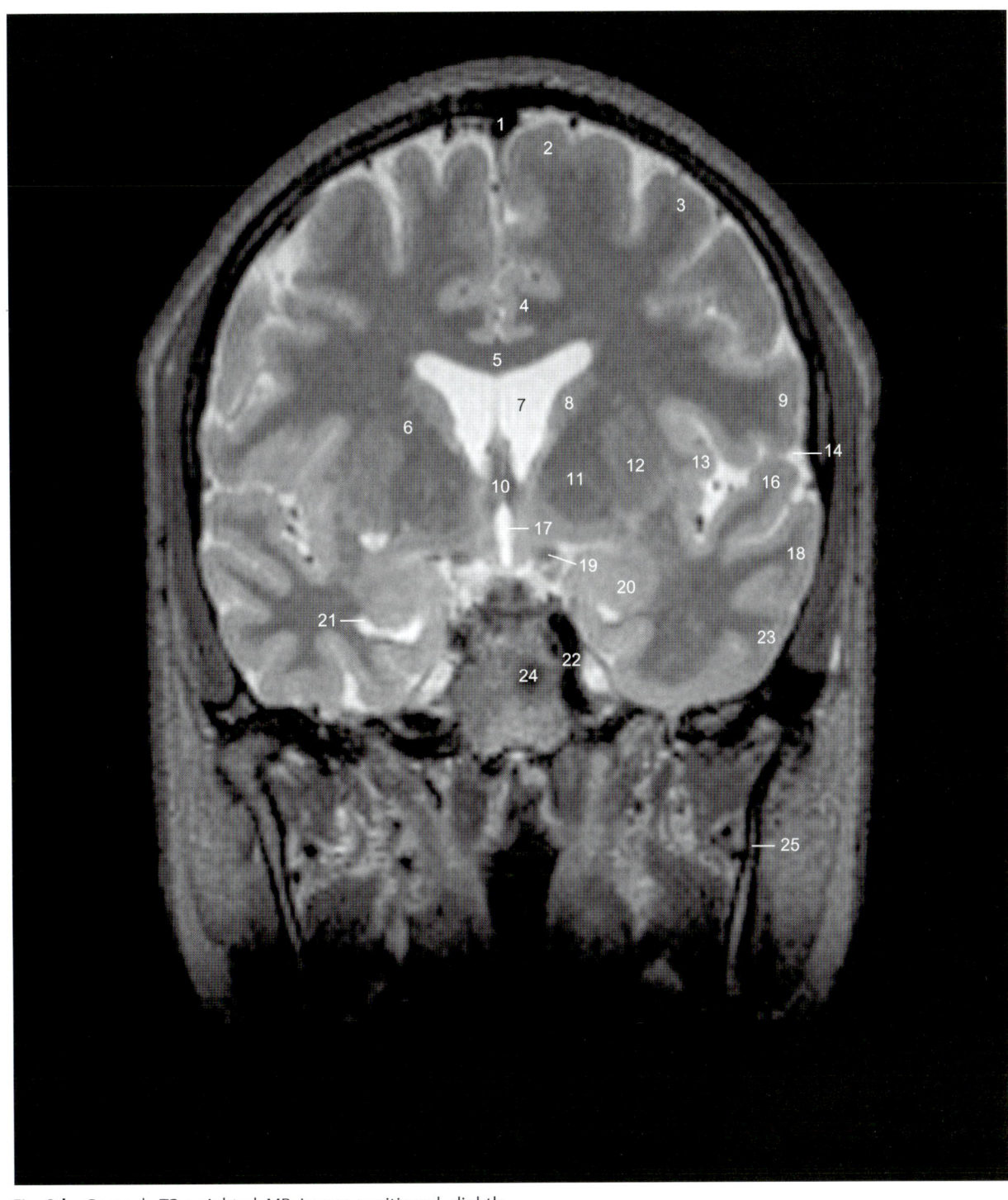

Coronal Slices

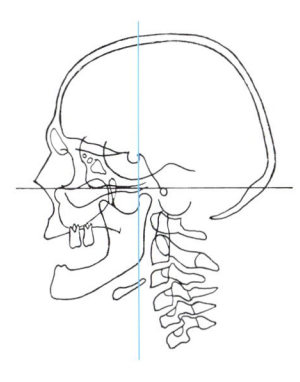

1 Superior sagittal sinus
2 Superior frontal gyrus
3 Middle frontal gyrus
4 Cingulate gyrus
5 Corpus callosum
6 Anterior limb of internal capsule
7 Frontal (anterior) horn of lateral ventricle
8 Caudate nucleus
9 Inferior frontal gyrus
10 Fornix
11 Globus pallidus
12 Putamen
13 Insula
14 Lateral sulcus (Sylvian fissure)
16 Superior temporal gyrus
17 Third ventricle
18 Middle temporal gyrus
19 Optic tract
20 Amygdaloid body
21 Temporal (inferior) horn of lateral ventricle
22 Internal carotid artery
23 Inferior temporal gyrus
24 Sphenoidal sinus
25 Ramus of mandible

Fig. 9d Coronal, T2-weighted MR image positioned slightly more posteriorly than the sectional plane of Figs. 9a and 9c.

46 Atlas

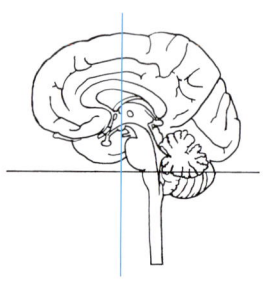

1 Superior frontal gyrus
2 Middle frontal gyrus
3 Falx cerebri
4 Cingulate gyrus
5 Precentral gyrus
6 Trunk (body) of corpus callosum
7 Septum pellucidum
8 Frontal (anterior) horn of lateral ventricle
9 Body of caudate nucleus
10 Fornix
11 Choroid plexus
12 Genu of internal capsule
13 Interventricular foramen (of Monro)
14 Anterior nuclei of thalamus
15 Globus pallidus
16 Putamen
17 Insula
18 Lateral sulcus (Sylvian fissure)
19 Superior temporal gyrus
20 External capsule
21 Extreme capsule
22 Claustrum
23 Basal nucleus (of Meynert)
24 Third ventricle
25 Mammillary body with fornix
26 Optic tract
27 Amygdaloid body
28 Middle temporal gyrus
29 Temporal (inferior) horn of lateral ventricle
30 Hippocampus
31 Oculomotor nerve
32 Trochlear nerve
33 Anterior petroclinoidal fold
34 Abducens nerve
35 Pons
36 Parahippocampal gyrus
37 Trigeminal nerve
38 Lateral occipitotemporal gyrus
39 Inferior temporal gyrus
40 Sphenoidal sinus, posterior wall
41 Superior cervical ganglion
42 Vagus nerve (within the slice)
43 Sympathetic trunk (within the slice)
44 Hypoglossal nerve
45 Superior laryngeal nerve

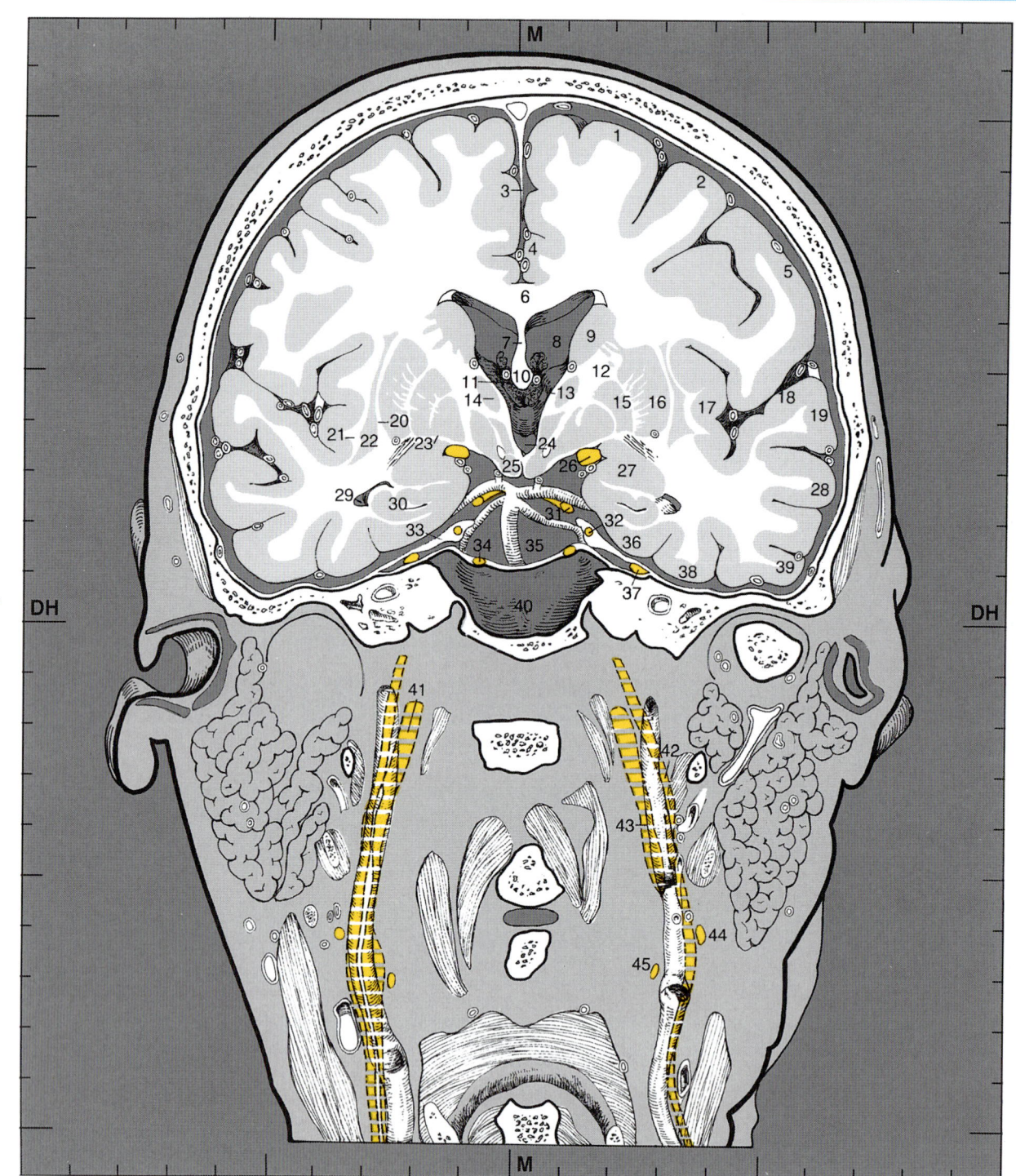

Fig. 10a Anterior section surface of the seventh coronal slice showing brain structures and cranial nerves. The interventricular foramina, the mammillary bodies and the frontal (anterior) horn of the lateral ventricles are positioned in this slice.

Coronal Slices

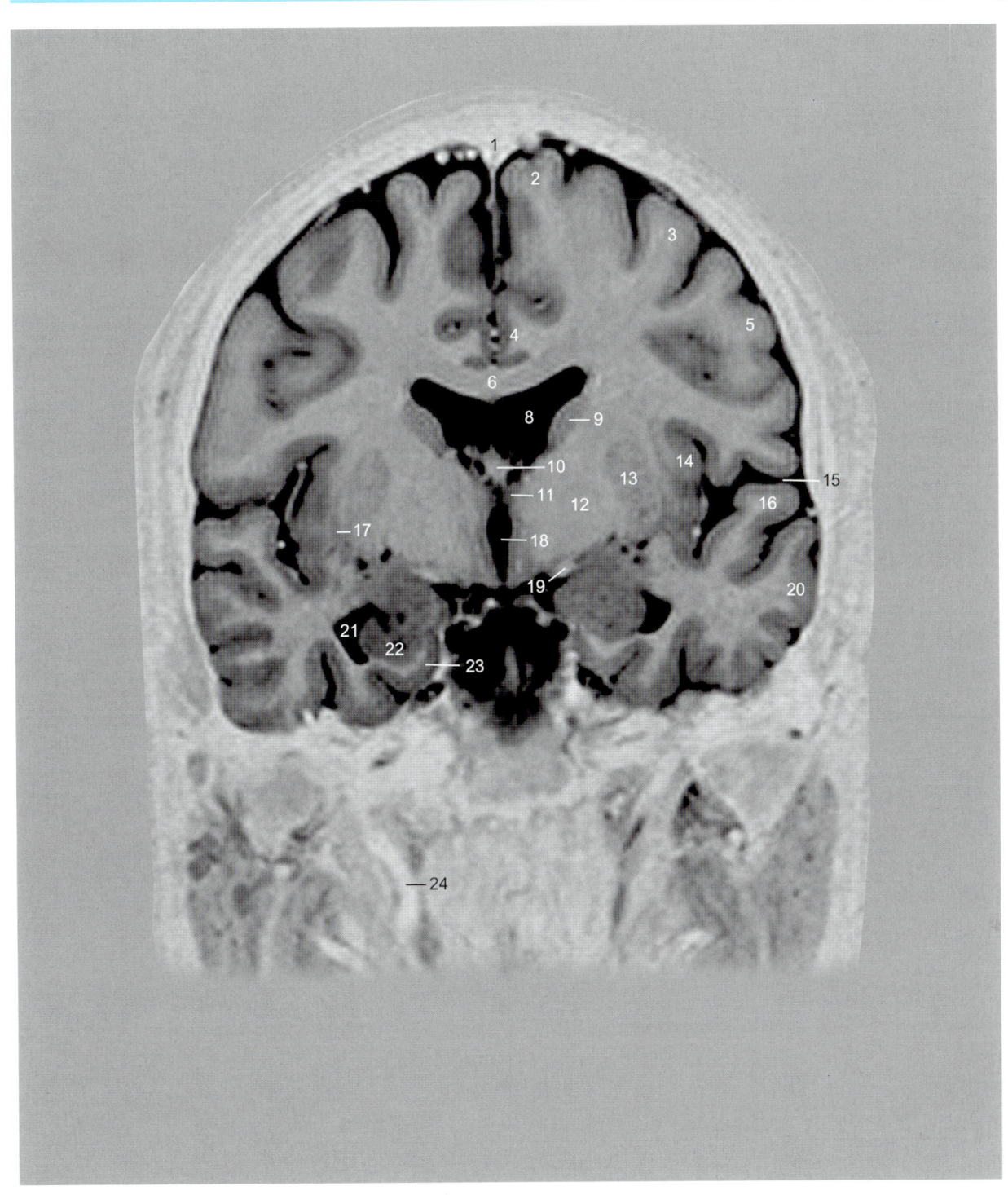

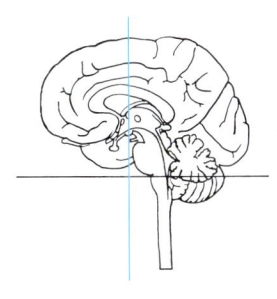

Fig. 10b Coronal, T1-weighted MR image corresponding approximately to the sectional plane of Figs. 10a and 10c.

1 Superior sagittal sinus
2 Superior frontal gyrus
3 Middle frontal gyrus
4 Cingulate gyrus
5 Precentral gyrus
6 Trunk (body) of corpus callosum
8 Frontal (anterior) horn of lateral ventricle
9 Body of caudate nucleus
10 Fornix
11 Interventricular foramen (of Monro)
12 Globus pallidus
13 Putamen
14 Insula
15 Lateral sulcus (Sylvian fissure)
16 Superior temporal gyrus
17 Claustrum
18 Third ventricle
19 Optic tract
20 Middle temporal gyrus
21 Temporal (inferior) horn of lateral ventricle
22 Hippocampus
23 Parahippocampal gyrus
24 Internal carotid artery

48   Atlas

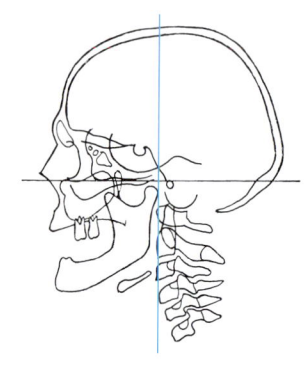

1 Superior sagittal sinus
2 Posteromedial frontal artery
3 Paracentral artery
4 Parietal bone
5 Artery of precentral sulcus
6 Pericallosal artery
7 Artery of central sulcus
8 Superior thalamostriate (terminal) vein
9 Insular arteries
10 Anterior choroidal artery
11 Posterior communicating artery
12 Basal vein (of Rosenthal)
13 Posterior cerebral artery
14 Oculomotor nerve
15 Temporalis
16 Temporal artery of middle cerebral artery
17 Basilar artery
18 Superior cerebellar artery
19 Middle meningeal artery
20 Temporal bone
21 Sphenoid
22 External acoustic meatus
23 Internal carotid artery
24 Head of mandible (cut)
25 Auricle (pinna)
26 Anterior arch of atlas
27 External carotid artery
28 Occipital artery
29 Stylohyoid ligament (ossified)
30 Parotid gland
31 Axis
32 Posterior belly of digastric
33 External carotid artery (cut)
34 Third cervical vertebra
35 Sternocleidomastoid
36 Constrictor of pharynx
37 Cricoid cartilage
38 Common carotid artery
39 Thyroid cartilage

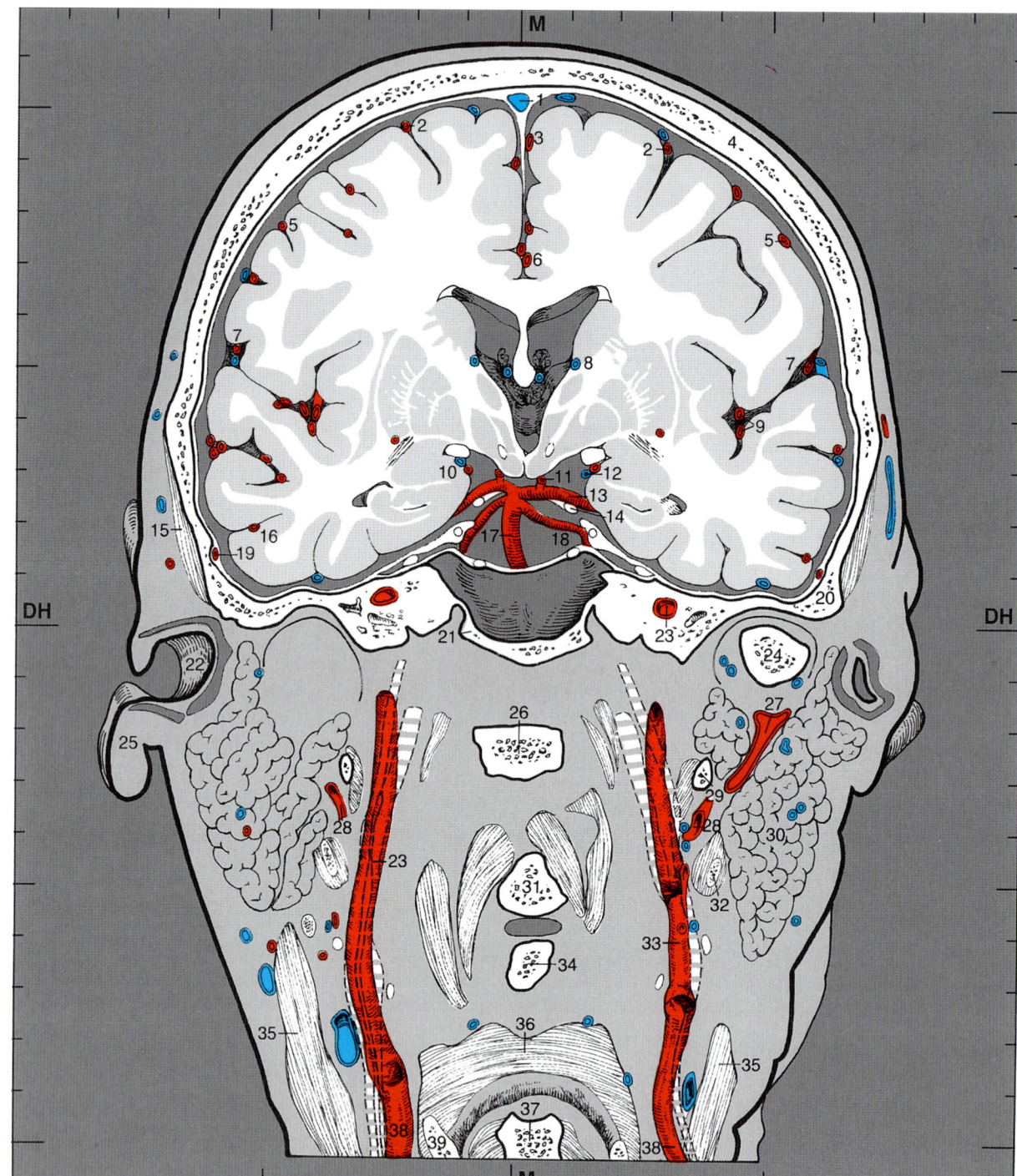

Fig. **10c** Anterior section surface of the seventh coronal slice showing bony structures, muscles, and blood vessels. The sectional plane lies at the level of the anterior wall of the cartilaginous external acoustic meatus. The cervical vertebral bodies are cut superficially. The internal carotid arteries take an upward course within the slice.

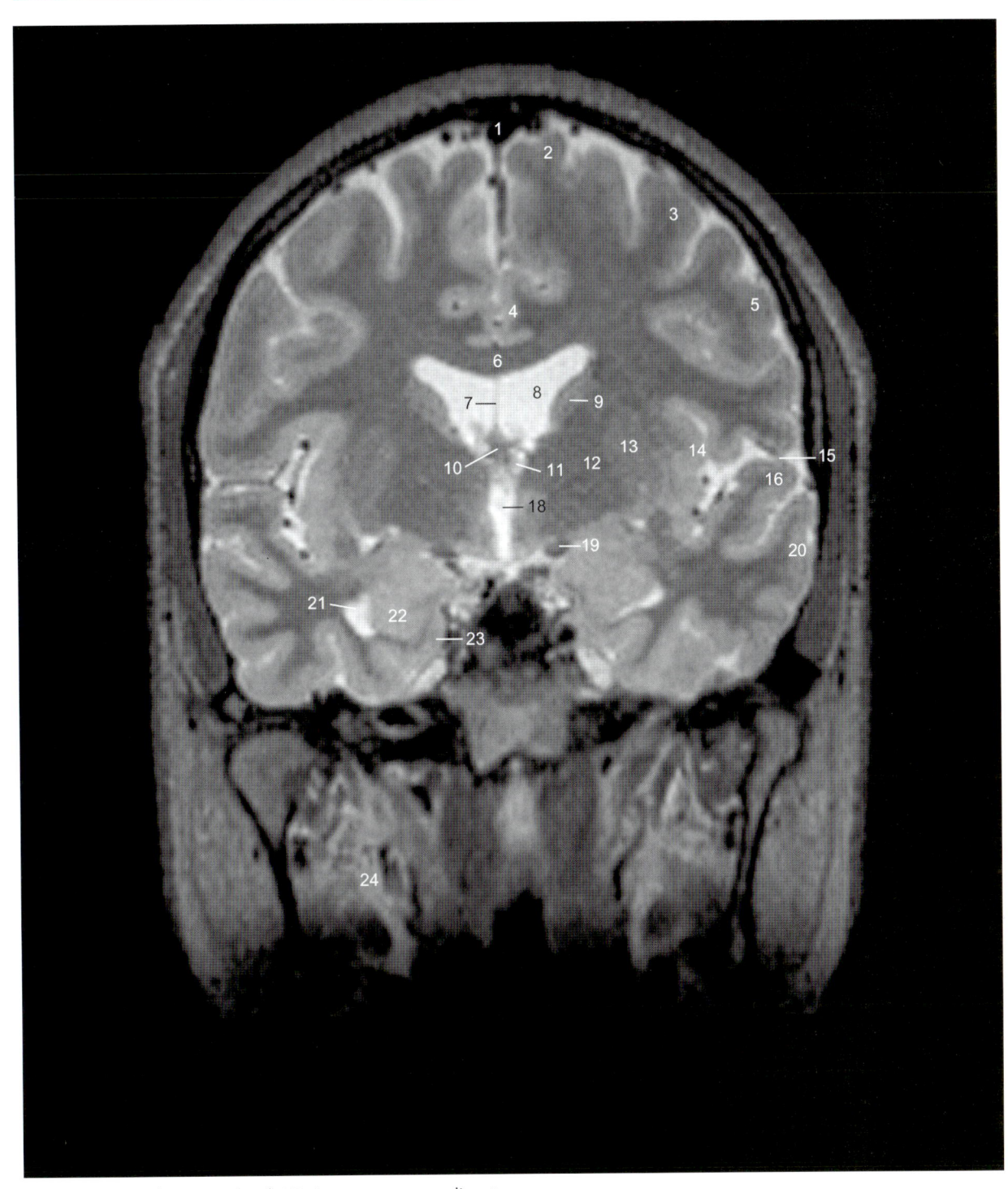

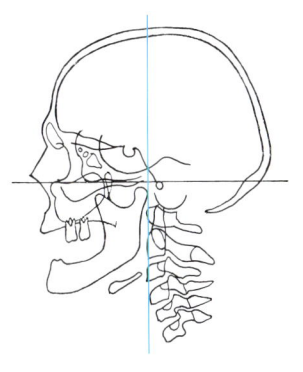

Coronal Slices

1 Superior sagittal sinus
2 Superior frontal gyrus
3 Middle frontal gyrus
4 Cingulate gyrus
5 Precentral gyrus
6 Trunk (body) of corpus callosum
7 Septum pellucidum
8 Frontal (anterior) horn of lateral ventricle
9 Body of caudate nucleus
10 Fornix
11 Interventricular foramen (of Monro)
12 Globus pallidus
13 Putamen
14 Insula
15 Lateral sulcus (Sylvian fissure)
16 Superior temporal gyrus
18 Third ventricle
19 Optic tract
20 Middle temporal gyrus
21 Temporal (inferior) horn of lateral ventricle
22 Hippocampus
23 Parahippocampal gyrus
24 Internal carotid artery

Fig. **10d** Coronal, T2-weighted MR image corresponding to the sectional plane of Figs. 10a and 10c.

Atlas

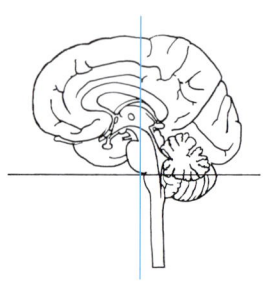

1 Superior frontal gyrus
2 Falx cerebri
3 Precentral gyrus
4 Central sulcus
5 Cingulate gyrus
6 Trunk (body) of corpus callosum
7 Postcentral gyrus
8 Central part (body) of lateral ventricle
9 Caudate nucleus
10 Choroid plexus of lateral ventricle
11 Lateral dorsal nucleus of thalamus
12 Fornix
13 Medial nuclei of thalamus
14 Ventral lateral nucleus of thalamus
15 Posterior limb of internal capsule
16 Putamen
17 Insula
18 Transverse temporal gyrus (of Heschl)
19 Lateral sulcus (Sylvian fissure)
20 Superior temporal gyrus
21 Third ventricle
22 Subthalamic nucleus
23 Globus pallidus
24 Temporal (inferior) horn of lateral ventricle
25 Red nucleus
26 Optic tract
27 Middle temporal gyrus
28 Substantia nigra
29 Tail of caudate nucleus
30 Interpeduncular cistern
31 Hippocampus
32 Parahippocampal gyrus
33 Trochlear nerve
34 Lateral occipitotemporal gyrus
35 Inferior temporal gyrus
36 Tentorium of cerebellum
37 Pons
38 Trigeminal nerve
39 Facial nerve and intermediate nerve
40 Vestibulocochlear nerve
41 Abducens nerve
42 Vagus nerve and glossopharyngeal nerve
43 Hypoglossal nerve
44 Facial nerve
45 Accessory nerve
46 Sympathetic trunk

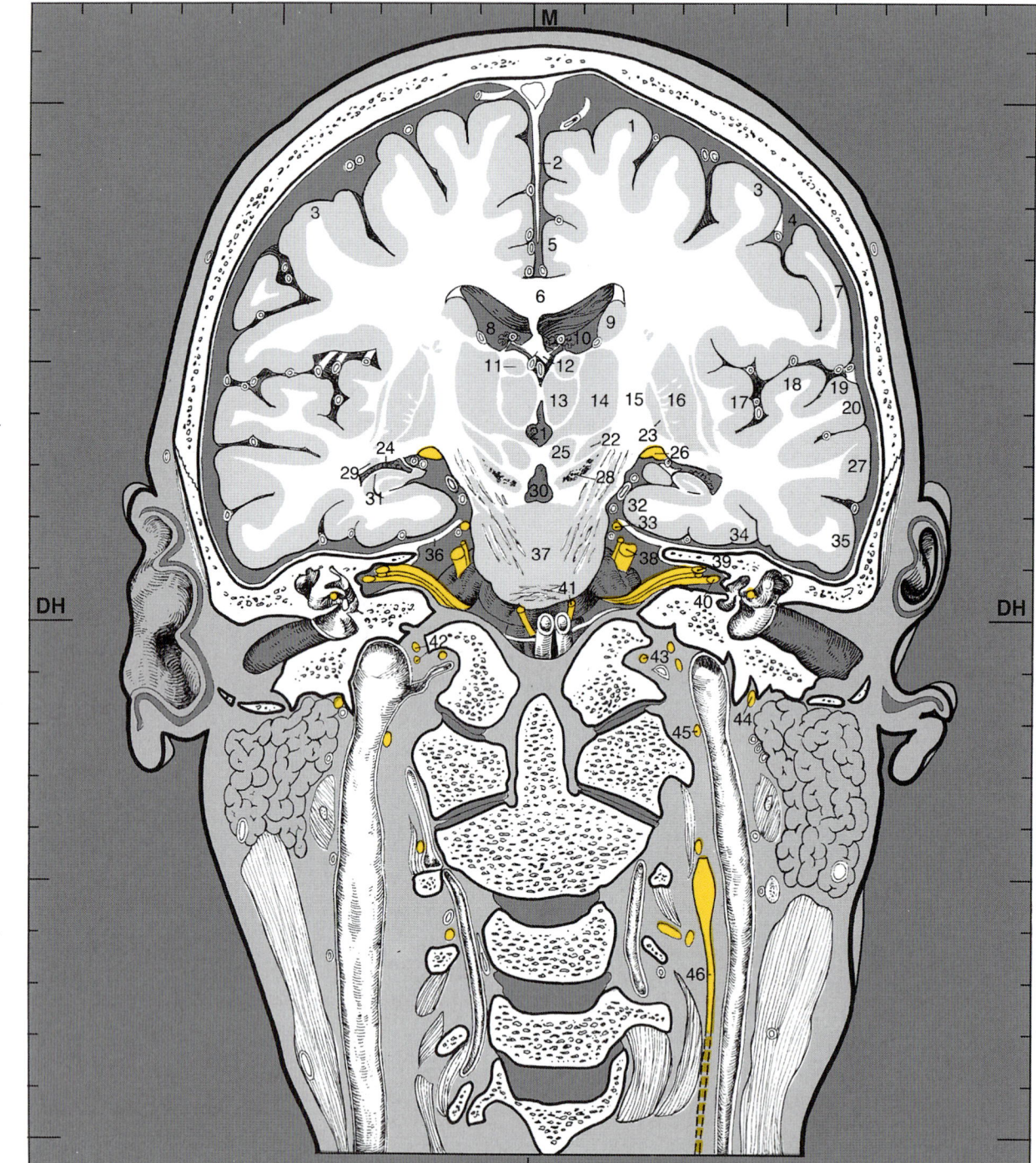

Fig. **11a** Anterior section surface of the eighth coronal slice showing brain structures and cranial nerves. The sectional plane runs through the telencephalon, diencephalon, midbrain, and pons at the level of the interpeduncular fossa. The fourth, fifth, sixth, seventh, and eighth cranial nerves are found in the cranial cavity, the seventh, ninth, eleventh, and twelfth cranial nerves outside the cranial cavity.

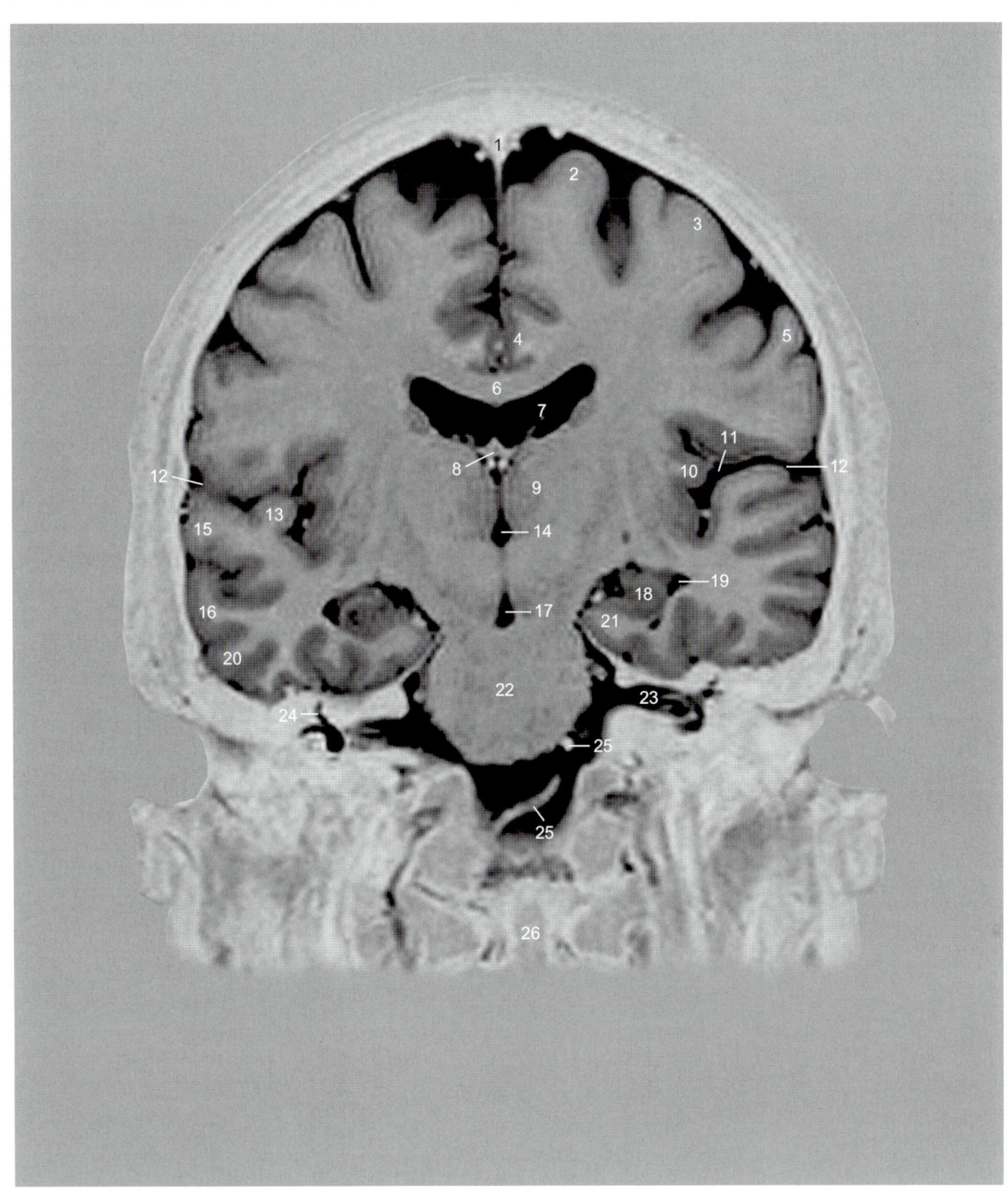

Fig. **11b** Coronal, T1-weighted MR image corresponding approximately to the sectional plane of Figs. 11a and 11c.

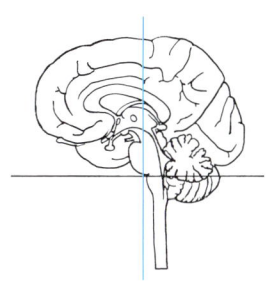

1 Superior sagittal sinus
2 Superior frontal gyrus
3 Precentral artery
4 Cingulate gyrus
5 Postcentral gyrus
6 Trunk (body) of corpus callosum
7 Central part (body) of lateral ventricle
8 Fornix and internal cerebral vein
9 Thalamus
10 Insula
11 Cistern of lateral cerebral fossa (cistern of Sylvian fissure)
12 Lateral sulcus (Sylvian fissure)
13 Transverse temporal gyrus
14 Third ventricle
15 Superior temporal gyrus
16 Middle temporal gyrus
17 Interpeduncular cistern
18 Hippocampus
19 Temporal (inferior) horn of lateral ventricle
20 Inferior temporal gyrus
21 Parahippocampal gyrus
22 Pons
23 Internal acoustic meatus with facial nerve (lies superior) and vestibulocochlear nerve (lies inferior)
24 Anterior semicircular canal
25 Vertebral artery (Var.)
26 Dens of axis

52 Atlas

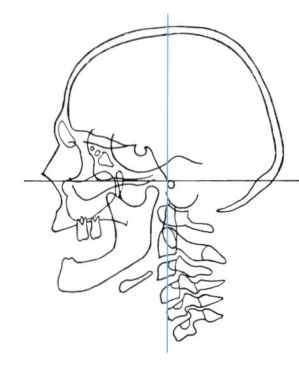

1 Superior sagittal sinus
2 Bridging vein
3 Paracentral artery
4 Artery of precentral sulcus
5 Parietal bone
6 Precuneal artery
7 Artery of central sulcus
8 Pericallosal artery
9 Superior thalamostriate (terminal) vein
10 Internal cerebral vein
11 Insular arteries
12 Temporal artery of middle cerebral artery
13 Posterior choroidal artery
14 Basal vein (of Rosenthal)
15 Posterior cerebral artery
16 Temporal artery of posterior cerebral artery
17 Superior cerebellar artery
18 Temporal bone
19 Auricle (pinna)
20 Internal acoustic meatus
21 Posterior inferior cerebellar artery (PICA)
22 Tympanic cavity
23 Tympanic membrane
24 External acoustic meatus
25 Vertebral artery
26 Occipital condyle
27 Styloid process
28 Stylomastoid foramen
29 Atlanto-occipital joint
30 Dens of axis
31 Lateral mass of atlas
32 Posterior belly of digastric
33 Axis
34 Lateral atlantoaxial joint
35 Occipital artery
36 Intervertebral disc
37 Internal jugular vein
38 Body of third cervical vertebra
39 Sternocleidomastoid
40 Fourth cervical vertebra
41 Fifth cervical vertebra

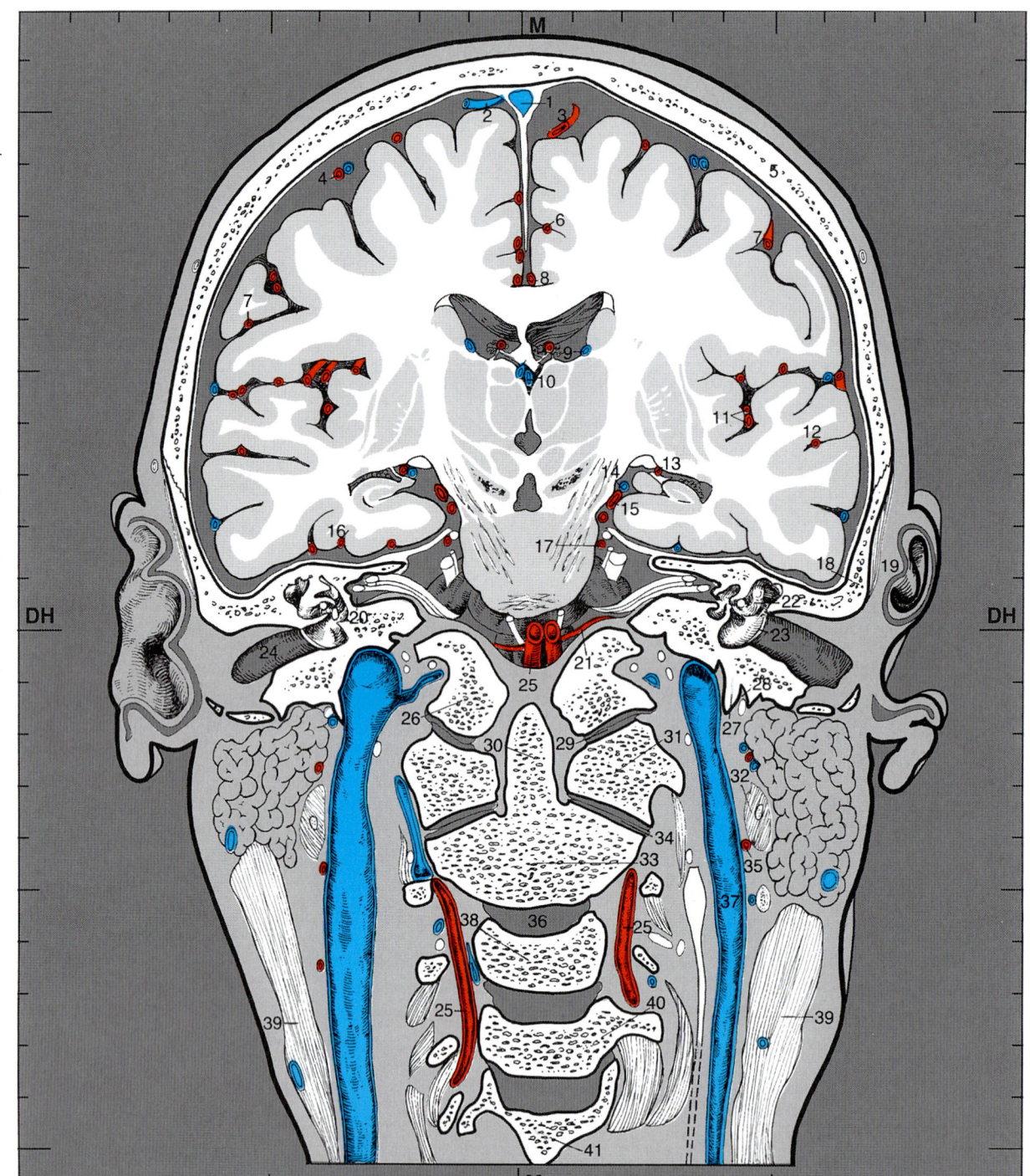

Fig. **11c** Anterior section surface of the eighth coronal slice showing bony structures, muscles, and blood vessels. The bony external acoustic meatus, the tympanic cavity, and the internal acoustic meatus are positioned in this slice. The internal jugular veins run laterally from the dens of axis and the cervical vertebral bodies.

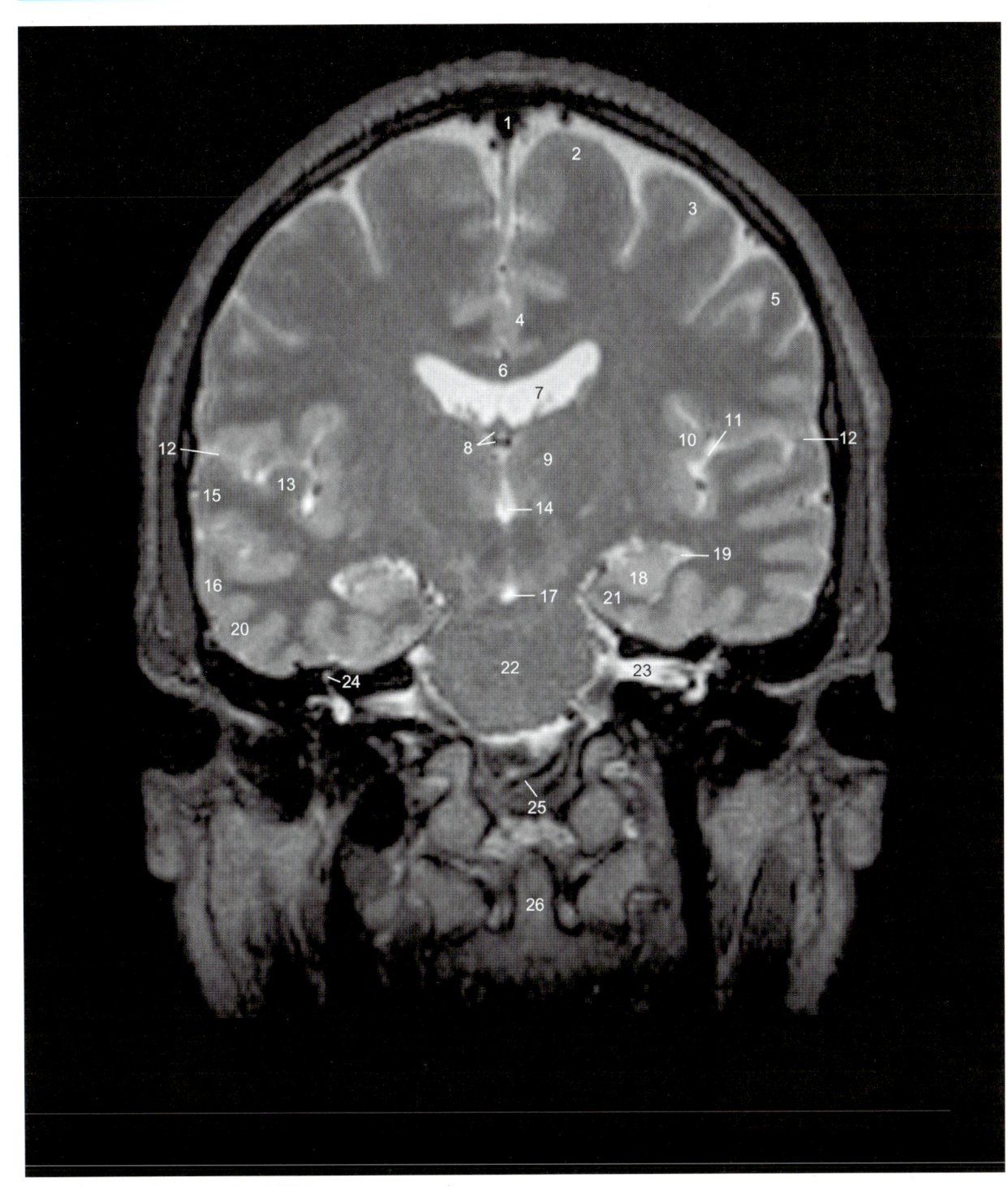

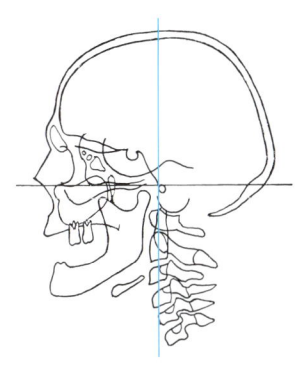

Coronal Slices

1. Superior sagittal sinus
2. Superior frontal gyrus
3. Precentral artery
4. Cingulate gyrus
5. Postcentral gyrus
6. Trunk (body) of corpus callosum
7. Central part (body) of lateral ventricle
8. Fornix and internal cerebral vein
9. Thalamus
10. Insula
11. Cistern of lateral cerebral fossa (cistern of Sylvian fissure)
12. Lateral sulcus (Sylvian fissure)
13. Transverse temporal gyrus (of Heschl)
14. Third ventricle
15. Superior temporal gyrus
16. Middle temporal gyrus
17. Interpeduncular cistern
18. Hippocampus
19. Temporal (inferior) horn of lateral ventricle
20. Inferior temporal gyrus
21. Parahippocampal gyrus
22. Pons
23. Internal acoustic meatus with facial nerve (lies superior) and vestibulocochlear nerve (lies inferior)
24. Anterior semicircular canal
25. Vertebral artery (Var.)
26. Dens of axis

Fig. **11d** Coronal, T2-weighted MR image corresponding approximately to the sectional plane of Figs. 11a and 11c.

Atlas

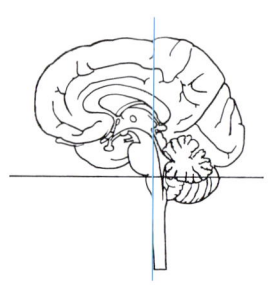

1 Superior frontal gyrus
2 Precentral gyrus
3 Postcentral gyrus
4 Central sulcus
5 Cingulate gyrus
6 Supramarginal gyrus
7 Central part (body) of lateral ventricle
8 Trunk (body) of corpus callosum
9 Caudate nucleus
10 Posterior transverse temporal gyrus
11 Anterior transverse temporal gyrus (of Heschl)
12 Fornix
13 Pulvinar of thalamus
14 Transverse temporal gyrus (of Heschl)
15 Superior temporal gyrus
16 Centromedian nucleus of thalamus
17 Posterior commissure
18 Medial geniculate body
19 Lateral geniculate body
20 Tail of caudate nucleus
21 Temporal (inferior) horn of lateral ventricle
22 Middle temporal gyrus
23 Aqueduct of midbrain
24 Periaqueductal gray substance
25 Trochlear nerve
26 Parahippocampal gyrus
27 Lateral occipitotemporal gyrus
28 Inferior temporal gyrus
29 Tentorium of cerebellum
30 Pons
31 Anterior lobe of cerebellum
32 Middle cerebellar peduncle
33 Primary fissure of cerebellum
34 Facial nerve and intermediate nerve
35 Vestibulocochlear nerve
36 Glossopharyngeal nerve and vagus nerve
37 Flocculus (H X)
38 Inferior olivary nucleus
39 Accessory nerve
40 Hypoglossal nerve
41 Pyramidal decussation
42 Anterior (ventral) root of first cervical spinal nerve
43 Spinal cord
44 Anterior (ventral) root of second spinal nerve
45 Second cervical spinal ganglion
46 Anterior median fissure
47 Anterior (ventral) root of fifth cervical spinal nerve

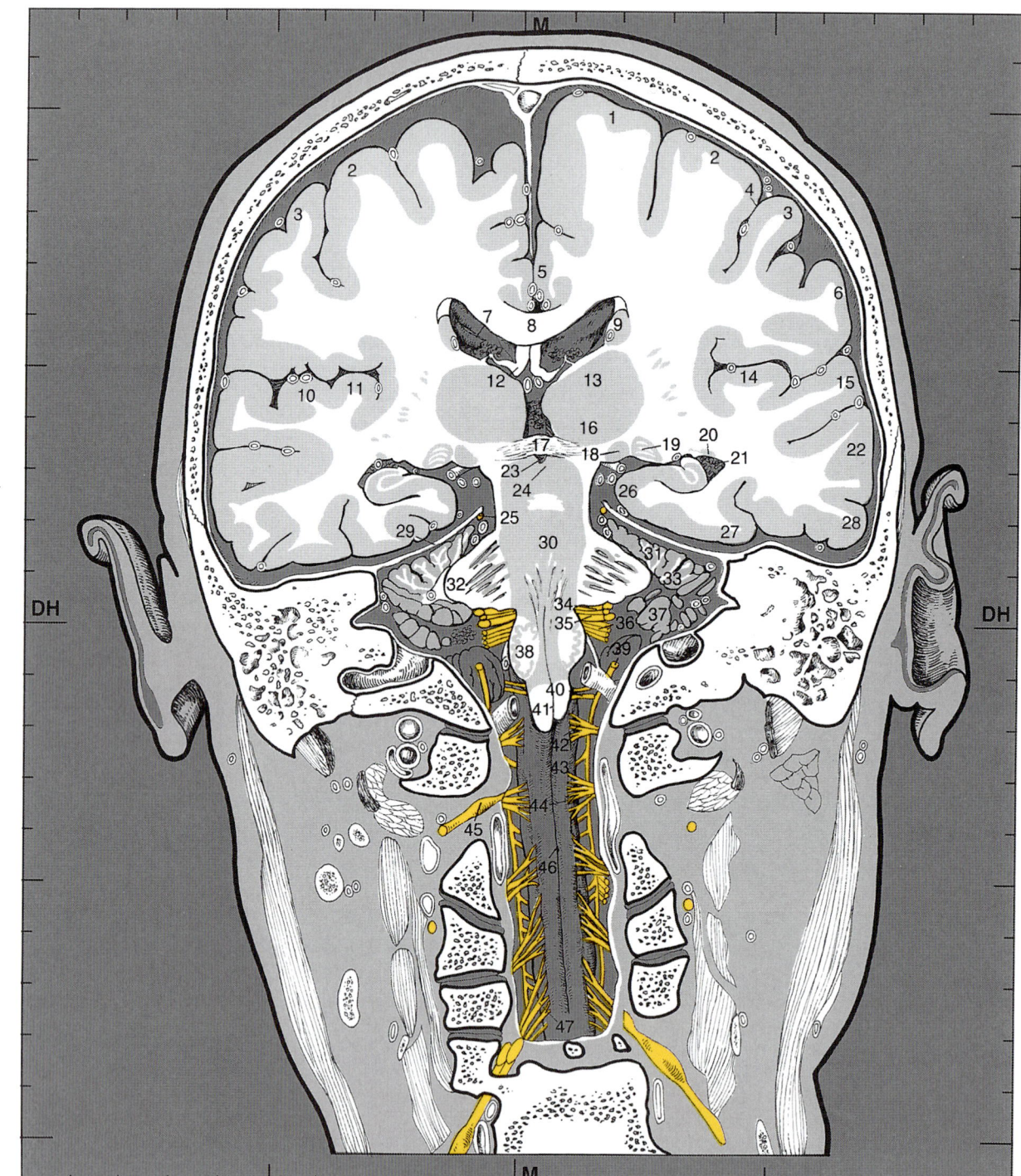

Fig. **12a** Anterior section surface of the ninth coronal slice. The posterior commissure is found on this sectional plane. Lateral ventricles with the central part (body) and the temporal (inferior) horn together with the first portion of the aqueduct of midbrain are demonstrated. The seventh, eighth, ninth, tenth, eleventh, and twelfth cranial nerves branch off from the brainstem. The tectal (quadrigeminal) plate lies within the section and is, therefore, not visible (Fig. 2b).

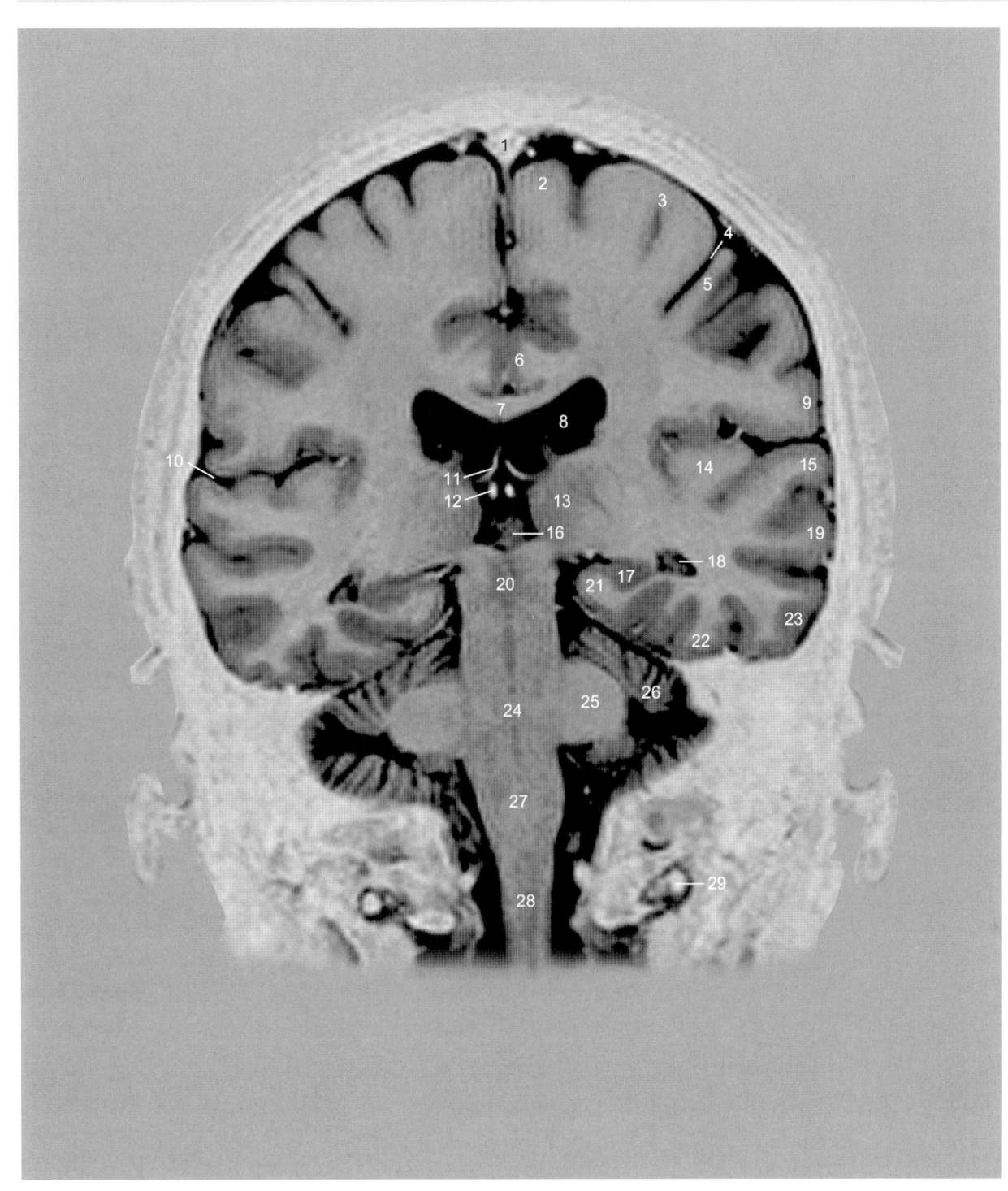

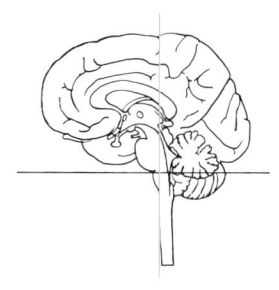

Coronal Slices

1 Superior sagittal sinus
2 Superior frontal gyrus
3 Precentral gyrus
4 Central sulcus
5 Postcentral gyrus
6 Cingulate gyrus
7 Trunk (body) of corpus callosum
8 Central part (body) of lateral ventricle
9 Supramarginal gyrus
10 Lateral sulcus (Sylvian fissure)
11 Fornix and blood vessel
12 Internal cerebral vein
13 Pulvinar of thalamus
14 Transverse temporal gyrus (of Heschl)
15 Superior temporal gyrus
16 Pineal gland
17 Hippocampus
18 Temporal (inferior) horn of lateral ventricle
19 Middle temporal gyrus
20 Midbrain
21 Parahippocampal gyrus
22 Lateral occipitotemporal gyrus
23 Inferior temporal gyrus
24 Pons
25 Middle cerebellar peduncle
26 Cerebellum
27 Medulla oblongata
28 Spinal cord
29 Vertebral artery

Fig. **12b** Coronal, T1-weighted MR image corresponding approximately to the sectional plane of Figs. 12a and 12c.

56 Atlas

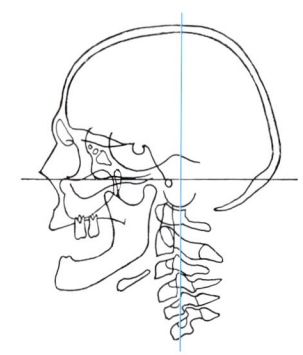

1 Superior sagittal sinus
2 Paracentral artery
3 Artery of central sulcus
4 Precuneal artery
5 Anterior parietal artery
6 Parietal bone
7 Pericallosal artery
8 Superior thalamostriate (terminal) vein
9 Angular artery
10 Internal cerebral vein
11 Temporal artery of middle cerebral artery
12 Posterior choroidal artery
13 Medial occipital artery
14 Basal vein (of Rosenthal)
15 Lateral occipital artery
16 Superior cerebellar artery
17 Auricle (pinna)
18 Temporal bone
19 Sigmoid sinus
20 Posterior inferior cerebellar artery (PICA)
21 Vertebral artery
22 Occipital bone
23 Mastoid process
24 Atlanto-occipital joint
25 Occipital artery
26 Posterior belly of digastric
27 Vertebral vein
28 Lateral mass of atlas
29 Articular process and arch of axis
30 Articular process and arch of third cervical vertebra
31 Articular process and arch of fourth cervical vertebra
32 Sternocleidomastoid
33 Fifth cervical vertebra

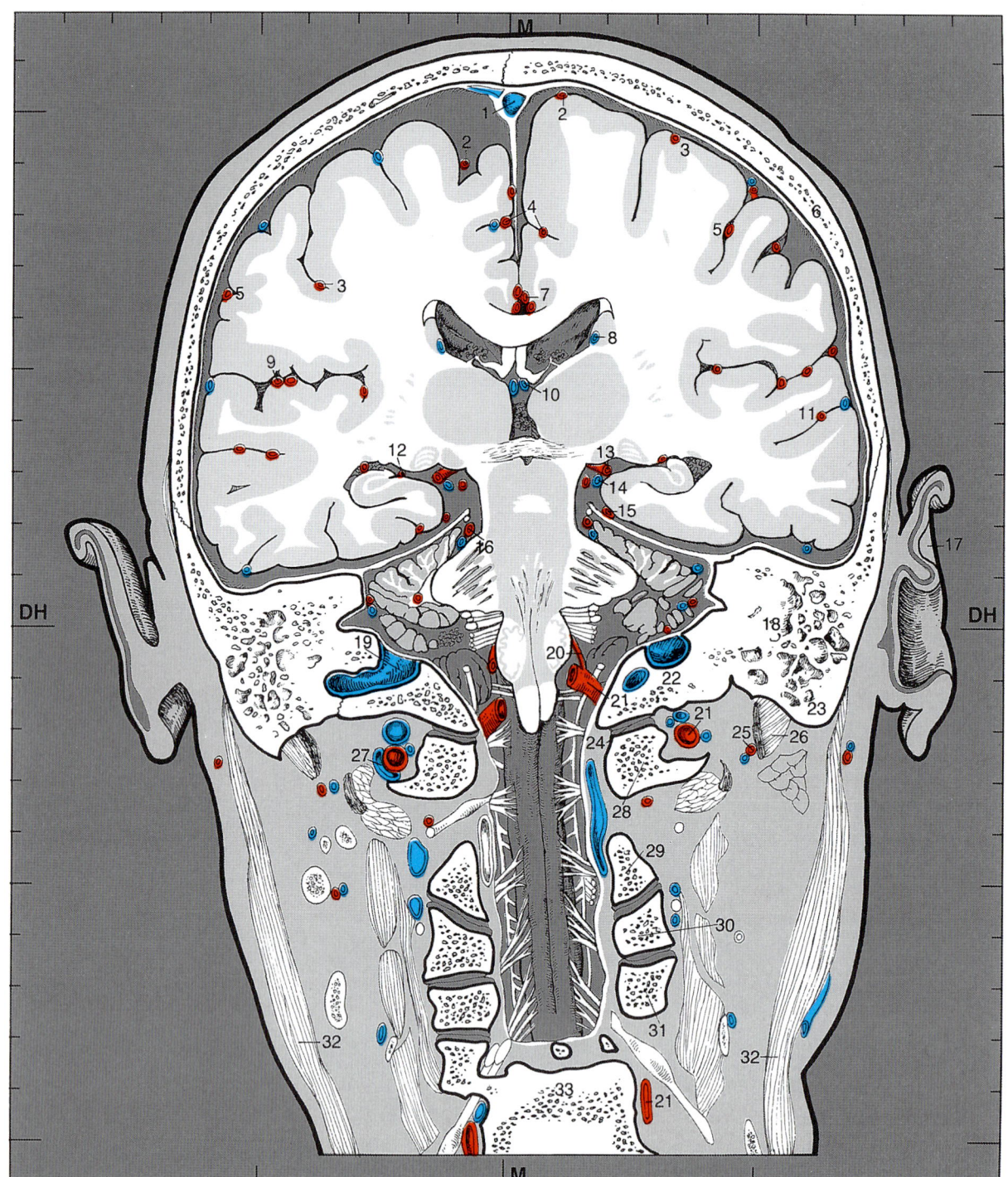

Fig. 12c Anterior section surface of the ninth coronal slice showing bony structures, muscles, and blood vessels. The sectional plane lies just within the middle of the mastoid process and exposes the posterior cranial fossa and the upper vertebral canal in the region of the first four cervical vertebrae.

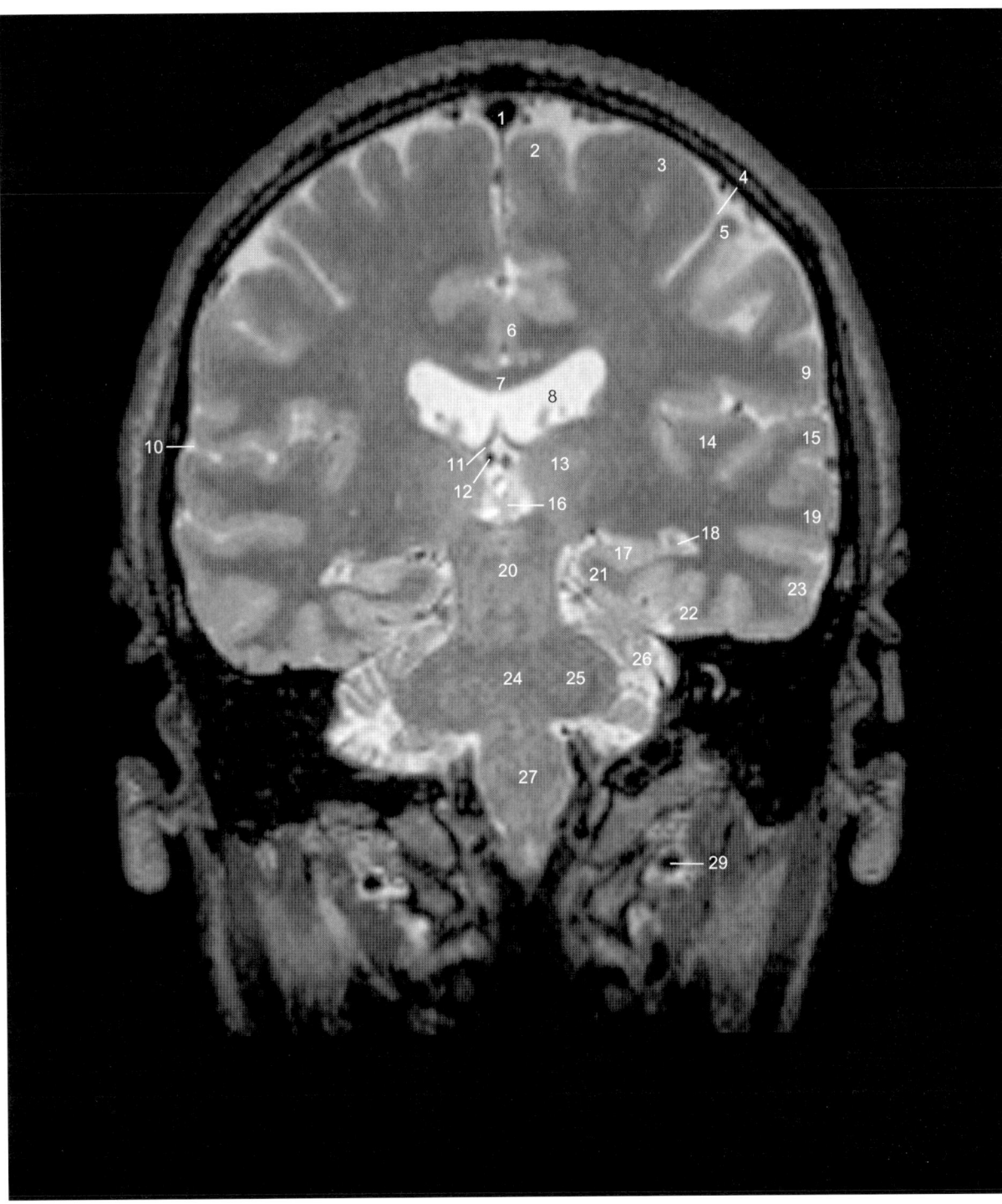

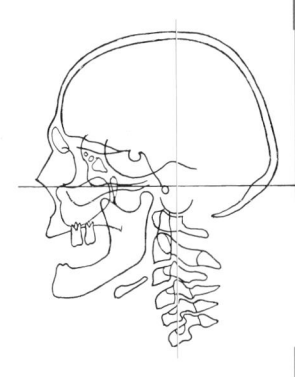

Coronal Slices

1 Superior sagittal sinus
2 Superior frontal gyrus
3 Precentral gyrus
4 Central sulcus
5 Postcentral gyrus
6 Cingulate gyrus
7 Trunk (body) of corpus callosum
8 Central part (body) of lateral ventricle
9 Supramarginal gyrus
10 Lateral sulcus (Sylvian fissure)
11 Fornix and blood vessel
12 Internal cerebral vein
13 Pulvinar of thalamus
14 Transverse temporal gyrus (of Heschl)
15 Superior temporal gyrus
16 Pineal gland
17 Hippocampus
18 Temporal (inferior) horn of lateral ventricle
19 Middle temporal gyrus
20 Midbrain
21 Parahippocampal gyrus
22 Lateral occipitotemporal gyrus
23 Inferior temporal gyrus
24 Pons
25 Middle cerebellar peduncle
26 Cerebellum
27 Medulla oblongata
29 Vertebral artery

Fig. **12d** Coronal, T2-weighted MR image corresponding approximately to the sectional plane of Figs. 12a and 12c.

58 Atlas

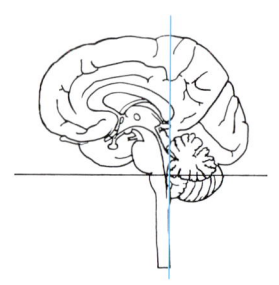

1 Precentral gyrus
2 Falx cerebri
3 Central sulcus
4 Paracentral lobule
5 Postcentral gyrus
6 Cingulate gyrus
7 Supramarginal gyrus
8 Lateral sulcus (Sylvian fissure)
9 Atrium of lateral ventricle
10 Splenium of corpus callosum
11 Tail of caudate nucleus
12 Superior temporal gyrus
13 Fornix
14 Pineal gland
15 Hippocampus
16 Middle temporal gyrus
17 Tentorium of cerebellum
18 Medial occipitotemporal gyrus
19 Lateral occipitotemporal gyrus
20 Inferior temporal gyrus
21 Anterior lobe of cerebellum
22 Primary fissure of cerebellum
23 Roof of fourth ventricle
24 Choroid plexus of fourth ventricle
25 Posterior lobe of cerebellum
26 Floor of rhomboid fossa (cut)
27 Cisterna magna (posterior cerebellomedullary cistern)
28 Suboccipital nerve
29 Greater occipital nerve
30 Third occipital nerve
31 Spinal cord

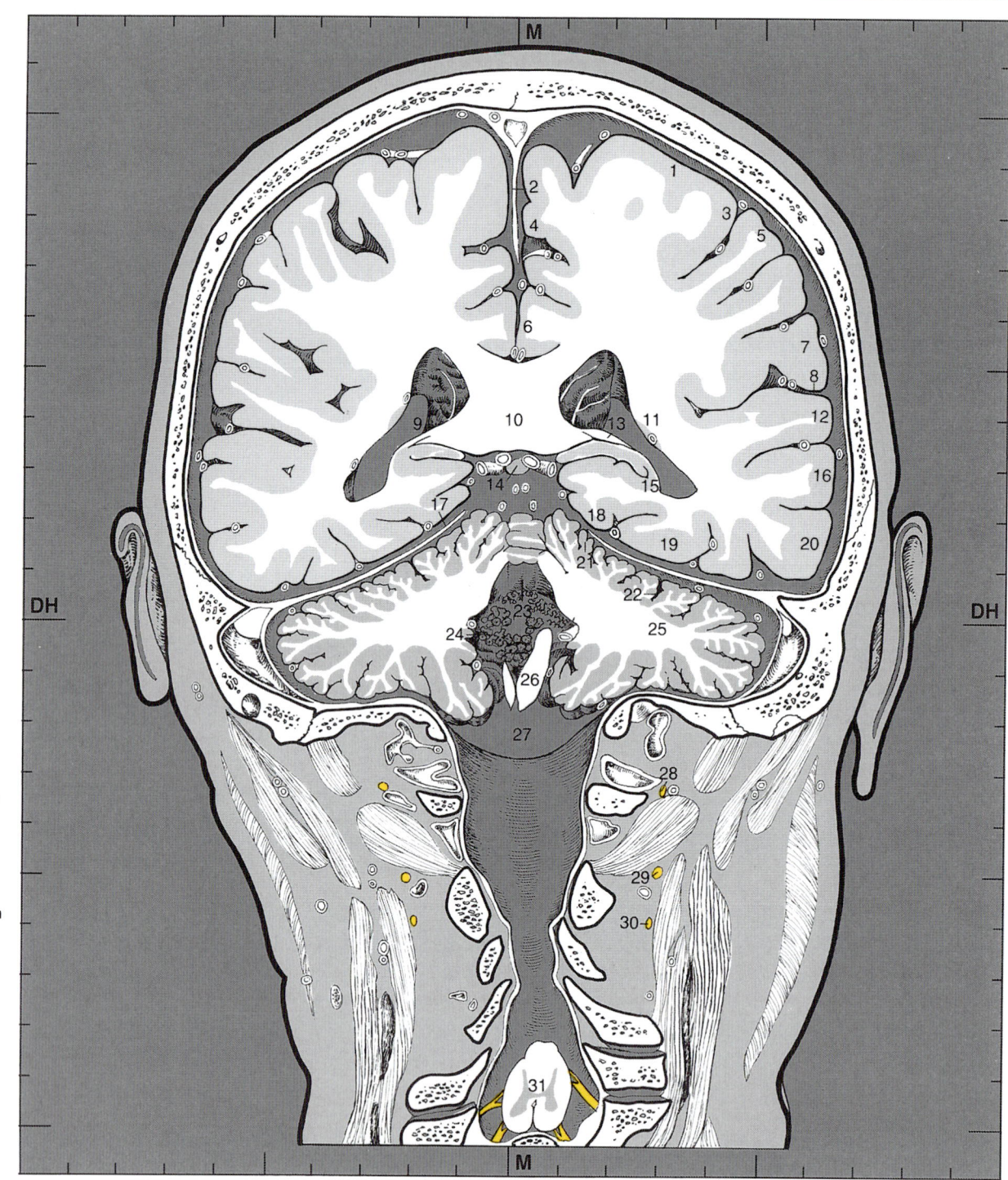

Fig. **13a** Anterior section surface of the tenth coronal slice showing brain structures and branches of spinal nerves. The sectional plane reveals the splenium of the corpus callosum, the atrium of the lateral ventricles, the pineal gland, the floor of the rhomboid fossa, and the cerebellum as the roof of the fourth ventricle.

Coronal Slices

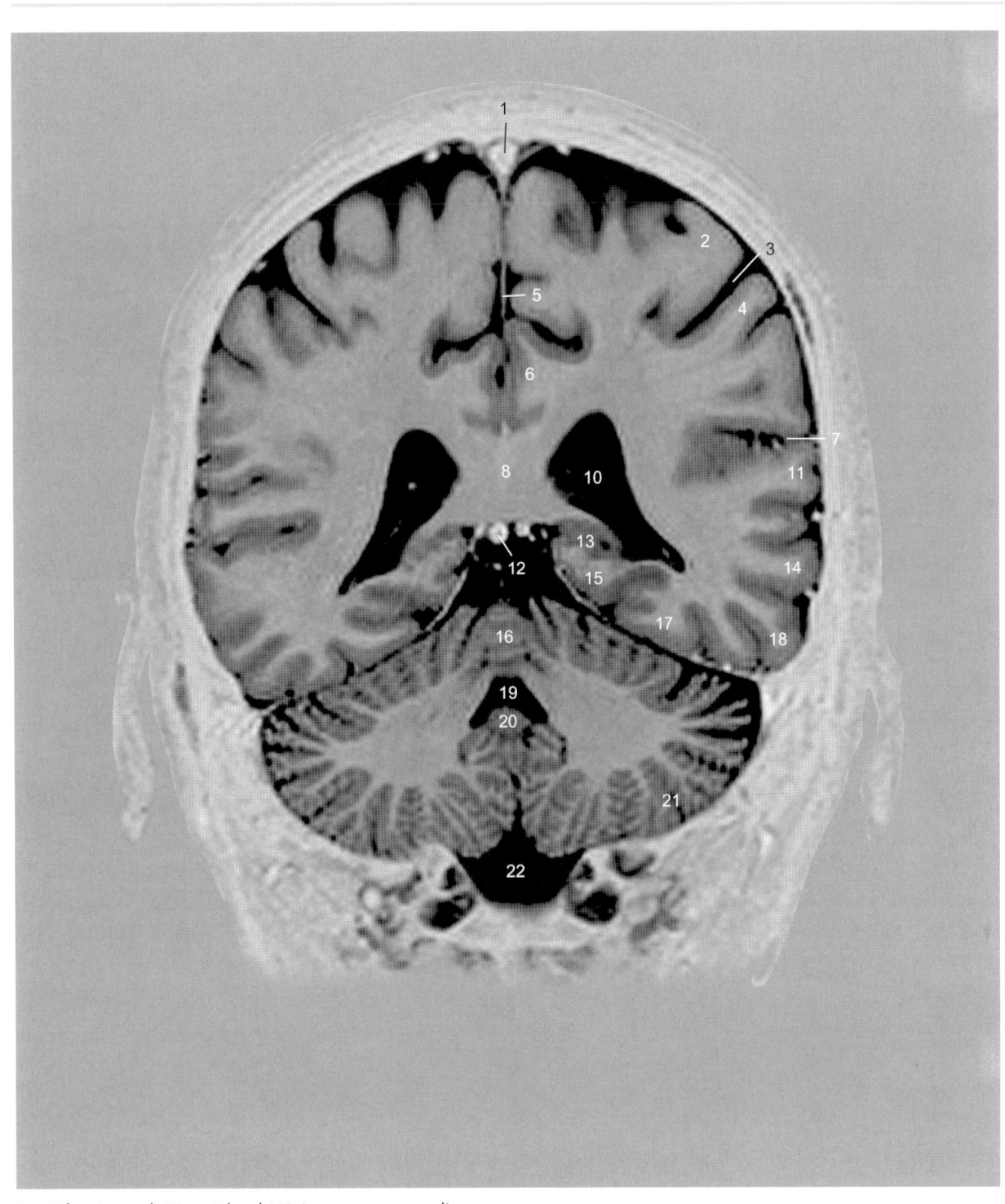

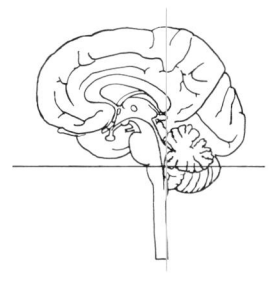

Fig. **13b** Coronal, T1-weighted MR image corresponding approximately to the sectional plane of Figs. 13a and 13c.

1 Superior sagittal sinus
2 Precentral gyrus
3 Central sulcus
4 Postcentral gyrus
5 Falx cerebri
6 Cingulate gyrus
7 Lateral sulcus (Sylvian fissure)
8 Splenium of corpus callosum
10 Atrium of lateral ventricle
11 Superior temporal gyrus
12 Internal cerebral vein
13 Hippocampus
14 Middle temporal gyrus
15 Medial occipitotemporal gyrus
16 Vermis of anterior lobe of cerebellum
17 Lateral occipitotemporal gyrus
18 Inferior temporal gyrus
19 Fourth ventricle
20 Nodule of vermis (X)
21 Posterior lobe of cerebellum
22 Cisterna magna (posterior cerebellomedullary cistern)

60 Atlas

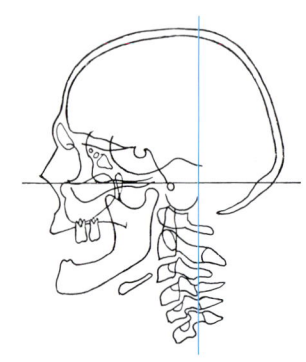

1 Superior sagittal sinus
2 Paracentral artery
3 Artery of central sulcus
4 Parietal bone
5 Precuneal artery
6 Anterior parietal artery
7 Angular artery
8 Superior thalamostriate (terminal) vein
9 Temporal artery of middle cerebral artery
10 Internal cerebral vein
11 Basal vein (of Rosenthal)
12 Medial occipital artery
13 Superior cerebellar artery
14 Lateral occipital artery
15 Temporal bone
16 Sigmoid sinus
17 Posterior inferior cerebellar artery (PICA)
18 Auricle (pinna)
19 Occipital bone
20 Vertebral vein (cut)
21 Vertebral artery (cut)
22 Obliquus capitis superior
23 Suboccipital venous plexus
24 Posterior arch of atlas
25 Occipital artery
26 Obliquus capitis inferior
27 Sternocleidomastoid
28 Arch of axis
29 Arch of third cervical vertebra
30 Arch of fourth cervical vertebra
31 Arch of fifth cervical vertebra

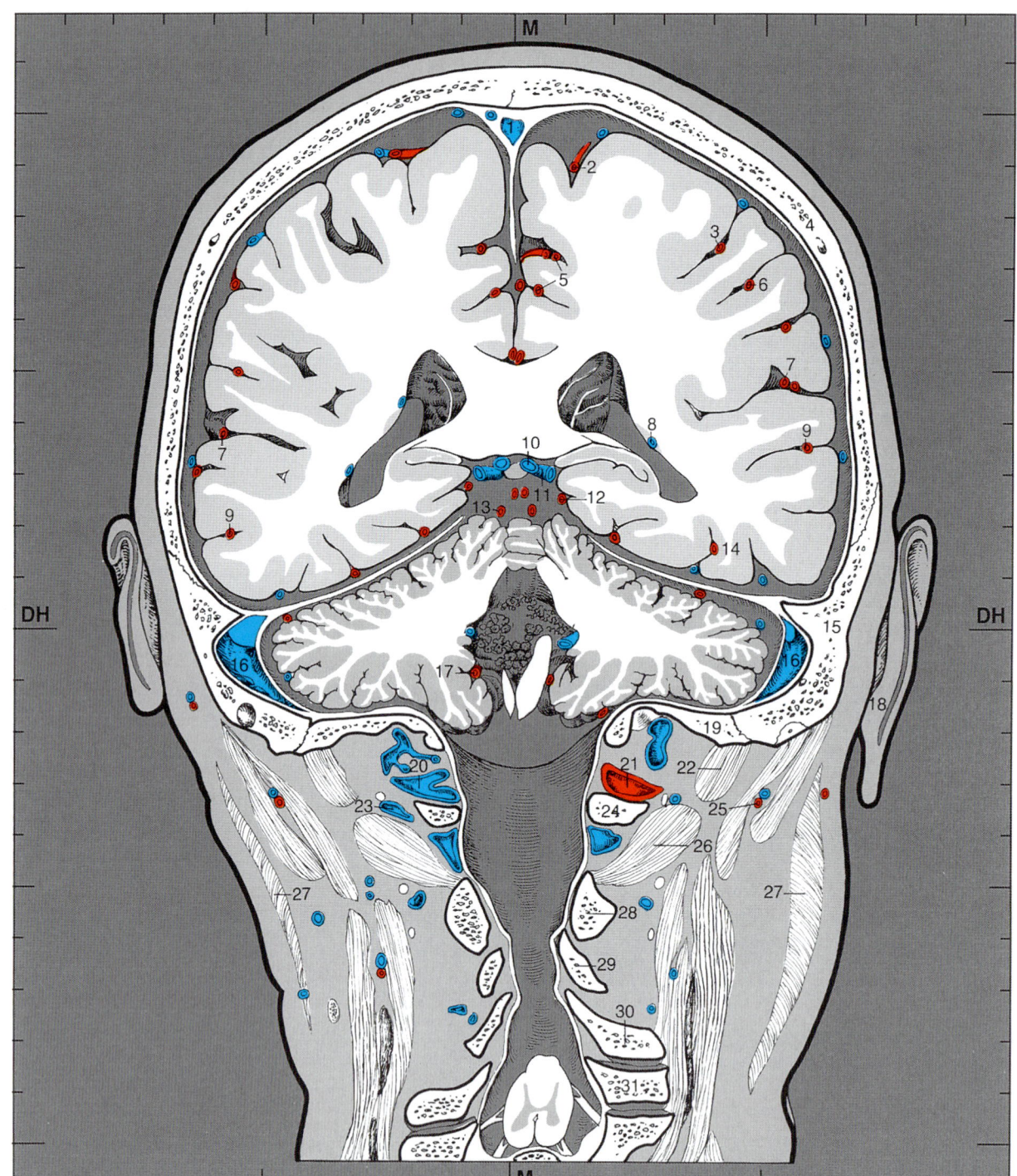

Fig. **13c** Anterior section surface of the tenth coronal slice showing bony structures, muscles, and blood vessels. The sectional plane lies in close proximity posteriorly to the petrous part of the temporal bone and runs just posterior to the middle of the foramen magnum (Fig. 2a). The arches of the upper cervical vertebrae are cut at this level.

Coronal Slices

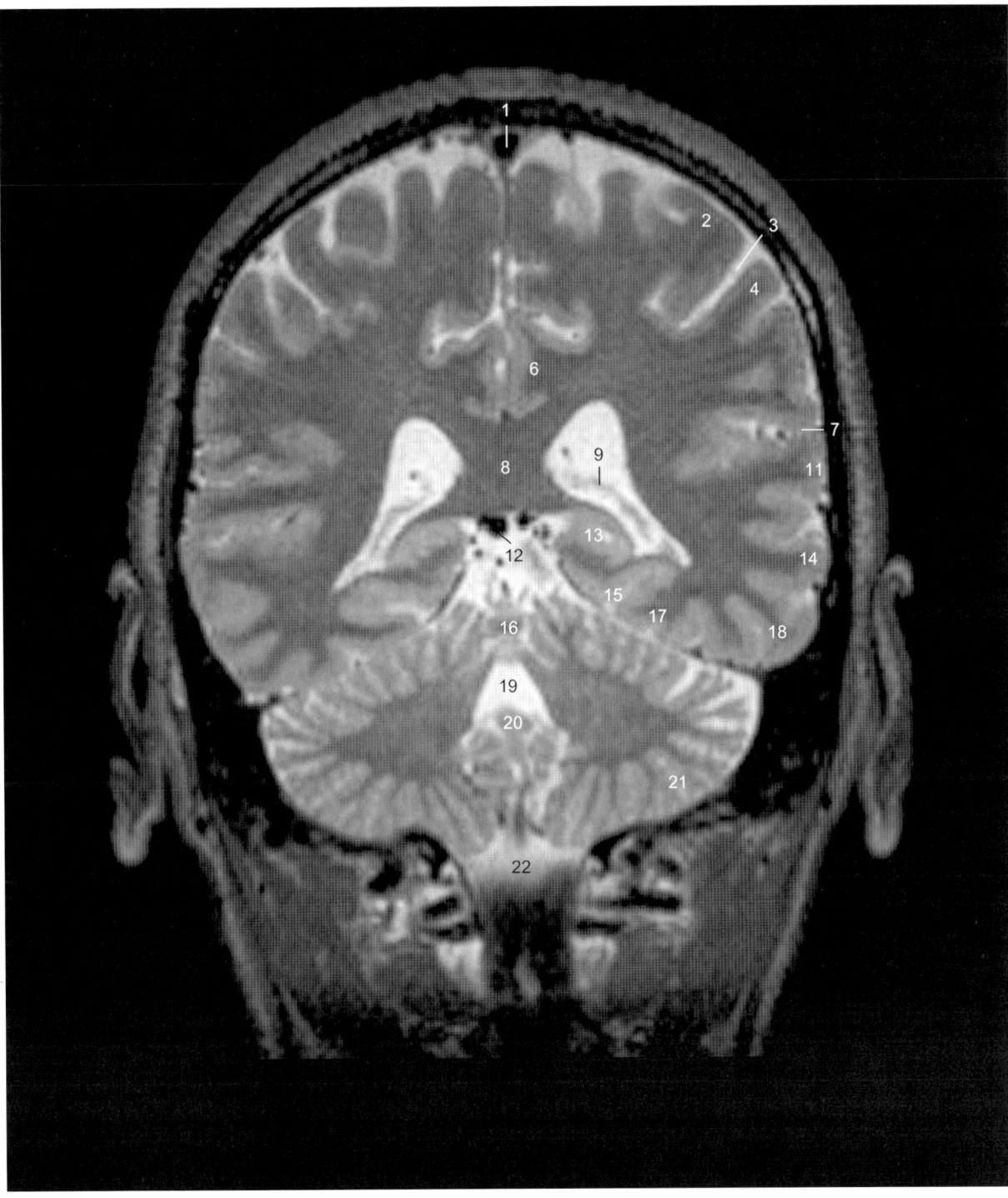

Fig. **13d** Coronal, T2-weighted MR image corresponding approximately to the sectional plane of Figs. 13a and 13c.

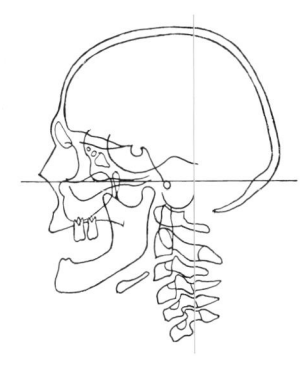

1 Superior sagittal sinus
2 Precentral gyrus
3 Central sulcus
4 Postcentral gyrus
6 Cingulate gyrus
7 Lateral sulcus (Sylvian fissure)
8 Splenium of corpus callosum
9 Choroid plexus of lateral ventricle
11 Superior temporal gyrus
12 Internal cerebral vein
13 Hippocampus
14 Middle temporal gyrus
15 Medial occipitotemporal gyrus
16 Vermis of anterior lobe of cerebellum
17 Lateral occipitotemporal gyrus
18 Inferior temporal gyrus
19 Fourth ventricle
20 Nodule of vermis (X)
21 Posterior lobe of cerebellum
22 Cisterna magna (posterior cerebellomedullary cistern)

62   Atlas

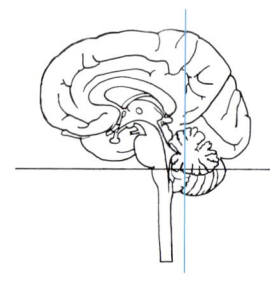

1 Precentral gyrus
2 Postcentral gyrus
3 Paracentral lobule
4 Falx cerebri
5 Supramarginal gyrus
6 Occipital (posterior) horn of lateral ventricle
7 Superior temporal sulcus
8 Superior temporal gyrus
9 Middle temporal gyrus
10 Anterior lobe of cerebellum
11 Medial occipitotemporal gyrus
12 Tentorium of cerebellum
13 Lateral occipitotemporal gyrus
14 Inferior temporal gyrus
15 Primary fissure of cerebellum
16 Uvula of vermis (IX)
17 Dentate nucleus
18 Posterior lobe of cerebellum
19 Cisterna magna (posterior cerebellomedullary cistern)
20 Greater occipital nerve
21 Third occipital nerve

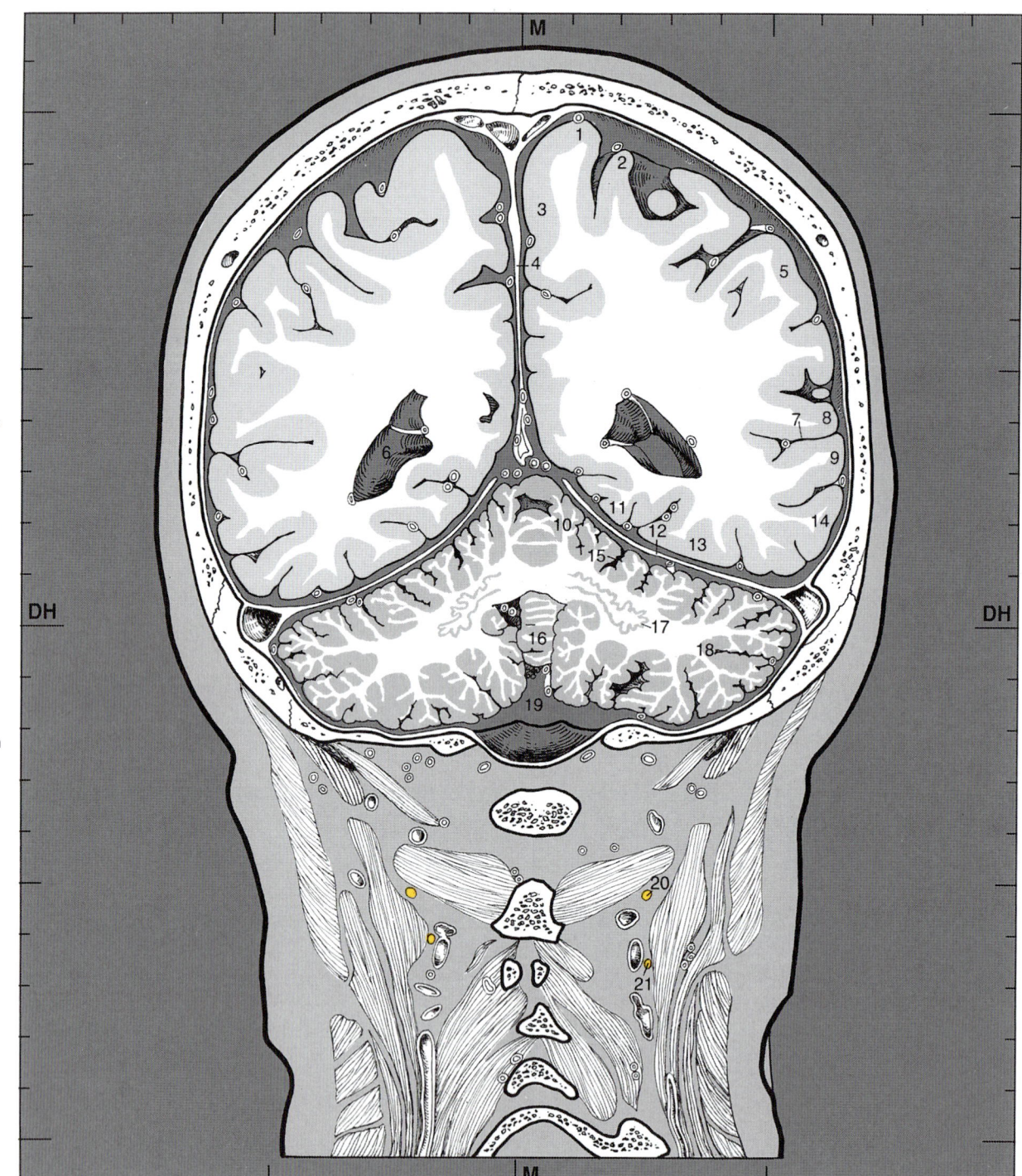

Fig. **14a** Anterior section surface of the eleventh coronal slice showing brain structures and branches of spinal nerves. In the supratentorial space the occipital (posterior) horns of the lateral ventricles serves as a guideline structure. The cerebellum together with the dentate nucleus are revealed in the infratentorial space.

Coronal Slices

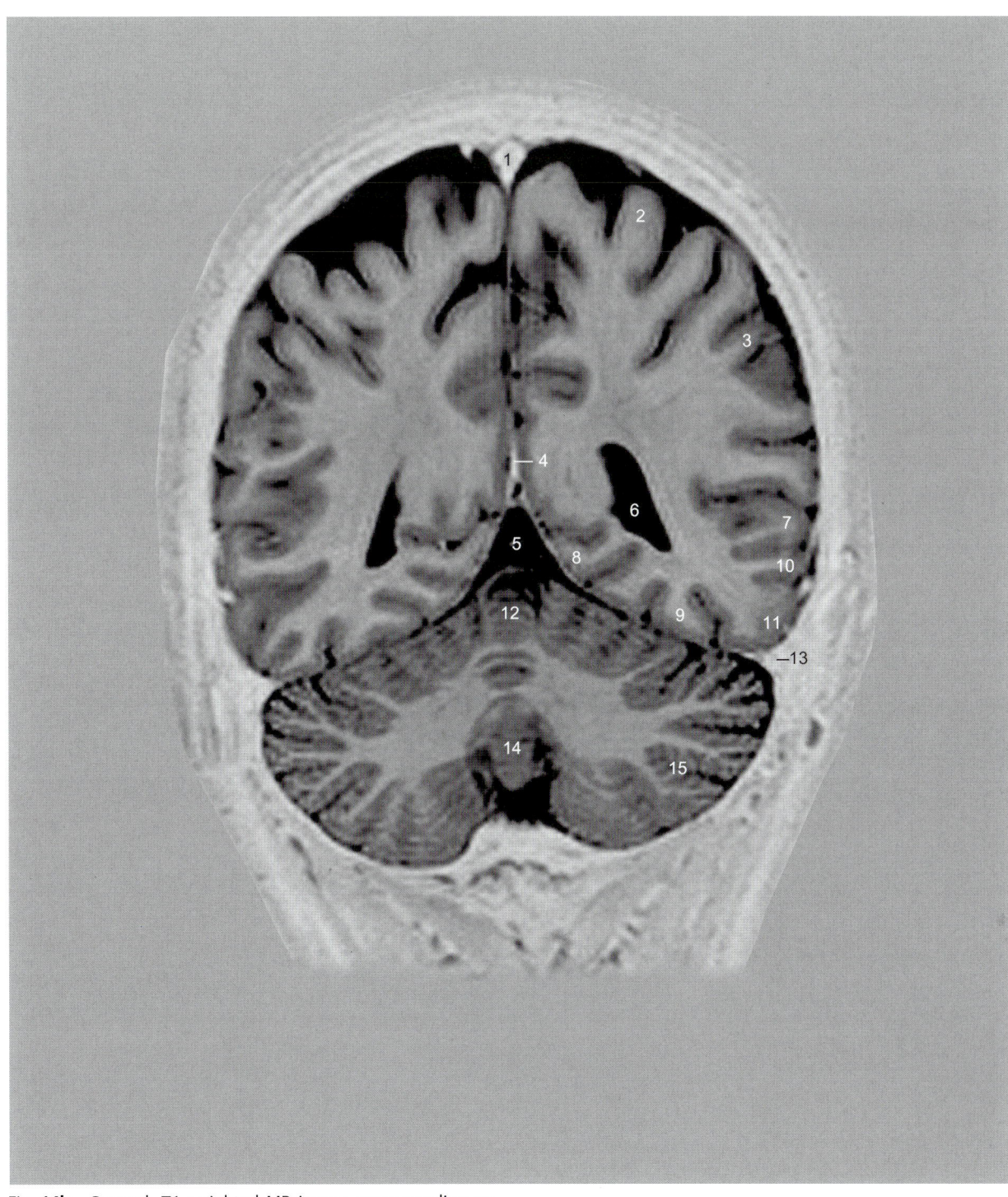

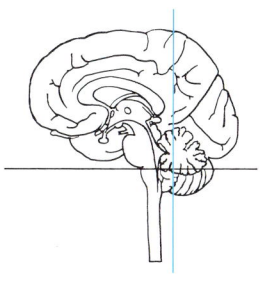

1 Superior sagittal sinus
2 Superior parietal lobule
3 Supramarginal gyrus
4 Straight sinus
5 Superior cerebellar cistern
6 Occipital (posterior) horn of lateral ventricle
7 Superior temporal gyrus
8 Medial occipitotemporal gyrus
9 Lateral occipitotemporal gyrus
10 Middle temporal gyrus
11 Inferior temporal gyrus
12 Vermis of anterior lobe of cerebellum
13 Transverse sinus
14 Vermis of cerebellum
15 Posterior lobe of cerebellum

Fig. **14b** Coronal, T1-weighted MR image corresponding approximately to the sectional plane of Figs. 14a and 14c.

64 Atlas

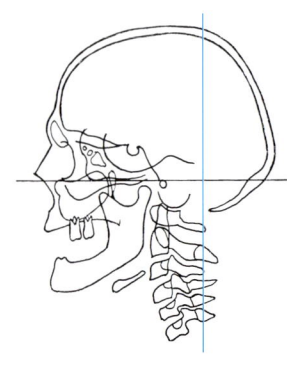

1 Superior sagittal sinus
2 Precuneal artery
3 Anterior parietal artery
4 Parietal bone
5 Posterior parietal artery
6 Angular artery
7 Straight sinus
8 Superior cerebellar artery
9 Medial occipital artery
10 Lateral occipital artery
11 Transverse sinus
12 Posterior inferior cerebellar artery (PICA)
13 Foramen magnum
14 Occipital bone
15 Rectus capitis posterior minor
16 Obliquus capitis superior
17 Posterior arch of atlas
18 Occipital artery
19 Splenius capitis
20 Obliquus capitis inferior
21 Spinous process of axis
22 Suboccipital venous plexus
23 Spinous process of third cervical vertebra
24 Spinous process of fourth cervical vertebra
25 Arch of fifth cervical vertebra
26 Arch of sixth cervical vertebra

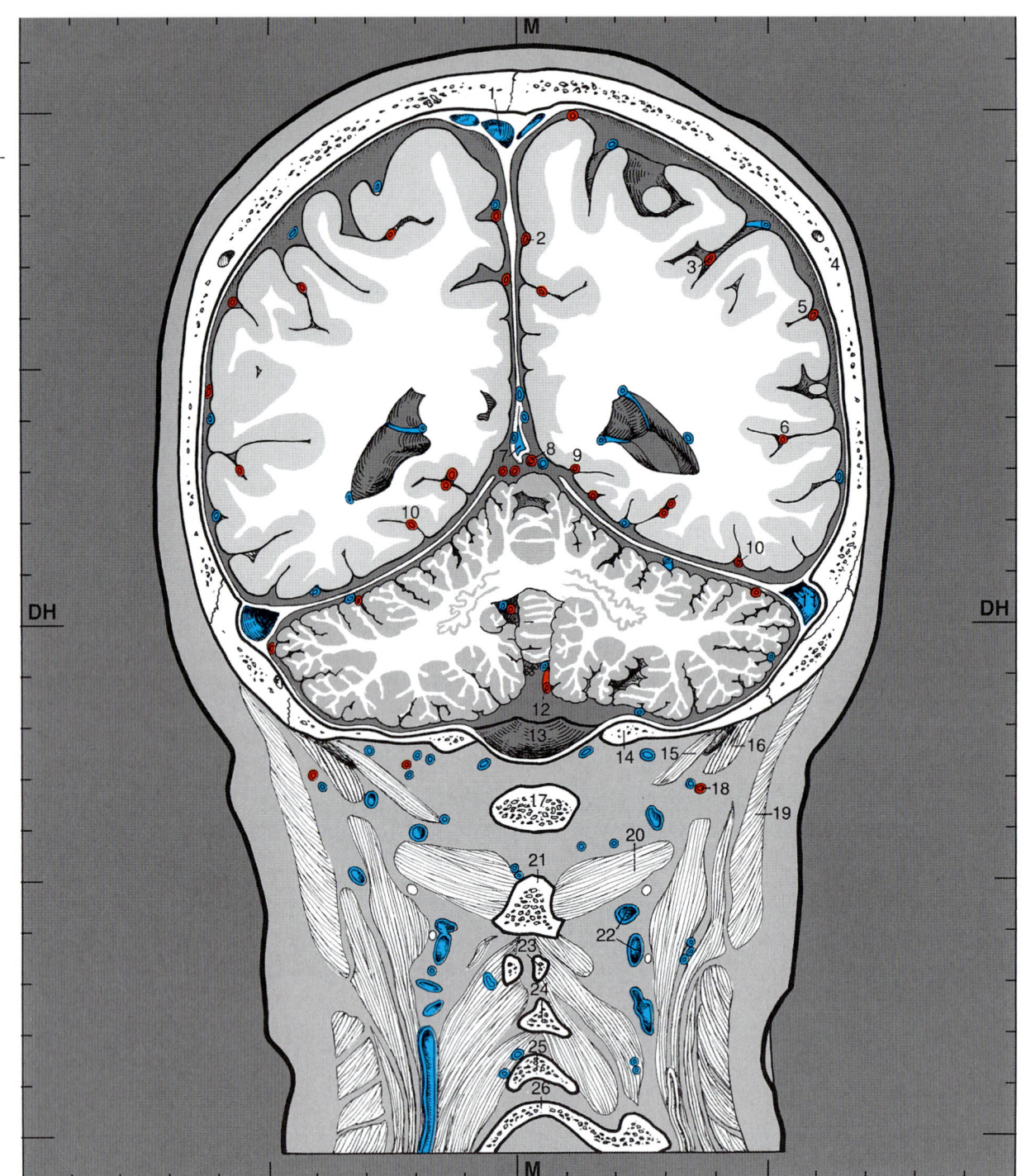

Fig. **14c** Anterior section surface of the eleventh coronal slice showing bony structures, cervical muscles, and blood vessels. The section reveals the dorsal part of the foramen magnum.

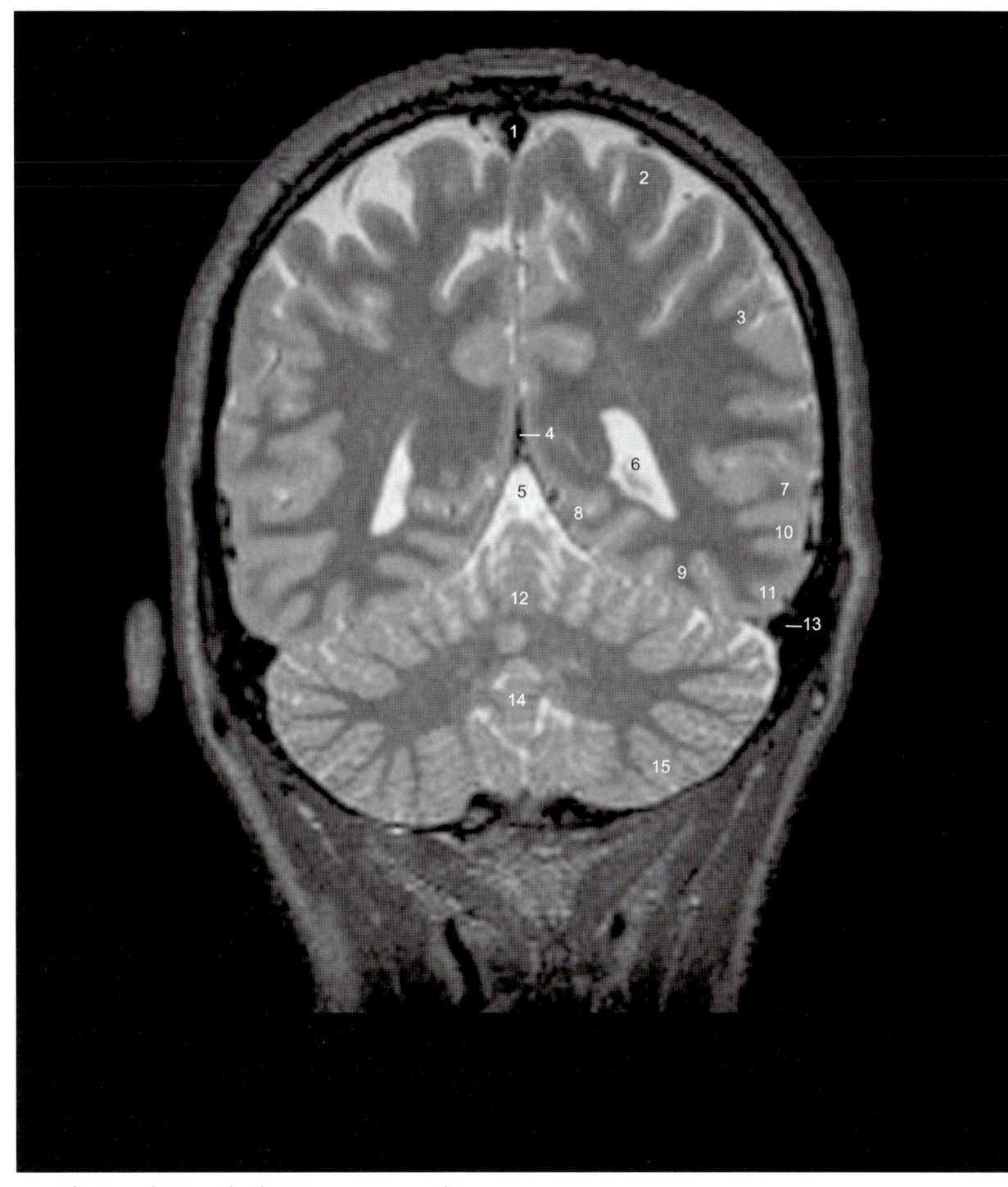

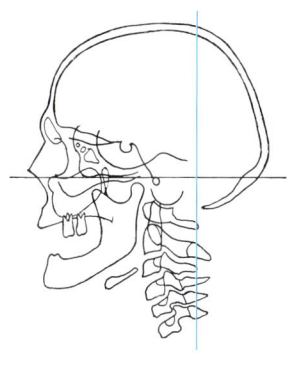

Coronal Slices

1 Superior sagittal sinus
2 Superior parietal lobule
3 Supramarginal gyrus
4 Straight sinus
5 Superior cerebellar cistern
6 Occipital (posterior) horn of lateral ventricle
7 Superior temporal gyrus
8 Medial occipitotemporal gyrus
9 Lateral occipitotemporal gyrus
10 Middle temporal gyrus
11 Inferior temporal gyrus
12 Vermis of anterior lobe of cerebellum
13 Transverse sinus
14 Vermis of cerebellum
15 Posterior lobe of cerebellum

Fig. **14d** Coronal, T2-weighted MR image corresponding approximately to the sectional plane of Figs. 14a and 14c.

Atlas

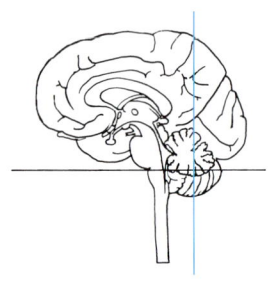

1 Superior parietal lobule
2 Longitudinal cerebral (interhemispheric) fissure
3 Falx cerebri
4 Precuneus
5 Angular gyrus
6 Parieto-occipital sulcus
7 Dura mater
8 Primary visual cortex
9 Cuneus
10 Occipital (posterior) horn of lateral ventricle
11 Middle temporal gyrus
12 Calcarine sulcus
13 Anterior lobe of cerebellum
14 Medial occipitotemporal gyrus
15 Lateral occipitotemporal gyrus
16 Inferior temporal gyrus
17 Tentorium of cerebellum
18 Primary fissure of cerebellum
19 Posterior lobe of cerebellum
20 Pyramis of vermis (VIII)
21 Cisterna magna (posterior cerebellomedullary cistern)
22 Greater occipital nerve
23 Third occipital nerve

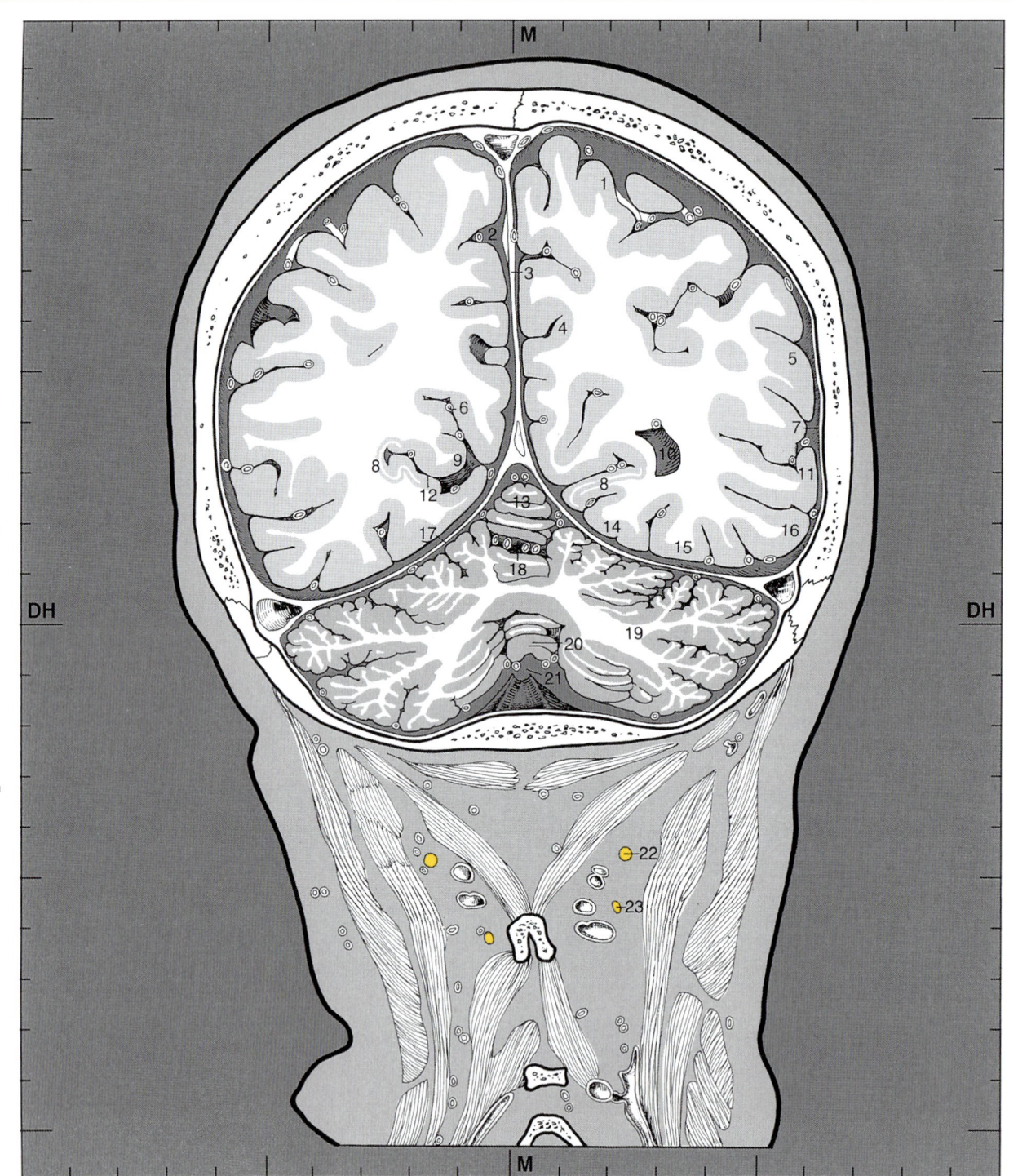

Fig. **15a** Anterior section surface of the twelfth coronal slice showing brain structures and branches of spinal nerves. The section reveals the posterior horn of the lateral ventricle, seen only in the left cerebral hemisphere. The tentorium cerebelli separates the supratentorial space from the infratentorial space.

Coronal Slices

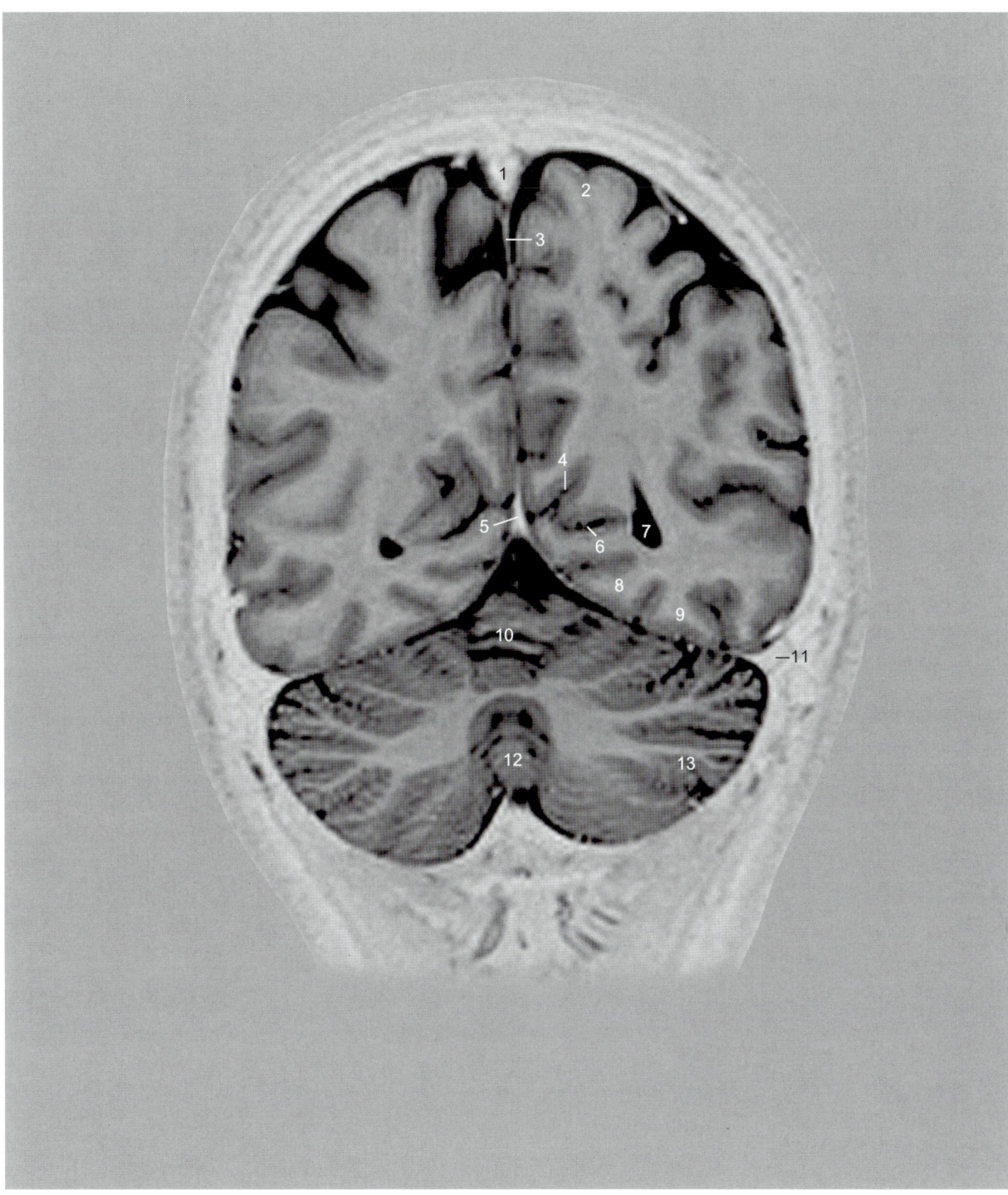

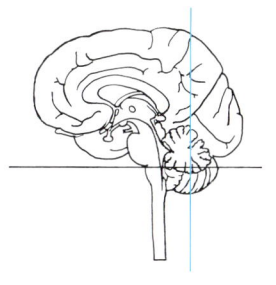

1 Superior sagittal sinus
2 Superior parietal lobule
3 Falx cerebri
4 Parieto-occipital sulcus
5 Straight sinus
6 Calcarine sulcus
7 Occipital (posterior) horn of lateral ventricle
8 Medial occipitotemporal gyrus
9 Lateral occipitotemporal gyrus
10 Vermis of anterior lobe of cerebellum
11 Transverse sinus
12 Vermis of cerebellum
13 Posterior lobe of cerebellum

Fig. **15b** Coronal, T1-weighted MR image corresponding approximately to the sectional plane of Figs. 15a and 15c.

68 Atlas

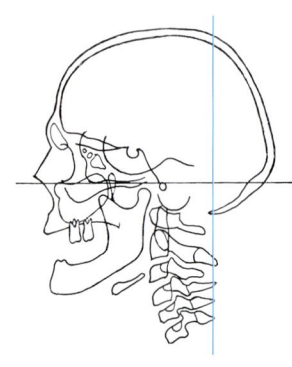

1 Superior sagittal sinus
2 Anterior parietal artery
3 Parietal bone
4 Precuneal artery
5 Posterior parietal artery
6 Falx cerebri
7 Parieto-occipital artery
8 Angular artery
9 Straight sinus
10 Temporo-occipital artery
11 Calcarine artery
12 Superior cerebellar artery
13 Lateral occipital artery
14 Tentorium of cerebellum
15 Transverse sinus
16 Posterior inferior cerebellar artery (PICA)
17 Occipital bone
18 Occipital artery
19 Rectus capitis posterior minor
20 Rectus capitis posterior major
21 Splenius capitis
22 Spinous process of axis
23 Suboccipital venous plexus
24 Spinous process of fourth cervical vertebra
25 Spinous process of fifth cervical vertebra

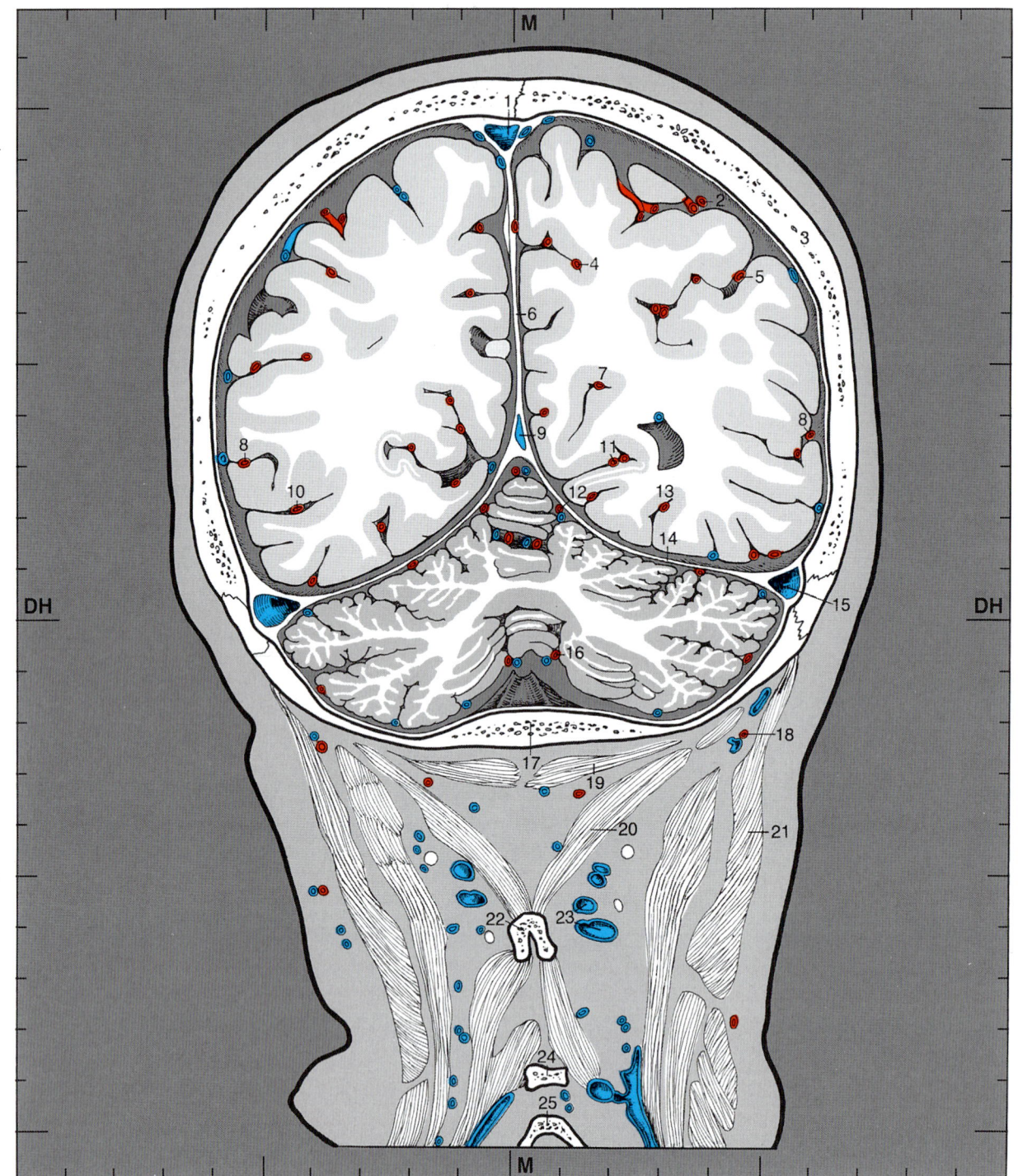

Fig. **15c** Anterior section surface of the twelfth coronal slice showing bony structures, cervical muscles, and blood vessels. The section lies posterior to the foramen magnum. Of the cervical vertebrae, only three spinous processes are revealed.

Coronal Slices

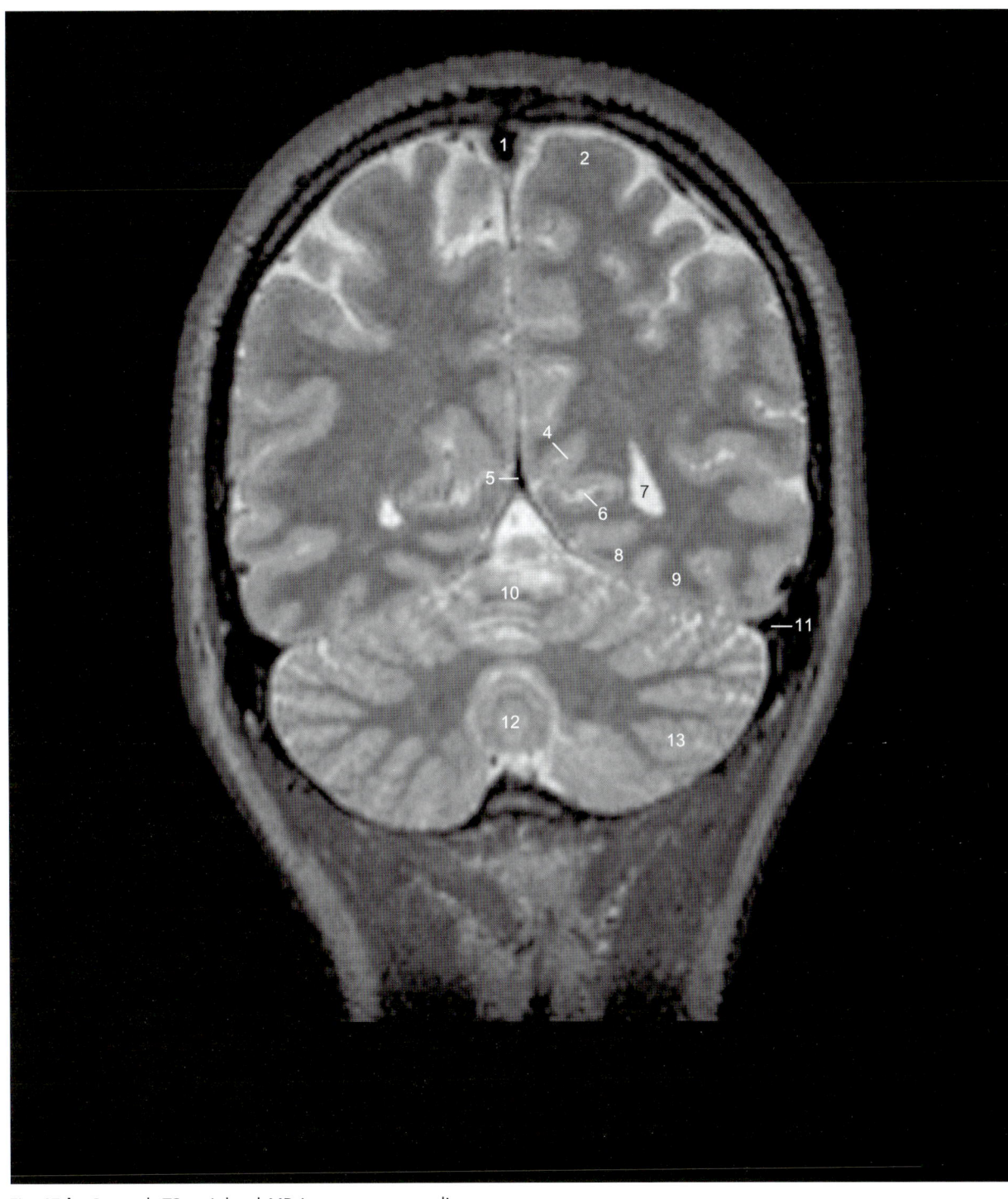

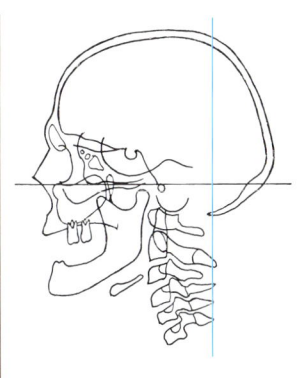

1 Superior sagittal sinus
2 Superior parietal lobule
4 Parieto-occipital sulcus
5 Straight sinus
6 Calcarine sulcus
7 Occipital (posterior) horn of lateral ventricle
8 Medial occipitotemporal gyrus
9 Lateral occipitotemporal gyrus
10 Vermis of anterior lobe of cerebellum
11 Transverse sinus
12 Vermis of cerebellum
13 Posterior lobe of cerebellum

Fig. **15d** Coronal, T2-weighted MR image corresponding approximately to the sectional plane of Figs. 15a and 15c.

70 Atlas

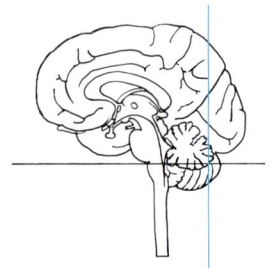

1 Superior parietal lobule
2 Longitudinal cerebral (inter-hemispheric) fissure
3 Precuneus
4 Angular gyrus
5 Falx cerebri
6 Parieto-occipital sulcus
7 Cuneus
8 Occipital gyri
9 Calcarine sulcus
10 Primary visual cortex
11 Dura mater
12 Medial occipitotemporal gyrus
13 Lateral occipitotemporal gyrus
14 Tentorium of cerebellum
15 Folium of vermis (VII A)
16 Posterior lobe of cerebellum
17 Greater occipital nerve
18 Third occipital nerve

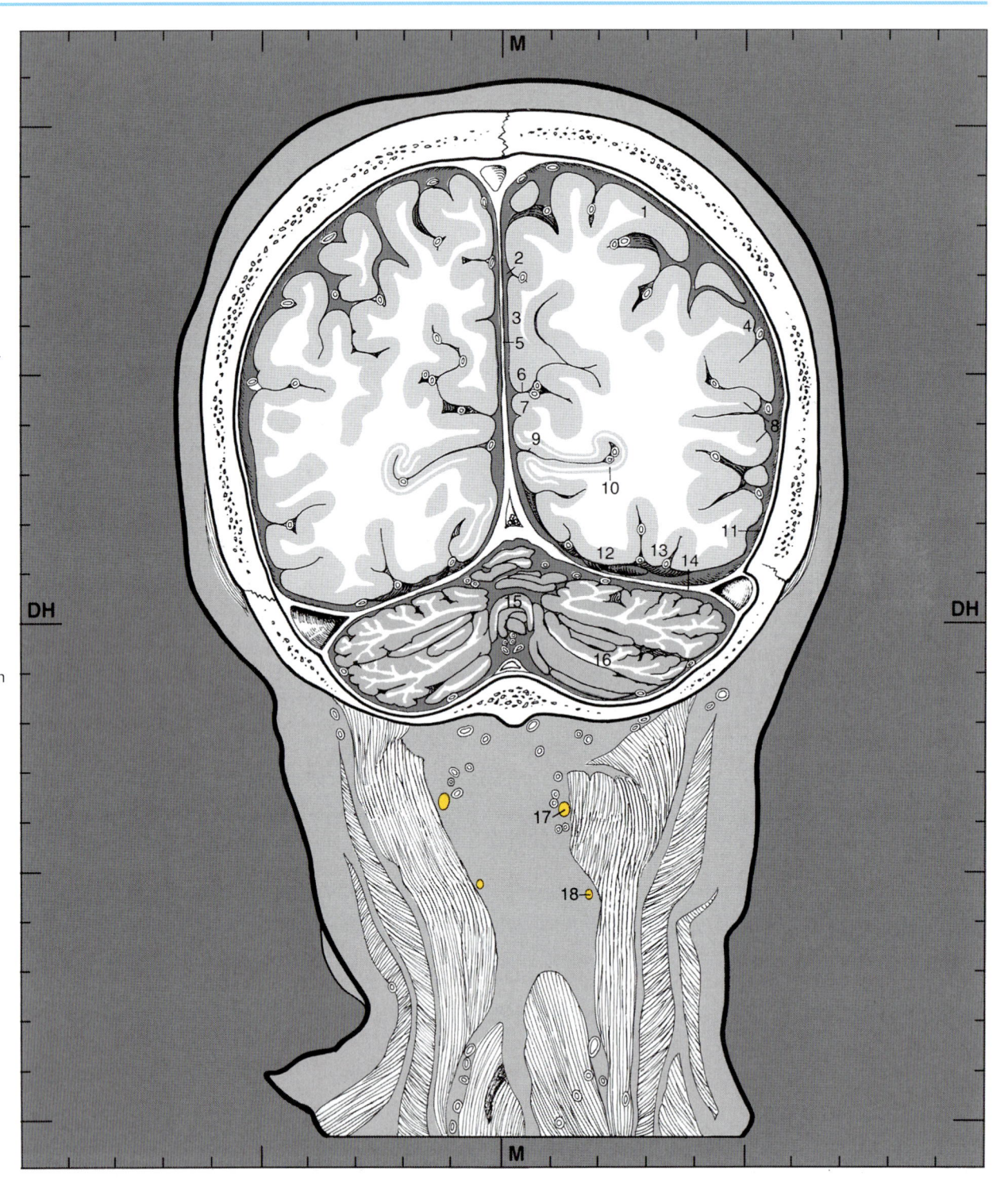

Fig. **16a** Anterior section surface of the thirteenth coronal slice showing brain structures and branches of spinal nerves. From the telencephalon only parts of the parietal and occipital lobes are cut. The cerebellum is sectioned tangentially.

Coronal Slices

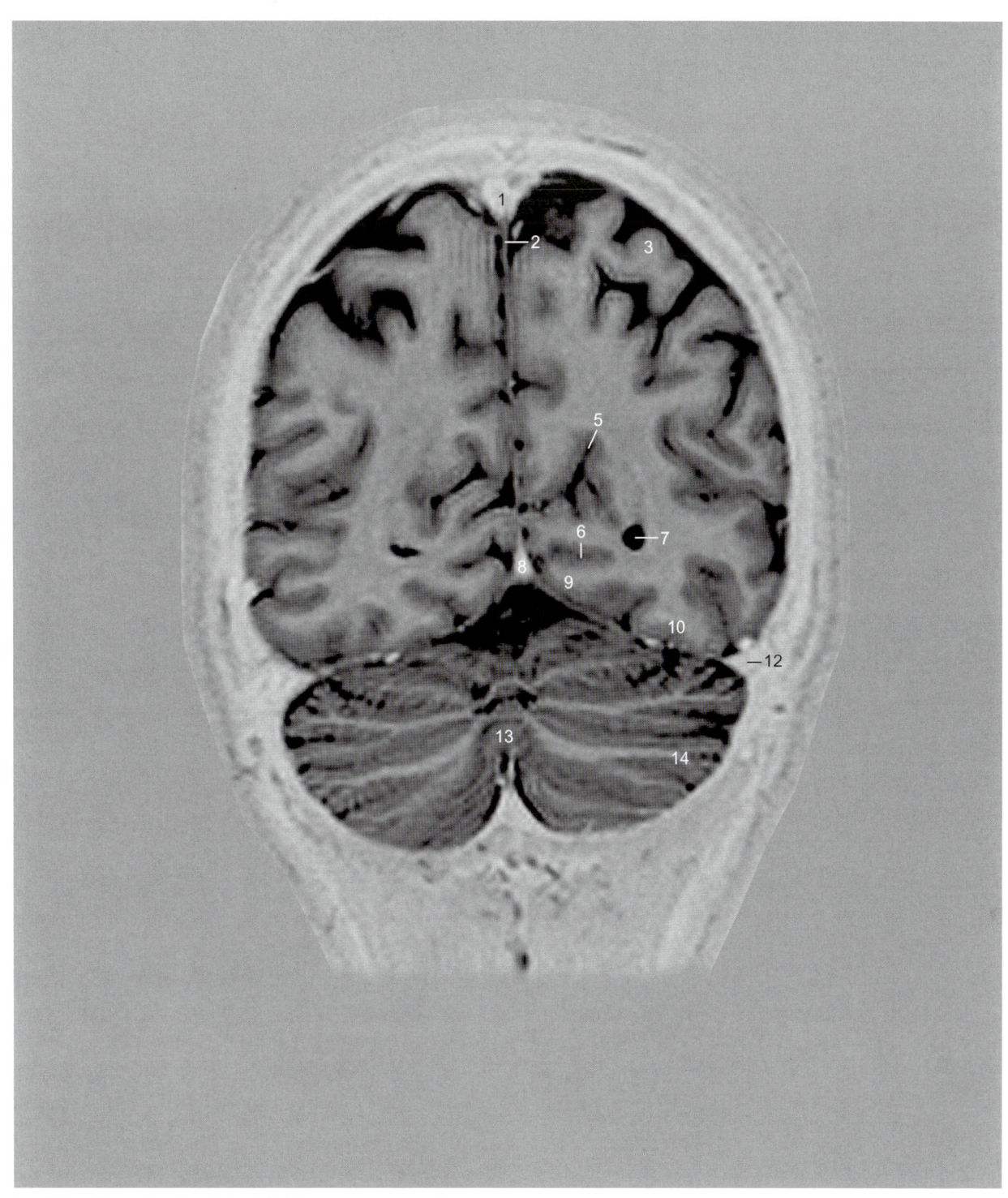

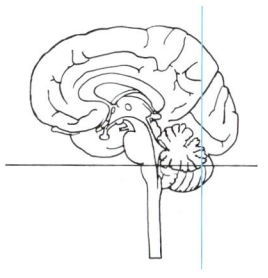

1 Superior sagittal sinus
2 Falx cerebri
3 Superior parietal lobule
5 Parieto-occipital sulcus
6 Calcarine sulcus
7 Occipital (posterior) horn of lateral ventricle
8 Straight sinus
9 Medial occipitotemporal gyrus
10 Lateral occipitotemporal gyrus
12 Transverse sinus
13 Vermis of anterior lobe of cerebellum
14 Hemisphere of posterior lobe of cerebellum

Fig. **16b** Coronal, T1-weighted MR image corresponding approximately to the sectional plane of Figs. 16a and 16c.

72　Atlas

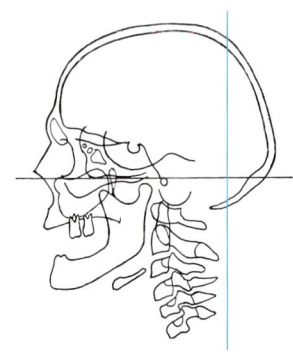

1 Superior sagittal sinus
2 Precuneal artery
3 Posterior parietal artery
4 Parietal bone
5 Falx cerebri
6 Parieto-occipital artery
7 Angular artery
8 Calcarine artery
9 Temporo-occipital artery
10 Straight sinus
11 Tentorium of cerebellum
12 Lateral occipital artery
13 Transverse sinus
14 Posterior inferior cerebellar artery (PICA)
15 Occipital bone
16 Occipital artery
17 Semispinalis capitis
18 Splenius capitis
19 Ligamentum nuchae
20 Trapezius

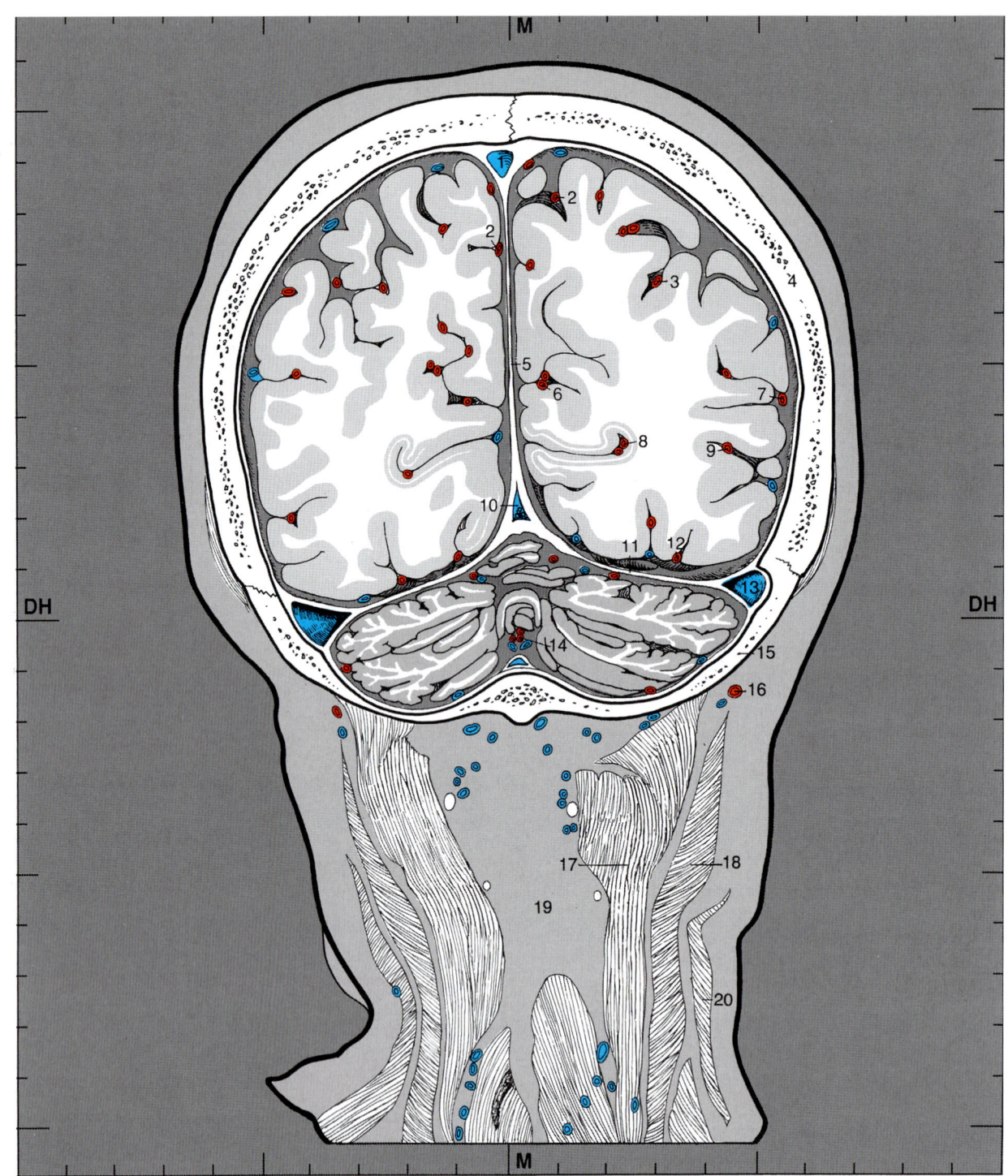

Fig. **16c**　Anterior section surface of the thirteenth coronal slice showing bony structures, cervical muscles, and blood vessels. The parietal and occipital bones form a circular bony ring.

Coronal Slices

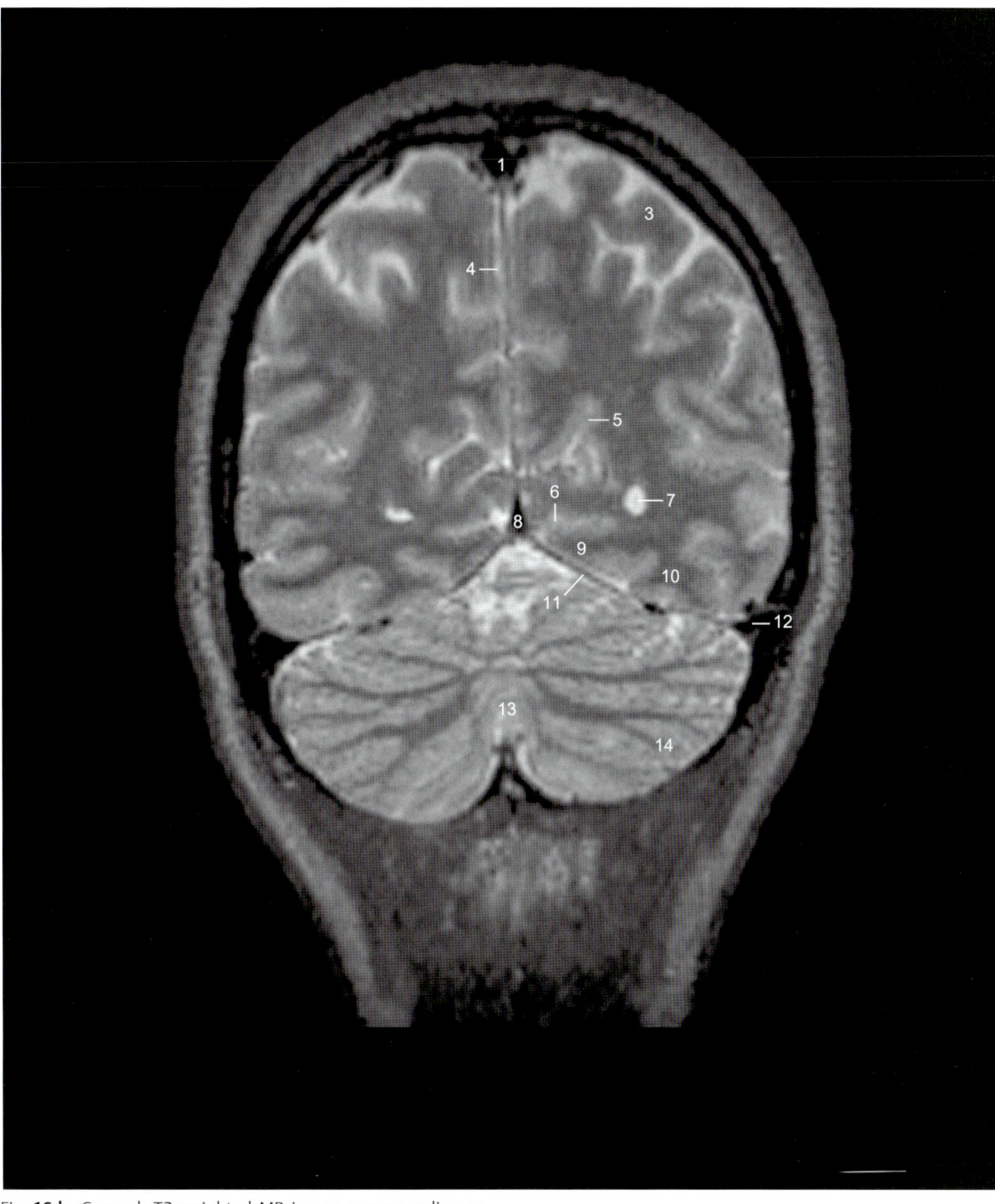

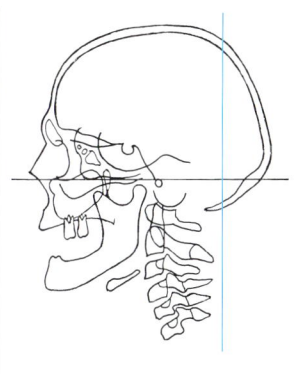

1 Superior sagittal sinus
3 Superior parietal lobule
4 Interhemispheric cistern
5 Parieto-occipital sulcus
6 Calcarine sulcus
7 Occipital (posterior) horn of lateral ventricle
8 Straight sinus
9 Medial occipitotemporal gyrus
10 Lateral occipitotemporal gyrus
11 Transverse cerebral fissure, tentorium of cerebellum
12 Transverse sinus
13 Vermis of anterior lobe of cerebellum
14 Hemisphere of posterior lobe of cerebellum

Fig. **16d** Coronal, T2-weighted MR image corresponding approximately to the sectional plane of Figs. 16a and 16c.

74   Atlas

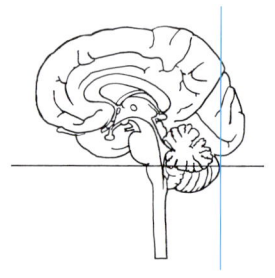

1 Precuneus
2 Longitudinal cerebral (interhemispheric) fissure
3 Parieto-occipital sulcus
4 Falx cerebri
5 Occipital gyri
6 Cuneus
7 Primary visual cortex
8 Calcarine sulcus
9 Dura mater
10 Medial occipitotemporal gyrus
11 Lateral occipitotemporal gyrus
12 Greater occipital nerve

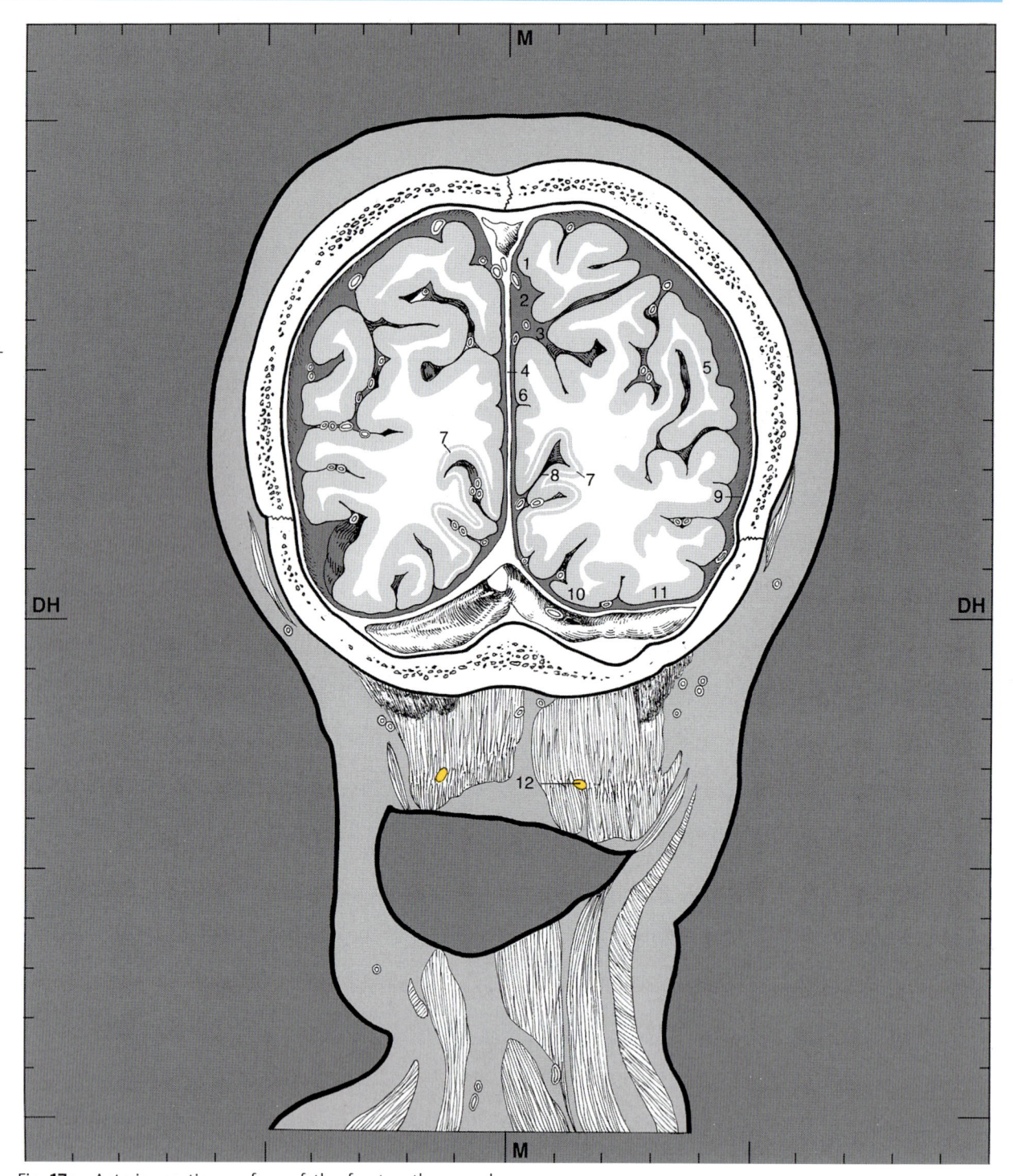

Fig. **17a** Anterior section surface of the fourteenth coronal slice showing brain structures and branches of the second spinal nerve. The posterior part of both cerebral hemispheres consists almost only of occipital lobes.

Coronal Slices

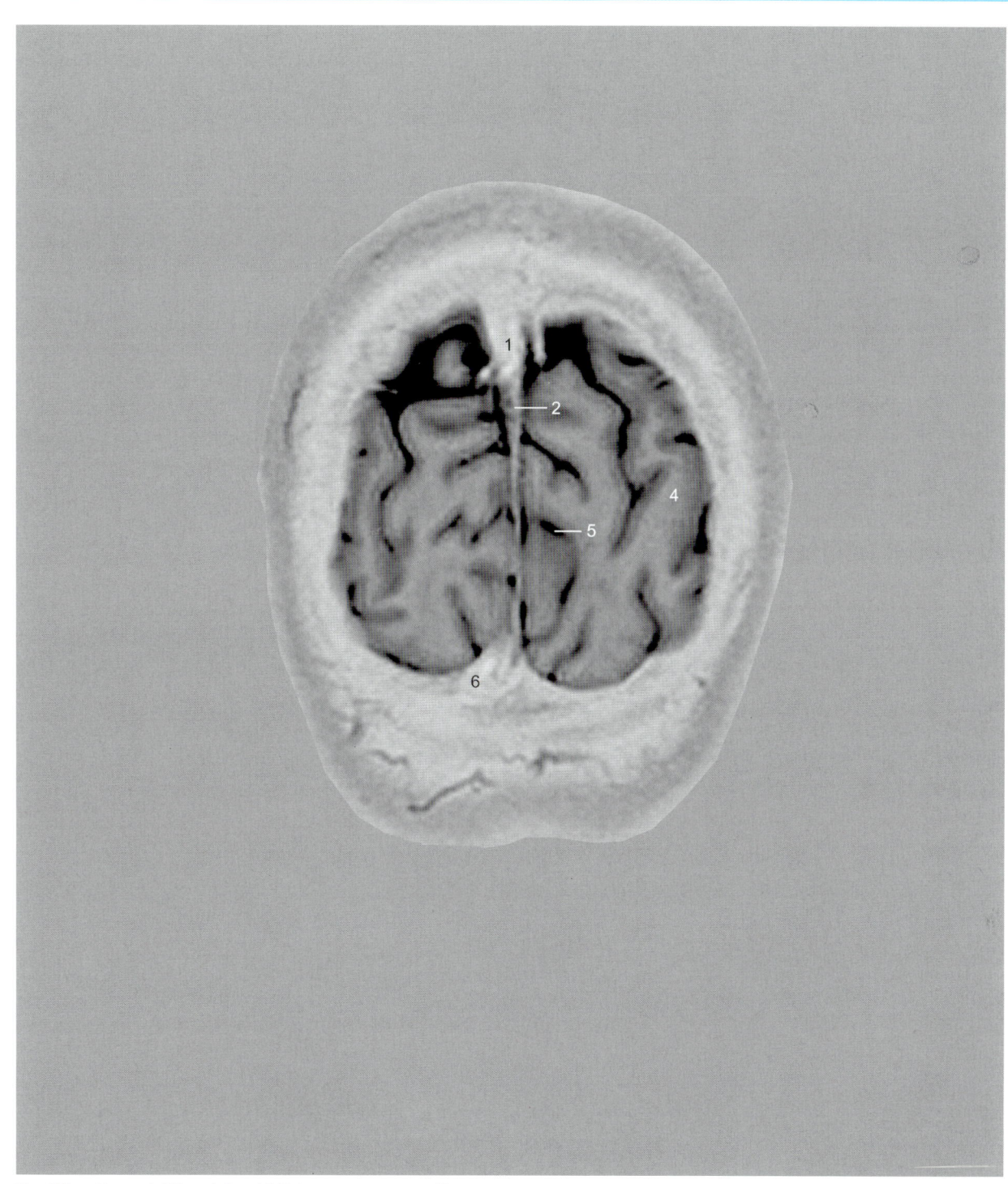

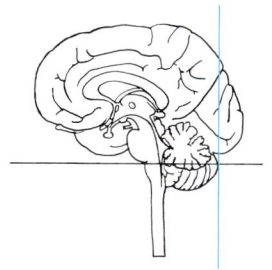

1 Superior sagittal sinus
2 Falx cerebri
4 Occipital gyrus
5 Calcarine sulcus
6 Transverse sinus

Fig. **17b** Coronal, T1-weighted MR image corresponding approximately to the sectional plane of Figs. 17a and 17c.

76   Atlas

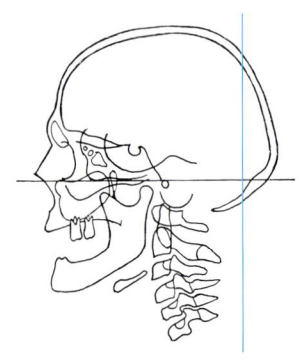

1 Superior sagittal sinus
2 Parieto-occipital artery
3 Parietal bone
4 Angular artery
5 Calcarine artery
6 Temporo-occipital artery
7 Lateral occipital artery
8 Confluence of sinuses
9 Transverse sinus
10 Occipital bone
11 Occipital artery
12 Semispinalis capitis
13 Splenius capitis
14 Ligamentum nuchae
15 Trapezius

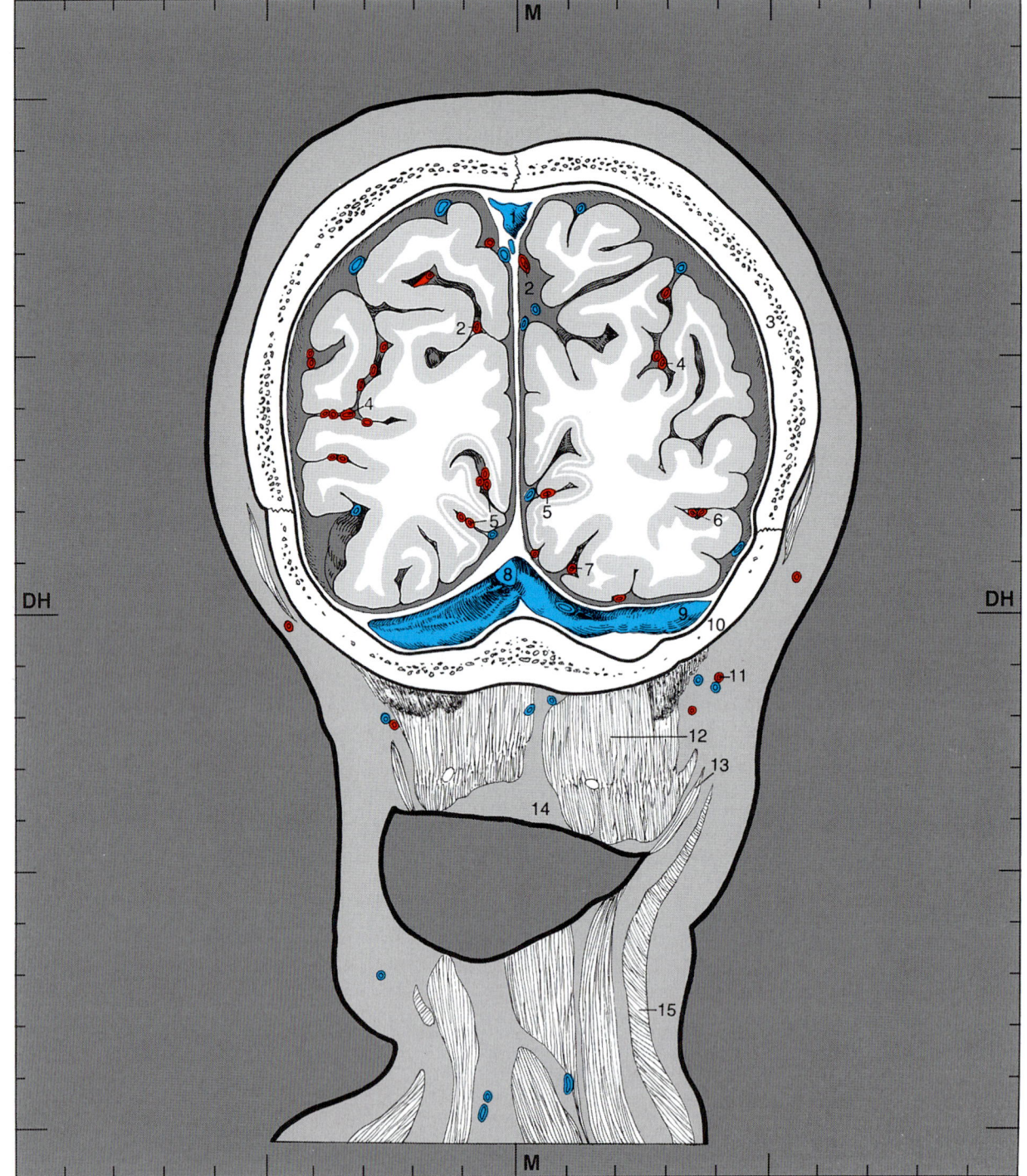

Fig. **17c** Anterior section surface of the fourteenth coronal slice showing bony structures, cervical muscles, and blood vessels. This slice reveals the confluence of the sinuses. On cutting, an opening was formed due to the curvature of the nape of the neck.

Coronal Slices

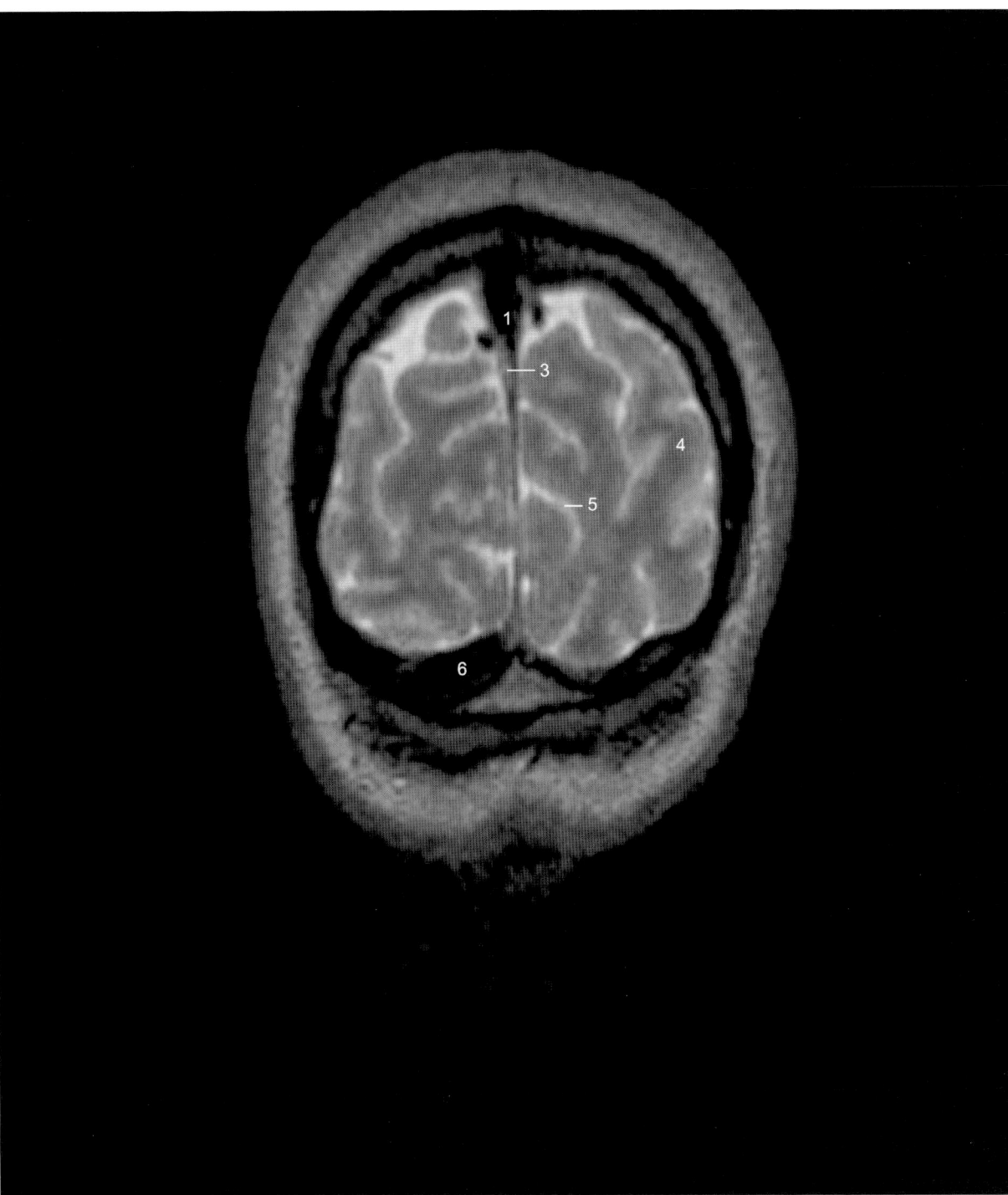

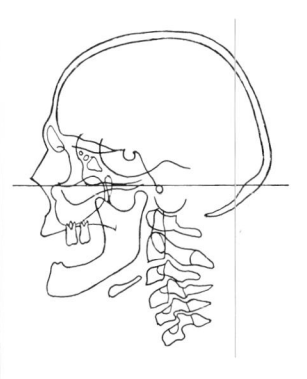

1 Superior sagittal sinus
3 Interhemispheric cistern
4 Occipital gyrus
5 Calcarine sulcus
6 Transverse sinus

Fig. **17d** Coronal, T2-weighted MR image corresponding approximately to the sectional plane of Figs. 17a and 17c.

78 Atlas

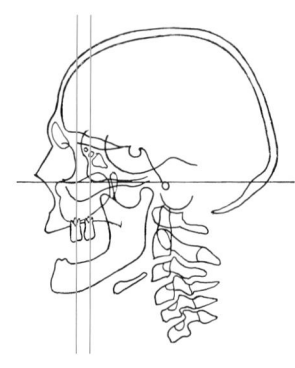

1 Frontal bone
2 Crista galli
3 Anterior cranial fossa
4 Roof of orbit
5 Frontozygomatic suture
6 Orbital plate
7 Ethmoidal cells
8 Orbit
9 Floor of orbit
10 Infraorbital canal
11 Zygomatic bone
12 Middle nasal concha
13 Nasal septum
14 Maxillary sinus
15 Inferior nasal concha
16 Hard palate
17 Maxilla
18 Second molar tooth
19 First molar tooth (cut)
20 Body of mandible
21 Mandibular canal

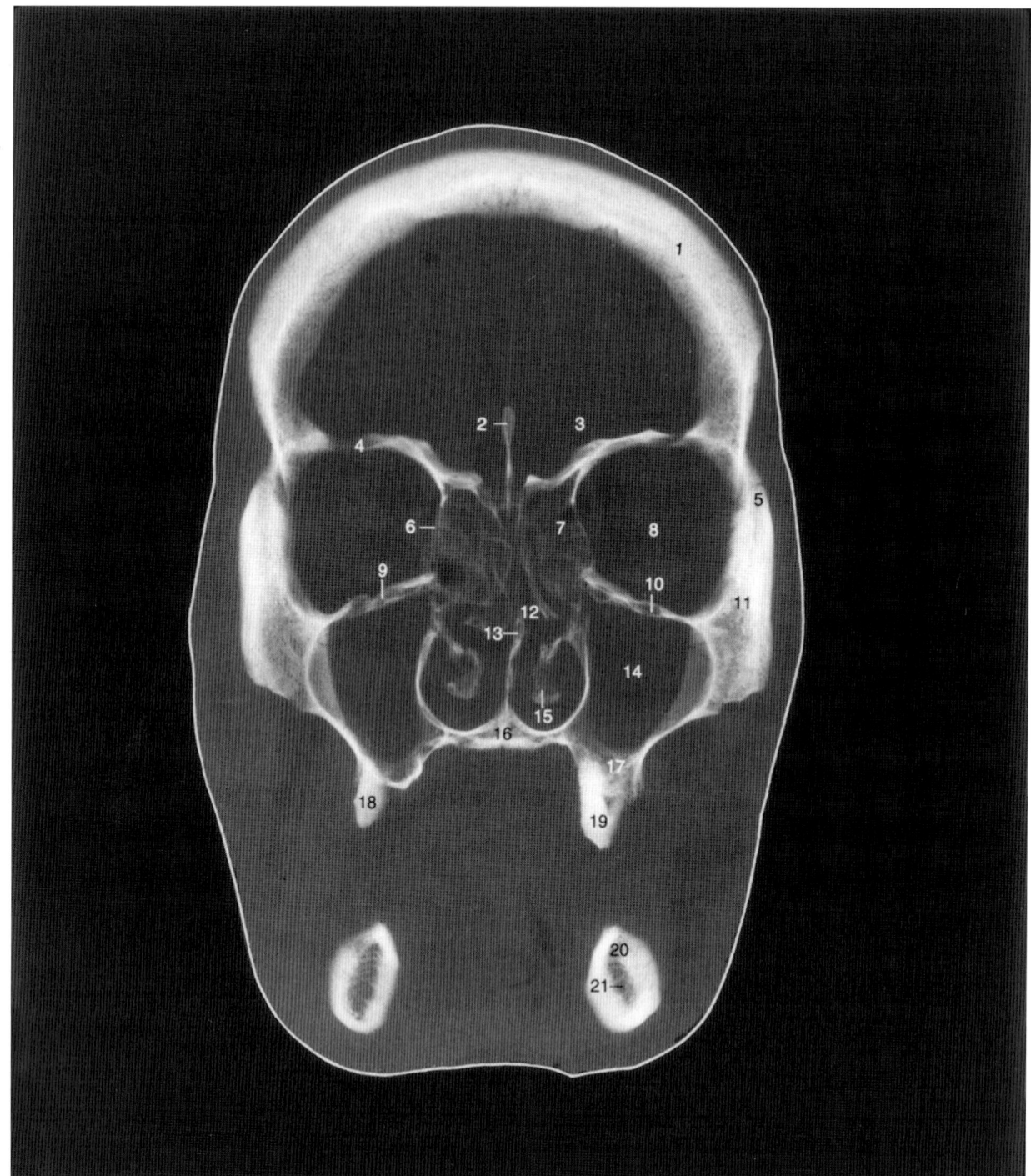

Fig. 18 Radiograph of the first coronal slice. The outer border of the head has been added. Guideline structures include the anterior cranial fossa, crista galli, orbits, ethmoidal cells, nasal conchae, maxillary sinuses, and mandible.

Coronal Slices

Fig. 19 Radiograph of the second coronal slice. The outer border of the head has been added. Bony guideline structures include the roof and the floor of the orbit, nasal conchae, maxillary sinuses, and mandible.

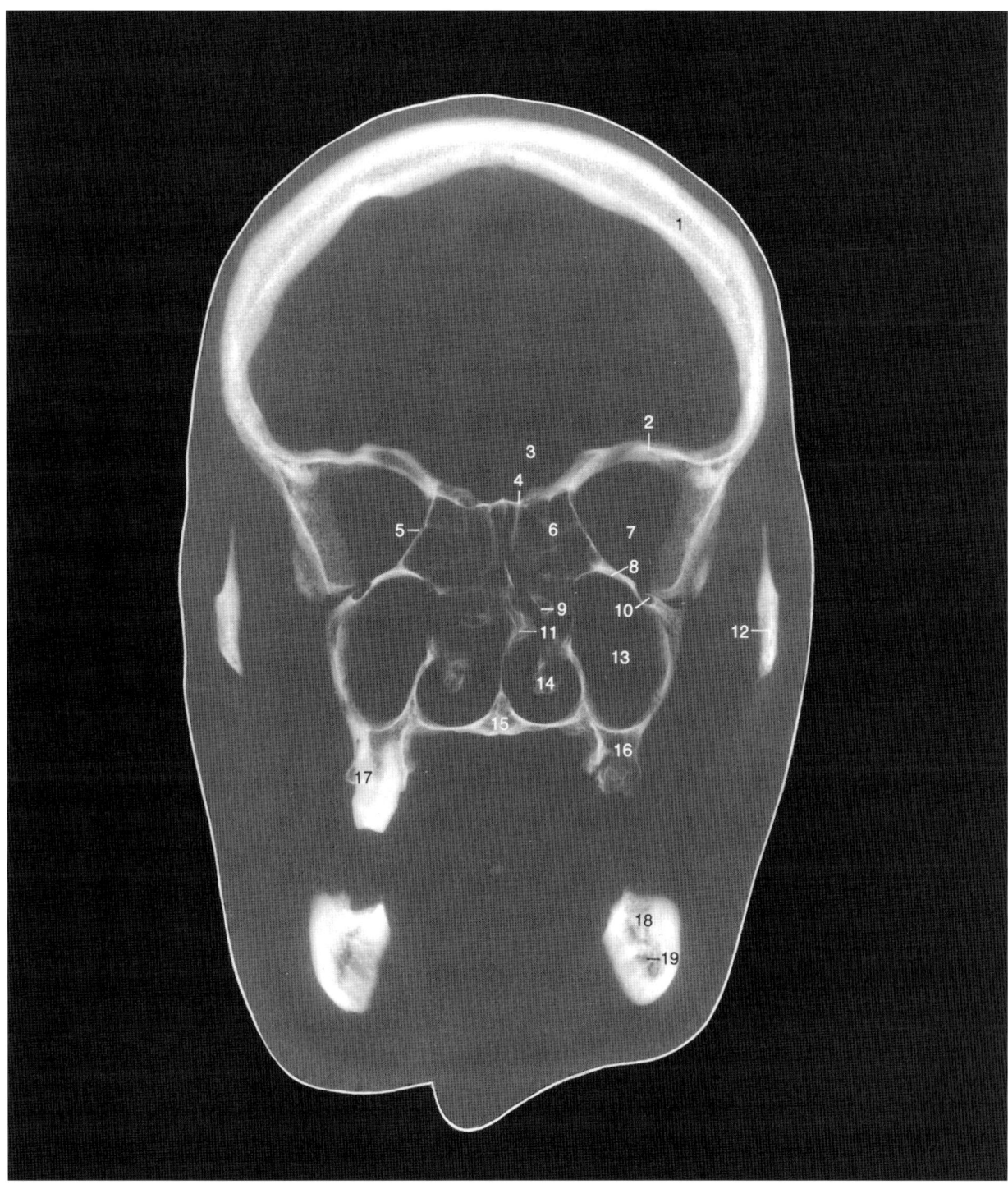

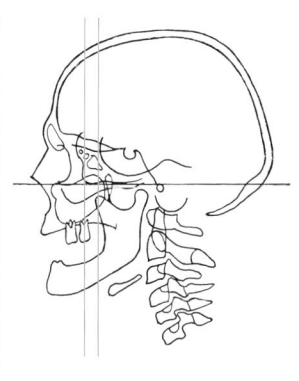

1 Frontal bone
2 Roof of orbit
3 Anterior cranial fossa
4 Cribriform plate of ethmoid
5 Orbital plate
6 Ethmoidal cells
7 Orbit
8 Floor of orbit
9 Middle nasal concha
10 Infraorbital canal
11 Nasal septum
12 Zygomatic bone
13 Maxillary sinus
14 Inferior nasal concha
15 Hard palate
16 Maxilla
17 Second molar tooth
18 Body of mandible
19 Mandibular canal

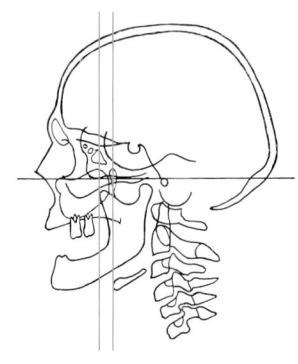

80 Atlas

1 Frontal bone
2 Anterior cranial fossa
3 Orbit
4 Superior orbital fissure
5 Greater wing of sphenoid
6 Ethmoidal cells and sphenoidal sinus
7 Pterygopalatine fossa
8 Middle nasal concha
9 Zygomatic arch
10 Maxillary sinus (cut)
11 Nasal septum
12 Maxilla
13 Inferior nasal concha
14 Coronoid process
15 Hard palate
16 Pterygoid hamulus
17 Ramus of mandible
18 Mandibular canal

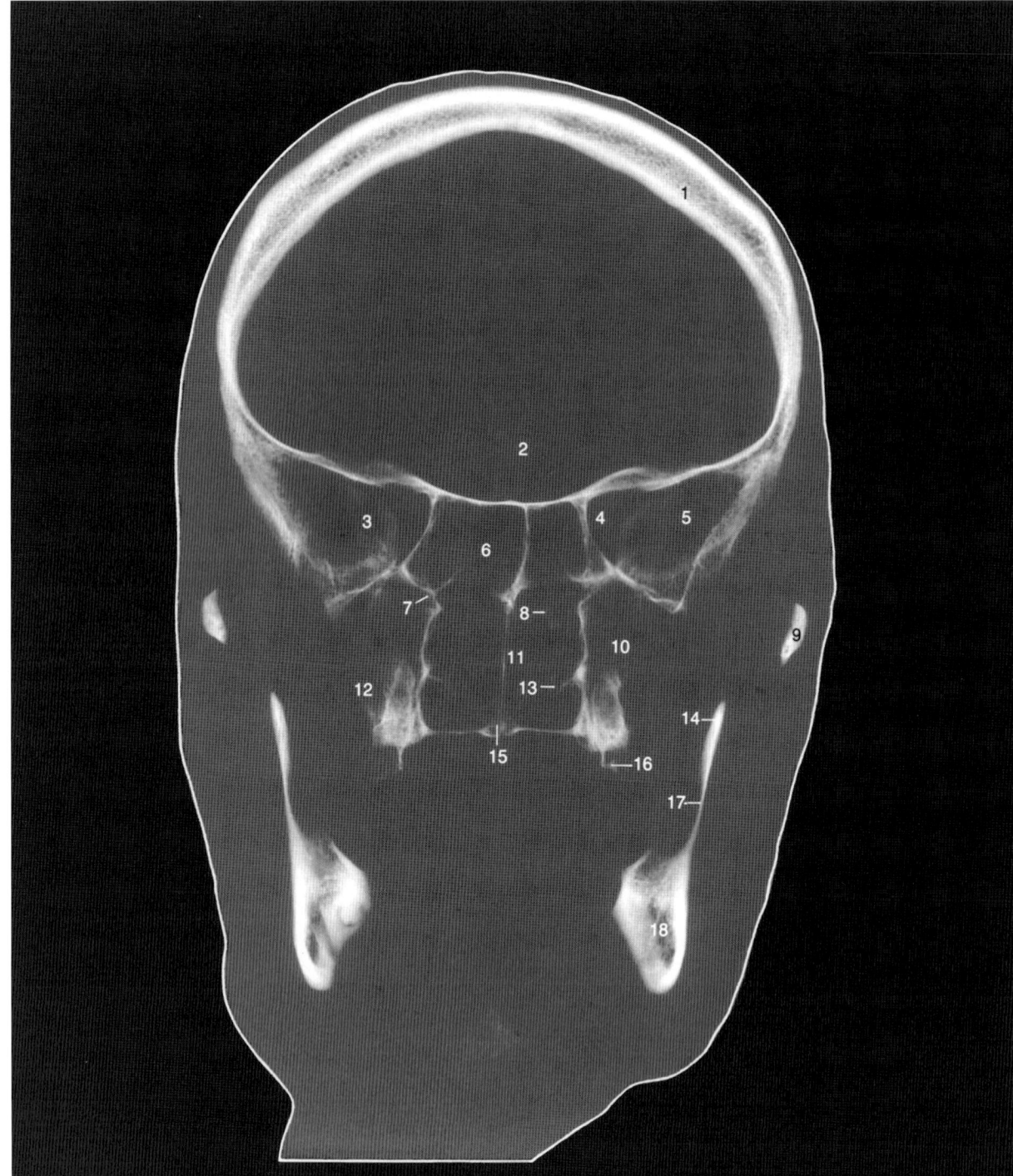

Fig. 20 Radiograph of the third coronal slice. The frontal bone forms the floor of the anterior cranial fossa and the roof of the orbit. Paranasal sinuses and nasal conchae are shown.

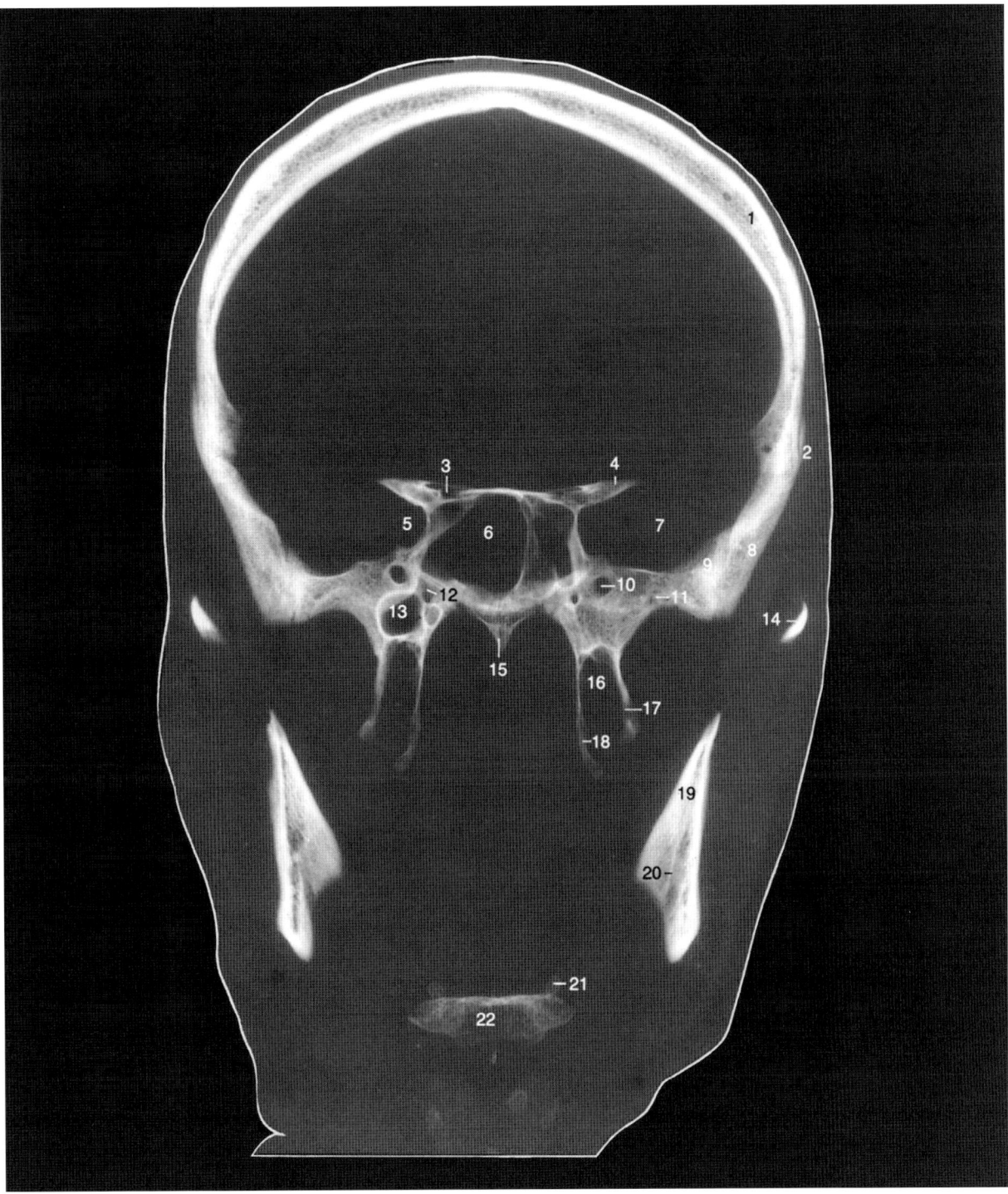

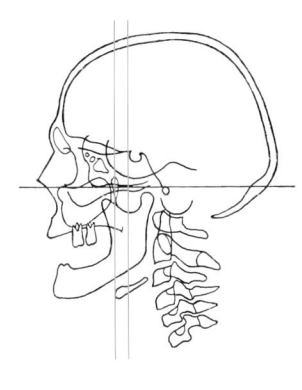

Coronal Slices

1 Parietal bone
2 Squamous suture
3 Optic canal
4 Lesser wing of sphenoid
5 Superior orbital fissure
6 Sphenoidal sinus
7 Middle cranial fossa
8 Temporal bone
9 Sphenosquamous suture
10 Foramen rotundum
11 Sphenoid
12 Pterygoid canal
13 Pterygopalatine fossa
14 Zygomatic arch
15 Nasal septum
16 Pterygoid fossa
17 Lateral pterygoid plate
18 Medial pterygoid plate
19 Ramus of mandible
20 Mandibular canal
21 Lesser cornu of hyoid bone
22 Body of hyoid bone

Fig. 21 Radiograph of the fourth coronal slice revealing the optic canal, the foramen rotundum, and the medial pterygoid plate of the sphenoid. The middle portion of the hyoid bone is also visible.

82 Atlas

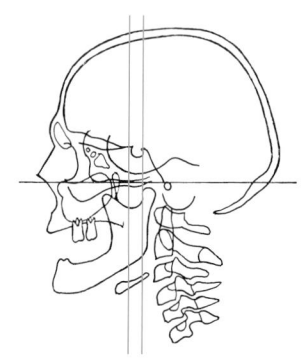

1 Parietal bone
2 Anterior clinoid process
3 Hypophysial fossa
4 Carotid sulcus
5 Middle cranial fossa
6 Temporal bone
7 Sphenoidal sinus
8 Sphenoid
9 Ramus of mandible
10 Mandibular canal
11 Stylohyoid ligament (ossified)
12 Greater cornu of hyoid bone
13 Thyroid cartilage (ossified)

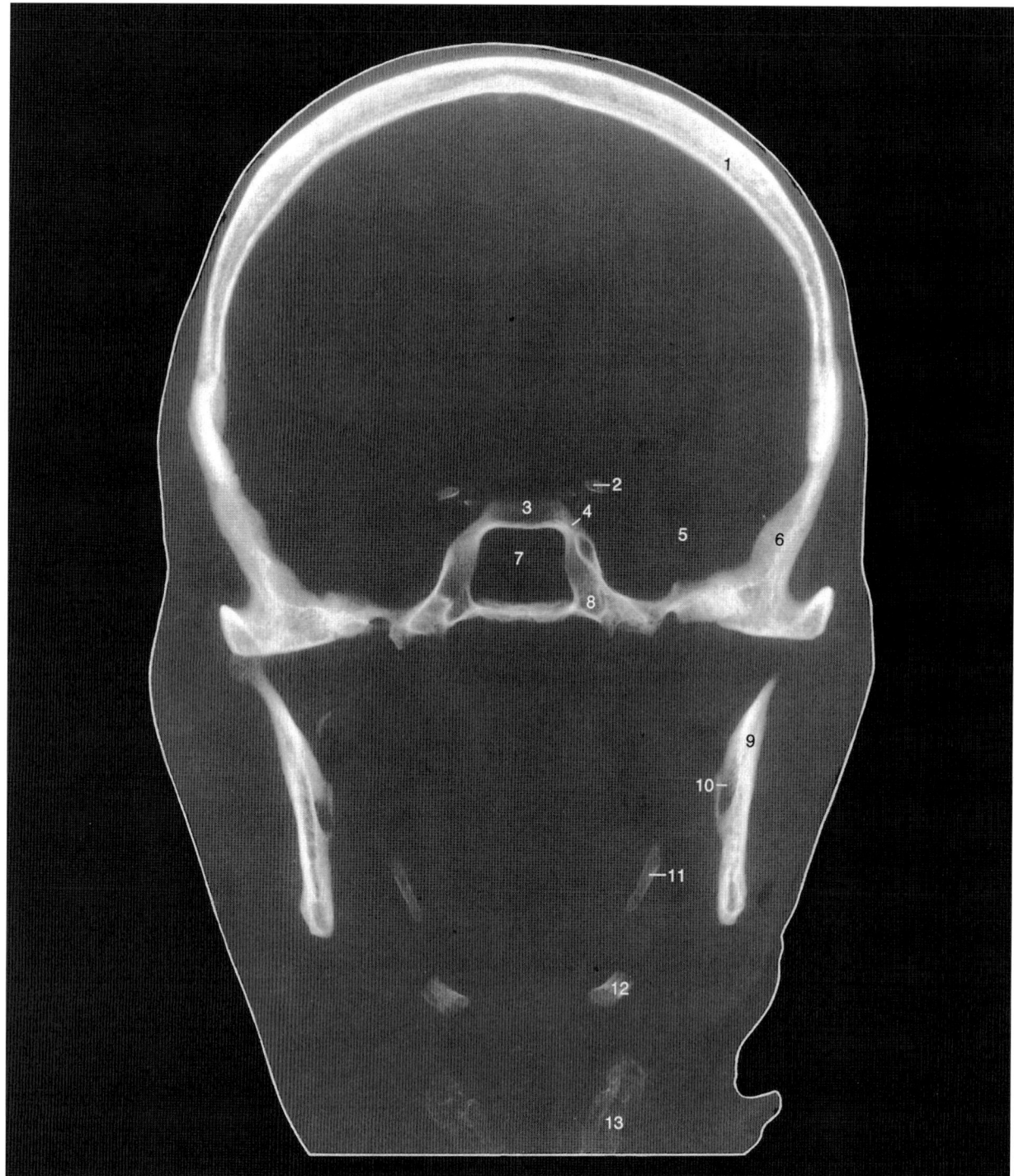

Fig. 22 Radiograph of the fifth coronal slice. The middle cranial fossa, sphenoidal sinus, ramus of the mandible, and the lateral portions of the hyoid bone are demonstrated.

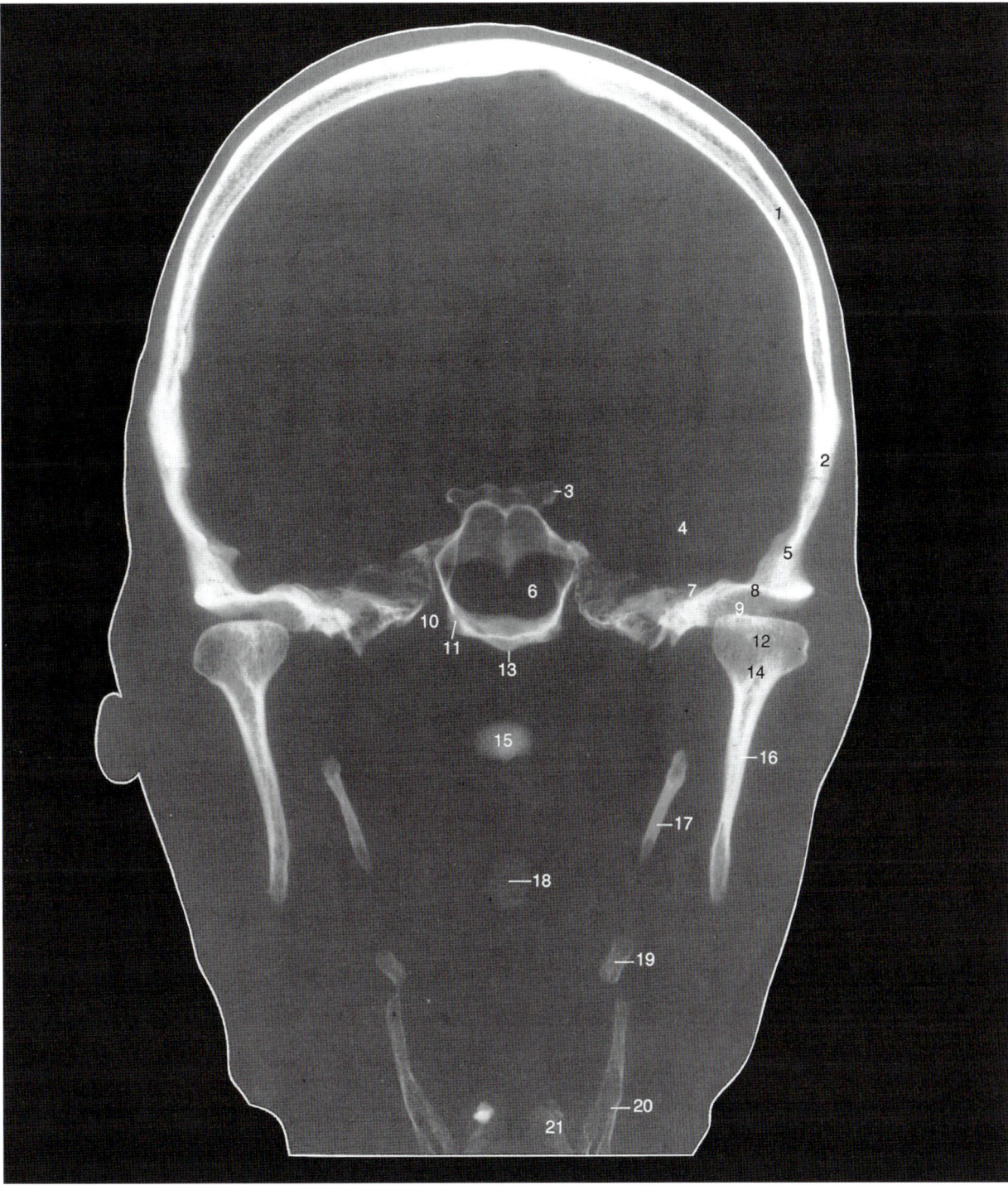

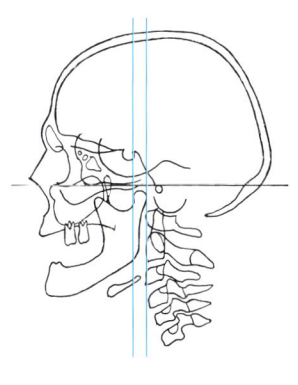

Coronal Slices

1 Parietal bone
2 Squamous suture
3 Posterior clinoid process
4 Middle cranial fossa
5 Temporal bone
6 Sphenoidal sinus
7 Sphenosquamous suture
8 Mandibular fossa
9 Temporomandibular joint
10 Carotid canal
11 Sphenoid
12 Head of mandible
13 Pharyngeal tubercle
14 Neck of mandible
15 Anterior arch of atlas
16 Ramus of mandible
17 Stylohyoid ligament (ossified)
18 Body of axis
19 Greater cornu of hyoid bone
20 Thyroid cartilage
21 Cricoid cartilage

Fig. 23 Radiograph of the sixth coronal slice. The middle cranial fossa at the level of the posterior clinoid processes, the temporomandibular joints, and the lateral portions of the hyoid bone are demonstrated.

84 Atlas

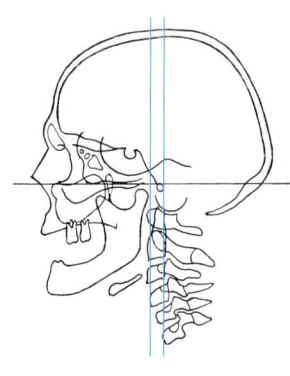

1 Parietal bone
2 Squamous suture
3 Superior margin of petrous part of temporal bone
4 Vestibule
5 Temporal bone
6 Cochlea
7 Sphenoid
8 External acoustic meatus
9 Spheno-occipital synchondrosis
10 Occipital bone
11 Styloid process
12 Anterior arch of atlas
13 Dens of axis
14 Stylohyoid ligament (ossified)
15 Lateral atlantoaxial joint
16 Axis
17 Third cervical vertebra
18 Fourth cervical vertebra

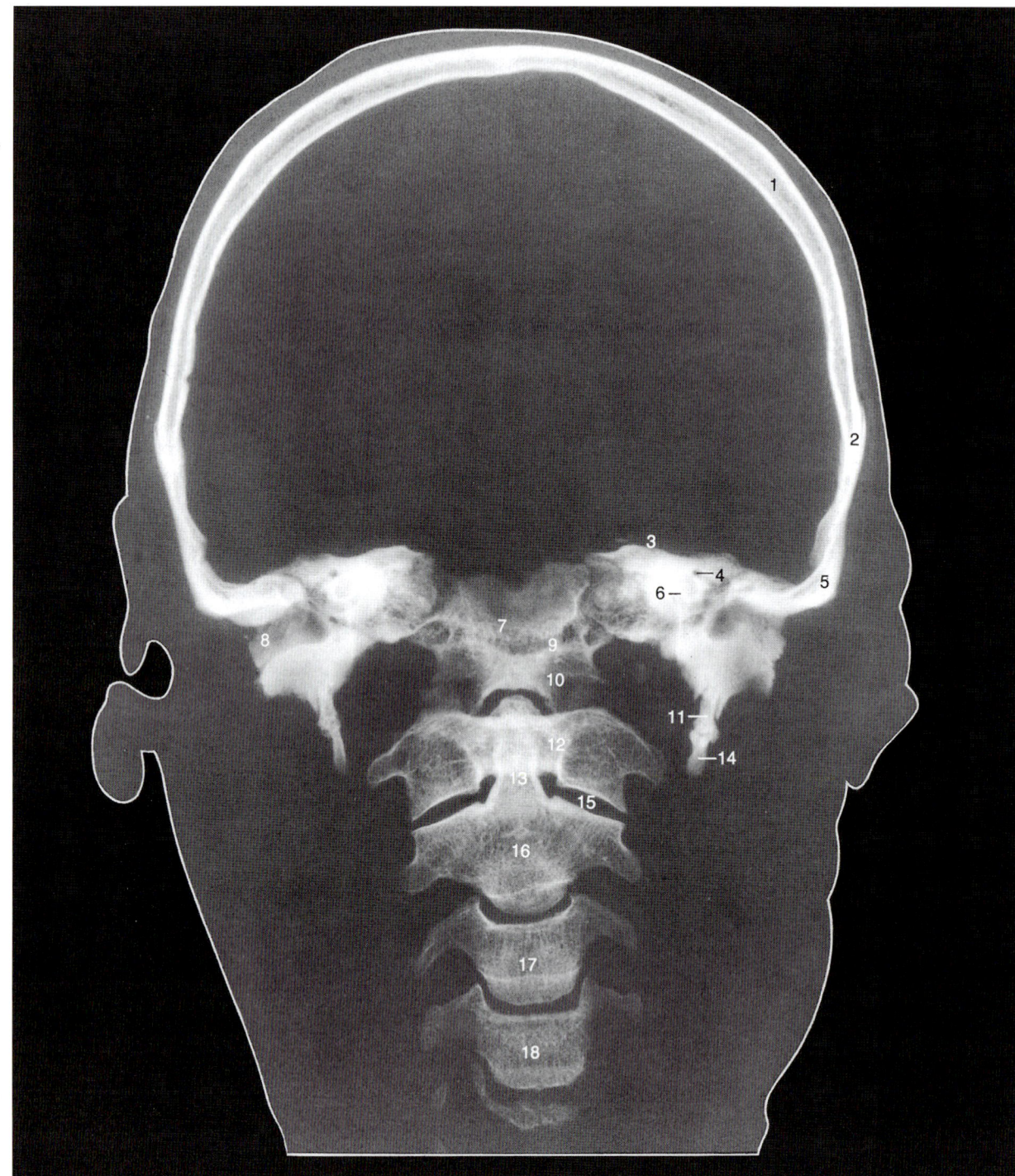

Fig. 24 Radiograph of the seventh coronal slice that reveals the petrous part of the temporal bone, the cochlea, and the styloid process, together with the anterior parts of the upper cervical vertebral column.

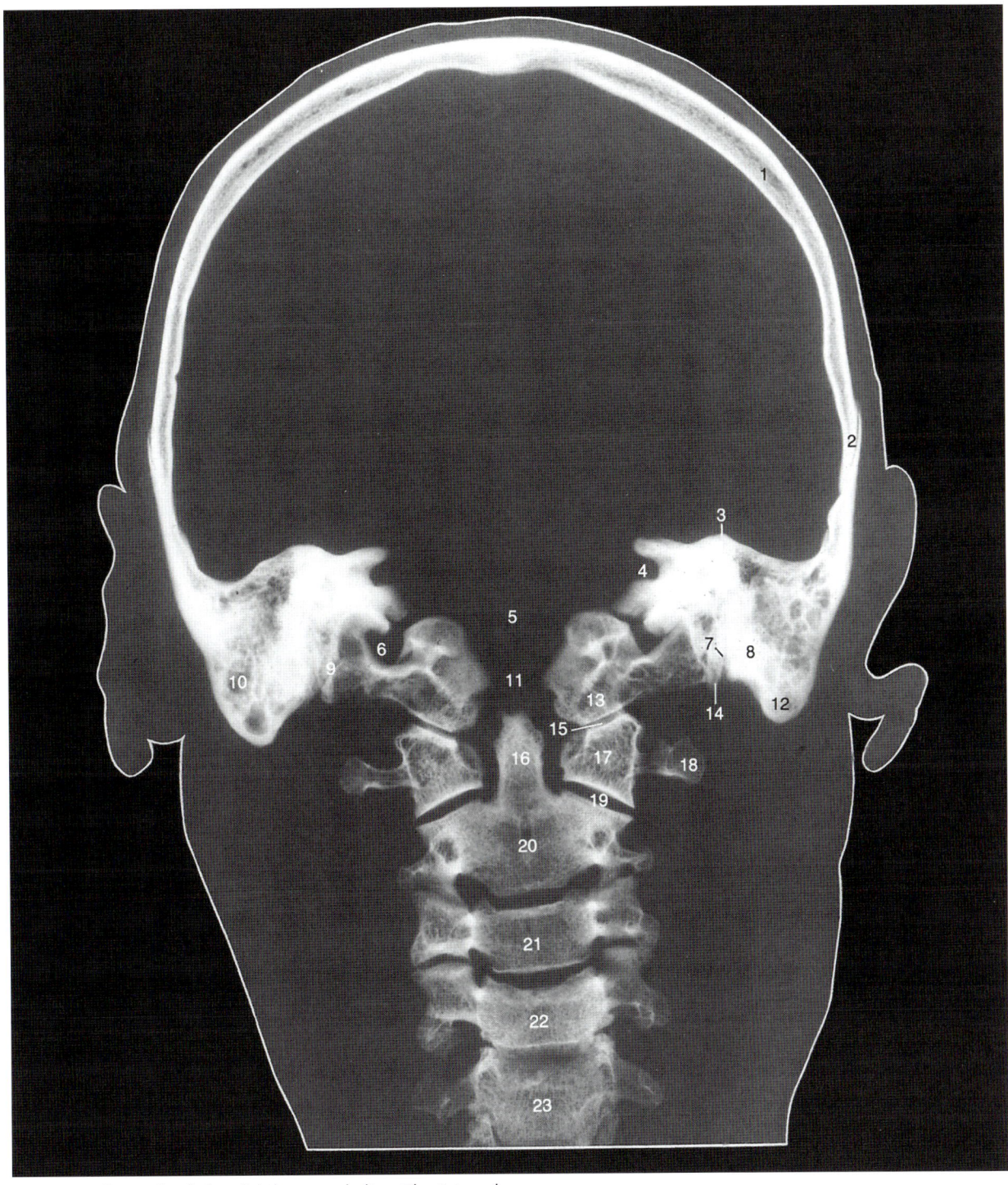

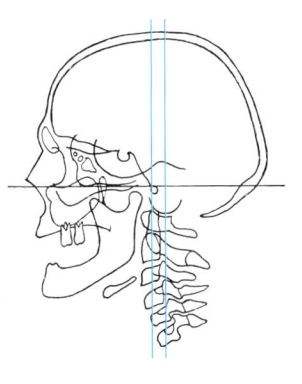

Coronal Slices 85

1 Parietal bone
2 Squamous suture
3 Arcuate eminence
4 Internal acoustic meatus
5 Posterior cranial fossa
6 Jugular foramen
7 Facial canal
8 Temporal bone
9 Petro-occipital synchondrosis
10 Mastoid cells
11 Foramen magnum
12 Mastoid process
13 Occipital condyle
14 Styloid process
15 Atlanto-occipital joint
16 Dens of axis
17 Lateral mass of atlas
18 Transverse process of atlas
19 Lateral atlantoaxial joint
20 Axis
21 Third cervical vertebra
22 Fourth cervical vertebra
23 Fifth cervical vertebra

Fig. 25 Radiograph of the eighth coronal slice. The internal acoustic meatus, facial canal, and the mastoid cells are seen in the petrous part of the temporal bone. The first five cervical vertebrae can be clearly seen.

86 Atlas

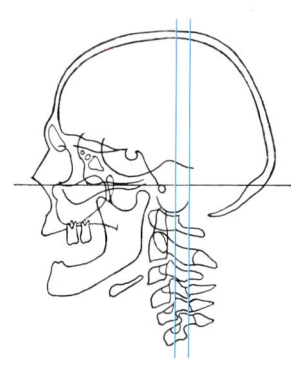

1 Parietal bone
2 Squamous suture
3 Posterior cranial fossa
4 Temporal bone
5 Sigmoid sinus
6 Occipital bone
7 Occipitomastoid suture
8 Mastoid process
9 Foramen magnum
10 Atlanto-occipital joint
11 Lateral mass of atlas
12 Articular process and arch of axis
13 Vertebral canal
14 Articular process and arch of third cervical vertebra
15 Articular process and arch of fourth cervical vertebra
16 Articular process and arch of fifth cervical vertebra

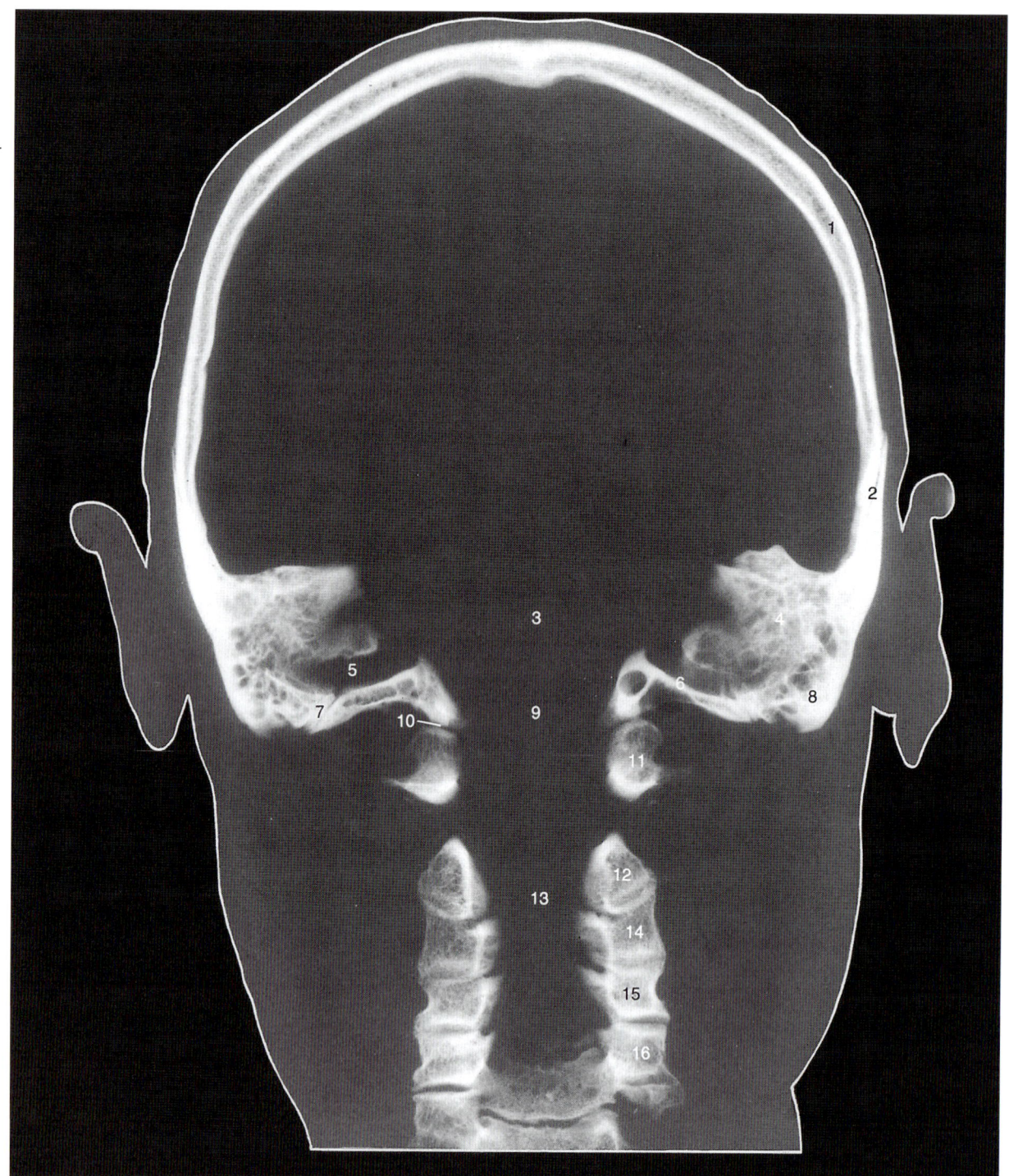

Fig. 26 Radiograph of the ninth coronal slice. The posterior cranial fossa is positioned medial to the petrous part of the temporal bones and joins the spinal canal at the level of the foramen magnum.

Coronal Slices   87

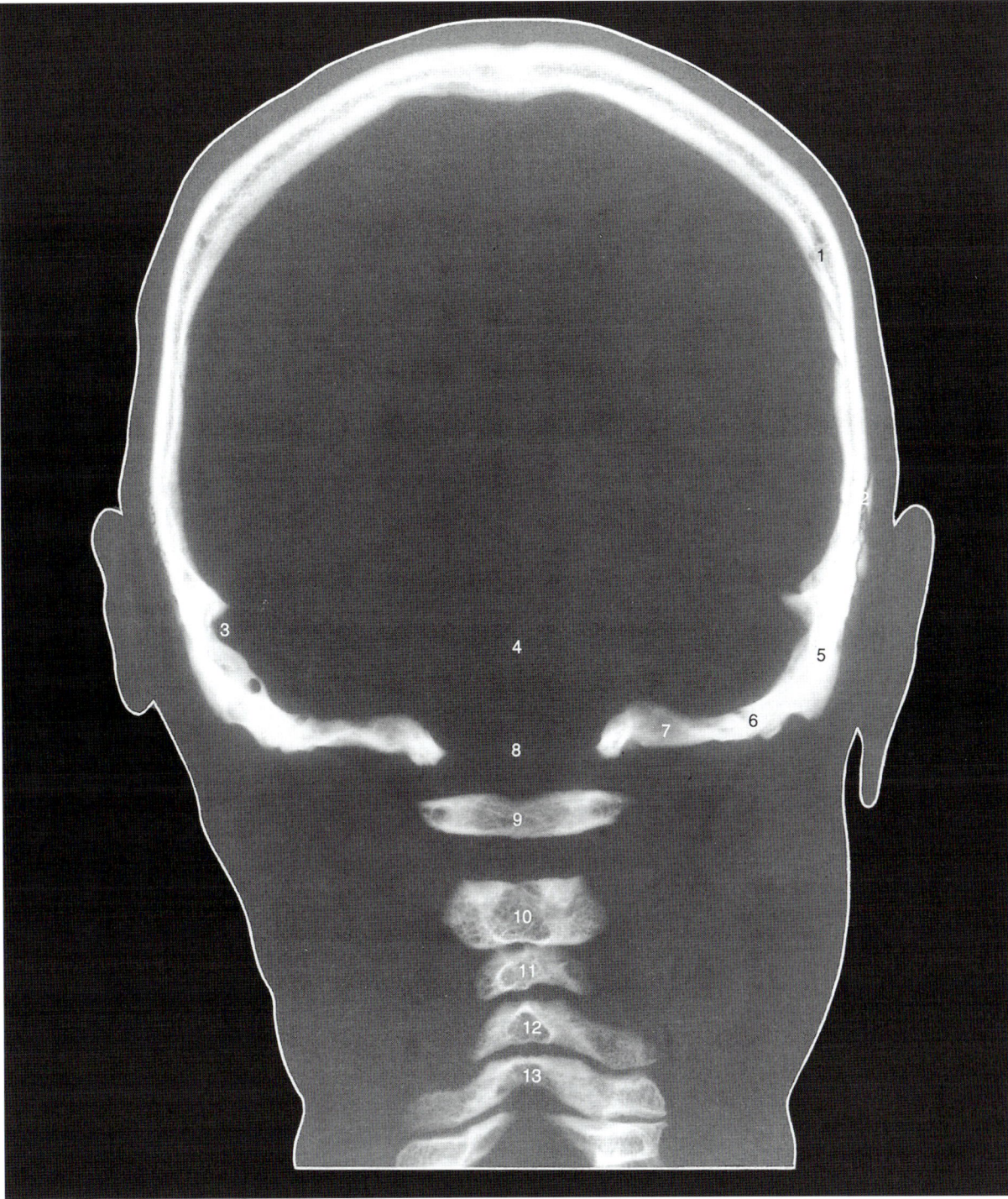

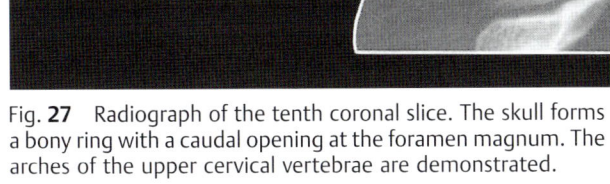

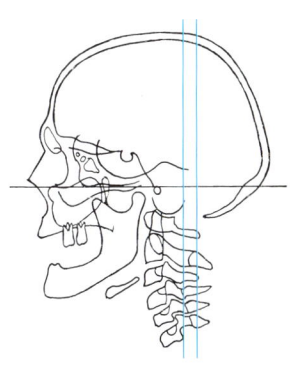

1 Parietal bone
2 Squamous suture
3 Groove for sigmoid sinus
4 Posterior cranial fossa
5 Temporal bone
6 Occipitomastoid suture
7 Occipital bone
8 Foramen magnum
9 Posterior arch of atlas
10 Arch of axis
11 Arch of third cervical vertebra
12 Arch of fourth cervical vertebra
13 Arch of fifth cervical vertebra

Fig. 27 Radiograph of the tenth coronal slice. The skull forms a bony ring with a caudal opening at the foramen magnum. The arches of the upper cervical vertebrae are demonstrated.

88 Atlas

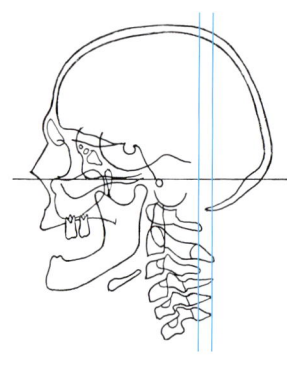

1 Parietal bone
2 Posterior cranial fossa
3 Occipital bone
4 Posterior arch of atlas
5 Spinous process of axis
6 Spinous process of third cervical vertebra
7 Spinous process of fourth cervical vertebra
8 Arch of fifth cervical vertebra
9 Arch of sixth cervical vertebra

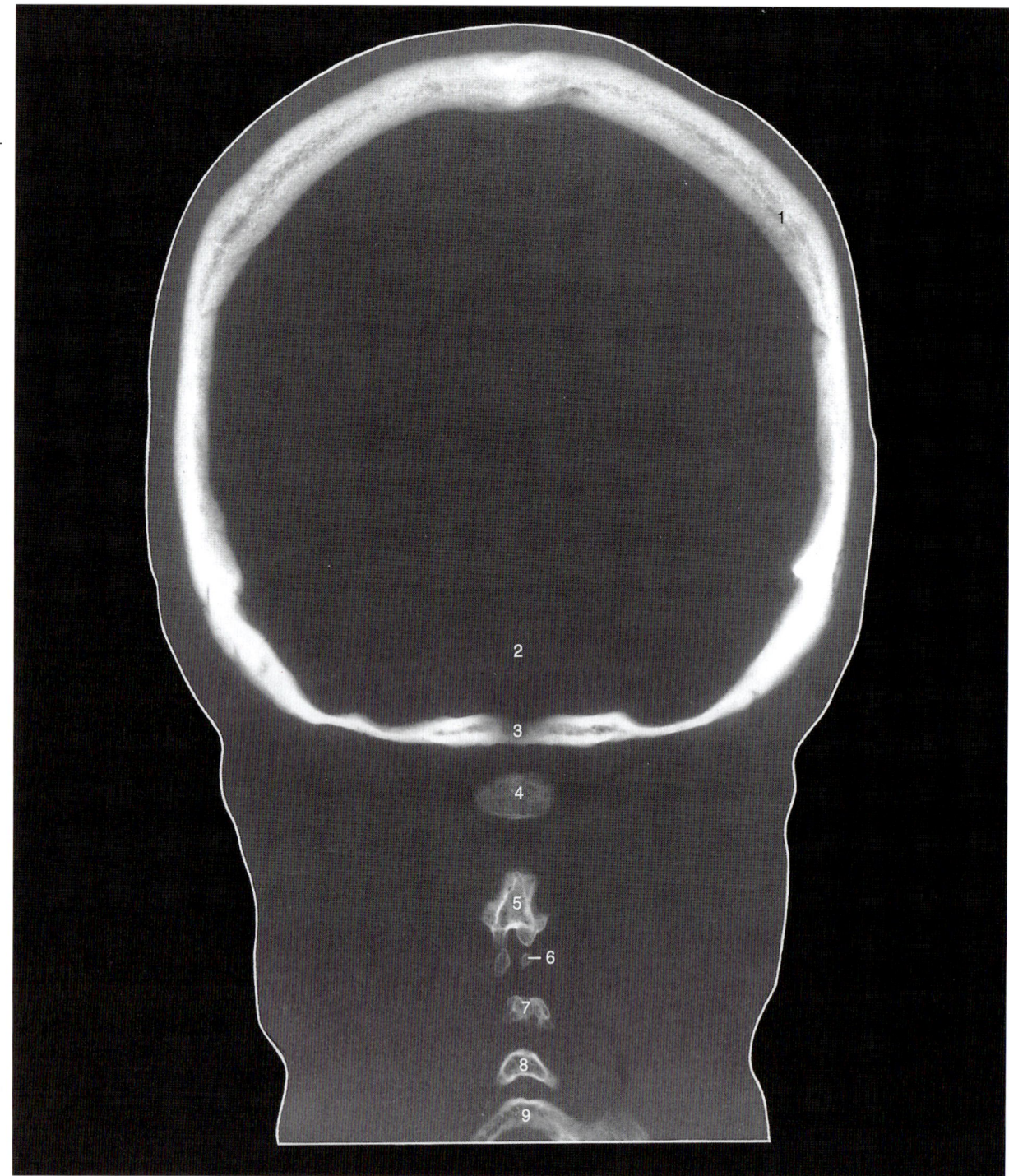

Fig. 28 Radiograph of the eleventh coronal slice. The parietal and occipital bones form a bony ring. Only the spinous processes or arches of the upper cervical vertebrae are seen.

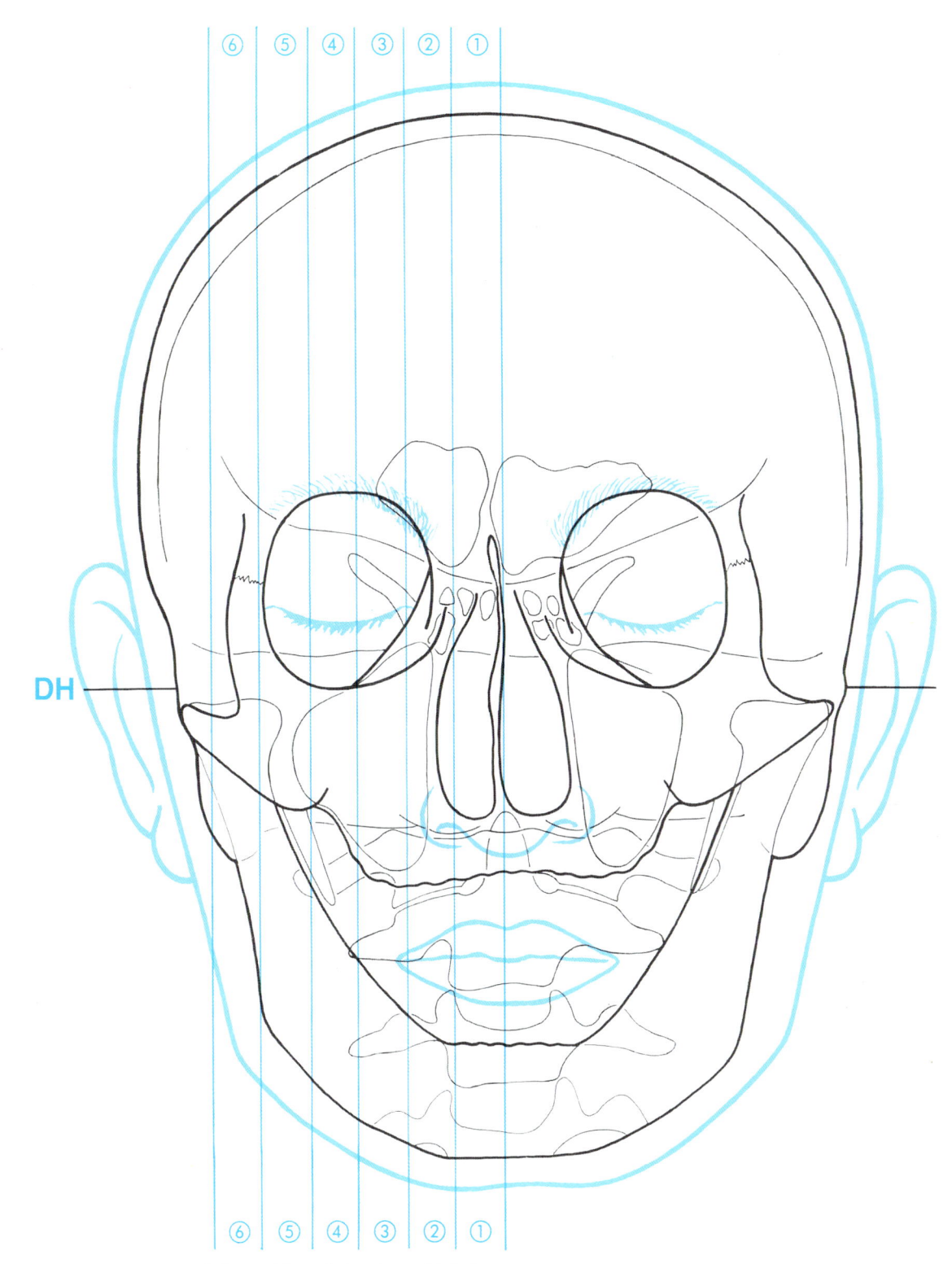

Fig. 29 Frontal view of the position of the six sagittal slices. These slices are portrayed from a medial aspect in the atlas portion (Figs. 32a,c–37a,c). The encircled numbers indicate the number of the 1-cm-thick slices. The illustrated surface of each slice, therefore, represents the line medial to the encircled number of the corresponding slice (Chap. 8).
DH Reid's base line

Atlas

1 Frontal bone
2 Roof of orbit
3 Left frontal sinus
4 Crista galli
5 Frontozygomatic suture
6 Orbit
7 Superior orbital fissure
8 Zygomatic bone
9 Ethmoidal cells
10 Superior margin of petrous part of temporal bone
11 Floor of orbit
12 Nasal septum
13 Head of mandible
14 Anterior nasal aperture
15 Maxillary sinus
16 Occipital condyle
17 Styloid process
18 Dens of axis
19 Mastoid process
20 Atlas
21 Transverse process of atlas
22 Ramus of mandible
23 Transverse process of axis
24 Third cervical vertebra
25 Body of mandible

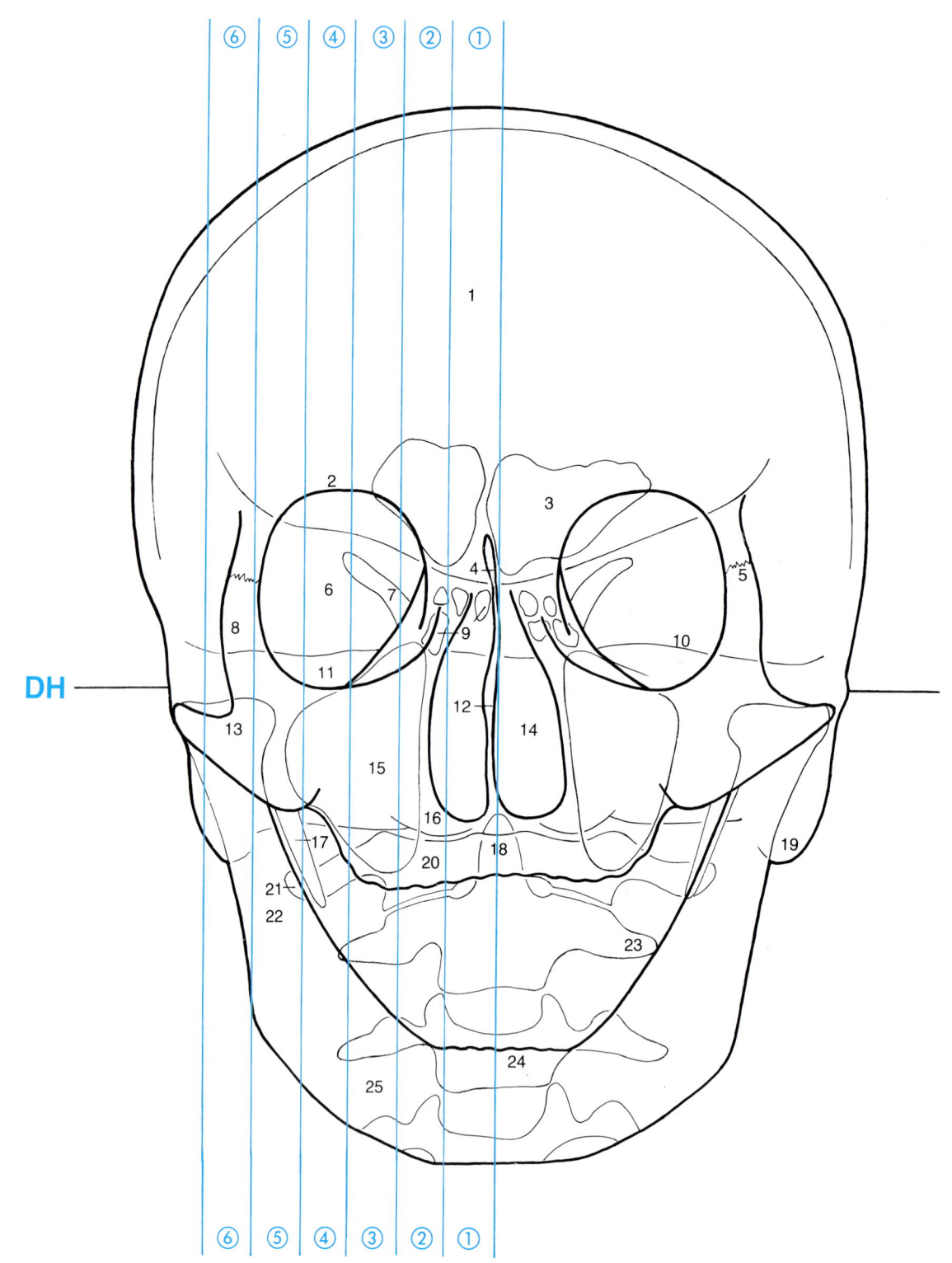

Fig. 30a Tracing of an anterior-posterior teleradiograph taken from the same head as in Fig. 29. The six sagittal slices were fitted together, illustrated, and numbered consecutively in medial to lateral sequence (Chap. 8).
DH Reid's base line

Sagittal Slices

1 Longitudinal cerebral (interhemispheric) fissure
2 Superior frontal sulcus
3 Middle frontal gyrus
4 Superior frontal gyrus
5 Inferior frontal sulcus
6 Inferior frontal gyrus
7 Lateral sulcus (Sylvian fissure)
8 Superior temporal gyrus
9 Superior temporal sulcus
10 Middle temporal gyrus
11 Olfactory bulb
12 Interpeduncular fossa
13 Oculomotor nerve
14 Pole of temporal lobe
15 Pons
16 Trigeminal nerve
17 Facial nerve and intermediate nerve
18 Abducens nerve
19 Inferior olive
20 Vestibulocochlear nerve
21 Flocculus (H X)
22 Glossopharyngeal nerve
23 Vagus nerve
24 Pyramid of medulla oblongata
25 Tonsil of cerebellum (H IX)
26 Accessory nerve
27 Hypoglossal nerve
28 Anterior (ventral) root of first cervical spinal nerve
29 Second cervical spinal nerve
30 Spinal cord

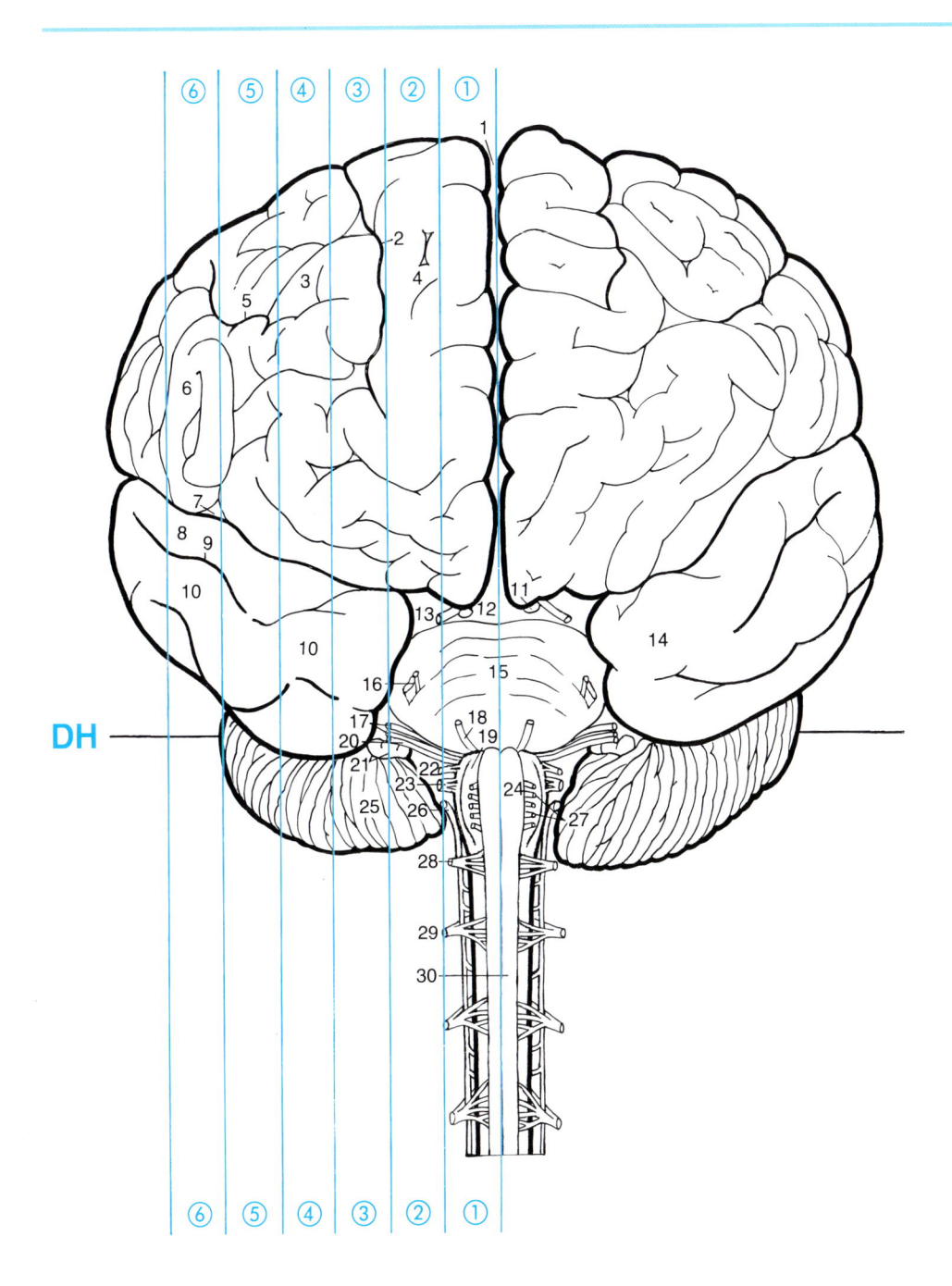

Fig. 30b Frontal view of the brain taken from the same head as in Fig. 30a. The frontal plane lies vertical to the Reid's base line. The sagittal slices were assembled and numbered as shown in Fig. 30a (Chap. 8).
DH Reid's base line

92 Atlas

1 Frontal pole
2 Longitudinal cerebral (interhemispheric) fissure
3 Superior frontal gyrus
4 Middle frontal gyrus
5 Inferior frontal gyrus
6 Inferior frontal sulcus
7 Superior frontal sulcus
8 Precentral sulcus
9 Central sulcus
10 Precentral gyrus
11 Supramarginal gyrus
12 Postcentral gyrus
13 Postcentral sulcus
14 Angular gyrus
15 Superior parietal lobule
16 Parieto-occipital sulcus
17 Occipital gyri
18 Occipital pole

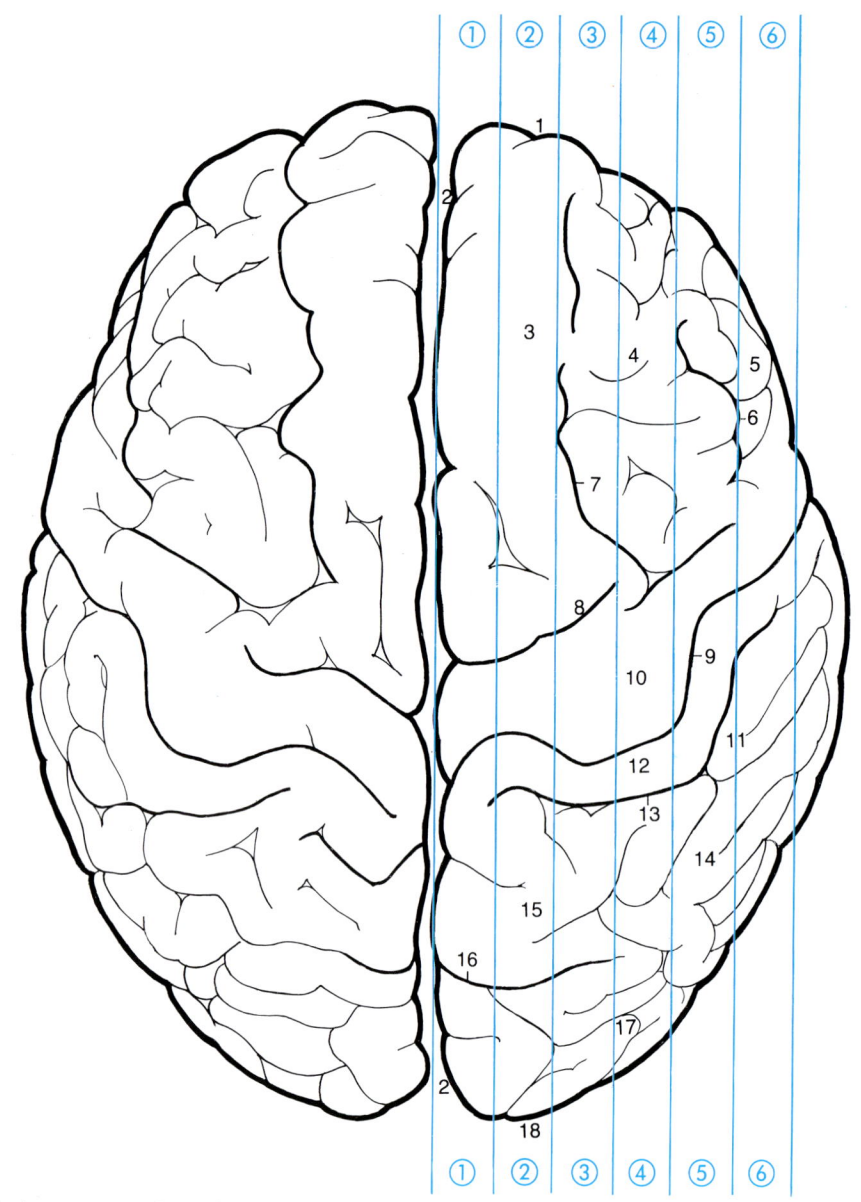

Fig. 31 View of the brain as seen from above taken from the same head as in Figs. 30a,b. The sagittal slices were assembled and numbered as shown in Fig. 30a (Chap. 8).

Sagittal Slices

MR images of the sagittal slices enable the simultaneous visualization of the facial skeleton and the neurocranium. The median plane clearly shows the:
- Brainstem (medulla oblongata, pons, midbrain)
- Cerebellum
- Forebrain (diencephalon, telencephalon)
- transition of the medulla oblongata into the spinal cord at the craniocervical junction.

The typical contour of the corpus callosum, lesions, aplasia, or atrophy are also depicted in this plane. The pituitary gland and its pathologic changes can be evaluated in this particular plane and in some of the paramedian planes. The bicommissural line is easily identified in the median plane (Chap. 1.2); therefore, by means of a bicommissurally oriented coordinate system, anatomic information from stereotactic brain atlases can be transferred onto the corresponding MR images of the patients. The sulci and gyri of the telencephalon are well defined in the median and lateral sagittal slices, since the sulci that run an almost vertical course to the sectional plane are seen more clearly than the sulci that are cut diagonally and tangentially, due to the partial volume effect.

The availability of sagittal slices is a major advantage in MRI. Abnormalities of the midline structures of the brain can be seen distinctly. Narrowing of the vertebral canal as a result of extradural tumors, disc herniation, or spinal injury (Chap. 4.2) can be diagnosed with accuracy.

Atlas

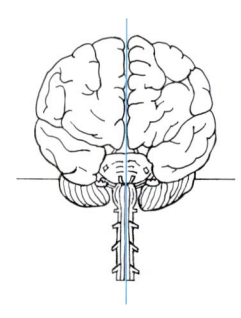

1 Cingulate sulcus
2 Parieto-occipital sulcus
3 Genu of corpus callosum
4 Septum pellucidum
5 Fornix
6 Splenium of corpus callosum
7 Paraterminal gyrus
8 Anterior commissure
9 Interthalamic adhesion
10 Third ventricle
11 Posterior commissure
12 Pineal gland
13 Left frontal sinus
14 Lamina terminalis
15 Mammillary body
16 Oculomotor nerve
17 Tegmentum of midbrain
18 Superior colliculus
19 Inferior colliculus
20 Culmen (IV, V)
21 Tentorium of cerebellum
22 Olfactory bulb and tract (within the slice)
23 Optic nerve
24 Optic chiasm
25 Infundibulum
26 Primary fissure of cerebellum
27 Pituitary gland
28 Pons
29 Declive (VI)
30 Folium of vermis (VII A)
31 Sphenoidal sinus
32 Fourth ventricle
33 Nodule of vermis (X)
34 Nasal septum
35 Abducens nerve (within the slice)
36 Medulla oblongata
37 Uvula of vermis (IX)
38 Pyramis of vermis (VIII)
39 Pharyngeal tonsil
40 Obex of medulla oblongata
41 Tonsil of cerebellum (H IX)
42 Nasopharynx
43 Central canal
44 Oral cavity
45 Spinal cord
46 Uvula of palate
47 Tongue
48 Oropharynx

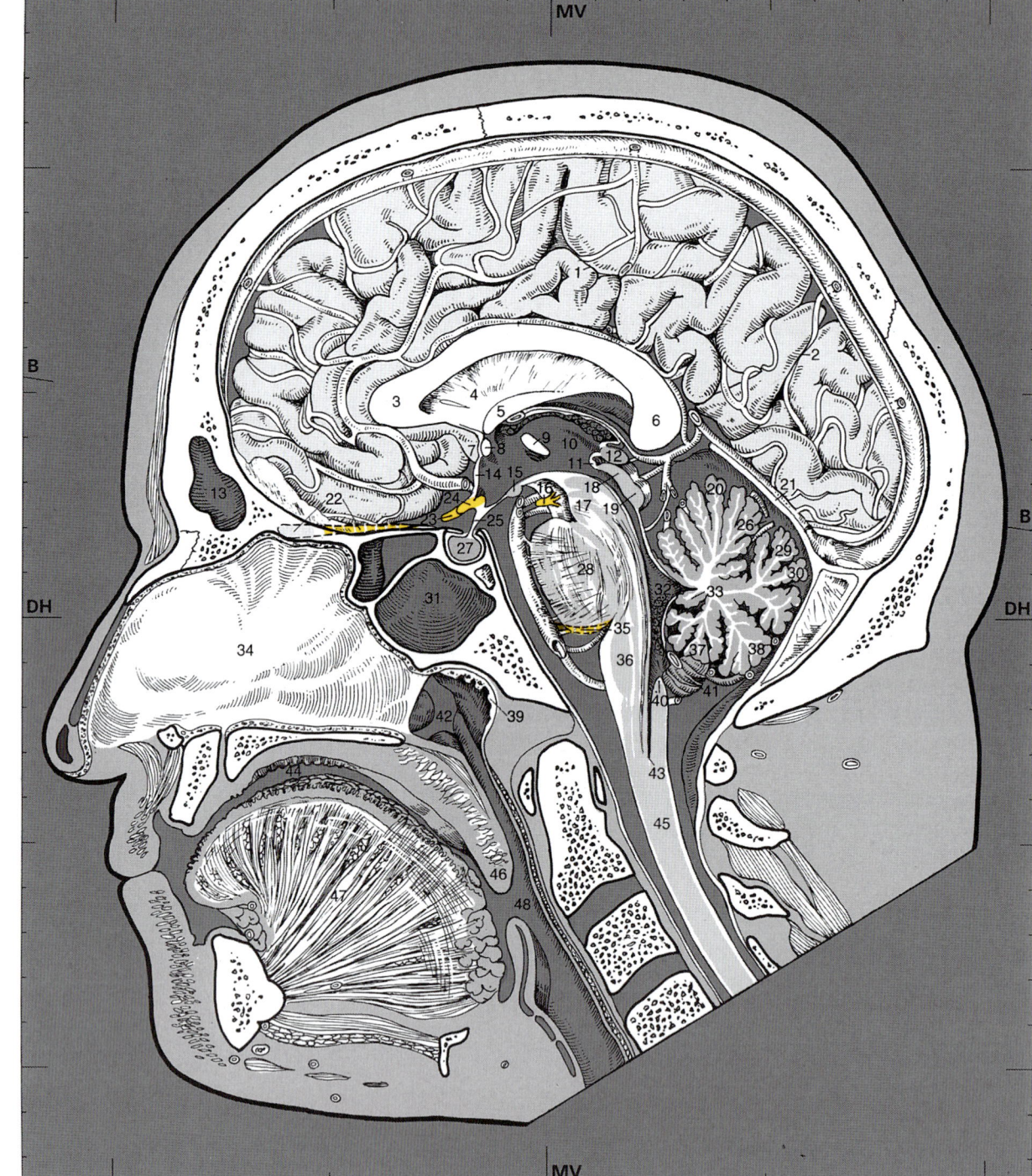

Fig. **32a** Medial view of the first sagittal slice showing nasal septum, paranasal sinuses, oral cavity, brain, and spinal cord structures. The falx cerebri was removed to reveal the medial surface of the telencephalon. Third ventricle, aqueduct, and fourth ventricle serve as guideline structures for the diencephalon and brainstem. The first, second, third, and sixth cranial nerves are graphically demonstrated although they are partially located within the slice.
B Bicommissural line, DH Reid's base line, MV Meatovertical line

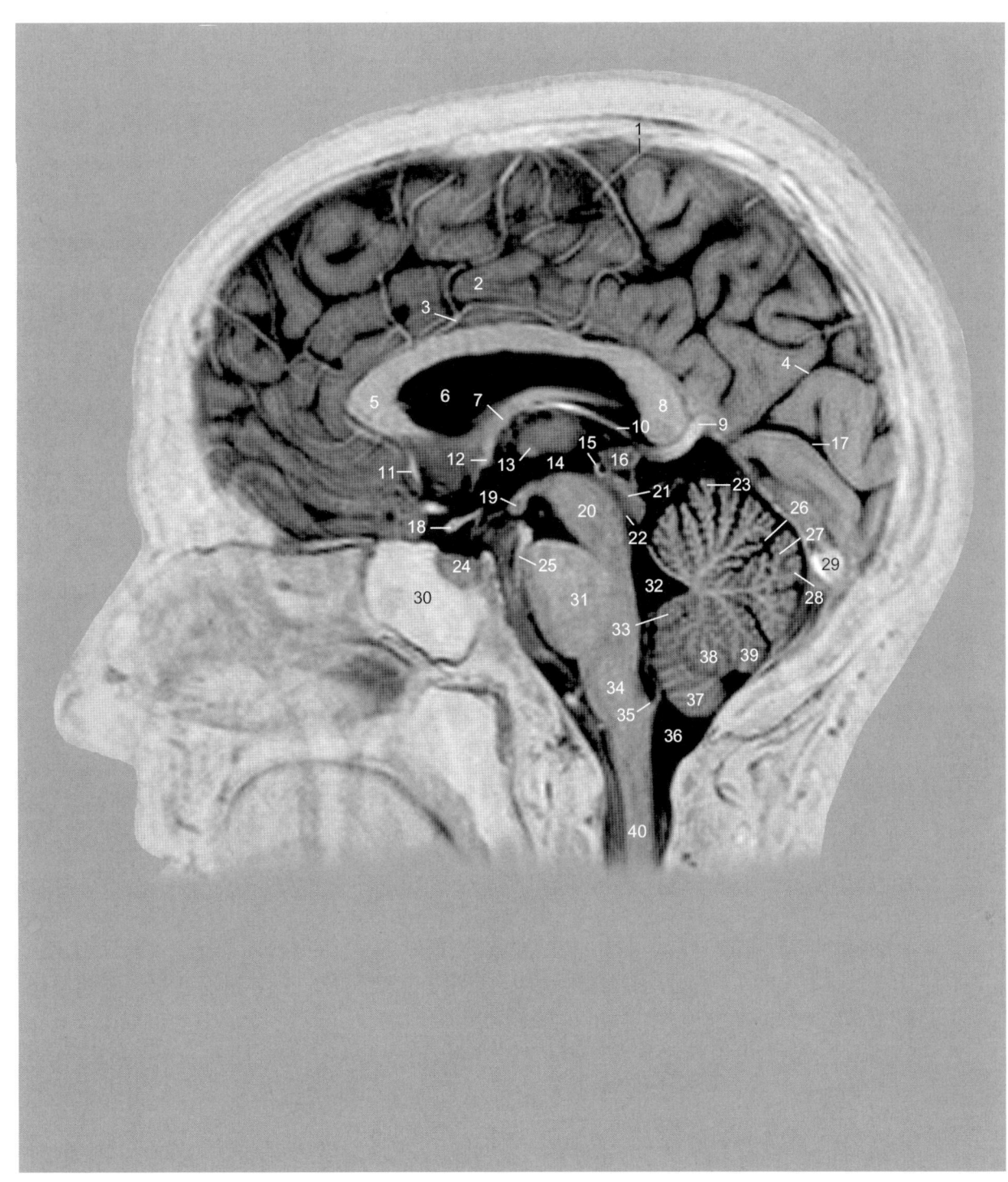

Sagittal Slices

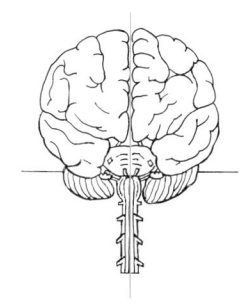

1 Superior sagittal sinus with bridging vein (indicating line)
2 Cingulate gyrus
3 Pericallosal artery
4 Parieto-occipital sulcus
5 Genu of corpus callosum
6 Lateral ventricle
7 Fornix
8 Splenium of corpus callosum
9 Great cerebral vein (of Galen)
10 Internal cerebral vein
11 Anterior cerebral artery
12 Anterior commissure
13 Interthalamic adhesion
14 Third ventricle
15 Posterior commissure
16 Pineal gland
17 Calcarine sulcus
18 Optic chiasm
19 Mammillary body
20 Tegmentum of midbrain
21 Tectal plate
22 Aqueduct of midbrain
23 Culmen (IV, V)
24 Pituitary gland
25 Basilar artery
26 Primary fissure of cerebellum
27 Declive (VI)
28 Folium of vermis (VII A)
29 Confluence of sinuses
30 Sphenoidal sinus
31 Pons
32 Fourth ventricle
33 Nodule of vermis (X)
34 Medulla oblongata
35 Obex of medulla oblongata
36 Cisterna magna (posterior cerebellomedullary cistern)
37 Tonsil of cerebellum (H IX)
38 Uvula of vermis (IX)
39 Pyramis of vermis (VIII)
40 Spinal cord

Fig. **32b** Sagittal, T1-weighted MR image (Turbo-Inversion-Recovery-Sequence) corresponding approximately to the sectional plane of Figs. 32a. The selected sequence emphasizes the brain structures and suppresses the surrounding soft tissues. A missing number with its label indicates here and in the following legends of MR images that this number can be found in the other corresponding MR illustrations. The two sagittal MR series (Figs. 32b–37b and 32d–37d) were obtained from a 38-year-old female. Technical data (Chap. 8).

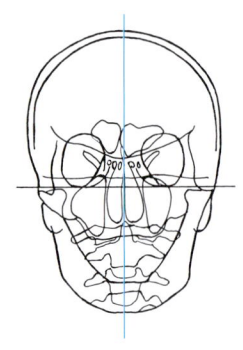

1 Coronal suture
2 Superior sagittal sinus
3 Parietal bone
4 Frontal bone
5 Posteromedial frontal artery
6 Paracentral artery
7 Precuneal artery
8 Intermediomedial frontal artery
9 Pericallosal artery
10 Lambdoid suture
11 Anteromedial frontal artery
12 Internal cerebral vein
13 Great cerebral vein (of Galen)
14 Parieto-occipital artery
15 Calcarine artery
16 Crista galli
17 Polar frontal artery
18 Origin of anterior communicating artery
19 Medial frontobasal artery
20 Anterior cerebral artery
21 Posterior cerebral artery
22 Superior cerebellar artery
23 Straight sinus
24 Nasal bone
25 Basilar artery
26 Confluence of sinuses
27 Internal occipital protuberance
28 Clivus
29 Anterior inferior cerebellar artery (AICA)
30 External occipital protuberance (inion)
31 Vertebral artery
32 Pharyngeal tubercle
33 Posterior inferior cerebellar artery (PICA)
34 Incisive canal of maxilla
35 Anterior arch of atlas
36 Dens of axis
37 Transverse ligament of atlas
38 Posterior arch of atlas
39 Spinous process of axis
40 Intervertebral disc
41 Genioglossus
42 Epiglottis
43 Third cervical vertebra
44 Body of mandible
45 Geniohyoid
46 Mylohyoid
47 Hyoid bone

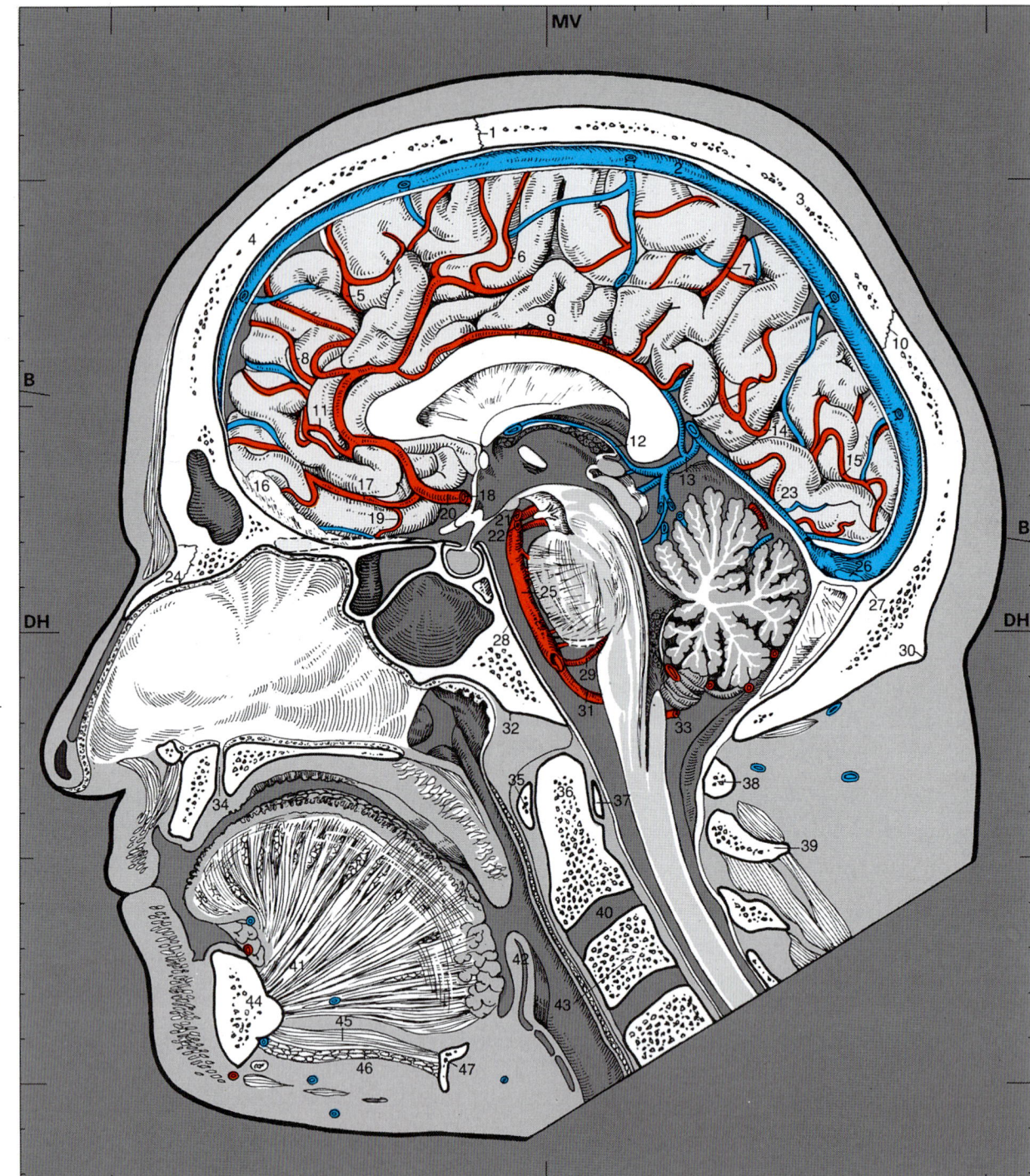

Fig. **32c** Medial view of the first sagittal slice of the right half of the head revealing bony structures, muscles, and blood vessels. The cranial cavity was opened on the plane of the crista galli and the internal occipital protuberance. The upper cervical vertebrae together with the vertebral canal were cut in half.
B Bicommissural line, DH Reid's base line, MV Meatovertical line

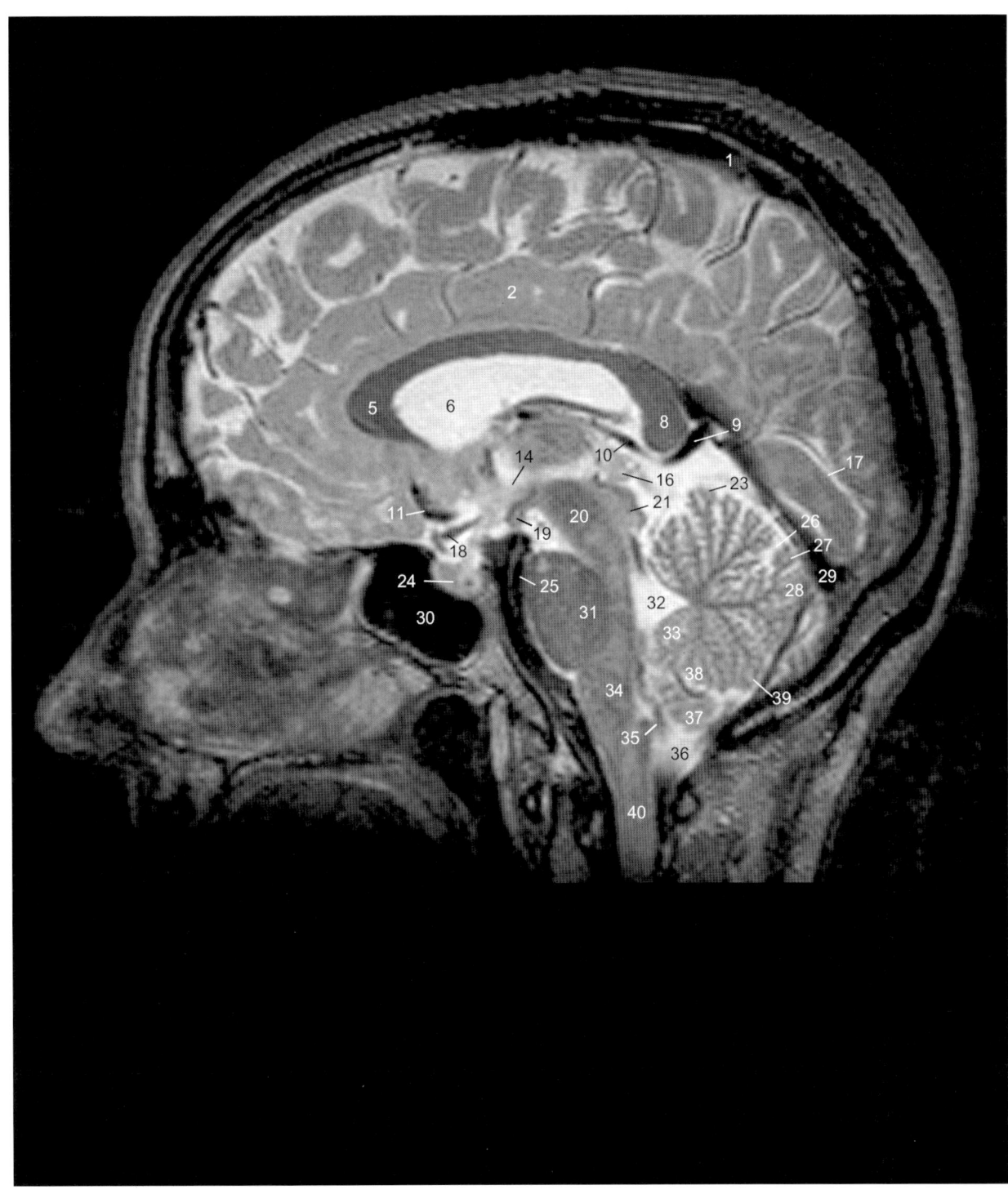

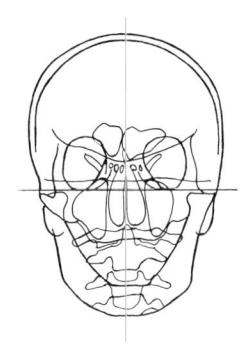

Sagittal Slices

1 Superior sagittal sinus
2 Cingulate gyrus
5 Genu of corpus callosum
6 Lateral ventricle
8 Splenium of corpus callosum
9 Great cerebral vein (of Galen)
10 Internal cerebral vein
11 Anterior cerebral artery
14 Third ventricle
16 Pineal gland
17 Calcarine sulcus
18 Optic chiasm
19 Mammillary body
20 Tegmentum of midbrain
21 Tectal plate
23 Culmen (IV, V)
24 Pituitary gland
25 Basilar artery
26 Primary fissure of cerebellum
27 Declive (VI)
28 Folium of vermis (VII A)
29 Confluence of sinuses
30 Sphenoidal sinus
31 Pons
32 Fourth ventricle
33 Nodule of vermis (X)
34 Medulla oblongata
35 Obex of medulla oblongata
36 Cisterna magna (posterior cerebellomedullary cistern)
37 Tonsil of cerebellum (H IX)
38 Uvula of vermis (IX)
39 Pyramis of vermis (VIII)
40 Spinal cord

Fig. **32d** Sagittal, T2-weighted MR image corresponding approximately to the sectional plane of Figs. 32c. A missing number with its label indicates here and in the following legends of MR images that this number can be found in the other corresponding T1-weighted MR image. The two sagittal MR series (Figs. 32b–37b and 32d–37d) were obtained from a 38-year-old female. Technical data (Chap. 8).

98 Atlas

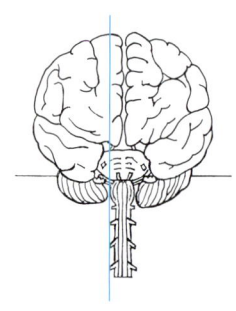

1 Precentral gyrus
2 Postcentral gyrus
3 Superior frontal gyrus
4 Precuneus
5 Cingulate gyrus
6 Parieto-occipital sulcus
7 Caudate nucleus
8 Medial nuclei of thalamus
9 Choroid plexus of lateral ventricle
10 Pulvinar of thalamus
11 Primary visual cortex
12 Occipital gyri
13 Frontal sinus
14 Anterior commissure
15 Subthalamic nucleus
16 Calcarine sulcus
17 Olfactory tract
18 Optic nerve
19 Optic tract
20 Substantia nigra
21 Tentorium of cerebellum
22 Ethmoidal cells
23 Oculomotor nerve
24 Pons
25 Sphenoidal sinus
26 Trigeminal nerve
27 Dentate nucleus
28 Semilunar hiatus
29 Facial nerve and intermediate nerve (within the slice)
30 Vestibulocochlear nerve (within the slice)
31 Abducens nerve
32 Middle nasal concha
33 Tonsil of cerebellum (H IX)
34 Glossopharyngeal nerve and vagus nerve
35 Inferior nasal concha
36 Hypoglossal nerve and hypoglossal canal
37 Nasal vestibule
38 Spinal root of accessory nerve
39 Anterior (ventral) root of first cervical spinal nerve
40 Posterior (dorsal) and anterior (ventral) roots of second cervical spinal nerve
41 Oral cavity
42 Palatine tonsil
43 Tongue
44 Lingual nerve
45 Oropharynx
46 Inferior alveolar nerve
47 Hypoglossal nerve

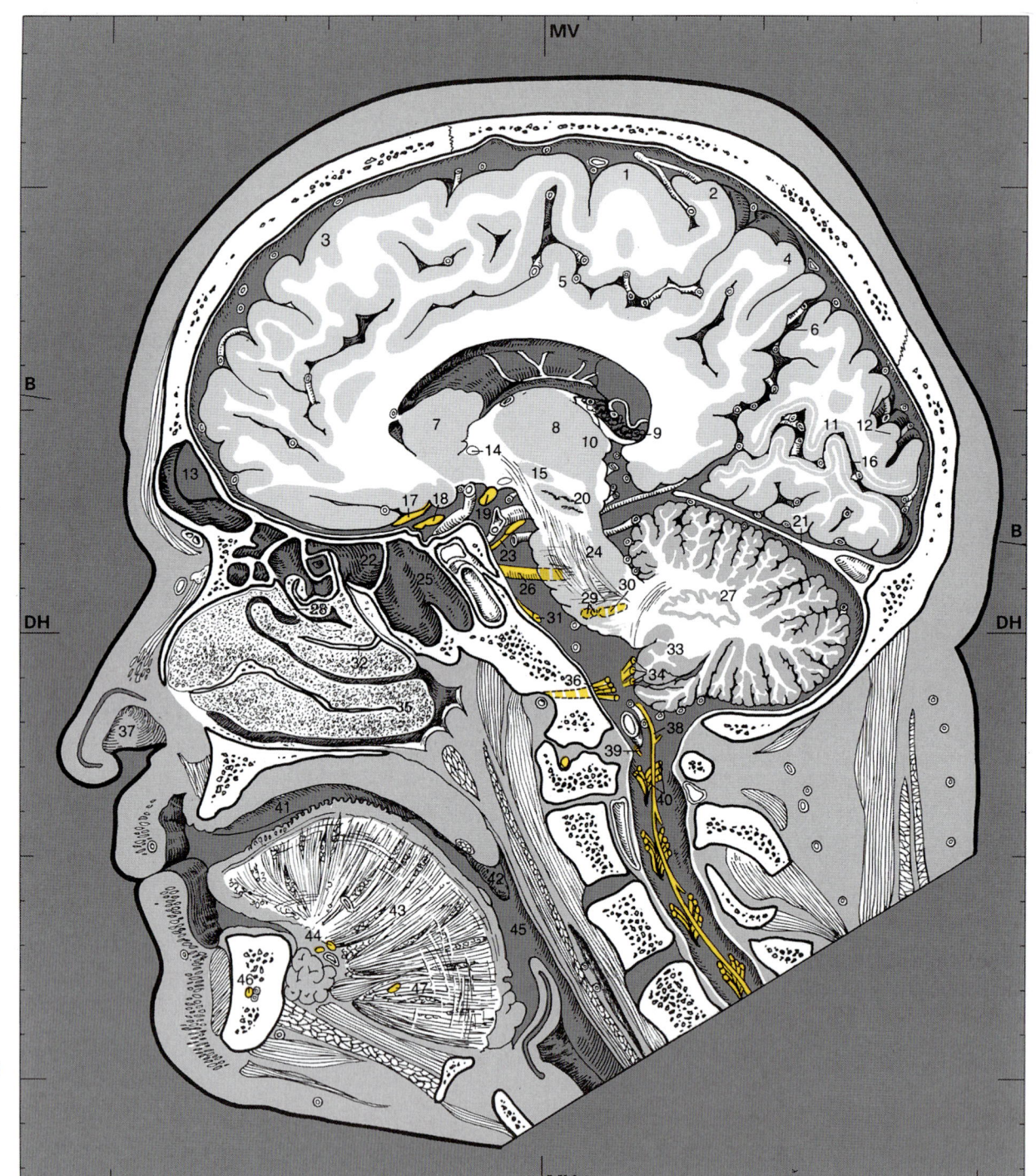

Fig. **33a** Medial view of the second sagittal slice representing the paranasal sinuses, oral cavity, brain structures, cranial and spinal nerves. The anterior and middle parts of the right lateral ventricle are visible. Only the lateral parts of the midbrain and pons are cut in this slice. The spinal roots of the eleventh cranial nerve and the roots of the first spinal nerves are seen in the vertebral canal. The enlarged nasal conchae are tangentially cut in the nasal cavity.

Sagittal Slices

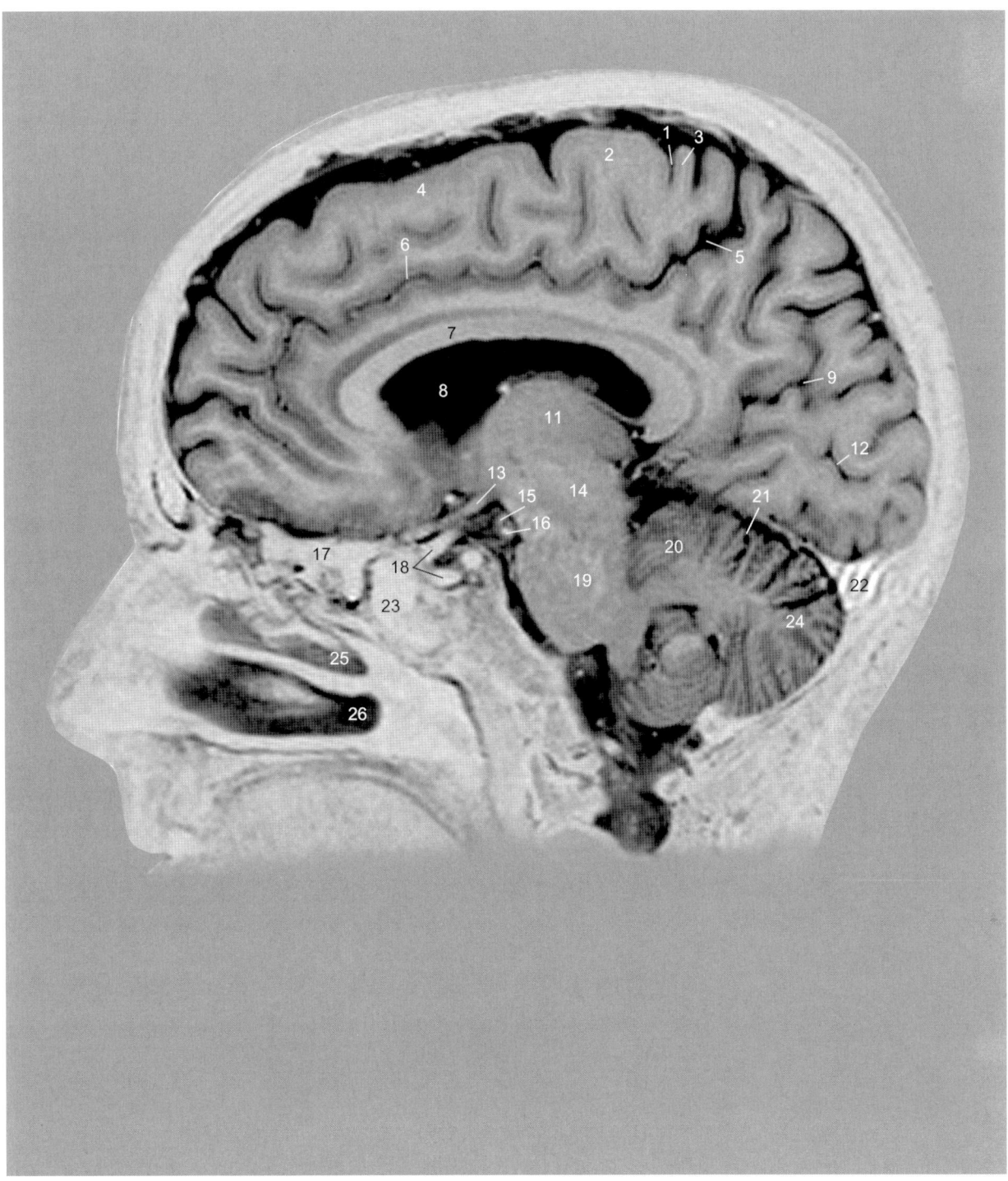

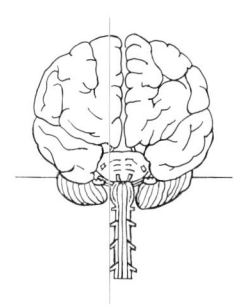

1 Central sulcus
2 Precentral gyrus
3 Postcentral gyrus
4 Superior frontal gyrus
5 Marginal branch of cingulate sulcus
6 Cingulate sulcus
7 Trunk (body) of corpus callosum
8 Lateral ventricle
9 Parieto-occipital sulcus
11 Thalamus
12 Calcarine sulcus
13 Optic tract
14 Midbrain
15 Posterior cerebral artery
16 Superior cerebellar artery
17 Ethmoidal cells
18 Carotid syphon
19 Pons
20 Anterior lobe of cerebellum
21 Primary fissure of cerebellum
22 Transverse sinus
23 Sphenoidal sinus
24 Posterior lobe of cerebellum
25 Middle nasal concha
26 Inferior nasal concha

Fig. **33b** Sagittal, T1-weighted MR image corresponding approximately to the sectional plane of Figs. 33a and 33c. Technical data (Chap. 8).

Atlas

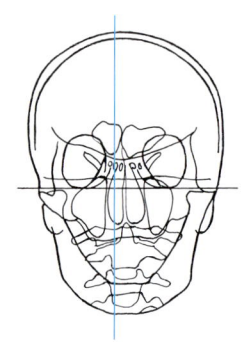

1 Coronal suture
2 Posteromedial frontal artery
3 Paracentral artery
4 Parietal bone
5 Frontal bone
6 Precuneal artery
7 Anteromedial frontal artery
8 Lambdoid suture
9 Intermediomedial frontal artery
10 Parieto-occipital artery
11 Polar frontal artery
12 Calcarine artery
13 Medial frontobasal artery
14 Anterior cerebral artery
15 Anterior choroidal artery
16 Medial occipital artery
17 Internal carotid artery
18 Posterior clinoid process
19 Posterior cerebral artery
20 Superior cerebellar artery
21 Cavernous sinus
22 Transverse sinus
23 Occipital bone
24 Pharyngeal opening of pharyngotympanic tube
25 Posterior inferior cerebellar artery (PICA)
26 Vertebral artery
27 Maxilla
28 Hard palate
29 Levator veli palatini
30 Longus capitis
31 Atlas
32 Semispinalis capitis
33 Trapezius
34 Orbicularis oris
35 Constrictor of pharynx
36 Palatoglossus
37 Axis
38 Splenius capitis
39 Body of mandible
40 Sublingual gland
41 Epiglottis
42 Geniohyoid
43 Mylohyoid
44 Anterior belly of digastric
45 Platysma
46 Hyoid bone

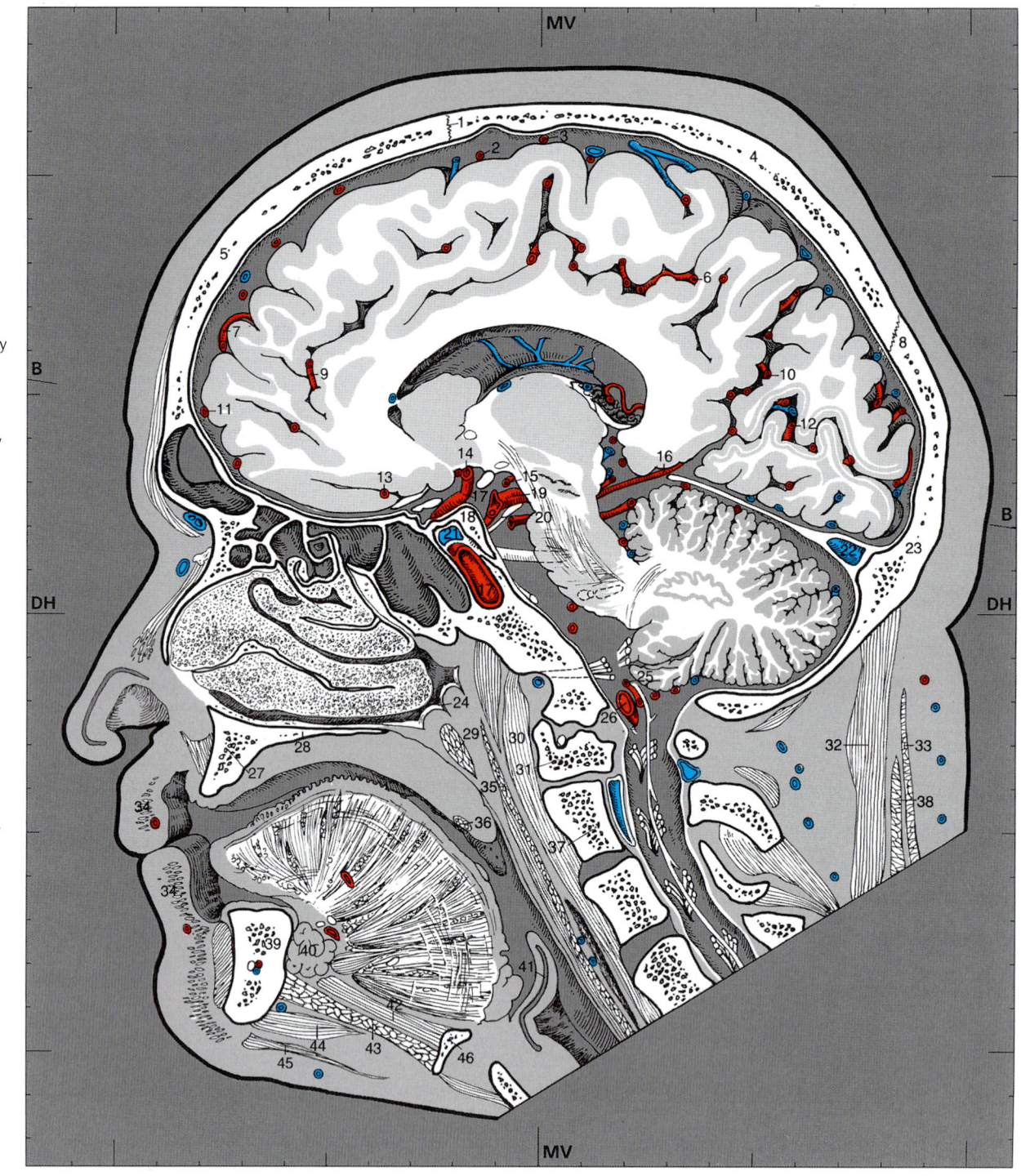

Fig. **33c** Medial view of the second sagittal slice depicting bony structures, muscles, and blood vessels. The sectional plane positioned 1 cm to the median plane lies lateral to the hypophysial fossa and extends through the cavernous sinus and the foramen magnum. The orbit is located lateral to the cut surface and is, therefore, not visible.

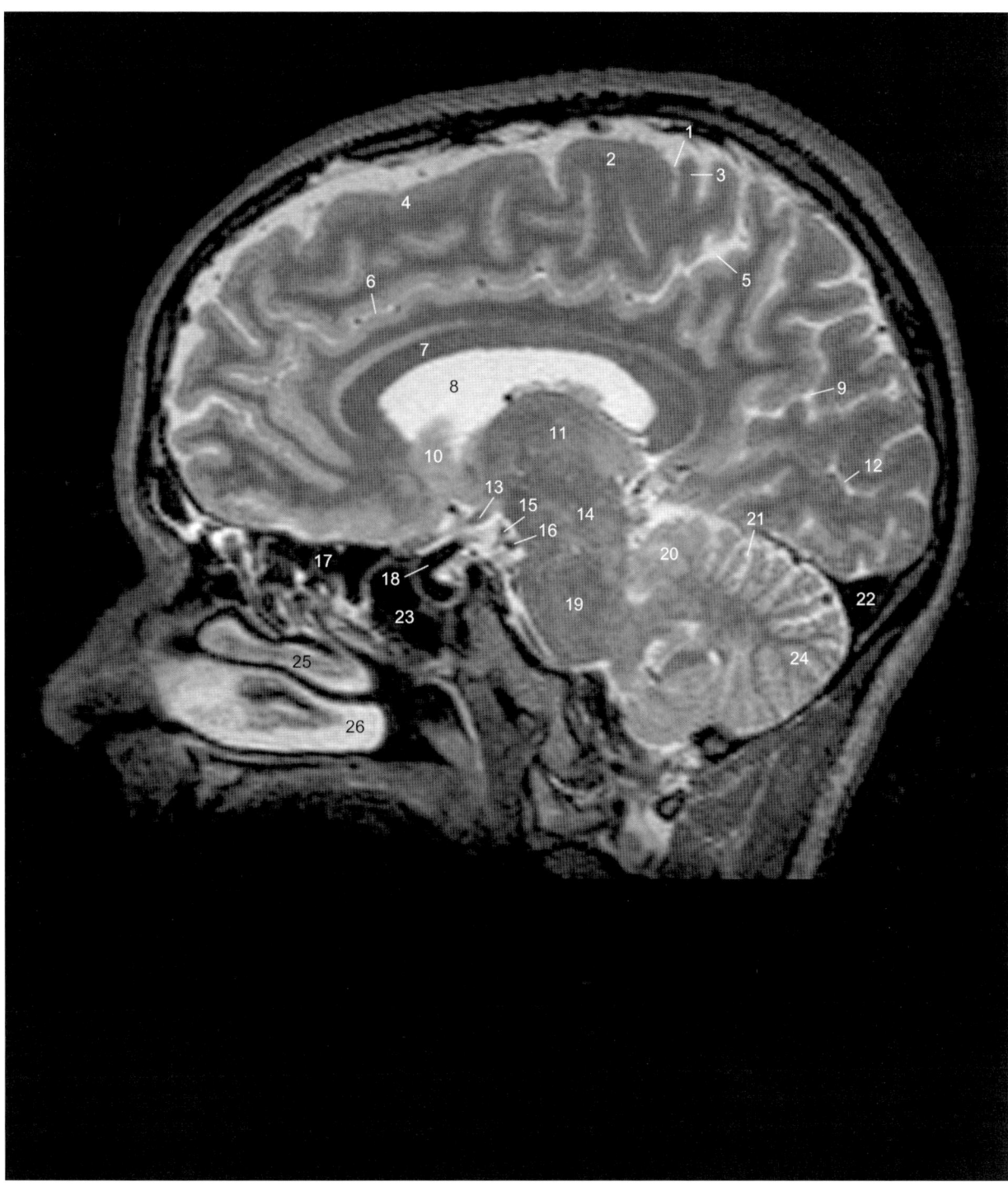

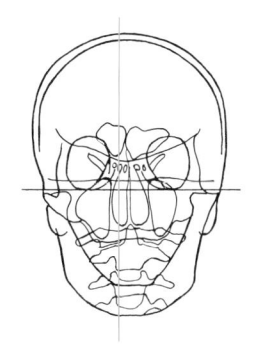

Sagittal Slices

1 Central sulcus
2 Precentral gyrus
3 Postcentral gyrus
4 Superior frontal gyrus
5 Marginal branch of cingulate sulcus
6 Cingulate sulcus
7 Trunk (body) of corpus callosum
8 Lateral ventricle
9 Parieto-occipital sulcus
10 Head of caudate nucleus
11 Thalamus
12 Calcarine sulcus
13 Optic tract
14 Midbrain
15 Posterior cerebral artery
16 Superior cerebellar artery
17 Ethmoidal cells
18 Carotid syphon
19 Pons
20 Anterior lobe of cerebellum
21 Primary fissure of cerebellum
22 Transverse sinus
23 Sphenoidal sinus
24 Posterior lobe of cerebellum
25 Middle nasal concha
26 Inferior nasal concha

Fig. **33d** Sagittal, T2-weighted MR image corresponding approximately to the sectional plane of Figs. 33a and 33c. Technical data (Chap. 8).

Atlas

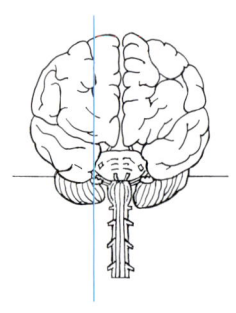

1 Superior frontal gyrus
2 Precentral gyrus
3 Postcentral gyrus
4 Parieto-occipital sulcus
5 Body of caudate nucleus
6 Occipital gyri
7 Putamen
8 Globus pallidus
9 Ventral posterolateral nucleus of thalamus
10 Pulvinar of thalamus
11 Frontal sinus
12 Anterior commissure
13 Optic tract
14 Posterior limb of internal capsule
15 Medial geniculate body
16 Fornix
17 Uncus of parahippocampal gyrus
18 Primary visual cortex
19 Medial occipitotemporal gyrus
20 Optic nerve
21 Oculomotor nerve
22 Trochlear nerve
23 Ophthalmic nerve
24 Abducens nerve
25 Trigeminal nerve
26 Palatine nerves
27 Maxillary nerve
28 Trigeminal (Gasserian) ganglion
29 Facial nerve and intermediate nerve
30 Vestibulocochlear nerve
31 Glossopharyngeal nerve, vagus nerve, accessory nerve
32 Maxillary sinus
33 Hypoglossal nerve
34 Anterior (ventral) root of first cervical spinal nerve
35 Oral cavity
36 Superior cervical ganglion (in the lateral part of the slice)
37 Tongue
38 Posterior (dorsal) and anterior (ventral) roots of third cervical spinal nerve and ganglion
39 Inferior alveolar nerve
40 Lingual nerve

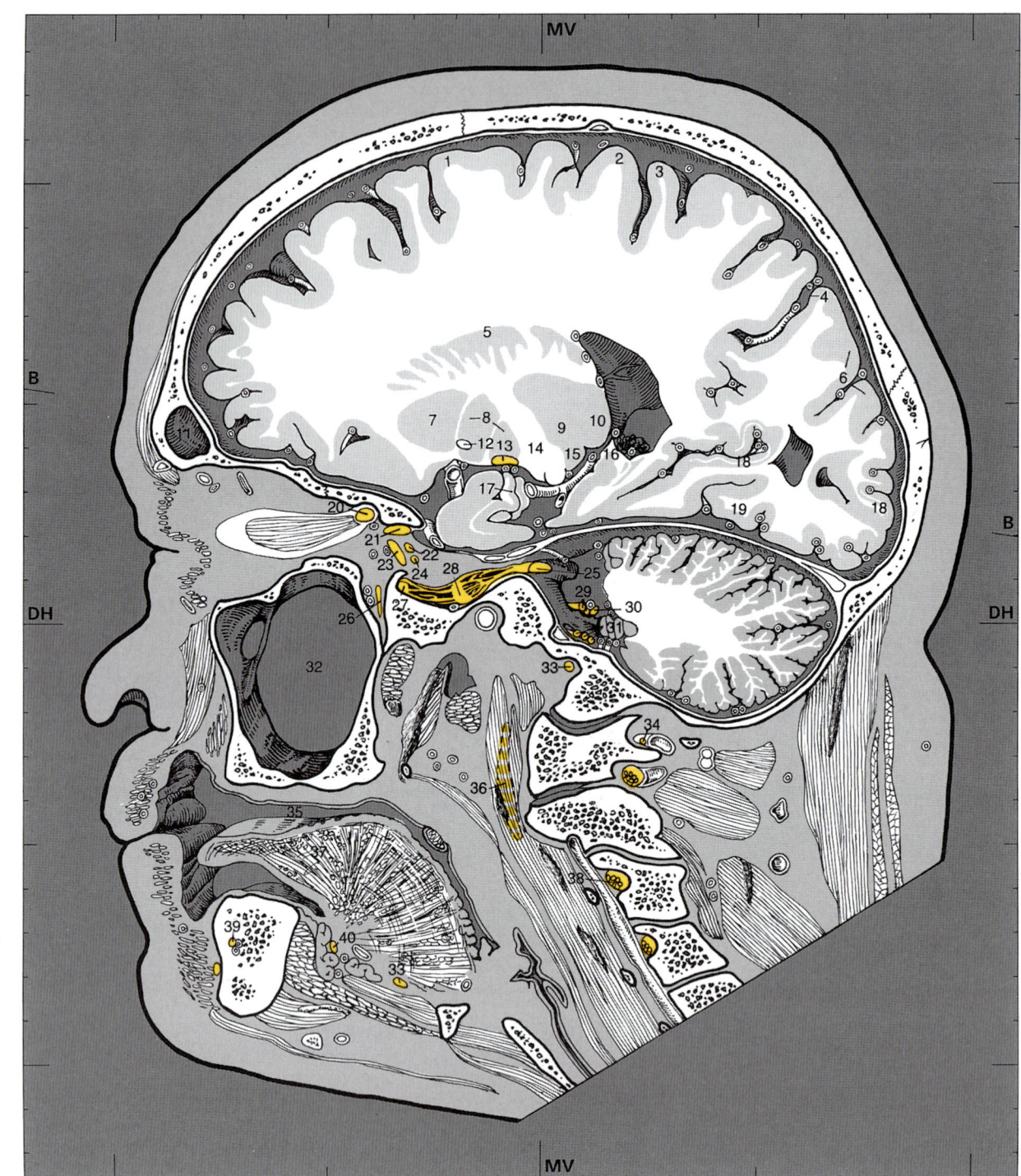

Fig. **34a** Medial view of the third sagittal slice representing paranasal sinuses, oral cavity, brain structures, cranial nerves, and the first spinal nerves. The cut surface is positioned laterally to the brainstem at the level of the medial geniculate body. The temporal lobe is tangentially cut.

Sagittal Slices

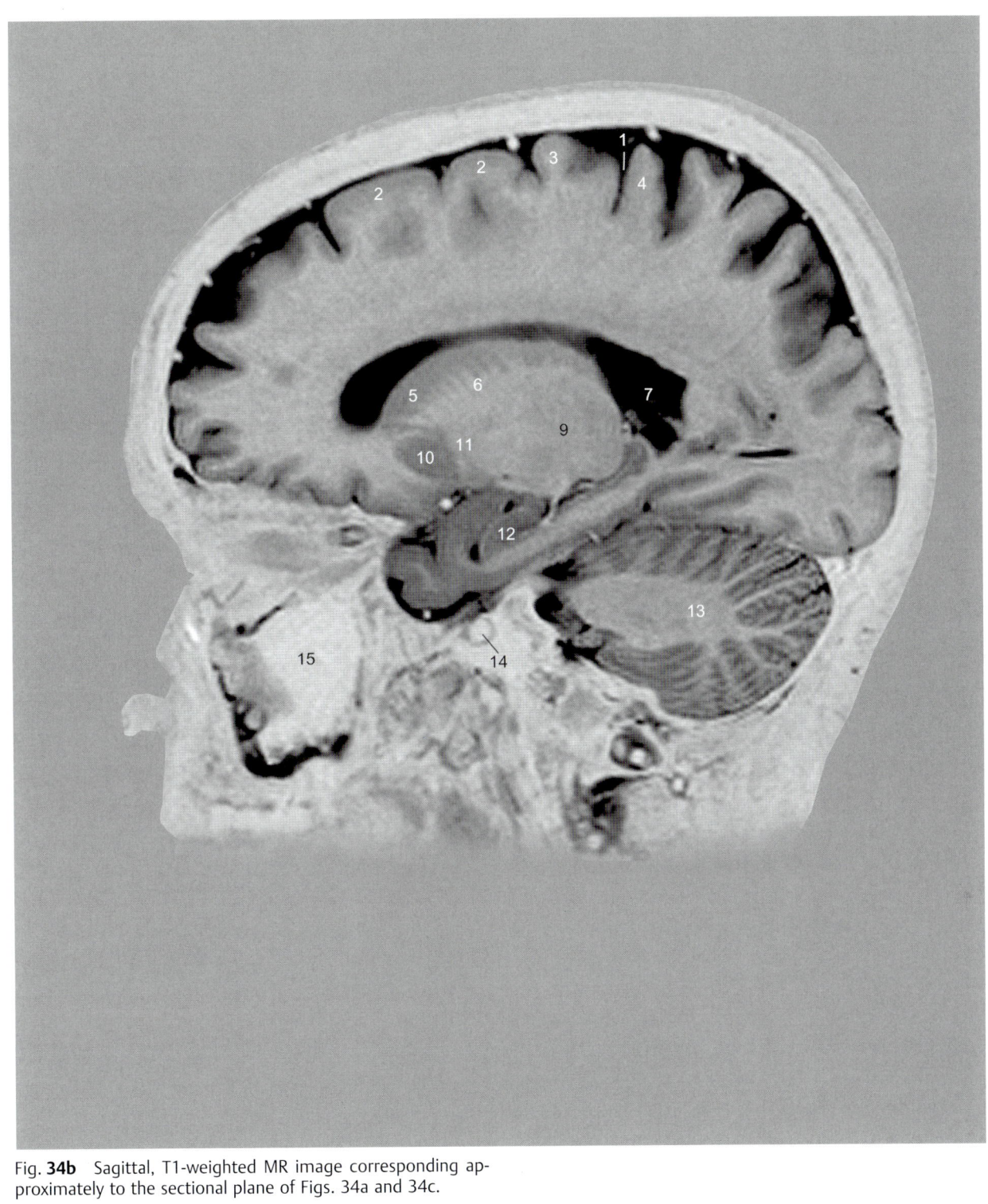

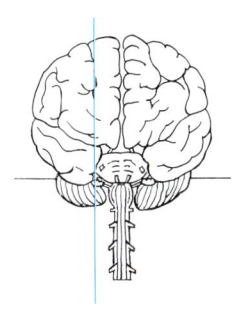

1 Central sulcus
2 Superior frontal gyrus
3 Precentral gyrus
4 Postcentral gyrus
5 Caudate nucleus
6 Internal capsule
7 Lateral ventricle
9 Thalamus
10 Putamen
11 Globus pallidus
12 Hippocampus
13 Cerebellum
14 Internal carotid artery
15 Maxillary sinus

Fig. **34b** Sagittal, T1-weighted MR image corresponding approximately to the sectional plane of Figs. 34a and 34c.

104 Atlas

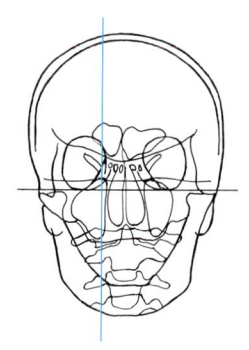

1 Coronal suture
2 Paracentral artery
3 Posteromedial frontal artery
4 Intermediomedial frontal artery
5 Anteromedial frontal artery
6 Parieto-occipital artery
7 Lambdoid suture
8 Occipitofrontalis
9 Polar frontal artery
10 Medial occipital artery
11 Calcarine artery
12 Roof of orbit
13 Middle cerebral artery
14 Posterior cerebral artery
15 Lateral occipital artery
16 Medial rectus
17 Superior orbital fissure
18 Superior cerebellar artery
19 Transverse sinus
20 Floor of orbit
21 Pterygopalatine fossa
22 Temporal bone
23 Internal carotid artery
24 Anterior inferior cerebellar artery (AICA)
25 Inferior petrosal sinus
26 Pharyngotympanic tube
27 Occipital condyle
28 Posterior inferior cerebellar artery (PICA)
29 Levator veli palatini
30 Atlanto-occipital joint
31 Tensor veli palatini
32 Orbicularis oris
33 Maxilla
34 Pterygoid hamulus
35 Lateral mass of atlas
36 Vertebral artery
37 Semispinalis capitis
38 Splenius capitis
39 Trapezius
40 Lateral atlantoaxial joint
41 Axis
42 Obliquus capitis inferior
43 Palatoglossus
44 Body of mandible
45 Anterior belly of digastric
46 Mylohyoid
47 Geniohyoid

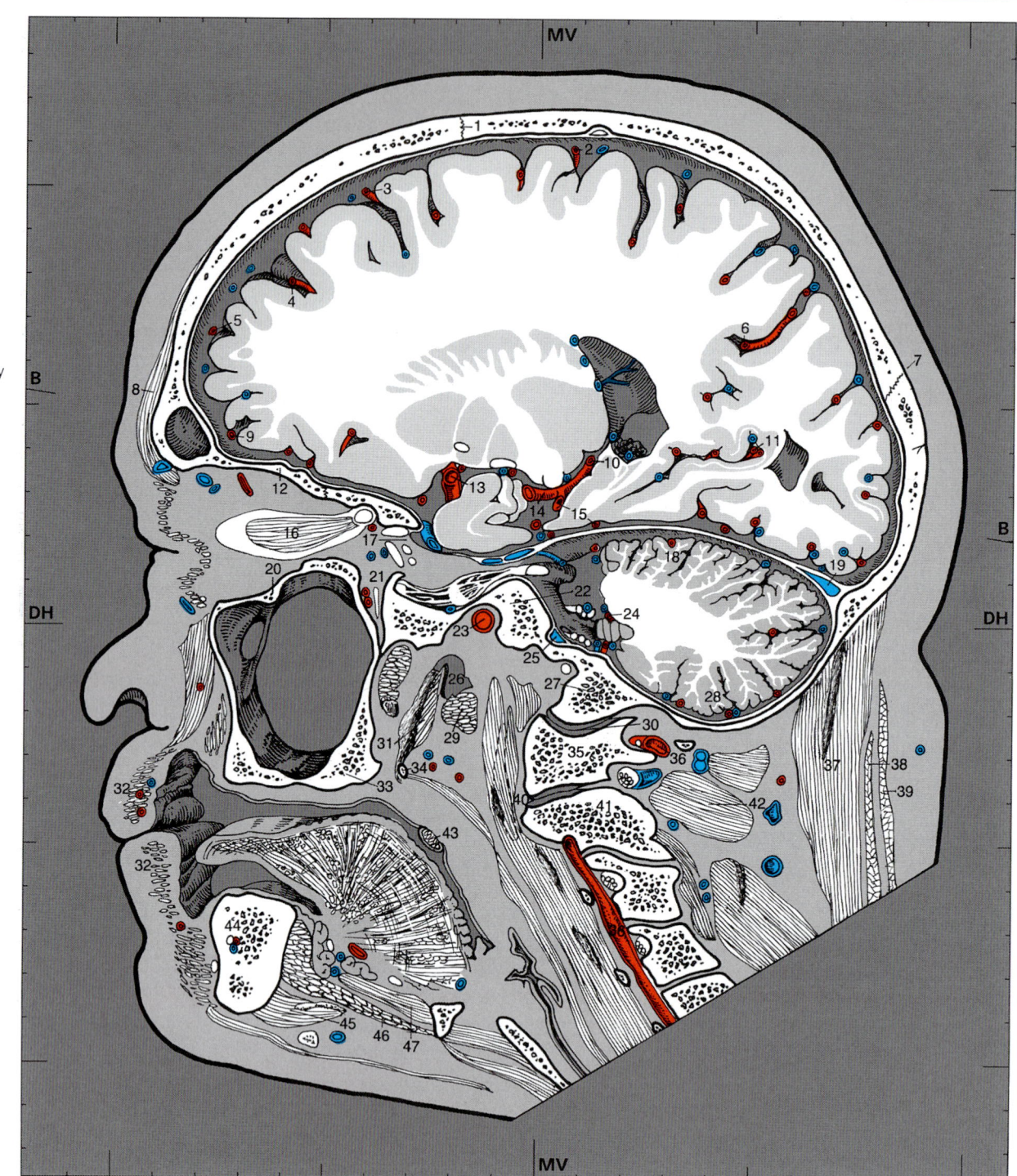

Fig. **34c** Medial view of the third sagittal slice revealing bony structures, muscles, and blood vessels. The cut surface runs through the orbital apex, the medial part of the superior orbital fissure, the middle cranial fossa, and the parapharyngeal space.

Sagittal Slices

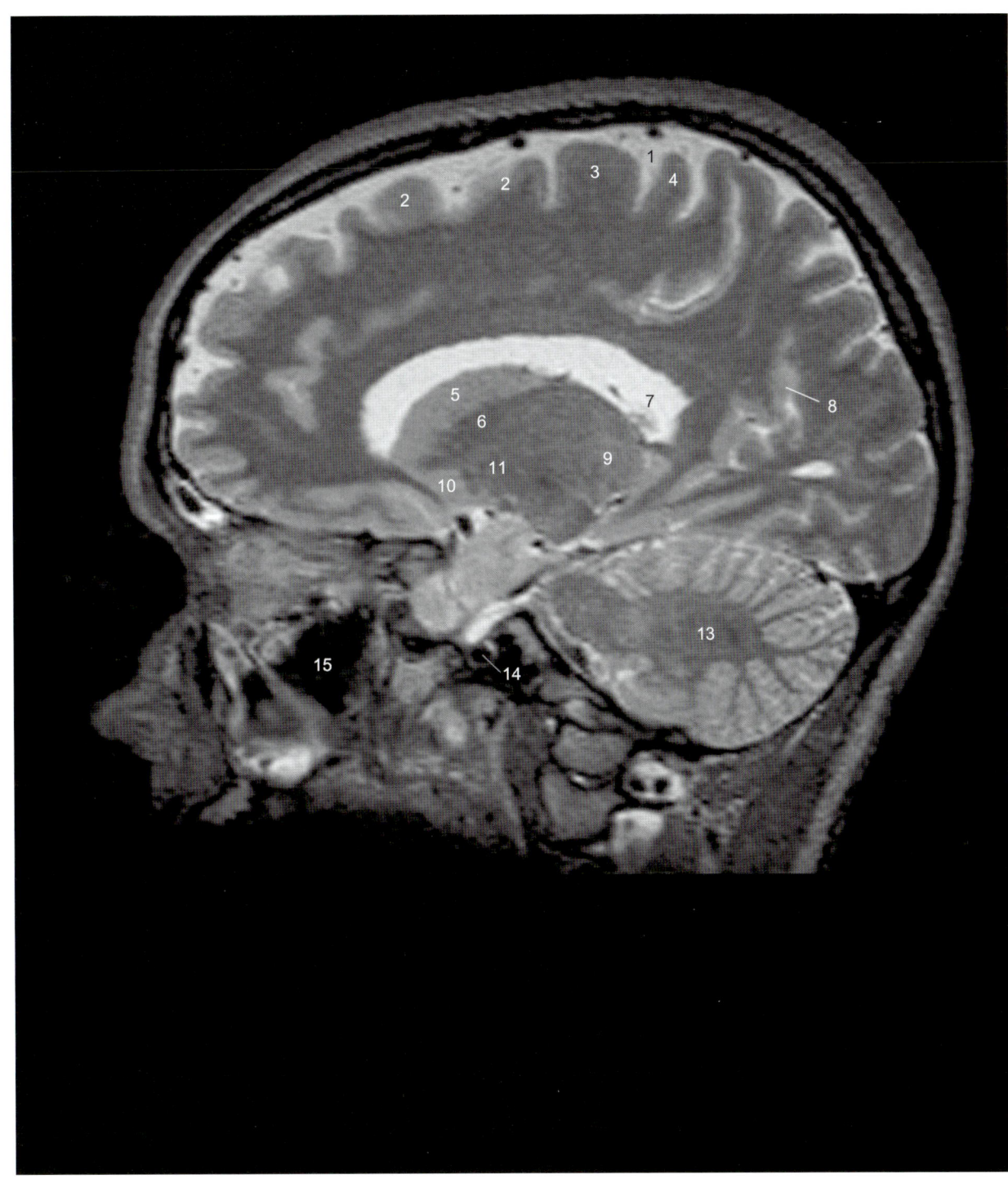

1 Central sulcus
2 Superior frontal gyrus
3 Precentral gyrus
4 Postcentral gyrus
5 Caudate nucleus
6 Internal capsule
7 Lateral ventricle
8 Parieto-occipital sulcus
9 Thalamus
10 Putamen
11 Globus pallidus
13 Cerebellum
14 Internal carotid artery
15 Maxillary sinus

Fig. **34d** Sagittal, T2-weighted MR image corresponding approximately to the sectional plane of Figs. 34a and 34c.

106 Atlas

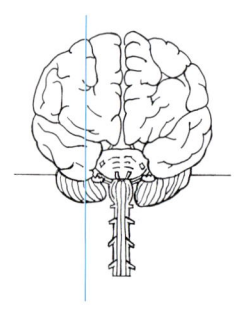

1 Middle frontal gyrus
2 Precentral gyrus
3 Postcentral gyrus
4 Angular gyrus
5 Extreme capsule
6 Cortex of insula
7 Occipital gyri
8 External capsule
9 Claustrum
10 Putamen
11 Tail of caudate nucleus
12 Frontal nerve
13 Anterior commissure
14 Choroid plexus of temporal (inferior) horn
15 Upper eyelid
16 Lens
17 Eyeball
18 Optic nerve
19 Abducens nerve
20 Middle temporal gyrus
21 Amygdaloid body
22 Hippocampus
23 Medial occipitotemporal gyrus
24 Lower eyelid
25 Infraorbital nerve
26 Inferior temporal gyrus
27 Facial nerve and intermediate nerve
28 Vestibulocochlear nerve
29 Mandibular nerve and otic ganglion
30 Vagus nerve
31 Glossopharyngeal nerve
32 Accessory nerve
33 Hypoglossal nerve
34 Superior cervical ganglion
35 Oral cavity
36 Sympathetic trunk (within the slice)
37 Inferior alveolar nerve
38 Lingual nerve

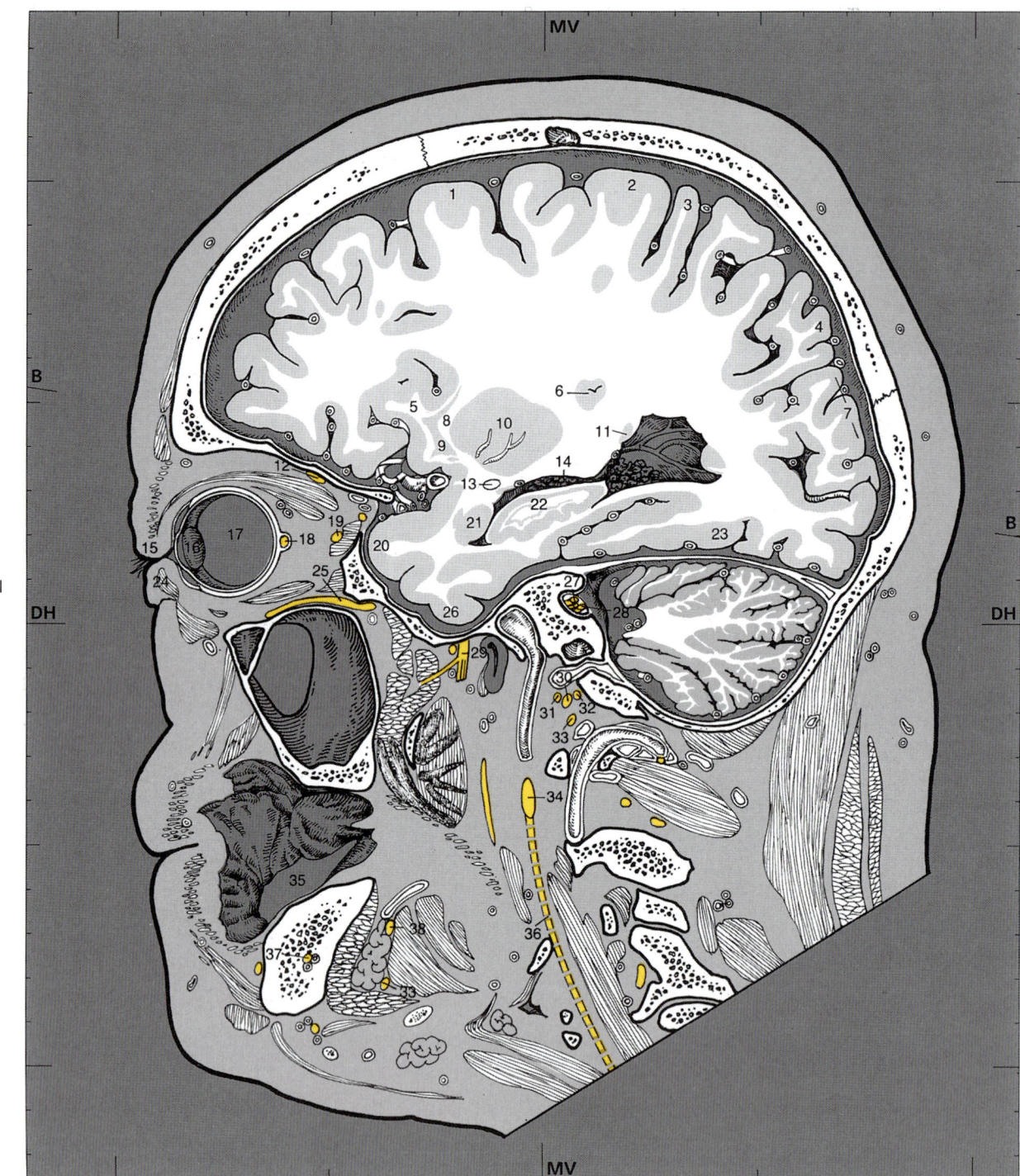

Fig. **35a** Medial view of the fourth sagittal slice showing brain structures and cranial nerves. Demonstrated in the supratentorial space are parts of the telencephalon that are positioned lateral to the frontal (anterior) horn and the central part (body) of the lateral ventricle. The hippocampus and the amygdaloid body are in close proximity to the temporal (inferior) horn. In the infratentorial space the cut runs through the cerebellar hemisphere.

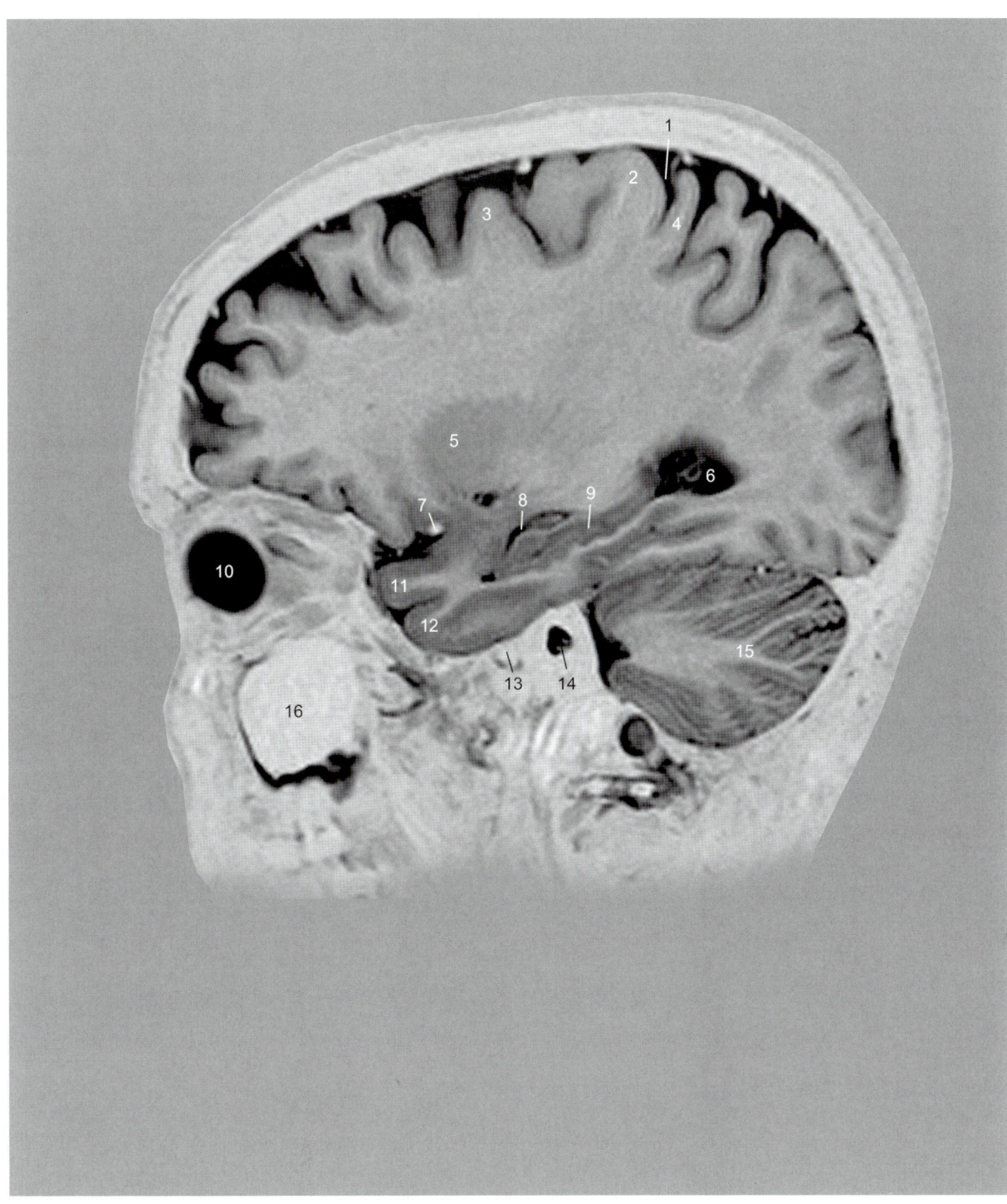

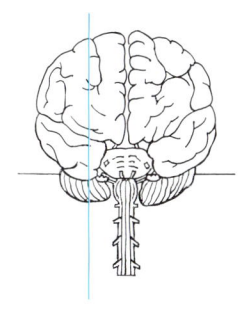

Sagittal Slices

1 Central sulcus
2 Precentral gyrus
3 Middle frontal gyrus
4 Postcentral gyrus
5 Putamen
6 Lateral ventricle
7 Middle cerebral artery
8 Temporal (inferior) horn of lateral ventricle
9 Hippocampus
10 Eyeball
11 Middle temporal gyrus
12 Inferior temporal gyrus
13 Internal carotid artery
14 Internal acoustic meatus with facial nerve (lies superior) and vestibulocochlear nerve (lies inferior)
15 Cerebellum
16 Maxillary sinus

Fig. **35b** Sagittal, T1-weighted MR image corresponding approximately to the sectional plane of Figs. 35a and 35c.

108 Atlas

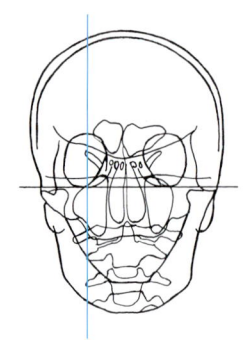

1 Coronal suture
2 Artery of precentral sulcus
3 Frontal bone
4 Prefrontal artery
5 Parietal bone
6 Artery of central sulcus
7 Parietal artery
8 Angular artery
9 Insular artery
10 Lateral frontobasal artery
11 Lambdoid suture
12 Roof of orbit
13 Levator palpebrae superioris
14 Middle cerebral artery
15 Temporo-occipital artery
16 Lens
17 Superior rectus
18 Lateral rectus
19 Temporal artery of posterior cerebral artery
20 Inferior oblique
21 Inferior rectus
22 Orbitalis
23 Internal acoustic meatus
24 Superior cerebellar artery
25 Transverse sinus
26 Occipital bone
27 Floor of orbit
28 Temporal bone
29 Cartilage of pharyngotympanic tube
30 Internal jugular vein near jugular foramen
31 Sigmoid sinus
32 Lateral pterygoid
33 Lateral pterygoid plate
34 Medial pterygoid
35 Internal carotid artery
36 Transverse process of atlas
37 Vertebral artery
38 Posterior inferior cerebellar artery (PICA)
39 Semispinalis capitis
40 Maxilla
41 Obliquus capitis inferior
42 Styloglossus
43 Axis
44 Splenius capitis
45 Trapezius
46 Mylohyoid
47 Digastric tendon

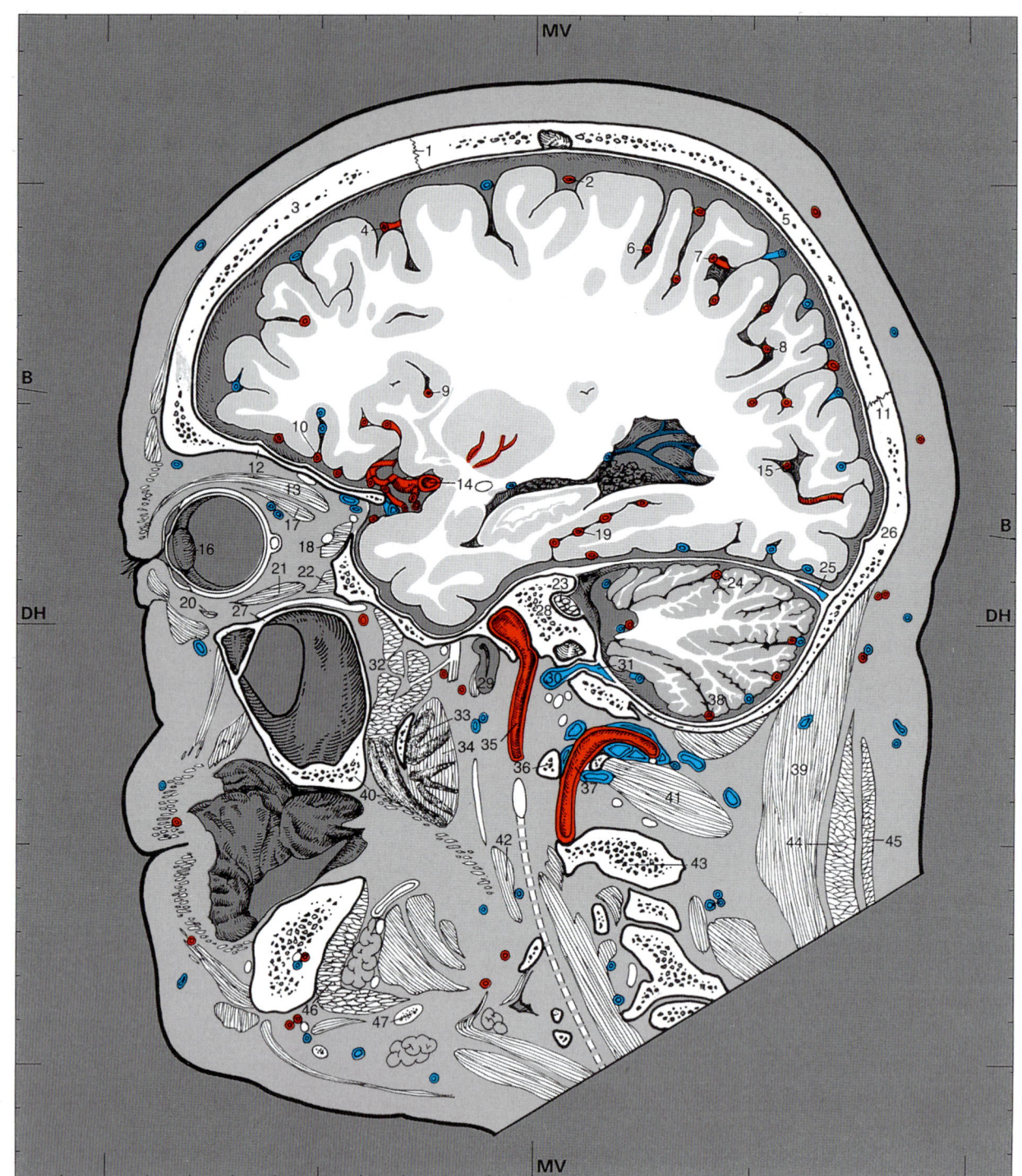

Fig. 35c Medial view of the fourth sagittal slice depicting bony structures, muscles, and blood vessels. The sectional plane lies close to the medial part of the mid plane of the eyeball cutting the lens, the superior rectus, and the inferior rectus. Demonstrated in this slice are the internal acoustic meatus, jugular foramen, and parapharyngeal space.

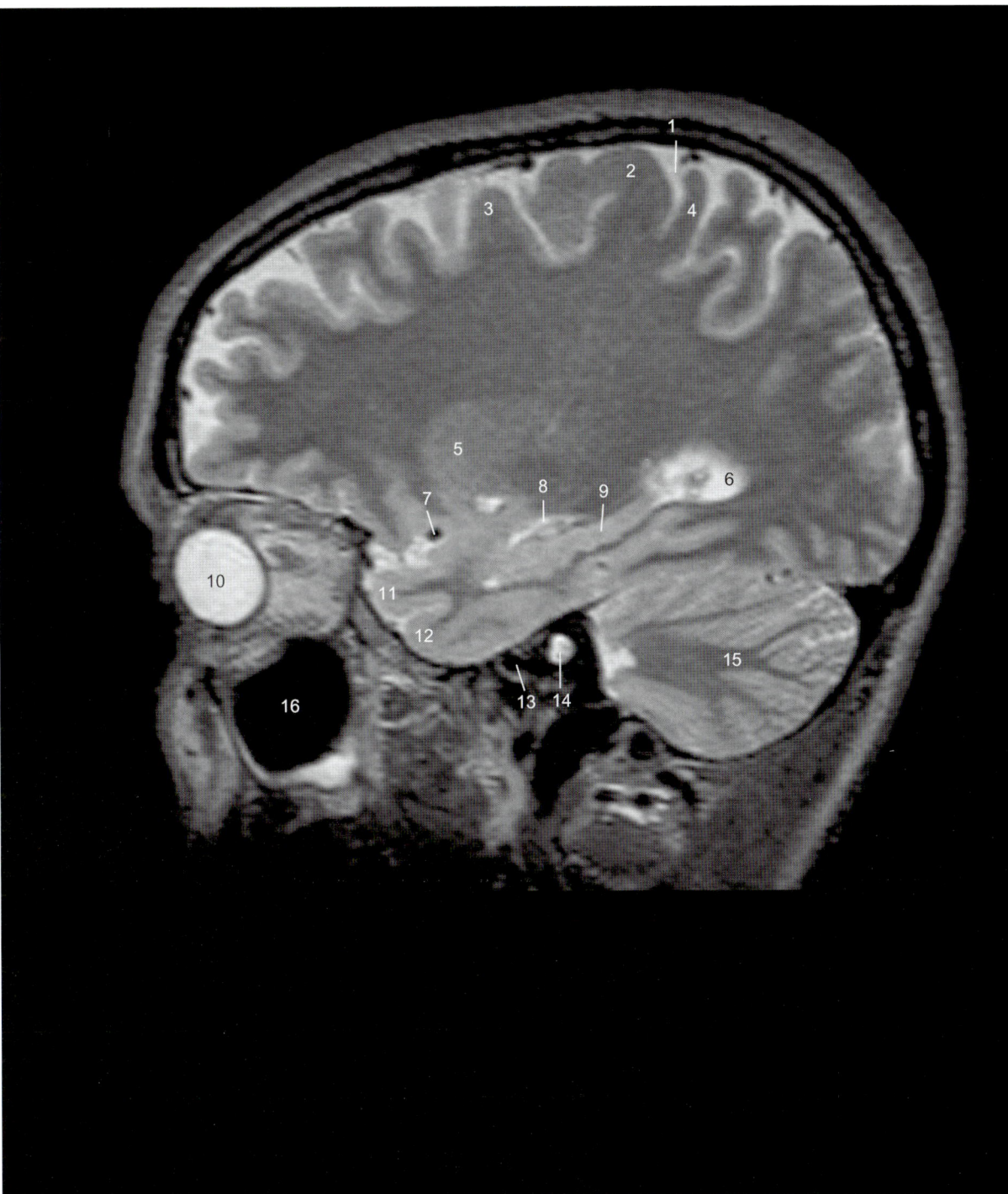

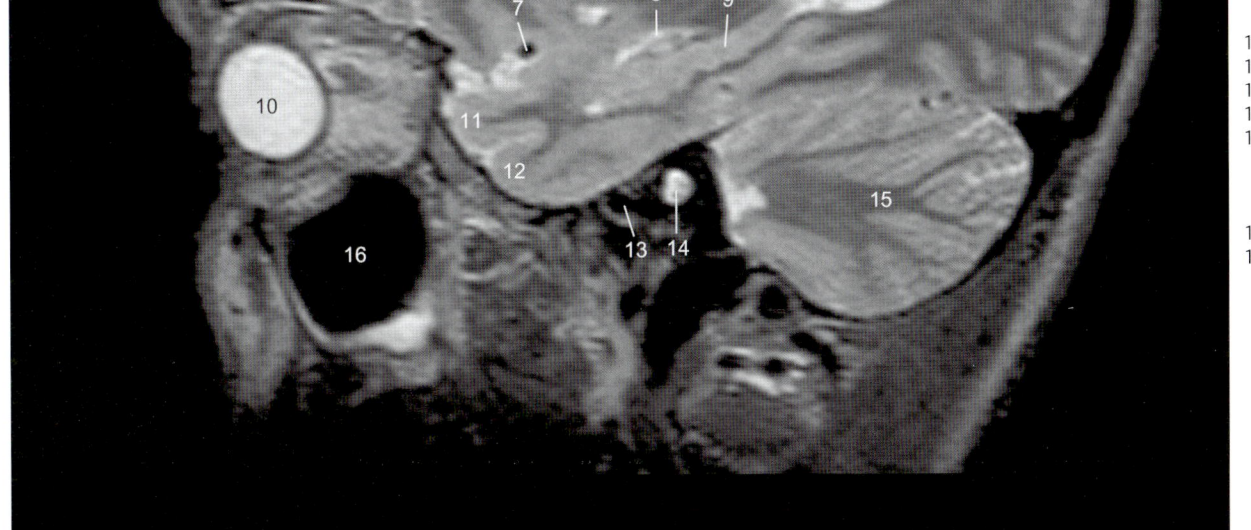

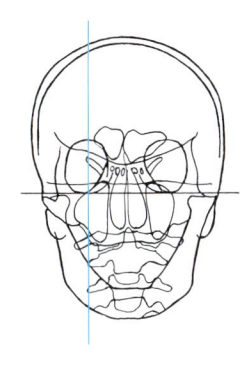

Sagittal Slices

1 Central sulcus
2 Precentral gyrus
3 Middle frontal gyrus
4 Postcentral gyrus
5 Putamen
6 Lateral ventricle
7 Middle cerebral artery
8 Temporal (inferior) horn of lateral ventricle
9 Hippocampus
10 Eyeball
11 Middle temporal gyrus
12 Inferior temporal gyrus
13 Internal carotid artery
14 Internal acoustic meatus with facial nerve (lies superior) and vestibulocochlear nerve (lies inferior)
15 Cerebellum
16 Maxillary sinus

Fig. **35d** Sagittal, T2-weighted MR image corresponding approximately to the sectional plane of Figs. 35a and 35c.

110 Atlas

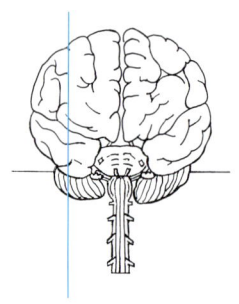

1 Dura mater
2 Precentral sulcus
3 Precentral gyrus
4 Central sulcus
5 Postcentral gyrus
6 Supramarginal gyrus
7 Inferior frontal gyrus
8 Lateral sulcus (Sylvian fissure)
9 Angular gyrus
10 Cortex of insula
11 Anterior transverse temporal gyrus (of Heschl)
12 Posterior transverse temporal gyrus
13 Superior temporal gyrus
14 Eyeball
15 Retina
16 Middle temporal gyrus
17 Occipital gyri
18 Lateral occipitotemporal gyrus
19 Inferior temporal gyrus
20 Tentorium of cerebellum
21 Maxillary sinus
22 Facial nerve and facial canal (within the slice)
23 Posterior lobe of cerebellum
24 Inferior alveolar nerve
25 Accessory nerve
26 Lingual nerve
27 Vagus nerve
28 Oral vestibule
29 Hypoglossal nerve

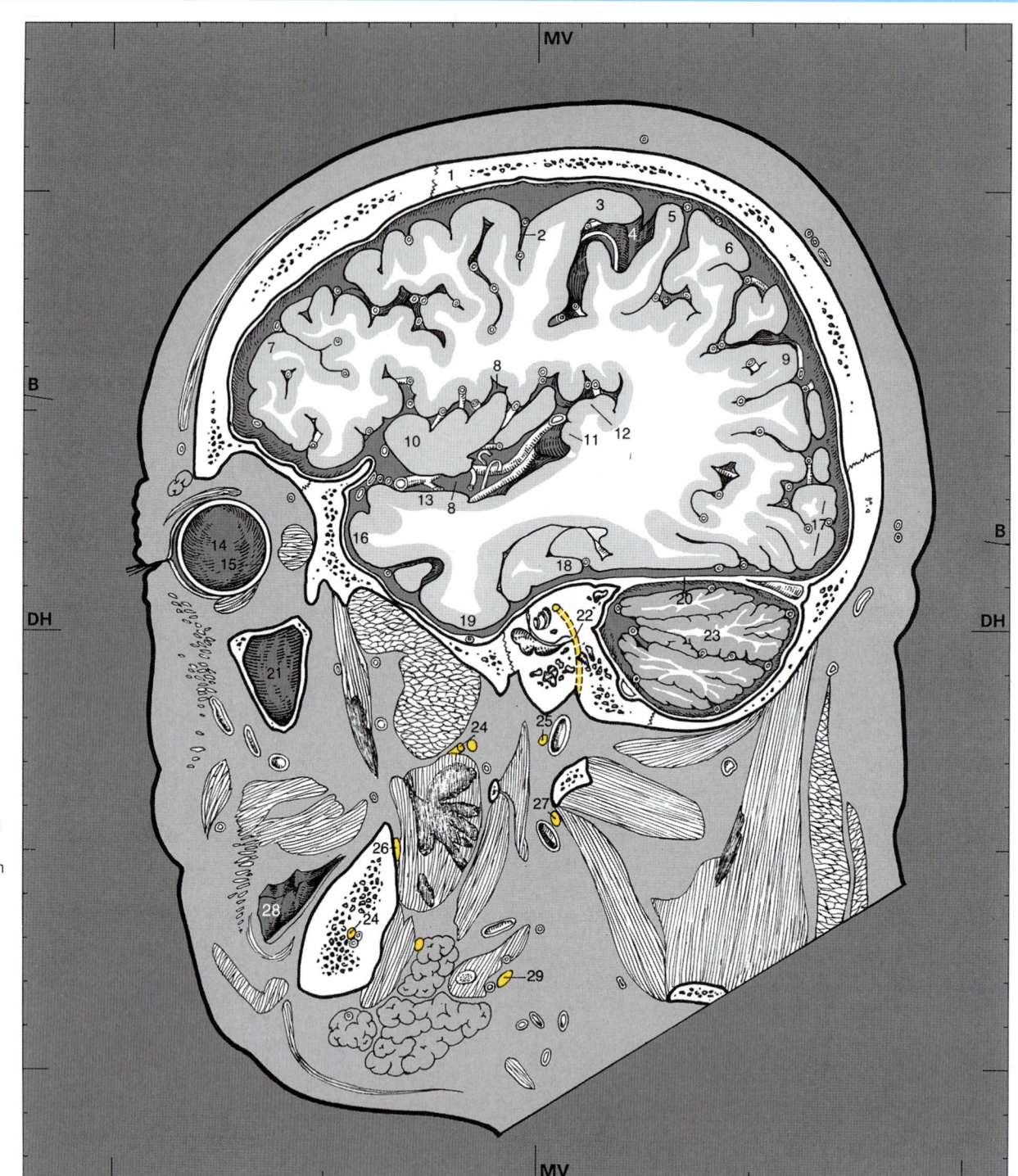

Fig. **36a** Medial view of the fifth sagittal slice demonstrating brain structures and cranial nerves. Superficial tangential separation of the cortex of insula which lies in the lateral sulcus surrounded by the insular arteries. Branches of the fifth, seventh, tenth, eleventh, and twelfth cranial nerves are visible.

Sagittal Slices

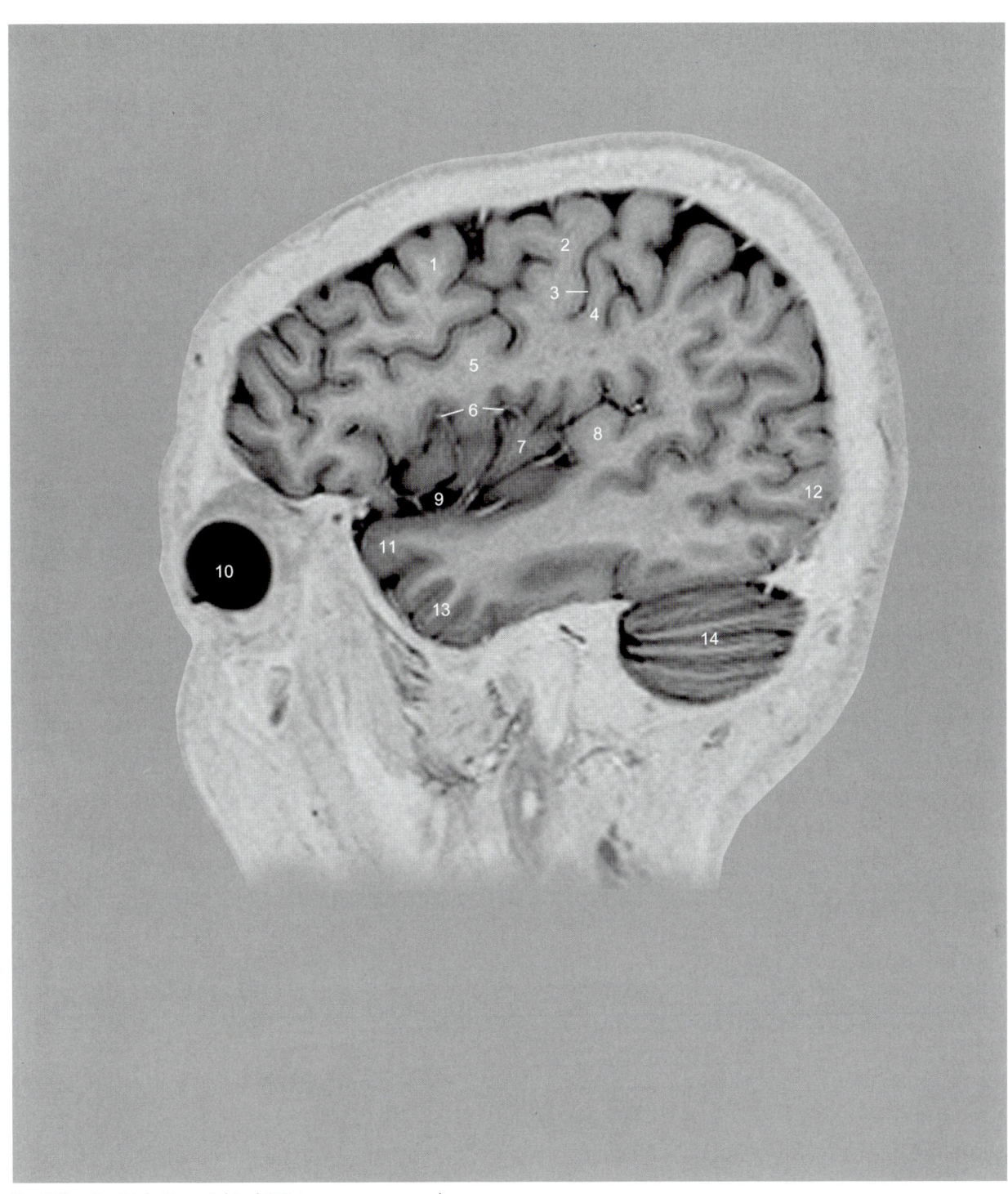

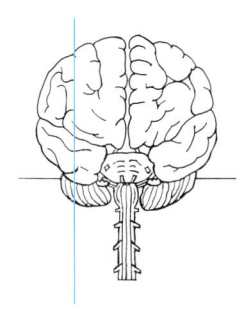

1 Middle frontal gyrus
2 Precentral gyrus
3 Central sulcus
4 Postcentral gyrus
5 Inferior frontal gyrus
6 Insular arteries
7 Insula
8 Transverse temporal gyrus (of Heschl)
9 Cistern of lateral cerebral fossa (cistern of Sylvian fissure)
10 Eyeball
11 Middle temporal gyrus
12 Occipital gyri
13 Inferior temporal gyrus
14 Posterior lobe of cerebellum

Fig. **36b** Sagittal, T1-weighted MR image corresponding approximately to the sectional plane of Figs. 36a and 36c.

112 Atlas

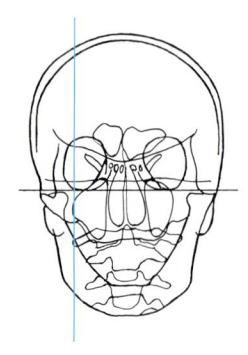

1 Coronal suture
2 Frontal bone
3 Artery of precentral sulcus
4 Artery of central sulcus
5 Parietal bone
6 Prefrontal artery
7 Parietal artery
8 Angular artery
9 Insular arteries
10 Lateral frontobasal artery
11 Lambdoid suture
12 Lacrimal gland
13 Levator palpebrae superioris
14 Temporo-occipital artery
15 Lateral rectus
16 Temporal artery of middle cerebral artery
17 Occipital bone
18 Inferior oblique
19 Cochlea
20 Transverse sinus
21 Superior cerebellar artery
22 Maxilla
23 Temporalis
24 Maxillary artery
25 Lateral pterygoid
26 Middle meningeal artery
27 Tympanic cavity
28 Facial canal (within the slice)
29 Temporal bone
30 Sigmoid sinus
31 Posterior inferior cerebellar artery (PICA)
32 Internal jugular vein
33 Styloid process
34 Transverse process of atlas
35 Obliquus capitis inferior
36 Medial pterygoid
37 Stylohyoid
38 Internal carotid artery
39 Semispinalis capitis
40 Splenius capitis
41 Trapezius
42 Mandible
43 Inferior alveolar artery and vein
44 Facial artery
45 Lingual artery
46 Posterior belly of digastric
47 Submandibular gland

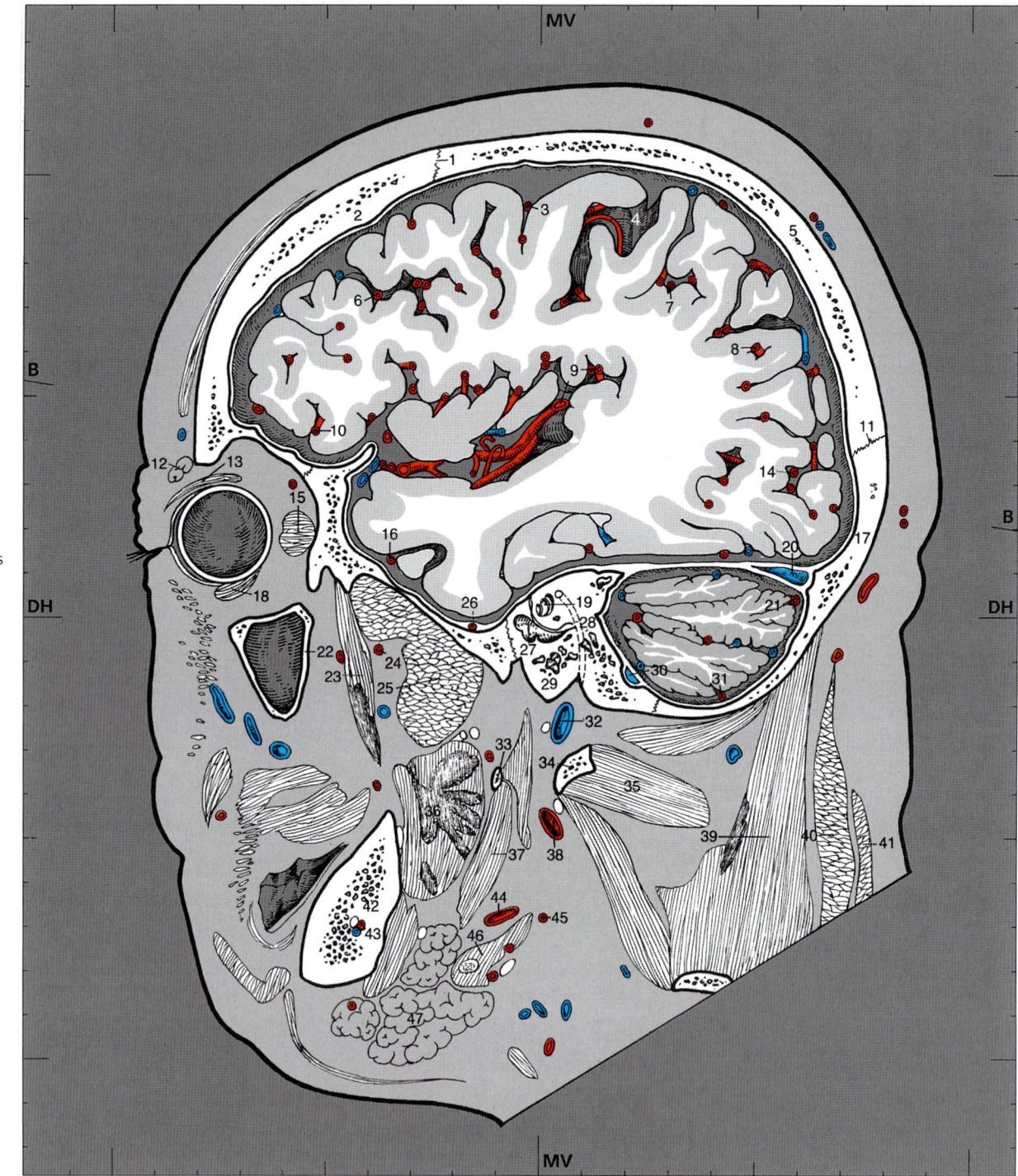

Fig. **36c** Medial view of the fifth sagittal slice showing bony structures, muscles, and blood vessels. The lateral part of the eyeball is cut. The skull base is cut at the level of the cochlea.

Sagittal Slices

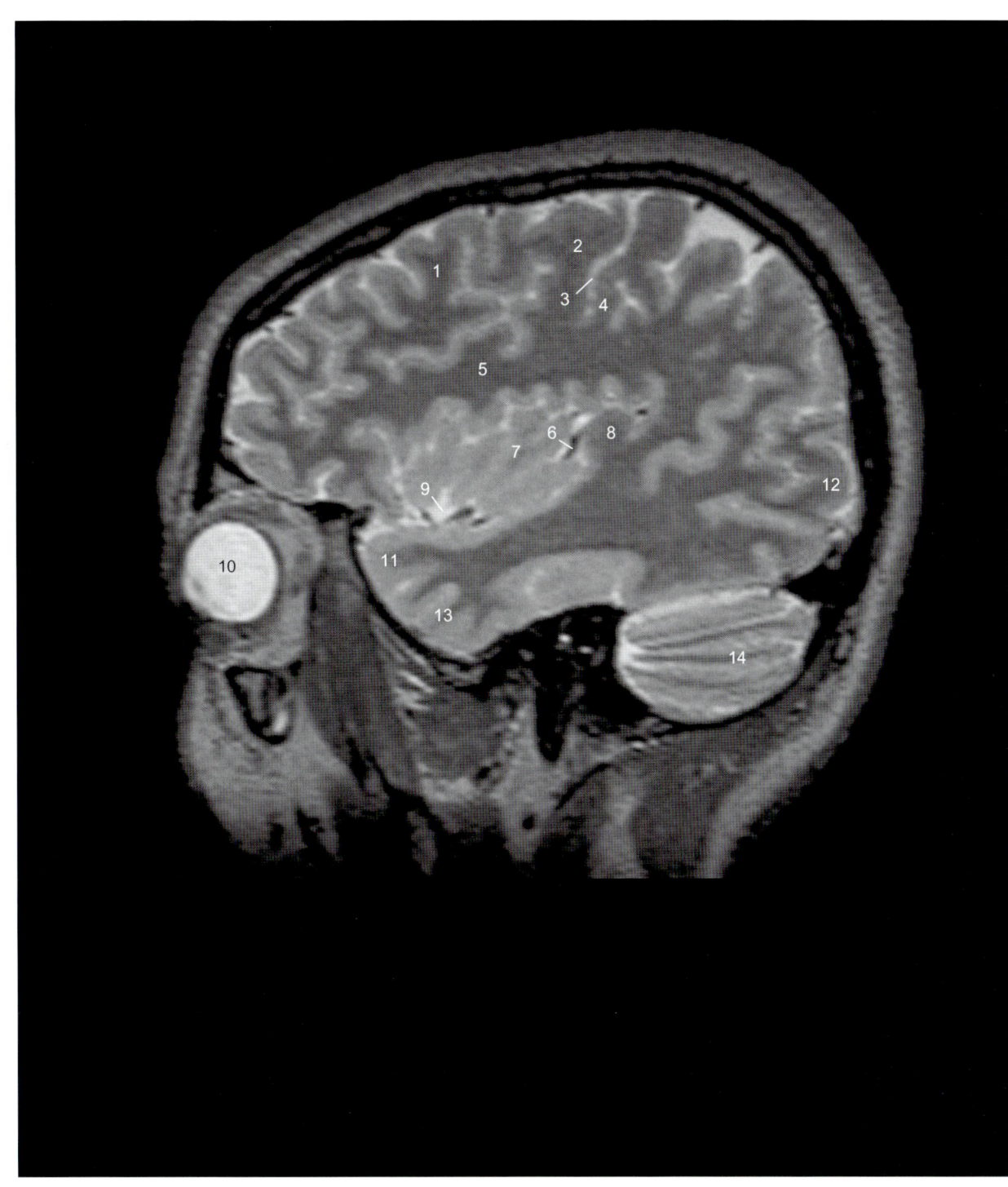

1 Middle frontal gyrus
2 Precentral gyrus
3 Central sulcus
4 Postcentral gyrus
5 Inferior frontal gyrus
6 Insular arteries
7 Insula
8 Transverse temporal gyrus (of Heschl)
9 Cistern of lateral cerebral fossa (cistern of Sylvian fissure)
10 Eyeball
11 Middle temporal gyrus
12 Occipital gyri
13 Inferior temporal gyrus
14 Posterior lobe of cerebellum

Fig. **36d** Sagittal, T2-weighted MR image corresponding approximately to the sectional plane of Figs. 36a and 36c.

114   Atlas

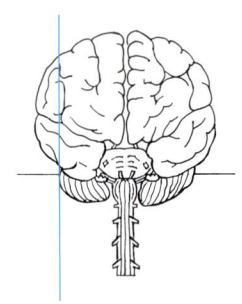

1 Dura mater
2 Precentral gyrus
3 Central sulcus
4 Postcentral gyrus
5 Precentral sulcus
6 Supramarginal gyrus
7 Inferior frontal gyrus
8 Angular gyrus
9 Lateral sulcus (Sylvian fissure)
10 Superior temporal gyrus
11 Anterior transverse temporal gyrus (of Heschl)
12 Posterior transverse temporal gyrus
13 Temporal plane
14 Superior temporal sulcus
15 Middle temporal gyrus
16 Inferior temporal gyrus
17 Posterior lobe of cerebellum (tangentially cut)
18 Facial nerve
19 Inferior alveolar nerve
20 Accessory nerve
21 Vagus nerve

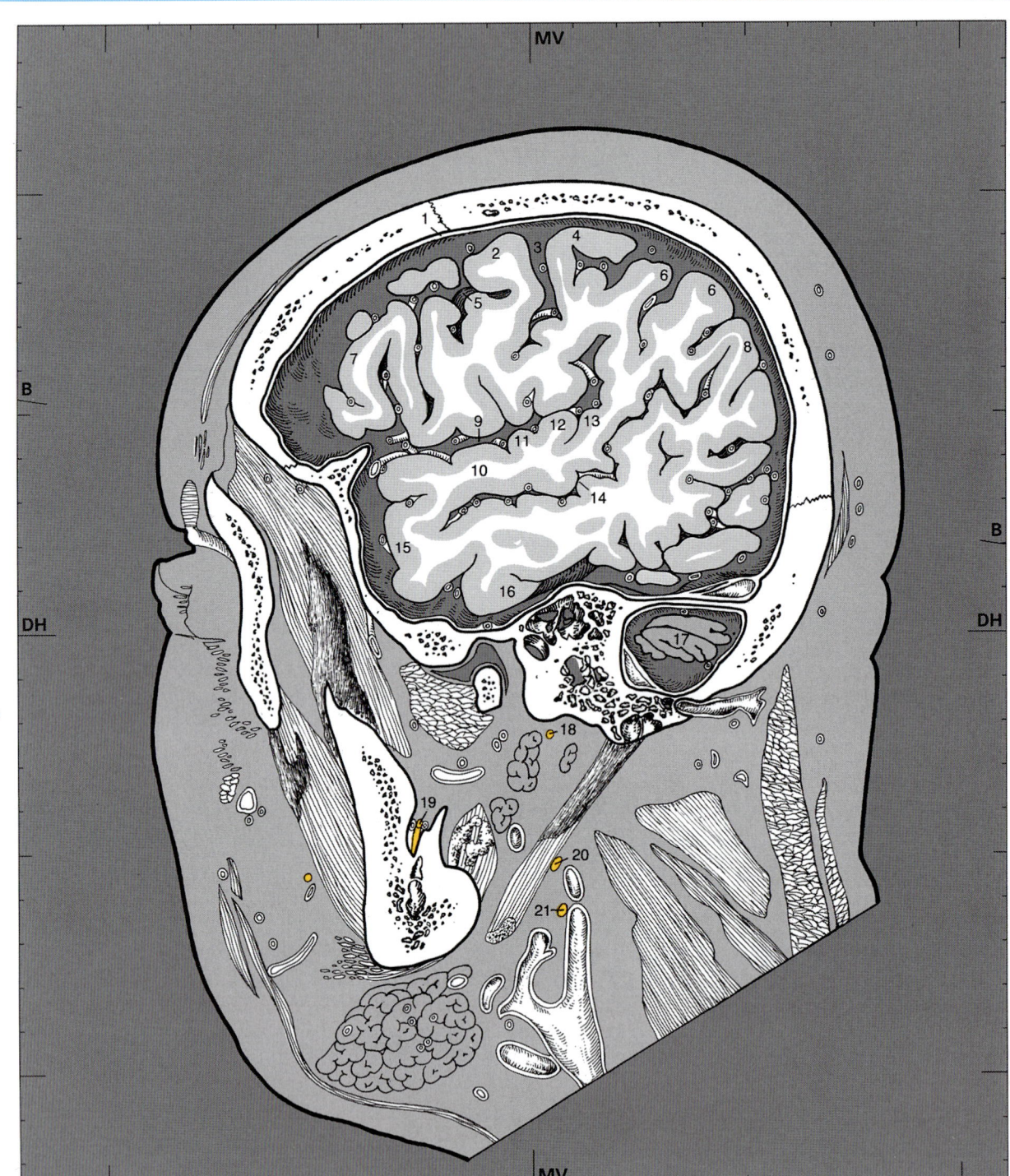

Fig. **37a** Medial view of the sixth sagittal slice representing brain structures and cranial nerves. The cerebral cortex is superficially cut and appears as the operculum around the lateral sulcus.

Sagittal Slices

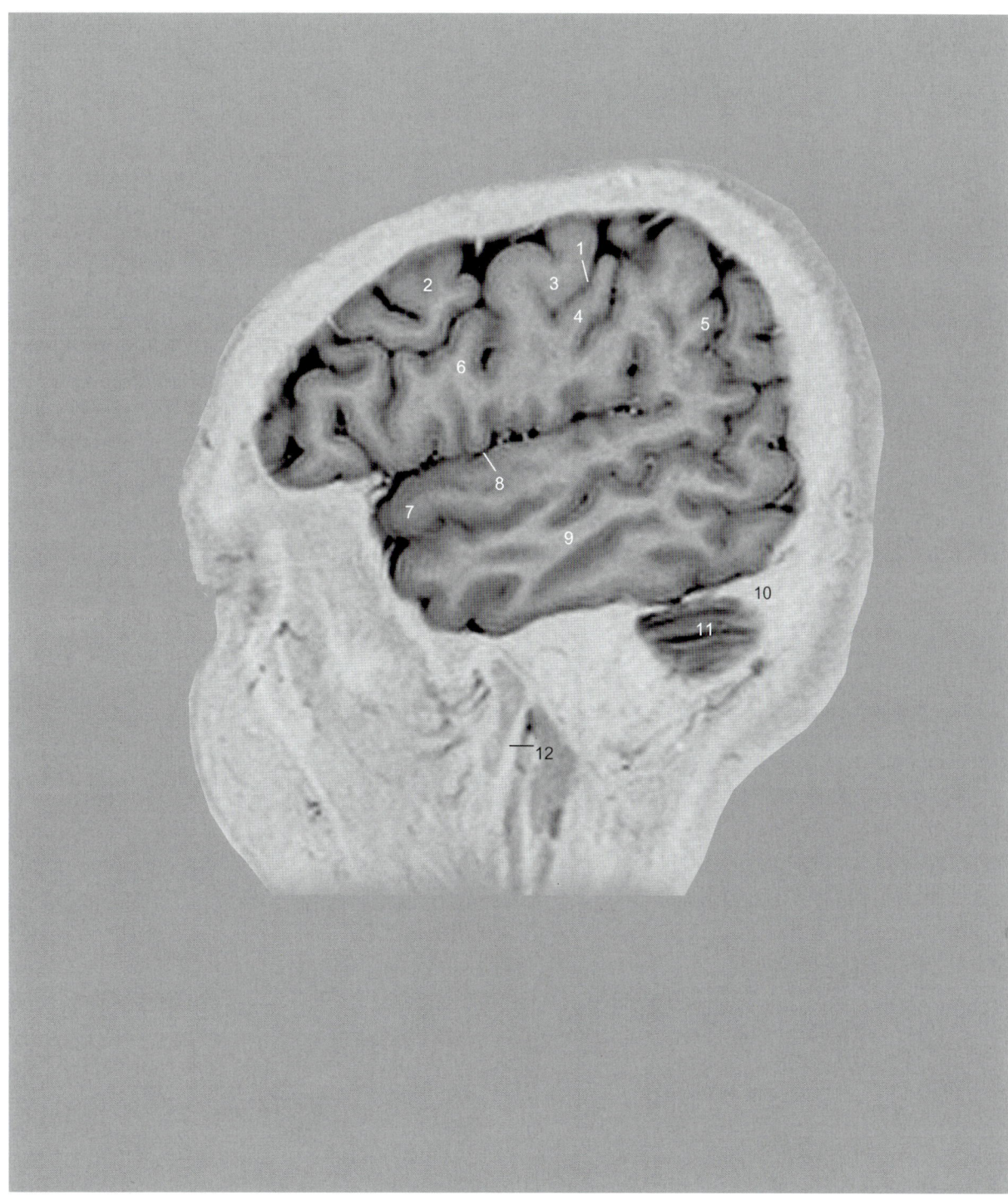

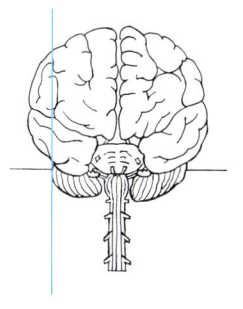

1 Central sulcus
2 Middle frontal gyrus
3 Precentral gyrus
4 Postcentral gyrus
5 Supramarginal gyrus
6 Inferior frontal gyrus
7 Superior temporal gyrus
8 Lateral sulcus (Sylvian fissure)
9 Middle temporal gyrus
10 Transverse sinus
11 Posterior lobe of cerebellum
12 Internal carotid artery

Fig. **37b** Sagittal, T1-weighted MR image corresponding approximately to the sectional plane of Figs. 37a and 37c.

116 Atlas

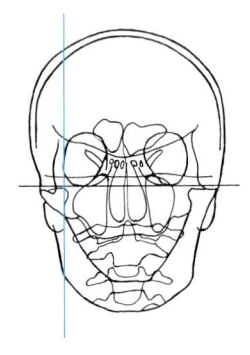

1 Coronal suture
2 Frontal bone
3 Parietal bone
4 Artery of central sulcus
5 Artery of precentral sulcus
6 Parietal artery
7 Prefrontal artery
8 Angular artery
9 Temporo-occipital artery
10 Temporalis
11 Temporal artey of middle cerebral artery
12 Lambdoid suture
13 Zygomatic bone
14 Transverse sinus
15 Occipital bone
16 Articular tubercle
17 Mandibular fossa
18 Articular disc of temporo-mandibular joint
19 Head of mandible
20 External acoustic meatus
21 Sigmoid sinus
22 Coronoid process
23 Lateral pterygoid
24 Mastoid process
25 Emissary vein
26 Maxillary artery
27 Pterygoid venous plexus
28 Parotid gland
29 Masseter
30 Ramus of mandible
31 Inferior alveolar artery and vein in mandibular foramen
32 Medial pterygoid
33 External carotid artery
34 Longissimus capitis
35 Splenius capitis
36 Trapezius
37 Posterior belly of digastric
38 Internal jugular vein
39 Levator scapulae
40 Facial artery
41 Internal carotid artery
42 Platysma
43 Submandibular gland
44 Common carotid artery

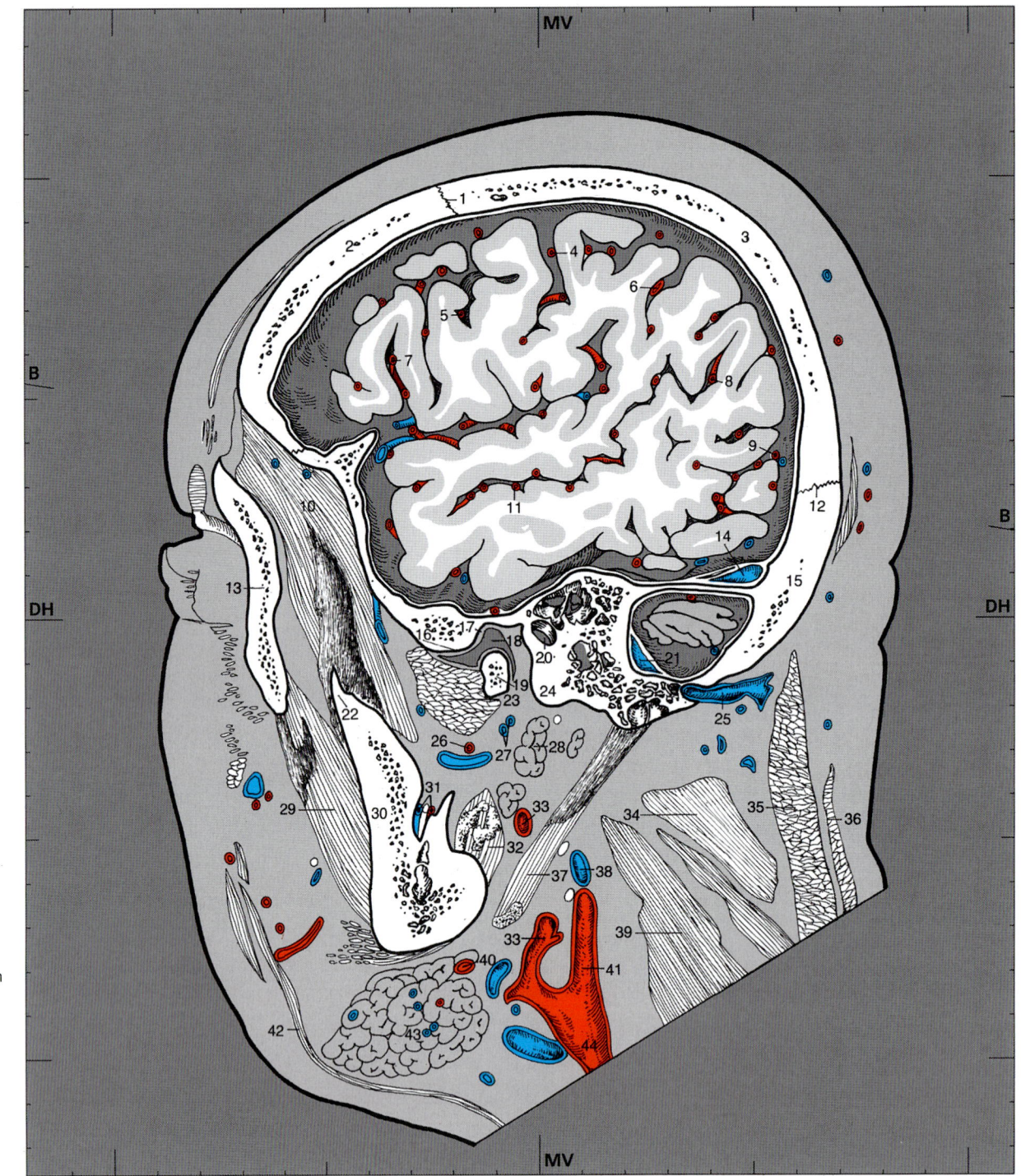

Fig. **37c** Medial view of the sixth sagittal slice revealing bony structures, muscles, and blood vessels. This slice lies close to the lateral part of the orbit and incorporates the bony external acoustic meatus and the bifurcation of the common carotid artery.

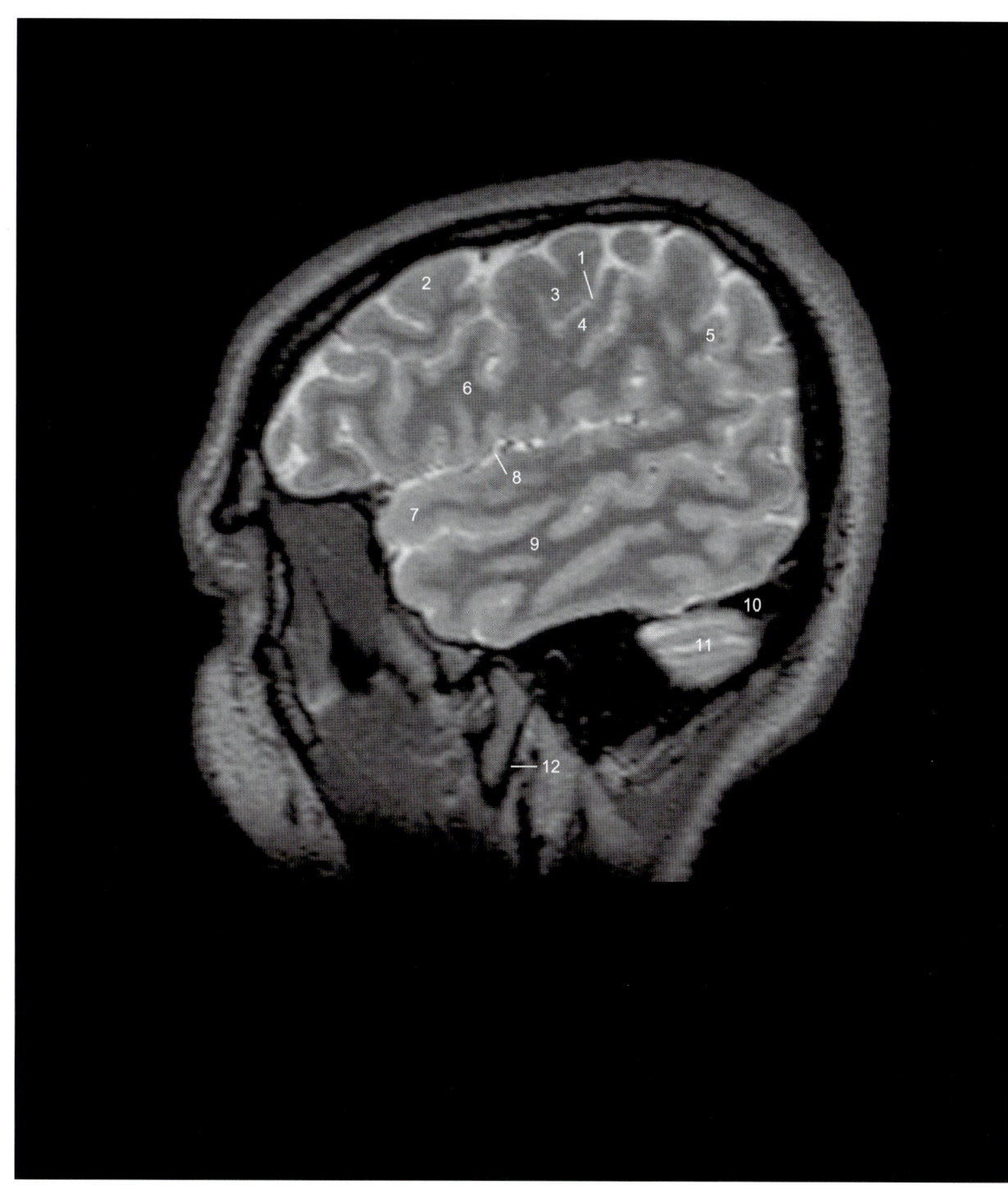

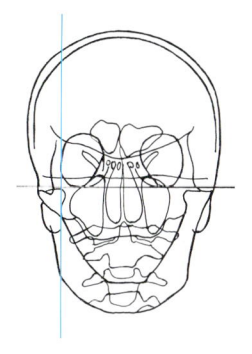

Sagittal Slices

1 Central sulcus
2 Middle frontal gyrus
3 Precentral gyrus
4 Postcentral gyrus
5 Supramarginal gyrus
6 Inferior frontal gyrus
7 Superior temporal gyrus
8 Lateral sulcus (Sylvian fissure)
9 Middle temporal gyrus
10 Transverse sinus
11 Posterior lobe of cerebellum
12 Internal carotid artery

Fig. **37d** Sagittal, T2-weighted MR image corresponding approximately to the sectional plane of Figs. 37a and 37c.

118   Atlas

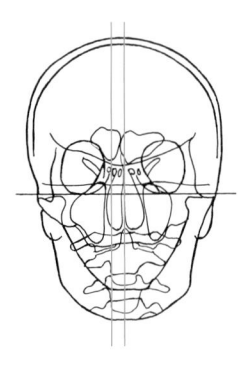

1   Coronal suture, bregma
2   Parietal bone
3   Frontal bone
4   Lambdoid suture
5   Saw cut
6   Frontal sinus
7   Crista galli
8   Anterior cranial fossa
9   Occipital bone
10 Tuberculum sellae
11 Dorsum sellae
12 Cribriform plate of ethmoid
13 Hypophysial fossa
14 Nasal bone
15 Internal occipital protuberance
16 Sphenoidal sinus
17 Sphenoid
18 Clivus
19 External occipital protuberance (inion)
20 Posterior cranial fossa
21 Nasal septum
22 Pharyngeal tubercle
23 Foramen magnum
24 Anterior nasal spine
25 Posterior nasal spine
26 Vertebral canal
27 Hard palate
28 Median atlantoaxial joint
29 Anterior arch of atlas
30 Posterior arch of atlas
31 Dens of axis
32 Incisive canal of maxilla
33 Alveolar process of maxilla
34 Spinous process of axis
35 Spinous process of third cervical vertebra
36 Third cervical vertebra
37 Body of mandible
38 Fourth cervical vertebra
39 Hyoid bone

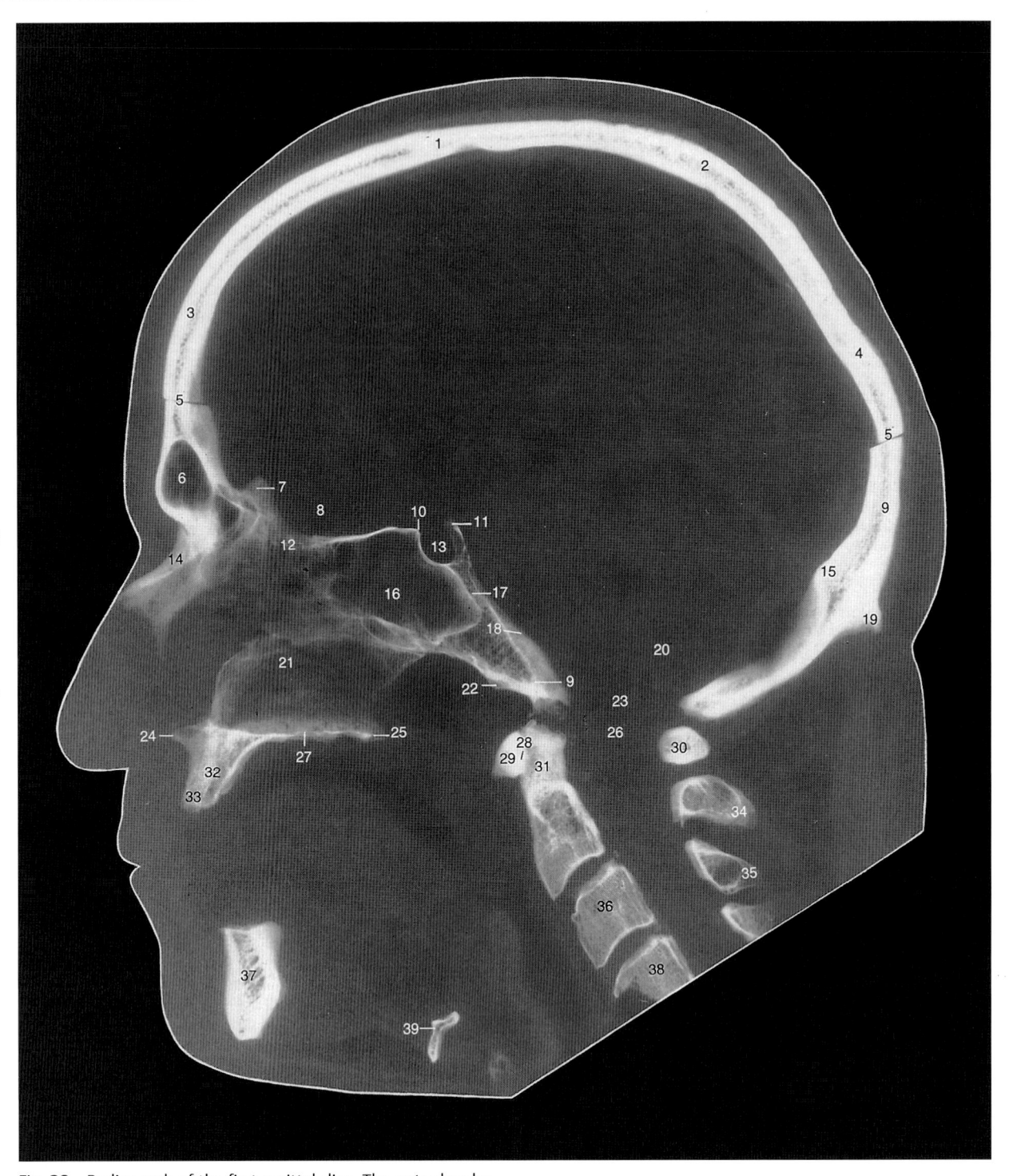

Fig. 38 Radiograph of the first sagittal slice. The outer border of the head has been added. Guideline structures include the hypophysial fossa, frontal sinus, sphenoidal sinus, atlas, and dens of axis.

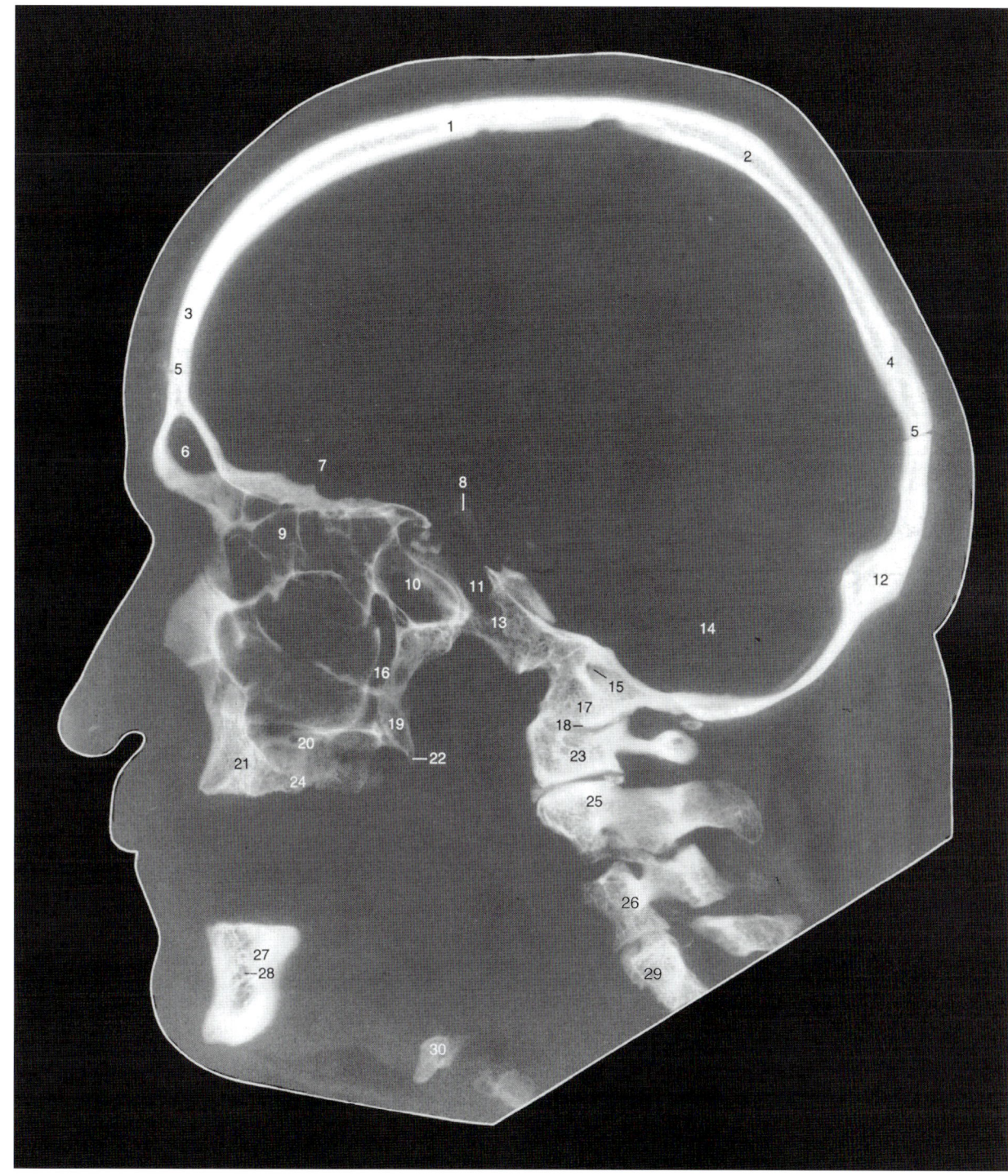

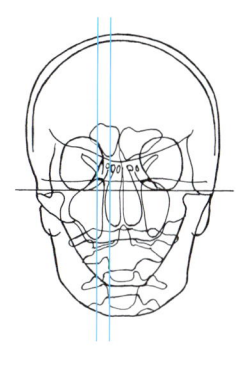

Sagittal Slices

1 Coronal suture
2 Parietal bone
3 Frontal bone
4 Lambdoid suture
5 Saw cut
6 Frontal sinus
7 Anterior cranial fossa
8 Posterior clinoid process
9 Ethmoidal cells
10 Sphenoidal sinus
11 Carotid canal
12 Occipital bone
13 Sphenoid
14 Posterior cranial fossa
15 Hypoglossal canal
16 Greater palatine canal
17 Occipital condyle
18 Atlanto-occipital joint
19 Medial pterygoid plate
20 Hard palate
21 Maxilla
22 Pterygoid hamulus
23 Lateral mass of atlas
24 Alveolar process of maxilla
25 Axis
26 Third cervical vertebra
27 Body of mandible
28 Mandibular canal
29 Fourth cervical vertebra
30 Hyoid bone

Fig. **39** Radiograph of the second sagittal slice. The floors of the anterior and posterior cranial fossae are shown. Guideline structures are the ethmoidal cells, hard palate, mandible, and the contours of the first four cervical vertebrae.

120   Atlas

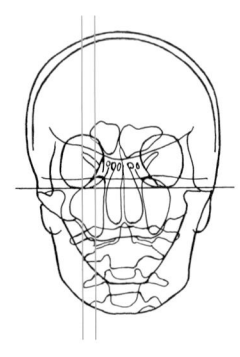

1 Coronal suture
2 Parietal bone
3 Frontal bone
4 Lambdoid suture
5 Frontal sinus
6 Anterior cranial fossa
7 Roof of orbit
8 Sphenofrontal suture
9 Sphenoid
10 Anterior clinoid process
11 Orbit
12 Foramen rotundum
13 Middle cranial fossa
14 Floor of orbit
15 Pterygopalatine fossa
16 Carotid canal
17 Temporal bone
18 Occipital bone
19 Posterior cranial fossa
20 Maxillary sinus
21 Pterygoid process
22 Occipital condyle
23 Atlanto-occipital joint
24 Maxilla
25 Pterygoid hamulus
26 Lateral mass of atlas
27 Lateral atlanto-axial joint
28 Axis
29 Third cervical vertebra
30 Body of mandible
31 Mandibular canal
32 Fourth cervical vertebra
33 Thyroid cartilage
34 Hyoid bone

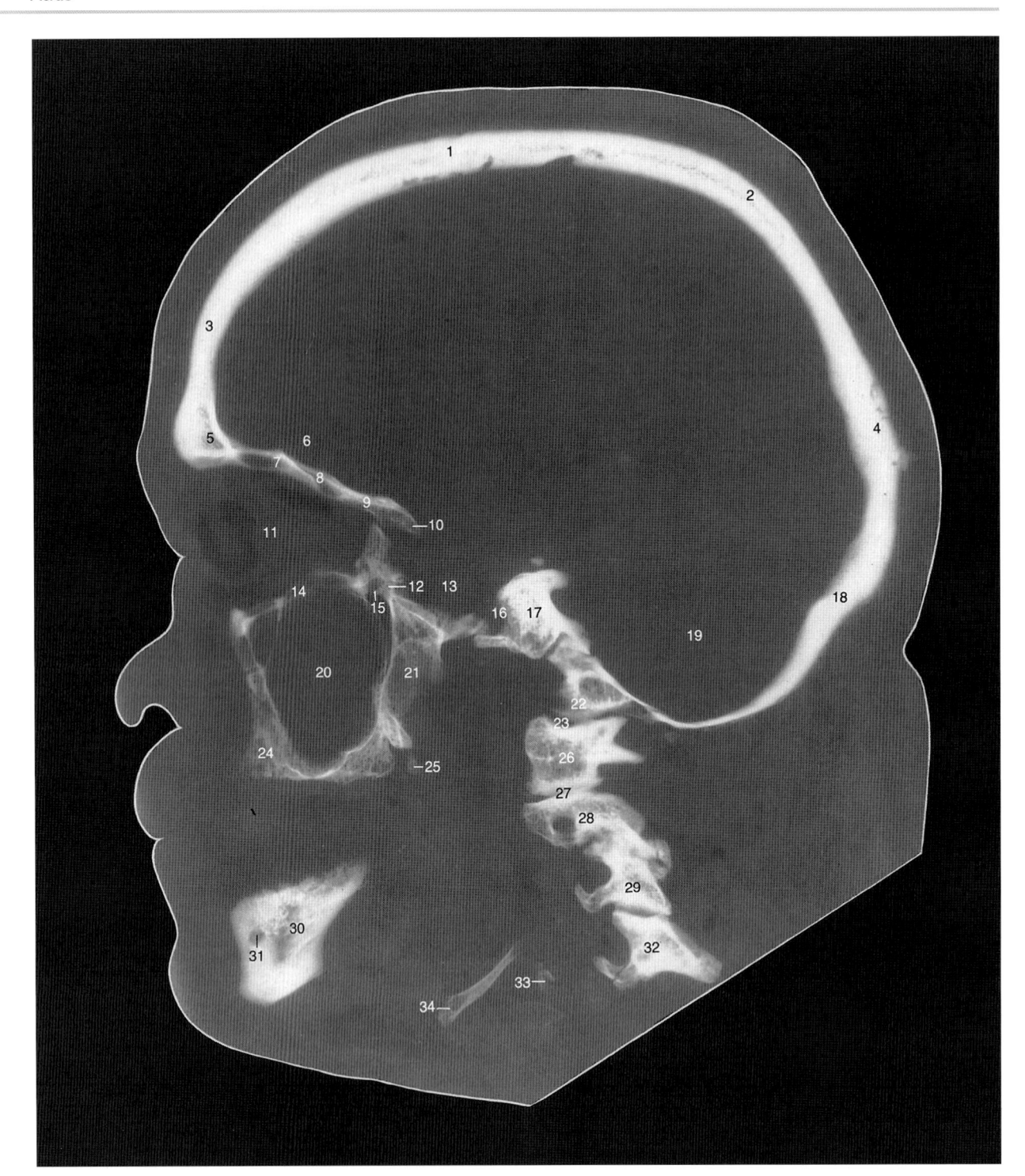

Fig. **40** Radiograph of the third sagittal slice. Guideline structures for the facial skeleton and the craniocervical junction are the roof and floor of the orbit, maxillary sinus, mandible, and the contours of the first four cervical vertebrae. The three terraces of the anterior, middle, and posterior cranial fossae are demonstrated in the cranial cavity.

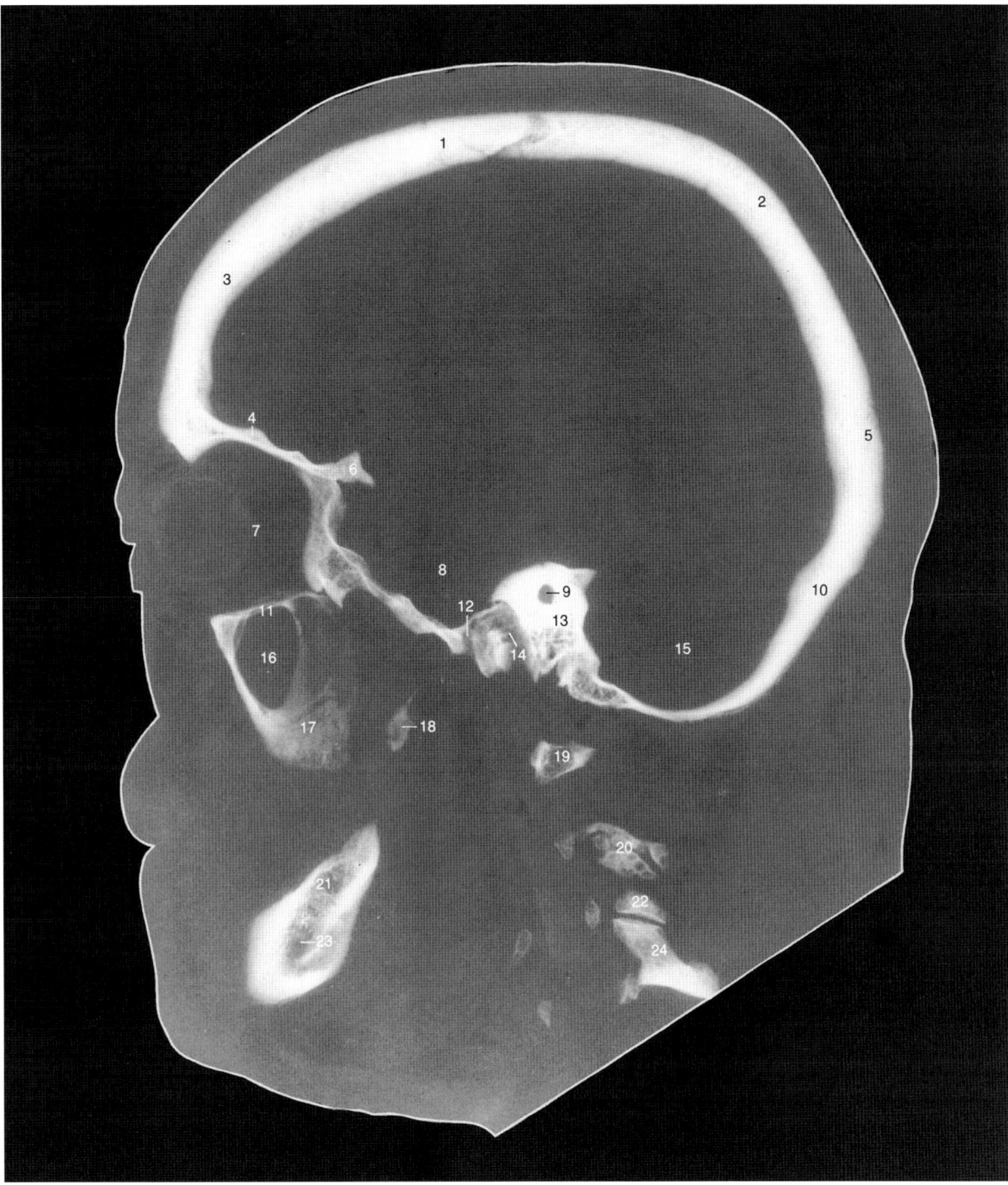

Fig. 41 Radiograph of the fourth sagittal slice. The terraces of the anterior, middle, and posterior cranial fossae are clearly shown.

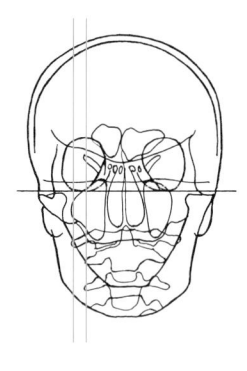

1 Coronal suture
2 Parietal bone
3 Frontal bone
4 Roof of orbit, floor of anterior cranial fossa
5 Lambdoid suture
6 Lesser wing of sphenoid
7 Orbit
8 Middle cranial fossa
9 Internal acoustic meatus
10 Occipital bone
11 Floor of orbit
12 Foramen ovale
13 Temporal bone
14 Carotid canal
15 Posterior cranial fossa
16 Maxillary sinus
17 Maxilla
18 Lateral pterygoid plate
19 Transverse process of atlas
20 Axis
21 Mandible
22 Third cervical vertebra
23 Mandibular canal
24 Fourth cervical vertebra

122   Atlas

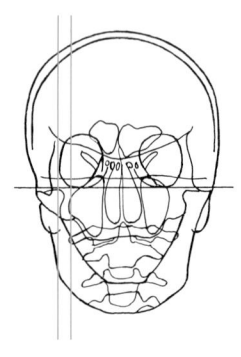

1 Coronal suture
2 Parietal bone
3 Frontal bone
4 Lambdoid suture
5 Occipital bone
6 Arcuate eminence
7 Middle cranial fossa
8 Tympanic cavity
9 Posterior cranial fossa
10 Maxilla
11 Facial canal
12 Temporal bone
13 Stylomastoid foramen
14 Styloid process
15 Transverse process of atlas
16 Ramus of mandible
17 Mandibular canal

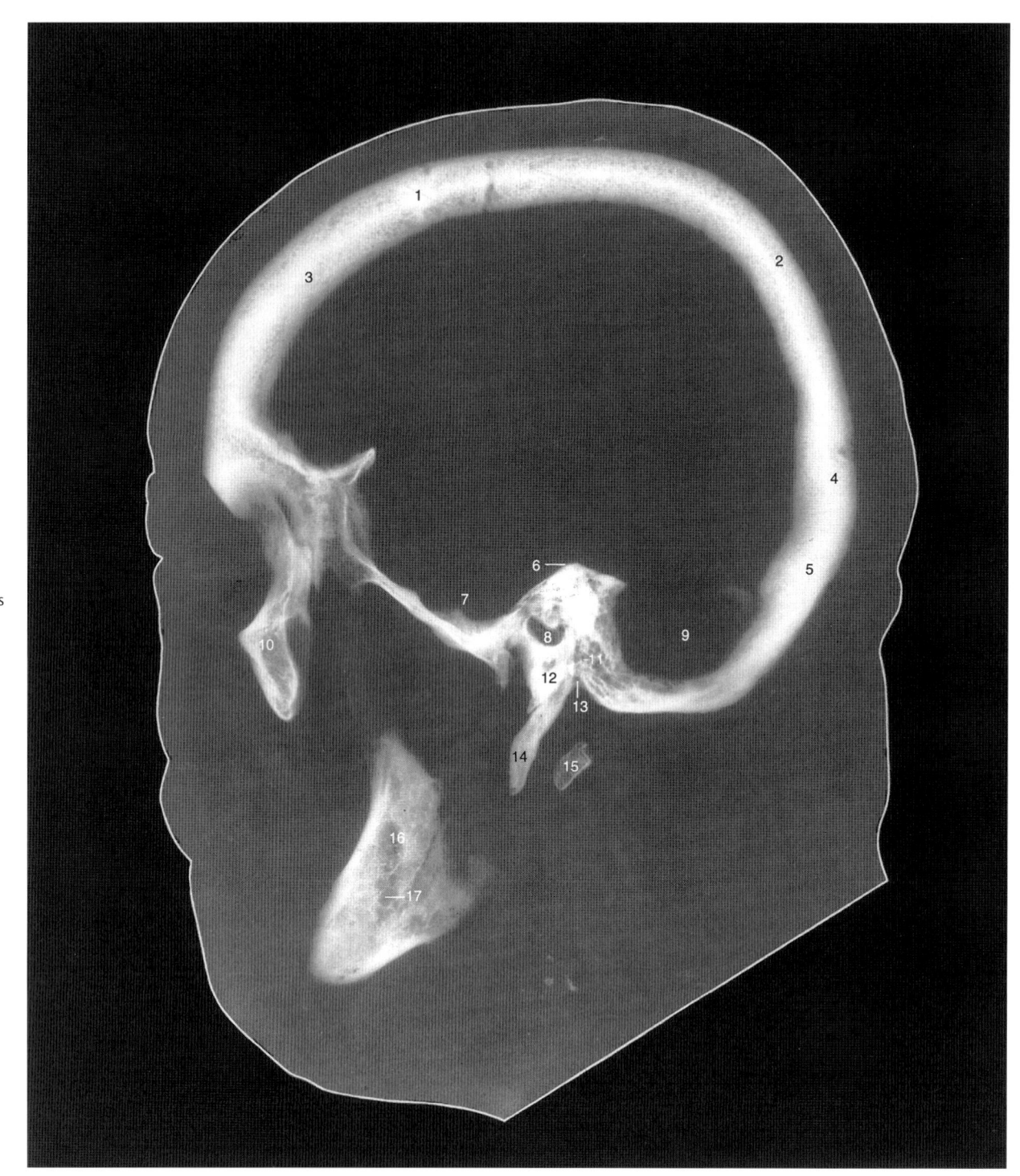

Fig. 42   Radiograph of the fifth sagittal slice. The skull base lies at the level of the anterior semicircular canal, the facial canal, the tympanic cavity, and the styloid process.

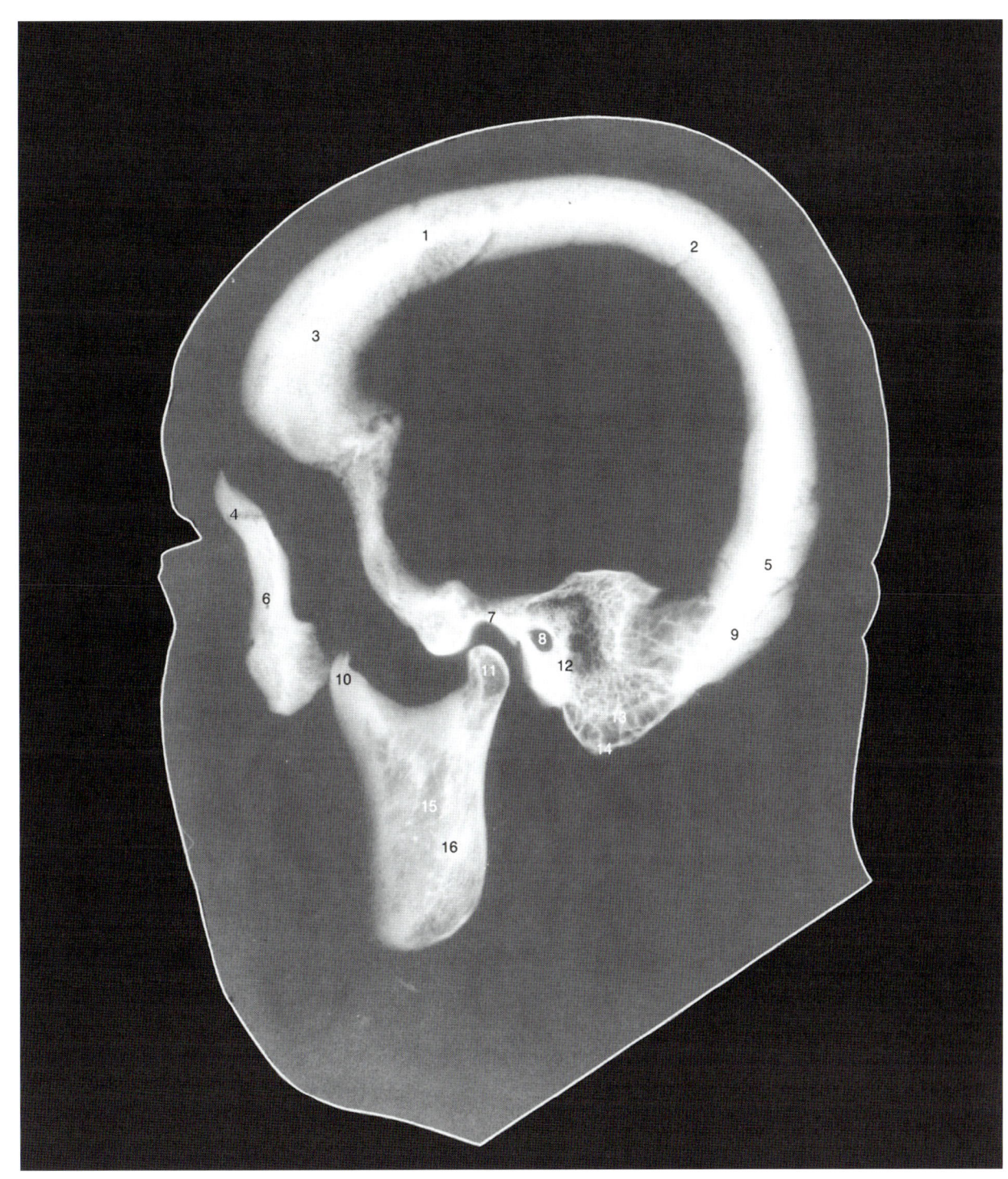

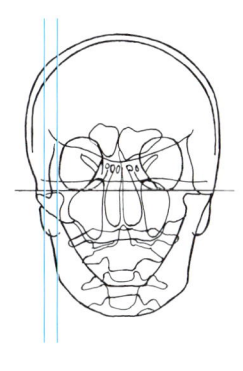

Sagittal Slices

1 Coronal suture
2 Parietal bone
3 Frontal bone
4 Frontozygomatic suture
5 Lambdoid suture
6 Zygomatic bone
7 Mandibular fossa
8 External acoustic meatus
9 Occipital bone
10 Coronoid process
11 Condylar process
12 Temporal bone
13 Mastoid cells
14 Mastoid process
15 Mandibular foramen
16 Ramus of mandible

Fig. 43 Radiograph of the sixth sagittal slice. The slice lies at the level of the temporomandibular joint and includes the mastoid process.

124 Atlas

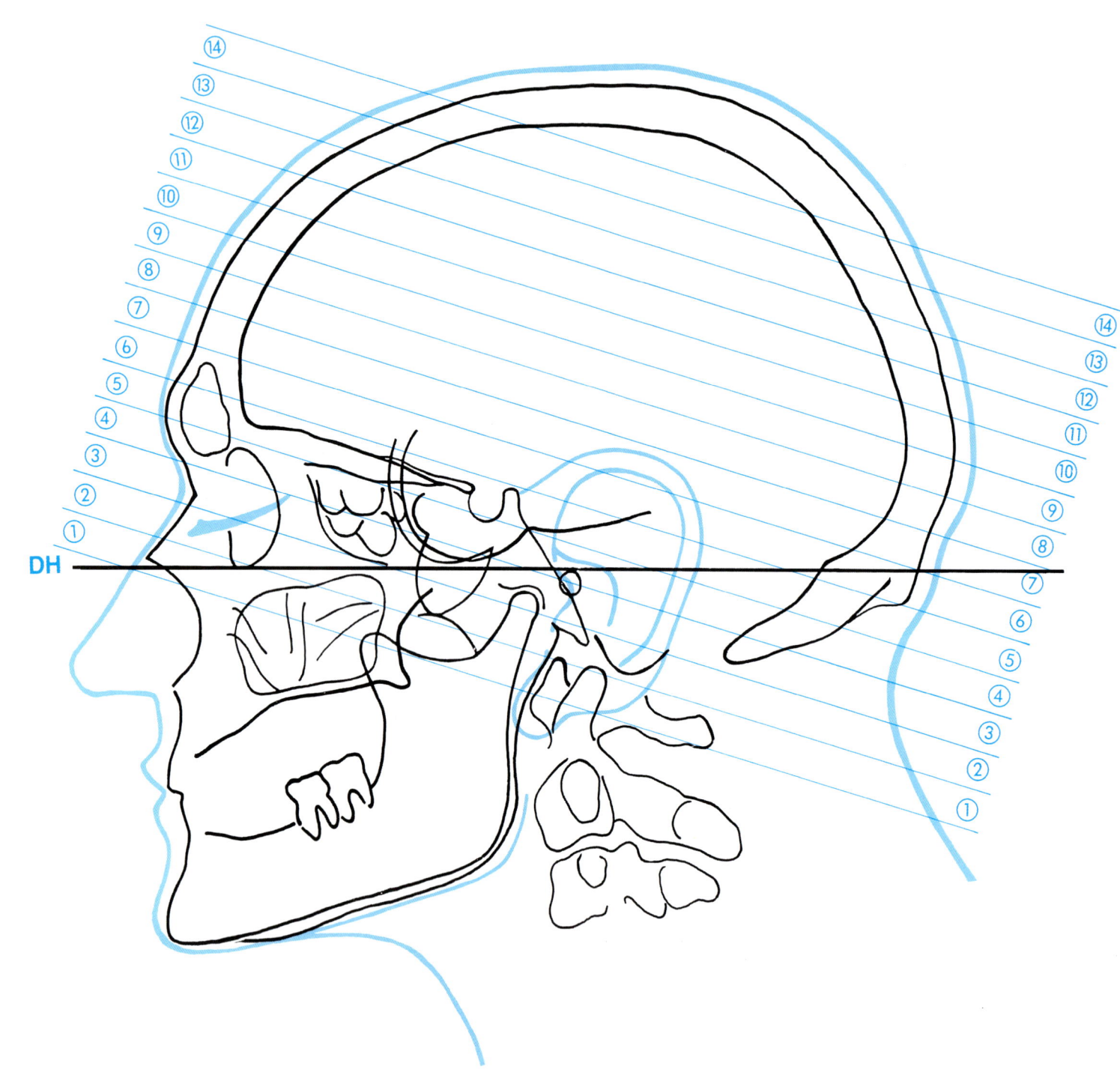

Fig. 44 Canthomeatal parallel planes are shown on the lateral surface of the head of a 44-year-old male (Chap. 8). The 14 slices are described in an inferior to superior order in the atlas portion of this book (Figs. 47a, 48a,c–60a,c). The encircled numbers indicate the numbers of 1-cm-thick slices that are illustrated in the atlas as seen from above. The illustrated surface of each section, therefore, represents the line above the encircled number of the corresponding slice. Technical data (Chap. 8).
DH Reid's base line

Canthomeatally Oriented Slices 125

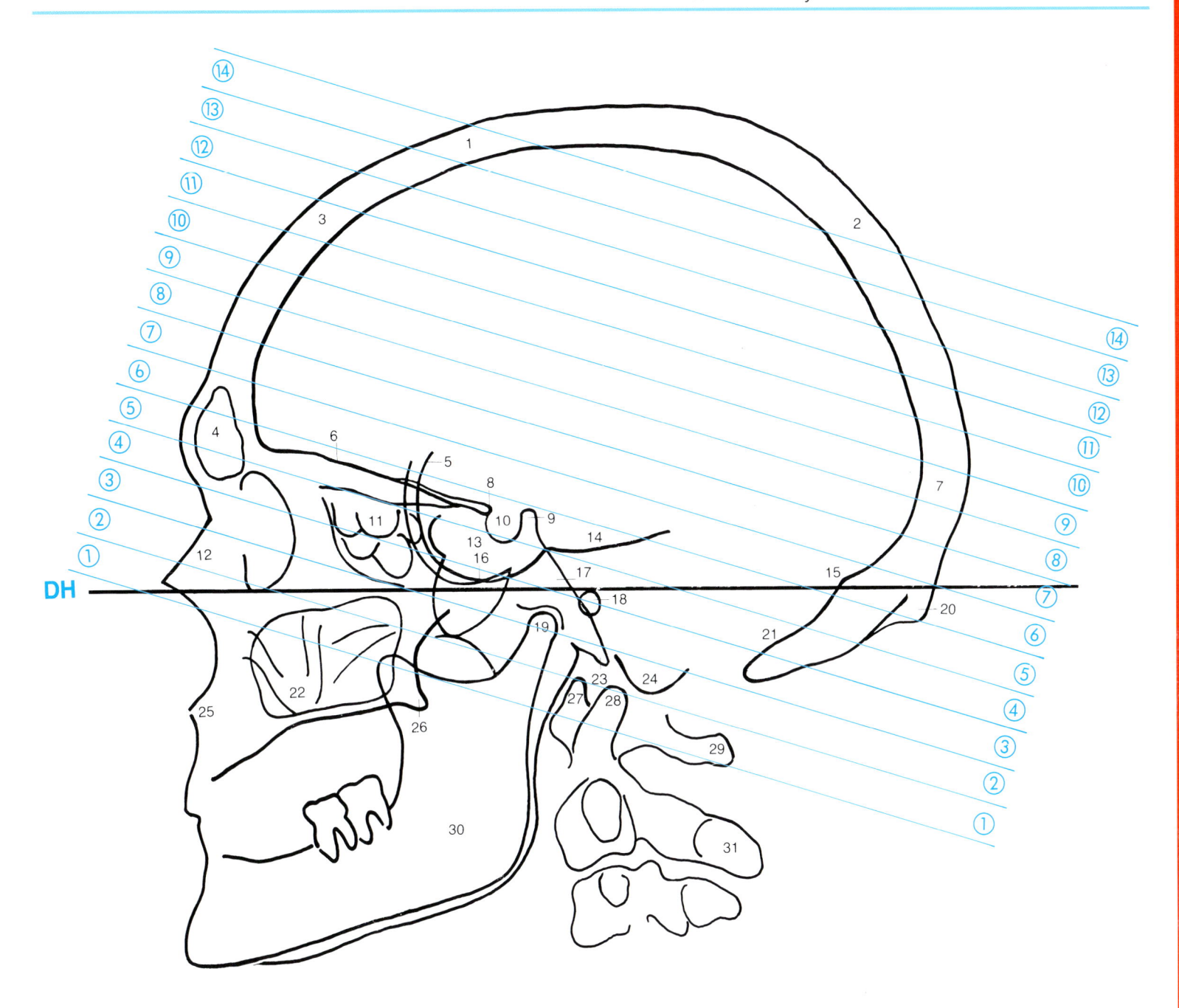

Fig. **45a** Tracing of the lateral radiograph of the same head demonstrated in Fig. 44. The 14 canthomeatally oriented slices were assembled in their original anatomic forms and numbered consecutively in an inferior to superior direction. The encircled number indicates the number of the slice. Technical data (Chap. 8).
DH Reid's base line

1 Bregma
2 Parietal bone
3 Frontal bone
4 Frontal sinus
5 Greater wing of sphenoid
6 Floor of anterior cranial fossa
7 Occipital bone
8 Anterior clinoid process
9 Dorsum sellae, posterior clinoid process
10 Sella turcica (hypophysial fossa)
11 Ethmoidal cells
12 Nasal bone
13 Sphenoidal sinus
14 Superior margin of petrous part of temporal bone
15 Internal occipital protuberance
16 Floor of middle cranial fossa
17 Clivus
18 External acoustic meatus
19 Head of mandible
20 External occipital protuberance (inion)
21 Floor of posterior cranial fossa
22 Maxillary sinus
23 Basion
24 Mastoid process
25 Anterior nasal spine
26 Posterior nasal spine
27 Anterior arch of atlas
28 Dens of axis
29 Posterior arch of atlas
30 Mandible
31 Spinous process of axis

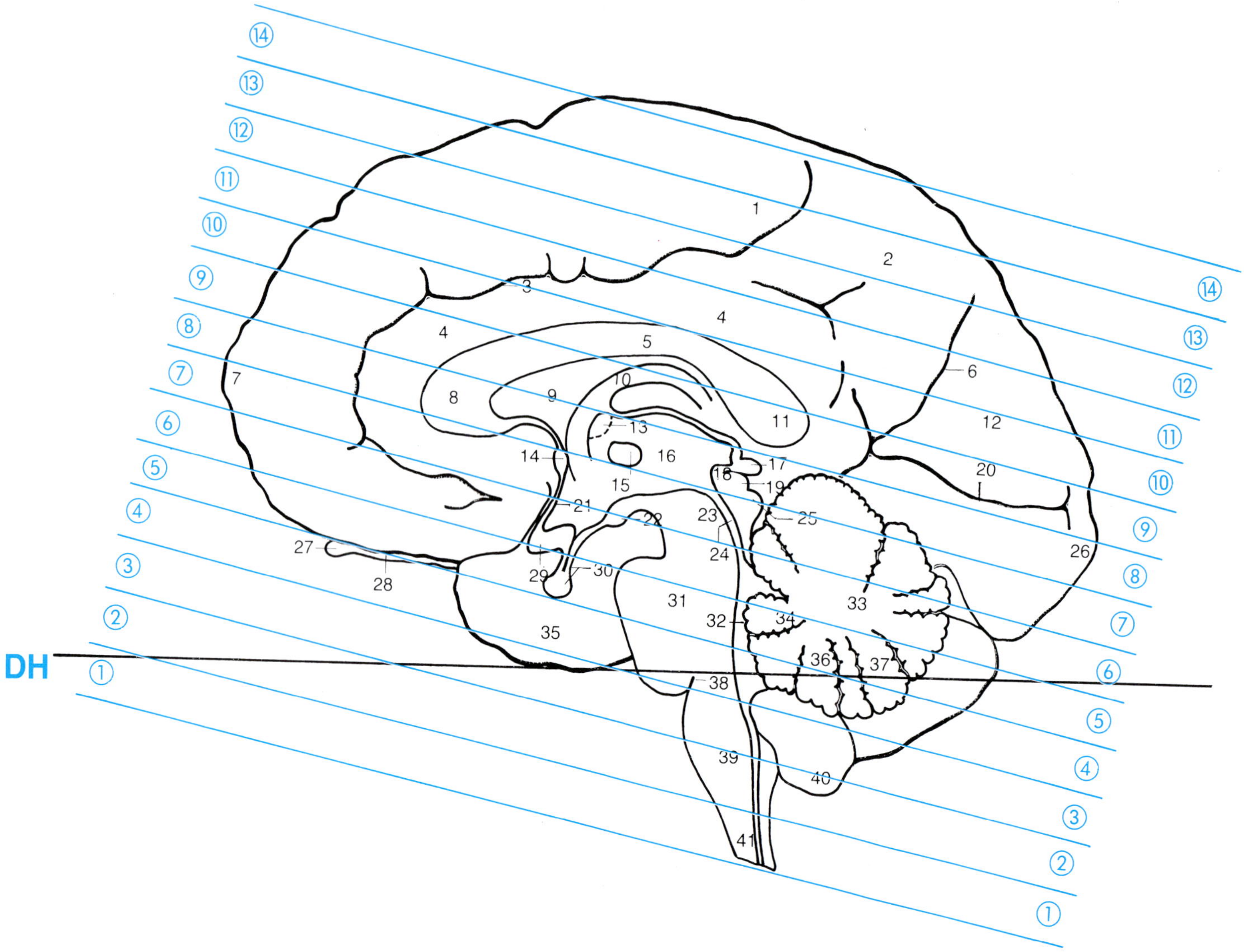

126 Atlas

Fig. **45b** Medial view of the brain of the same head as demonstrated in Fig. 45a (Chap. 8). The canthomeatally oriented slices were fitted back together and numbered as shown in Fig. 45a. DH Reid's base line

1 Paracentral lobule
2 Precuneus
3 Cingulate sulcus
4 Cingulate gyrus
5 Trunk (body) of corpus callosum
6 Parieto-occipital sulcus
7 Frontal pole
8 Genu of corpus callosum
9 Septum pellucidum
10 Fornix
11 Splenium of corpus callosum
12 Cuneus
13 Interventricular foramen (of Monro)
14 Anterior commissure
15 Interthalamic adhesion
16 Third ventricle
17 Pineal gland
18 Posterior commissure
19 Superior colliculus
20 Calcarine sulcus
21 Lamina terminalis
22 Mammillary body
23 Midbrain
24 Aqueduct of midbrain
25 Inferior colliculus
26 Occipital pole
27 Olfactory bulb
28 Olfactory tract
29 Optic chiasm
30 Infundibulum and pituitary gland
31 Pons
32 Fourth ventricle
33 Cerebellum
34 Nodule of vermis (X)
35 Temporal lobe
36 Uvula of vermis (IX)
37 Pyramis of vermis (VIII)
38 Foramen cecum
39 Medulla oblongata
40 Tonsil of cerebellum (H IX)
41 Spinal cord

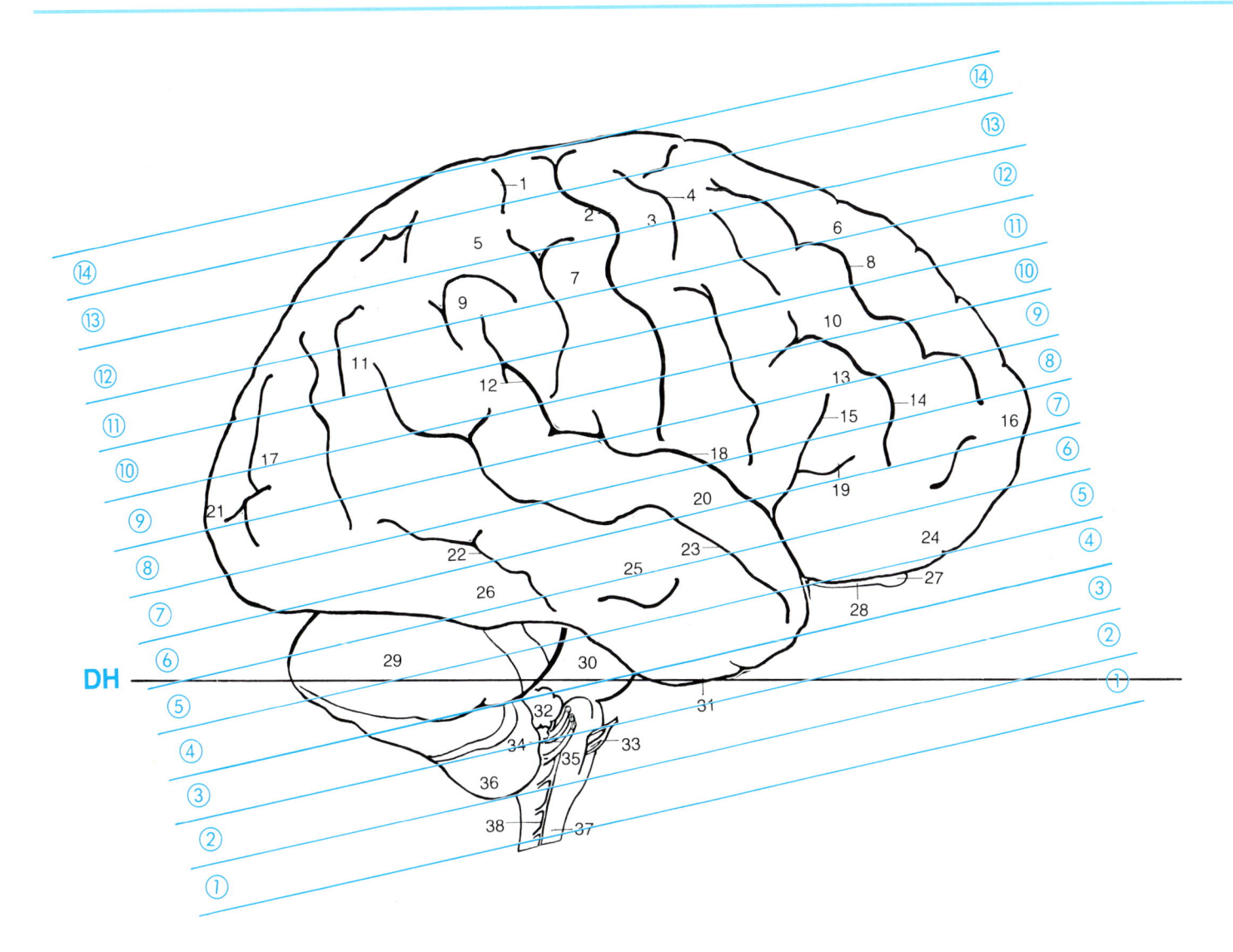

Fig. 46 Lateral view of the brain of the same head as demonstrated in Figs. 45a,b (Chap. 8). The canthomeatally oriented slices were fitted back together and numbered as shown in Fig. 45a.
DH Reid's base line

1 Postcentral sulcus
2 Central sulcus
3 Precentral gyrus
4 Precentral sulcus
5 Superior parietal lobule
6 Superior frontal gyrus
7 Postcentral gyrus
8 Superior frontal sulcus
9 Supramarginal gyrus
10 Middle frontal gyrus
11 Angular gyrus
12 Posterior ramus of lateral sulcus (Sylvian fissure)
13 Inferior frontal gyrus
14 Inferior frontal sulcus
15 Ascending ramus of lateral sulcus (Sylvian fissure)
16 Frontal pole
17 Occipital gyri
18 Lateral sulcus (Sylvian fissure)
19 Anterior ramus of lateral sulcus (Sylvian fissure)
20 Superior temporal gyrus
21 Occipital pole
22 Inferior temporal sulcus
23 Superior temporal sulcus
24 Orbital gyri
25 Middle temporal gyrus
26 Inferior temporal gyrus
27 Olfactory bulb
28 Olfactory tract
29 Cerebellum
30 Pons
31 Base of temporal lobe
32 Flocculus (H X)
33 Hypoglossal nerve
34 Glossopharyngeal nerve, vagus nerve, accessory nerve
35 Medulla oblongata
36 Tonsil of cerebellum (H IX)
37 Spinal cord
38 Spinal root of accessory nerve

128   Atlas

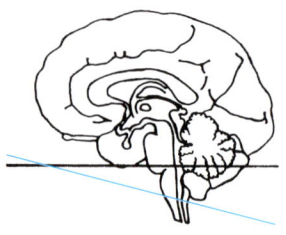

1 Nasal bone
2 Nasal septum
3 Maxilla
4 Orbit
5 Zygomatic bone
6 Infraorbital canal
7 Maxillary sinus
8 Palatine bone
9 Lateral pterygoid plate
10 Mandible
11 Internal carotid artery
12 Styloid process
13 Internal jugular vein
14 Anterior arch of atlas
15 Dens of axis
16 Occipital condyle
17 Lateral mass of atlas
18 Auricle (pinna)
19 Anterior median fissure
20 Anterior (ventral) root of first cervical spinal nerve
21 Spinal cord
22 Posterior (dorsal) funiculus
23 Spinal root of accessory nerve
24 Vertebral artery, V3 segment
25 Spinal dura mater
26 Posterior arch of atlas

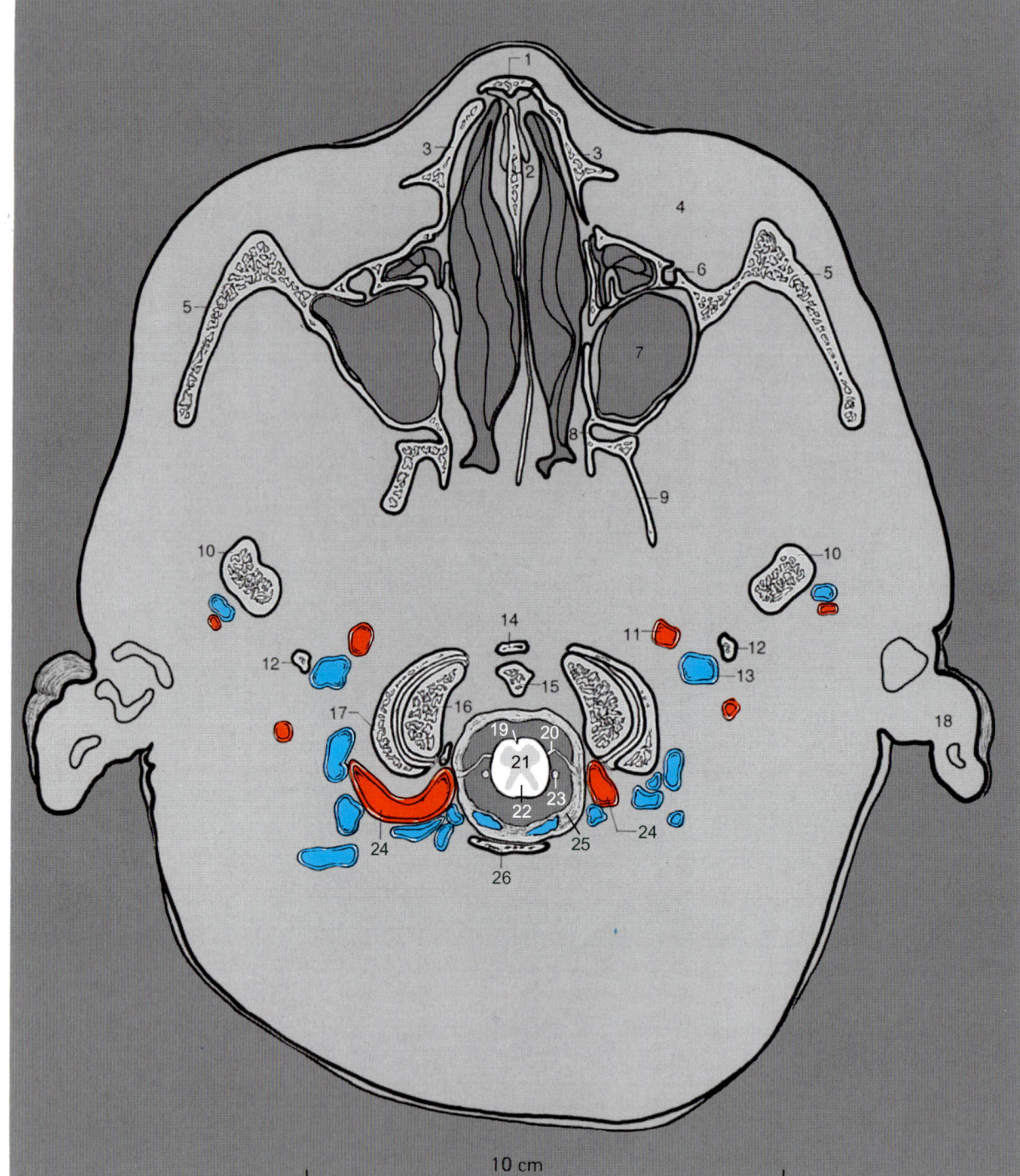

Fig. **47a** View of the superior surface of the first slice of the canthomeatal series. In the upper left corner the blue line demonstrates the sectional plane through the spinal cord (Fig. 45b). Spinal cord and spinal nerves, bony structures and blood vessels.

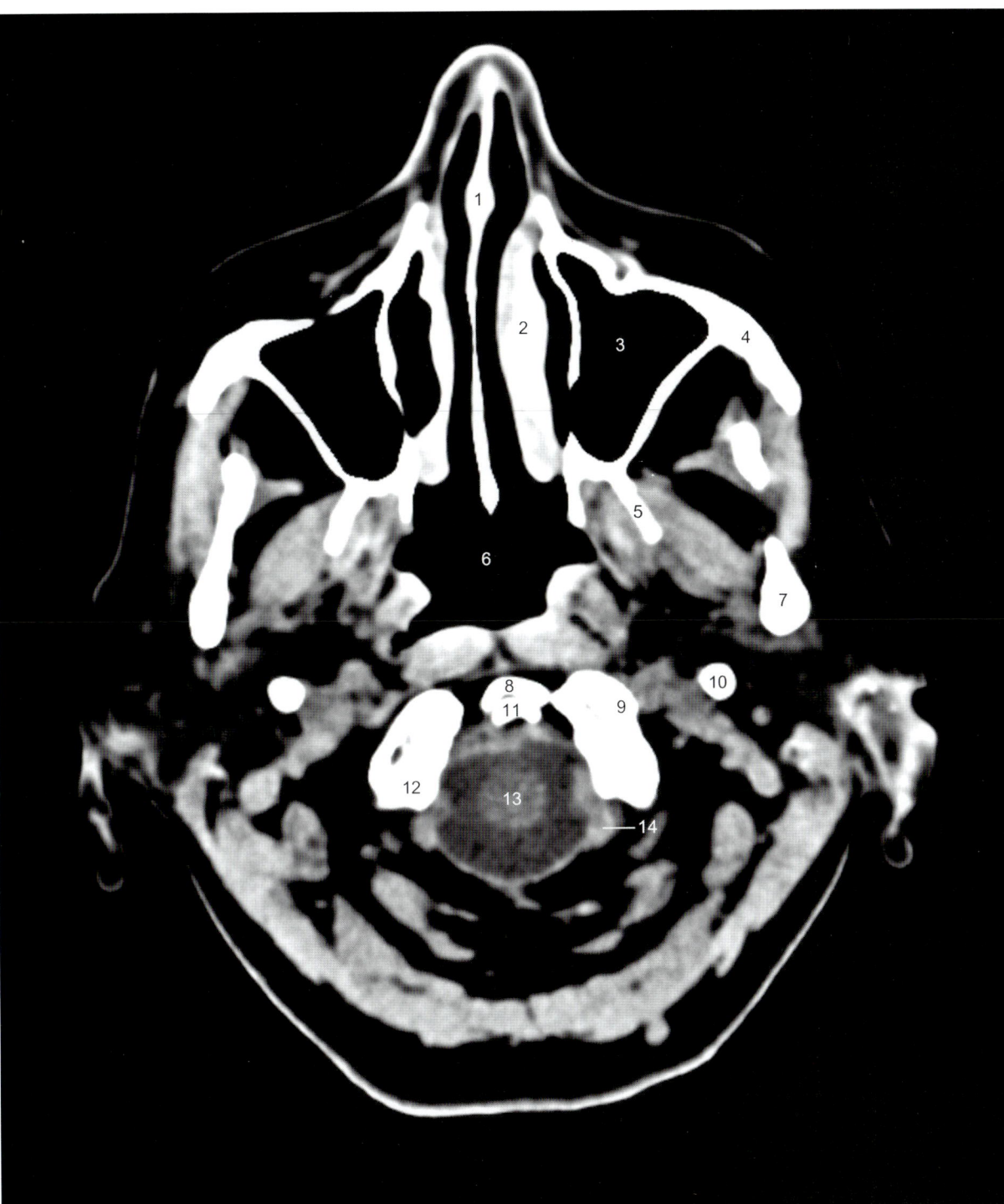

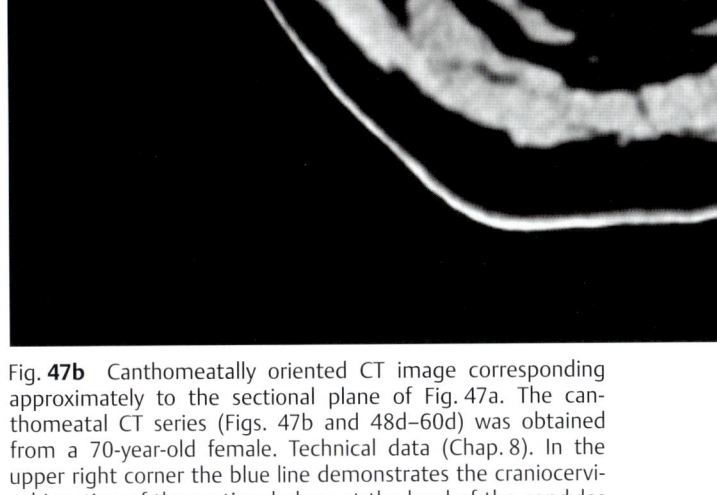

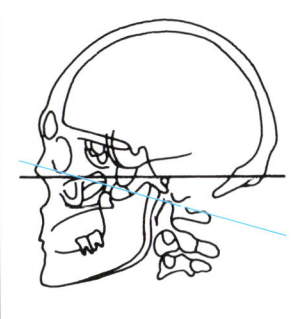

Canthomeatally Oriented Slices

1 Nasal septum
2 Inferior nasal concha
3 Maxillary sinus
4 Zygomatic bone
5 Lateral pterygoid plate
6 Nasopharynx
7 Mandible
8 Anterior arch of atlas
9 Lateral mass of atlas
10 Styloid process
11 Dens of axis (cut)
12 Occipital condyle
13 Spinal cord
14 Vertebral artery (entry into subarachnoid space)

Fig. **47b** Canthomeatally oriented CT image corresponding approximately to the sectional plane of Fig. 47a. The canthomeatal CT series (Figs. 47b and 48d–60d) was obtained from a 70-year-old female. Technical data (Chap. 8). In the upper right corner the blue line demonstrates the craniocervical junction of the sectional plane at the level of the condyles and the atlas (Fig. 45a).

130 Atlas

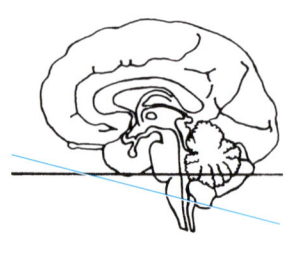

1 Eyeball
2 Anterior median fissure
3 Pyramid of medulla oblongata
4 Inferior olivary nucleus
5 Hypoglossal nerve
6 Spinal root of accessory nerve
7 Gracile tubercle
8 Cuneate tubercle
9 Tonsil of cerebellum (H IX)
10 Dura mater

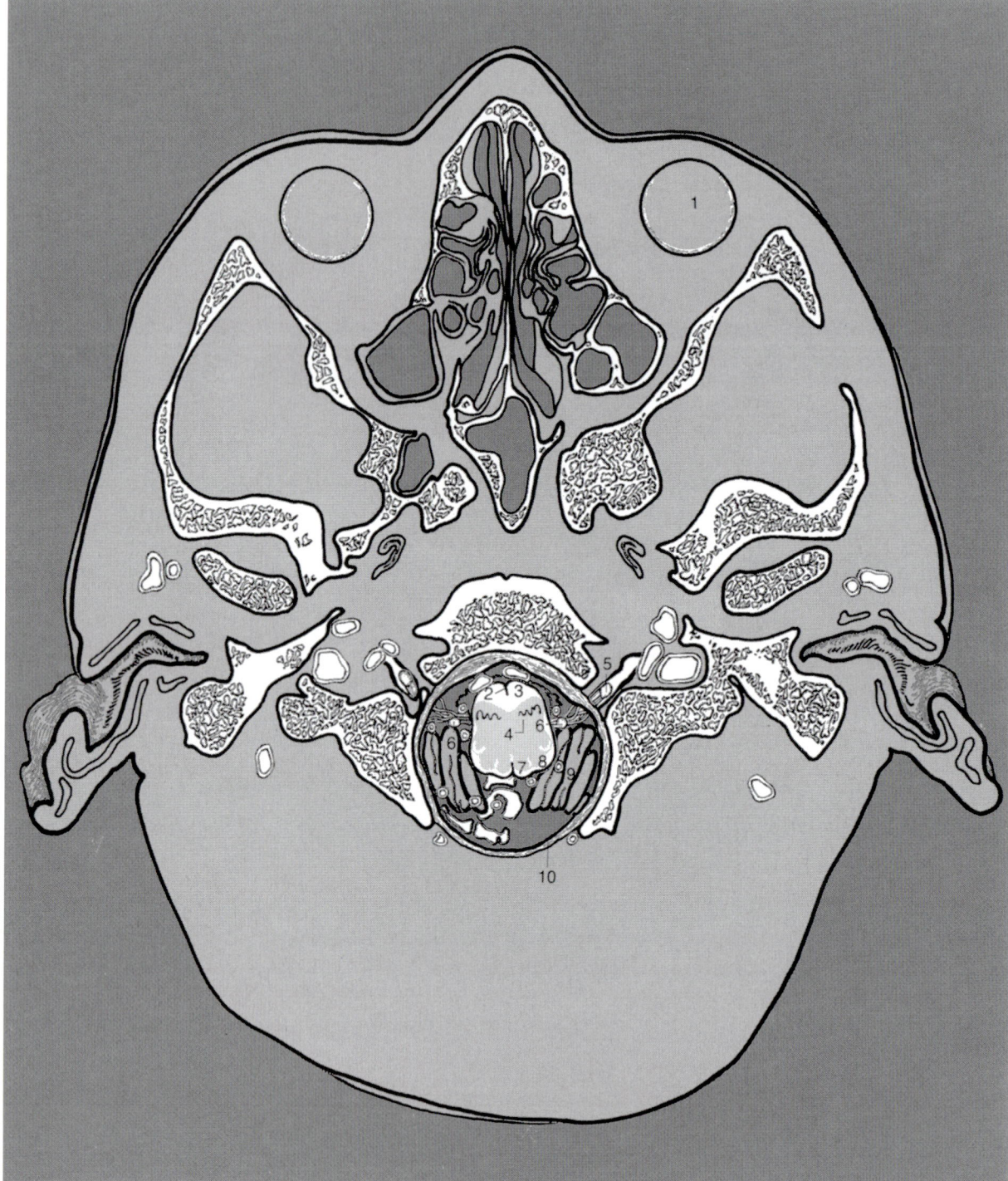

Fig. 48a Superior section surface of the second canthomeatally oriented slice depicting brain structures and meninges. The posterior cranial fossa is cut just above the foramen magnum. The medulla oblongata and cerebellar tonsils are dissected.

Canthomeatally Oriented Slices

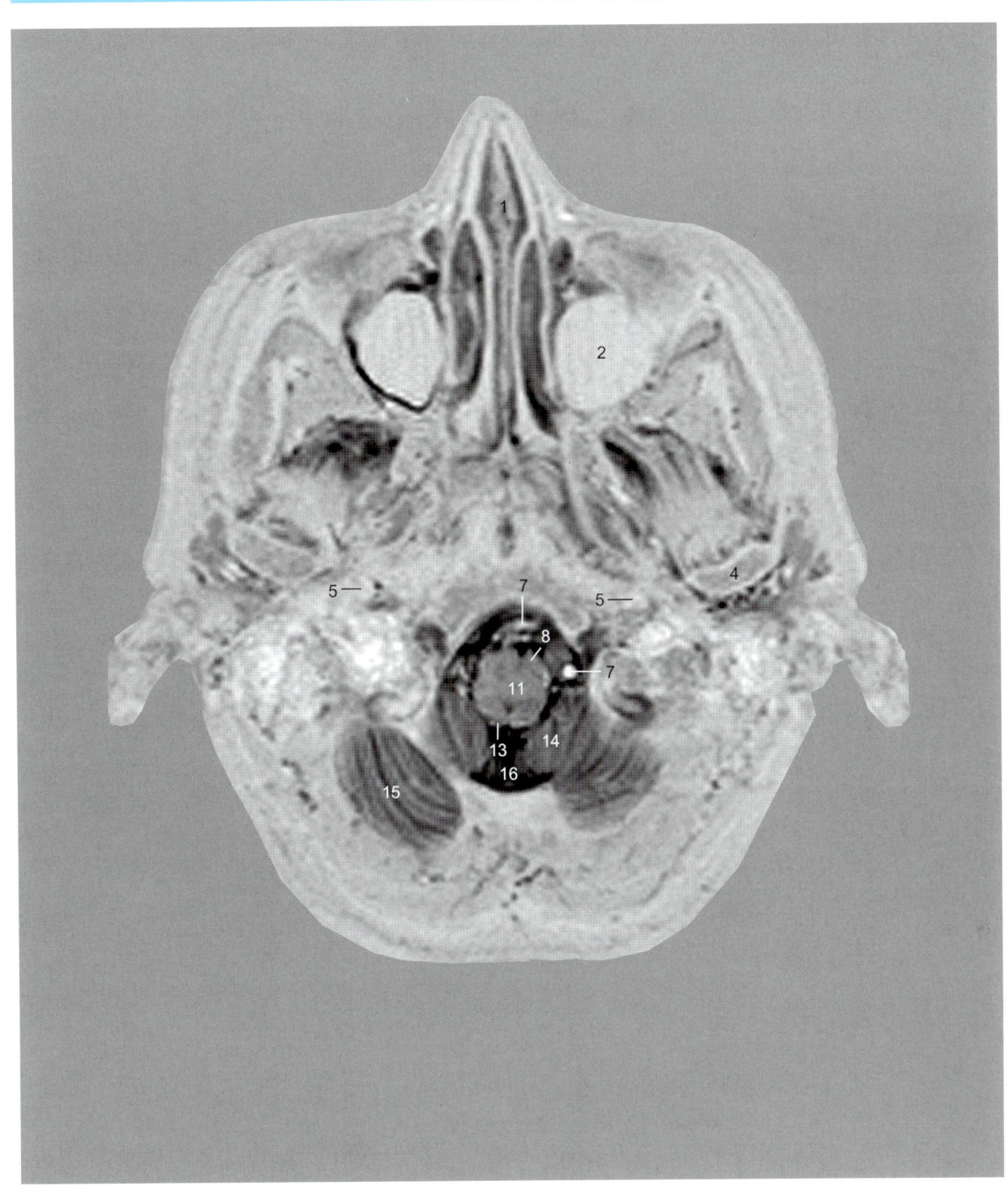

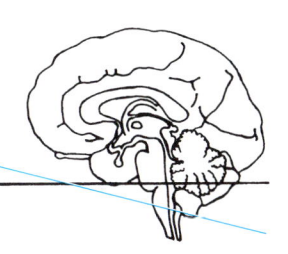

1 Nasal septum
2 Maxillary sinus
4 Mandible
5 Internal carotid artery
7 Vertebral artery
8 Pyramid of medulla oblongata
11 Medulla oblongata
13 Gracile tubercle
14 Tonsil of cerebellum (H IX)
15 Hemisphere of cerebellum (cut)
16 Cisterna magna (posterior cerebellomedullary cistern)

Fig. **48b** Canthomeatally oriented, T1-weighted MR image (Turbo-Inversion-Recovery-Sequence) corresponding closely to the sectional plane of Figs. 48a and 48c. The selected sequence emphasizes the brain structures and suppresses the surrounding soft tissues. The canthomeatally oriented MR series was obtained from a 38-year-old female. A missing number with its label indicates here and in the following legends of MR images that this number can be found in the other corresponding CT images. See following page (Fig. 48d). Technical data (Chap. 8).

Special note: These and the following MR and CT images (Figs. 48b–60b and 48d–60d) taken from the canthomeatal series were obtained from two different individuals.

Atlas

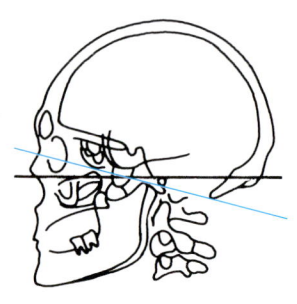

1 Nasal bone
2 Nasal septum
3 Zygomatic bone
4 Ethmoidal cells
5 Orbit
6 Maxillary sinus
7 Zygomatic arch
8 Sphenoidal sinus
9 Cartilage of pharyngotympanic tube
10 Mandible
11 Basilar part of occipital bone
12 Internal carotid artery
13 Internal jugular vein
14 Floor of external acoustic meatus
15 Vertebral artery
16 Hypoglossal canal
17 Mastoid process
18 Posterior inferior cerebellar artery (PICA)
19 Auricle (pinna)
20 Foramen magnum

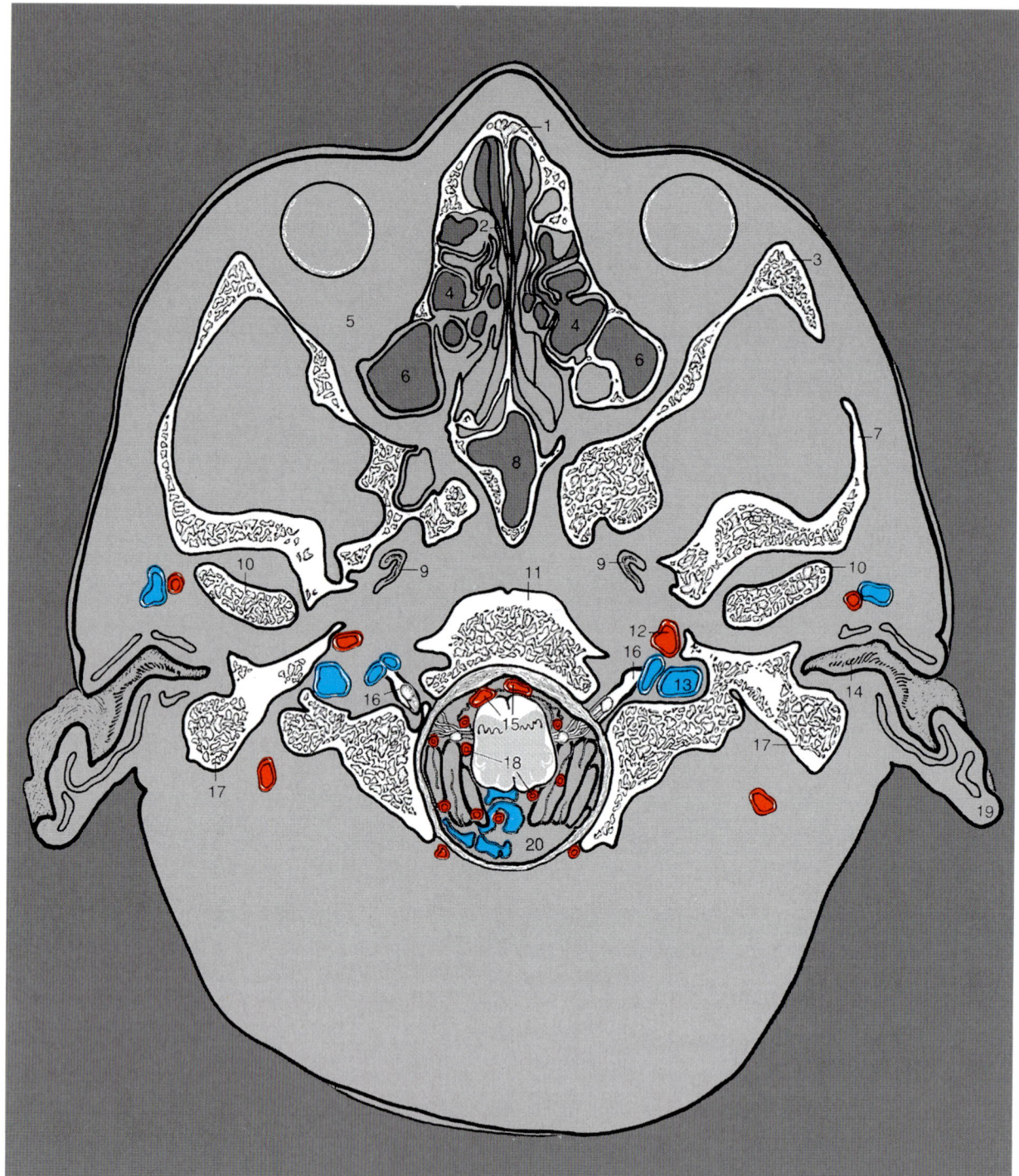

Fig. **48c** Superior section surface of the second canthomeatally oriented slice revealing bony structures and blood vessels. The sectional plane runs diagonally to the foramen magnum (see text) at the level of the hypoglossal canal. The floor of the lateral portion of the external acoustic meatus is cut horizontally.

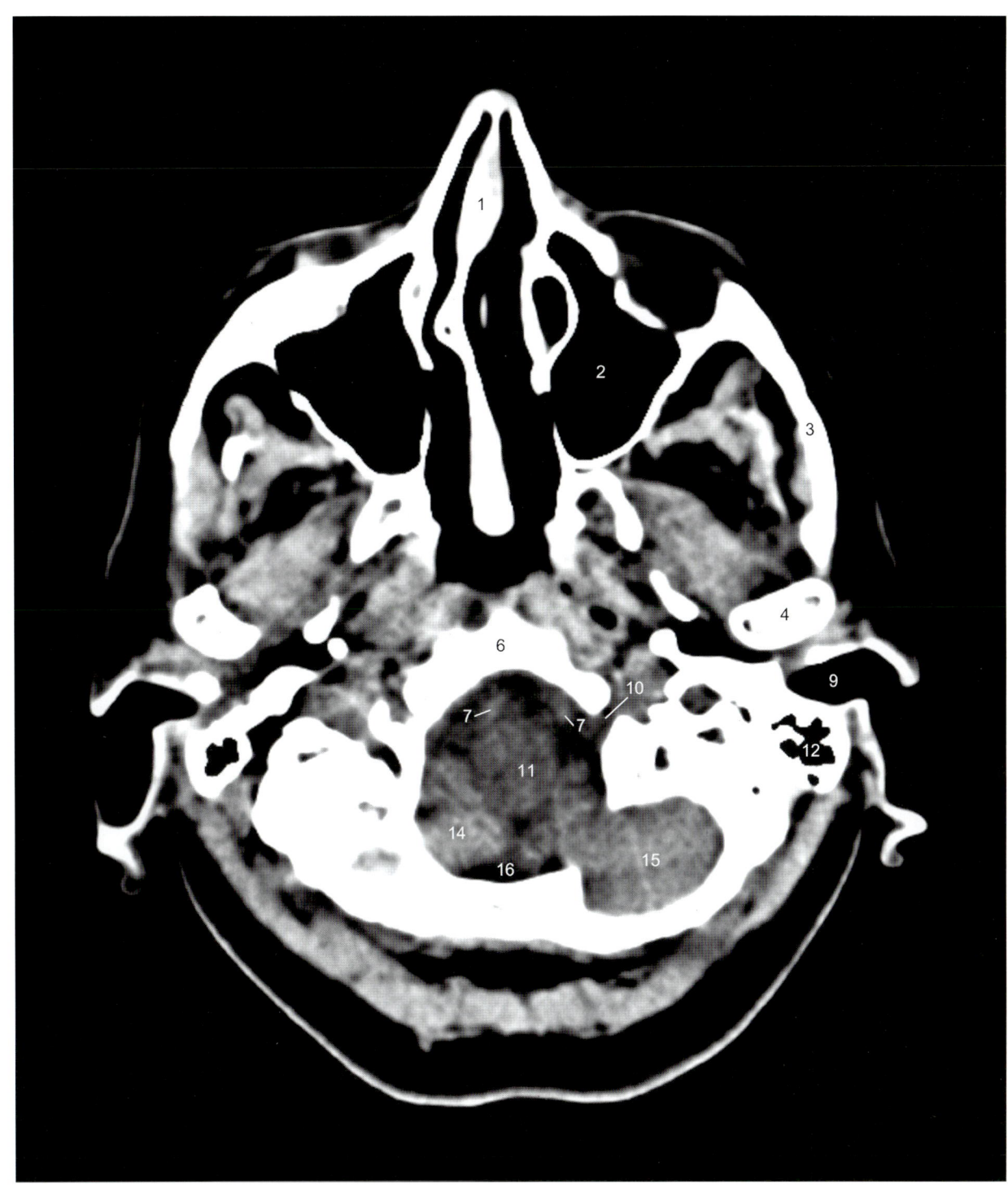

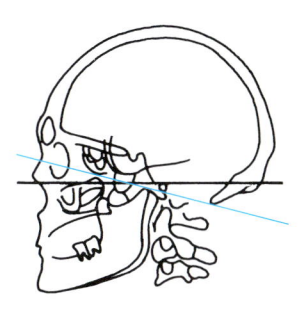

Canthomeatally Oriented Slices

1 Nasal septum
2 Maxillary sinus
3 Zygomatic arch
4 Mandible
6 Basilar part of occipital bone
7 Vertebral artery
9 External acoustic meatus
10 Hypoglossal canal
11 Medulla oblongata
12 Mastoid cells
14 Tonsil of cerebellum (H IX)
15 Hemisphere of cerebellum (cut)
16 Cisterna magna (posterior cerebellomedullary cistern)

Fig. **48d** Canthomeatally oriented CT image of a 70-year-old female corrresponding closely to Figs. 48a and 48c. A missing number with its label indicates here and in the following legends of CT images that this number can be found in the other corresponding MR image. See previous page (Fig. 48b).

134 Atlas

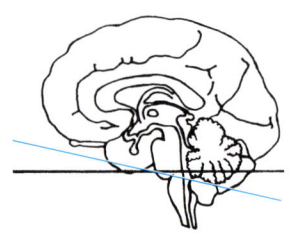

1 Eyeball
2 Optic nerve
3 Base of temporal lobe
4 Maxillary nerve and mandibular nerve
5 Abducens nerve
6 Pons
7 Foramen cecum
8 Inferior olivary nucleus
9 Glossopharyngeal nerve and vagus nerve
10 Accessory nerve
11 Spinal root of accessory nerve
12 Flocculus (H X)
13 Facial nerve
14 Medulla oblongata
15 Cuneate tubercle
16 Gracile tubercle
17 Tonsil of cerebellum (H IX)
18 Hemisphere of posterior lobe of cerebellum
19 Dura mater

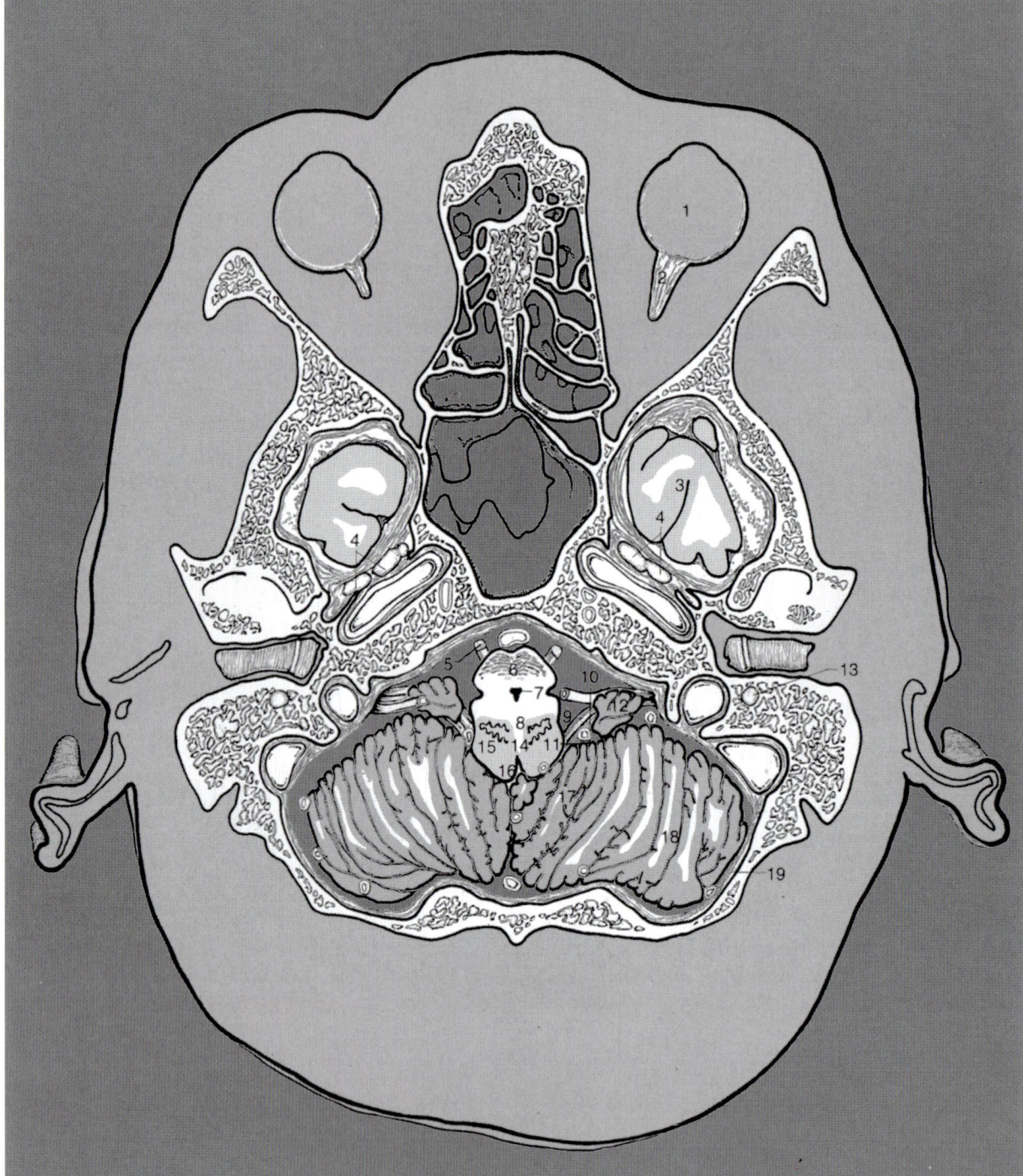

Fig. **49a** Superior section surface of the third canthomeatally oriented slice revealing brain structures and meninges. The sectional plane intersects the middle of the eyeballs and the base of both temporal lobes and cuts diagonally through the border between pons and medulla oblongata. The facial nerve is cut in the bony canal of the petrous part of the temporal bone.

Canthomeatally Oriented Slices

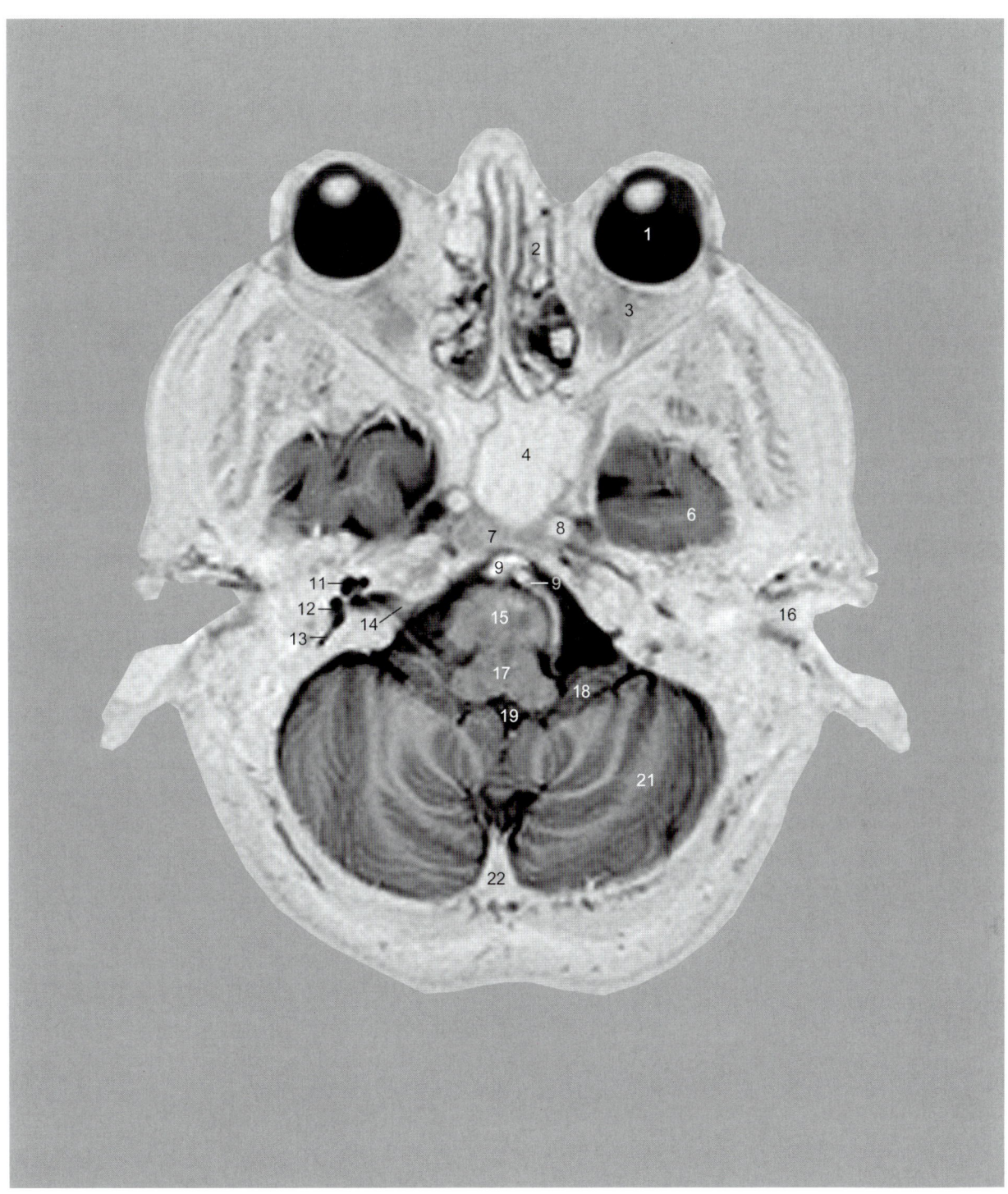

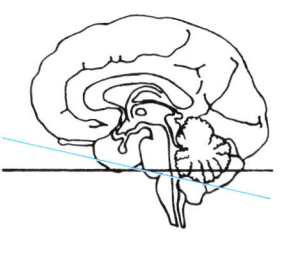

1 Lens within eyeball
2 Ethmoidal cells
3 Retrobulbar space
4 Sphenoidal sinus
6 Base of temporal lobe
7 Clivus
8 Internal carotid artery
9 Vertebral artery (Var.)
11 Cochlea
12 Vestibule
13 Posterior semicircular canal
14 Internal acoustic meatus
15 Pons
16 External acoustic meatus
17 Medulla oblongata
18 Flocculus (H X)
19 Fourth ventricle
21 Hemisphere of posterior lobe of cerebellum
22 Occipital sinus

Fig. **49b** Canthomeatally oriented, T1-weighted MR image corresponding closely to the sectional plane of Figs. 49a and 49c. The canthomeatally oriented MR series was obtained from a 38-year-old female.

136   Atlas

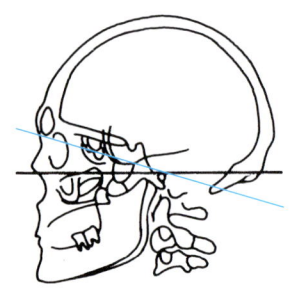

1 Ethmoidal cells
2 Zygomatic bone
3 Ethmoid
4 Orbit
5 Sphenoid
6 Frontal branch of middle
   meningeal artery
7 Sphenoidal sinus
8 Temporal bone
9 Internal carotid artery
10 Clivus
11 Basilar artery
12 Tympanic cavity
13 Tympanic membrane
14 External acoustic meatus
15 Anterior inferior cerebellar
   artery (AICA)
16 Jugular foramen
17 Internal jugular vein
18 Facial canal
19 Sigmoid sinus
20 Mastoid cells
21 Auricle (pinna)
22 Occipital sinus
23 Occipital bone

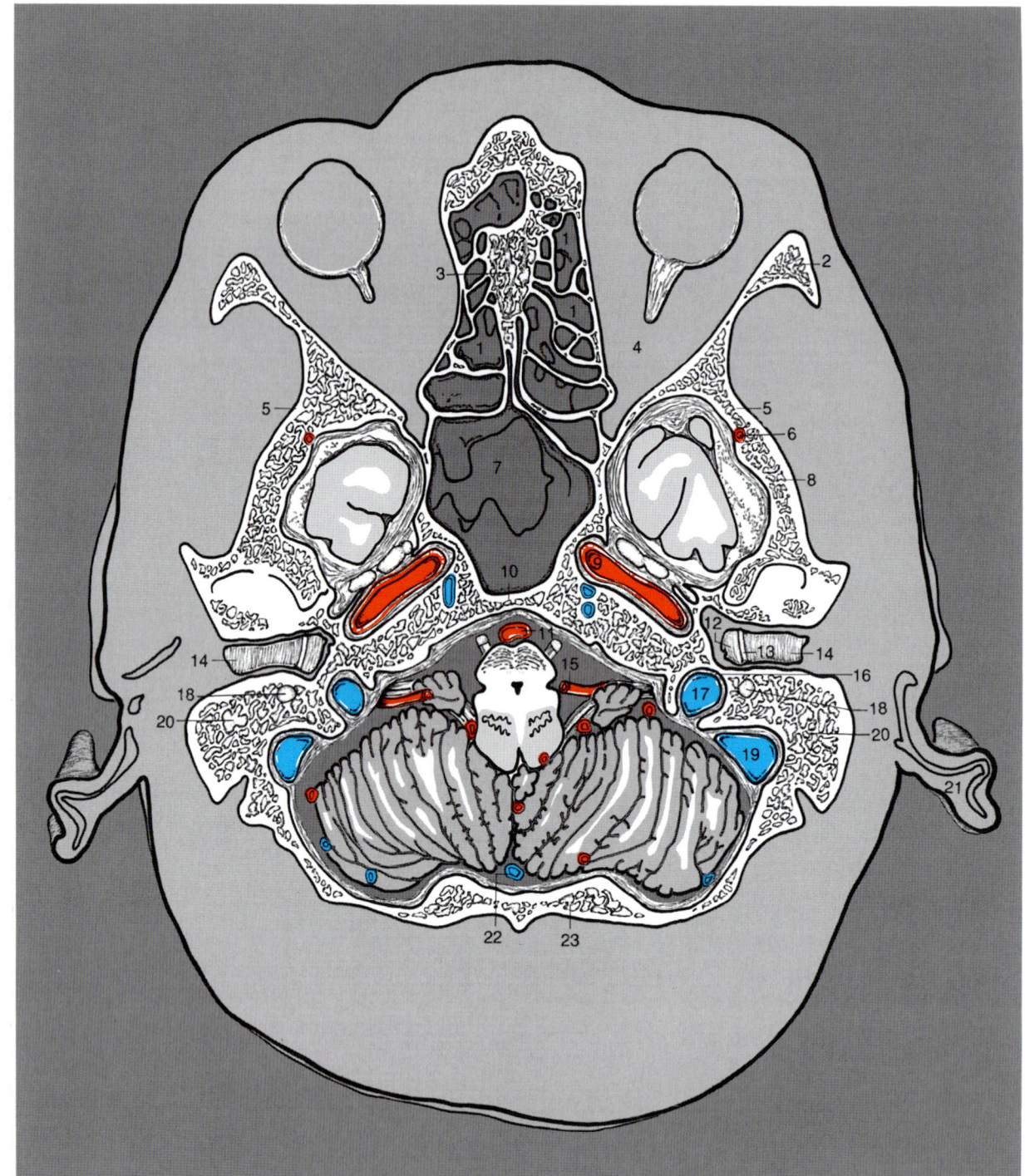

Fig. **49c** Superior section surface of the third canthomeatally oriented slice showing bony structures and blood vessels. The sectional plane runs through the middle of the eyeballs and medial portion of the external acoustic meatus. This corresponds to the canthomeatal plane. The floor of the middle cranial fossa lies in the section just below the sectional plane. The radiograph of this section shows the foramen ovale and the foramen spinosum (Figs. 63.8 and 63.11).

Canthomeatally Oriented Slices

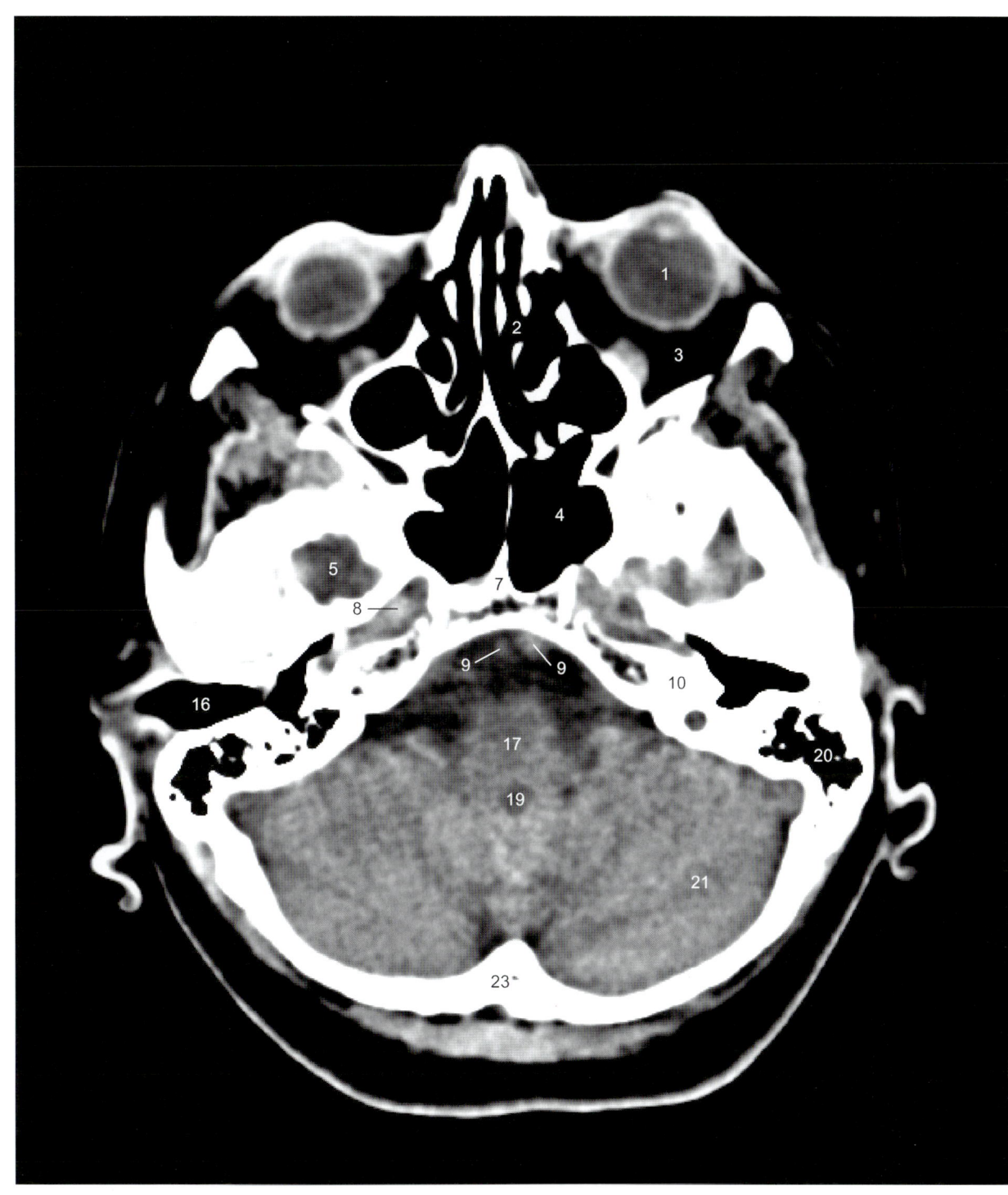

1 Eyeball with lens
2 Ethmoidal cells
3 Retrobulbar space
4 Sphenoidal sinus
5 Base of middle cranial fossa
7 Clivus
8 Internal carotid artery
9 Vertebral artery
10 Petrous part of temporal bone
16 External acoustic meatus
17 Medulla oblongata
19 Fourth ventricle
20 Mastoid cells
21 Hemisphere of posterior lobe of cerebellum
23 Occipital bone

Fig. **49d** Canthomeatally oriented CT image of a 70-year-old female corresponding closely to the sectional plane of Figs. 49a and 49c.

138 Atlas

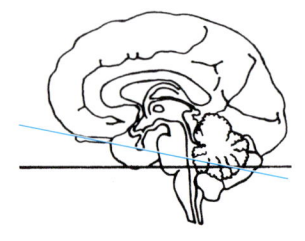

1 Eyeball
2 Straight gyrus
3 Olfactory bulb
4 Olfactory tract
5 Optic nerve
6 Temporal lobe
7 Pituitary gland
8 Inferior temporal gyrus
9 Abducens nerve
10 Trigeminal nerve near the opening of trigeminal cave
11 Abducens nerve near opening of dura mater
12 Basilar sulcus
13 Pons
14 Facial nerve and intermediate nerve
15 Vestibulocochlear nerve
16 Fourth ventricle
17 Middle cerebellar peduncle
18 Uvula of vermis (IX)
19 Vermis of cerebellum
20 Hemisphere of posterior lobe of cerebellum
21 Dura mater

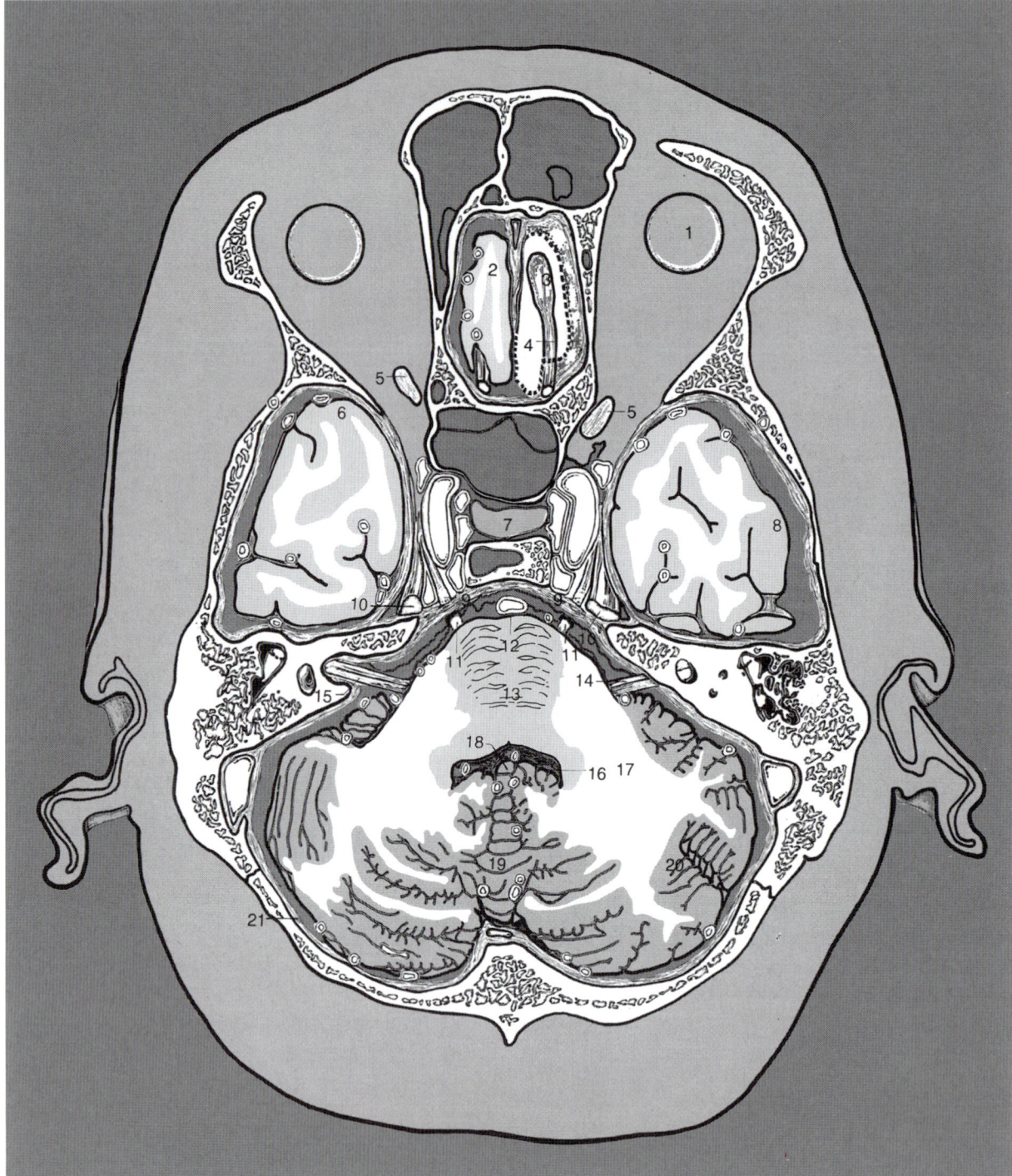

Fig. **50a** Superior section surface of the fourth canthomeatally oriented slice representing brain structures and meninges. The frontal cortex covering the right half of the anterior cranial fossa was removed to demonstrate the olfactory bulb and tract. These parts of the olfactory system are illustrated in the olfactory groove. The temporal lobes are shown in the middle cranial fossa. The pons and cerebellum are seen in the posterior cranial fossa.

Canthomeatally Oriented Slices 139

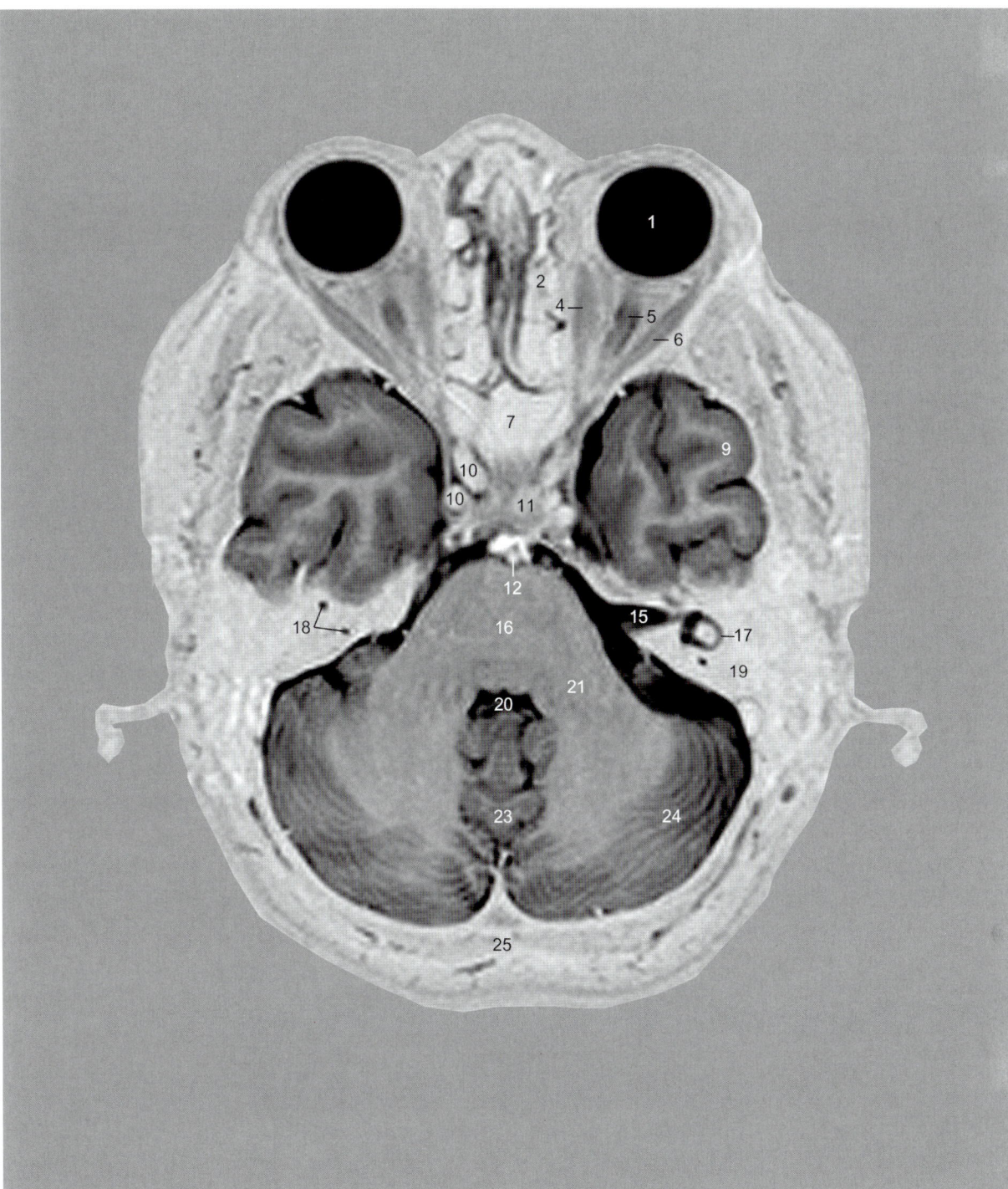

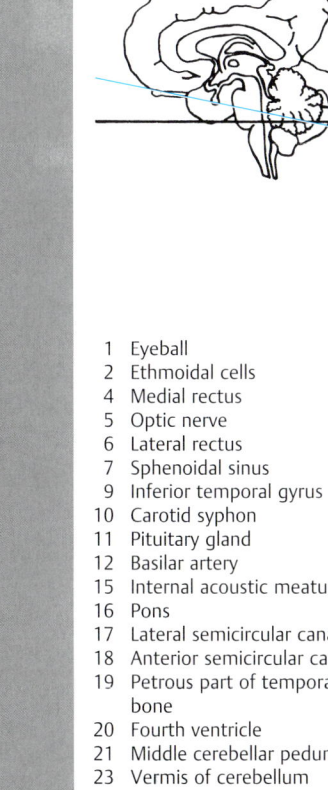

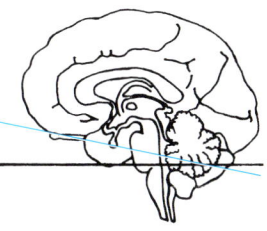

1 Eyeball
2 Ethmoidal cells
4 Medial rectus
5 Optic nerve
6 Lateral rectus
7 Sphenoidal sinus
9 Inferior temporal gyrus
10 Carotid syphon
11 Pituitary gland
12 Basilar artery
15 Internal acoustic meatus
16 Pons
17 Lateral semicircular canal
18 Anterior semicircular canal
19 Petrous part of temporal bone
20 Fourth ventricle
21 Middle cerebellar peduncle
23 Vermis of cerebellum
24 Hemisphere of posterior lobe of cerebellum
25 Occipital bone

Fig. **50b** Canthomeatally oriented, T1-weighted MR image corresponding approximately to the sectional plane of Figs. 50a and 50c. The canthomeatally oriented MR series was obtained from a 38-year-old female.

140 Atlas

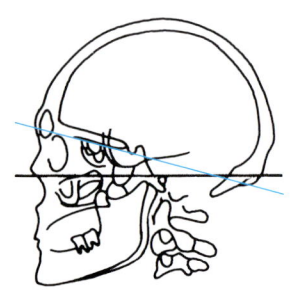

1 Frontal bone
2 Frontal sinus
3 Crista galli
4 Orbit
5 Sphenoid
6 Superior orbital fissure
7 Frontal branch of middle meningeal artery
8 Sphenoidal sinus
9 Cavernous sinus
10 Internal carotid artery
11 Dorsum sellae (cut)
12 Basilar artery
13 Malleus (hammer)
14 Incus (anvil)
15 Internal acoustic opening
16 Tympanic cavity
17 Anterior semicircular canal
18 Anterior inferior cerebellar artery (AICA)
19 Temporal bone
20 Sigmoid sinus
21 Auricle (pinna)
22 Lambdoid suture
23 Occipital sinus
24 Occipital bone

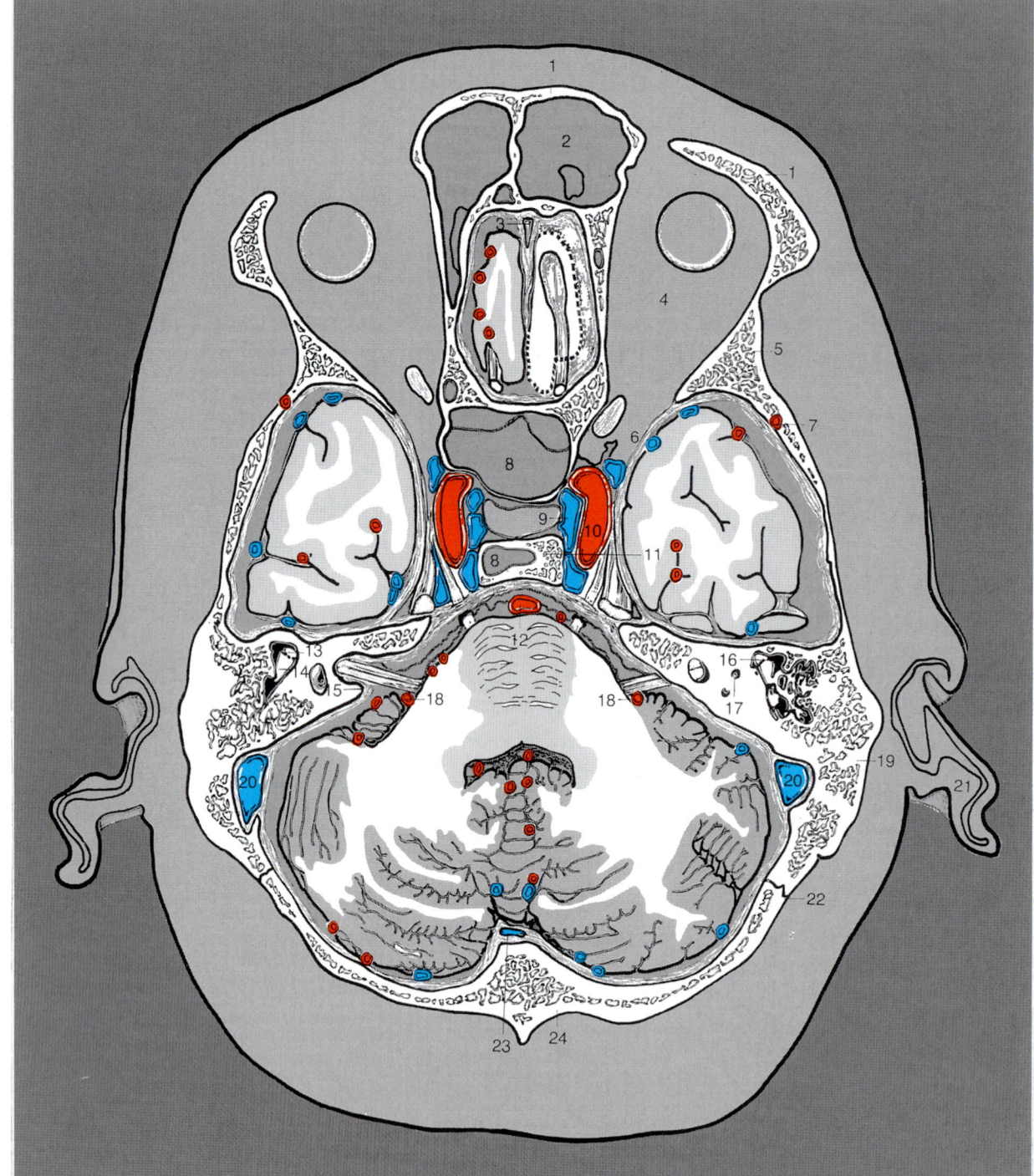

Fig. **50c** Superior section surface of the fourth canthomeatally oriented slice showing bony structures and blood vessels. The recess in the anterior cranial fossa in the region of the cribriform plate is cut with basal portions of the telencephalon. The sectional plane cuts through the sella turcica and dissects the dorsum sellae. The posterior cranial fossa is shown with the internal acoustic meatus.

Canthomeatally Oriented Slices

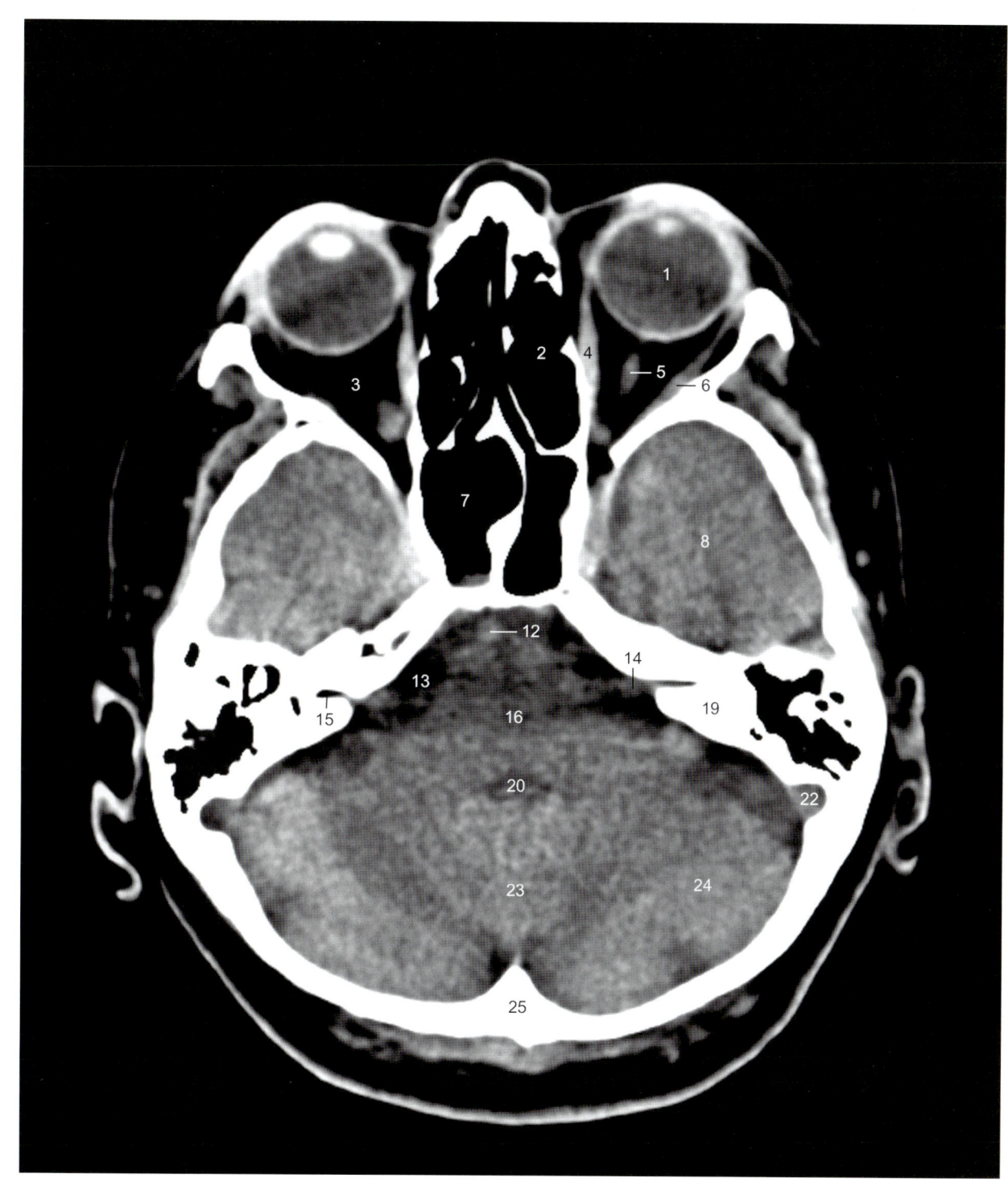

1 Eyeball
2 Ethmoidal cells
3 Retrobulbar space
4 Medial rectus
5 Optic nerve (tangentially cut)
6 Lateral rectus
7 Sphenoidal sinus
8 Temporal lobe
12 Basilar artery
13 Cerebellopontine cistern
14 Vestibulocochlear nerve, facial nerve
15 Internal acoustic meatus
16 Pons
19 Petrous part of temporal bone
20 Fourth ventricle
22 Sigmoid sinus
23 Vermis of cerebellum
24 Hemisphere of posterior lobe of cerebellum
25 Occipital bone

Fig. **50d** Canthomeatally oriented CT image corresponding to the sectional plane of Figs. 50a and 50c. The canthomeatally oriented CT series was obtained from a 70-year-old female. Slight deviations can be seen in the anterior cranial fossa and the sella turcica.

142   Atlas

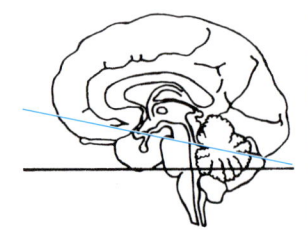

1 Falx cerebri
2 Orbital gyri
3 Straight gyrus
4 Superior temporal gyrus
5 Olfactory sulcus
6 Middle temporal gyrus
7 Olfactory tract
8 Optic chiasm
9 Infundibulum
10 Posterior clinoid process (covered)
11 Oculomotor nerve
12 Amygdaloid body
13 Temporal (inferior) horn of lateral ventricle
14 Hippocampus
15 Parahippocampal gyrus
16 Trochlear nerve
17 Inferior temporal gyrus
18 Pons
19 Tentorium of cerebellum
20 Cerulean nucleus
21 Fourth ventricle
22 Superior cerebellar peduncle
23 Fastigial nucleus
24 Dentate nucleus
25 Vermis of cerebellum
26 Falx cerebelli
27 Dura mater

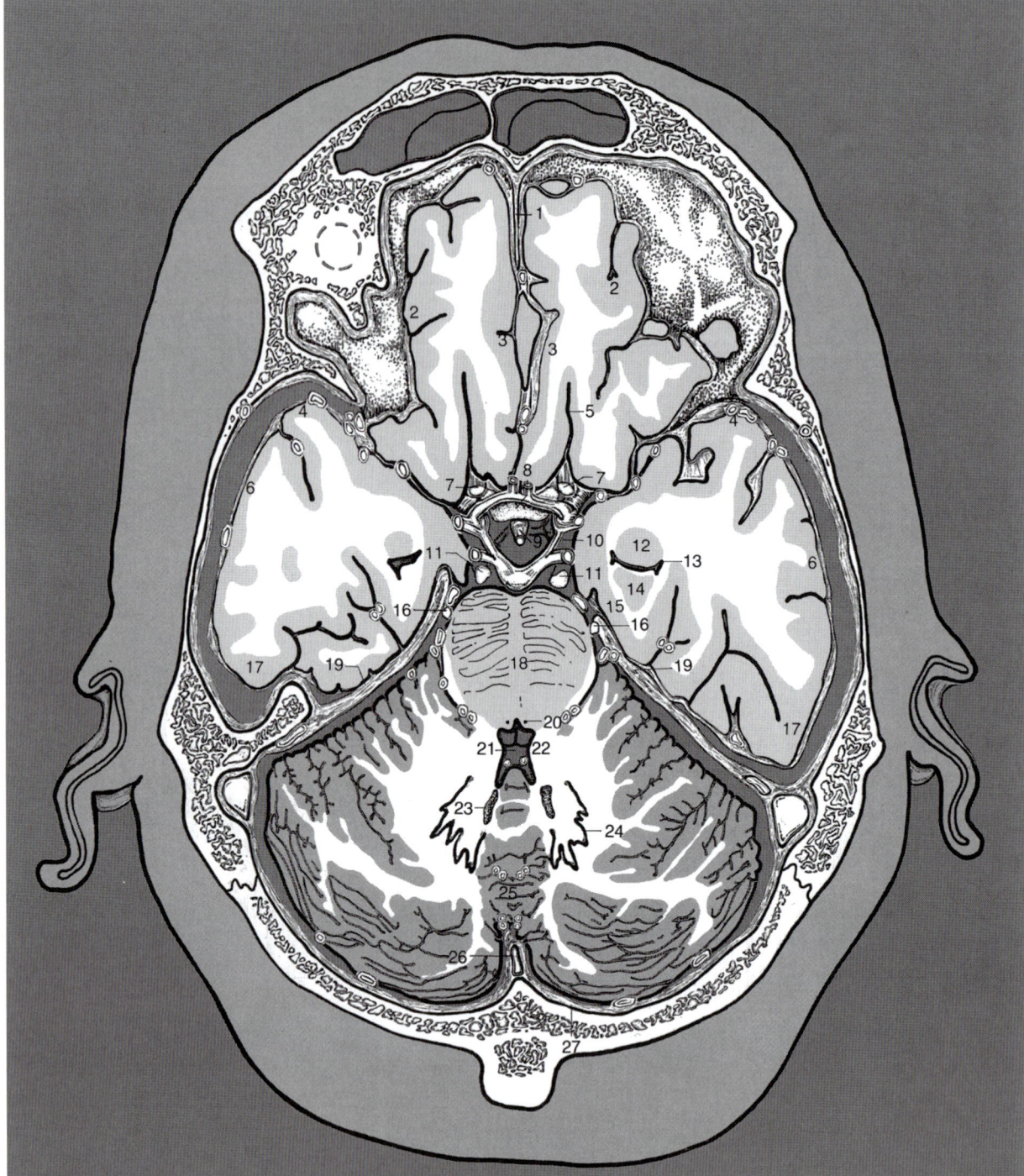

Fig. **51a** Superior section surface of the fifth canthomeatally oriented slice depicting brain structures and meninges. The sectional plane lies at the level of the entrance to the sella. The frontal and temporal lobes, infundibulum, pons, and cerebellum are shown.

Canthomeatally Oriented Slices

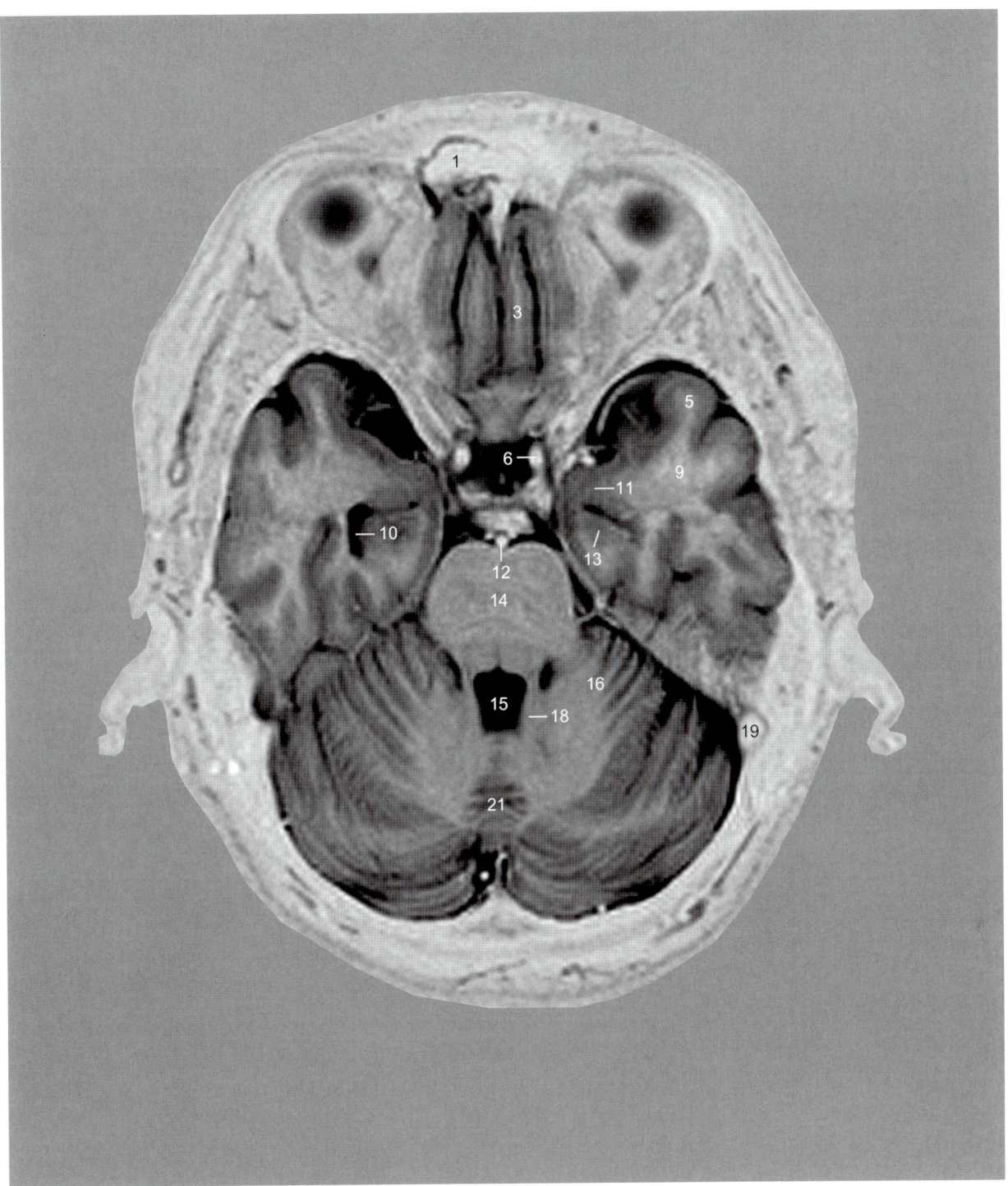

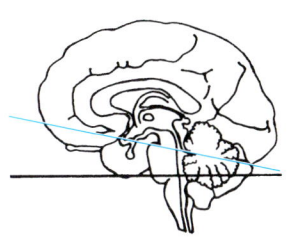

1 Frontal sinus
3 Straight gyrus
5 Superior temporal gyrus
6 Internal carotid artery
9 Temporal lobe
10 Temporal (inferior) horn of lateral ventricle
11 Amygdaloid body
12 Basilar artery
13 Hippocampus
14 Pons
15 Fourth ventricle
16 Anterior lobe of cerebellum
18 Superior cerebellar peduncle
19 Sigmoid sinus
21 Vermis of cerebellum

Fig. **51b** Canthomeatally oriented, T1-weighted MR image positioned slightly below the sectional plane of Figs. 51a and 51c.

144 Atlas

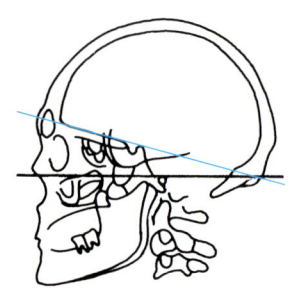

1 Frontal bone
2 Frontal sinus
3 Opened orbit
4 Anterior cranial fossa
5 Medial frontobasal artery
6 Sphenoid
7 Frontal branch of middle meningeal artery
8 Temporal artery of middle cerebral artery
9 Anterior communicating artery
10 Anterior cerebral artery
11 Middle cerebral artery
12 Posterior communicating artery
13 Posterior cerebral artery
14 Basilar artery
15 Basal vein (of Rosenthal)
16 Superior cerebellar artery
17 Tentorium of cerebellum
18 Temporal bone
19 Superior petrosal sinus
20 Sigmoid sinus
21 Auricle (pinna)
22 Lambdoid suture
23 Occipital sinus
24 Internal occipital protuberance
25 Occipital bone
26 External occipital protuberance (inion)

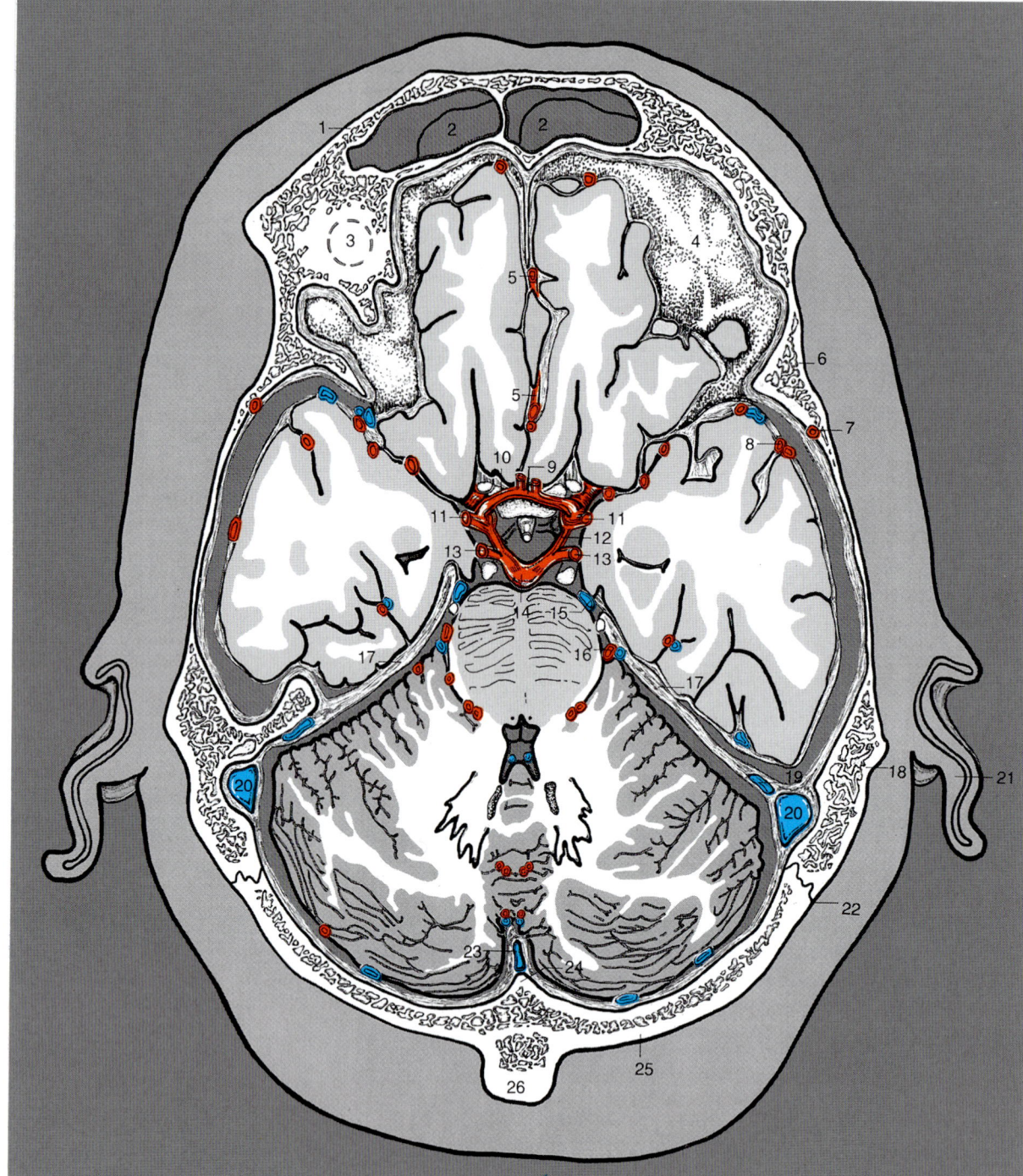

Fig. **51c** Superior section surface of the fifth canthomeatally oriented slice revealing bony structures and blood vessels. The cerebral arterial circle (circle of Willis) was dissected and graphically reconstructed. On the left side the sectional plane runs through the roof of the orbit and just above the dorsum sellae. The insertion of the tentorium of cerebellum covers both sides of the anterior portion of the superior margins of the petrous part of the temporal bones.

Canthomeatally Oriented Slices 145

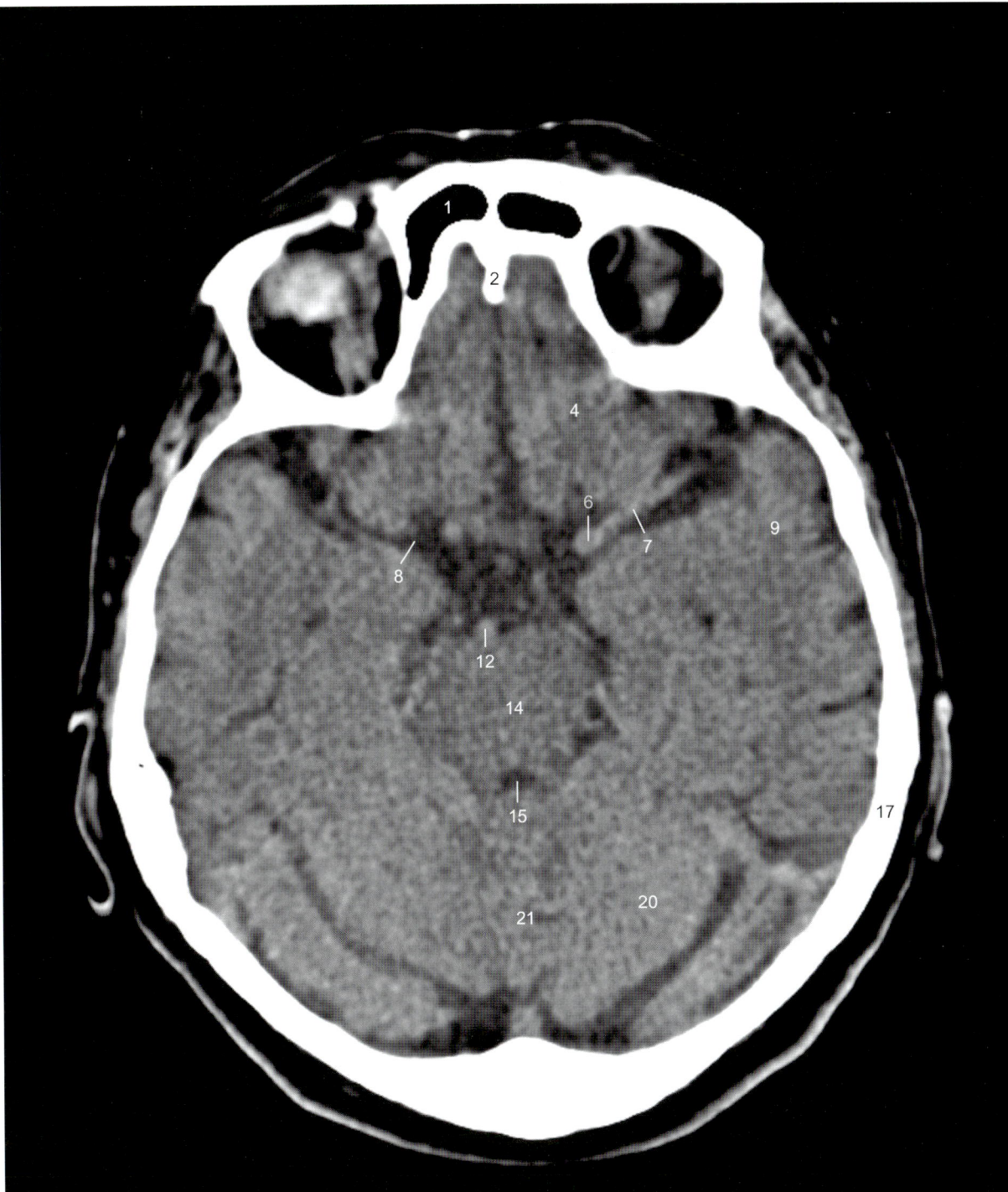

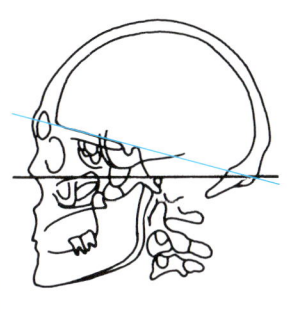

1 Frontal sinus
2 Crista galli
4 Base of frontal lobe
6 Internal carotid artery
7 Middle cerebral artery
8 Cistern of vallecula cerebri
9 Temporal lobe
12 Basilar artery
14 Pons
15 Fourth ventricle
17 Temporal bone
20 Hemisphere of cerebellum
21 Vermis of cerebellum

Fig. **51d** Canthomeatally oriented CT image positioned slightly below the sectional plane of Figs. 51a and 51c.

146   Atlas

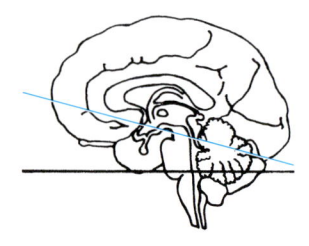

1 Superior frontal gyrus
2 Frontal pole
3 Falx cerebri
4 Middle frontal gyrus
5 Inferior frontal gyrus
6 Cingulate gyrus
7 Lateral sulcus (Sylvian fissure)
8 Temporal lobe
9 Circular sulcus of insula
10 Superior temporal gyrus
11 Subcallosal area
12 Floor of striatum, nucleus accumbens
13 Claustrum
14 Insula
15 Gyrus semilunaris
16 Lamina terminalis
17 Hypothalamus
18 Third ventricle
19 Fornix
20 Optic tract
21 Amygdaloid body
22 Middle temporal gyrus
23 Alveus
24 Hippocampus
25 Uncus of parahippocampal gyrus
26 Hippocampal sulcus
27 Parahippocampal gyrus
28 Cerebral crus
29 Substantia nigra
30 Tegmentum of midbrain
31 Temporal (inferior) horn of lateral ventricle
32 Inferior temporal gyrus
33 Transition of aqueduct into fourth ventricle
34 Cerulean nucleus
35 Trochlear nerve
36 Collateral sulcus
37 Lateral occipitotemporal gyrus
38 Vermis of anterior lobe of cerebellum
39 Hemisphere of anterior lobe of cerebellum
40 Tentorium of cerebellum
41 Primary fissure of cerebellum
42 Hemisphere of posterior lobe of cerebellum
43 Dura mater

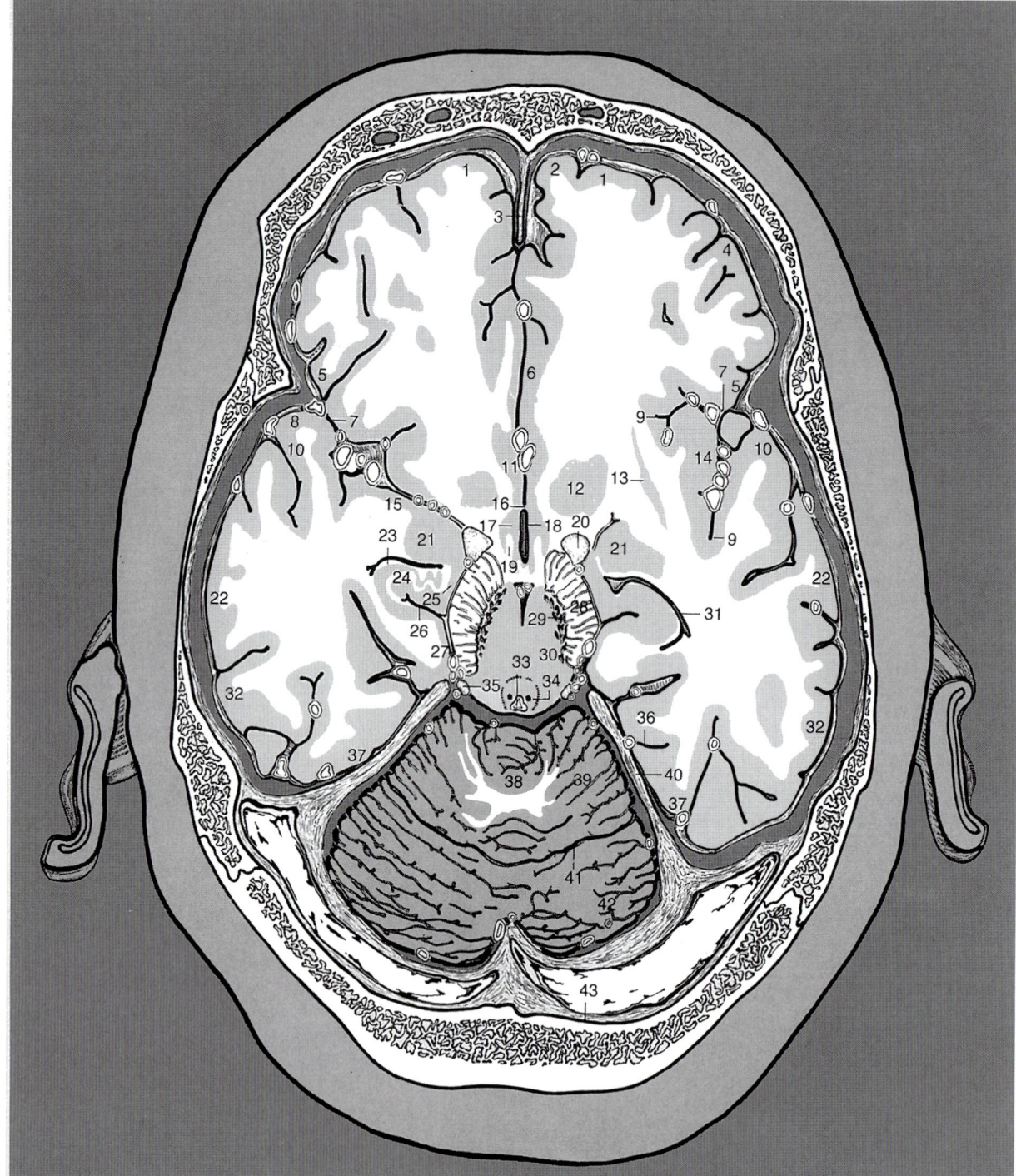

Fig. **52a** Superior section surface of the sixth canthomeatally oriented slice showing the frontal and temporal lobes, hypothalamus, midbrain, and cerebellum. Brain structures and meninges are described.

Canthomeatally Oriented Slices

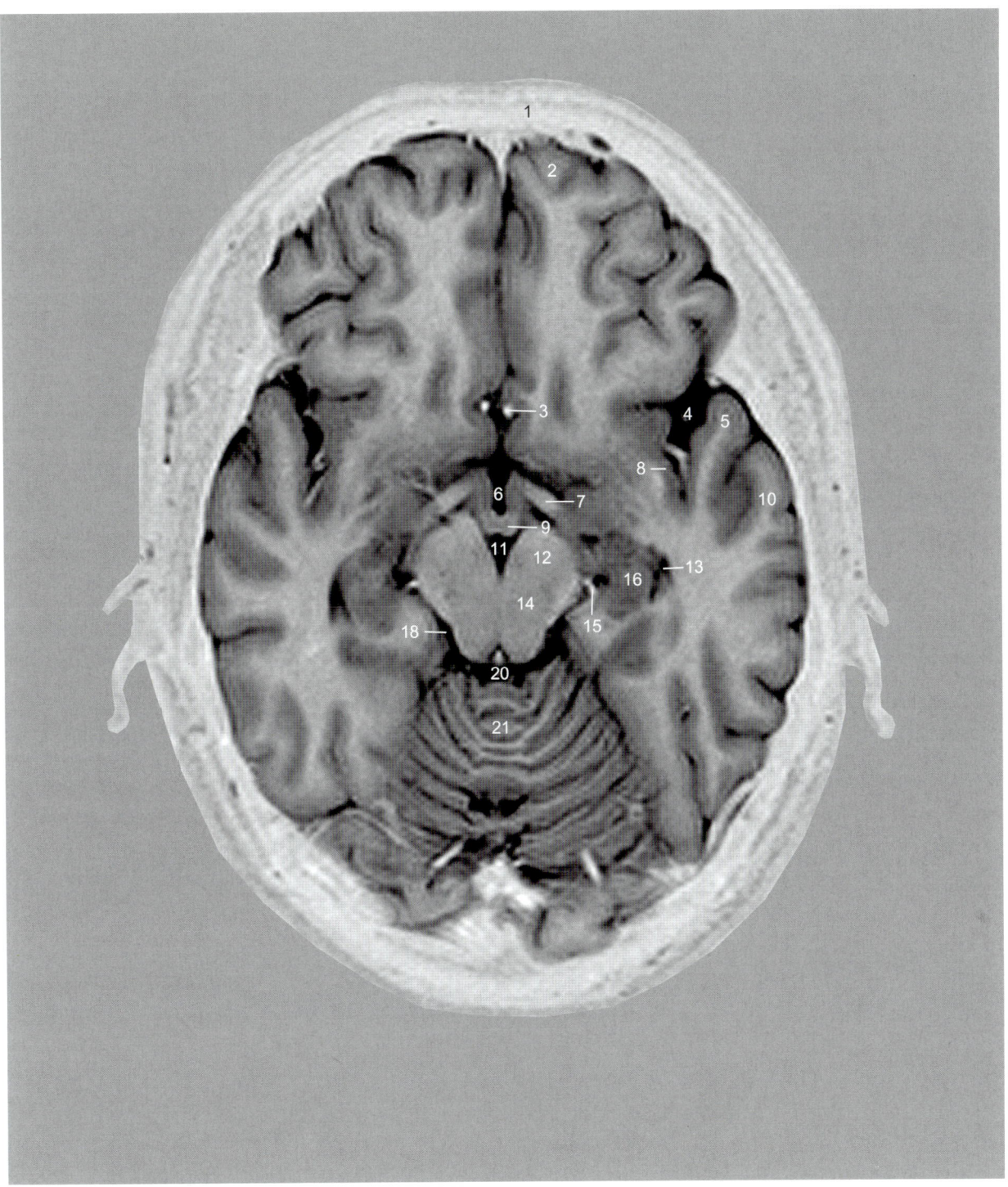

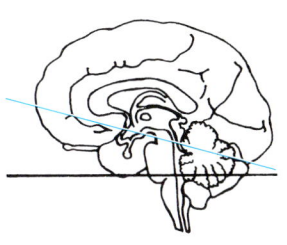

1 Frontal bone
2 Superior frontal gyrus
3 Anterior cerebral artery
4 Cistern of lateral cerebral fossa (cistern of Sylvian fissure)
5 Superior temporal gyrus
6 Third ventricle
7 Optic tract
8 Insula
9 Mammillary body
10 Middle temporal gyrus
11 Interpeduncular cistern
12 Cerebral crus
13 Temporal (inferior) horn of lateral ventricle
14 Tegmentum of midbrain
15 Posterior cerebral artery
16 Hippocampus
18 Ambient cistern
20 Quadrigeminal cistern (cistern of great cerebral vein)
21 Vermis of anterior lobe of cerebellum

Fig. **52b** Canthomeatally oriented, T1-weighted MR image corresponding approximately to the sectional plane of Figs. 52a and 52c.

148 Atlas

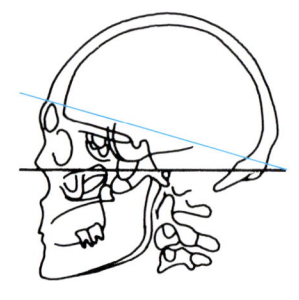

1 Frontal bone
2 Frontal sinus
3 Polar frontal artery
4 Branch of middle meningeal artery
5 Superficial middle cerebral vein
6 Anterior cerebral artery
7 Insular arteries
8 Temporal artery of middle cerebral artery
9 Anterolateral central arteries
10 Anterolateral and anteromedial central arteries
11 Temporal bone
12 Medial occipital artery
13 Lateral occipital artery
14 Posterior medial and posterior lateral choroidal arteries
15 Basal vein (of Rosenthal)
16 Auricle (pinna)
17 Tentorium of cerebellum
18 Lambdoid suture
19 Transverse sinus
20 Occipital bone

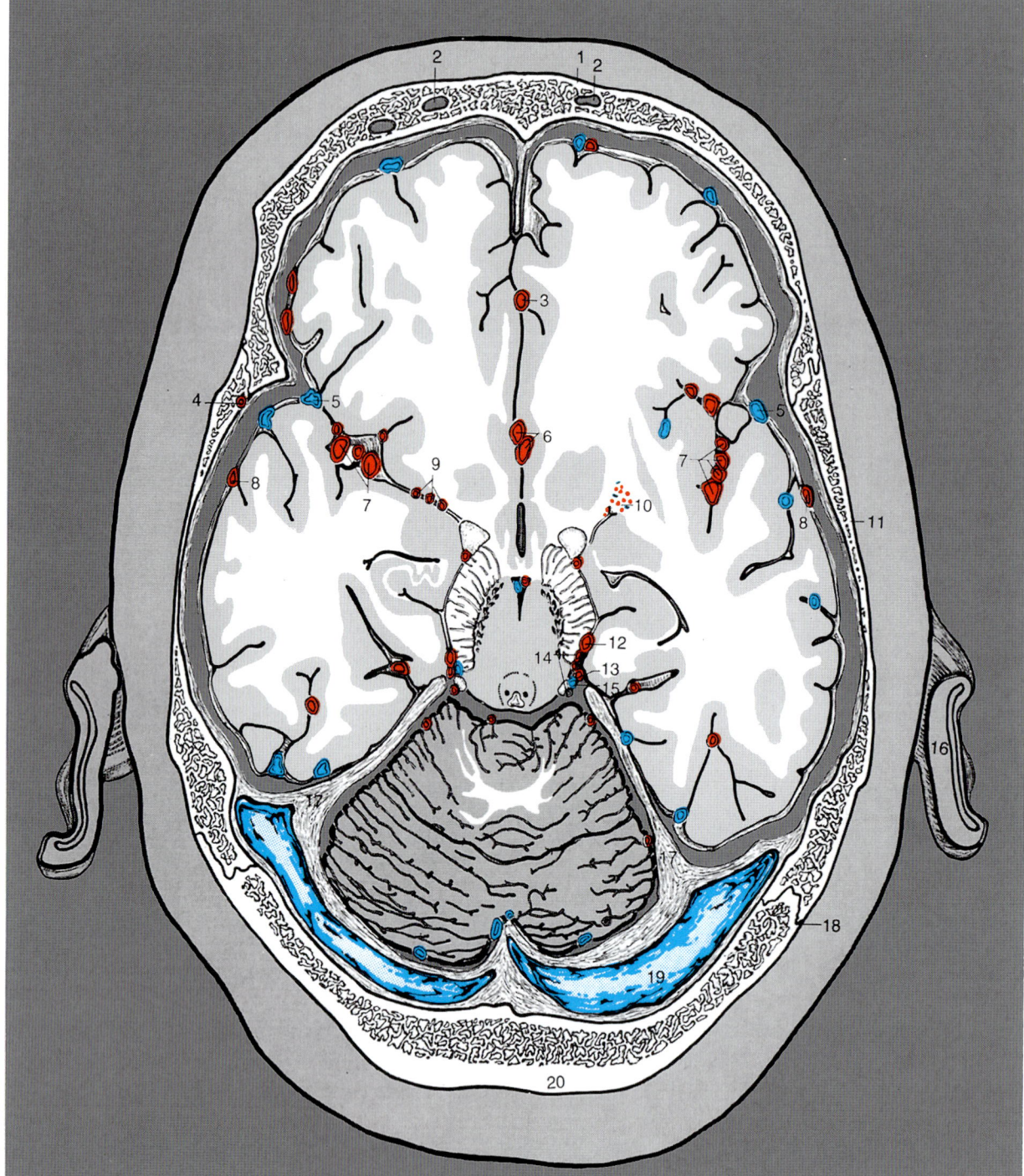

Fig. **52c** Superior section surface of the sixth canthomeatally oriented slice showing the anterior, middle, and posterior cranial fossae with their brain structures and blood vessels. The tentorium of cerebellum forms the anterior border of the posterior cranial fossa.

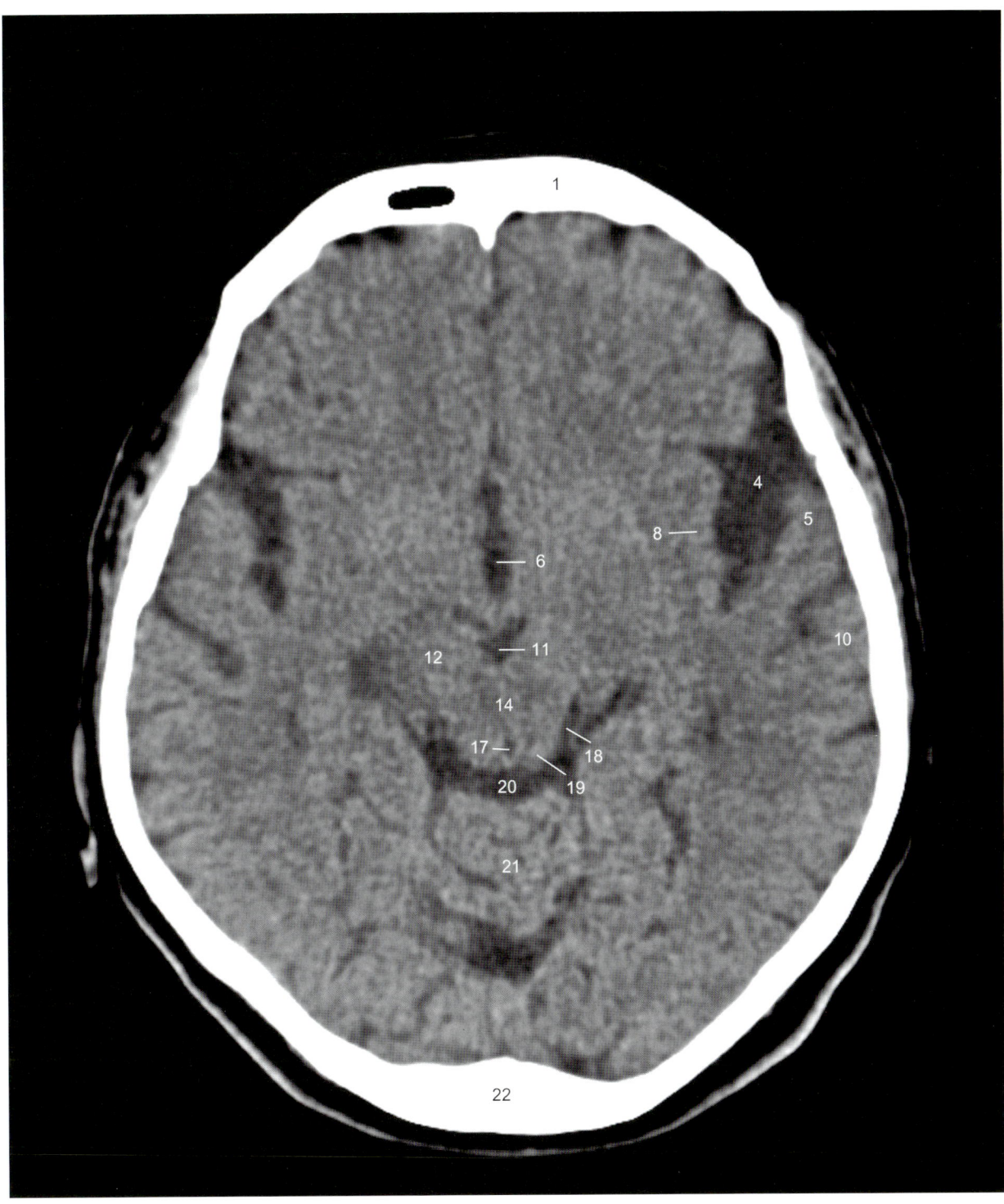

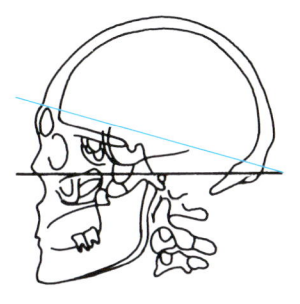

Canthomeatally Oriented Slices

1 Frontal bone
4 Cistern of lateral cerebral fossa (cistern of Sylvian fissure)
5 Superior temporal gyrus
6 Third ventricle
8 Insula
10 Middle temporal gyrus
11 Interpeduncular cistern
12 Cerebral crus
14 Tegmentum of midbrain
17 Aqueduct of midbrain
18 Ambient cistern
19 Inferior colliculus
20 Quadrigeminal cistern (cistern of great cerebral vein)
21 Vermis of anterior lobe of cerebellum
22 Occipital bone

Fig. **52d** Canthomeatally oriented CT image positioned slightly above the sectional plane of Figs. 52a and 52c.

150   Atlas

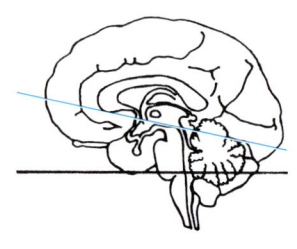

1 Superior frontal gyrus at the frontal pole
2 Middle frontal gyrus
3 Falx cerebri
4 Cingulate gyrus
5 Inferior frontal gyrus
6 Genu of corpus callosum
7 Frontal (anterior) horn of lateral ventricle
8 Circular sulcus of insula
9 Insula
10 Extreme capsule
11 Claustrum
12 External capsule
13 Putamen
14 Lateral part of globus pallidus
15 Medial part of globus pallidus
16 Head of caudate nucleus
17 Anterior limb of internal capsule
18 Genu of internal capsule
19 Posterior limb of internal capsule
20 Septal nuclei
21 Column of fornix
22 Hypothalamus
23 Mammillothalamic fasciculus (of Vicq d'Azyr)
24 Ascending ramus of lateral sulcus (Sylvian fissure)
25 Posterior ramus of lateral sulcus (Sylvian fissure)
26 Temporal lobe
27 Superior temporal gyrus
28 Third ventricle
29 Reticular nucleus of thalamus
30 Ventral posterolateral nucleus of thalamus
31 Medial geniculate body
32 Lateral geniculate body
33 Tail of caudate nucleus
34 Aqueduct of midbrain
35 Alveus
36 Hippocampus
37 Parahippocampal gyrus
38 Middle temporal gyrus
39 Inferior colliculus
40 Tentorium of cerebellum
41 Vermis of anterior lobe of cerebellum
42 Lateral occipitotemporal gyrus
43 Collateral sulcus
44 Medial occipitotemporal gyrus
45 Occipital gyri
46 Dura mater

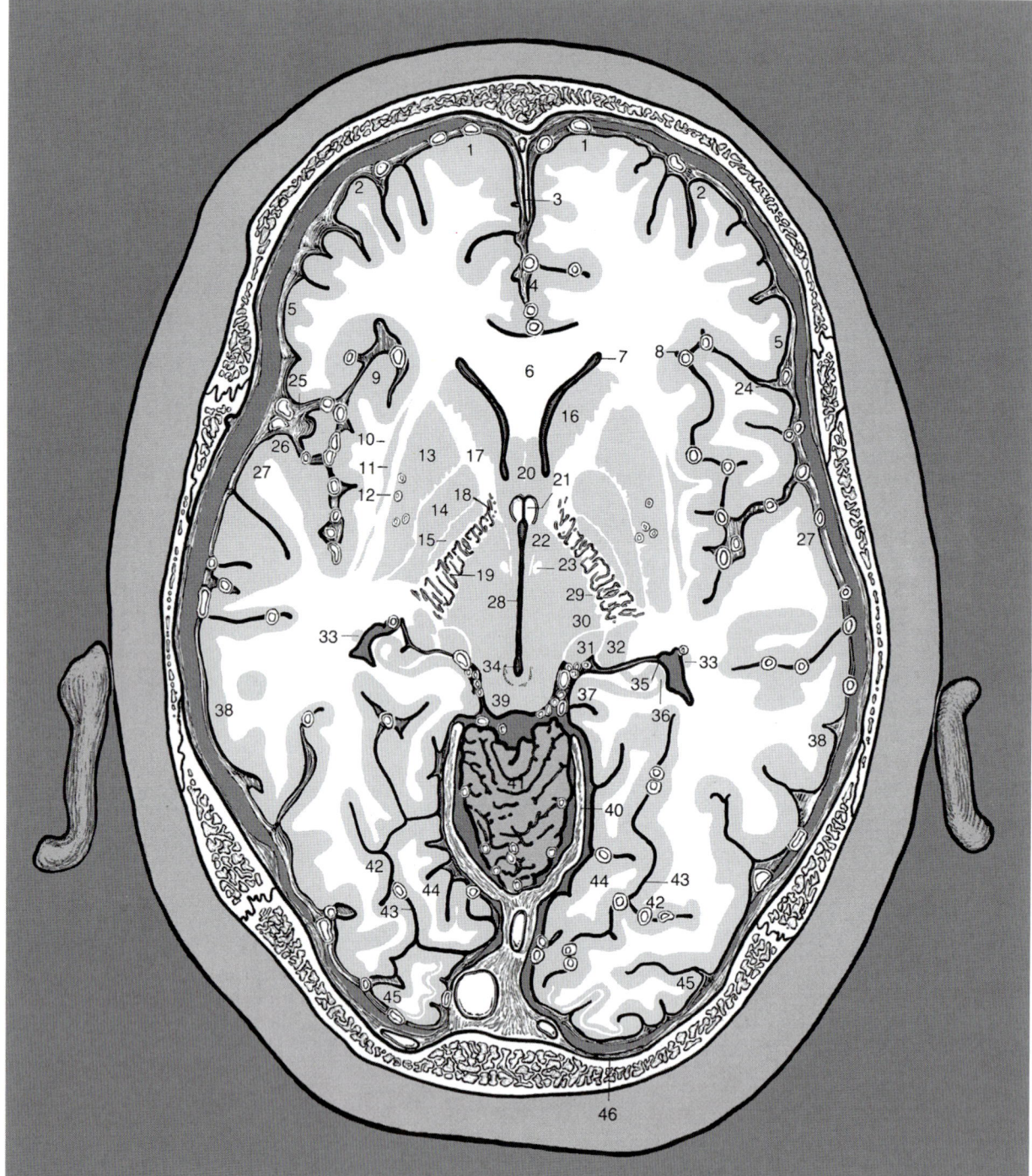

Fig. 53a Superior section surface of the seventh canthomeatally oriented slice representing brain structures and meninges. In this plane, the insula is seen at its longest extension. The striatum (putamen and caudate nucleus), internal capsule, hypothalamus, and thalamus are depicted. In the infratentorial space, the cerebellum only is shown.

Canthomeatally Oriented Slices

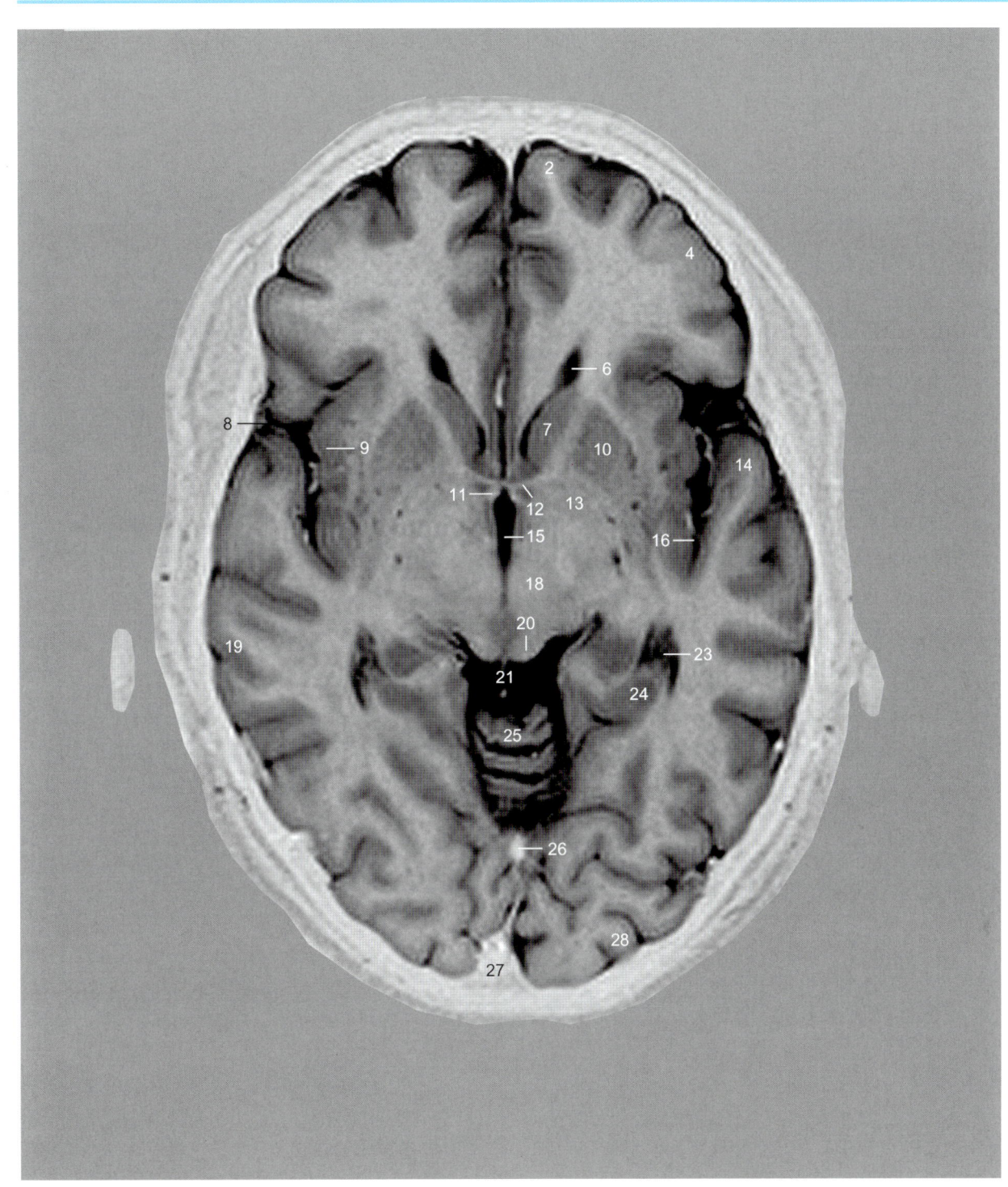

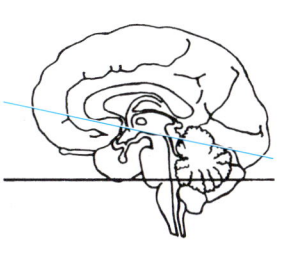

2 Superior frontal gyrus
4 Middle frontal gyrus
6 Frontal (anterior) horn of lateral ventricle
7 Head of caudate nucleus
8 Lateral sulcus (Sylvian fissure)
9 Insula
10 Putamen
11 Column of fornix
12 Anterior commissure
13 Globus pallidus
14 Superior temporal gyrus
15 Third ventricle
16 Cistern of lateral cerebral fossa (cistern of Sylvian fissure)
18 Thalamus
19 Middle temporal gyrus
20 Superior colliculus
21 Quadrigeminal cistern (cistern of great cerebral vein)
23 Lateral ventricle
24 Hippocampus
25 Vermis of anterior lobe of cerebellum
26 Straight sinus
27 Superior sagittal sinus
28 Occipital gyri

Fig. **53b** Canthomeatally oriented, T1-weighted MR image corresponding approximately to the sectional plane of Figs. 53a and 53c.

Atlas

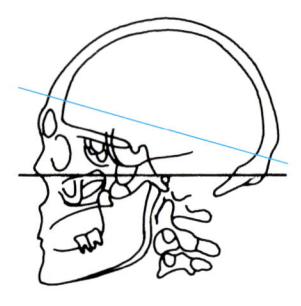

1 Frontal bone
2 Superior sagittal sinus
3 Bridging vein
4 Anteromedial frontal artery
5 Anterior cerebral artery
6 Insular arteries
7 Coronal suture
8 Parietal bone
9 Superficial middle cerebral vein
10 Temporal artery of middle cerebral artery
11 Frontal (anterior) horn of lateral ventricle
12 Anterolateral central arteries
13 Third ventricle
14 Temporal bone
15 Medial occipital artery
16 Posterior medial and posterior lateral choroidal arteries
17 Aqueduct of midbrain
18 Lateral occipital artery
19 Basal vein (of Rosenthal)
20 Auricle (pinna)
21 Tentorium of cerebellum
22 Branch of lateral occipital artery
23 Straight sinus
24 Lambdoid suture
25 Confluence of sinuses (blue dotted line within the slice)
26 Occipital bone

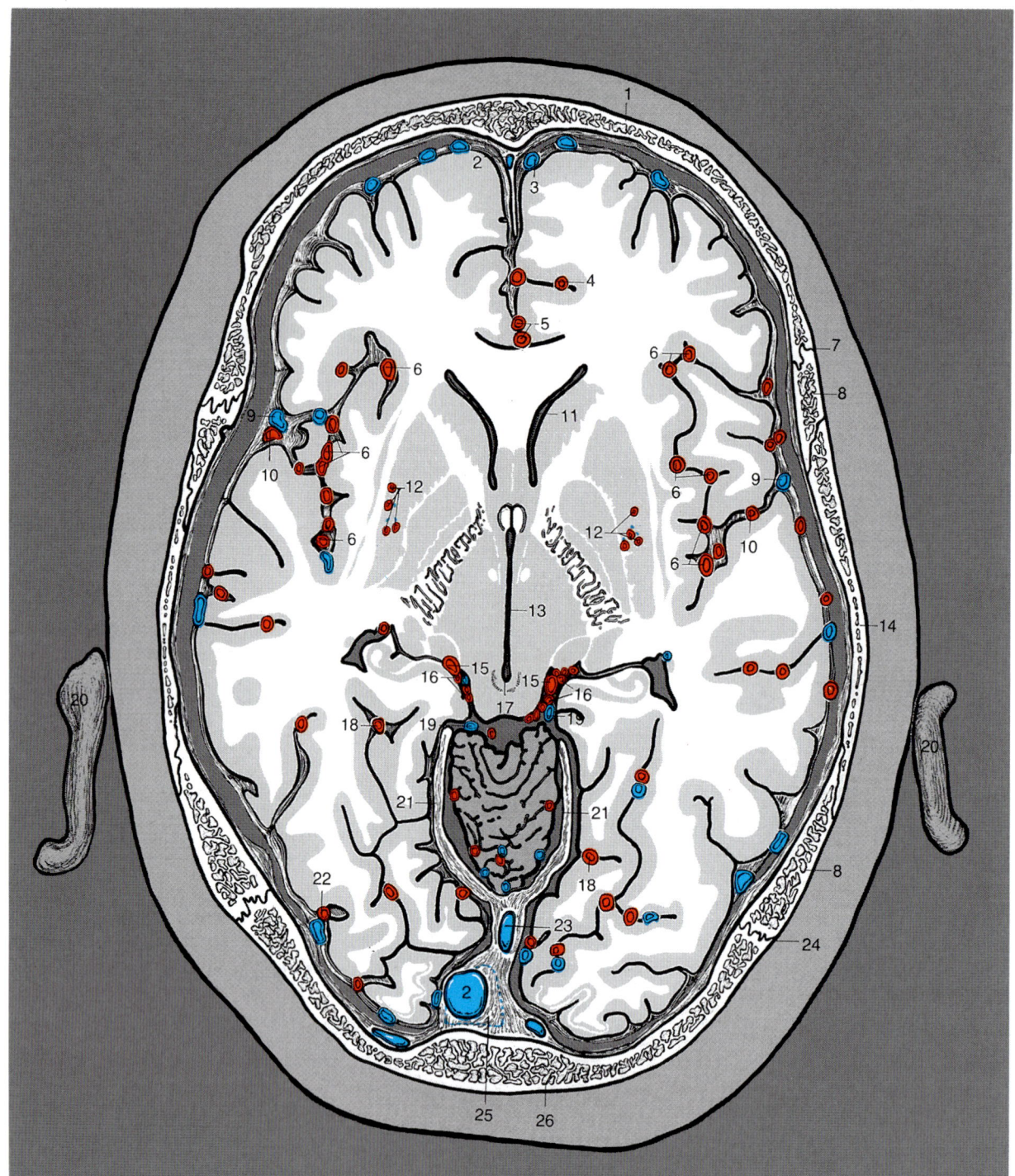

Fig. **53c** Superior section surface of the seventh canthomeatally oriented slice portraying bony structures and blood vessels together with basal portions of the frontal (anterior) horns of the lateral ventricles. The third ventricle is cut as it merges into the aqueduct of midbrain. The temporal (inferior) horns of the lateral ventricles are also depicted. The anterior portion of the tentorium of cerebellum is dissected.

Canthomeatally Oriented Slices

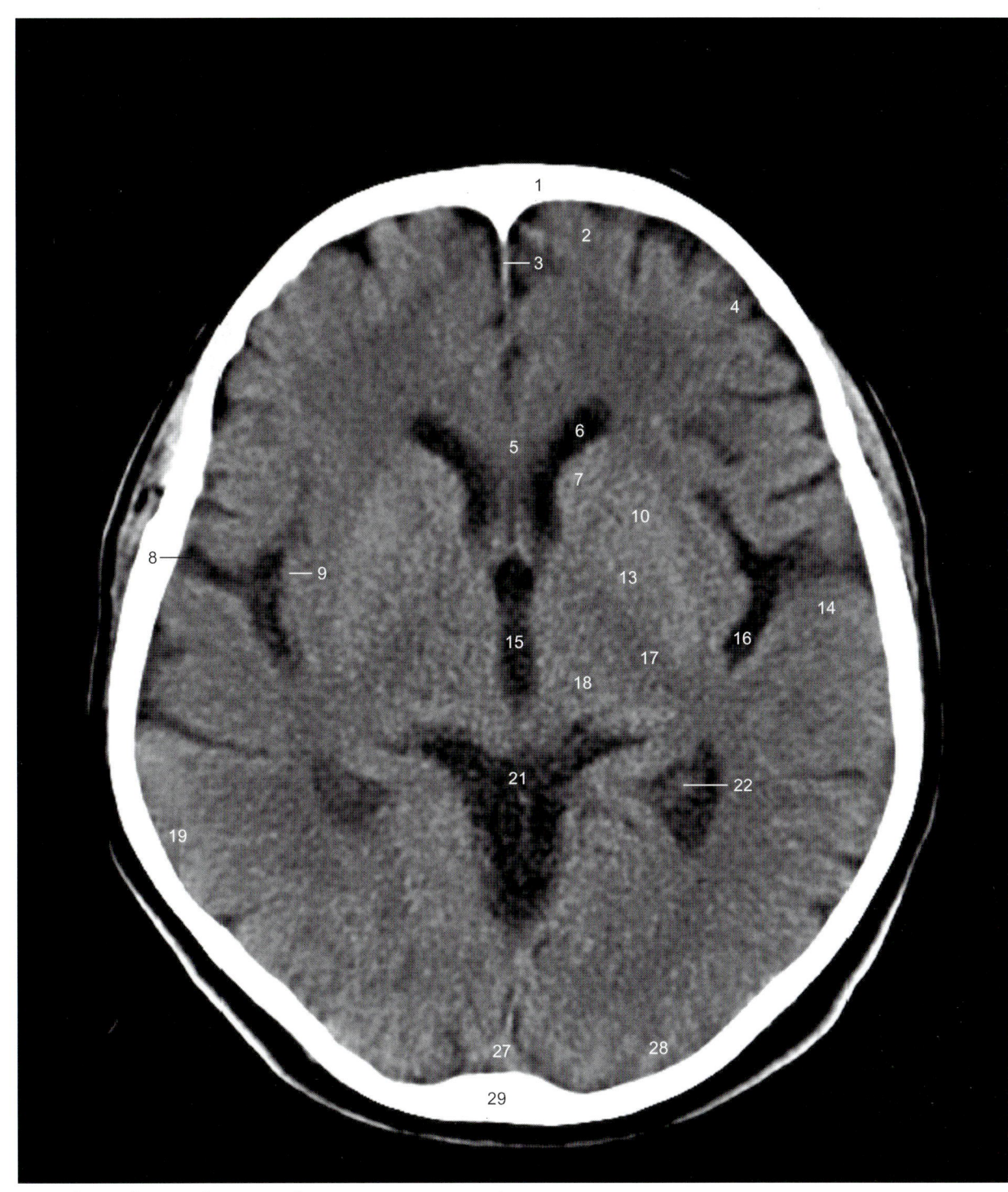

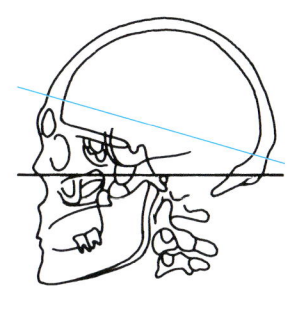

1 Frontal bone
2 Superior frontal gyrus
3 Falx cerebri
4 Middle frontal gyrus
5 Genu of corpus callosum
6 Frontal (anterior) horn of lateral ventricle
7 Head of caudate nucleus
8 Lateral sulcus (Sylvian fissure)
9 Insula
10 Putamen
13 Globus pallidus
14 Superior temporal gyrus
15 Third ventricle
16 Cistern of lateral cerebral fossa (cistern of Sylvian fissure)
17 Posterior limb of internal capsule
18 Thalamus
19 Middle temporal gyrus
21 Quadrigeminal cistern (cistern of great cerebral vein)
22 Choroid plexus of lateral ventricle
27 Superior sagittal sinus
28 Occipital gyri
29 Occipital bone

Fig. **53d** Canthomeatally oriented CT image positioned slightly above the sectional plane of Figs. 53a and 53c.

154 Atlas

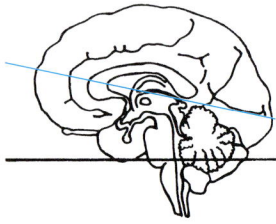

1 Superior frontal gyrus
2 Middle frontal gyrus
3 Falx cerebri
4 Inferior frontal gyrus
5 Cingulate gyrus
6 Corpus callosum
7 Anterior limb of internal capsule
8 Frontal (anterior) horn of lateral ventricle
9 Cave of septum pellucidum
10 Head of caudate nucleus
11 Precentral gyrus
12 Posterior ramus of lateral sulcus (Sylvian fissure)
13 Insula
14 Extreme capsule
15 Claustrum
16 External capsule
17 Putamen
18 Globus pallidus
19 Genu of internal capsule
20 Posterior limb of internal capsule
21 Fornix
22 Interventricular foramen (of Monro)
23 Anterior nuclei of thalamus
24 Medial nuclei of thalamus
25 Ventral lateral nucleus of thalamus
26 Lateral posterior nucleus of thalamus
27 Habenular nuclei
28 Pulvinar of thalamus
29 Central sulcus
30 Postcentral gyrus
31 Superior temporal gyrus
32 Transverse temporal gyri (of Heschl)
33 Circular sulcus of insula
34 Tail of caudate nucleus
35 Third ventricle
36 Fimbria of hippocampus
37 Hippocampus
38 Middle temporal gyrus
39 Parieto-occipital sulcus
40 Tentorium of cerebellum
41 Vermis of anterior lobe of cerebellum (from above)
42 Occipital gyri
43 Primary visual cortex
44 Calcarine sulcus
45 Occipital pole

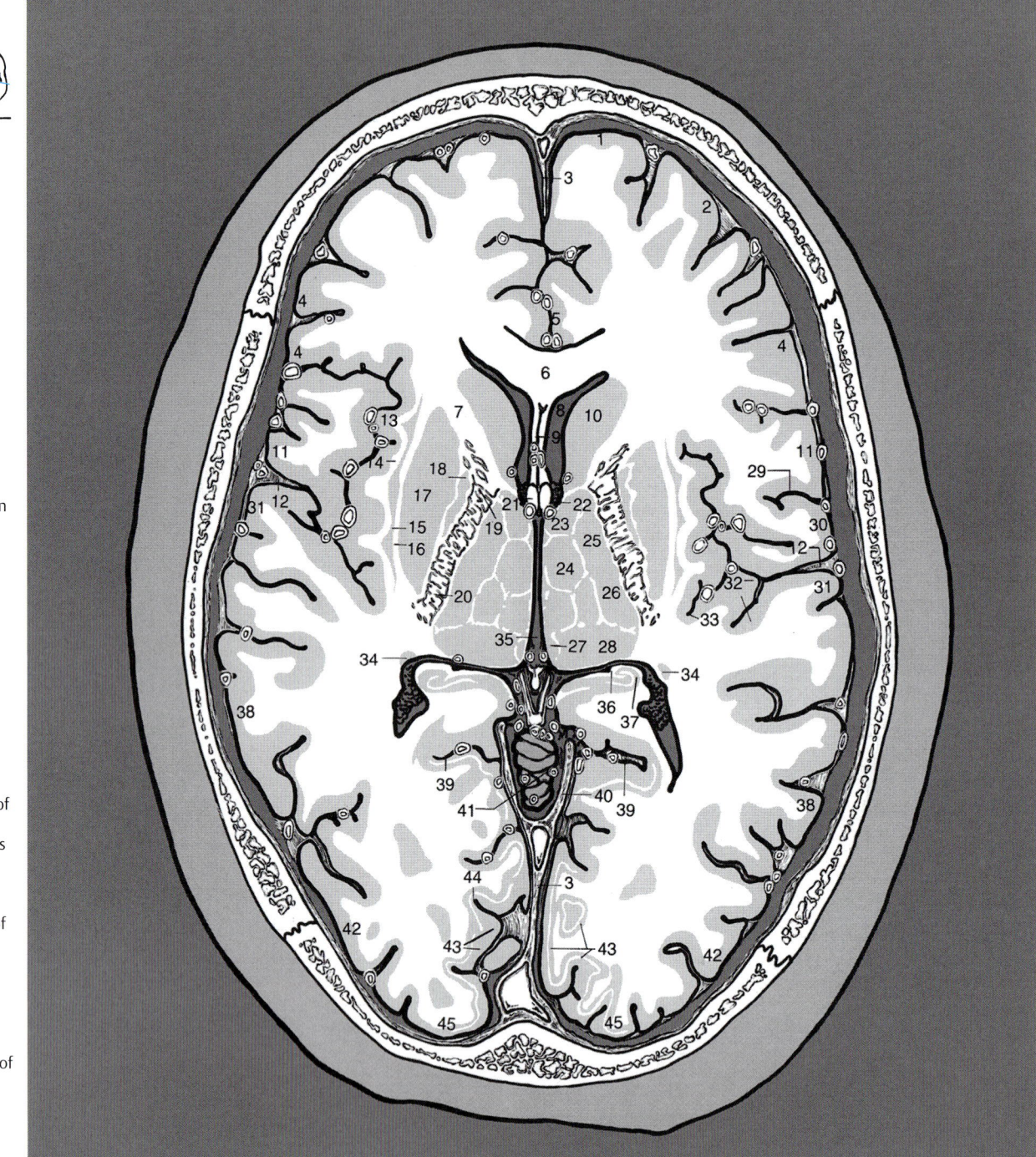

Fig. **54a** Superior section surface of the eighth canthomeatally oriented slice revealing brain structures and meninges. The sectional plane passes through the insula, striatum (putamen and caudate nucleus), internal capsule, and thalamus. Lying inferior to the sectional plane, and therefore not shown, are the superior colliculi, which are located between the third ventricle and the cerebellar vermis.

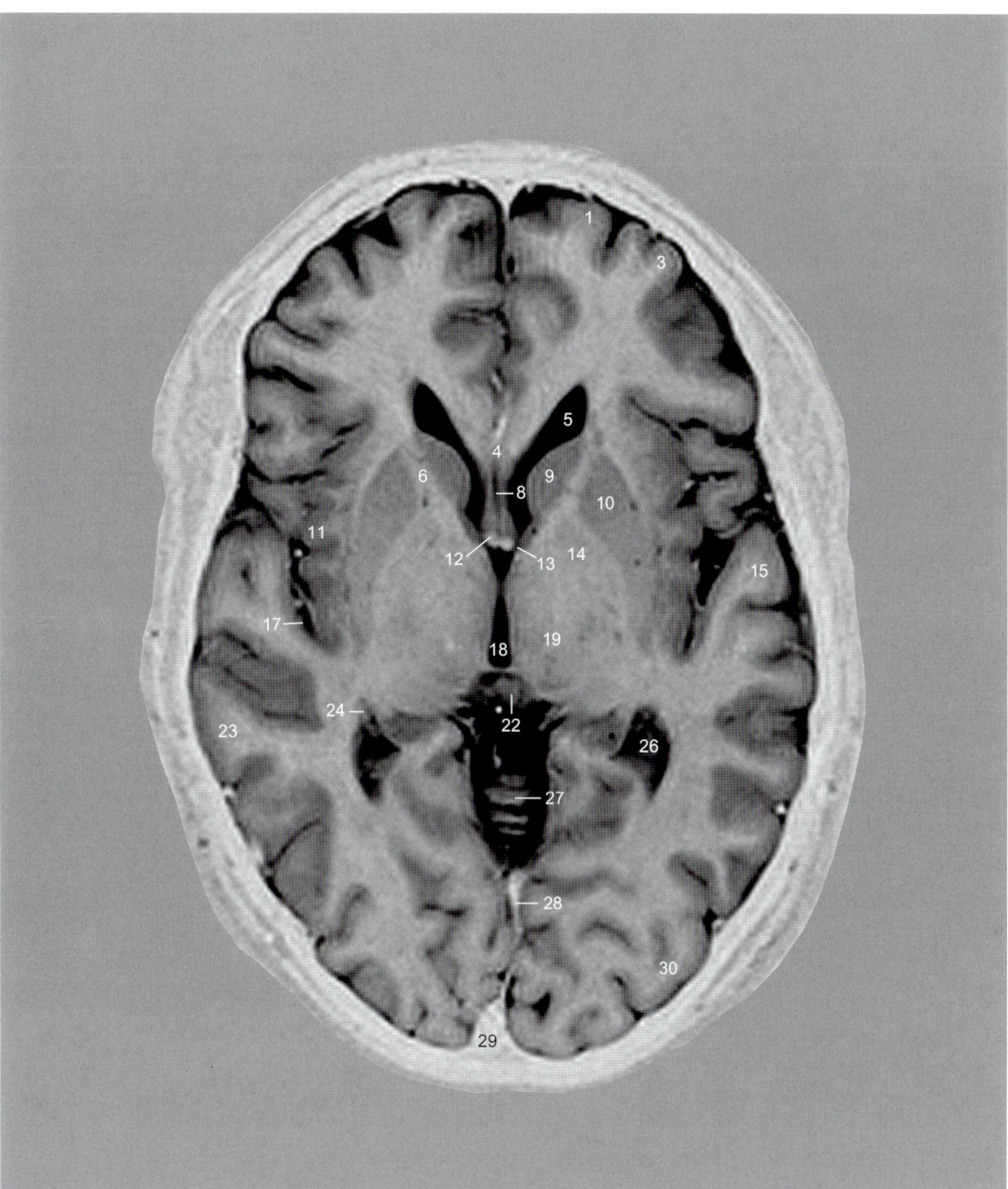

Fig. **54b** Canthomeatally oriented, T1-weighted MR image corresponding approximately to the sectional plane of Figs. 54a and 54c.

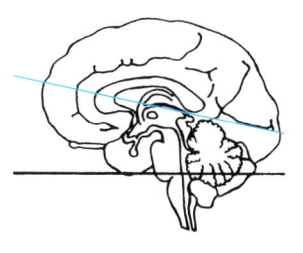

1 Superior frontal gyrus
3 Middle frontal gyrus
4 Genu of corpus callosum
5 Frontal (anterior) horn of lateral ventricle
6 Anterior limb of internal capsule
8 Cave of septum pellucidum
9 Head of caudate nucleus
10 Putamen
11 Insula
12 Column of fornix
13 Interventricular foramen (of Monro)
14 Globus pallidus
15 Superior temporal gyrus
17 Cistern of lateral cerebral fossa (cistern of Sylvian fissure)
18 Third ventricle
19 Thalamus
22 Pineal gland
23 Middle temporal gyrus
24 Tail of caudate nucleus
26 Atrium of lateral ventricle,
27 Vermis of anterior lobe of cerebellum
28 Straight sinus
29 Superior sagittal sinus
30 Occipital gyri

156 Atlas

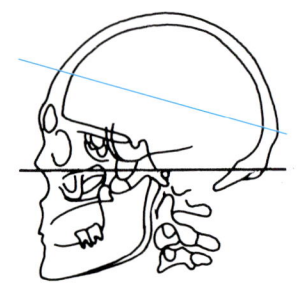

1 Frontal bone
2 Superior sagittal sinus
3 Superior cerebral vein
4 Anteromedial frontal artery
5 Callosomarginal artery
6 Coronal suture
7 Anterior cerebral artery
8 Artery of precentral sulcus
9 Insular arteries
10 Frontal (anterior) horn of lateral ventricle
11 Anterior vein of septum pellucidum
12 Internal cerebral vein
13 Third ventricle
14 Parietal bone
15 Temporo-occipital artery
16 Posterior lateral choroidal artery
17 Posterior medial choroidal artery
18 Pineal gland
19 Great cerebral vein (of Galen)
20 Choroid plexus in atrium of lateral ventricle
21 Medial occipital artery
22 Calcarine artery
23 Tentorium of cerebellum
24 Straight sinus
25 Lambdoid suture
26 Occipital bone

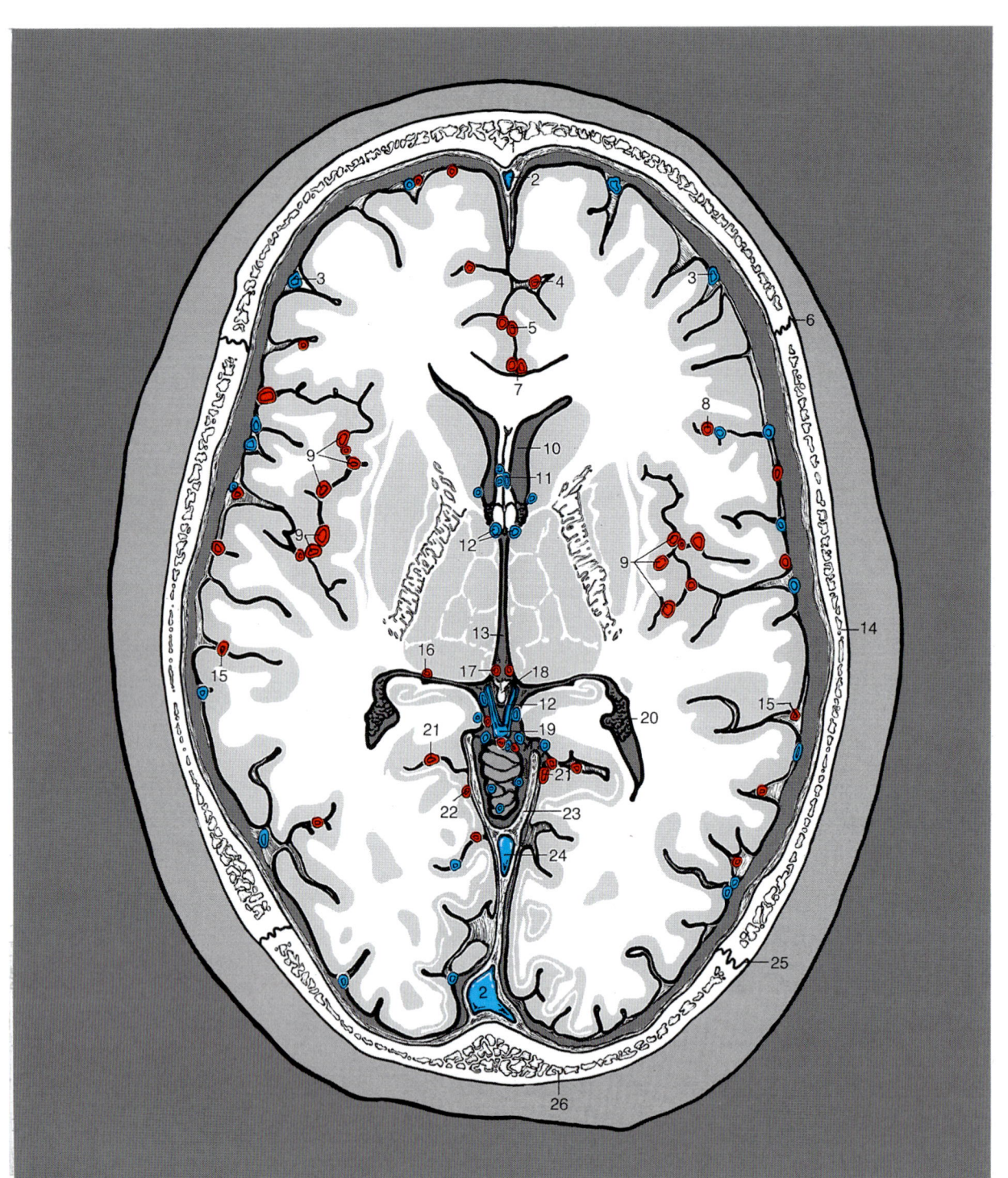

Fig. **54c** Superior section surface of the eighth canthomeatally oriented slice showing bony structures and blood vessels. The pineal gland lies between the upper and lower surfaces of this slice. The internal cerebral veins cover the pineal gland. Only a small portion of its superior surface can be seen. The sectional plane runs through the lateral and third ventricles. The ridge of the tentorium of cerebellum is dissected.

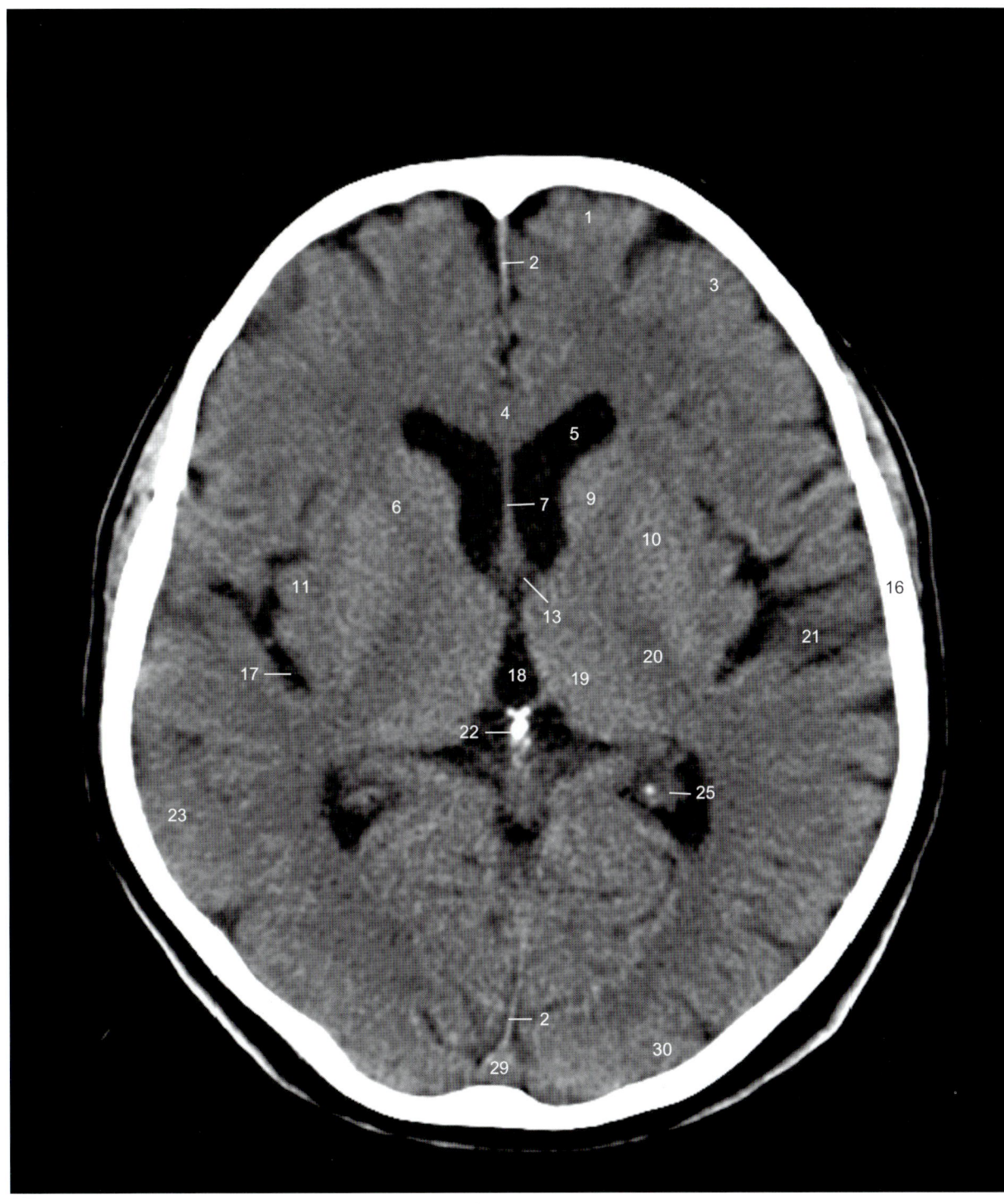

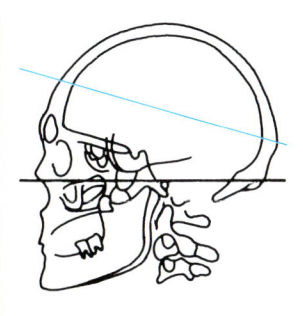

Canthomeatally Oriented Slices

1 Superior frontal gyrus
2 Falx cerebri
3 Middle frontal gyrus
4 Genu of corpus callosum
5 Frontal (anterior) horn of lateral ventricle
6 Anterior limb of internal capsule
7 Septum pellucidum
9 Head of caudate nucleus
10 Putamen
11 Insula
13 Interventricular foramen (of Monro)
16 Parietal bone
17 Cistern of lateral cerebral fossa (cistern of Sylvian fissure)
18 Third ventricle
19 Thalamus
20 Posterior limb of internal capsule
21 Transverse temporal gyrus (of Heschl)
22 Pineal gland
23 Middle temporal gyrus
25 Choroid plexus in atrium of lateral ventricle
29 Superior sagittal sinus
30 Occipital gyri

Fig. **54d** Canthomeatally oriented CT image corresponding closely to the sectional plane of Figs. 54a and 54c.

Atlas

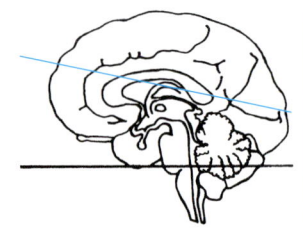

1 Superior frontal gyrus
2 Middle frontal gyrus
3 Falx cerebri
4 Cingulate sulcus
5 Cingulate gyrus
6 Minor (frontal) forceps
7 Inferior frontal gyrus
8 Trunk (body) of corpus callosum
9 Precentral gyrus
10 Frontal (anterior) horn of lateral ventricle
11 Central sulcus
12 Head of caudate nucleus
13 Claustrum
14 Insula
15 Postcentral gyrus
16 Corona radiata
17 Posterior ramus of lateral sulcus (Sylvian fissure)
18 Thalamus
19 Fornix
20 Superior temporal gyrus
21 Transverse temporal gyri (of Heschl)
22 Tail of caudate nucleus
23 Splenium of corpus callosum
24 Major (occipital) forceps
25 Parieto-occipital sulcus
26 Cuneus
27 Occipital gyri
28 Primary visual cortex

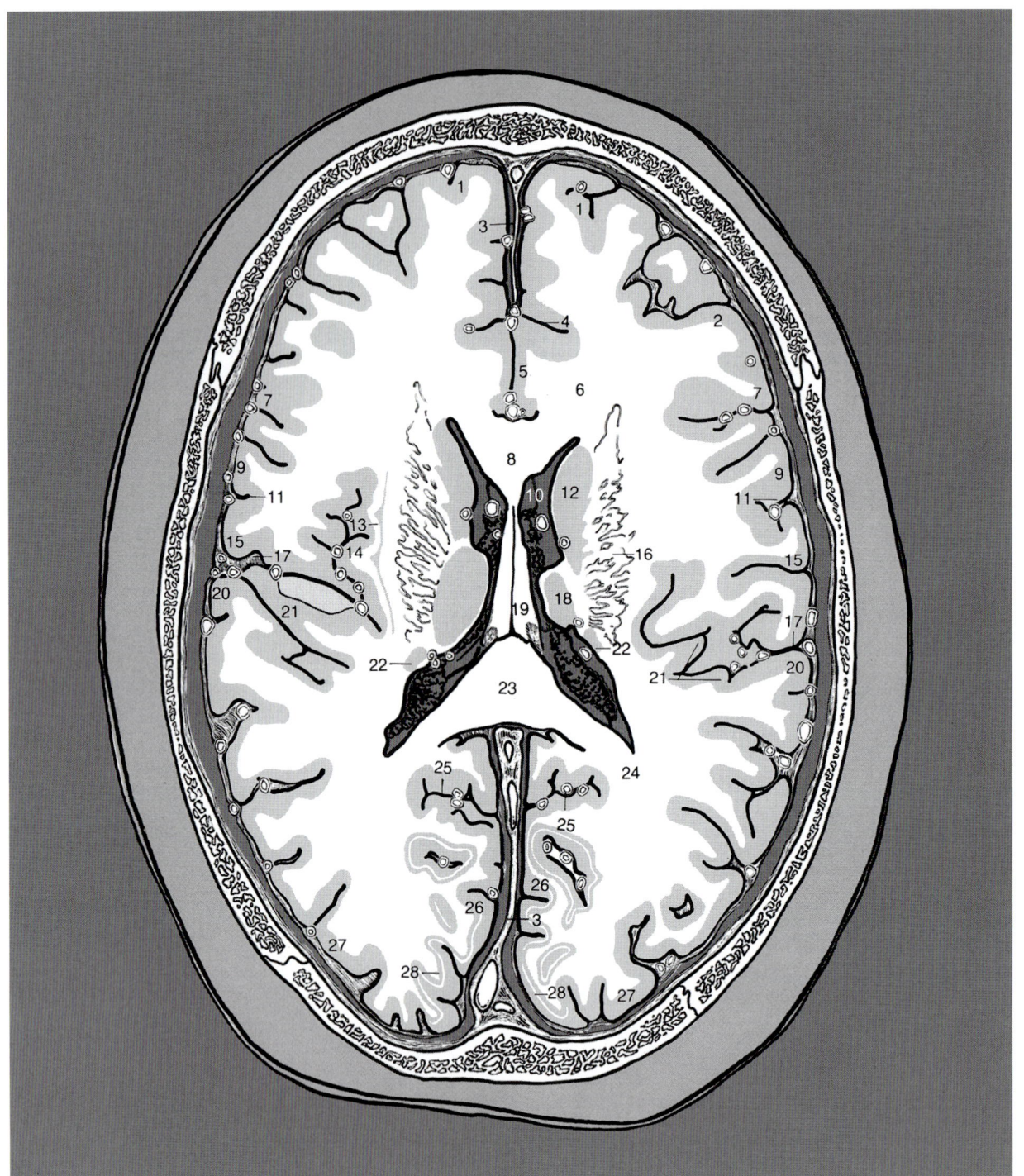

Fig. **55a** Superior section surface of the ninth canthomeatally oriented slice portraying brain structures and meninges. The sectional plane divides the cerebral falx into an anterior and a posterior part. The superior portion of the insula is seen. The splenium of the corpus callosum lies between the atrium of the right and left ventricles.

Canthomeatally Oriented Slices 159

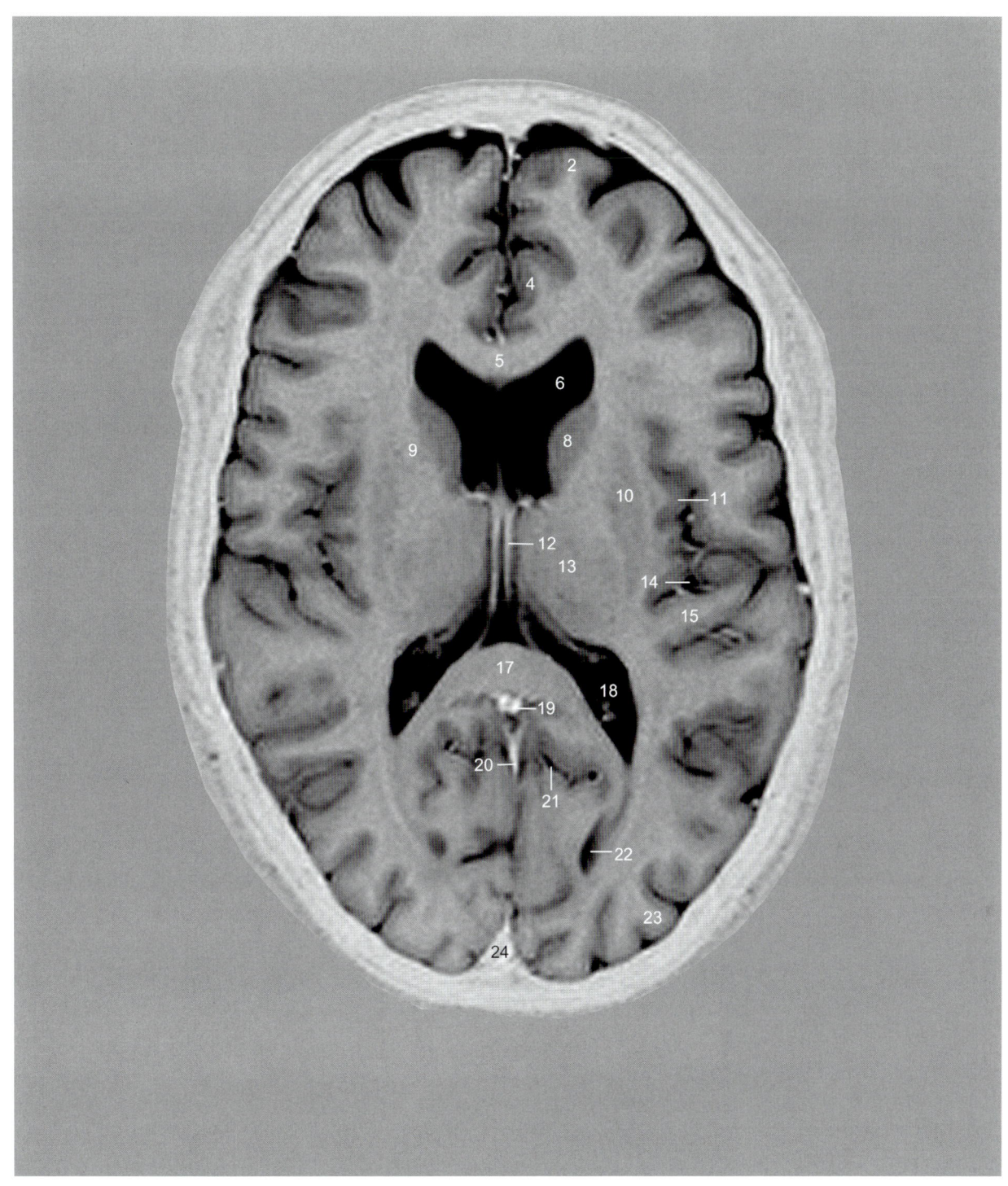

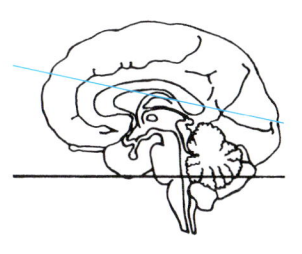

2 Superior frontal gyrus
4 Cingulate gyrus
5 Corpus callosum
6 Frontal (anterior) horn of lateral ventricle
8 Head of caudate nucleus
9 Anterior limb of internal capsule
10 Putamen
11 Insula
12 Fornix
13 Thalamus
14 Cistern of lateral cerebral fossa (cistern of Sylvian fissure)
15 Transverse temporal gyrus (of Heschl)
17 Splenium of corpus callosum
18 Lateral ventricle
19 Internal cerebral vein
20 Straight sinus
21 Parieto-occipital sulcus
22 Occipital (posterior) horn of lateral ventricle
23 Occipital gyri
24 Superior sagittal sinus

Fig. **55b** Canthomeatally oriented, T1-weighted MR image corresponding approximately to the sectional plane of Figs. 55a and 55c.

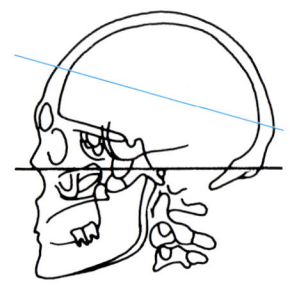

Atlas

1 Frontal bone
2 Superior sagittal sinus
3 Superior cerebral vein
4 Intermediomedial frontal artery
5 Prefrontal artery
6 Callosomarginal artery
7 Coronal suture
8 Pericallosal artery
9 Artery of precentral sulcus
10 Insular arteries
11 Superior thalamostriate vein and stria terminalis
12 Superior choroid vein
13 Central part (body) of lateral ventricle
14 Artery of central sulcus
15 Posterior lateral choroidal artery
16 Atrium of lateral ventricle and choroid plexus
17 Parietal artery
18 Parietal bone
19 Angular artery
20 Great cerebral vein (of Galen)
21 Parieto-occipital artery
22 Straight sinus
23 Calcarine artery
24 Lambdoid suture
25 Occipital bone

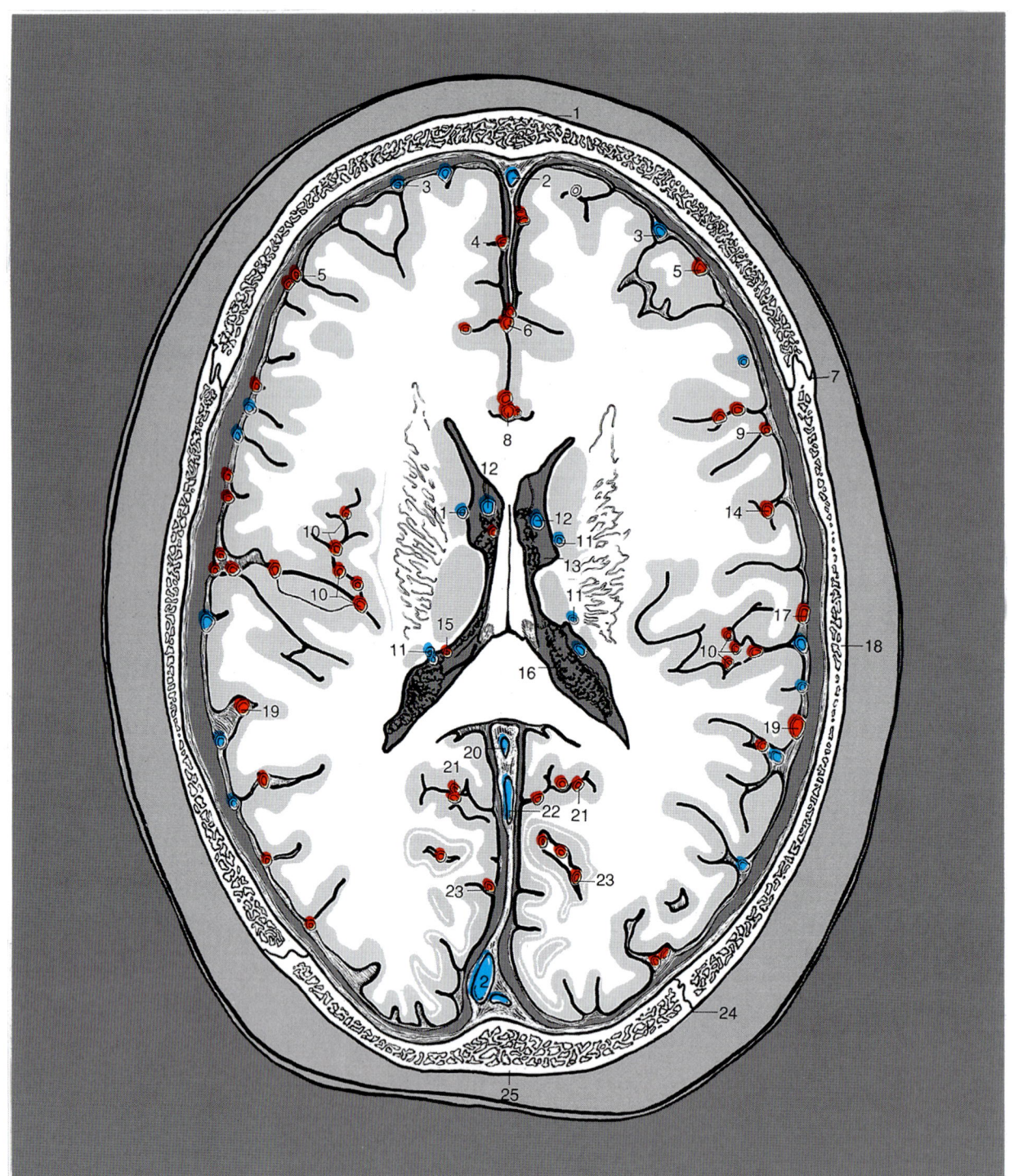

Fig. **55c** Superior section surface of the ninth canthomeatally oriented slice depicting bony structures and blood vessels. The sectional plane passes through the central parts of the lateral ventricles and lies just above the atrium of the lateral ventricles.

Canthomeatally Oriented Slices   **161**

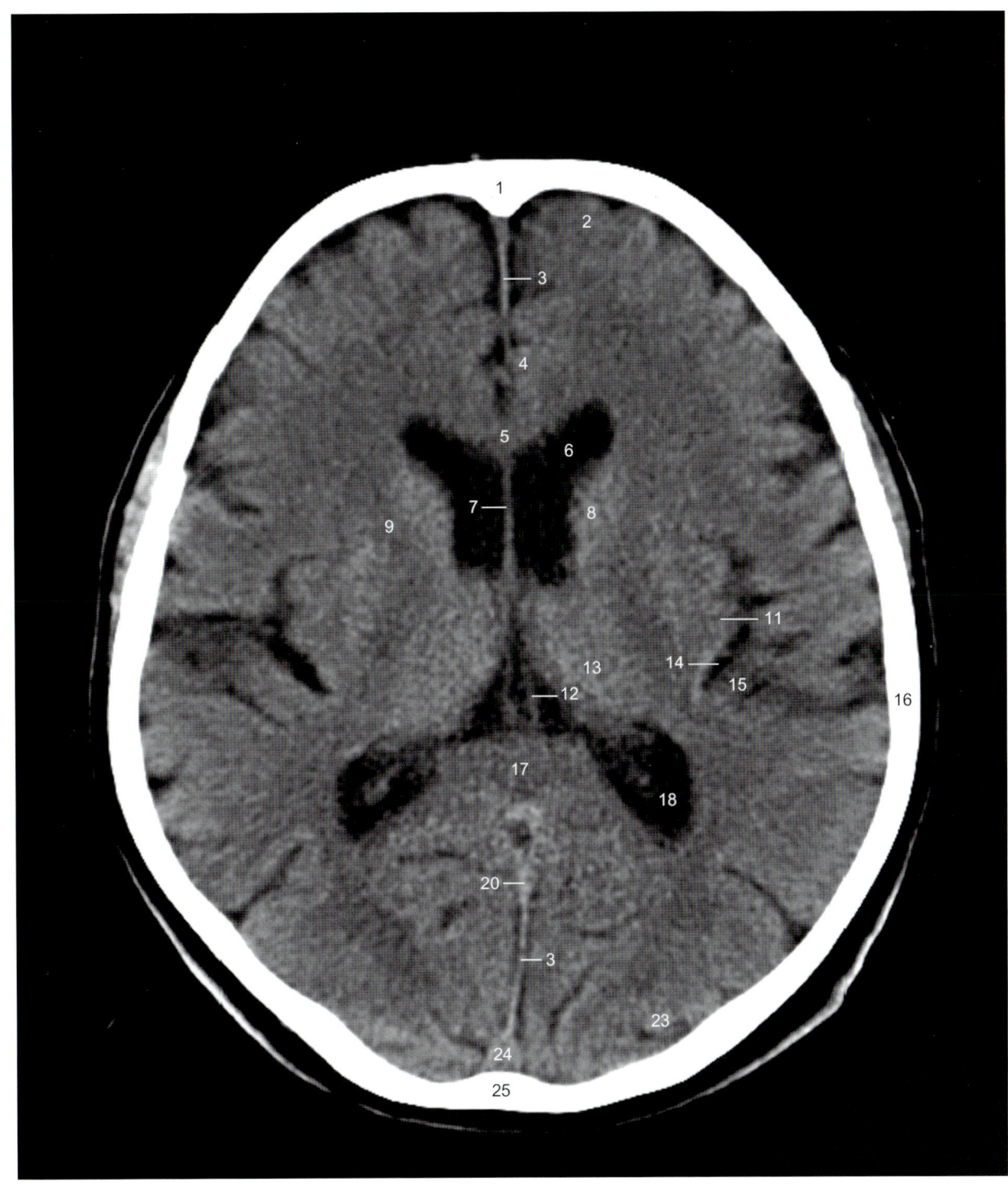

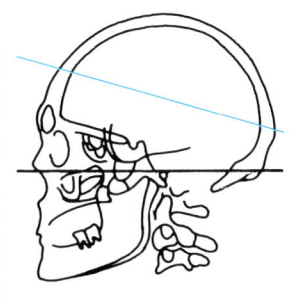

1 Frontal bone
2 Superior frontal gyrus
3 Falx cerebri
4 Cingulate gyrus
5 Corpus callosum
6 Frontal (anterior) horn of lateral ventricle
7 Septum pellucidum
8 Head of caudate nucleus
9 Anterior limb of internal capsule
11 Insula
12 Fornix
13 Thalamus
14 Cistern of lateral cerebral fossa (cistern of Sylvian fissure)
15 Transverse temporal gyrus (of Heschl)
16 Parietal bone
17 Splenium of corpus callosum
18 Lateral ventricle
20 Straight sinus
23 Occipital gyri
24 Superior sagittal sinus
25 Occipital bone

Fig. **55d** Canthomeatally oriented CT image positioned slightly below the sectional plane of Figs. 55a and 55c.

162   Atlas

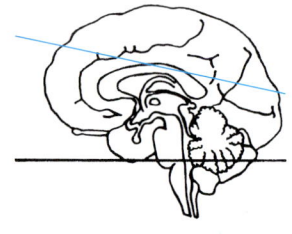

1   Superior frontal gyrus
2   Middle frontal gyrus
3   Falx cerebri
4   Cingulate sulcus
5   Precentral sulcus
6   Precentral gyrus
7   Central sulcus
8   Cingulate gyrus
9   Cingulum
10 Postcentral gyrus
11 Postcentral sulcus
12 Central part (body) of lateral ventricle
13 Supramarginal gyrus
14 Semioval center
15 Angular gyrus
16 Precuneus
17 Parieto-occipital sulcus
18 Dura mater
19 Occipital gyri
20 Cuneus

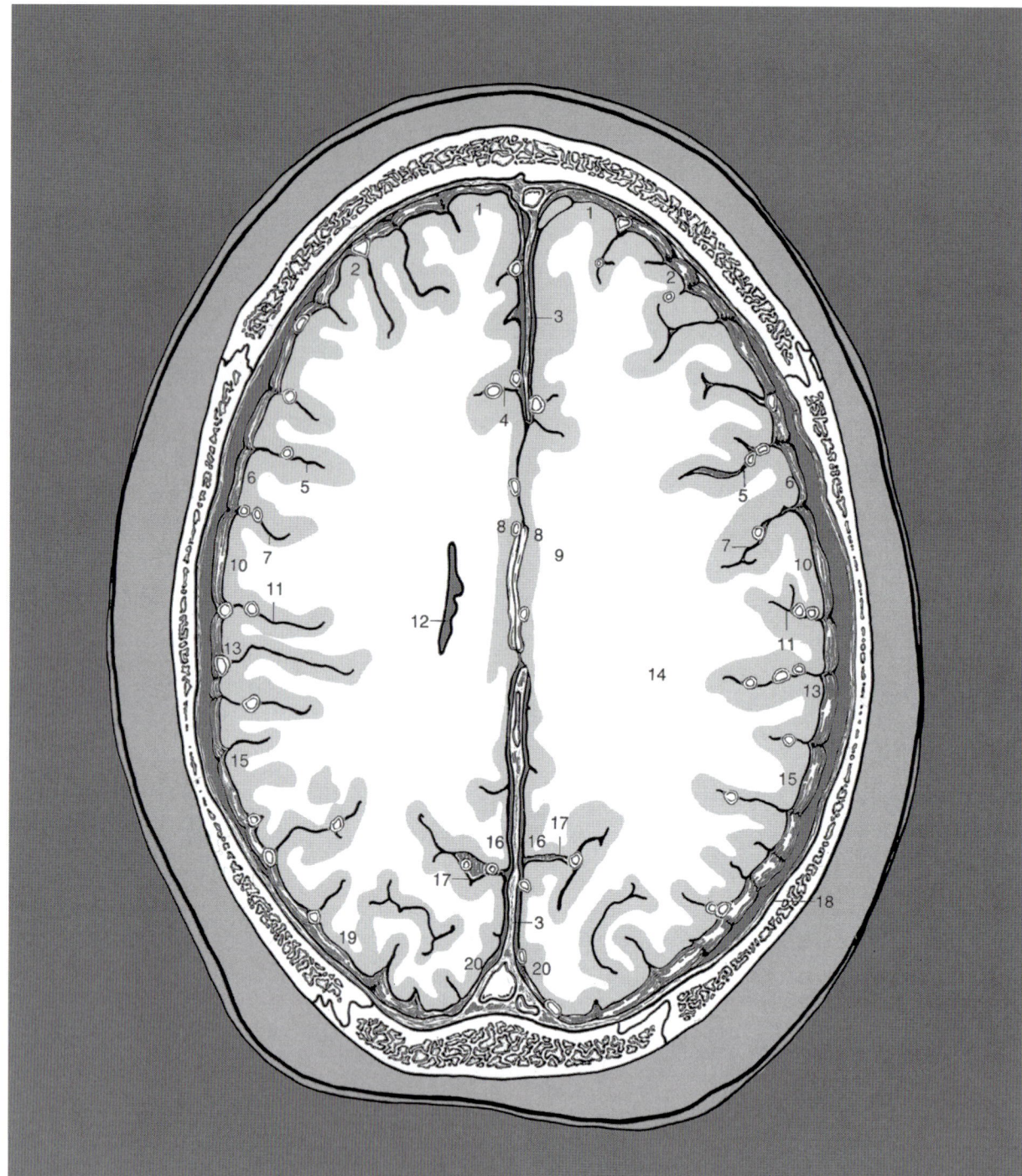

Fig. **56a** Superior section surface of the tenth canthomeatally oriented slice representing brain structures and meninges. The sectional plane divides the cerebral falx into an anterior and a posterior part. Between these two parts lies the supracommissural portion of the cingulate gyrus that covers the corpus callosum.

Canthomeatally Oriented Slices

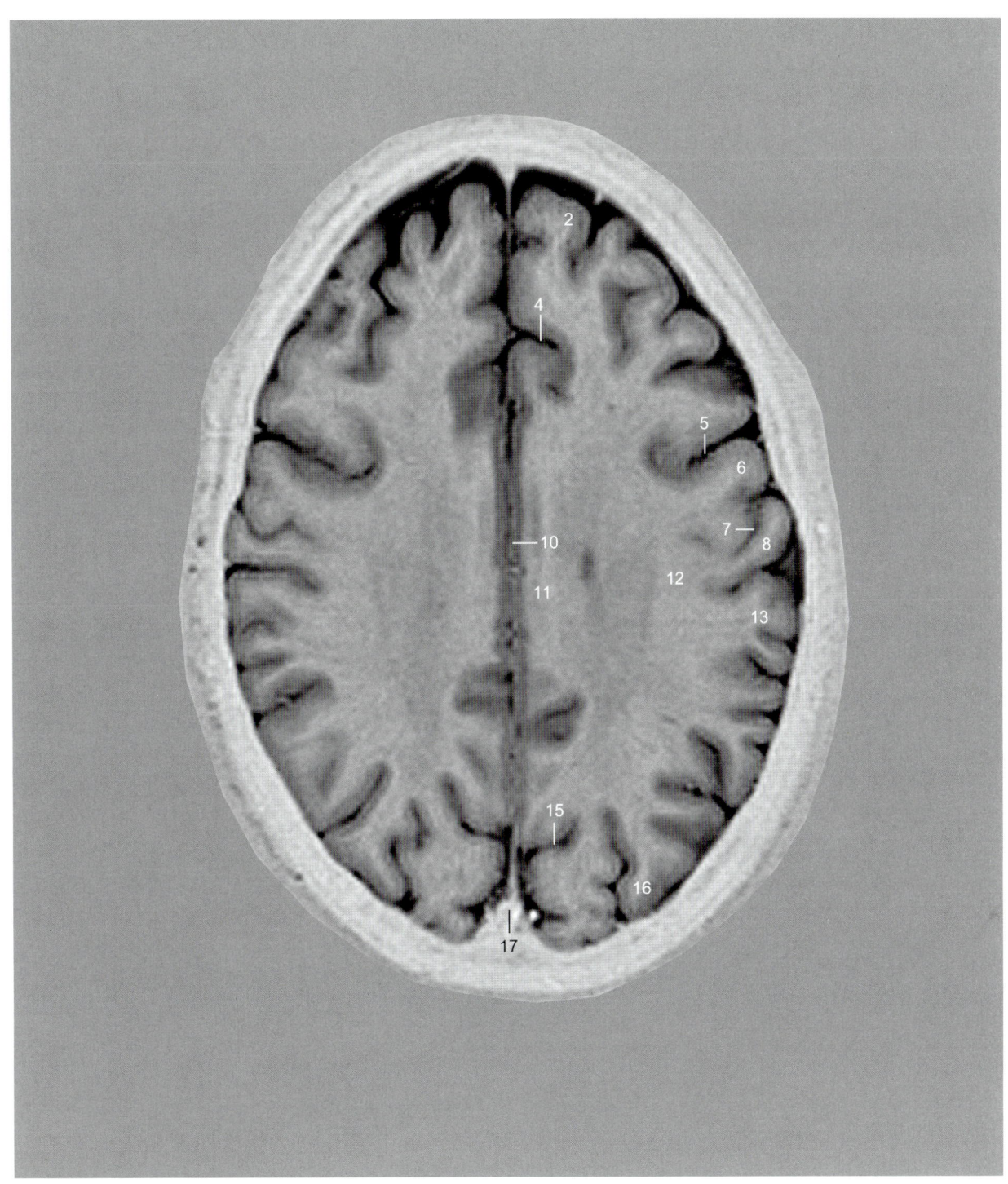

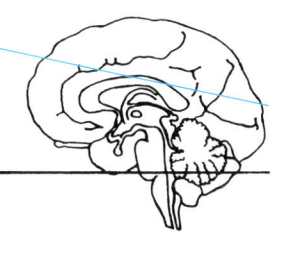

2 Superior frontal gyrus
4 Cingulate sulcus
5 Precentral sulcus
6 Precentral gyrus
7 Central sulcus
8 Postcentral gyrus
10 Cingulate gyrus
11 Cingulum
12 Semioval center
13 Supramarginal gyrus
15 Parieto-occipital sulcus
16 Occipital gyri
17 Superior sagittal sinus

Fig. **56b** Canthomeatally oriented, T1-weighted MR image corresponding approximately to the sectional plane of Figs. 56a and 56c.

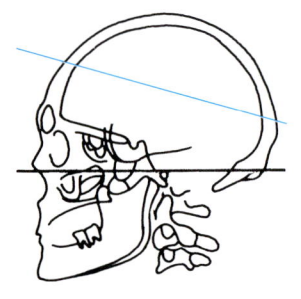

164 Atlas

1 Frontal bone
2 Superior sagittal sinus
3 Superior cerebral vein
4 Intermediomedial frontal artery
5 Prefrontal artery
6 Coronal suture
7 Callosomarginal artery
8 Artery of precentral sulcus
9 Artery of central sulcus
10 Pericallosal artery
11 Parietal artery
12 Central part (body) of lateral ventricle
13 Parietal bone
14 Inferior sagittal sinus
15 Angular artery
16 Parieto-occipital artery
17 Lambdoid suture
18 Occipital bone

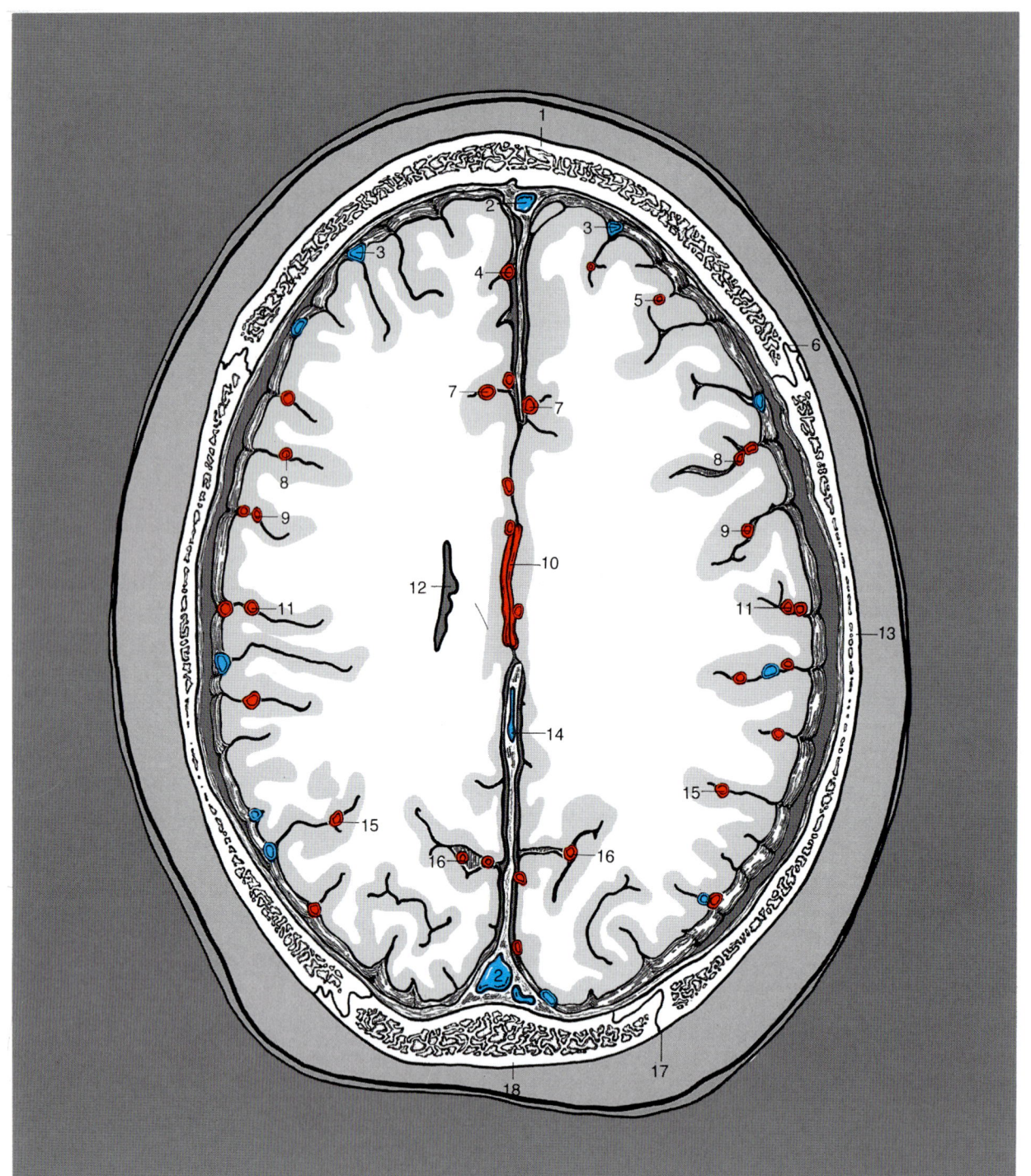

Fig. **56c** Superior section surface of the tenth canthomeatally oriented slice showing bony structures and blood vessels. The corpus callosum, which is not seen, forms the roof of the frontal (anterior) horns and central part (body) of lateral ventricles. On the left side the lateral ventricle is cut open.

Canthomeatally Oriented Slices 165

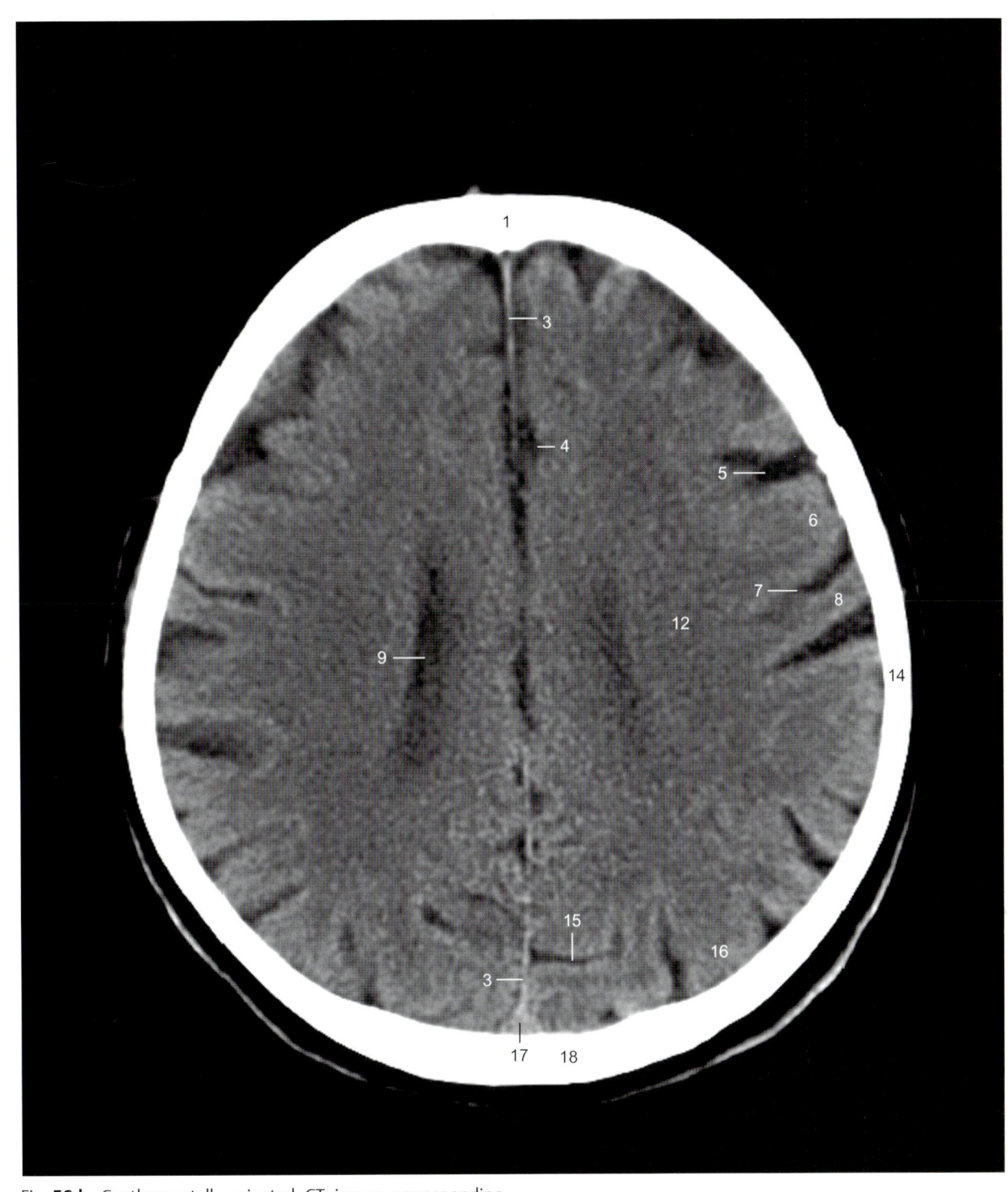

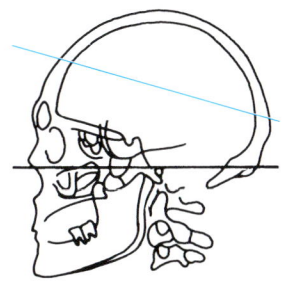

1 Frontal bone
3 Falx cerebri
4 Cingulate sulcus
5 Precentral sulcus
6 Precentral gyrus
7 Central sulcus
8 Postcentral gyrus
9 Central part (body) of lateral ventricle
12 Semioval center
14 Parietal bone
15 Parieto-occipital sulcus
16 Occipital gyri
17 Superior sagittal sinus
18 Occipital bone

Fig. **56d** Canthomeatally oriented CT image corresponding closely to the sectional plane of Figs. 56a and 56c.

166 Atlas

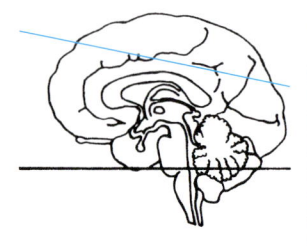

1 Superior frontal gyrus
2 Middle frontal gyrus
3 Precentral gyrus
4 Central sulcus
5 Cingulate sulcus
6 Cingulate gyrus
7 Postcentral gyrus
8 Semioval center
9 Supramarginal gyrus
10 Angular gyrus
11 Precuneus
12 Parieto-occipital sulcus
13 Dura mater
14 Falx cerebri
15 Cuneus

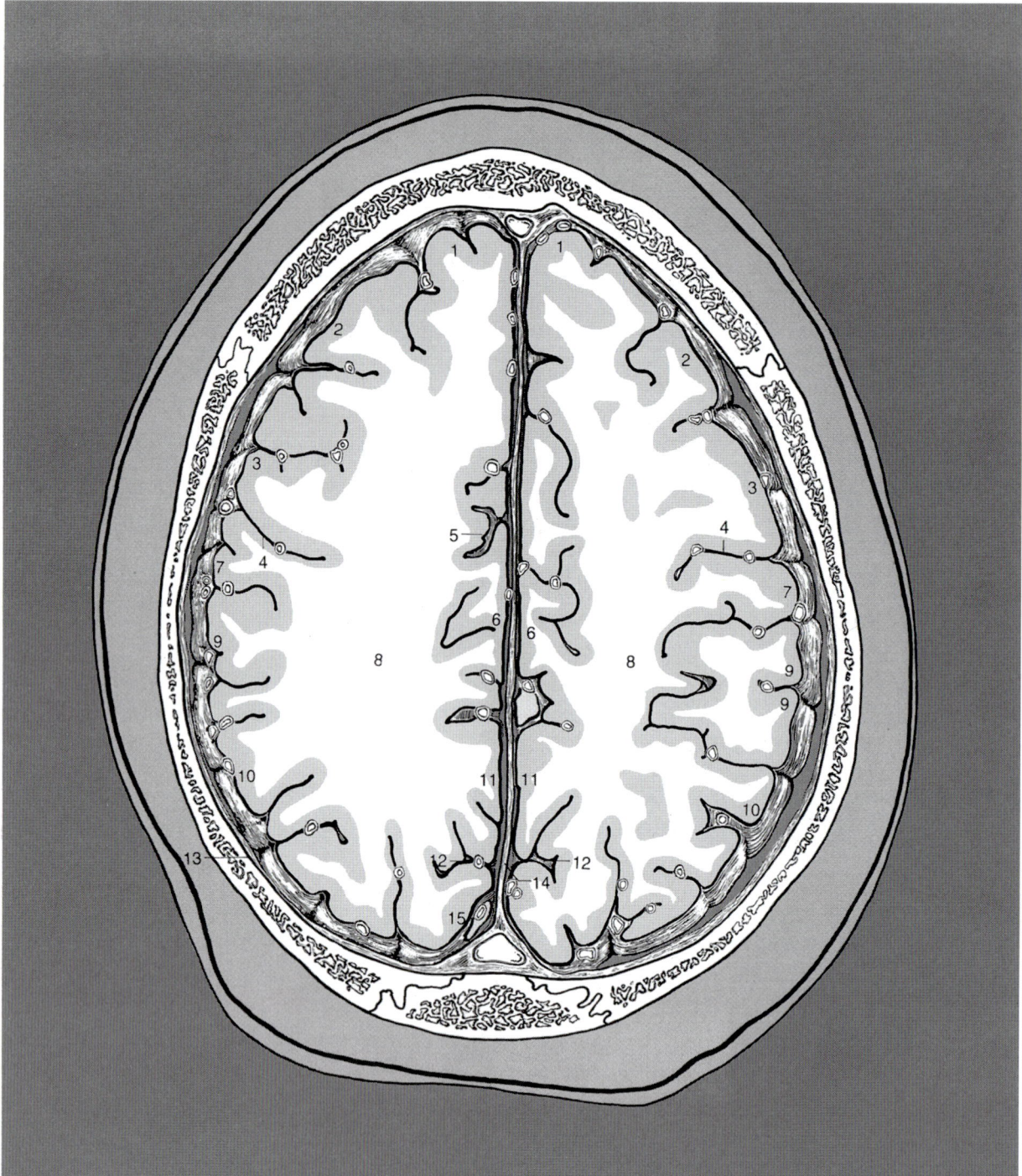

Fig. **57a** Superior section surface of the eleventh canthomeatally oriented slice depicting brain structures and meninges. The sectional plane cuts the cingulate sulcus tangentially. The cerebral falx separates the right and left hemispheres. The inferior edge of the cerebral falx is located in the middle of the section and, therefore, is not visible.

Canthomeatally Oriented Slices

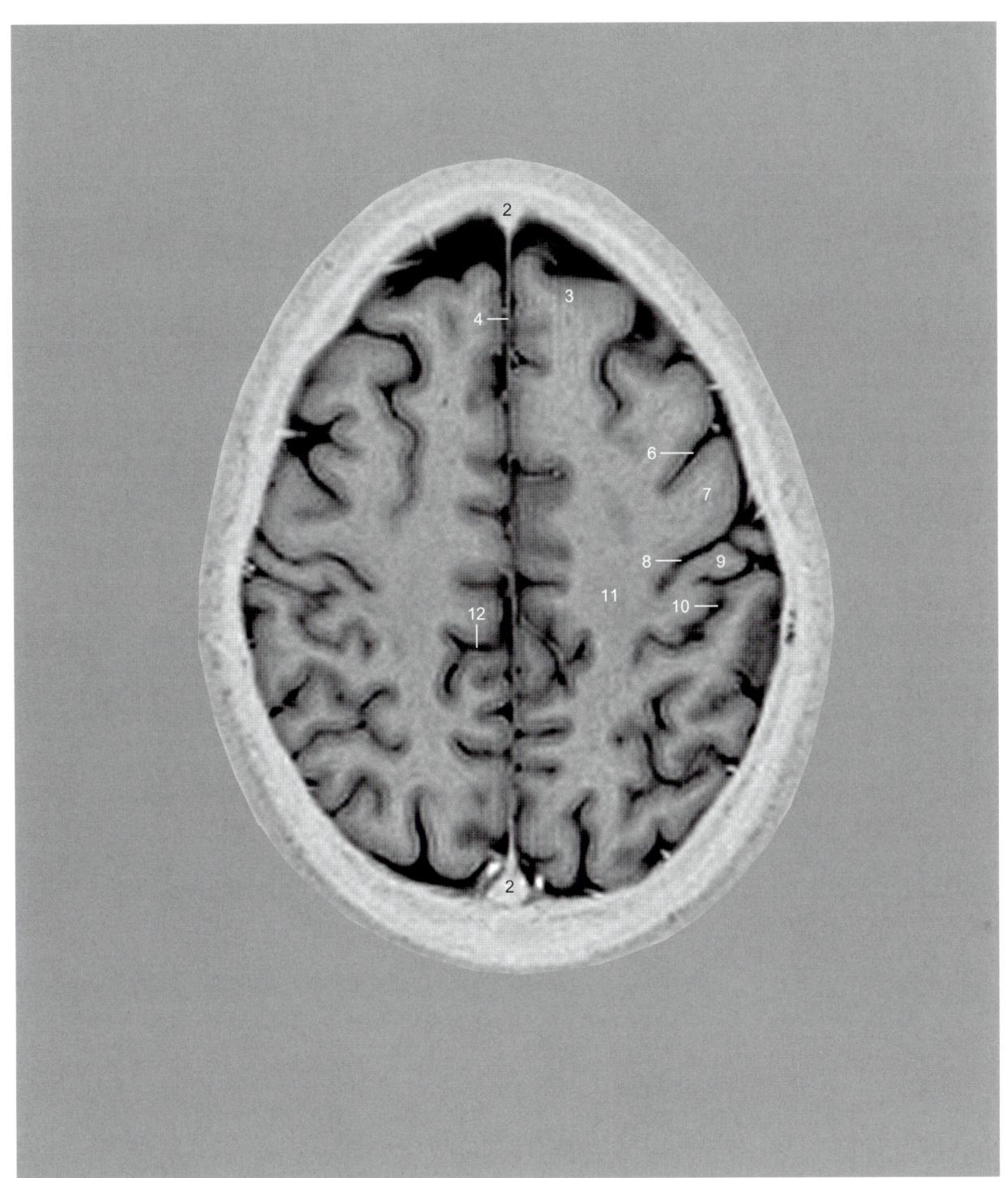

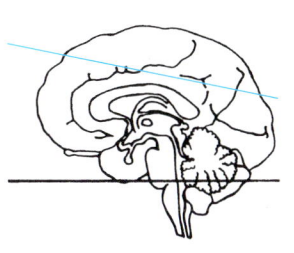

2 Superior sagittal sinus
3 Superior frontal gyrus
4 Falx cerebri
6 Precentral sulcus
7 Precentral gyrus
8 Central sulcus
9 Postcentral gyrus
10 Postcentral sulcus
11 Semioval center
12 Marginal branch of cingulate sulcus

Fig. **57b** Canthomeatally oriented, T1-weighted MR image corresponding approximately to the sectional plane of Figs. 57a and 57c.

168 Atlas

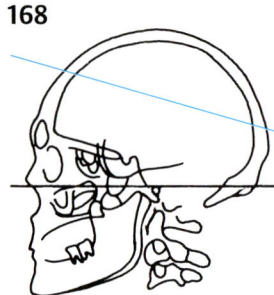

1 Frontal bone
2 Superior sagittal sinus
3 Superior cerebral vein
4 Intermediomedial frontal artery
5 Prefrontal artery
6 Coronal suture
7 Callosomarginal artery
8 Artery of precentral sulcus
9 Artery of central sulcus
10 Paracentral artery
11 Parietal bone
12 Parietal artery
13 Precuneal artery
14 Angular artery
15 Parieto-occipital artery
16 Occipital bone
17 Lambdoid suture

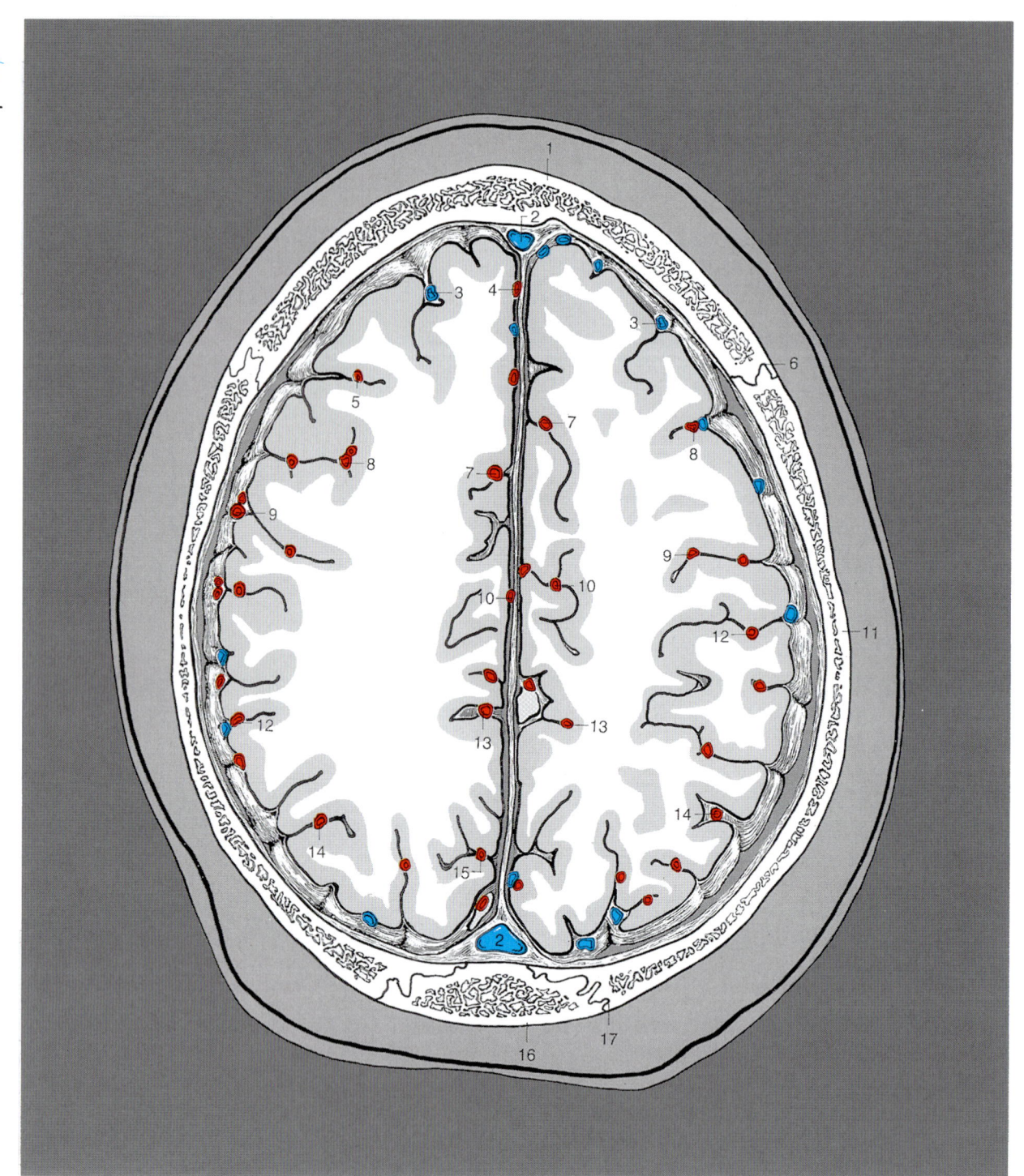

Fig. **57c** Superior section surface of the eleventh canthomeatally oriented slice demonstrating bony structures and blood vessels. The sectional plane lies in a supraventricular position.

Canthomeatally Oriented Slices

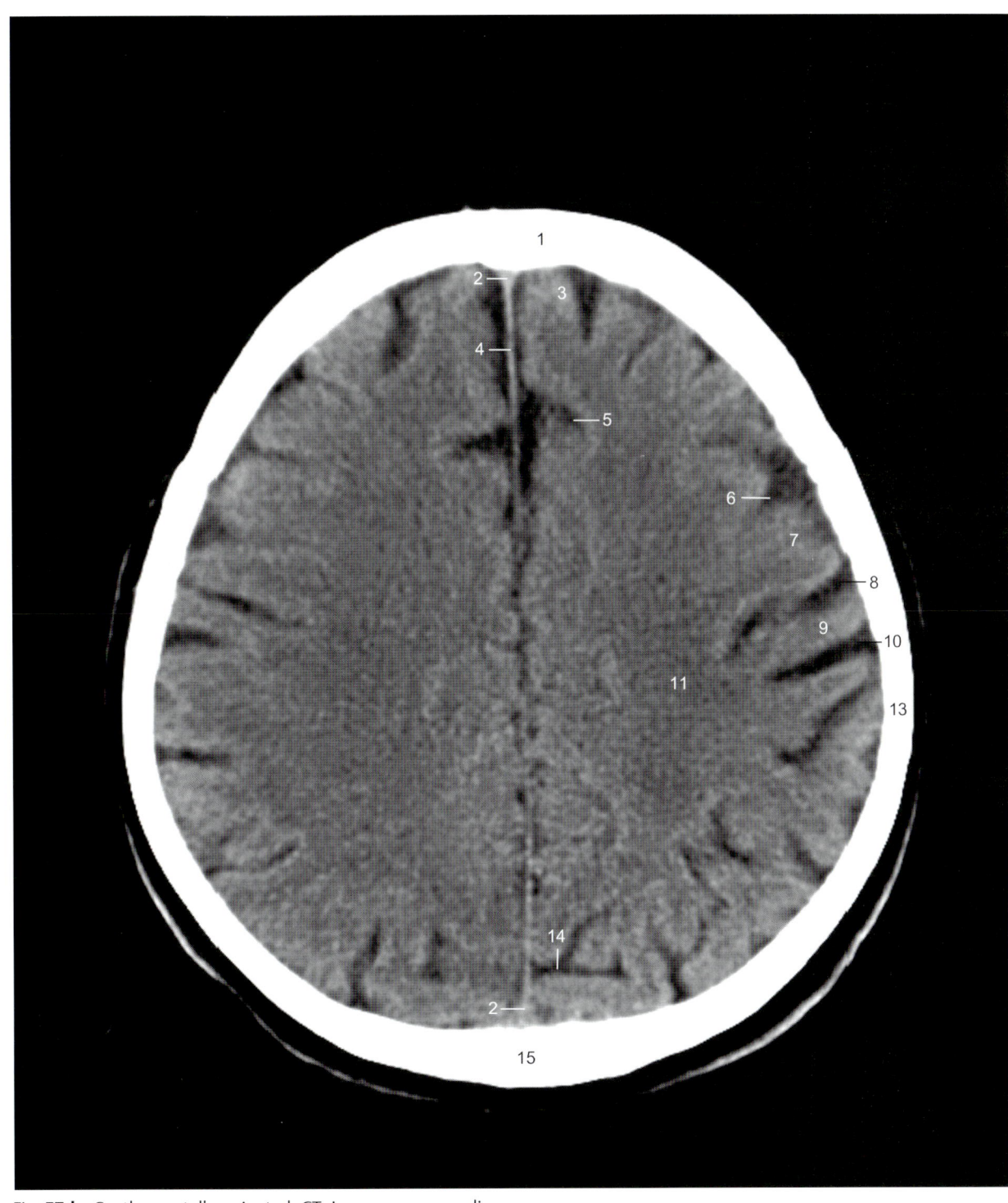

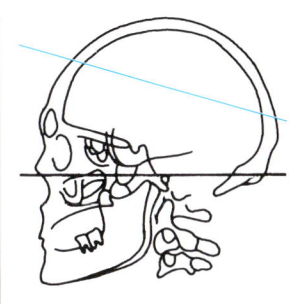

1 Frontal bone
2 Superior sagittal sinus
3 Superior frontal gyrus
4 Falx cerebri
5 Cingulate sulcus
6 Precentral sulcus
7 Precentral gyrus
8 Central sulcus
9 Postcentral gyrus
10 Postcentral sulcus
11 Semioval center
13 Parietal bone
14 Parieto-occipital sulcus
15 Occipital bone

Fig. **57d** Canthomeatally oriented CT image corresponding closely to the sectional plane of Figs. 57a and 57c.

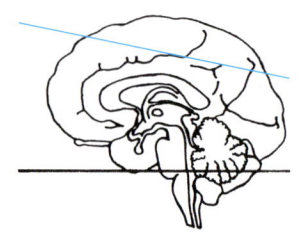

1 Superior frontal gyrus
2 Middle frontal gyrus
3 Precentral sulcus
4 Precentral gyrus
5 Central sulcus
6 Postcentral gyrus
7 Semioval center
8 Paracentral lobule
9 Superior parietal lobule
10 Falx cerebri
11 Precuneus
12 Parieto-occipital sulcus
13 Dura mater

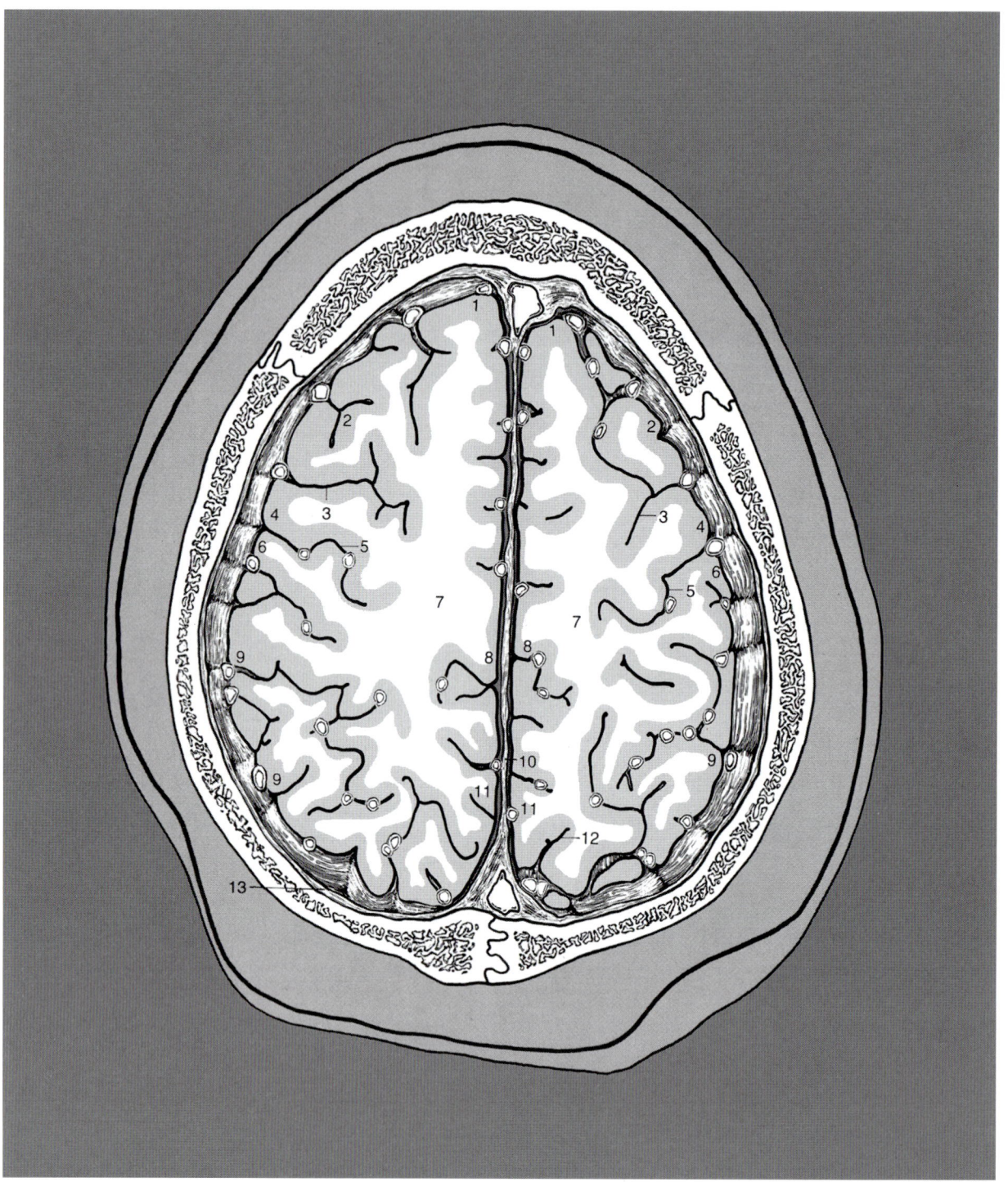

Fig. **58a** Superior section surface of the twelfth canthomeatally oriented slice portraying brain structures and meninges. The cerebral falx extends straight through the entire section, separating the left from the right hemisphere. The sectional plane lies above the cingulate gyrus.

Canthomeatally Oriented Slices 171

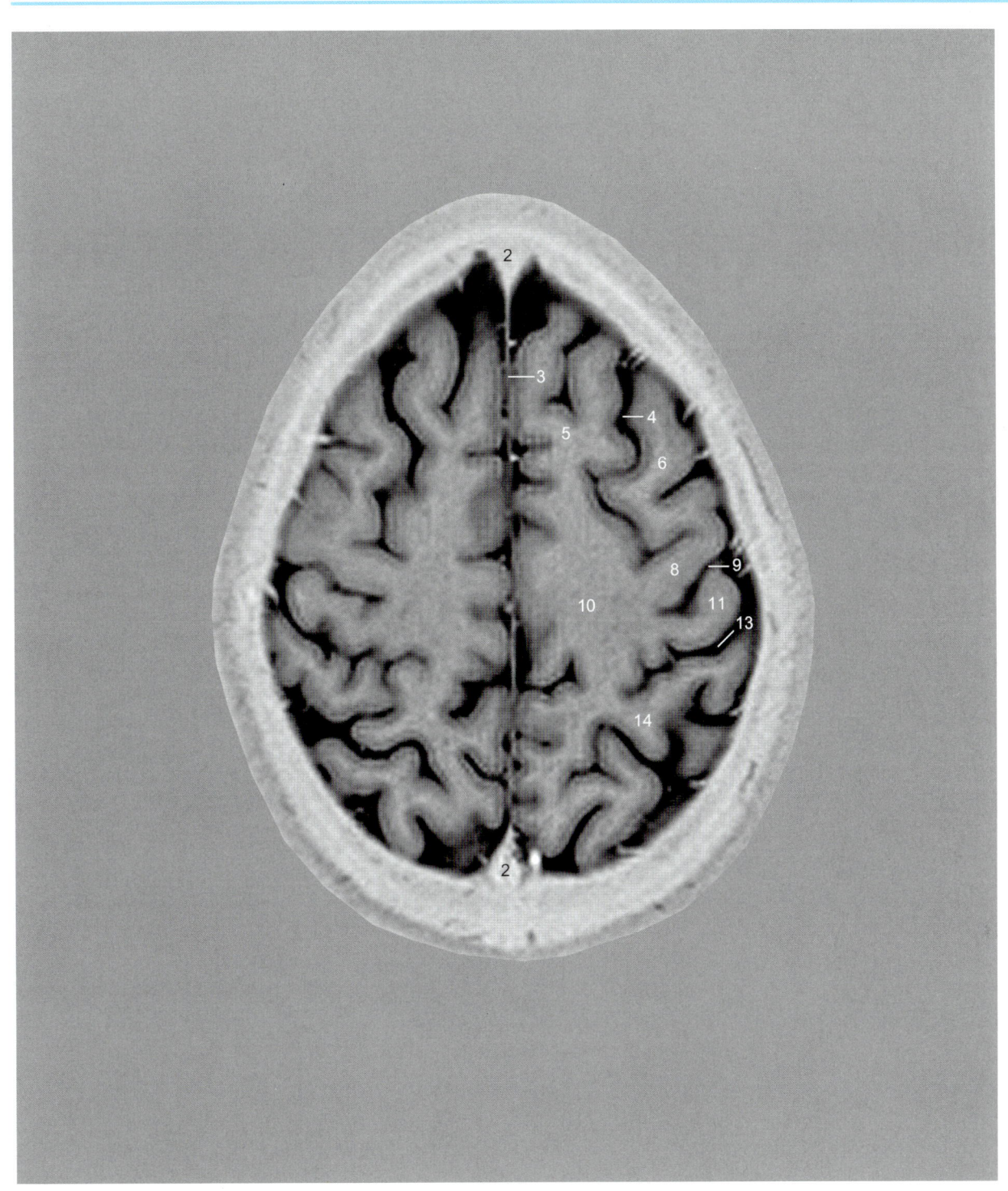

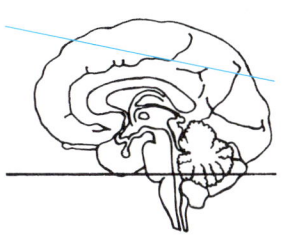

2 Superior sagittal sinus
3 Falx cerebri
4 Superior frontal sulcus
5 Superior frontal gyrus
6 Middle frontal gyrus
8 Precentral gyrus
9 Central sulcus
10 Semioval center
11 Postcentral gyrus
13 Postcentral sulcus
14 Superior parietal lobule

Fig. **58b** Canthomeatally oriented, T1-weighted MR image corresponding approximately to the sectional plane of Figs. 58a and 58c.

172 Atlas

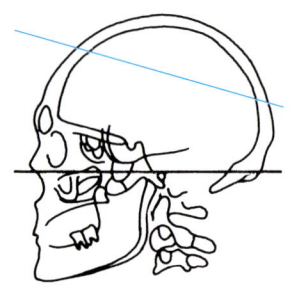

1 Frontal bone
2 Superior sagittal sinus
3 Posteromedial frontal artery
4 Superior cerebral vein
5 Coronal suture
6 Parietal bone
7 Paracentral artery
8 Precuneal artery
9 Sagittal suture
10 Scalp
11 Skin of the head

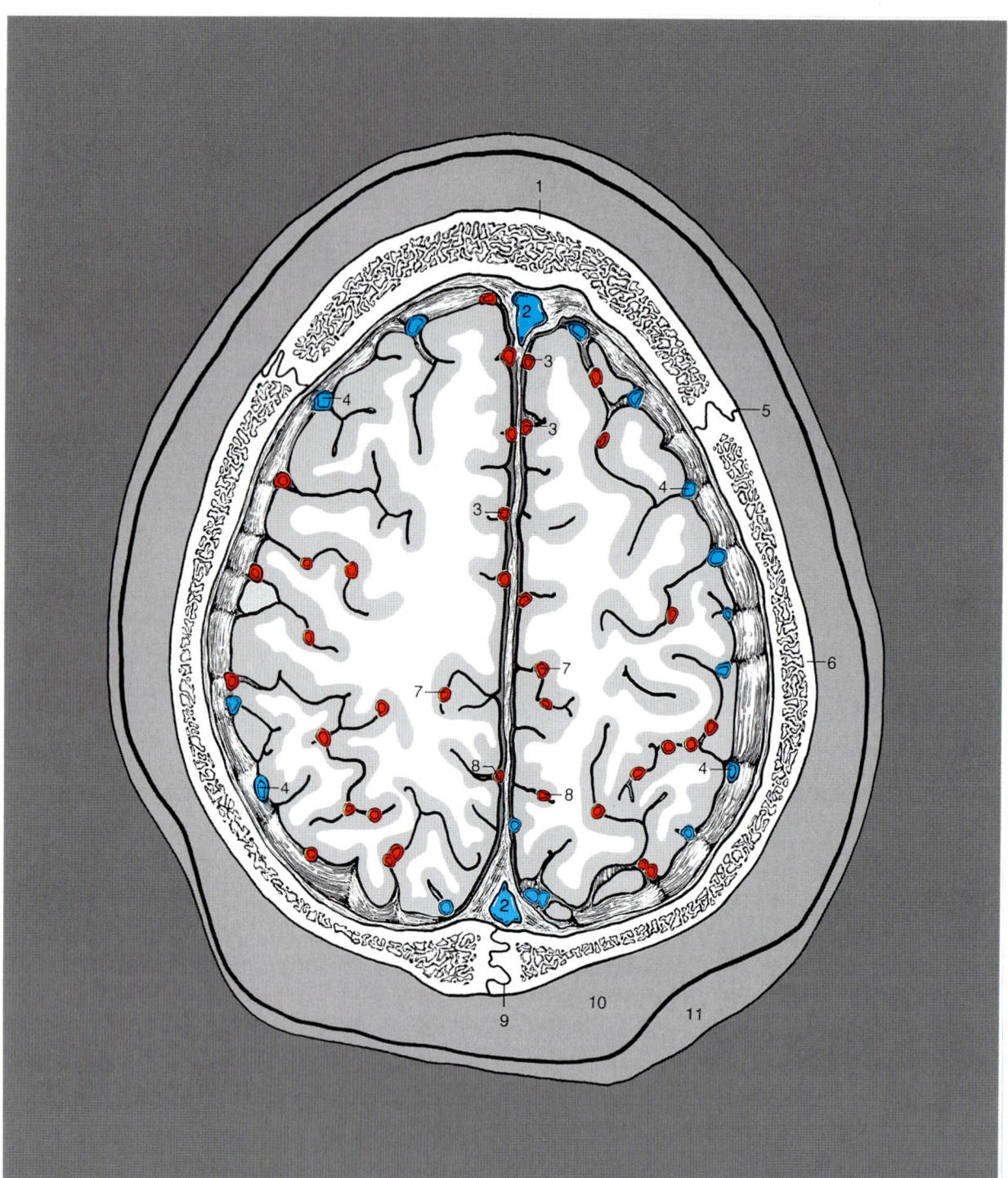

Fig. **58c** Superior section surface of the twelfth canthomeatally oriented slice revealing bony structures and blood vessels. The sectional plane lies in a supraventricular position.

Canthomeatally Oriented Slices 173

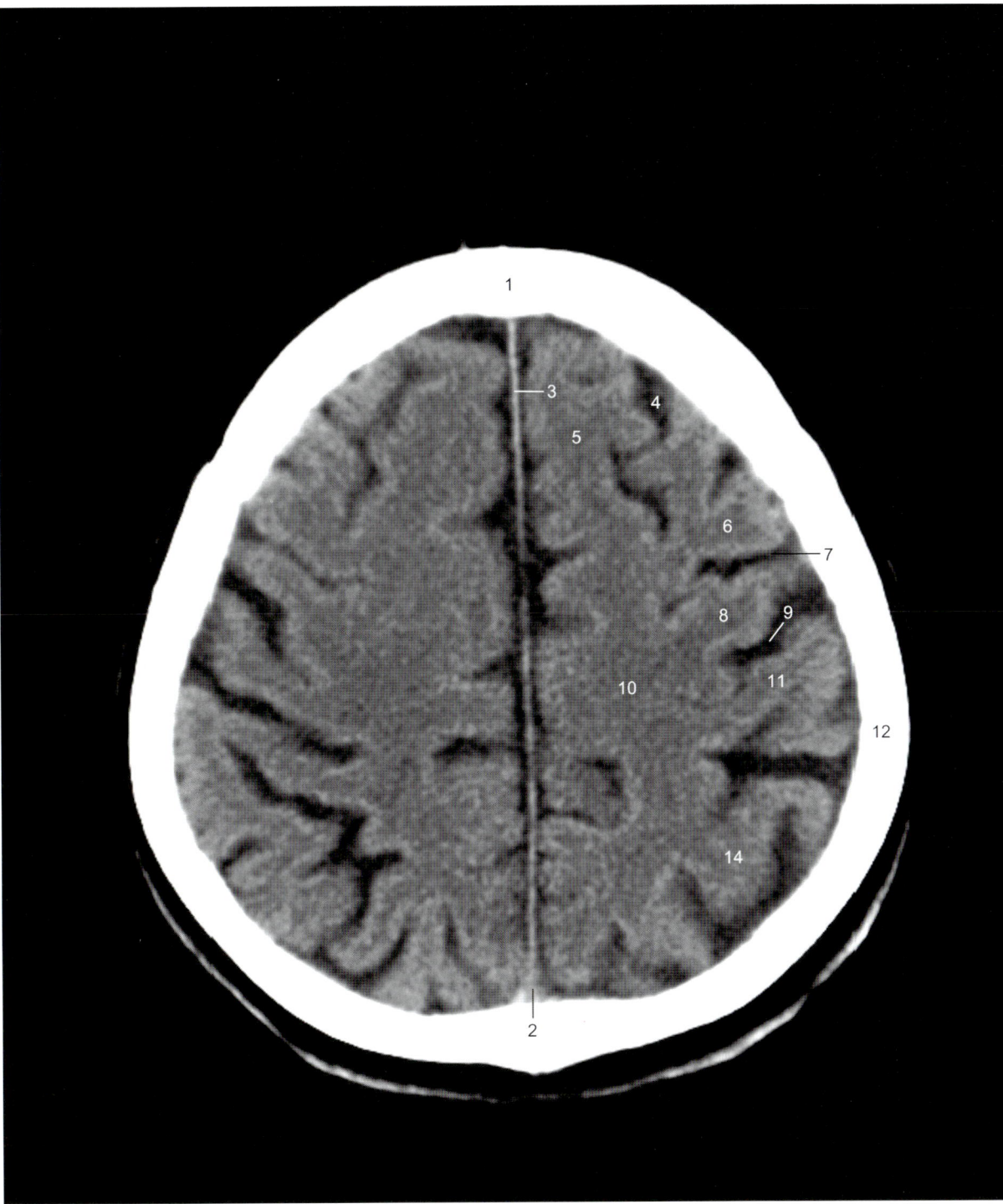

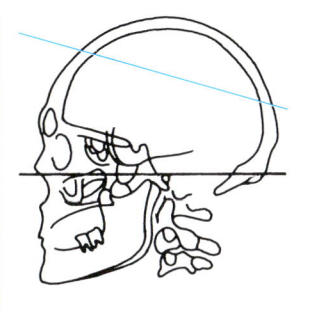

1 Frontal bone
2 Superior sagittal sinus
3 Falx cerebri
4 Superior frontal sulcus
5 Superior frontal gyrus
6 Middle frontal gyrus
7 Precentral sulcus
8 Precentral gyrus
9 Central sulcus
10 Semioval center
11 Postcentral gyrus
12 Parietal bone
14 Superior parietal lobule

Fig. **58d** Canthomeatally oriented CT image corresponding closely to the sectional plane of Figs. 58a and 58c.

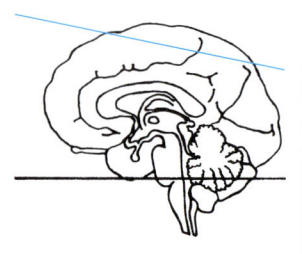

174 Atlas

1 Superior frontal gyrus
2 Precentral sulcus
3 Precentral gyrus
4 Central sulcus
5 Postcentral gyrus
6 Paracentral lobule
7 Falx cerebri
8 Dura mater
9 Superior parietal lobule
10 Precuneus

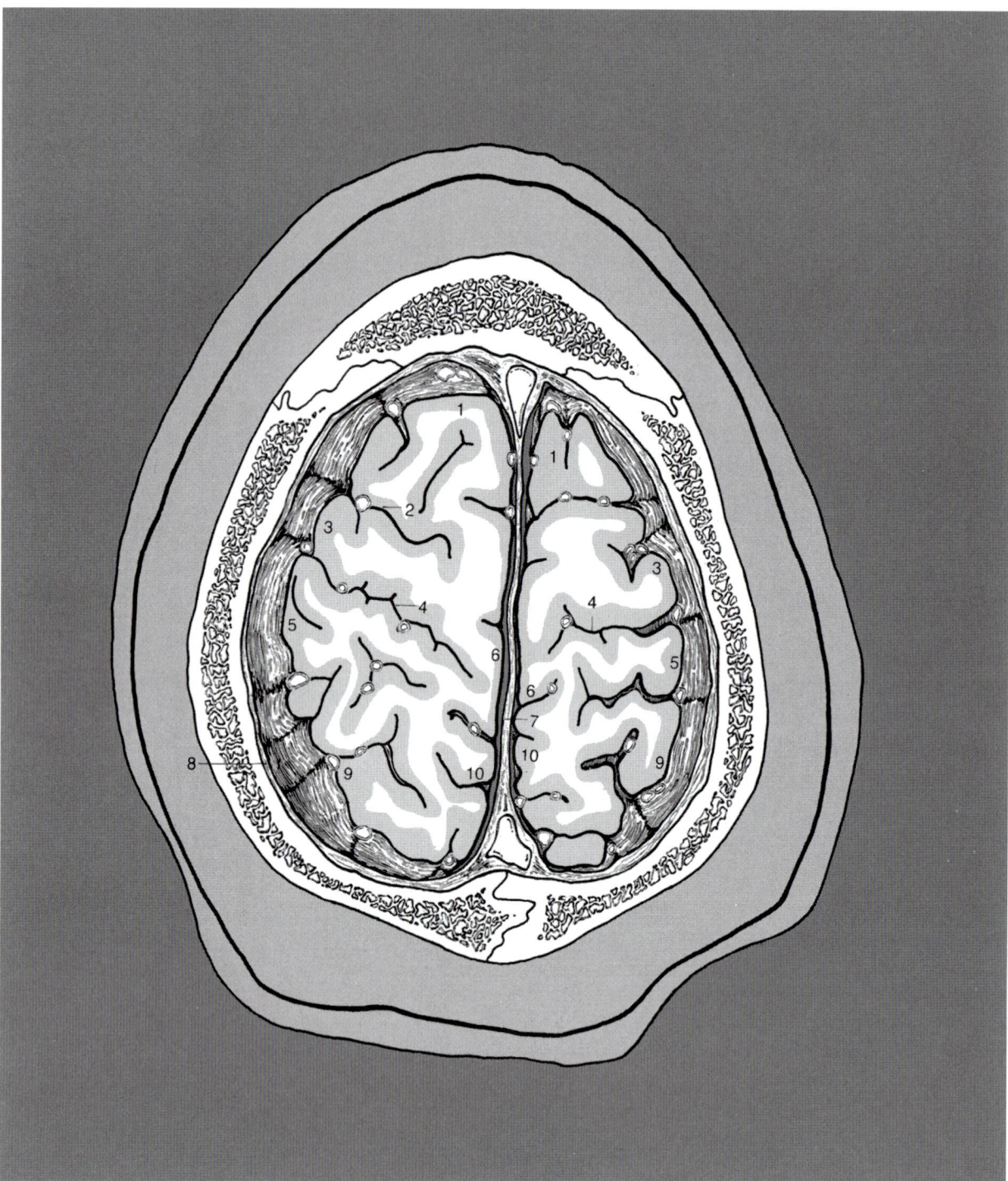

Fig. **59a** Superior section surface of the thirteenth canthomeatally oriented slice representing brain structures and meninges. The central sulcus separates the frontal from the parietal lobe.

Canthomeatally Oriented Slices 175

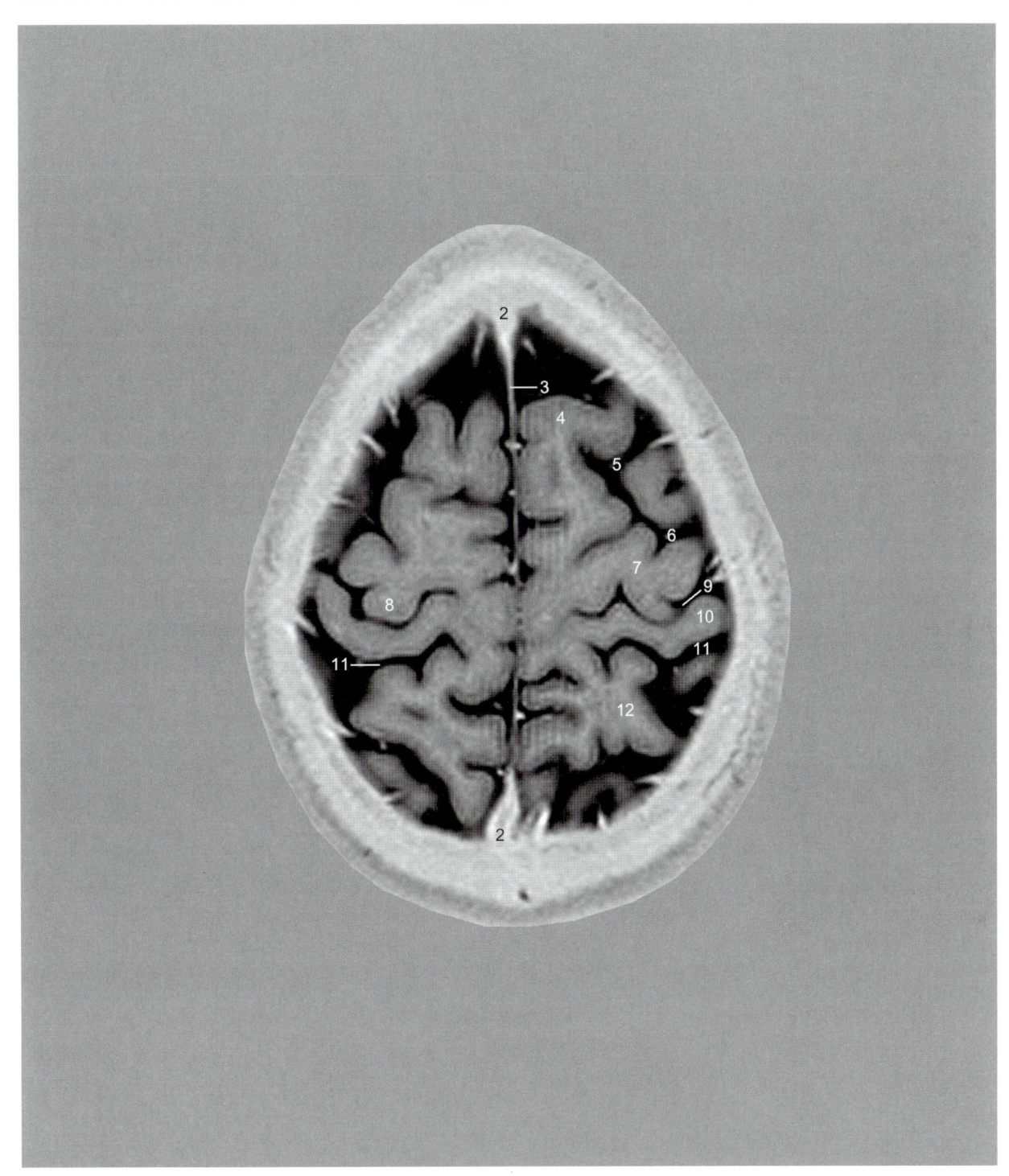

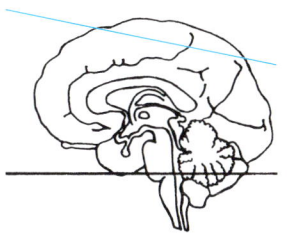

2 Superior sagittal sinus
3 Falx cerebri
4 Superior frontal gyrus
5 Superior frontal sulcus
6 Precentral sulcus
7 Precentral gyrus
8 Precentral gyrus
9 Central sulcus
10 Postcentral gyrus
11 Postcentral sulcus
12 Superior parietal lobule

Fig. **59b** Canthomeatally oriented, T1-weighted MR image corresponding approximately to the sectional plane of Figs. 59a and 59c.

176 Atlas

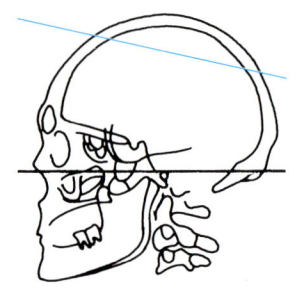

1 Frontal bone
2 Superior sagittal sinus
3 Coronal suture
4 Posteromedial frontal artery
5 Superior cerebral vein
6 Parietal bone
7 Paracentral artery
8 Precuneal artery
9 Sagittal suture

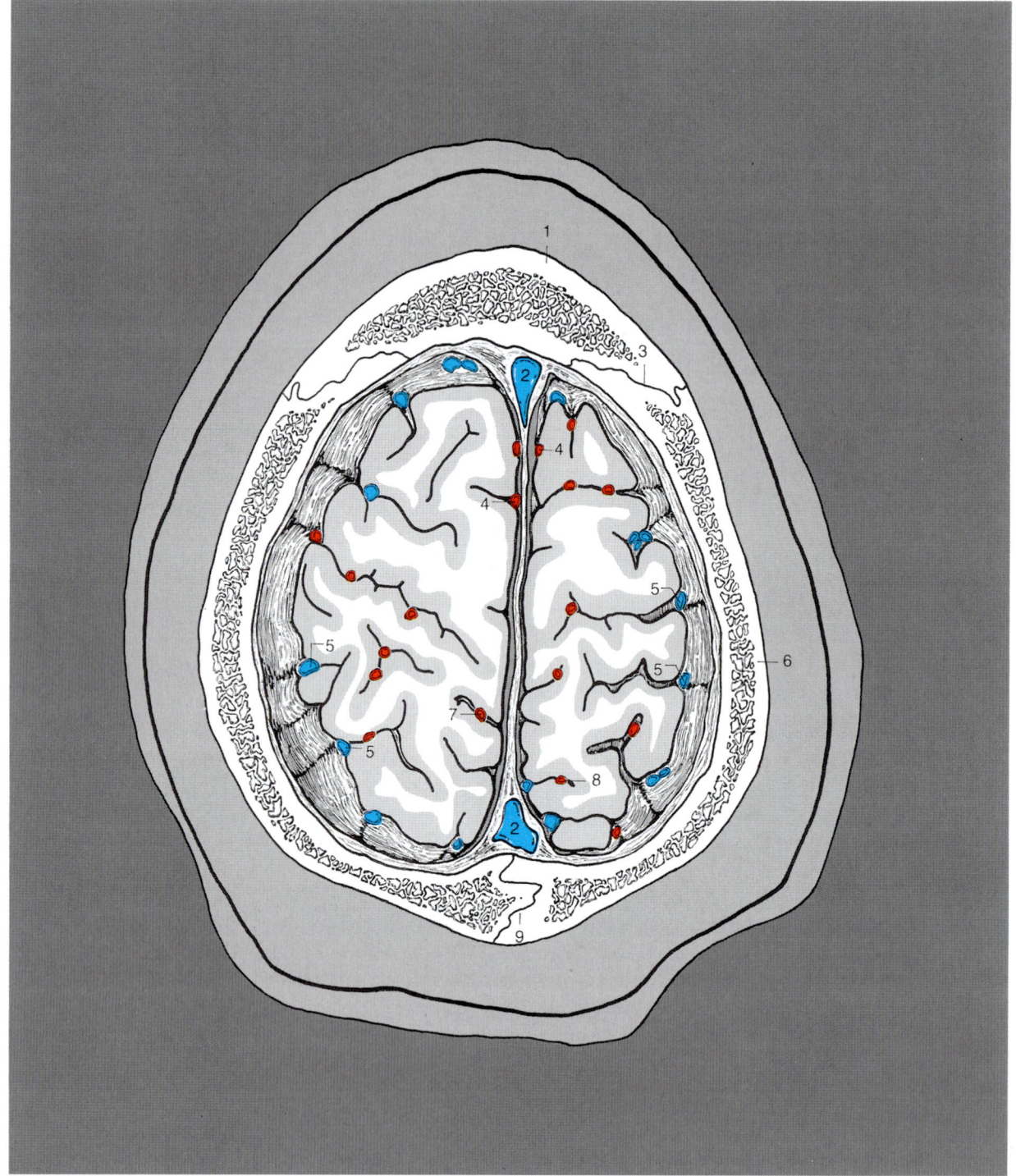

Fig. **59c** Superior section surface of the thirteenth canthomeatally oriented slice showing bony structures and blood vessels. The sectional plane lies in a supraventricular position.

Canthomeatally Oriented Slices 177

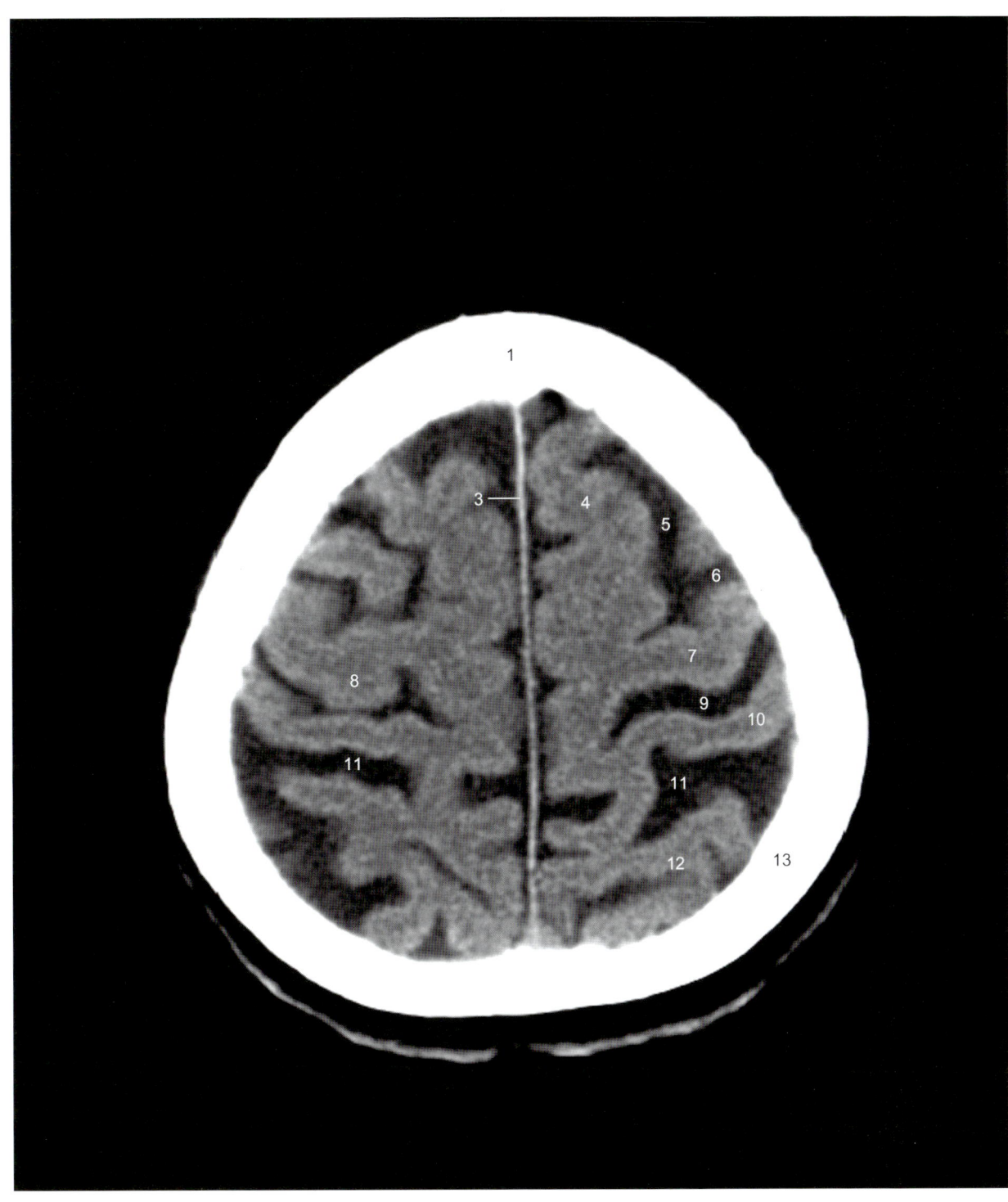

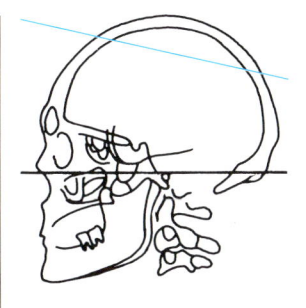

1 Frontal bone
3 Falx cerebri
4 Superior frontal gyrus
5 Superior frontal sulcus
6 Precentral sulcus
7 Precentral gyrus
8 Precentral gyrus
9 Central sulcus
10 Postcentral gyrus
11 Postcentral sulcus
12 Superior parietal lobule
13 Parietal bone

Fig. **59d** Canthomeatally oriented CT image corresponding closely to the sectional plane of Figs. 59a and 59c.

178   Atlas

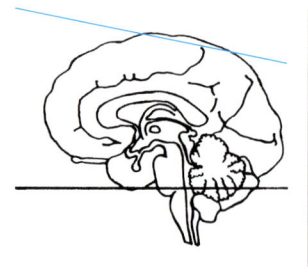

1 Precentral gyrus
2 Central sulcus
3 Postcentral gyrus
4 Dura mater

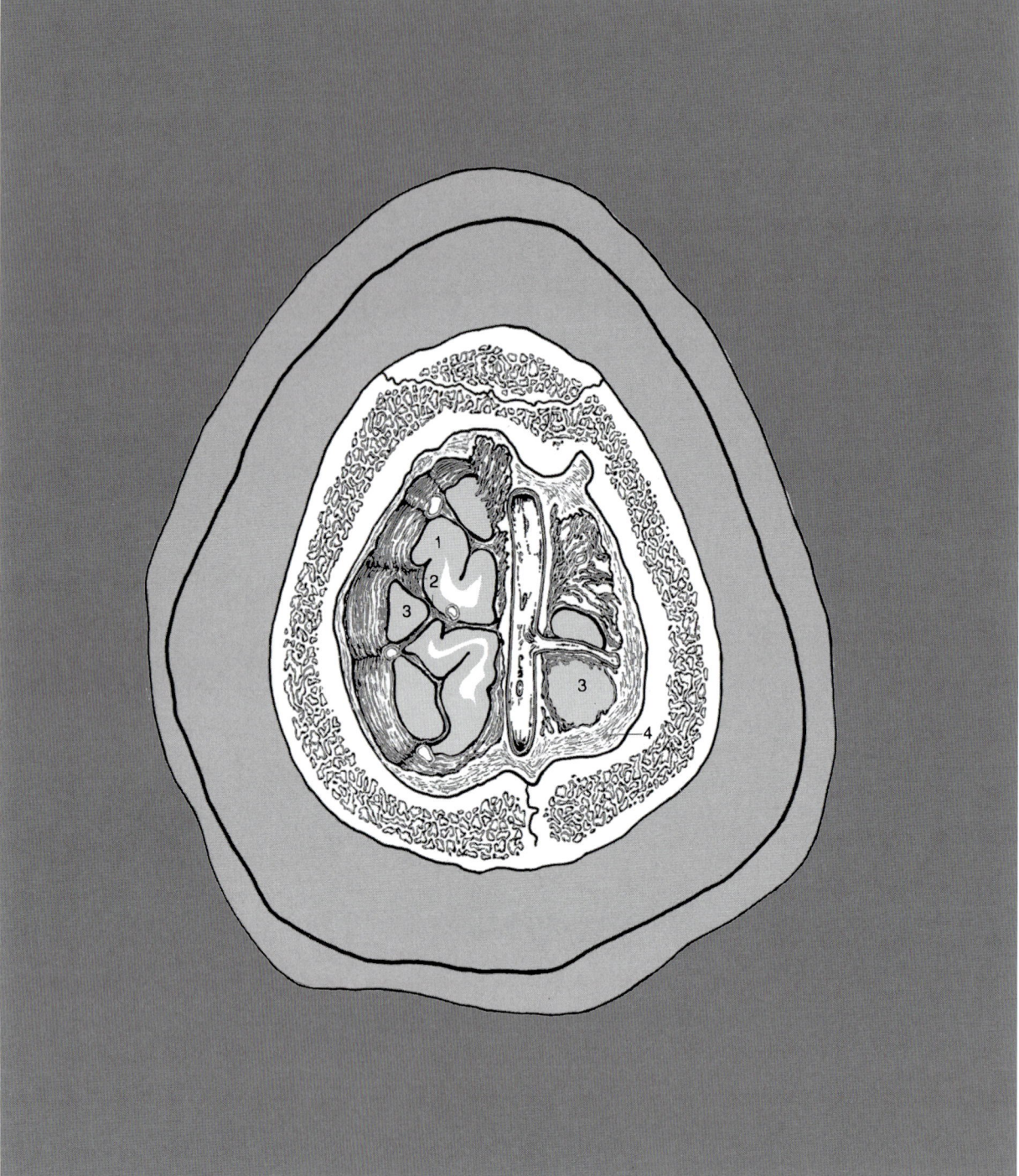

Fig. **60a** Superior section surface of the fourteenth canthomeatally oriented slice depicting brain structures and meninges. The central sulcus lies approximately 5 cm posterior to the bregma.

Canthomeatally Oriented Slices

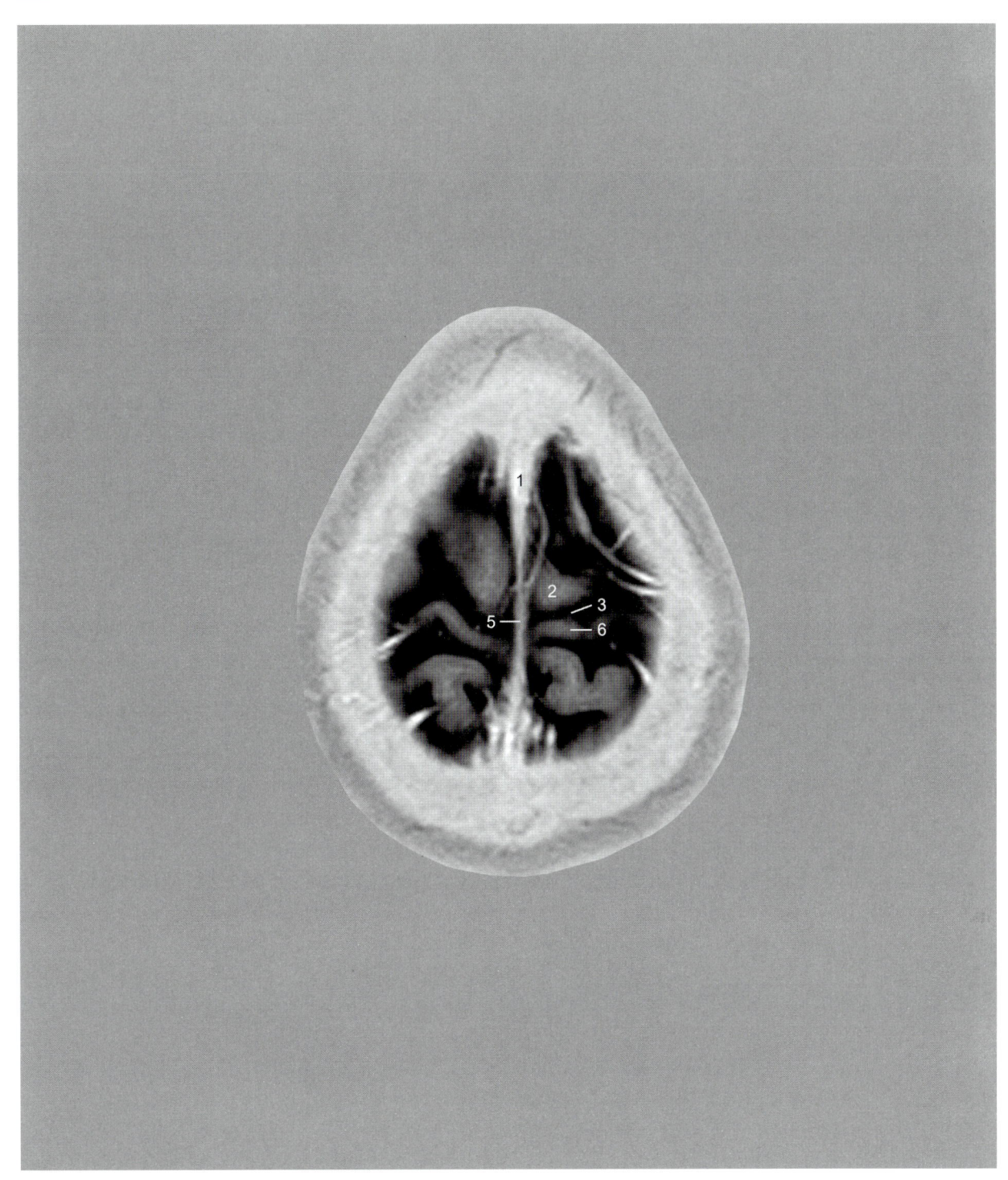

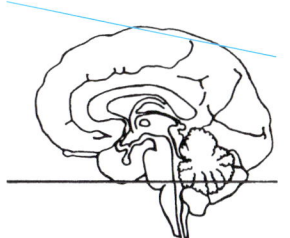

1 Superior sagittal sinus
2 Precentral gyrus
3 Central sulcus
5 Falx cerebri
6 Postcentral gyrus

Fig. **60b** Canthomeatally oriented, T1-weighted MR image positioned slightly below the sectional plane of Figs. 60a and 60c.

180 Atlas

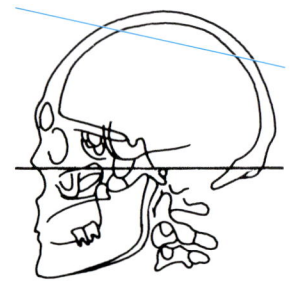

1 Frontal bone
2 Bregma
3 Coronal suture
4 Superior cerebral vein
5 Superior sagittal sinus
6 Parietal bone
7 Sagittal suture
8 Scalp
9 Skin of the head

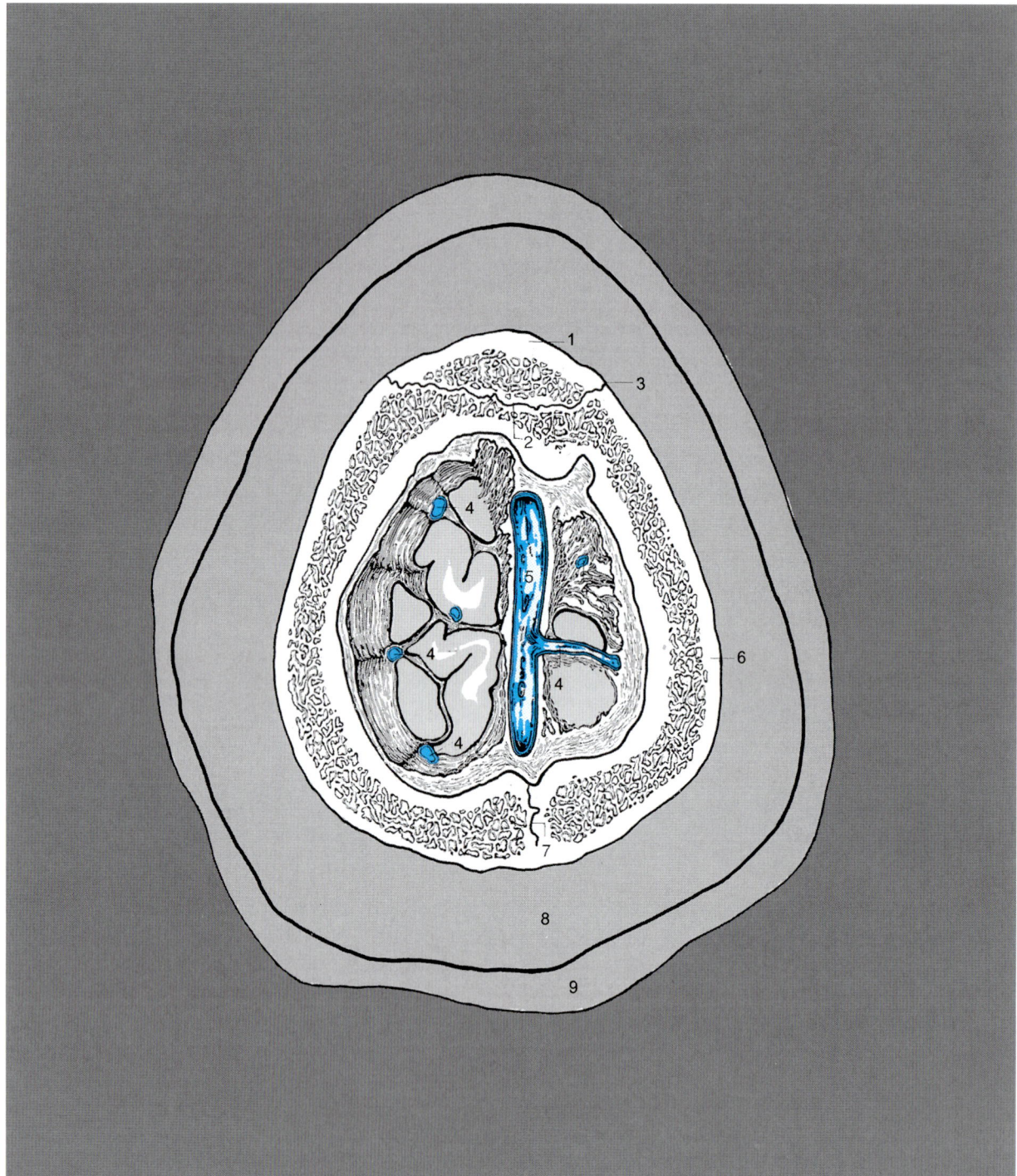

Fig. **60c** Superior section surface of the fourteenth canthomeatally oriented slice demonstrating bony structures and blood vessels. The sectional plane lies in a supraventricular position just beneath the top of the skullcap.

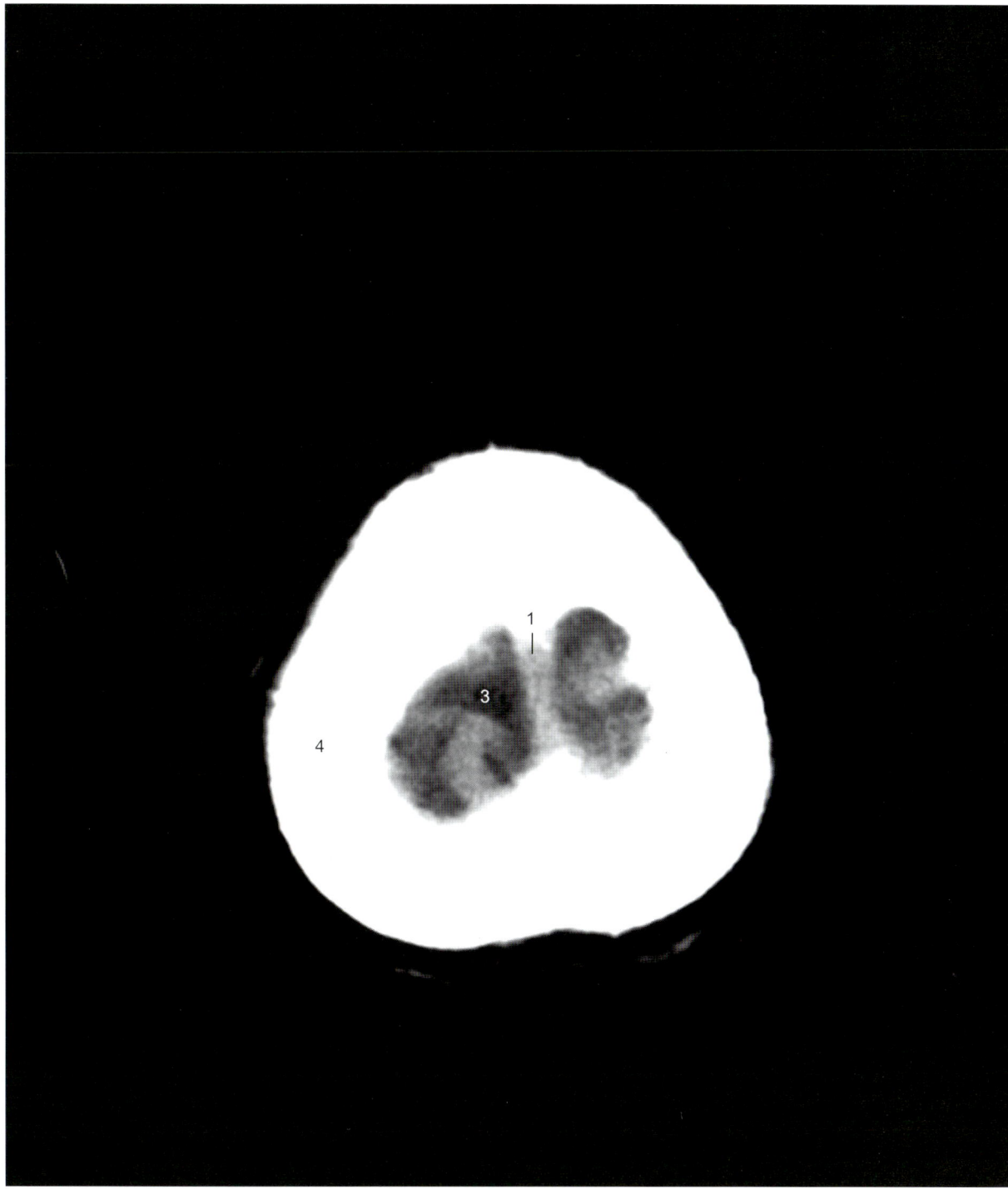

Canthomeatally Oriented Slices 181

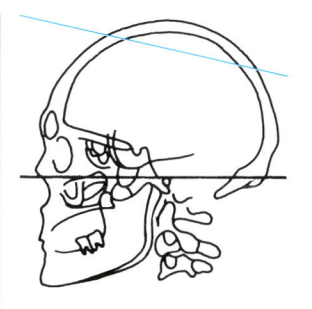

1 Superior sagittal sinus
3 Central sulcus
4 Parietal bone

Fig. **60d** Canthomeatally oriented CT image positioned slightly above the sectional plane of Figs. 60a and 60c.

182 Atlas

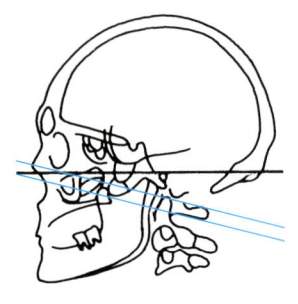

1 Nasal bone
2 Maxilla
3 Nasal septum
4 Infraorbital canal
5 Zygomatic bone
6 Maxillary sinus
7 Palatine bone
8 Lateral pterygoid plate
9 Mandible
10 Anterior arch of atlas
11 Styloid process
12 Dens of axis
13 Foramen transversarium
14 Lateral mass of atlas
15 Vertebral canal
16 Auricle (pinna)
17 Posterior arch of atlas

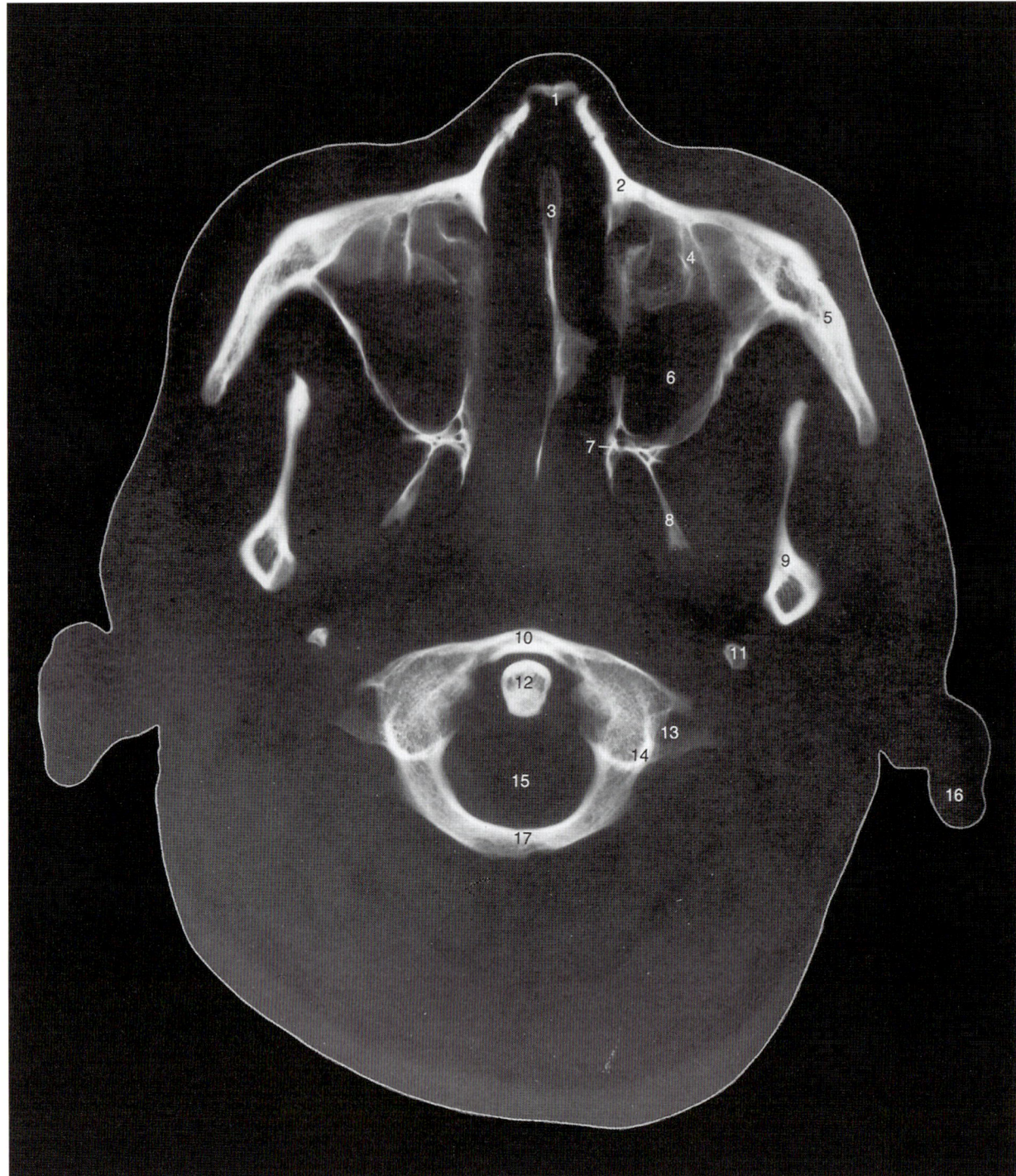

Fig. 61 Radiograph of the first canthomeatally oriented slice. The outer border of the head has been added. Guideline structures include the maxillary sinuses, atlas, and dens of axis.

Canthomeatally Oriented Slices

1 Nasal bone
2 Nasal septum
3 Ethmoidal cells
4 Orbit
5 Zygomatic bone
6 Maxillary sinus
7 Zygomatic arch
8 Foramen spinosum
9 Mandible
10 Basilar part of occipital bone
11 Basion
12 Jugular foramen
13 Hypoglossal canal
14 Mastoid process
15 Foramen magnum
16 Auricle (pinna)

Fig. 62 Radiograph of the second canthomeatally oriented slice. The outer border of the head has been added. Bony guideline structures include the nasal bone, nasal septum, and foramen magnum.

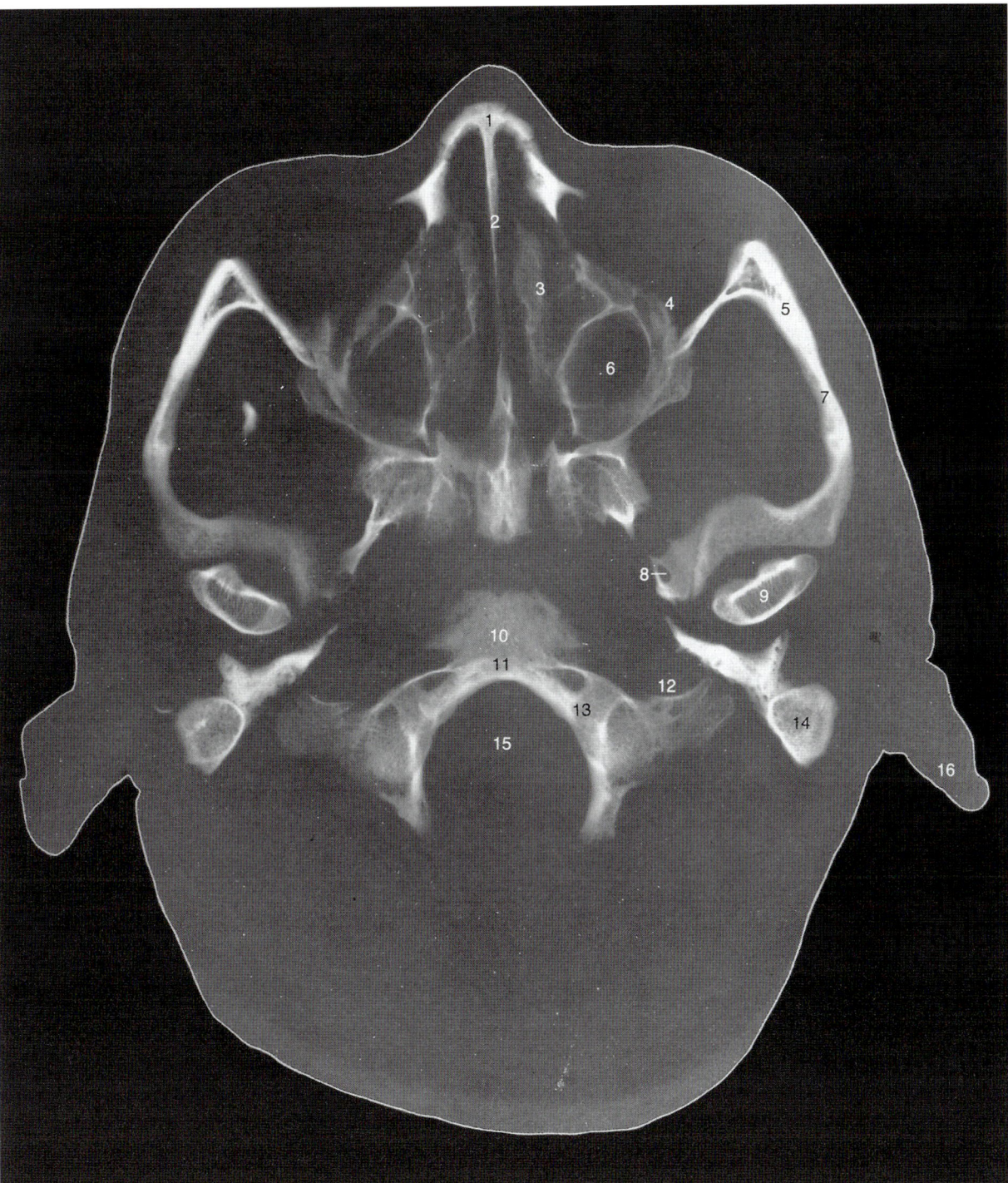

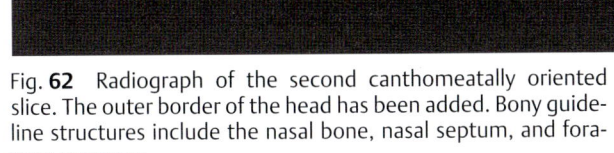

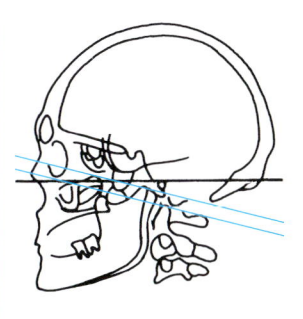

184   Atlas

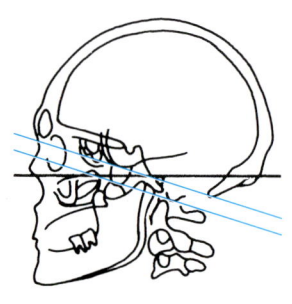

1 Ethmoidal cells
2 Orbit
3 Zygomatic bone
4 Ethmoid
5 Foramen rotundum
6 Sphenoidal sinus
7 Sphenoid, floor of middle cranial fossa
8 Foramen ovale
9 Temporal bone
10 Foramen lacerum
11 Foramen spinosum
12 Clivus
13 Head of mandible
14 Carotid canal
15 External acoustic meatus
16 Jugular foramen
17 Facial canal
18 Mastoid process
19 Occipital bone, floor of posterior cranial fossa

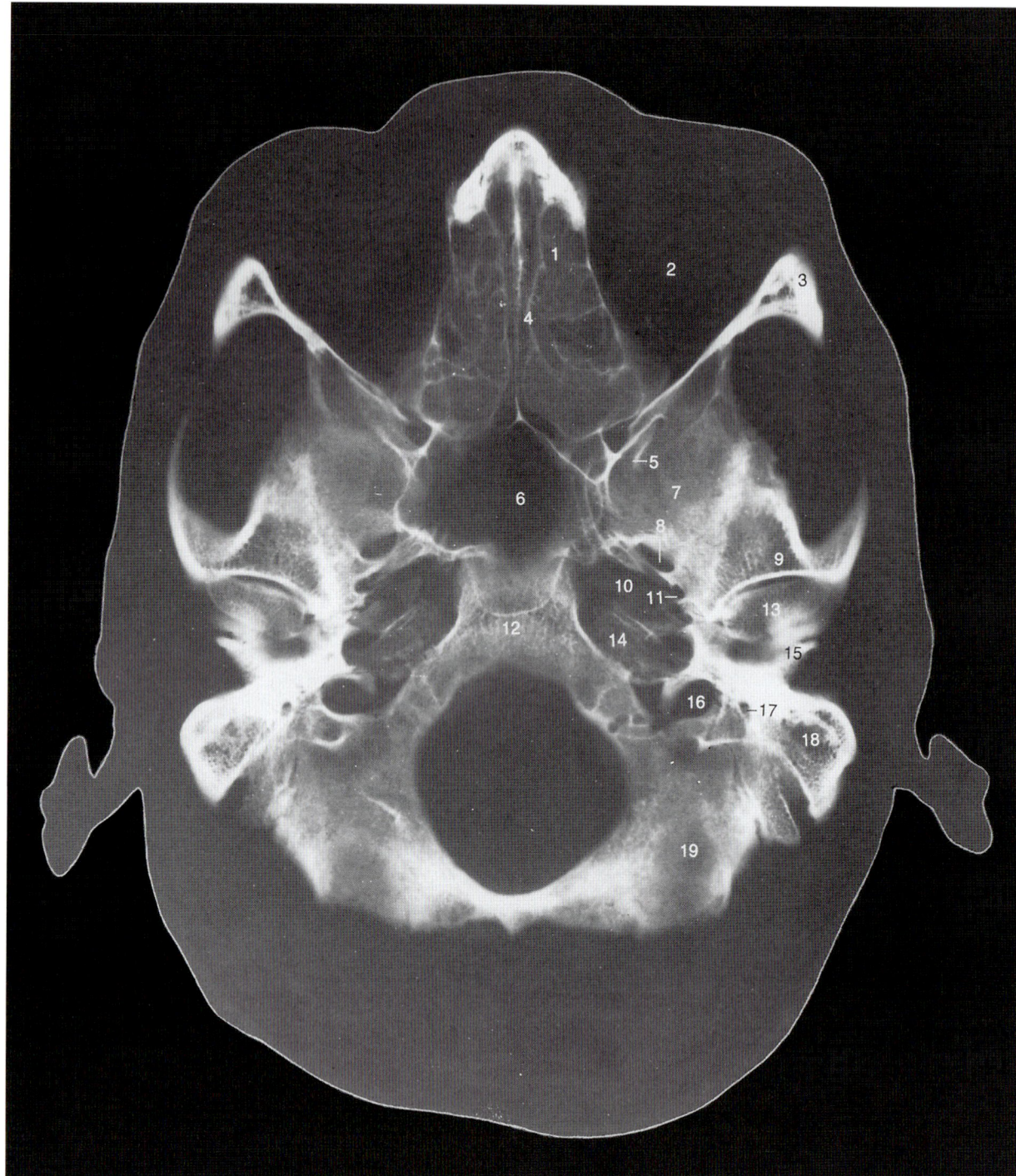

Fig. 63 Radiograph of the third canthomeatally oriented slice. The medial and lateral walls of the orbits are shown. The sphenoid forms the floor of the middle cranial fossa. The occipital bone encloses the posterior cranial fossa. The openings for the internal carotid arteries, internal jugular veins, middle meningeal arteries, as well as those for cranial nerves V/2, V/3, VII, IX, X, XI are shown.

Canthomeatally Oriented Slices 185

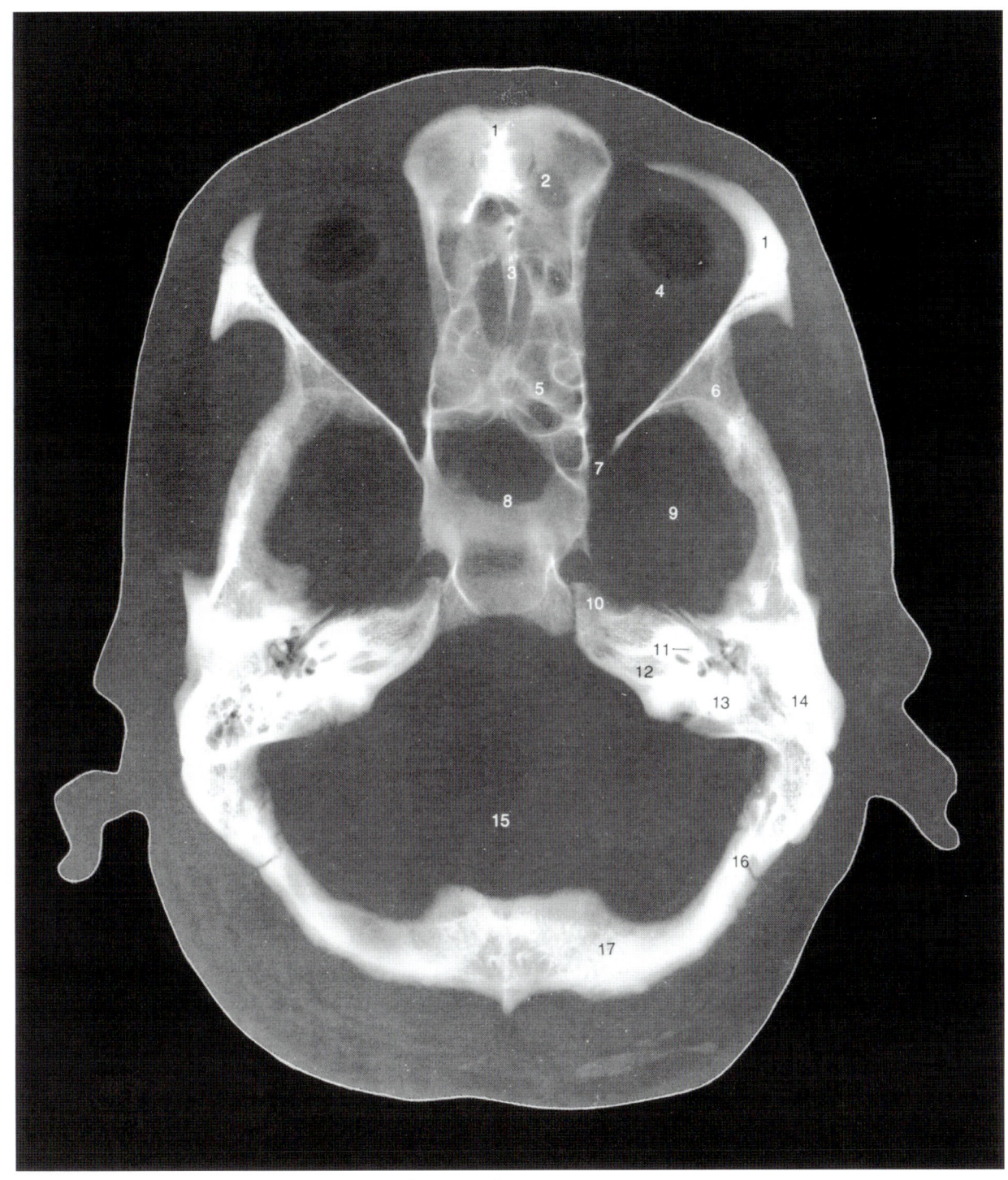

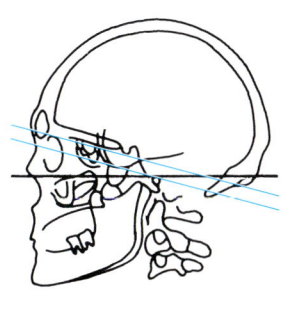

1 Frontal bone
2 Floor of frontal sinus
3 Crista galli
4 Orbit
5 Ethmoidal cells
6 Sphenoid
7 Superior orbital fissure
8 Sphenoid sinus
9 Middle cranial fossa
10 Apex of petrous part of temporal bone
11 Cochlea
12 Internal acoustic meatus
13 Petrous part of temporal bone
14 Temporal bone
15 Posterior cranial fossa
16 Lambdoid suture
17 Occipital bone

Fig. 64 Radiograph of the fourth canthomeatally oriented slice showing the upper portion of the orbits, sphenoidal sinus, middle cranial fossa, petrous part of the temporal bones, and posterior cranial fossa.

186 Atlas

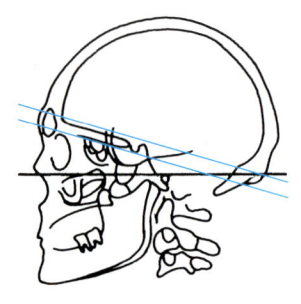

1 Frontal bone
2 Frontal sinus
3 Roof of orbit
4 Anterior cranial fossa
5 Sphenoid
6 Optic canal
7 Anterior clinoid process
8 Sella turcica (hypophysial fossa)
9 Middle cranial fossa
10 Posterior clinoid process
11 Dorsum sellae
12 Anterior semicircular canal
13 Posterior semicircular canal
14 Temporal bone
15 Posterior cranial fossa
16 Lambdoid suture
17 Internal occipital protuberance
18 Occipital bone
19 External occipital protuberance (inion)

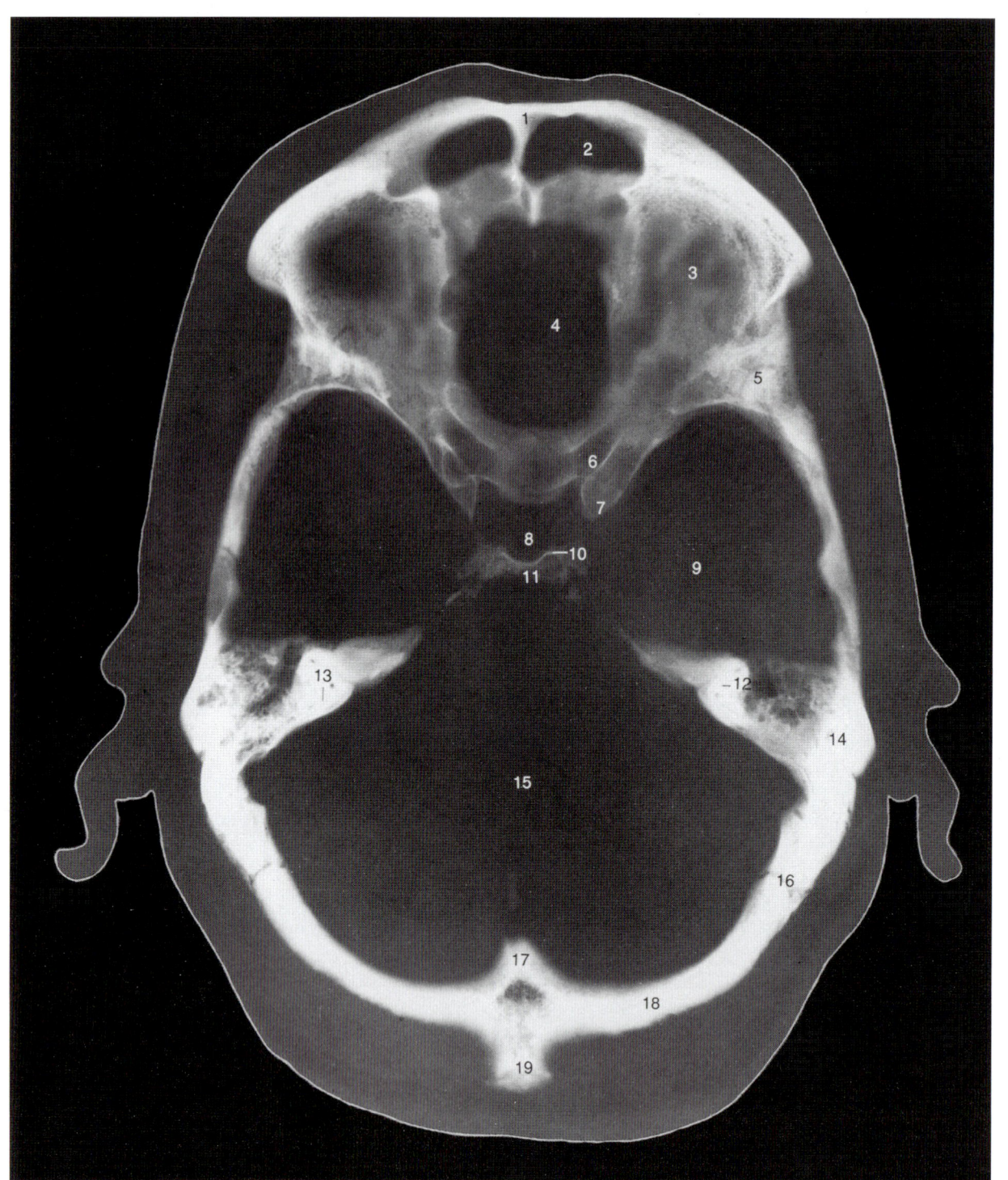

Fig. 65 Radiograph of the fifth canthomeatally oriented slice showing the floor of the anterior cranial fossa, anterior clinoid processes, dorsum sellae, and superior portion of the petrous part of the temporal bones.

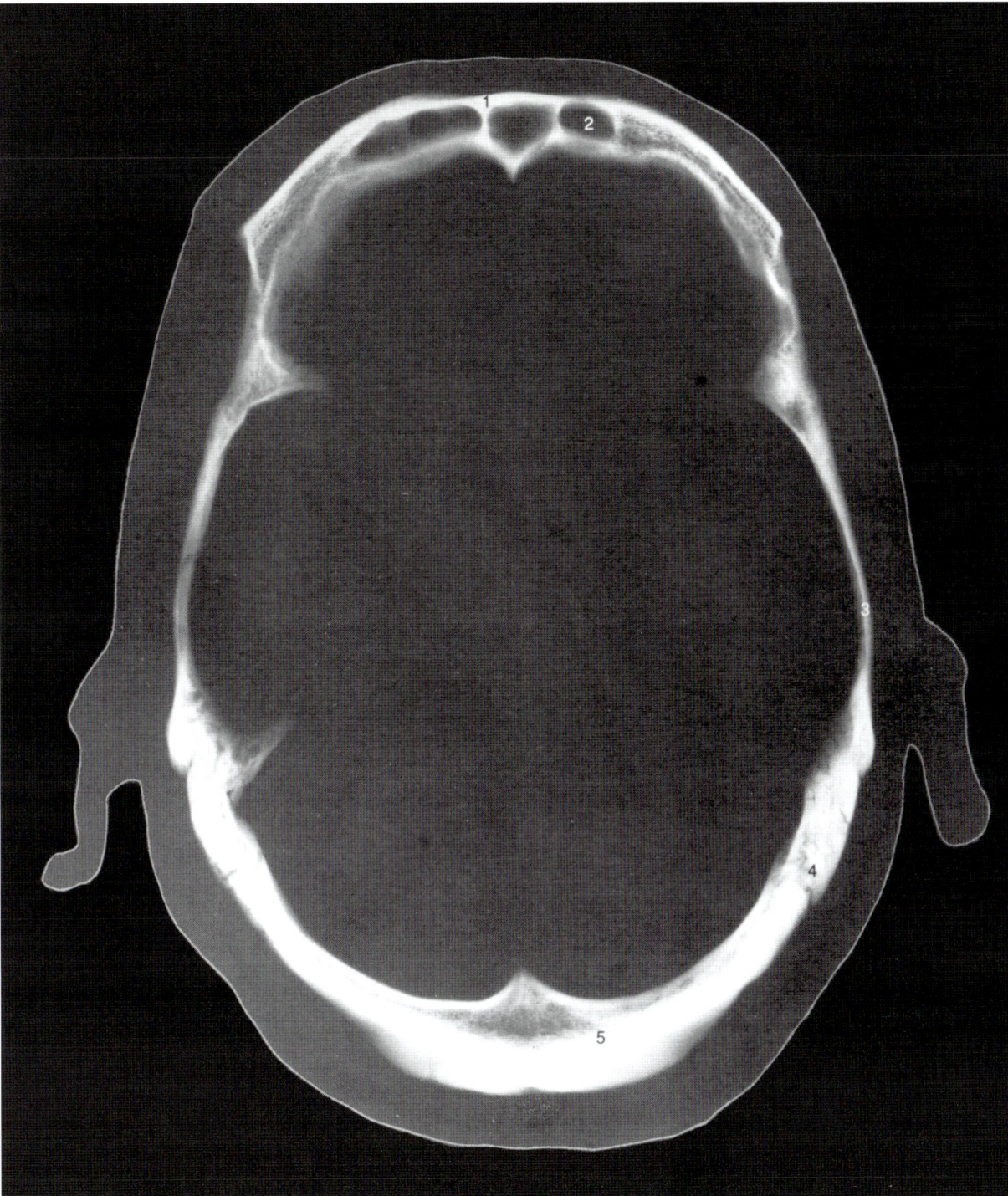

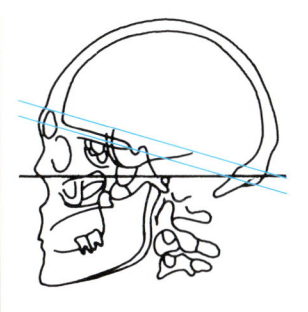

Canthomeatally Oriented Slices

1 Frontal bone
2 Frontal sinus
3 Temporal bone
4 Lambdoid suture
5 Occipital bone

Fig. **66** Radiograph of the sixth canthomeatally oriented slice. The skull forms an oval bony ring. Its inner processes, marking the borders of the anterior, middle, and posterior cranial fossae, are seen more clearly to the left.

Atlas

1. Corpus callosum
2. Fornix
3. Parieto-occipital sulcus
4. Interthalamic adhesion
5. Anterior commissure
6. Third ventricle
7. Pineal gland
8. Posterior commissure
9. Lamina terminalis
10. Frontal sinus
11. Hypothalamus
12. Superior colliculus
13. Culmen (IV, V)
14. Optic chiasm
15. Tegmentum of midbrain
16. Aqueduct of midbrain
17. Inferior colliculus
18. Mammillary body
19. Infundibulum
20. Primary fissure of cerebellum
21. Ethmoidal cells

22. Pituitary gland
23. Calcarine sulcus
24. Sphenoidal sinus
25. Pons
26. Declive (VI)
27. Clivus
28. Fastigium of fourth ventricle
29. Nodule of vermis (X)
30. Folium of vermis (VII A)
31. Tuber of vermis (VII B)
32. Uvula of vermis (IX)
33. Pyramis of vermis (VIII)
34. External acoustic meatus
35. Medulla oblongata
36. Head of mandible
37. Obex of medulla oblongata
38. Tonsil of cerebellum (H IX)
39. Foramen magnum
40. Maxillary sinus
41. Cisterna magna (posterior cerebellomedullary cistern)
42. Atlas
43. Spinal cord

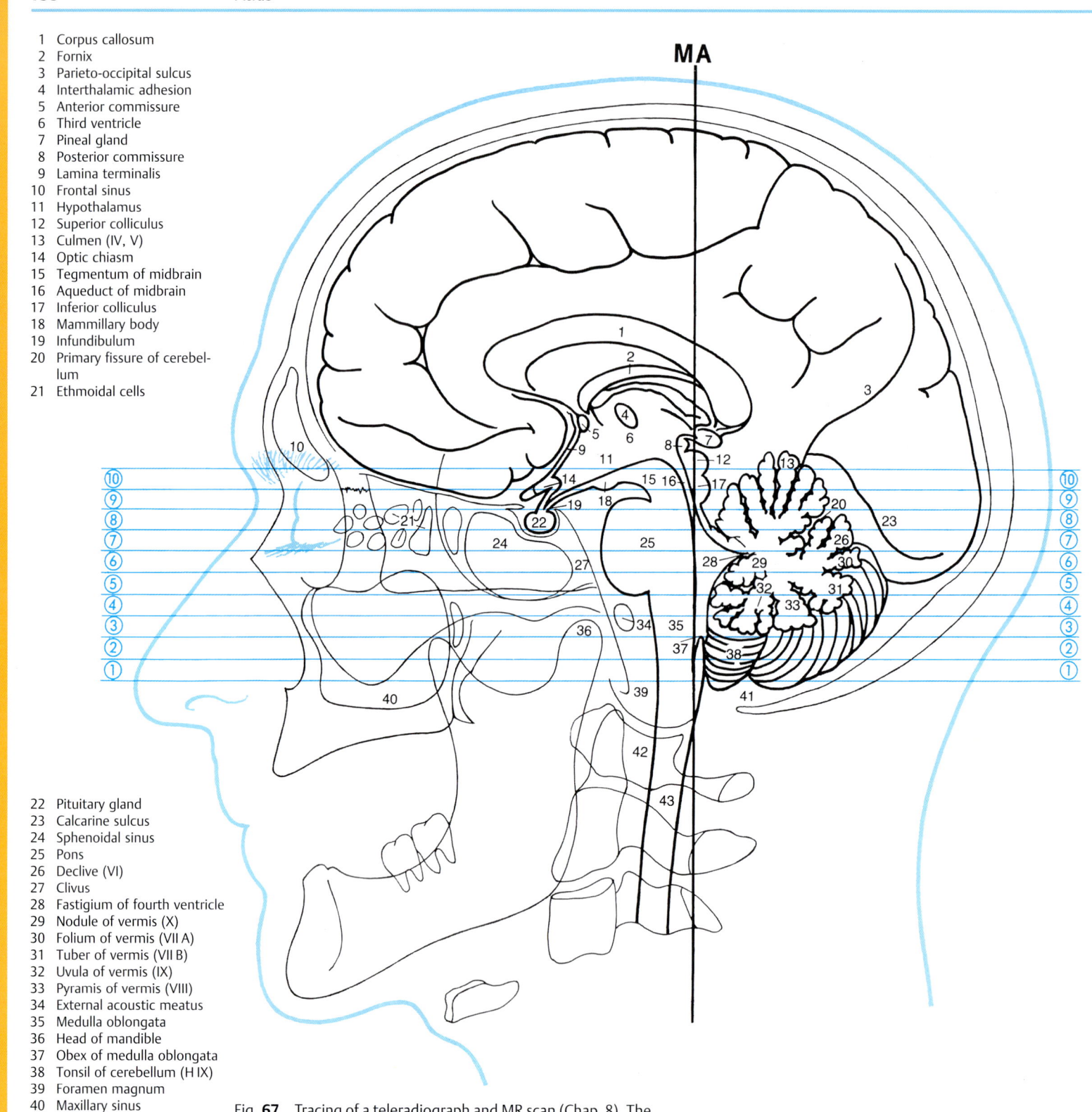

Fig. **67** Tracing of a teleradiograph and MR scan (Chap. 8). The 5-mm-thick slices of the brainstem series are cut vertically to Meynert's axis (MA). Meynert's axis runs tangentially through the floor of the rhomboid fossa and along the median plane. The slices are numbered consecutively in an inferior to superior order (Chap. 1.2 Three-dimensional coordinate systems for the localization of brain structures). The sectional plane always corresponds to the line positioned above the encircled number of the respective slice.

Brainstem Slices 189

1 Mesencephalic tract of trigeminal nerve
2 Mesencephalic nucleus of trigeminal nerve
3 Principal sensory nucleus of trigeminal nerve
4 Spinal tract of trigeminal nerve
5 Spinal nucleus of trigeminal nerve
6 Vestibular nuclei
7 Posterior (dorsal) and anterior (ventral) cochlear nuclei
8 Solitary nucleus
9 Accessory nucleus of oculomotor nerve (of Edinger–Westphal)
10 Oculomotor nucleus
11 Trochlear nucleus
12 Motor nucleus of trigeminal nerve
13 Genu of facial nerve
14 Abducens nucleus
15 Facial nucleus
16 Superior and inferior salivatory nuclei
17 Nucleus ambiguus
18 Posterior (dorsal) nucleus of vagus nerve
19 Hypoglossal nucleus
20 Spinal nucleus of accessory nerve
Vm Motor root of trigeminal nerve

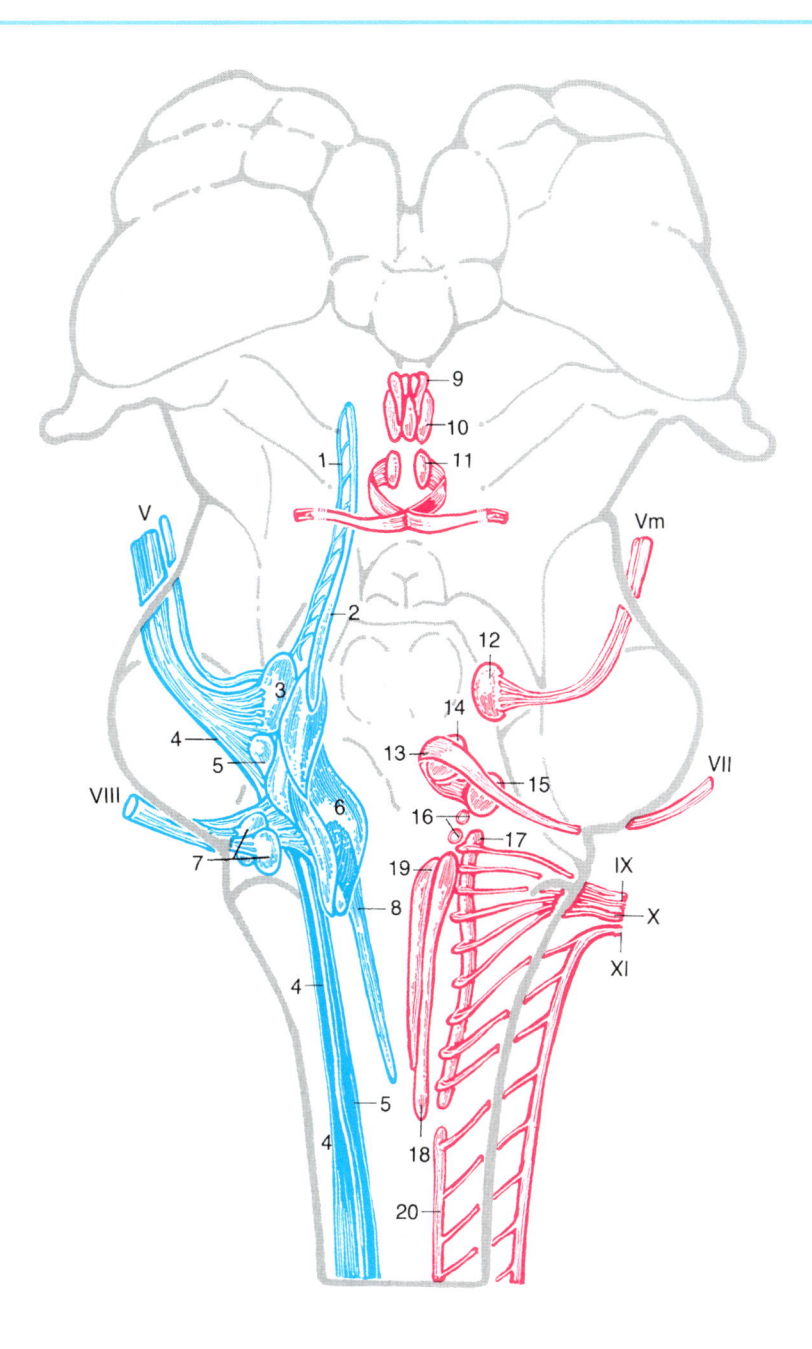

Fig. 68 Cranial nerve nuclei III–XII in the spinal cord, medulla oblongata, pons, and midbrain. The left side illustrates the sensory nuclei with two afferent nerves and fiber bundles. On the right are the motor and parasympathetic nuclei with efferent nerves. Roman numerals indicate the cranial nerves. According to (332).

190 Atlas

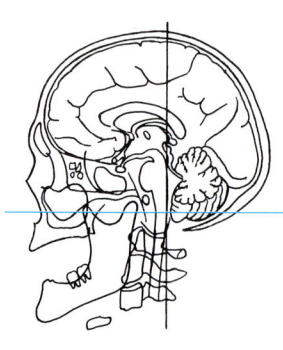

1 Maxilla
2 Inferior nasal concha
3 Maxillary sinus
4 Zygomatic bone
5 Nasal cavity
6 Nasal septum
7 Coronoid process
8 Temporalis
9 Masseter
10 Nasopharynx
11 Lateral pterygoid
12 Pharyngotympanic tube
13 Head of mandible
14 Internal carotid artery
15 Facial nerve
16 Hypoglossal canal
17 Jugular foramen
18 Mastoid cells
19 Medulla oblongata
20 Mastoid process
21 Sigmoid sinus, left–right asymmetry (Var.)
22 Tonsil of cerebellum (H IX)
23 Auricle (pinna)
24 Cisterna magna (posterior cerebellomedullary cistern)
25 Posterior lobe of cerebellum
26 Occipital bone

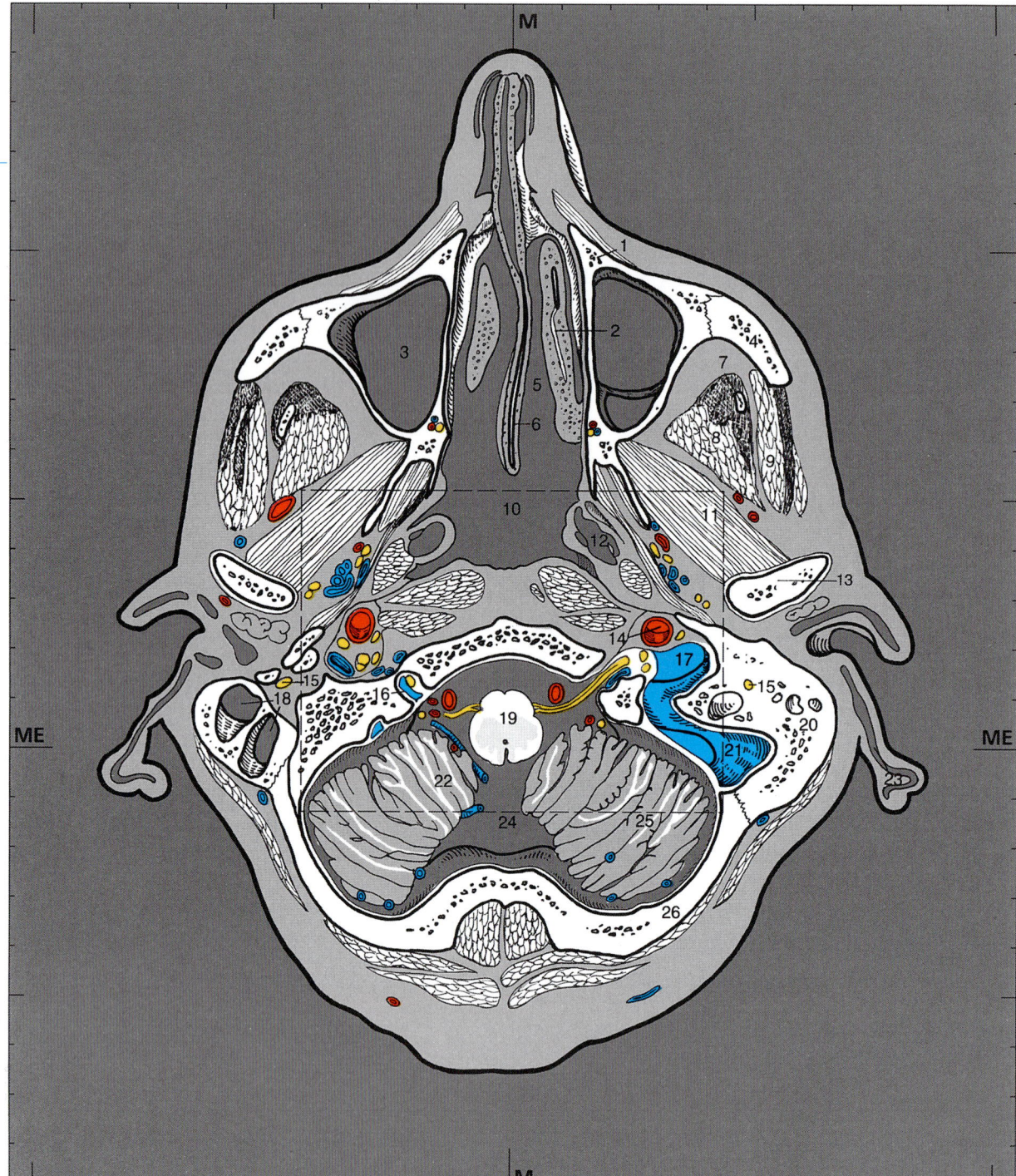

Fig. **69a** Superior section surface of the first slice of the brainstem. These serial slices were cut vertically to the median plane and Meynert's axis (Fig. 67). In the upper left corner, the blue line indicates the position of the sectional plane through the coronoid and articular processes of the mandible and the inferior part of the posterior cranial fossa. The slice lies almost 1 cm above the foramen magnum and includes the maxillary sinus, nasopharynx, the inferior part of the medulla oblongata, and the tonsil of cerebellum. The position of the median plane (M) and the Meynert's plane (ME) is shown on the frame of coordinates.

Figs. **69c** and **69d**   MR images positioned vertical to Meynert's axis, corresponding approximately to the sectional plane of Figs. 69a and 69b. These MR series were obtained from a 38-year-old female (Figs. 69c–78c and 69d–78d). The T1- and T2-weighted pair of images (Figs. 69c–78c and 69d–78d) have been described in the same legend. Should a structure be seen in one of the MR pair of images only, this will be indicated with a **c** or **d** at the end of the line.

Brainstem Slices

1 Medial pterygoid plate
2 Lateral pterygoid plate
3 Pharyngeal opening of pharyngotympanic tube
4 Nasopharynx
5 Cartilage of pharyngotympanic tube
6 Maxillary artery
7 Pterygoid venous plexus
8 Longus capitis
9 Rectus capitis anterior
10 Glossopharyngeal nerve
11 Internal jugular vein, left–right asymmetry (Var.)
12 Vagus nerve
13 Dura mater
14 Internal carotid artery
15 Bulb of internal jugular vein
16 Hypoglossal canal
17 Hypoglossal nerve
18 Vertebral artery
19 Pyramid of medulla oblongata
20 Anterior median fissure
21 Corticospinal tract
22 Medial longitudinal fasciculus
23 Anterior spinocerebellar tract
24 Spinothalamic tract
25 Reticular formation
26 Central canal
27 Posterior spinocerebellar tract
28 Caudal part of spinal nucleus of trigeminal nerve
29 Cuneate nucleus (of Burdach)
30 Gracile nucleus (of Goll)
31 Spinal root of accessory nerve
32 Sigmoid sinus, left–right asymmetry (Var.)
33 Tonsil of cerebellum (H IX)
34 Cisterna magna (posterior cerebellomedullary cistern)

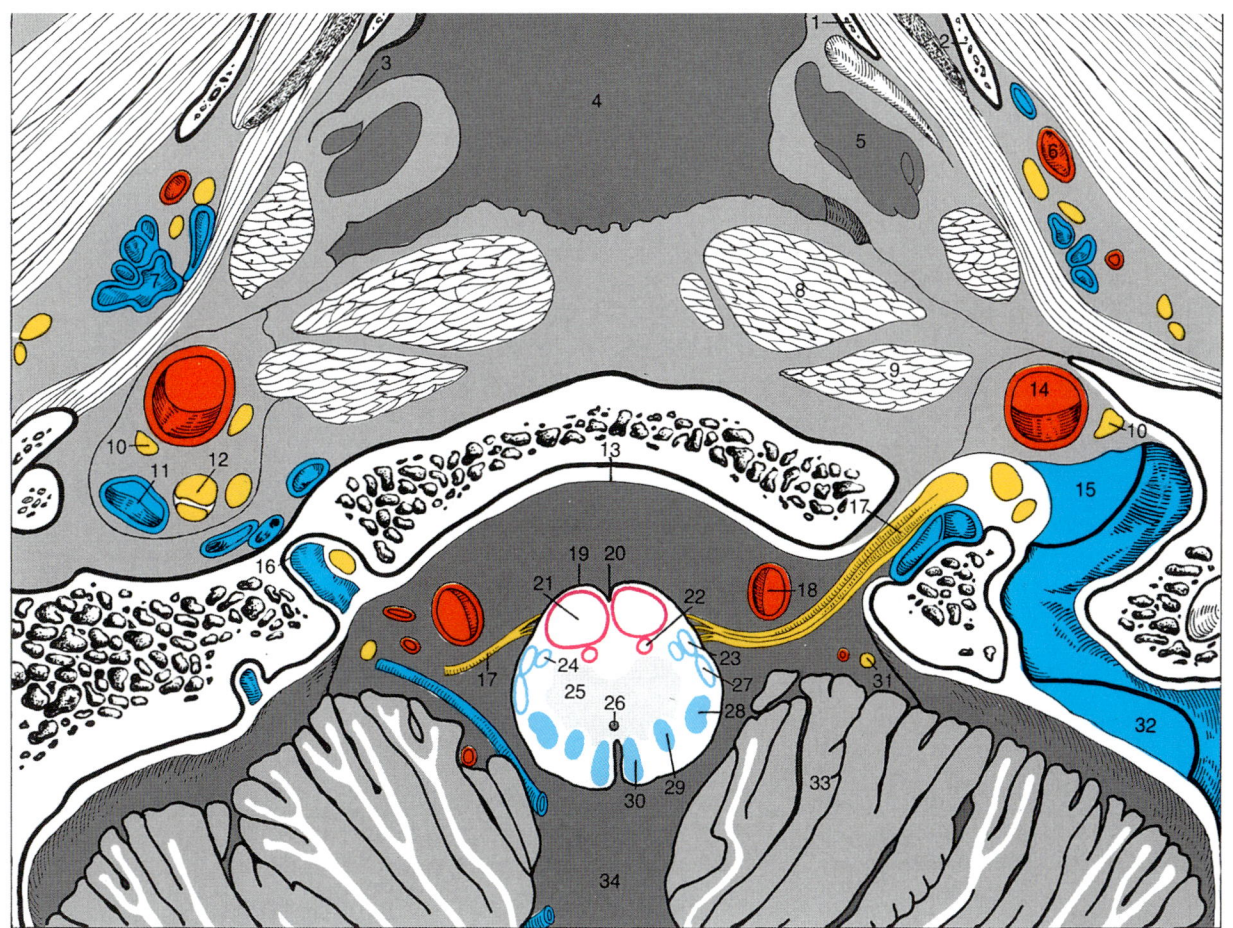

Fig. 69b Detail magnification of Fig. 69a. The opening of the pharyngotympanic tube into the nasopharynx is shown. The inferior portion of the medulla oblongata, the rootlets of the hypoglossal nerves, and the hypoglossal canal are included.

1 Maxillary sinus
2 Inferior nasal concha
3 Nasopharynx
4 Lateral pterygoid
5 Internal carotid artery
6 Vertebral artery
7 Pyramid of medulla oblongata
8 Closed portion of medulla oblongata
9 Central canal c
10 Gracile tubercle
11 Tonsil of cerebellum (H IX)
12 Cisterna magna (posterior cerebellomedullary cistern)
13 Hemisphere of posterior lobe of cerebellum

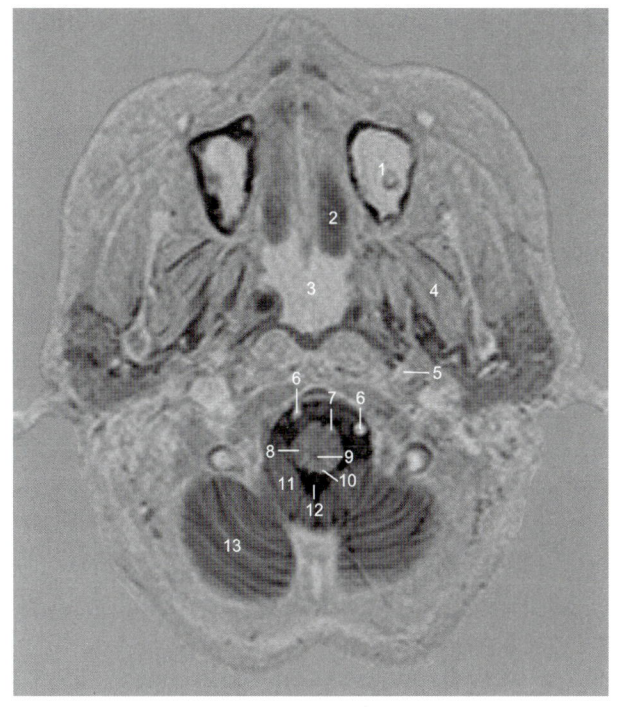

Fig. 69c T1-weighted MR image (Turbo-Inversion-Recovery-Sequence). The selected sequence emphasizes the brain structures and suppresses the surrounding soft tissue. Technical data (Chap. 8).

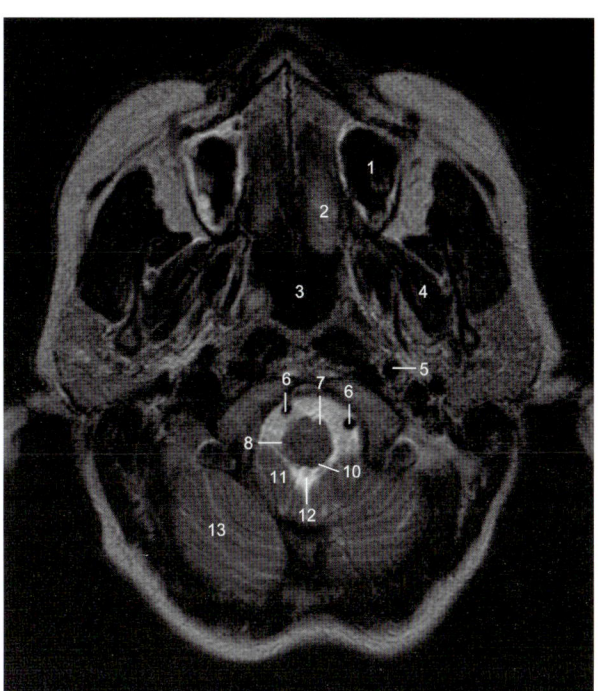

Fig. 69d T2-weighted MR image. Technical data (Chap. 8).

192   Atlas

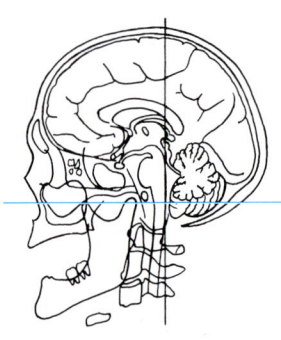

1 Maxilla
2 Inferior nasal concha
3 Nasal septum
4 Maxillary sinus
5 Zygomatic bone
6 Nasal cavity
7 Temporalis
8 Pterygoid process
9 Nasopharynx
10 Lateral pterygoid
11 Articular disc of temporomandibular joint
12 Head of mandible
13 Clivus
14 External acoustic meatus
15 Jugular foramen
16 Internal jugular vein (Var.)
17 Accessory nerve near opening of dura mater
18 Medulla oblongata
19 Bulb of internal jugular vein
20 Facial nerve
21 Sigmoid sinus
22 Temporal bone
23 Auricle (pinna)
24 Posterior lobe of cerebellum
25 Cisterna magna (posterior cerebellomedullary cistern)
26 Occipital bone

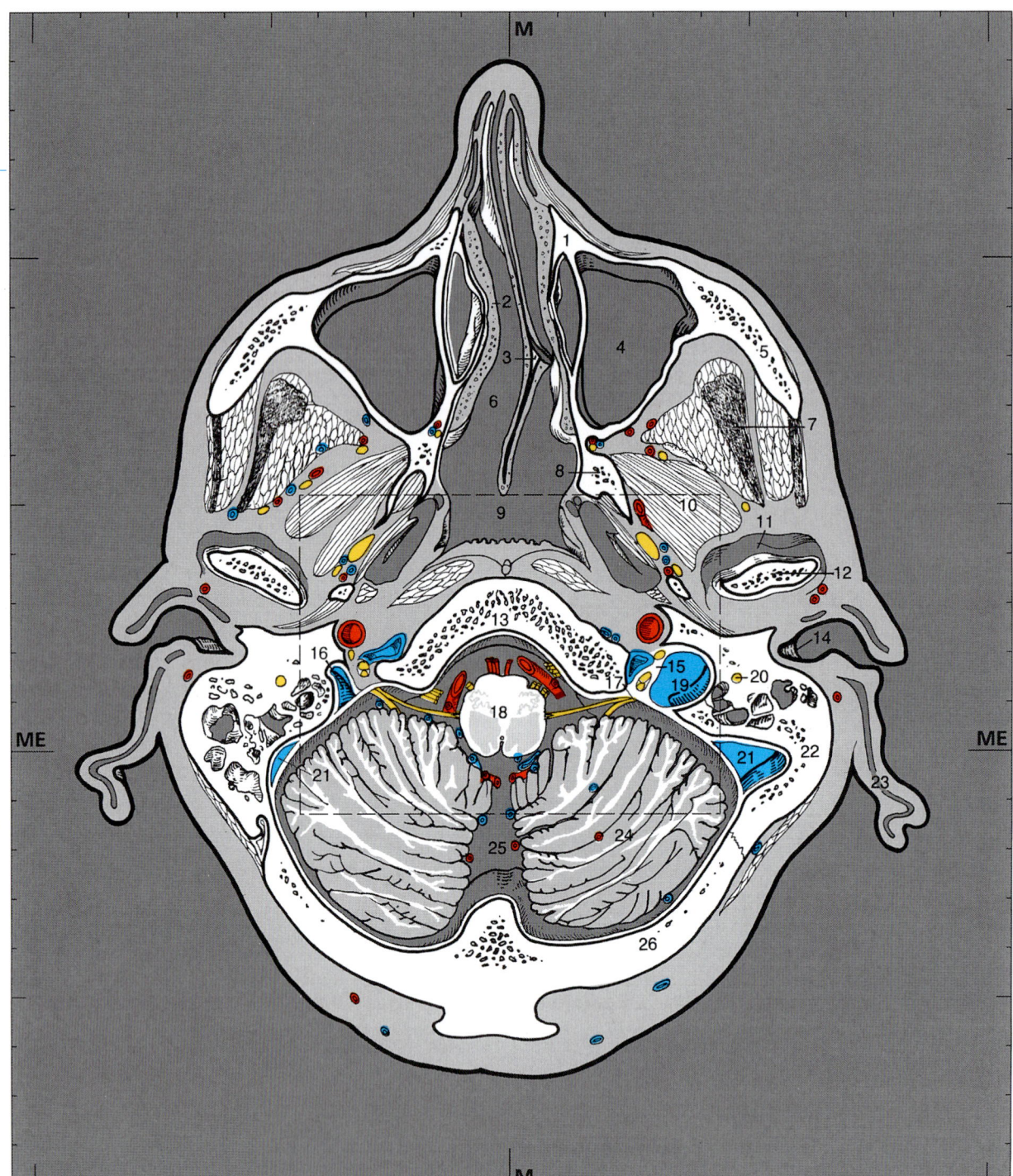

Fig. **70a** Superior section surface of the second slice of the brainstem series (Fig. 67). The sectional plane runs through the inferior nasal concha, temporomandibular joint, head of mandible, and the jugular foramen. In the posterior cranial fossa, the medulla oblongata is cut near the opening of the dura mater for the accessory nerve.

Figs. **70c** and **70d**   MR images positioned vertical to Meynert's axis corresponding approximately to the sectional plane of Figs. 70a and 70b.

Brainstem Slices

1 Nasopharynx
2 Cartilage of pharyngotympanic tube
3 Internal carotid artery
4 Glossopharyngeal nerve
5 Vagus nerve
6 Internal jugular vein (Var.)
7 Superior bulb of internal jugular vein
8 Vertebral artery
9 Hypoglossal nerve
10 Pyramid of medulla oblongata
11 Anterior median fissure
12 Corticospinal tract
13 Posterior inferior cerebellar artery (PICA)
14 Medial lemniscus
15 Hypoglossal nerve (within the slice)
16 Inferior olivary nucleus
17 Spinothalamic tract
18 Reticular formation
19 Medial longitudinal fasciculus
20 Nucleus ambiguus
21 Anterior spinocerebellar tract
22 Cranial and spinal roots of accessory nerve
23 Solitary nucleus
24 Hypoglossal nucleus
25 Posterior (dorsal) nucleus of vagus nerve
26 Posterior spinocerebellar tract
27 Cuneate nucleus (of Burdach)
28 Gracile nucleus (of Goll)
29 Obex of medulla oblongata
30 Central canal
31 Caudal part of spinal nucleus of trigeminal nerve

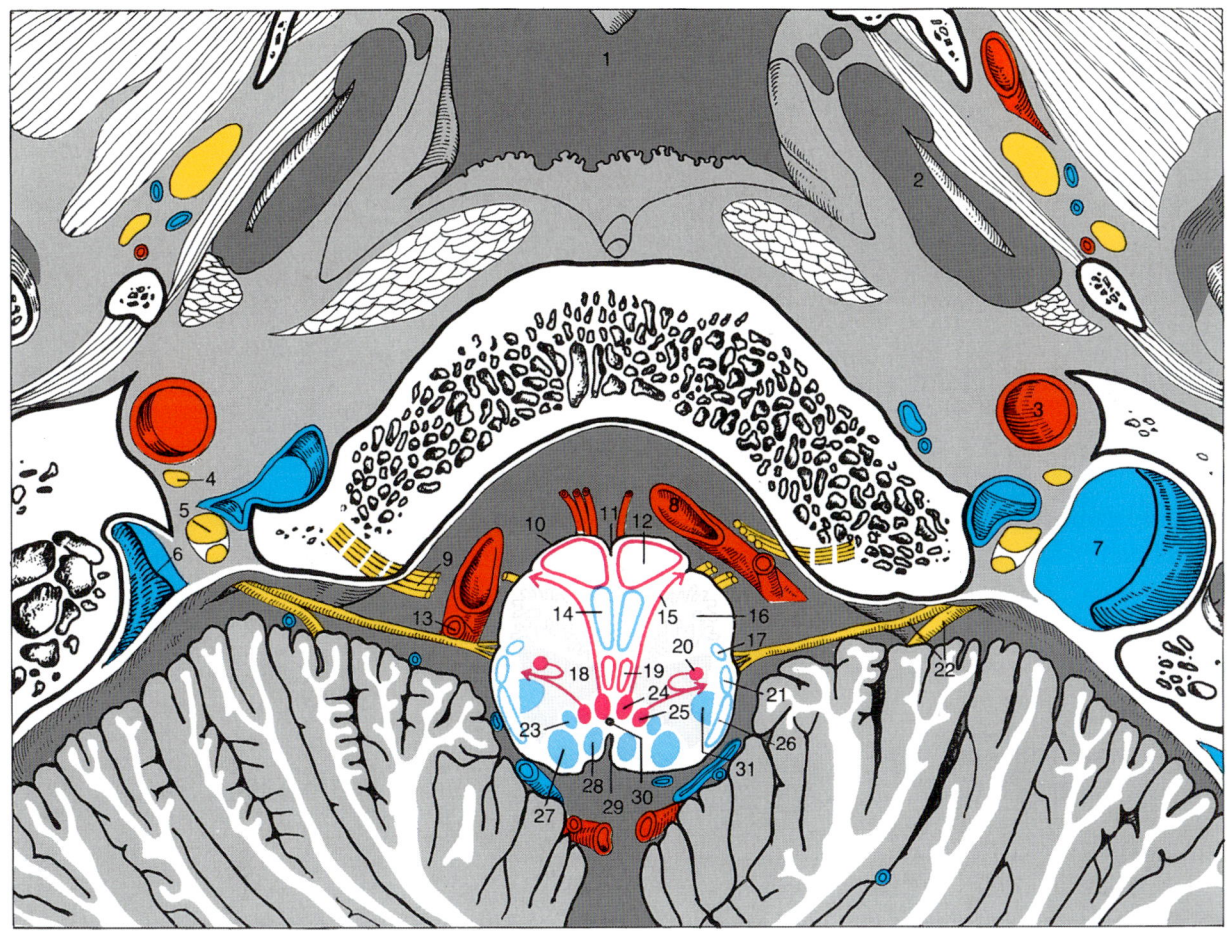

Fig. **70b** Detail magnification of Fig. 70a. The sectional plane cuts through the cartilaginous part of the pharyngotympanic tube, the inferior part of the inferior olivary nucleus, and the origin of the posterior inferior cerebellar artery (PICA) from the vertebral artery. Both internal jugular veins are asymmetric. The right side shows the jugular foramen to be extended with an enlarged bulb of the internal jugular vein (variant).

1 Nasal septum
2 Maxillary sinus
3 Nasopharynx
4 Clivus
5 Internal carotid artery **d**
6 Vertebral artery
7 Pyramid of medulla oblongata
8 Inferior olive
9 Obex of medulla oblongata
10 Tonsil of cerebellum (H IX)
11 Posterior lobe of cerebellum

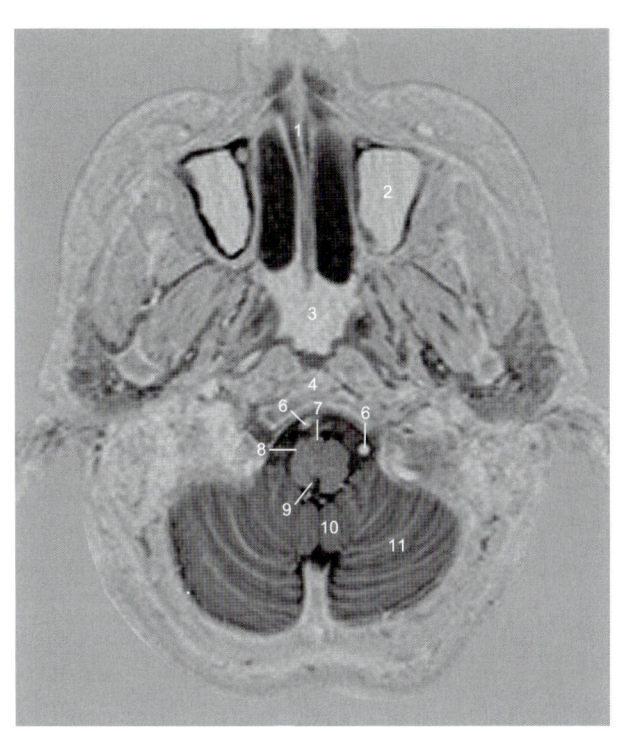

Fig. **70c** T1-weighted MR image. Technical data (Chap. 8).

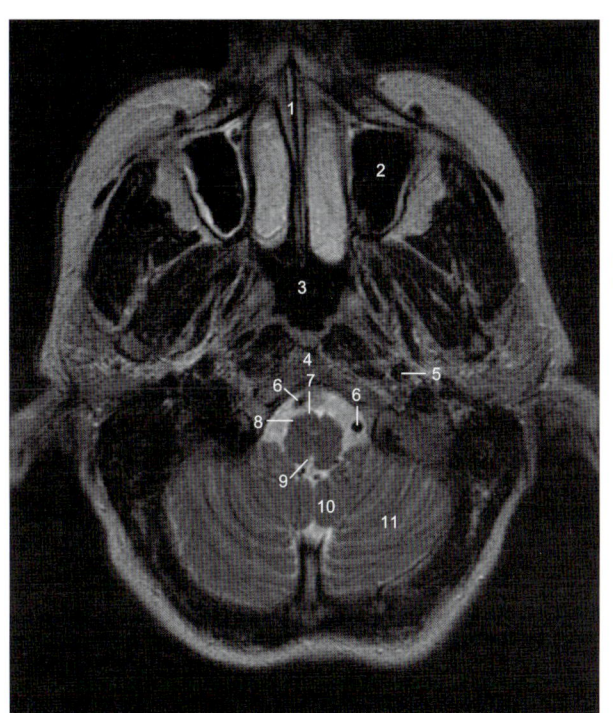

Fig. **70d** T2-weighted MR image. Technical data (Chap. 8).

194 Atlas

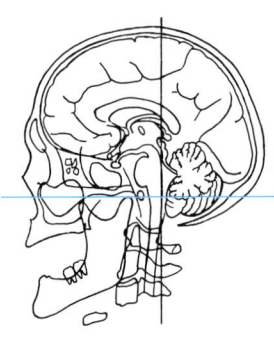

1 Maxilla
2 Nasolacrimal duct
3 Maxillary sinus
4 Zygomatic bone
5 Nasal cavity
6 Nasal septum
7 Temporalis
8 Lateral pterygoid
9 Mandibular nerve
10 Temporomandibular joint
11 Articular disc of temporomandibular joint
12 External acoustic meatus
13 Inferior petrosal sinus
14 Hypoglossal nerve
15 Facial nerve
16 Medulla oblongata
17 Inferior olive
18 Temporal bone
19 Floor of rhomboid fossa
20 Fourth ventricle
21 Sigmoid sinus
22 Auricle (pinna)
23 Uvula of vermis (IX)
24 Posterior lobe of cerebellum
25 Pyramis of vermis (VIII)
26 Occipital bone

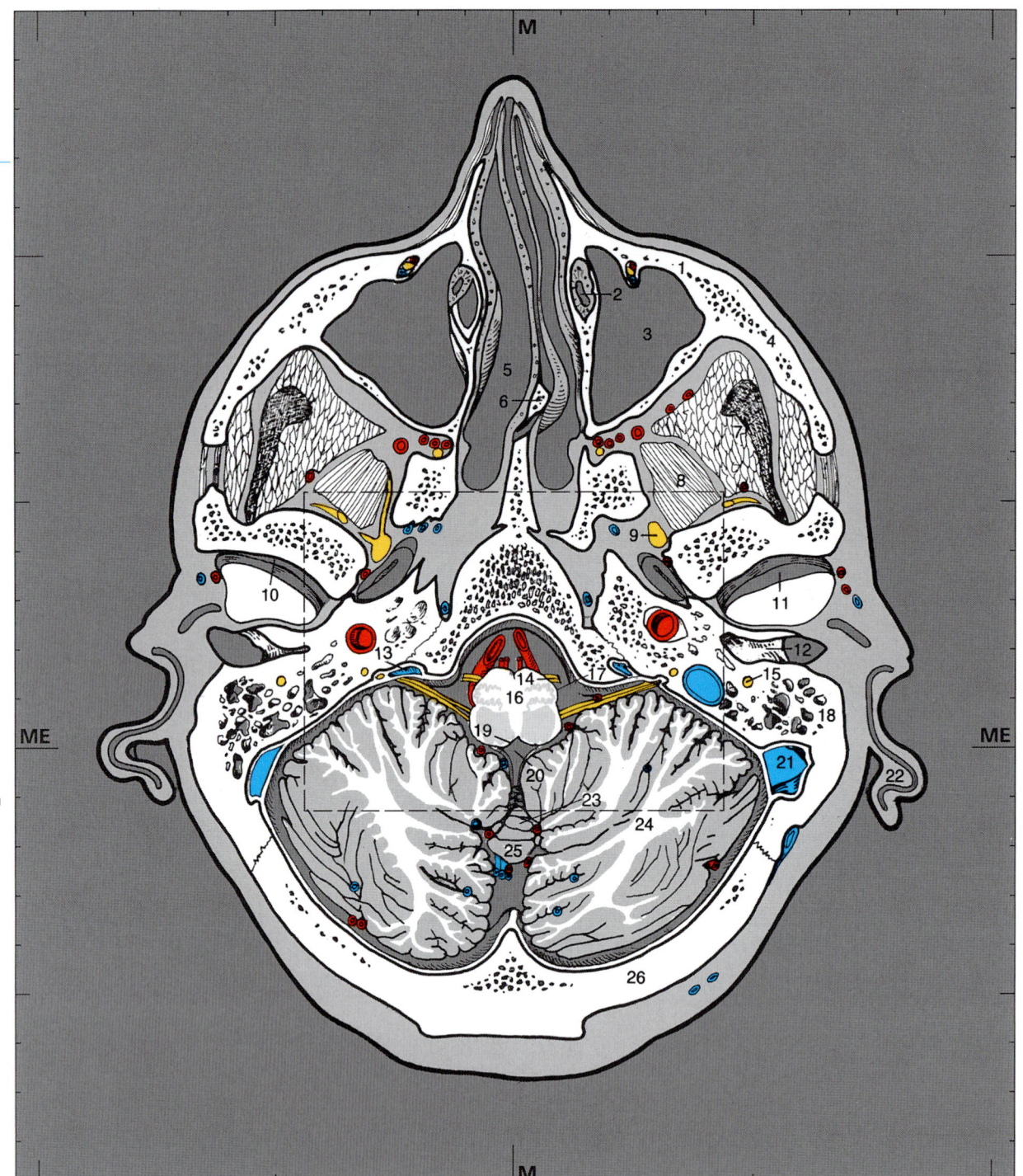

Fig. **71a** Superior section surface of the third slice of the brainstem series. The sectional plane lies at the level of the external acoustic meatus and the attachment of the inferior nasal concha to the lateral wall of the nasal cavity. In the posterior cranial fossa the medulla oblongata is cut at the inferior end of the rhomboid fossa.

Figs. **71c** and **71d** MR images positioned vertical to Meynert's axis corresponding approximately to the sectional plane of Figs. 71a and 71b.

Brainstem Slices

1 Mandibular nerve
2 Pharyngotympanic tube
3 Middle meningeal artery
4 Clivus
5 Internal carotid artery
6 Vertebral artery
7 Hypoglossal nerve
8 Pyramid of medulla oblongata
9 Anterior median fissure
10 Corticospinal tract
11 Glossopharyngeal nerve
12 Superior bulb of internal jugular vein
13 Medial lemniscus
14 Inferior olivary nucleus
15 Hypoglossal nerve (within the slice)
16 Nucleus ambiguus
17 Spinothalamic tract
18 Vagus nerve
19 Reticular formation
20 Medial longitudinal fasciculus
21 Anterior spinocerebellar tract
22 Cuneate nucleus (of Burdach)
23 Solitary nucleus
24 Median sulcus
25 Hypoglossal nucleus
26 Posterior (dorsal) nucleus of vagus nerve
27 Interpolar part of spinal nucleus of trigeminal nerve
28 Inferior cerebellar peduncle

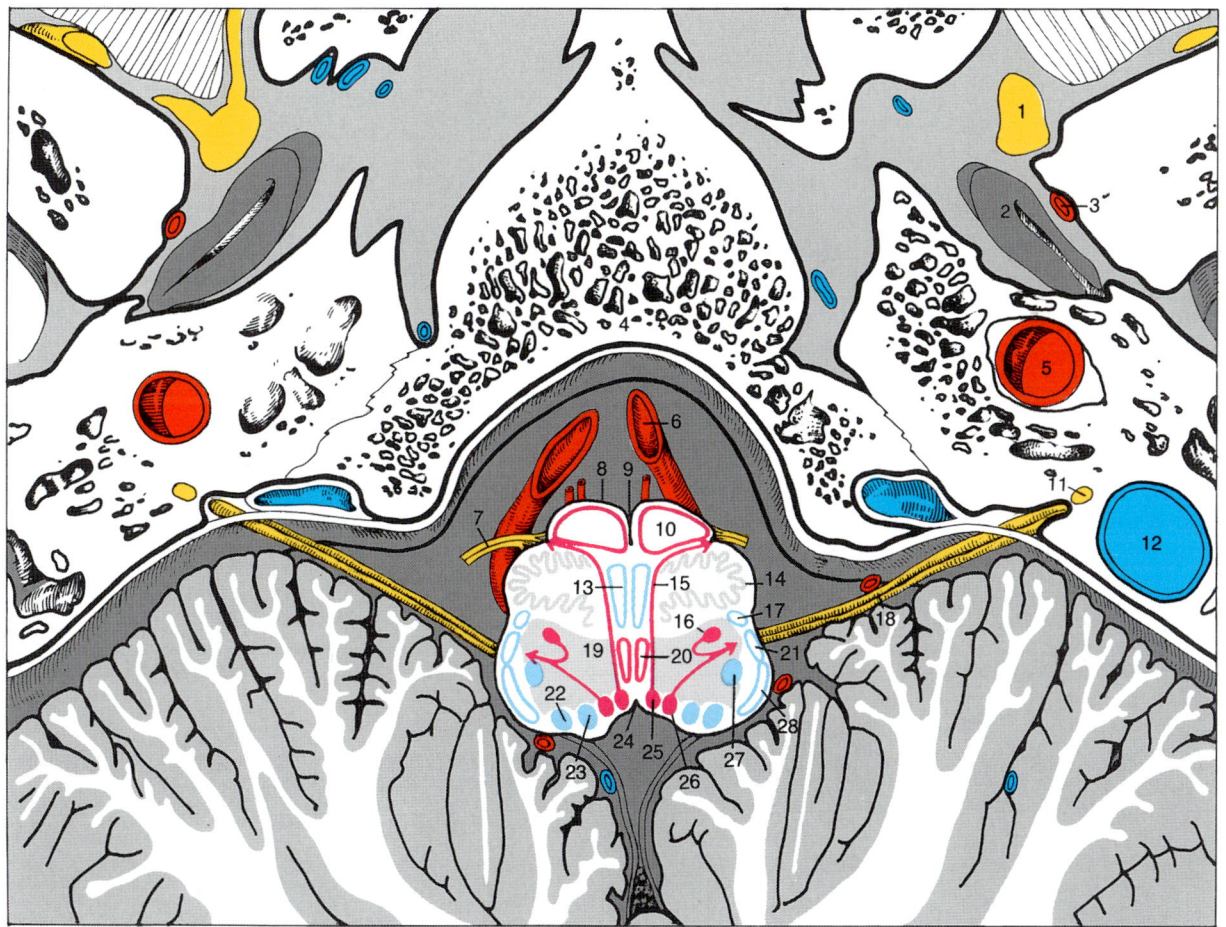

Fig. 71b Detail magnification of Fig. 71a. The mandibular nerve lies just below the foramen ovale. The roots of the vagus nerve branch off the medulla oblongata.

1 Nasal septum
2 Clivus
3 Head of mandible
4 Vertebral artery
5 Pyramid of medulla oblongata
6 Inferior olivary nucleus
7 Vagus nerve
8 Floor of rhomboid fossa
9 Uvula of vermis (IX)
10 Hemisphere of cerebellum
11 Pyramis of vermis (VIII)

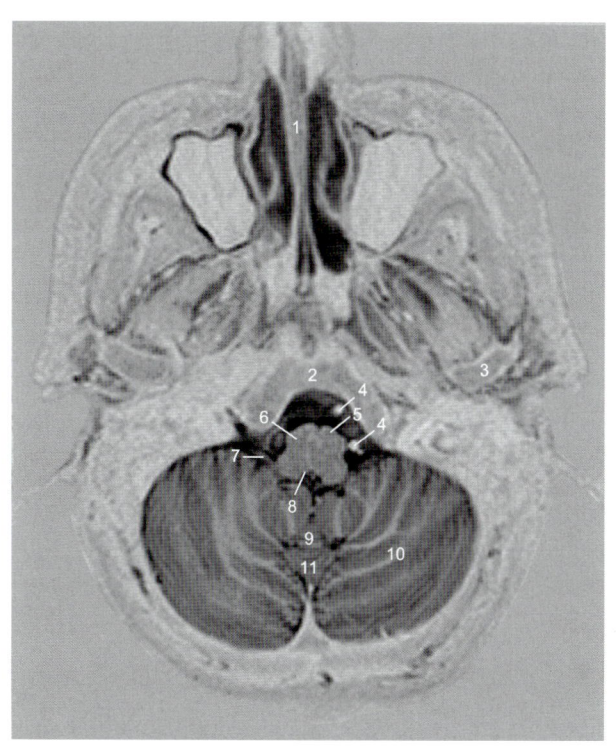

Fig. 71c T1-weighted MR image. Technical data (Chap. 8).

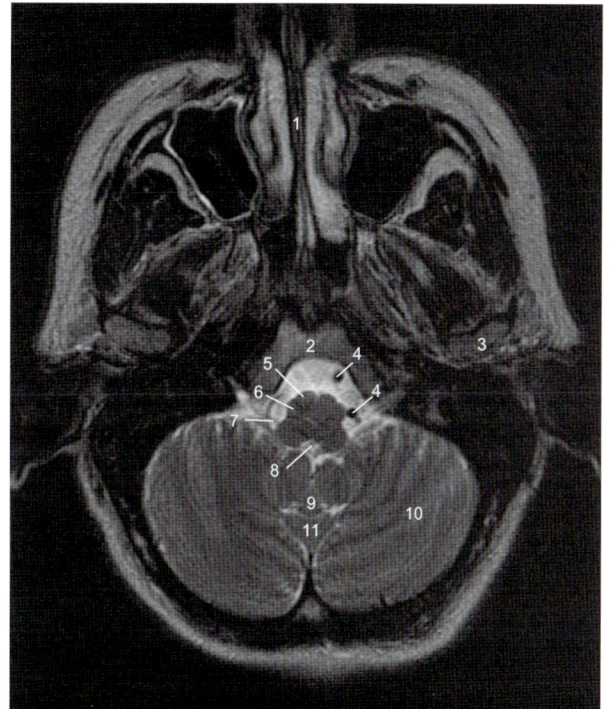

Fig. 71d T2-weighted MR image. Technical data (Chap. 8).

196   Atlas

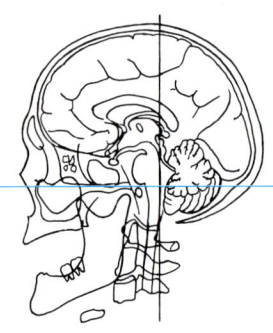

1 Nasal cavity
2 Nasolacrimal duct
3 Nasal septum
4 Maxillary sinus
5 Zygomatic bone
6 Middle nasal concha
7 Zygomatic arch
8 Temporalis
9 Floor of middle cranial fossa
10 Middle meningeal artery
11 Clivus
12 Temporal bone
13 Medulla oblongata
14 Flocculus (H X)
15 Lateral aperture (of Luschka) of fourth ventricle
16 Sigmoid sinus
17 Auricle (pinna)
18 Uvula of vermis (IX)
19 Pyramis of vermis (VIII)
20 Posterior lobe of cerebellum
21 Occipital bone

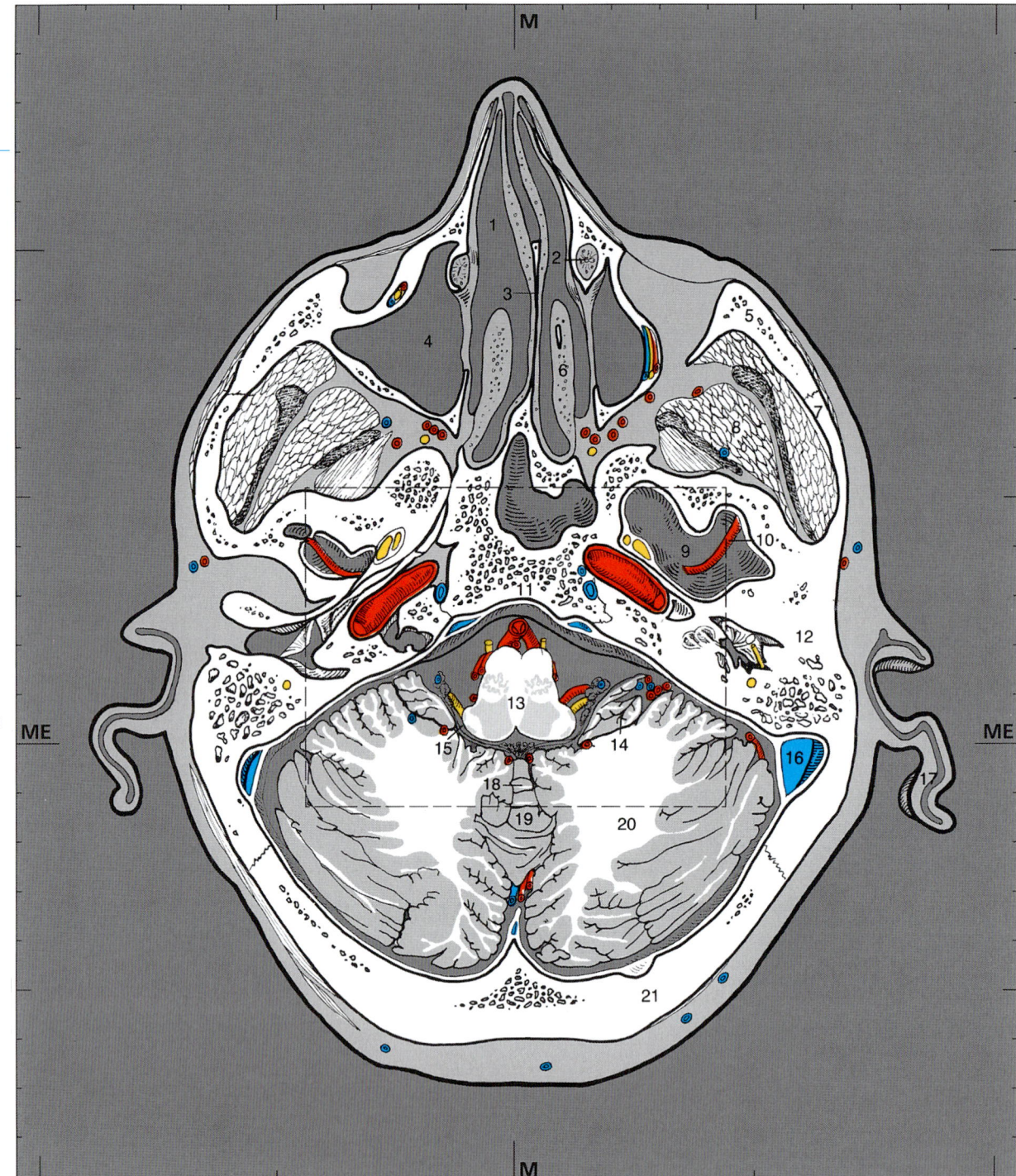

Fig. **72a** Superior section surface of the fourth slice of the brainstem series. The middle nasal concha is cut in the nasal cavity. The section surface runs through the floor of the middle cranial fossa, through the tympanic cavity of the temporal bone, and in the posterior cranial fossa through the superior portion of the medulla oblongata at the level of the lateral aperture of the fourth ventricle.

Figs. **72c** and **72d**   MR images positioned vertical to Meynert's axis corresponding approximately to the sectional plane of Figs. 72a and 72b.

Brainstem Slices

1	Sphenoidal sinus
2	Mandibular nerve
3	Middle meningeal artery
4	Internal carotid artery
5	Basilar artery
6	Vertebral artery
7	Pyramid of medulla oblongata
8	Abducens nerve
9	Corticospinal tract
10	Abducens nerve (within the slice)
11	Medial lemniscus
12	Flocculus (H X)
13	Choroid plexus
14	Inferior olivary nucleus
15	Reticular formation
16	Medial longitudinal fasciculus
17	Nucleus ambiguus
18	Spinothalamic tract
19	Oral part of spinal nucleus of trigeminal nerve
20	Vestibulocochlear nerve
21	Lateral aperture (of Luschka) of fourth ventricle
22	Prepositus nucleus
23	Floor of rhomboid fossa and fourth ventricle
24	Vestibular nuclei
25	Inferior cerebellar peduncle
26	Posterior (dorsal) and anterior (ventral) cochlear nuclei
27	Uvula of vermis (IX)

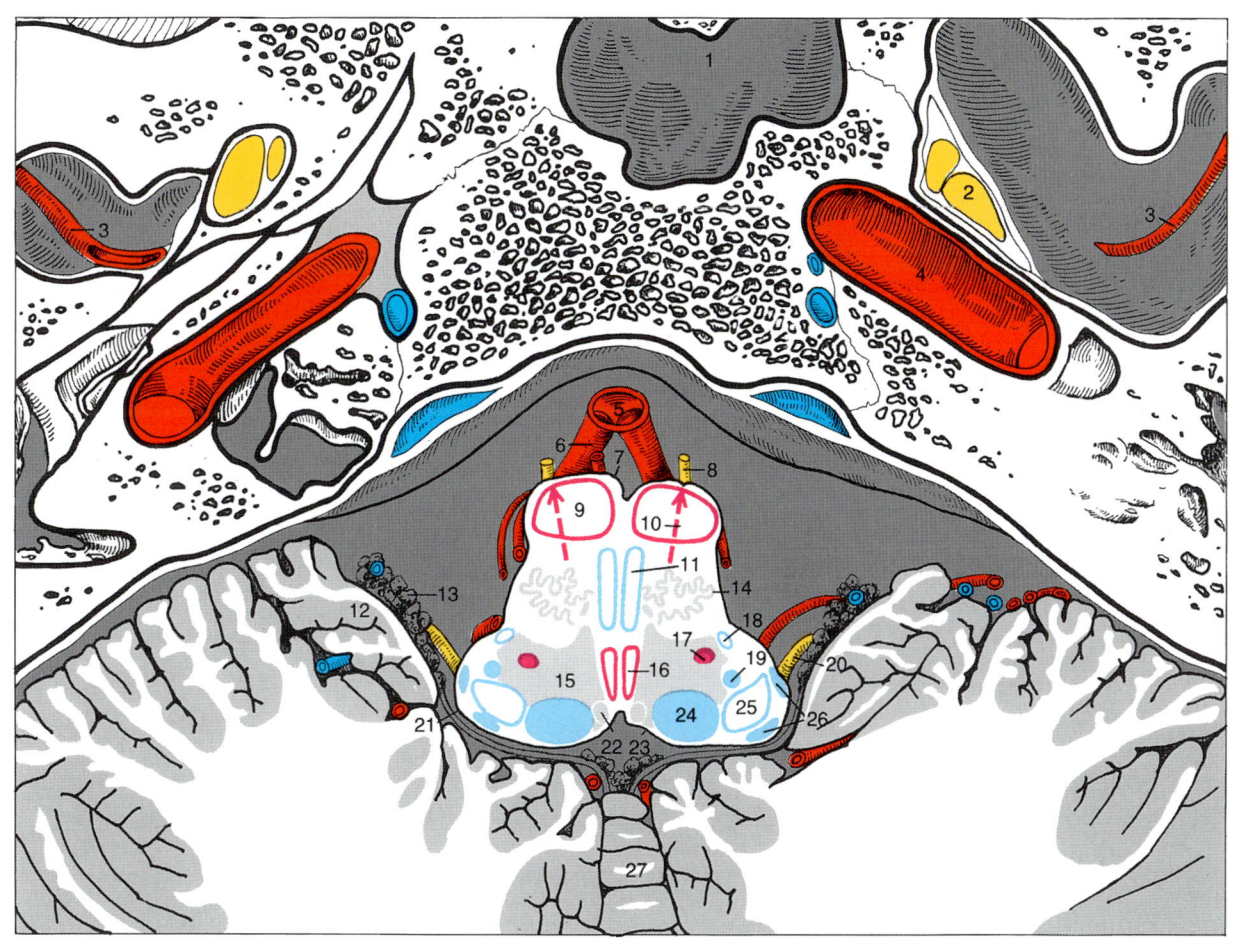

Fig. 72b The detail magnification of Fig. 72a reveals the junction of the vertebral arteries to the basilar artery. The roots of the abducens nerve arise at the border between the medulla oblongata and pons. The upper part of the inferior olivary nucleus is positioned in the medulla oblongata.

1	Nasal septum
2	Clivus
3	Vertebral artery (Var.)
4	Pyramid of medulla oblongata c
5	Flocculus (H X)
6	Lateral aperture (of Luschka) of fourth ventricle c
7	Floor of rhomboid fossa
8	Uvula of vermis (IX)
9	Pyramis of vermis (VIII)
10	Hemisphere of cerebellum

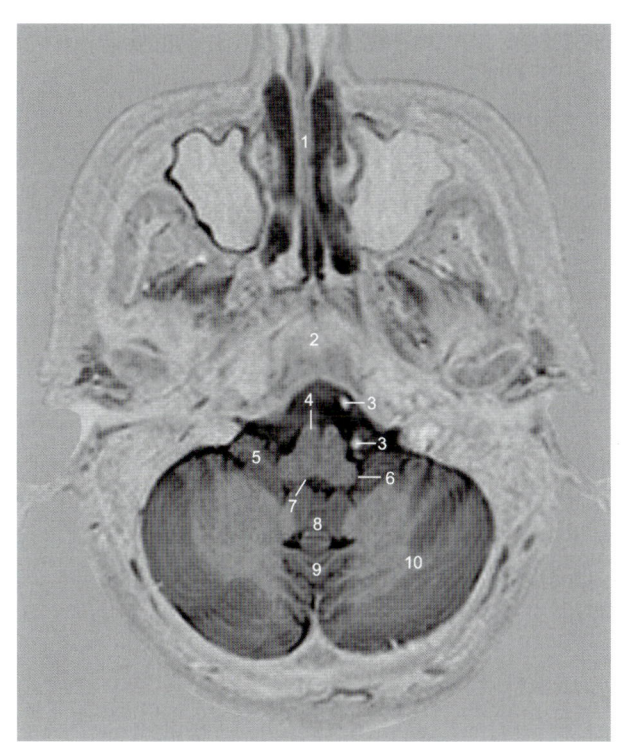

Fig. 72c T1-weighted MR image. Technical data (Chap. 8).

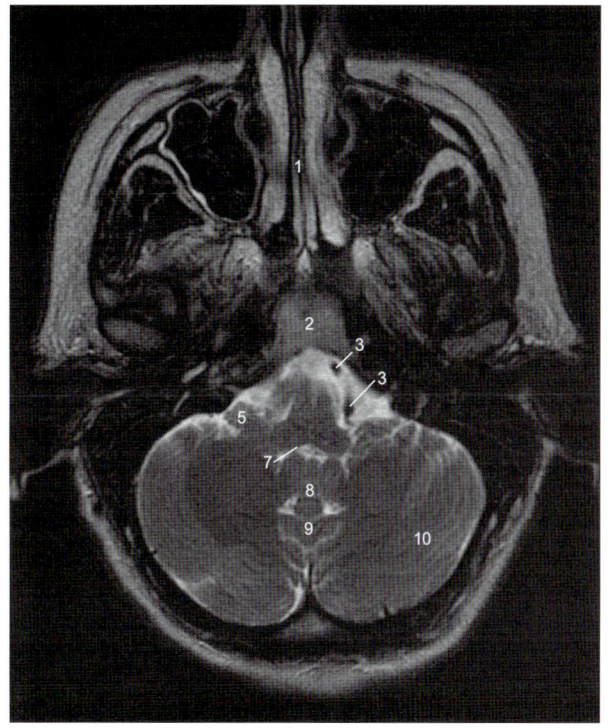

Fig. 72d T2-weighted MR image. Technical data (Chap. 8).

198 Atlas

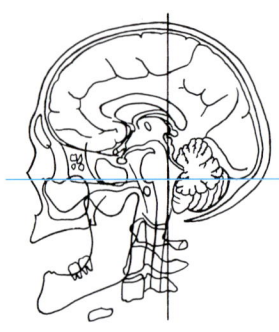

1 Nasal cavity
2 Semilunar hiatus
3 Middle nasal concha
4 Inferior oblique
5 Zygomatic bone
6 Nasal septum
7 Inferior rectus
8 Sphenoid
9 Temporalis
10 Maxillary nerve
11 Sphenoidal sinus
12 Middle meningeal artery
13 Base of temporal lobe
14 Malleus (hammer)
15 Internal acoustic meatus
16 Pons
17 Posterior semicircular canal
18 Temporal bone
19 Auricle (pinna)
20 Sigmoid sinus
21 Dentate nucleus
22 Uvula of vermis (IX)
23 Pyramis of vermis (VIII)
24 Posterior lobe of cerebellum
25 Tentorium of cerebellum
26 Transverse sinus
27 Base of occipital lobe
28 Internal occipital protuberance
29 Occipital bone

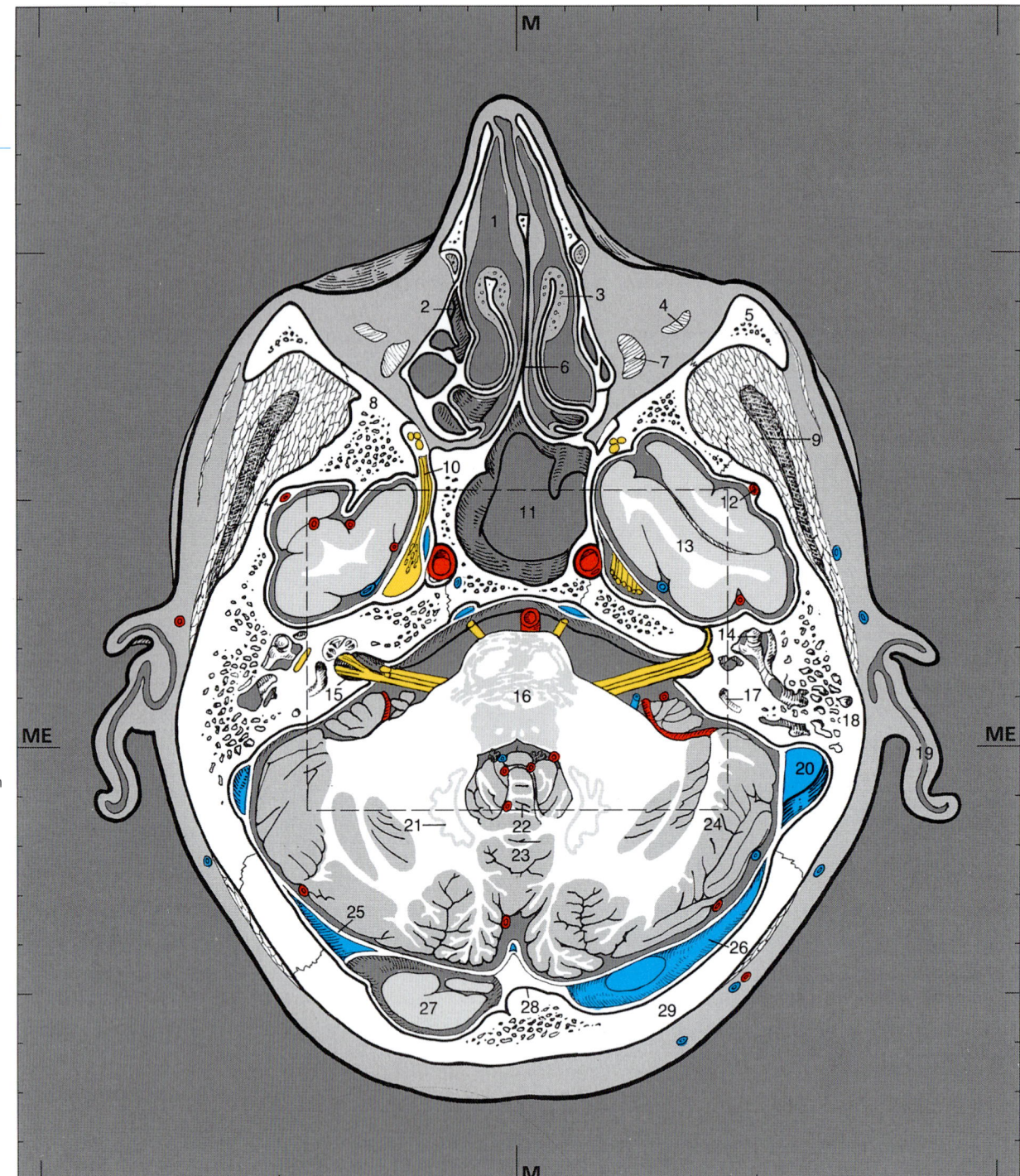

Fig. **73a** Superior section surface of the fifth slice of the brainstem series. The section surface runs just above the floor of the orbit. The bases of the temporal lobes lie in the middle cranial fossae. The malleus and the incus are revealed in the tympanic cavity. The posterior cranial fossa is seen at the level of the internal acoustic meatus, the pons, the dentate nucleus, and the internal occipital protuberance. The pole of the left occipital lobe is demonstrated on the left side.

Figs. **73c** and **73d** MR images positioned vertical to Meynert's axis and slightly superior to the sectional plane of Figs. 73a and 73b.

Brainstem Slices

1 Sphenoidal sinus
2 Internal carotid artery
3 Trigeminal (Gasserian) ganglion
4 Trigeminal nerve
5 Cochlea
6 Basilar artery
7 Abducens nerve
8 Greater petrosal nerve
9 Internal acoustic meatus
10 Pontine nuclei
11 Corticospinal tract
12 Facial nerve and intermediate nerve
13 Abducens nerve (within the slice)
14 Facial nerve (within the slice)
15 Vestibulocochlear nerve
16 Cerebellopontine cistern
17 Medial lemniscus
18 Spinothalamic tract
19 Superior olivary nucleus
20 Reticular formation
21 Facial nucleus
22 Oral part of spinal nucleus of trigeminal nerve
23 Flocculus (H X)
24 Middle cerebellar peduncle
25 Medial longitudinal fasciculus
26 Vestibular nuclei
27 Inferior cerebellar peduncle
28 Anterior inferior cerebellar artery (AICA)
29 Fourth ventricle
30 Nodule of vermis (X)
31 Posterior recess of fourth ventricle
32 Dentate nucleus

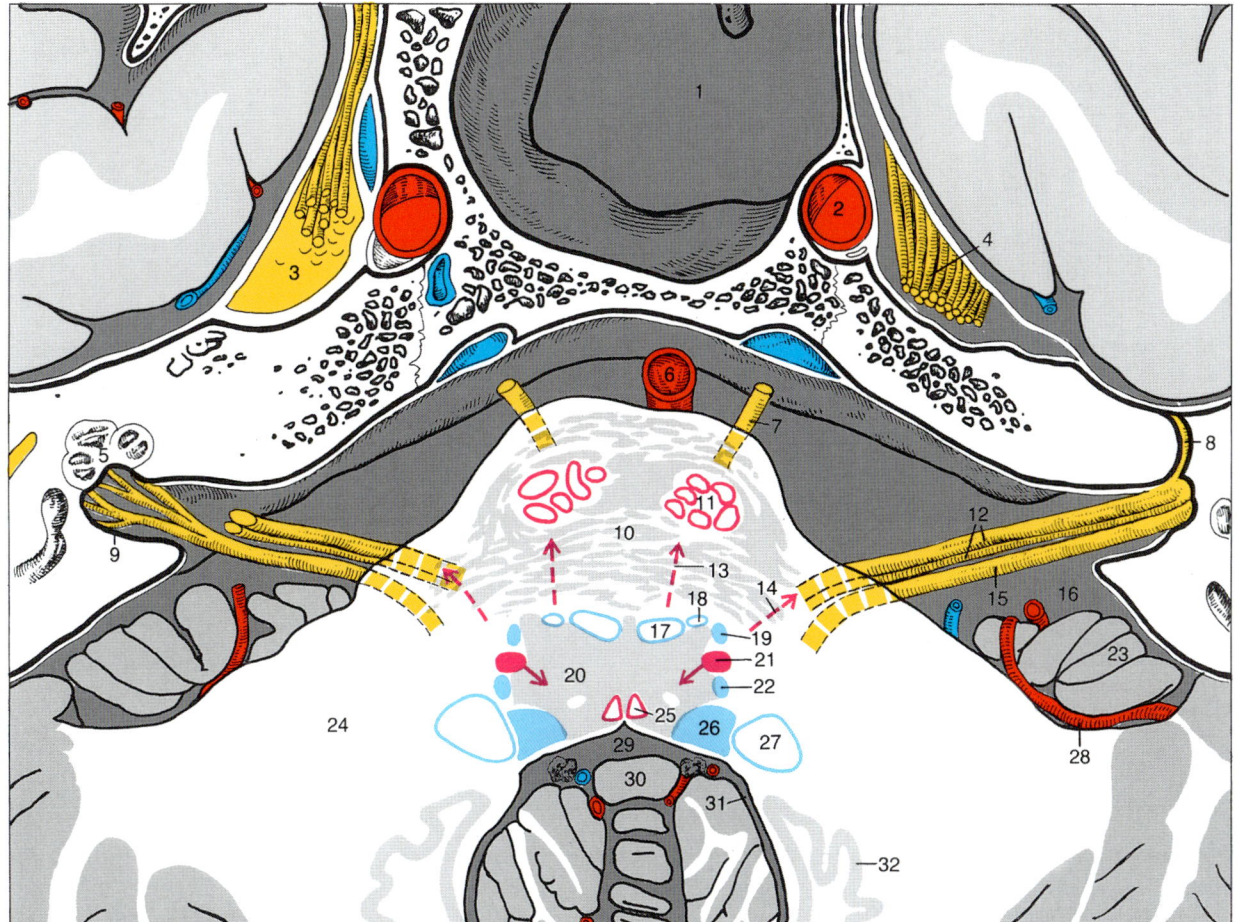

Fig. **73b** The detail magnification of Fig. 73a demonstrates the sphenoidal sinus together with the adjoining trigeminal ganglion (left) and the trigeminal nerve (right). The cross-section through the inferior pons portion reveals the middle peduncles of the cerebellum. The seventh and eighth cranial nerves enter the internal acoustic meatus.

1 Sphenoidal sinus
2 Base of temporal lobe
3 Clivus
4 Internal carotid artery
5 Basilar artery
6 Internal acoustic meatus
7 Inferior portion of pons
8 Facial nerve, vestibulocochlear nerve
9 Cerebellopontine cistern
10 Fourth ventricle
11 Nodule of vermis (X)
12 Middle cerebellar peduncle
13 Posterior recess of fourth ventricle

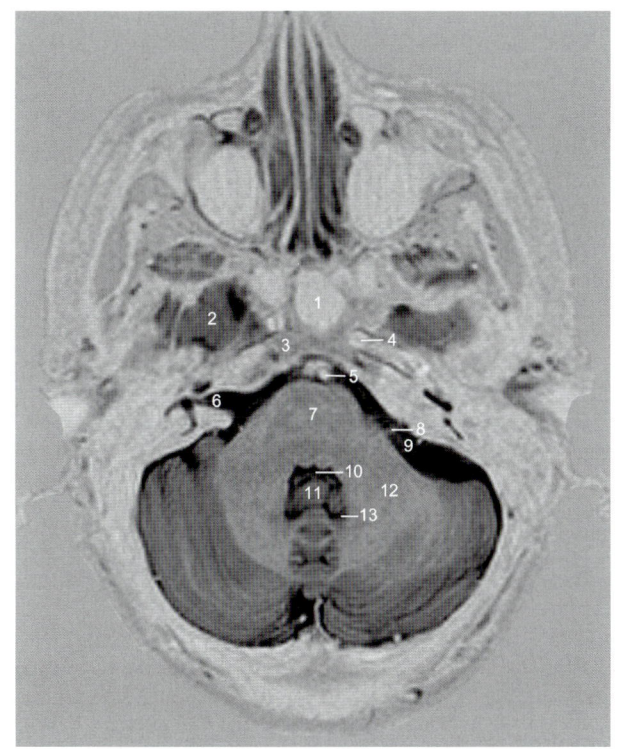

Fig. **73c** T1-weighted MR image. Technical data (Chap. 8).

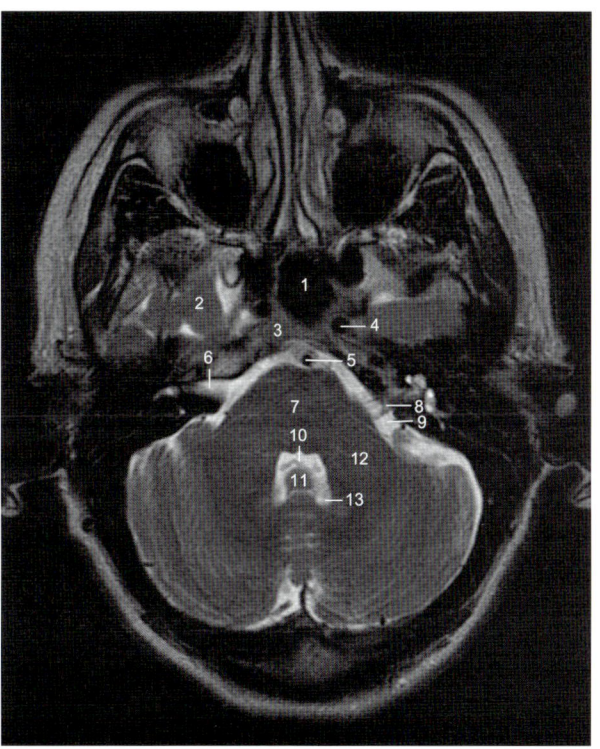

Fig. **73d** T2-weighted MR image. Technical data (Chap. 8).

200   Atlas

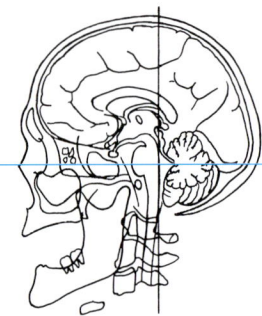

1 Nasal septum
2 Lower eyelid
3 Semilunar hiatus
4 Eyeball
5 Zygomatic bone
6 Ethmoidal bulla
7 Ethmoidal cells
8 Sphenoid
9 Inferior rectus
10 Sphenoidal sinus
11 Middle meningeal artery
12 Temporal lobe
13 Temporalis
14 Anterior semicircular canal
15 Pons
16 Anterior lobe of cerebellum
17 Primary fissure of cerebellum
18 Arcuate eminence
19 Auricle (pinna)
20 Temporal bone
21 Dentate nucleus
22 Transverse sinus
23 Posterior lobe of cerebellum
24 Tentorium of cerebellum
25 Lambdoid suture
26 Confluence of sinuses (Var.)
27 Base of occipital lobe
28 Occipital pole
29 Occipital bone

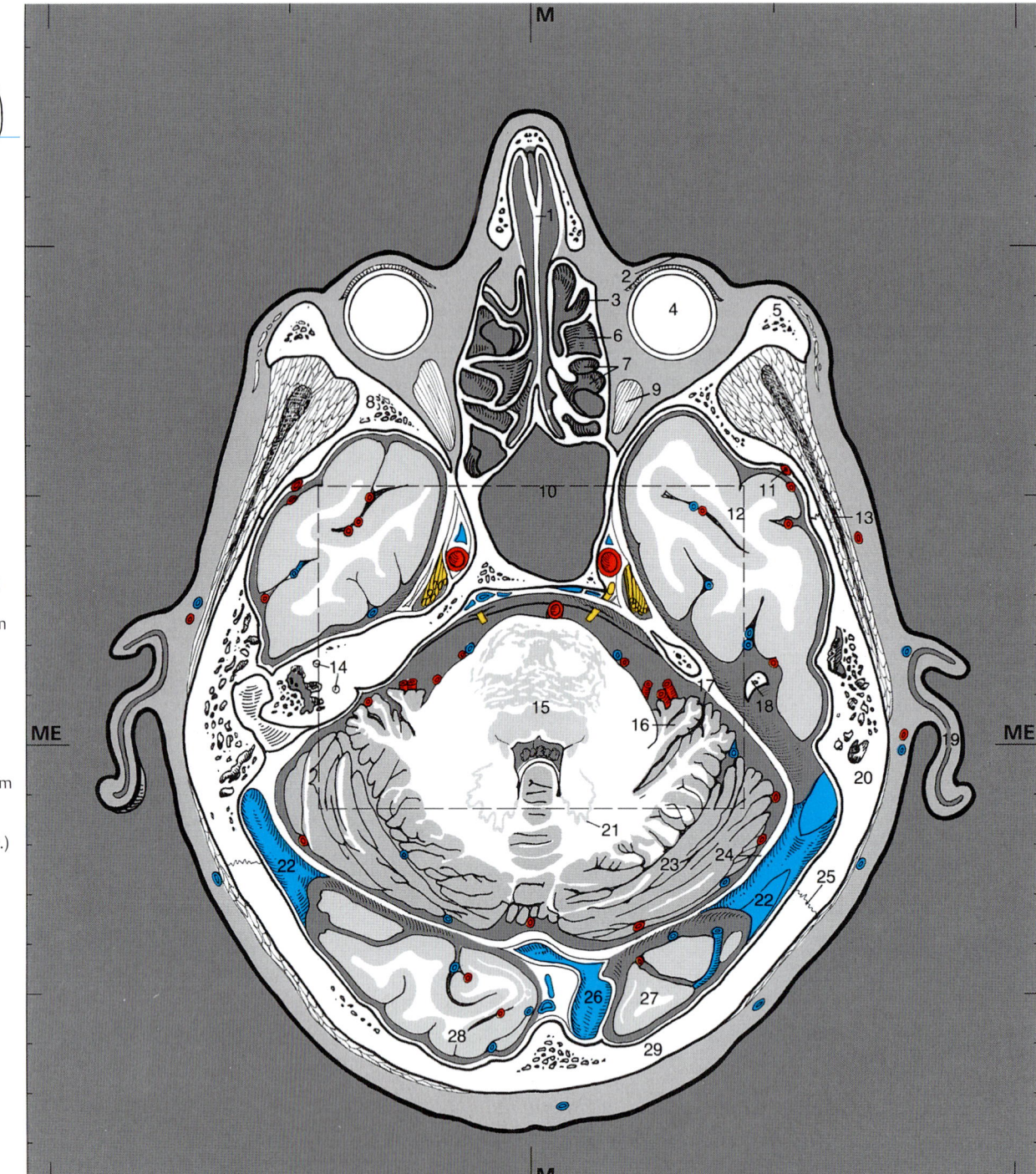

Fig. 74a Superior section surface of the sixth slice of the brainstem series. The section surface lies at the level of the ethmoidal cells, the sphenoidal sinus, and the upper part of the petrous part of the temporal bones. The pons and the cerebellum are revealed in the infratentorial space of this slice, the bases of both occipital lobes of the telencephalon in the supratentorial space. The two spaces are separated by the tentorium of cerebellum.

Figs. 74c and 74d MR images positioned vertical to Meynert's axis corresponding approximately to the sectional plane of Figs. 74a and 74b. The MR images show small right–left asymmetries that can be recognized in the pontomedullary junction at the outlet and along the course of the cranial nerves and at the skull base.

Brainstem Slices 201

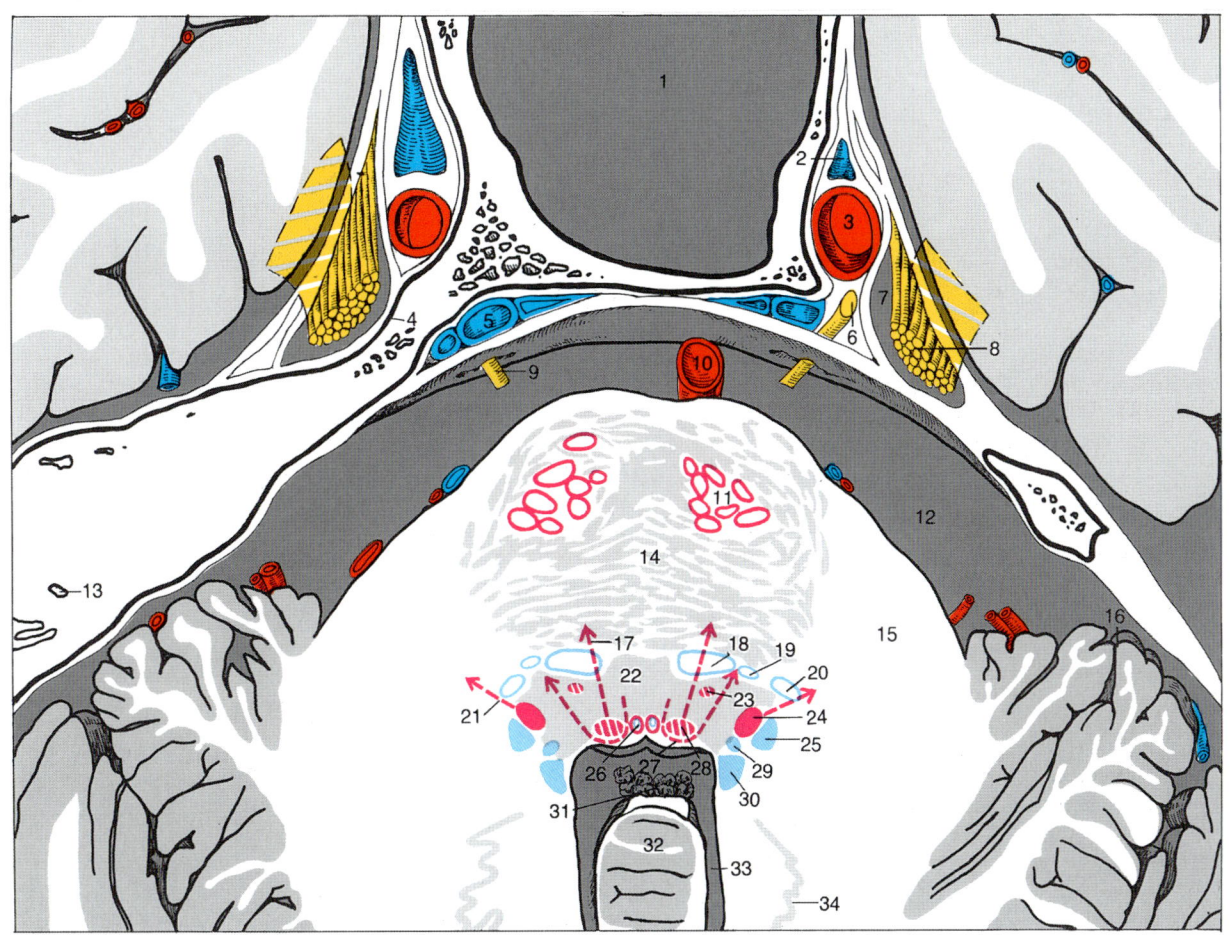

Fig. 74b The detail magnification of Fig. 74a shows the triangular part of the fifth cranial nerve and the sixth cranial nerve at the dura mater. The middle portion of the pons is cut.

1 Sphenoidal sinus
2 Cavernous sinus
3 Internal carotid artery
4 Trigeminal impression
5 Inferior petrosal sinus
6 Abducens nerve
7 Opening of trigeminal cistern
8 Triangular part of trigeminal nerve
9 Abducens nerve near opening of dura mater
10 Basilar artery
11 Corticospinal tract
12 Cerebellopontine cistern
13 Anterior semicircular canal
14 Pontine nuclei
15 Middle cerebellar peduncle
16 Primary fissure of cerebellum
17 Abducens nerve (within the slice)
18 Medial lemniscus
19 Spinothalamic tract
20 Lateral lemniscus
21 Motor root of trigeminal nerve (within the slice)
22 Reticular formation
23 Facial nucleus (in the inferior part of the slice)
24 Motor nucleus of trigeminal nerve
25 Principal sensory nucleus of trigeminal nerve
26 Medial longitudinal fasciculus
27 Genu of facial nerve
28 Abducens nucleus (within the slice)
29 Mesencephalic nucleus of trigeminal nerve
30 Superior vestibular nucleus
31 Choroid plexus of fourth ventricle
32 Nodule of vermis (X)
33 Posterior recess of fourth ventricle
34 Dentate nucleus

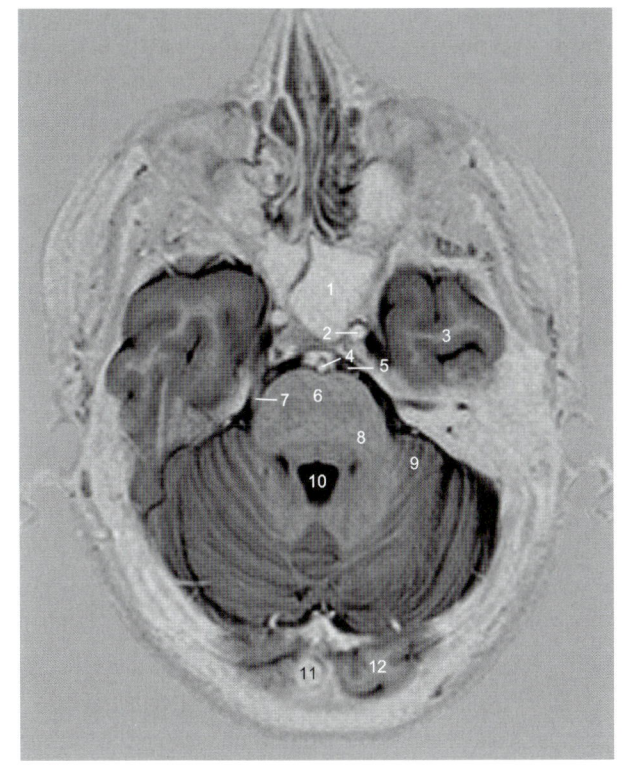

Fig. 74c T1-weighted MR image.

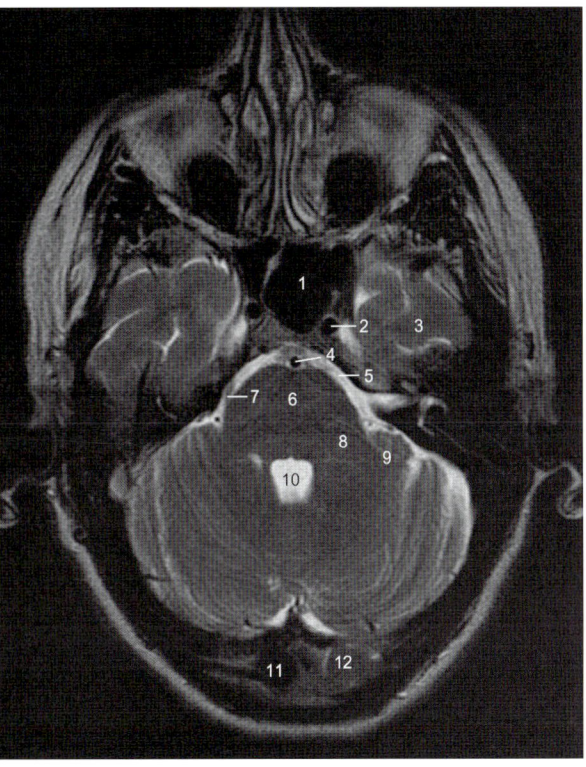

Fig. 74d T2-weighted MR image.

1 Sphenoidal sinus
2 Internal carotid artery
3 Temporal lobe
4 Basilar artery
5 Pontine cistern
6 Pons
7 Trigeminal nerve
8 Middle cerebellar peduncle
9 Anterior lobe of cerebellum
10 Fourth ventricle
11 Confluence of sinuses
12 Base of occipital lobe

202　Atlas

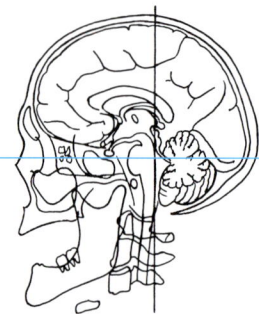

1 Upper eyelid
2 Lens
3 Orbital plate
4 Eyeball
5 Nasal septum
6 Ethmoidal cells
7 Sphenoid
8 Medial rectus
9 Optic nerve
10 Lateral rectus
11 Superior orbital fissure
12 Sphenoidal sinus
13 Pituitary gland
14 Temporalis
15 Trigeminal nerve
16 Pons
17 Anterior lobe of cerebellum
18 Primary fissure of cerebellum
19 Temporal bone
20 Auricle (pinna)
21 Posterior lobe of cerebellum
22 Tentorium of cerebellum
23 Parietal bone
24 Straight sinus
25 Lambdoid suture
26 Superior sagittal sinus
27 Occipital bone

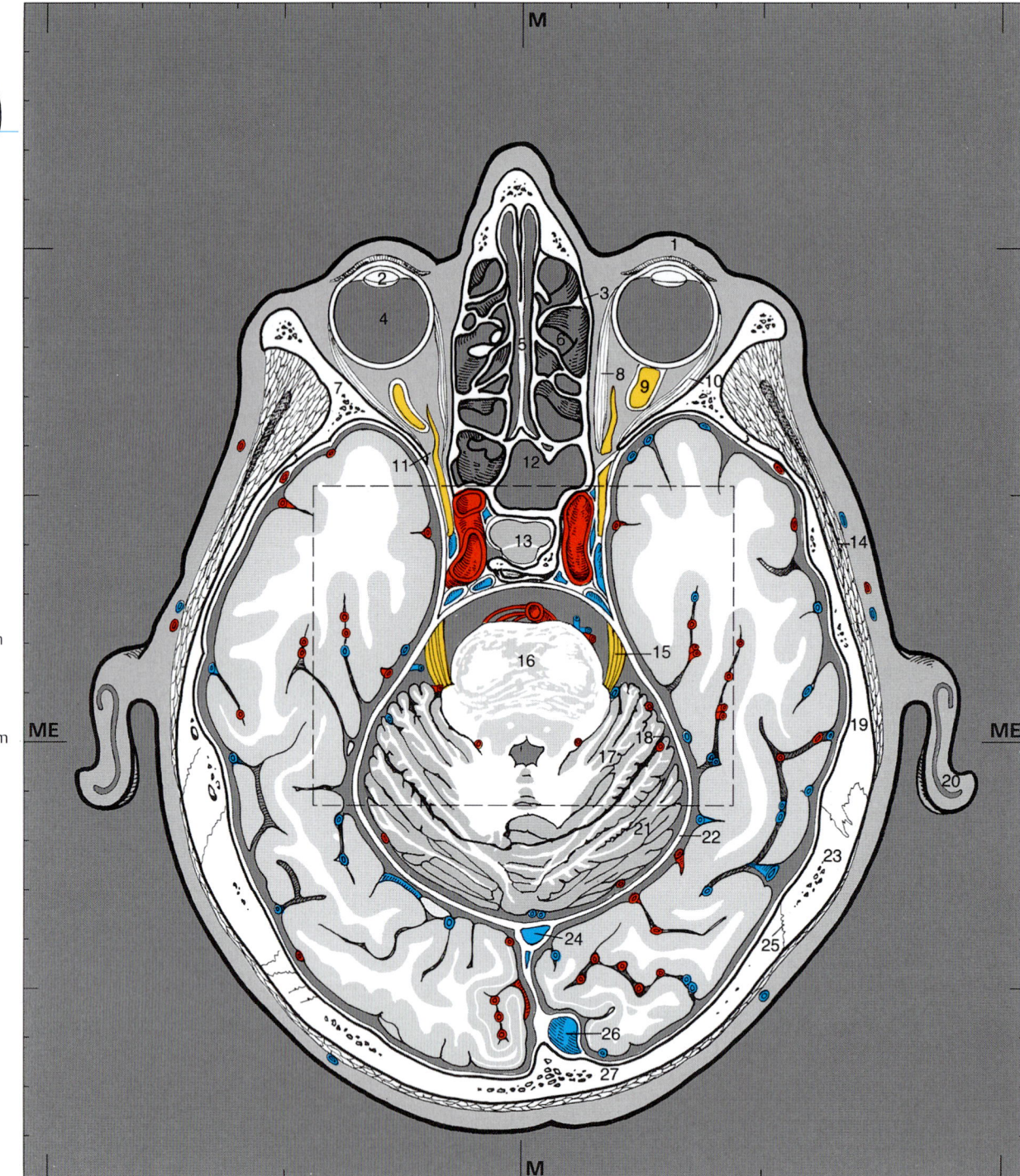

Fig. **75a** Superior section surface of the seventh slice of the brainstem series. The sectional plane runs through the superior orbital fissure, the sella turcica with the pituitary gland, and through the basal parts of the temporal and occipital lobes. The pons is positioned at the level of exit of the trigeminal nerve.

Figs. **75c** and **75d** MR images positioned vertical to Meynert's axis corresponding approximately to the sectional plane of Figs. 75a and 75b.

Brainstem Slices

1 Sphenoidal sinus
2 Adenohypophysis
3 Internal carotid artery
4 Cavernous sinus
5 Neurohypophysis
6 Dorsum sellae
7 Superior petrosal sinus
8 Basilar artery
9 Corticospinal tract
10 Pontine nuclei
11 Trigeminal nerve
12 Cerebellopontine cistern
13 Trigeminal nerve (within the slice)
14 Reticular formation
15 Paramedian pontine reticular formation (PPRF)
16 Medial lemniscus
17 Spinothalamic tract
18 Lateral lemniscus
19 Tentorium of cerebellum
20 Primary fissure of cerebellum
21 Medial longitudinal fasciculus
22 Cerulean nucleus
23 Fourth ventricle
24 Mesencephalic nucleus of trigeminal nerve
25 Superior cerebellar peduncle

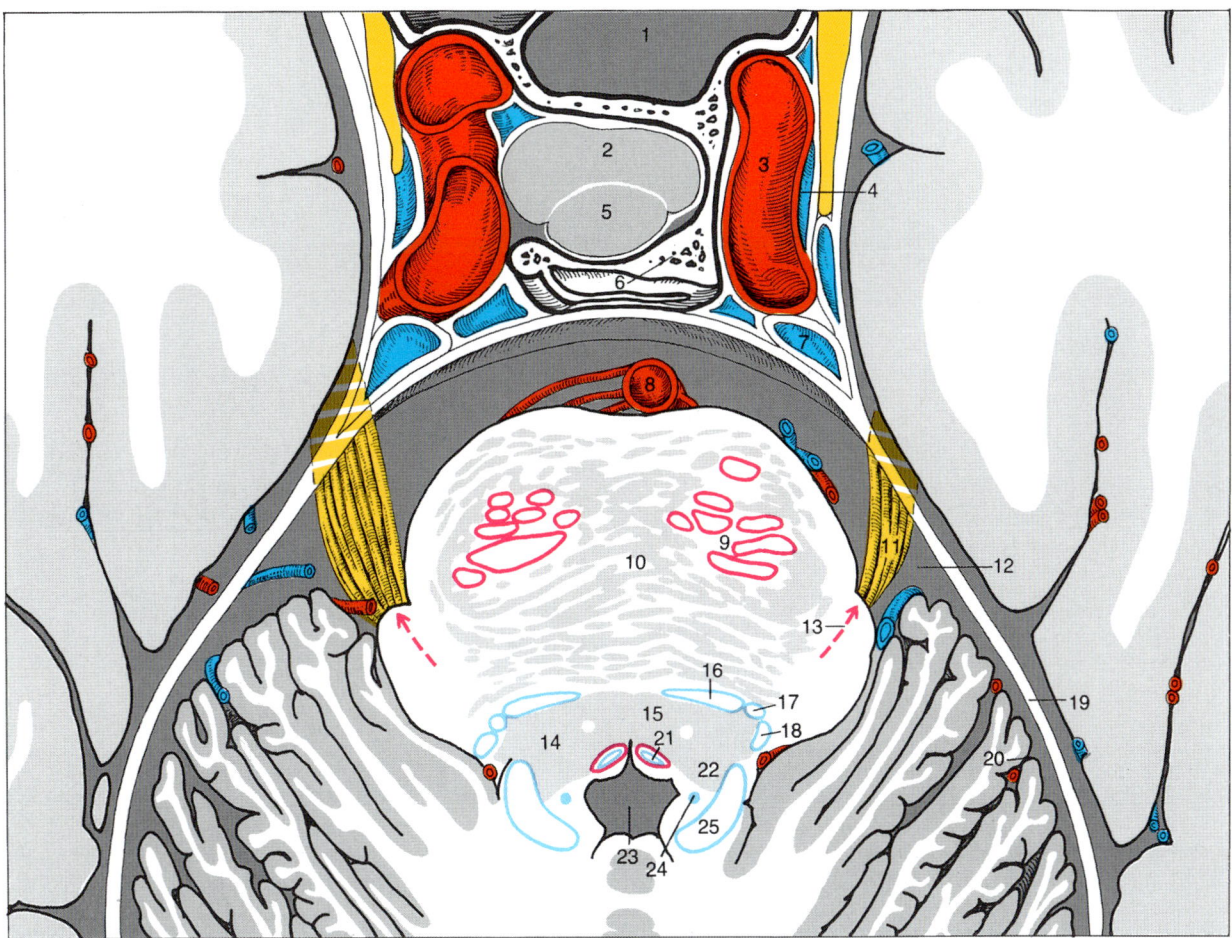

Fig. **75b** The detail magnification of Fig. 75a demonstrates the adenohypophysis and the neurohypophysis with the laterally positioned detail magnifications of the internal carotid arteries. The superior peduncles of the cerebellum lie lateral to the fourth ventricle.

1 Eyeball
2 Ethmoidal cells
3 Inferior rectus (cut) **d**
4 Pole of temporal lobe
5 Pituitary gland
6 Internal carotid artery
7 Basilar artery
8 Pons
9 Trigeminal nerve
10 Fourth ventricle
11 Anterior lobe of cerebellum
12 Pole of occipital lobe

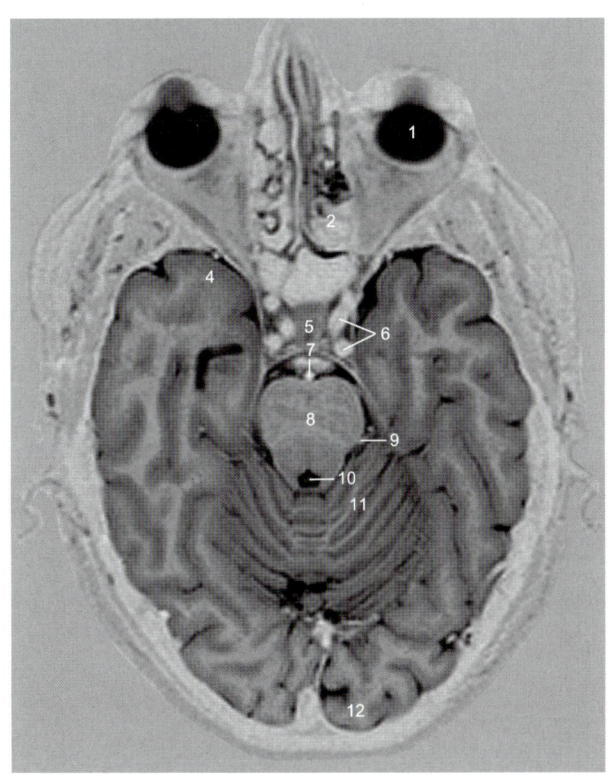

Fig. **75c** T1-weighted MR image.

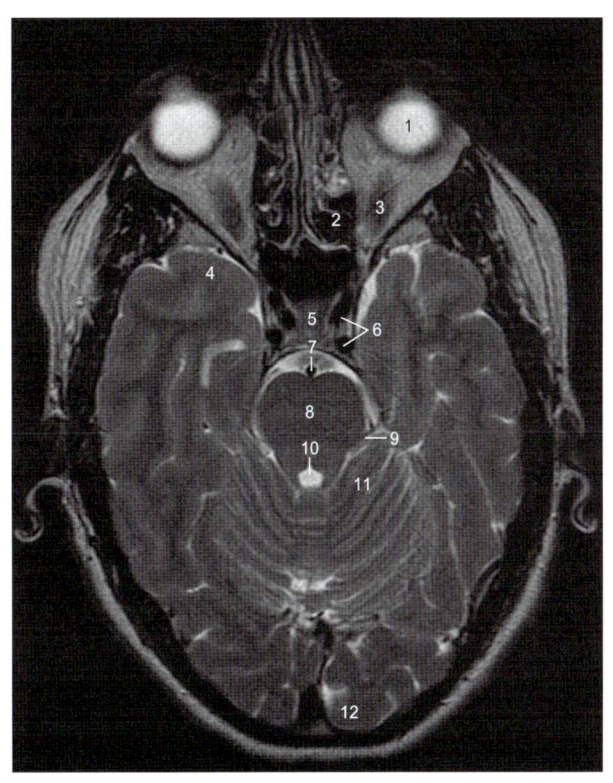

Fig. **75d** T2-weighted MR image.

204 Atlas

1 Upper eyelid
2 Lens
3 Eyeball
4 Lacrimal gland
5 Superior oblique
6 Olfactory bulb
7 Medial rectus
8 Ophthalmic artery
9 Lateral rectus
10 Superior rectus
11 Levator palpebrae superioris
12 Olfactory tract
13 Optic canal (within the slice)
14 Optic nerve
15 Middle meningeal artery
16 Temporalis
17 Temporal bone
18 Pons
19 Anterior lobe of cerebellum
20 Primary fissure of cerebellum
21 Posterior lobe of cerebellum
22 Tentorium of cerebellum
23 Straight sinus
24 Parietal bone
25 Falx cerebri
26 Lambdoid suture
27 Superior sagittal sinus
28 Occipital bone

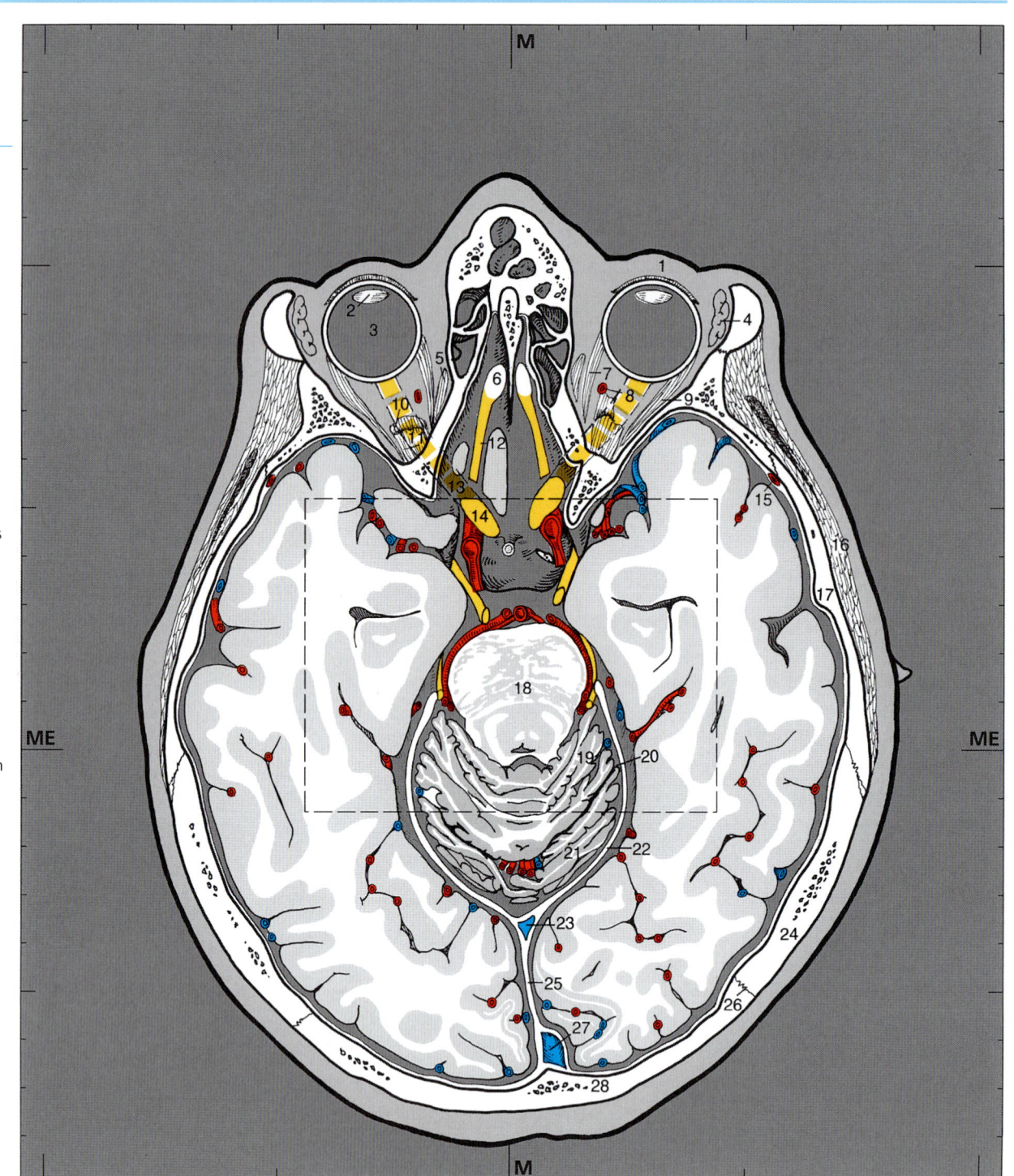

Fig. **76a** Superior section surface of the eighth slice of the brainstem series. The olfactory bulb and tract are in the anterior cranial fossa. The optic nerve runs into the optic canal. In this slice the supratentorial space with the temporal and occipital lobes of the telencephalon is considerably larger than the infratentorial space with the pons and the cerebellum.

Figs. **76c** and **76d**   MR images positioned vertical to Meynert's axis and slightly superior to the sectional plane of Figs. 76a and 76b.

Brainstem Slices

1 Optic nerve
2 Internal carotid artery
3 Posterior communicating artery
4 Infundibulum
5 Amygdaloid body
6 Dorsum sellae
7 Oculomotor nerve
8 Temporal (inferior) horn of lateral ventricle
9 Basilar artery
10 Superior cerebellar artery
11 Hippocampus
12 Pontine nuclei
13 Corticospinal tract
14 Trochlear nerve
15 Reticular formation
16 Medial lemniscus
17 Spinothalamic tract
18 Lateral lemniscus
19 Paramedian pontine reticular formation (PPRF)
20 Medial longitudinal fasciculus
21 Superior cerebellar peduncle
22 Fourth ventricle
23 Cerulean nucleus
24 Mesencephalic nucleus of trigeminal nerve
25 Tentorium of cerebellum

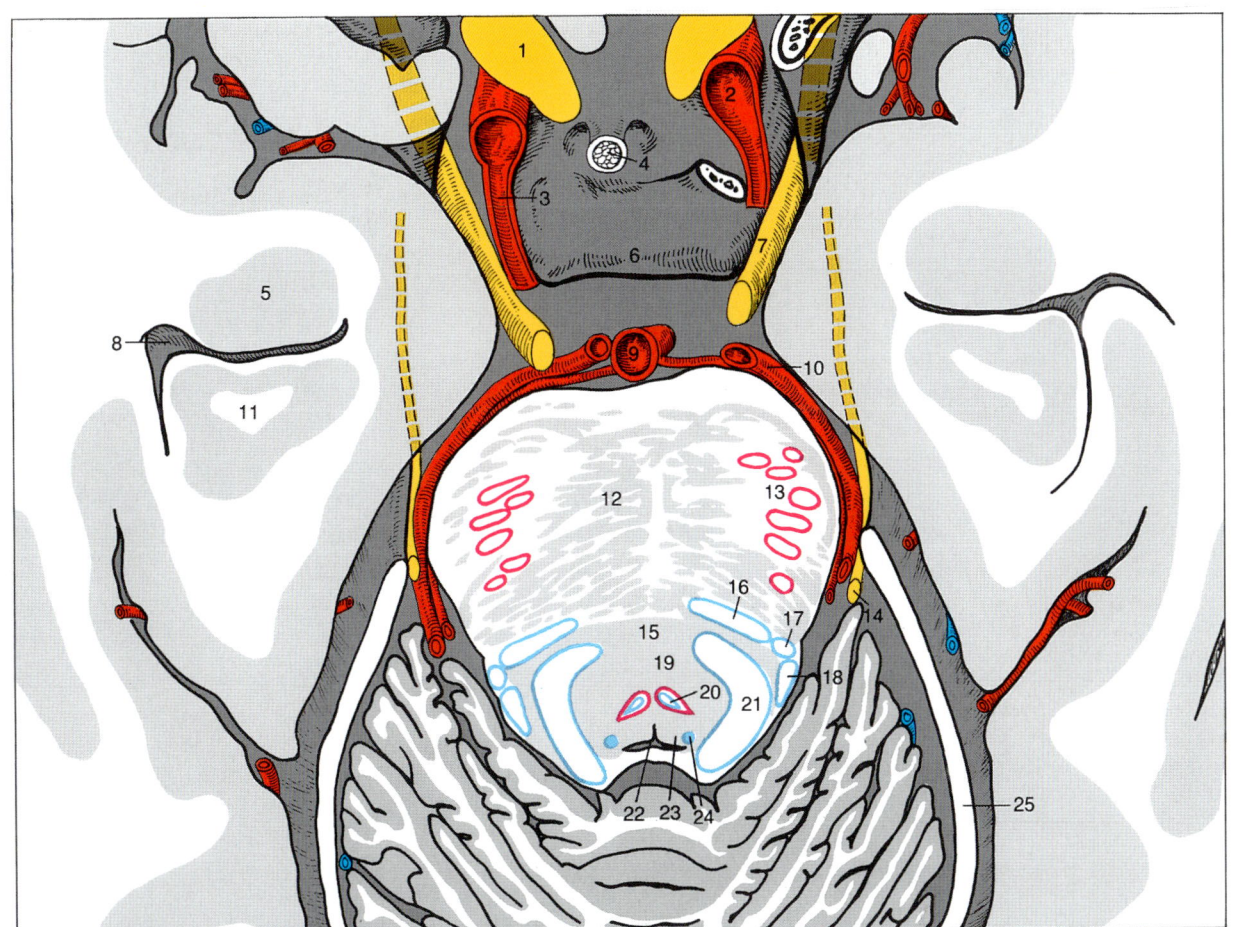

Fig. **76b** The detail magnification of Fig. 76a shows an almost horizontal path of the third and fourth cranial nerves. The roof of the sella turcica is penetrated by the infundibulum. The fourth ventricle narrows in the superior portion of the pons in the direction of the aqueduct of midbrain.

1 Lens
2 Eyeball
3 Retrobulbar space
4 Lateral rectus
5 Internal carotid artery
6 Infundibulum
7 Temporal (inferior) horn of lateral ventricle
8 Basilar artery
9 Pons
10 Anterior lobe of cerebellum
11 Interhemispheric cistern d
12 Superior sagittal sinus

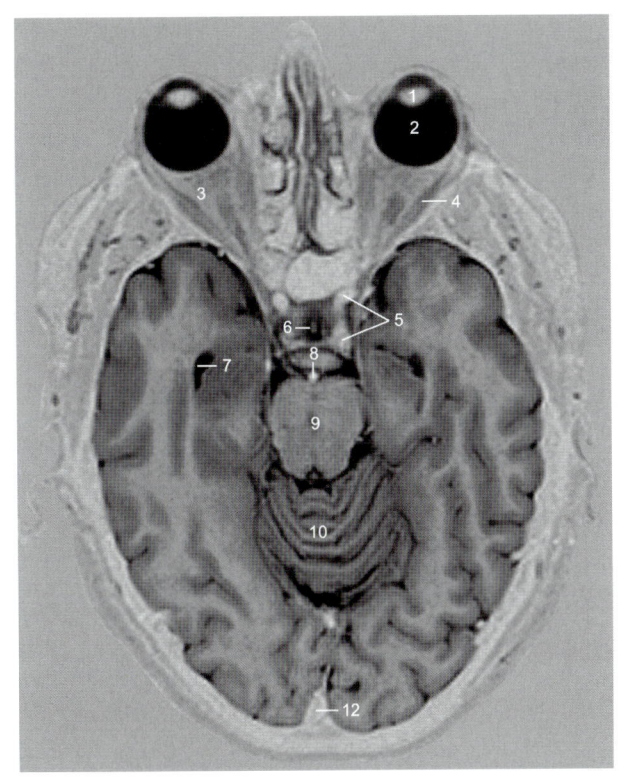

Fig. **76c** T1-weighted MR image.

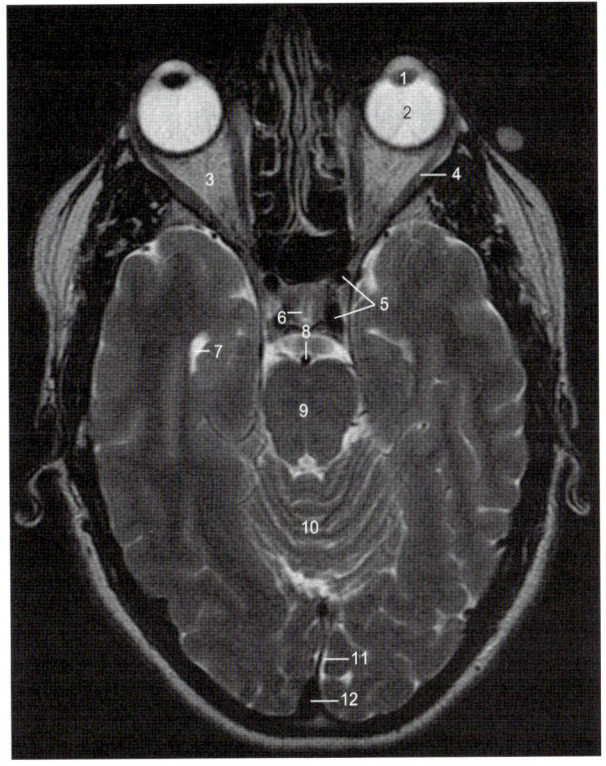

Fig. **76d** T2-weighted MR image.

206   Atlas

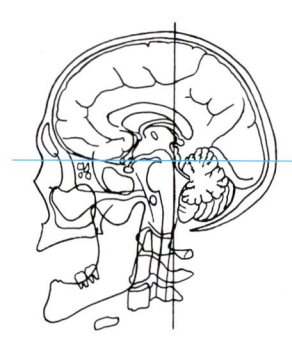

1 Frontal bone
2 Frontal sinus
3 Trochlea
4 Crista galli
5 Superior oblique
6 Superior rectus
7 Levator palpebrae superioris
8 Sphenoid
9 Straight gyrus
10 Temporalis
11 Temporal bone
12 Mammillary body
13 Interpeduncular cistern
14 Cerebral crus
15 Tegmentum of midbrain
16 Ambient cistern
17 Aqueduct of midbrain
18 Anterior lobe of cerebellum
19 Tentorium of cerebellum
20 Straight sinus
21 Parietal bone
22 Longitudinal cerebral (inter-hemispheric) fissure
23 Primary visual cortex
24 Falx cerebri
25 Calcarine sulcus
26 Lambdoid suture
27 Superior sagittal sinus
28 Occipital bone

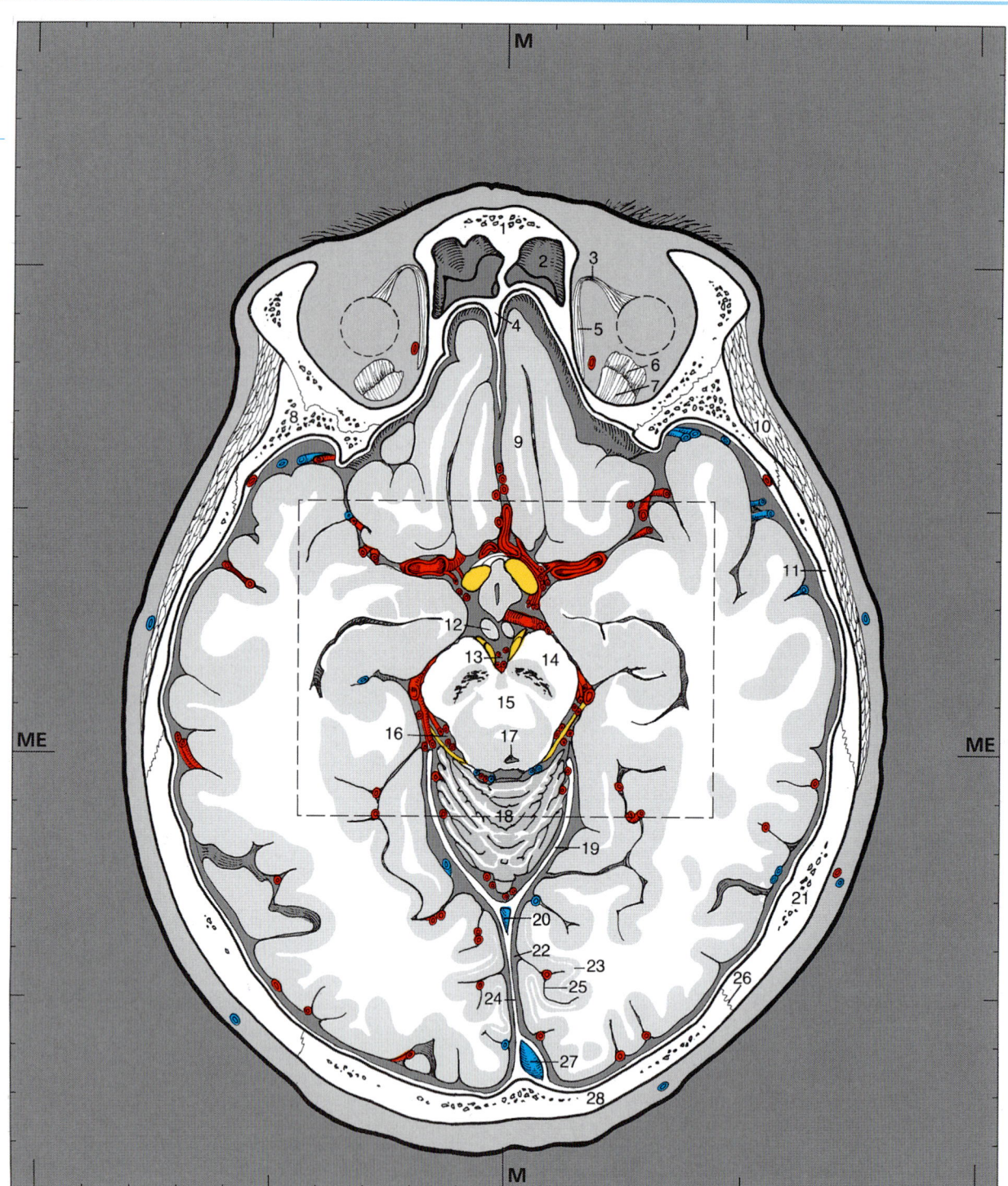

Fig. **77a** Superior section surface of the ninth slice of the brainstem series. The sectional plane is positioned anteriorly just below the roof of the orbit and medially in a posterior aspect to the straight gyrus above the anterior cranial fossa. The slice includes the mammillary bodies and the midbrain at the level of the inferior colliculus.

Figs. **77c** and **77d** MR images positioned vertical to Meynert's axis and slightly inferior to the sectional plane of Figs. 77a and 77b.

Brainstem Slices

1	Anterior cerebral artery
2	Optic nerve (within the slice)
3	Optic chiasm (within the slice)
4	Anteromedial central artery
5	Anterolateral central arteries
6	Optic tract
7	Middle cerebral artery
8	Infundibular recess
9	Hypothalamus
10	Mammillary body
11	Posterior cerebral artery
12	Posteromedial central arteries
13	Oculomotor nerve and its roots (arrow)
14	Interpeduncular fossa
15	Frontopontine tract
16	Corticonuclear tract
17	Corticospinal tract
18	Occipitopontine and temporopontine tracts
19	Hippocampus
20	Temporal (inferior) horn of lateral ventricle
21	Substantia nigra
22	Decussation of superior cerebellar peduncles
23	Medial lemniscus
24	Trochlear nerve
25	Reticular formation
26	Medial longitudinal fasciculus
27	Trochlear nucleus
28	Cerulean nucleus
29	Spinothalamic tract
30	Lateral lemniscus
31	Mesencephalic nucleus of trigeminal nerve
32	Aqueduct of midbrain
33	Decussation of trochlear nerves (within the slice)
34	Inferior colliculus

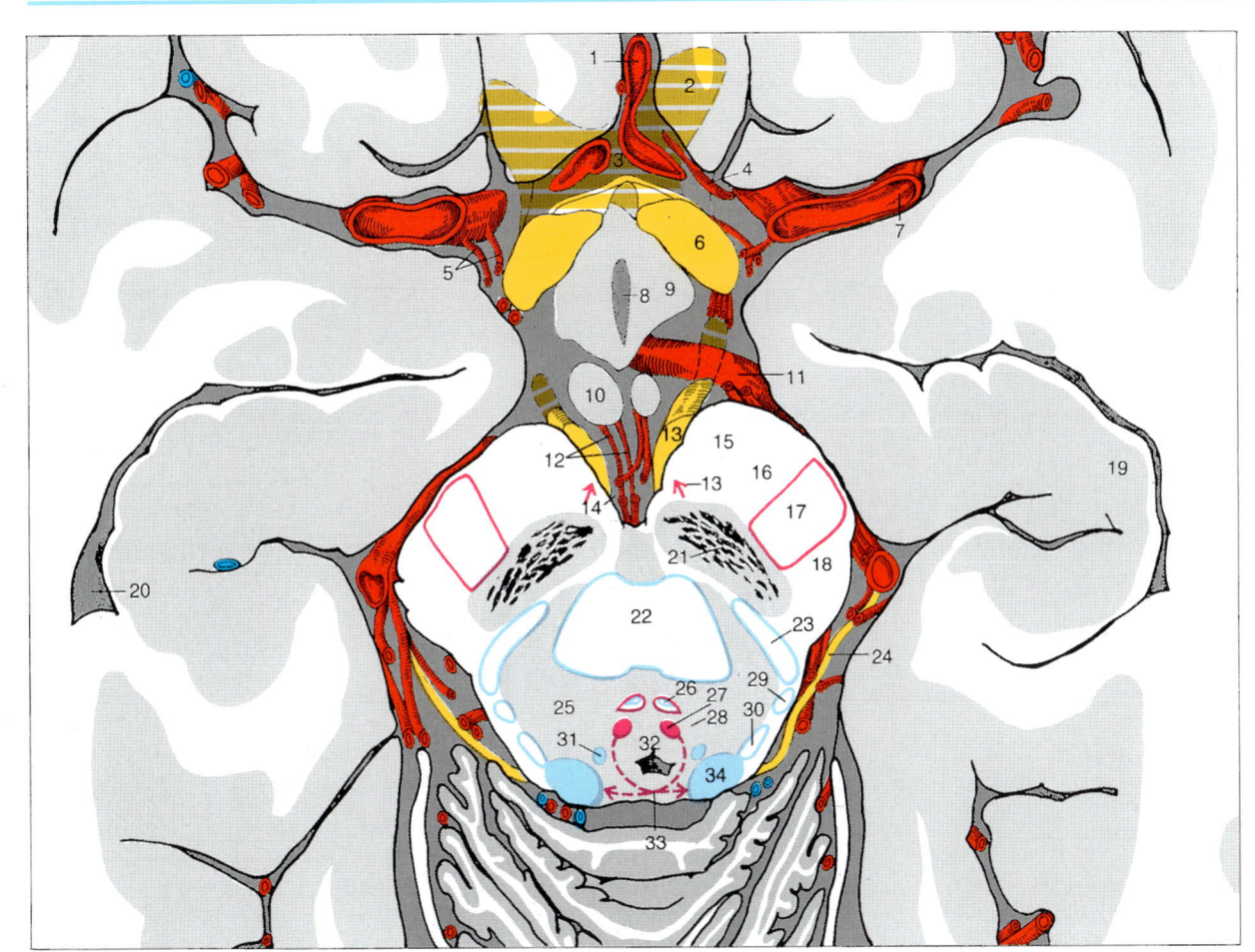

Fig. **77b** The detail magnification of Fig. 77a reveals the optic tract. The optic chiasm lies within the ninth slice (interrupted yellow markings). Positioned posteriorly is the hypothalamus with the mammillary bodies. Within this slice the trochlear nerve emerges from the midbrain lying posteriorly to the inferior colliculus.

1	Optic nerve
2	Straight gyrus
3	Temporalis **d**
4	Optic chiasm
5	Middle cerebral artery
6	Infundibulum
7	Mammillary body **c**
8	Oculomotor nerve **d**
9	Interpeduncular cistern
10	Cerebral crus
11	Tegmentum of midbrain
12	Aqueduct of midbrain
13	Ambient cistern
14	Inferior colliculus
15	Vermis of anterior lobe of cerebellum
16	Superior sagittal sinus **c**

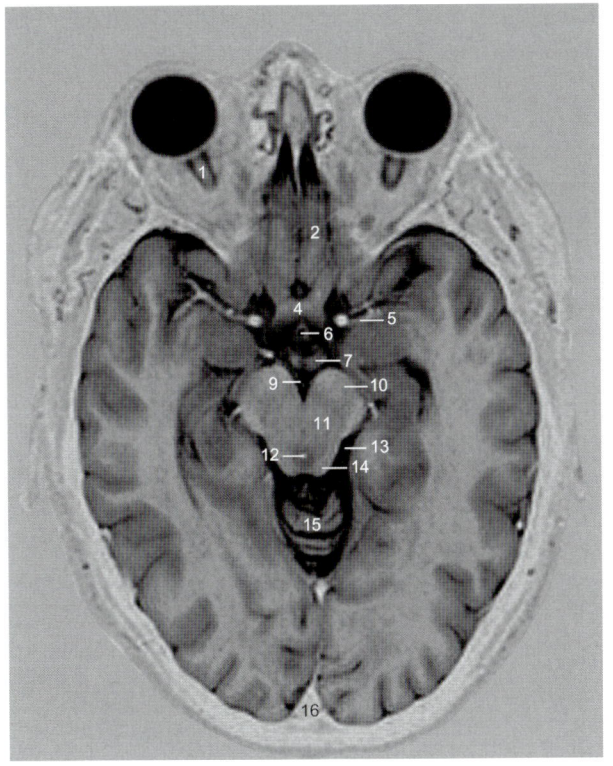

Fig. **77c** T1-weighted MR image.

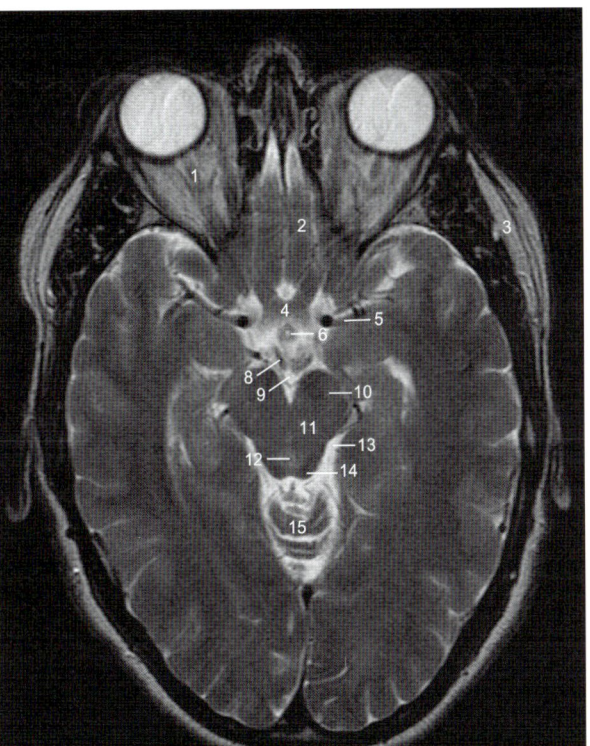

Fig. **77d** T2-weighted MR image.

208   Atlas

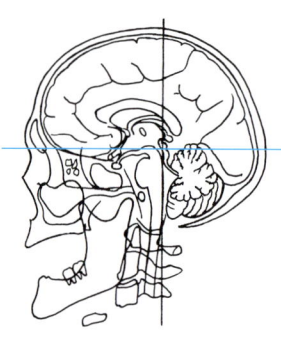

1 Frontal sinus
2 Crista galli
3 Frontal bone
4 Longitudinal cerebral (interhemispheric) fissure
5 Temporalis
6 Insular arteries
7 Hypothalamus
8 Temporal bone
9 Tegmentum of midbrain
10 Aqueduct of midbrain
11 Anterior lobe of cerebellum
12 Occipital (posterior) horn of
   lateral ventricle
13 Tentorium of cerebellum
14 Straight sinus
15 Primary visual cortex
16 Parietal bone
17 Falx cerebri
18 Calcarine sulcus
19 Lambdoid suture
20 Superior sagittal sinus
21 Occipital bone

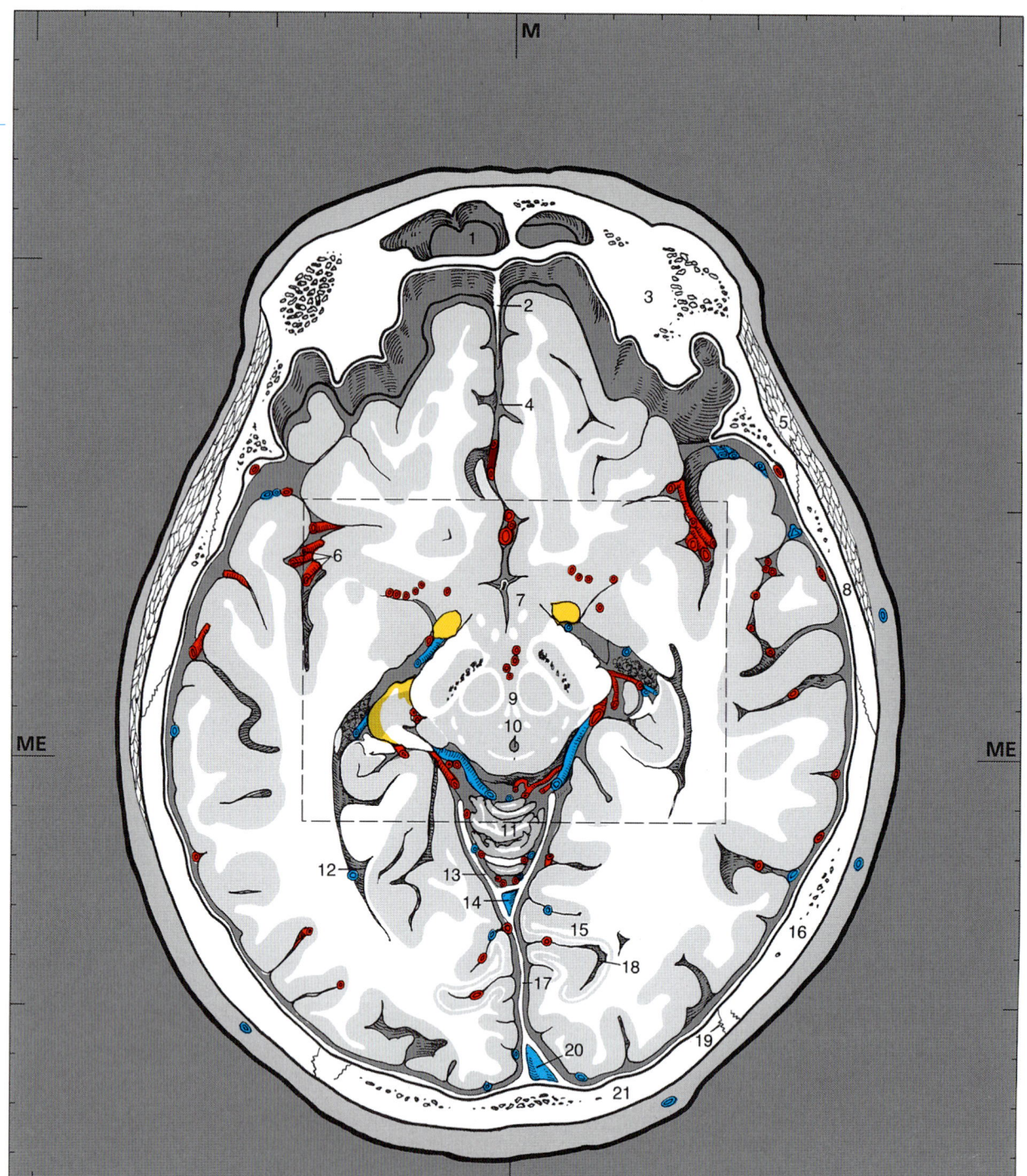

Fig. 78a Superior section surface of the tenth slice of the brainstem series. The frontal and temporal lobes, hypothalamus, and midbrain at the level of the superior colliculus and the hippocampus are demonstrated in this section.

Figs. 78c and 78d MR images positioned vertical to Meynert's axis and slightly inferior to the sectional plane of Figs. 78a and 78b.

Brainstem Slices

1 Anterior cerebral artery
2 Insular arteries
3 Lamina terminalis
4 Third ventricle
5 Hypothalamus
6 Optic tract
7 Fornix
8 Mammillothalamic fasciculus (of Vicq d'Azyr)
9 Cerebral crus
10 Frontopontine tract
11 Corticonuclear tract
12 Corticospinal tract
13 Occipitopontine and temporopontine tracts
14 Oculomotor nerve (within the slice)
15 Substantia nigra
16 Red nucleus
17 Lateral geniculate body
18 Medial geniculate body
19 Reticular formation
20 Oculomotor nucleus
21 Medial longitudinal fasciculus
22 Medial lemniscus
23 Posterior cerebral artery
24 Dentate gyrus
25 Hippocampus
26 Temporal (inferior) horn of lateral ventricle
27 Aqueduct of midbrain
28 Mesencephalic nucleus of trigeminal nerve
29 Spinothalamic tract
30 Ambient cistern
31 Superior colliculus
32 Basal vein (of Rosenthal)
33 Posterior lateral choroidal artery

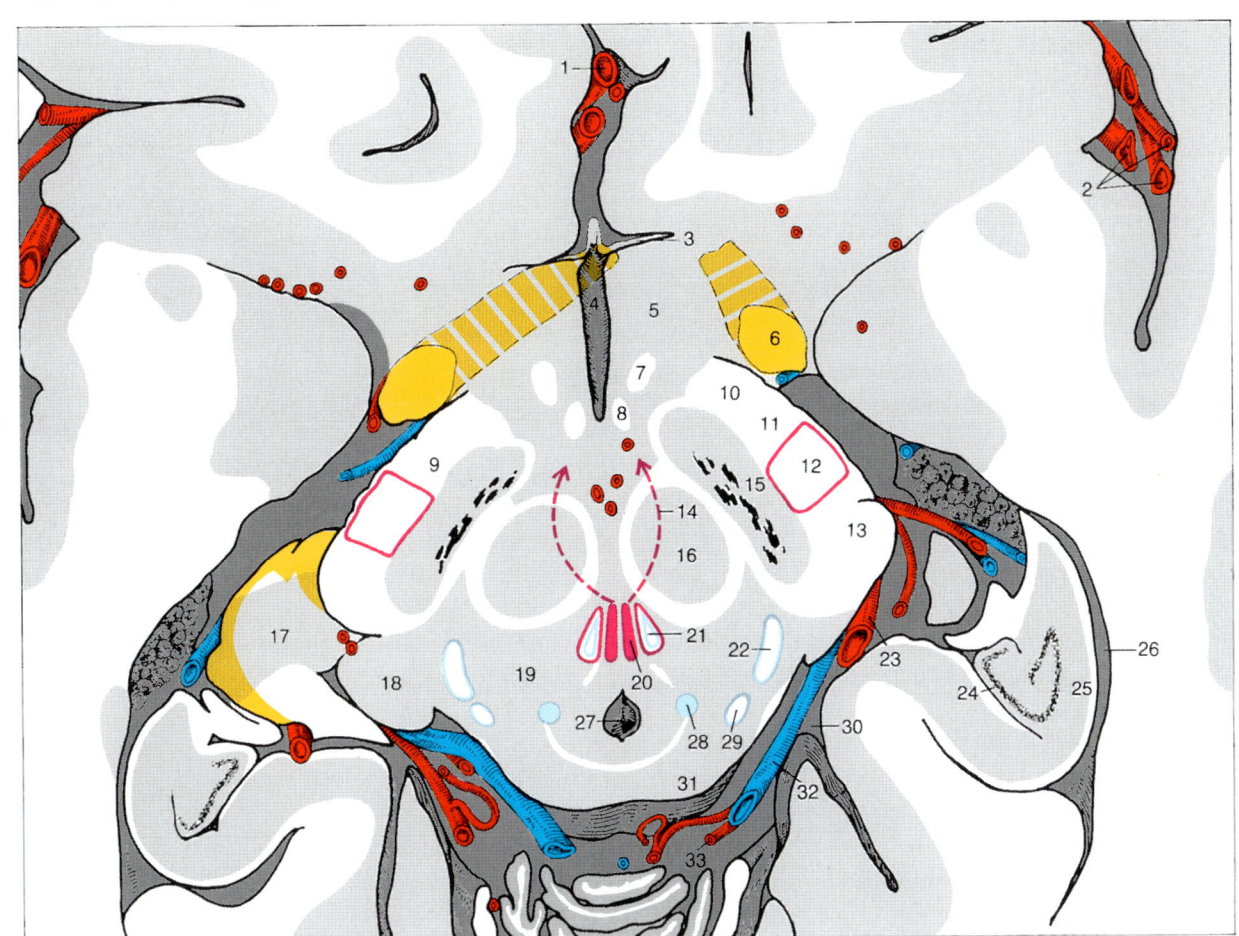

Fig. **78b** The detail magnification of Fig. 78a shows the neighboring structures of the optic tract, namely the hypothalamus, midbrain at the level of the superior colliculus, and the hippocampus.

1 Interhemispheric cistern
2 Anterior cerebral artery
3 Cistern of vallecula cerebri
4 Middle cerebral artery
5 Optic tract
6 Third ventricle
7 Mammillary body
8 Cerebral crus
9 Tegmentum of midbrain
10 Aqueduct of midbrain
11 Ambient cistern
12 Superior colliculus
13 Temporal (inferior) horn of lateral ventricle
14 Straight sinus
15 Calcarine sulcus
16 Superior sagittal sinus

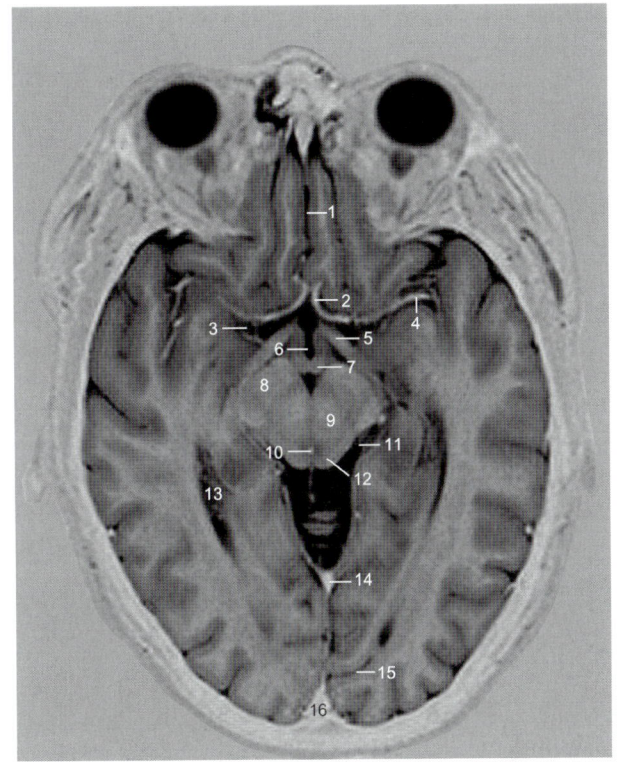

Fig. **78c** T1-weighted MR image. Technical data (Chap. 8).

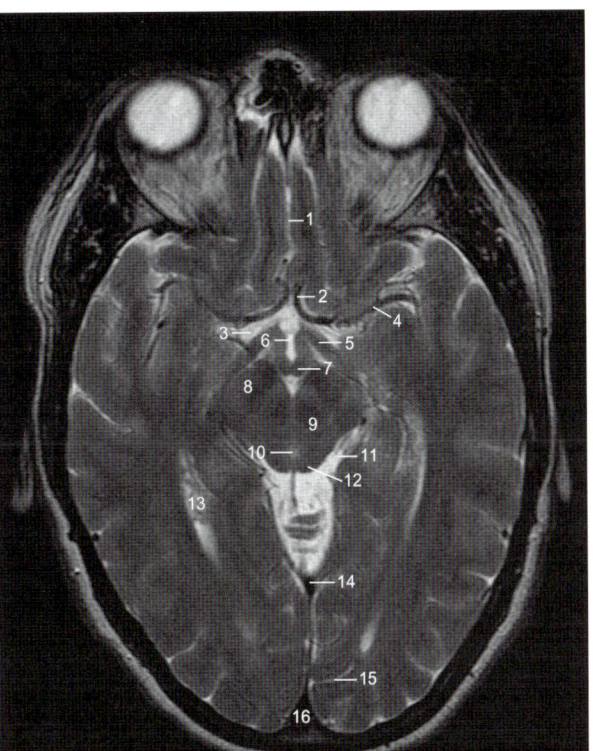

Fig. **78d** T2-weighted MR image. Technical data (Chap. 8).

3 Topography of the Facial Skeleton and its Cavities in Multiplanar Parallel Slices

Topography describes the positional relationships of anatomic structures in space. The standard textbooks of cranial topography, before the era of the new imaging procedures, favored the portrayal of anatomic structures as conceived from the individual layers and components of a dissected head and brain. Much practical knowledge was acquired from the surgical specialities.

The use of computed tomography (CT) and magnetic resonance imaging (MRI) requires a special **three-dimensional knowledge of anatomic structures** in order to interpret parallel brain slices. The equidistant serial CT and MR images of the head provide the neurologist with a view similar to the architect's renditions of an entire building and its subunits, using the plans of sequential floors. However, unlike the precise architectural drawings in which right angles predominate, CT and MR scans yield highly variable contours due to the complex shapes of anatomic structures.

The exact **position of the slices** is important in neuroanatomy. For the coronal series the positions are indicated in lateral views in Figures 1-3. For the sagittal series the positions are seen in frontal views in Figures 29 and 30. For the canthomeatal and brainstem slices they are indicated in the lateral views in Figures 44, 45, 46, 67. In the coronal series the slices are viewed anteriorly (from the front) in Figures 4-17. The depicted surface of each section represents the line to the left of the encircled number of the corresponding slice in Figures 1-3. The individual sagittal slices are viewed from the medial side (Figs. 32-37). The canthomeatal slices (Figs. 47-60) and the brainstem slices (Figs. 69-78) are viewed from above. Therefore, the line above the encircled number represents the depicted surface of each slice (Figs. 44, 45, 46, 67).

3.1 Facial Skeleton

The **facial skeleton** forms the bony walls of the first portion of the breathing and digestive apparatus, as well as of the orbital cavities. The nasal skeleton is formed by five bones. Four bones make up the skeleton of the jaws. Owing to their close proximity, individual bones may be related to two or more of the cavities. For example, the hard palate forms the floor of the nasal cavity and the roof of the oral cavity.

Bones of the Nasal Skeleton

The **ethmoid** is an unpaired bone derived from the cartilaginous nasal capsule. In coronal sections a T-shaped middle portion and paired lateral portions can be identified:
- The cribriform plate (Figs. 5c.13, 19.4, 38.12), forming the horizontal limb of the T
- The perpendicular plate, corresponding to the vertical limb of the T
- The ethmoidal cells (Figs. 2a.9, 4a.7, 18.7, 30a.9, 33a.22, 39.9, 45a.11, 49c.1, 63.1, 74a.7) lying between the nasal cavity and the orbits, as well as below the anterior cranial fossa.

The cribriform plate is inserted into the frontal bone medially and paramedially. This thin bony plate is perforated by numerous small holes through which the olfactory nerves run. The olfactory nerves run from the olfactory epithelium to the olfactory bulb. In the median plane the crista galli (Figs. 4c.7, 18.2, 30a.4, 32c.16, 38.7, 50c.3, 51d.2, 77a.4) projects upward from the lamina cribrosa into the cranial cavity. The falx cerebri is attached to this bony process.

The perpendicular plate is a continuation of the crista galli below the cribriform plate and forms the upper part of the bony nasal septum. The orbital plate (Figs. 4c.16, 5c.17, 18.6, 19.5, 75a.3) separates the ethmoidal cells laterally from the orbital cavity. The **ethmoidal cells** are hollow air sinus spaces in communication with the nasal cavity. The anterior and middle ethmoidal cells drain below the middle nasal concha, the posterior ethmoidal cells above it. The volume of the entire ethmoid labyrinth amounts to about 10 ml (260). On its medial side are the superior and middle nasal conchae projecting into the nasal cavity. Beneath the middle nasal concha is the middle nasal meatus (Figs. 4a.13, 5a.15, 6a.19) containing a half-moon shaped opening, the semilunar hiatus (Figs. 4a.12, 5a.13, 33a.28, 73a.2, 74a.3). The anterior and middle ethmoidal cells and the frontal and maxillary sinuses drain through this hiatus.

The independent **inferior nasal concha** is larger than the other turbinates and is about 4 cm long. In the coronal slices, the inferior turbinate with its hooklike appearance above the palate is a guideline structure (Figs. 4a.20, 4b.8, 4d.8, 5a.20, 18.15, 33a.35, 69a.2, 69c.2, 69d.2).

The **vomer** (ploughshare) is an unpaired bone that forms a lower part of the bony nasal septum. In addition to two bony portions, the nasal septum is also partly cartilaginous.

The **nasal bones** are paired. They are two small four-sided bones in the upper part of the bridge of the nose.

The tiny, four-sided, paired lacrimal bone is situated within the medial wall of the orbit and also forms part of the lateral wall of the nasal cavity.

Bones of the Upper and Lower Jaws

The **maxilla** is the central bone of the facial skeleton. It borders on the orbits, nasal and oral cavities, and forms the main part of the bony palate. The maxilla consists of a middle portion (the body) and four processes.

The large middle portion of the maxilla contains the **maxillary sinus**. It is the largest air-filled paranasal sinus, as can be seen in the coronal slices (Figs. 2a.24, 4a.19, 5a.19, 6a.22, 18.14), the sagittal slices (Figs. 30a.15, 34a.32, 36a.21, 40.20), and the axial slices (Figs. 45a.22, 47a.7, 48c.6, 61.6).

The frontal process of the maxilla runs between the nasal and the lacrimal bones, up to the frontal bone. The zygomatic process adjoins the zygomatic bone. The palatal process is a horizontal bony plate that joins the anterior end of the palatal bone, both of them forming the hard palate (Figs. 2a.30, 4c.25, 5c.24, 6c.23, 18.16, 19.15, 33c.28, 38.27). The alveolar process forms the alveoli, which bear the teeth of the upper jaw. After the teeth have been lost the alveolar process is absorbed; this is clearly seen in the maxilla in the sagittal series. In the part where the upper teeth were located, the maxilla is narrow, lacking the powerful alveolar process (Fig. 39.24) that projects into the oral cavity.

The **palatine bone** consists of the already described horizontal plate for the hard palate and an almost vertical plate forming the medial boundary of the pterygopalatine fossa.

The **zygomatic bone** is located between the maxilla, the temporal and the frontal bones (Figs. 2a.19, 4c.17, 18.11, 30a.8, 37c.13, 43.6, 47a.5, 48c.3, 61.5).

The **mandible** or lower jaw is the only moveable bone in the facial skeleton. It articulates with the base of the skull. The anterior part shaped like a bent open horse-shoe is known as the body (Figs. 2a.37, 4c.33, 5c.31, 18.20, 30a.25, 32c.44, 34c.44, 38.37). From this an ascending process, the ramus, runs upward (Figs. 2a.33, 7c.27, 8c.31, 21.19, 30a.22, 37c.30, 43.16).

The alveolar part of the body contains the teeth. After loss of the teeth the alveolar part is absorbed. As a result the mandibular canal comes to lie nearer to the toothless margin of the jaw (Figs. 39.28, 40.31). The ramus of the mandible runs upward from the body of the mandible at the angle of the jaw and then ends above in two processes, the coronoid (muscular) process, anteriorly (Fig. 2a.21), and the condylar (articular) process, posteriorly. The coronoid process receives the tendon of the temporalis and can be regarded as a tendon ossification (Fig. 37c.22). The condylar process first forms the narrower neck of the mandible (Figs. 2a.22, 23.14) and then ascends to the transversely protruding head of the mandible (Figs. 2a.20, 23.12). On the inner side of the ramus is the mandibular foramen through which the inferior alveolar nerve, artery, and vein enter the mandibular canal (Figs. 37c.31, 37a.19).

Pathologic changes in the facial skeleton (fractures, erosions) are often inadequately demonstrated by routine plain films, due to the complicated spatial relationships. In these cases it is necessary to take radiographs with special views and CT scans with high-resolution technique and thin slices (287). The **CT investigation** should be done in axial and coronal planes. For the axial series, slices parallel to the infraorbitomeatal plane are preferred (194, 287). The angle of the coronal series depends on the status of the patient to be examined. (How mobile is the cervical spine? Might filled teeth produce artifacts?) A "wide" window should always be used for imaging bony structures, and a "narrow" window for imaging the soft tissues.

3.2 Nasal Cavity and Paranasal Sinuses
(Figs. 79, 80)

The paired nasal cavities start at the nostrils that lead into the vestibule, then the true nasal cavity. At the posterior nasal apertures, the choanae, the nasal cavity passes into the nasopharynx. The nasal septum separates the right and left cavities.

All paranasal sinuses are connected with the main nasal cavities. The paranasal sinuses include:
- Ethmoidal cells
- Maxillary sinus
- Sphenoidal sinus
- Frontal sinus.

The central position of the nasal cavities and the paranasal sinuses, which extend above and below Reid's base line, are easily recognizable in the coronal and sagittal series (Figs. 4–10, 32–36). Posteriorly the sphenoidal sinus may extend almost to the meatovertical line (MV). In Figures 79, 80 the nasal cavities and the paranasal sinuses underneath the anterior cranial fossa, medial to and below the orbits and the middle cranial fossa, and above the oral cavity, are displayed in color. Posteriorly, within the fifth coronal slice, the transition from the nasal cavity through the choanae into the pharynx can be seen. In the sixth coronal slice the sphenoidal sinus (Fig. 9a.34) is located above the pharynx (Fig. 9c.29).

The medial wall of the nasal cavity is formed by the nasal septum (Figs. 4a.17, 5a.17, 18.13, 30a.12, 32a.34, 38.21, 47a.2, 48c.2, 62.2), which only approximates to the midline and can be bent to one side or the other in the anterior or posterior part (septal deviation) (Fig. 5a.17).

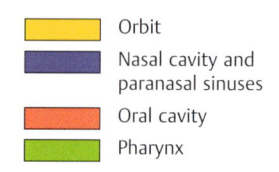

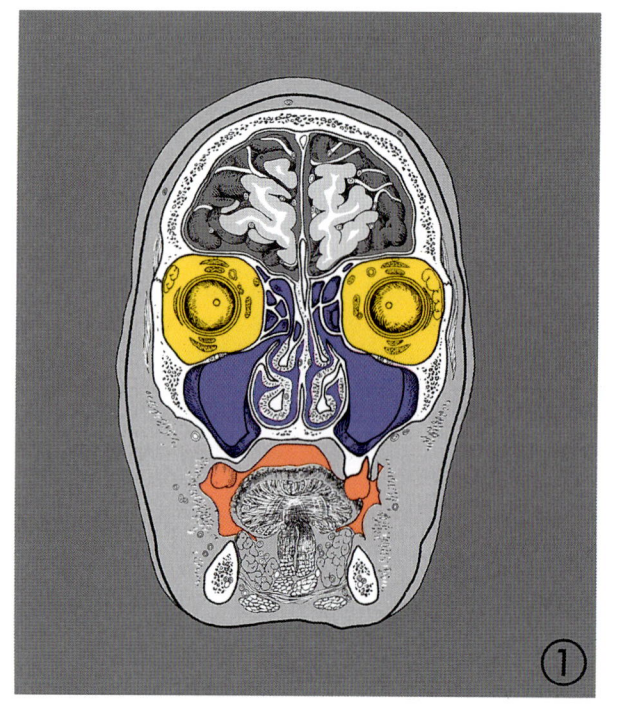

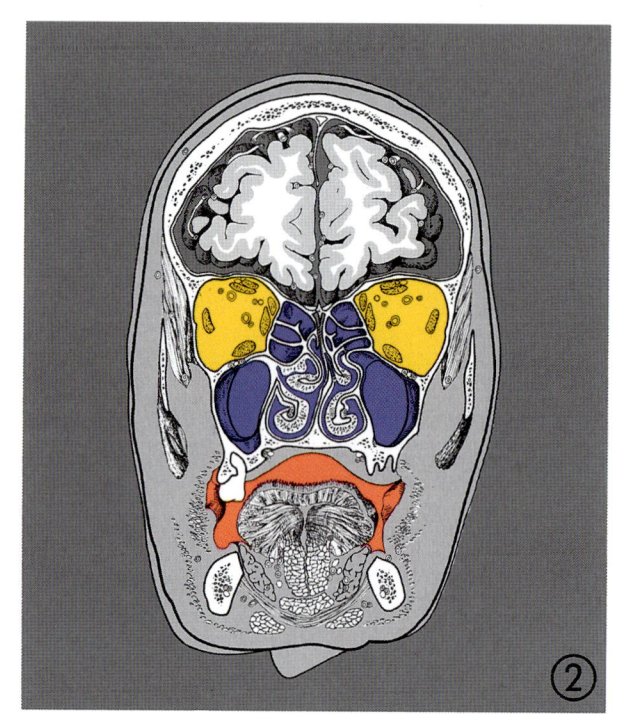

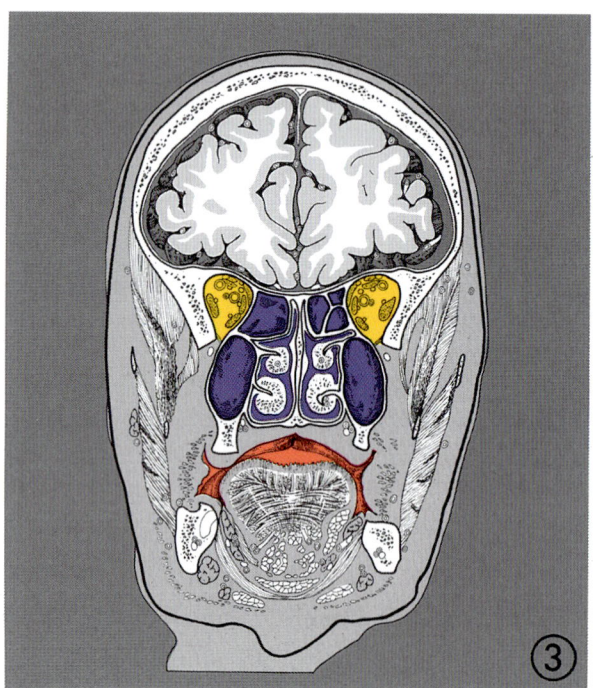

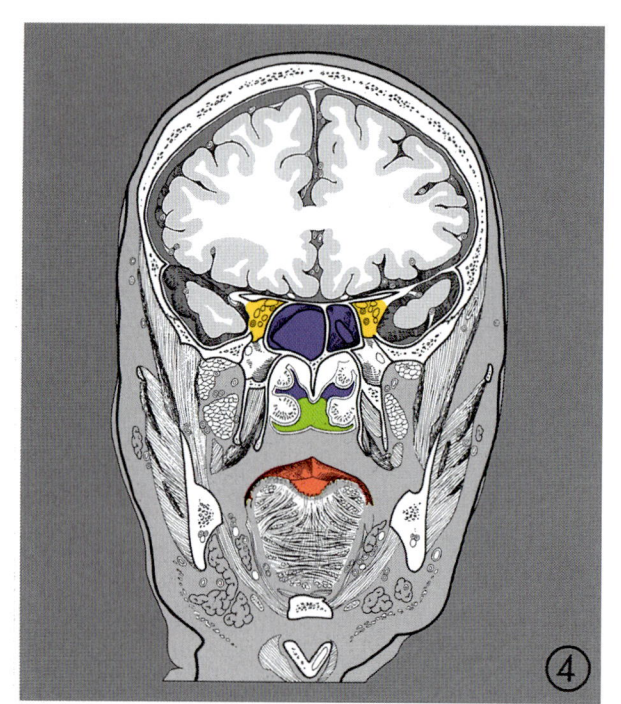

212   3   Topography of the Facial Skeleton and its Cavities in Multiplanar Parallel Slices

☐ Orbit
☐ Nasal cavity and paranasal sinuses
☐ Oral cavity
☐ Pharynx

Fig. 79 Coronal serial illustrations showing the compartments of the facial skeleton and the craniocervical junction. The encircled numbers (1–8) indicate the number of the respective slices (Figs. 1a, 2a,b, 3).

3.2 Nasal Cavity and Paranasal Sinuses

- Paranasal sinus
- Pharynx
- Oral cavity
- Parapharyngeal space
- Bones and muscles of craniocervical junction

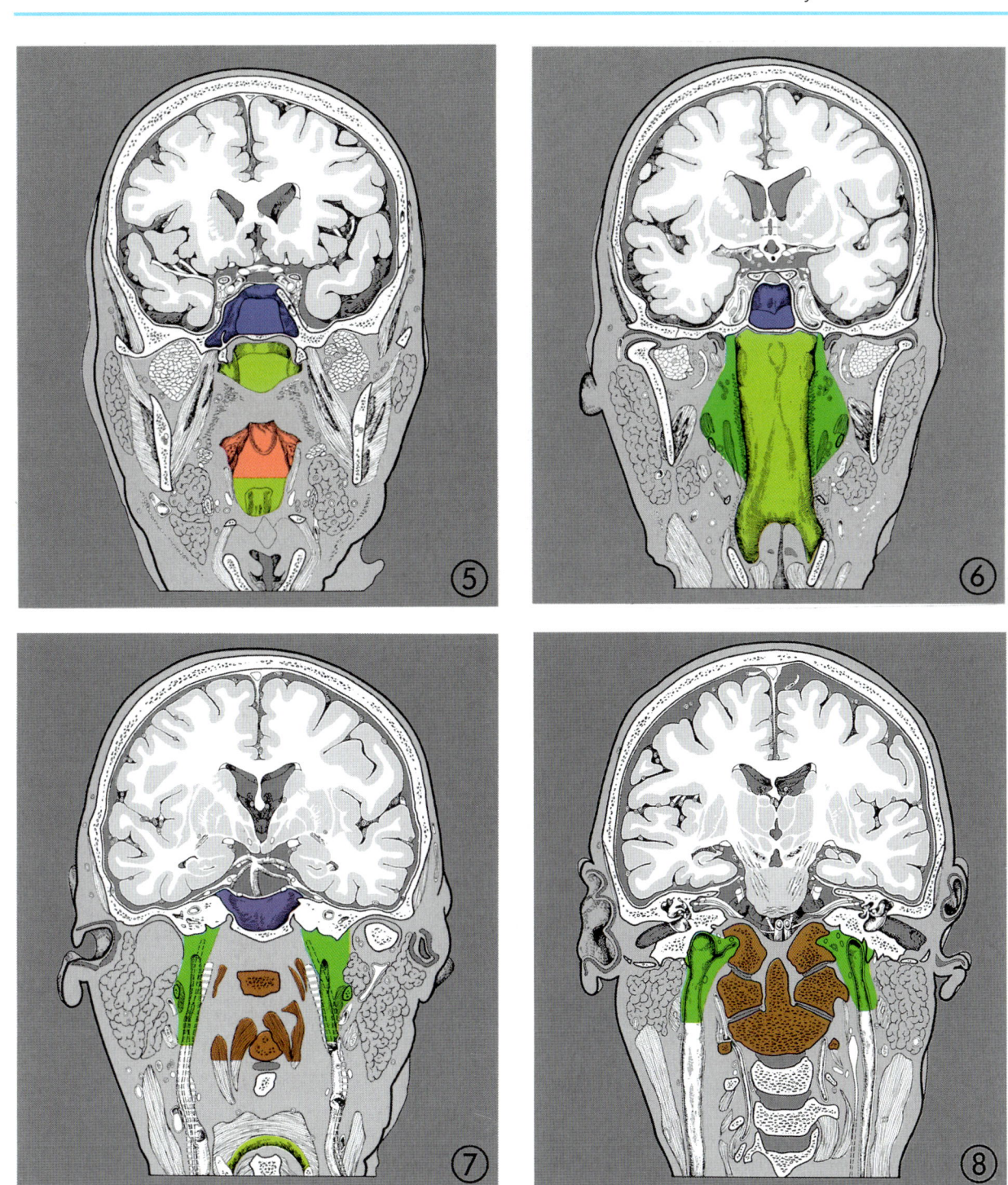

214   3 Topography of the Facial Skeleton and its Cavities in Multiplanar Parallel Slices

■ Bones and muscles of craniocervical junction

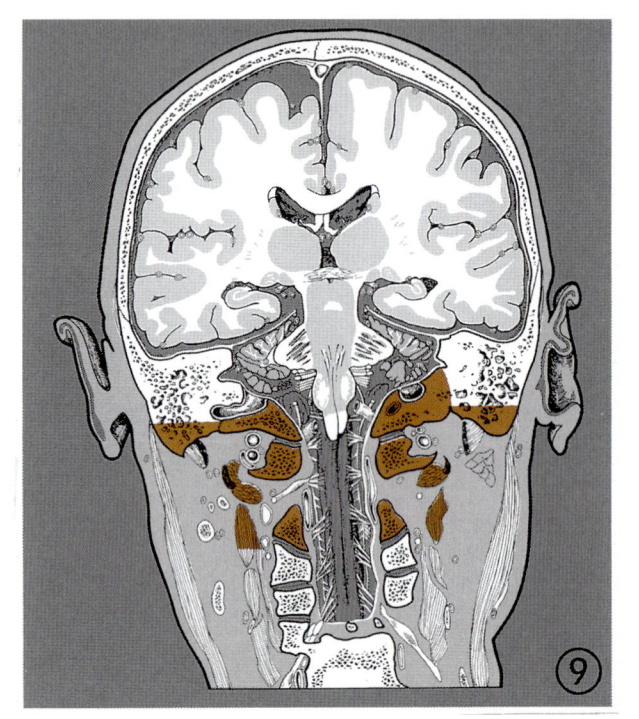

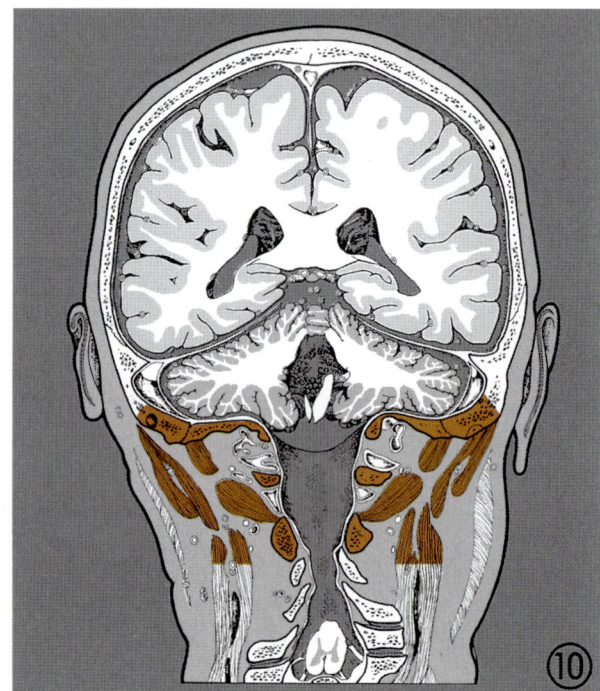

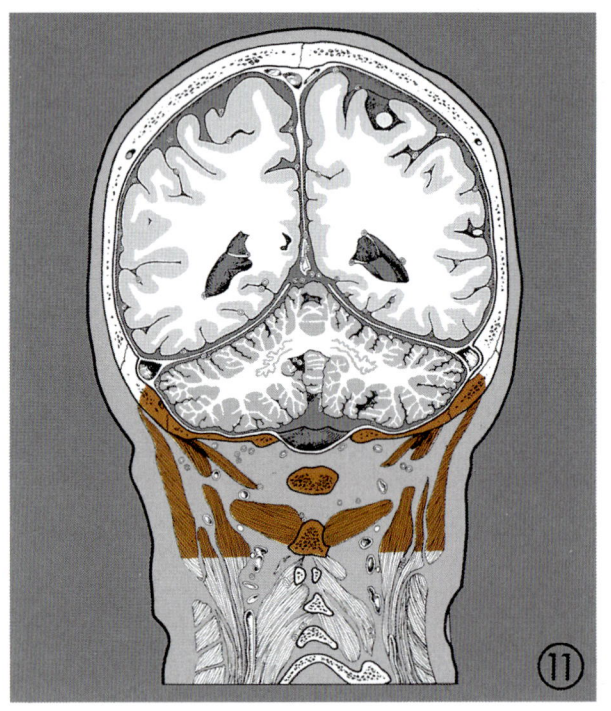

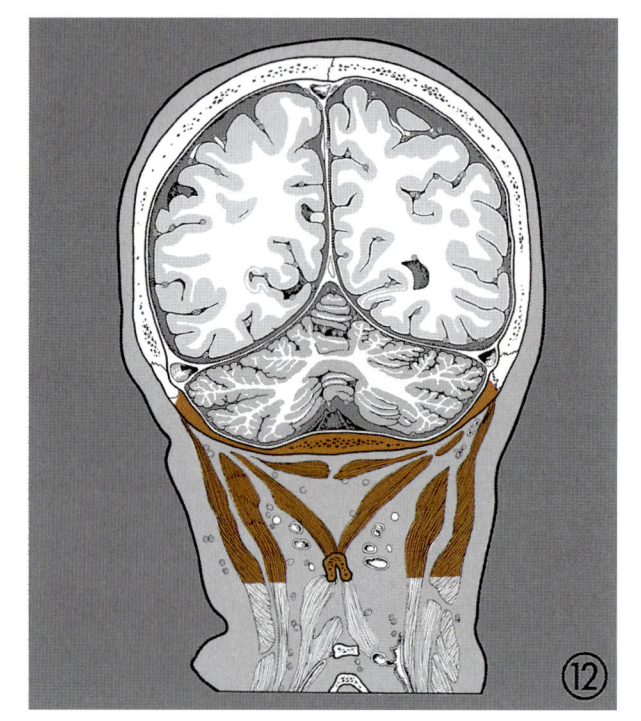

Fig. 79 Coronal serial illustrations showing the compartments of the facial skeleton and the craniocervical junction. The encircled numbers (9–14) indicate the number of the respective slices (Figs. 1a, 2a,b, 3).

3.2 Nasal Cavity and Paranasal Sinuses

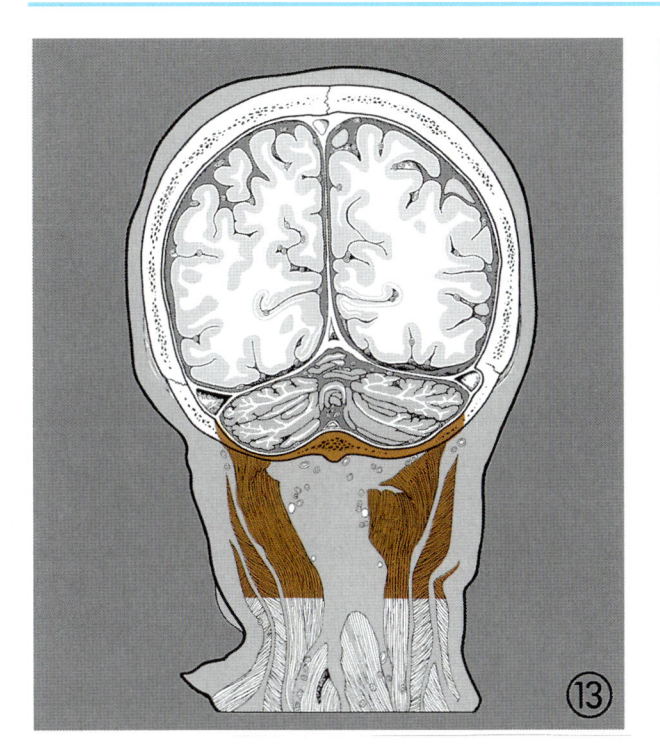

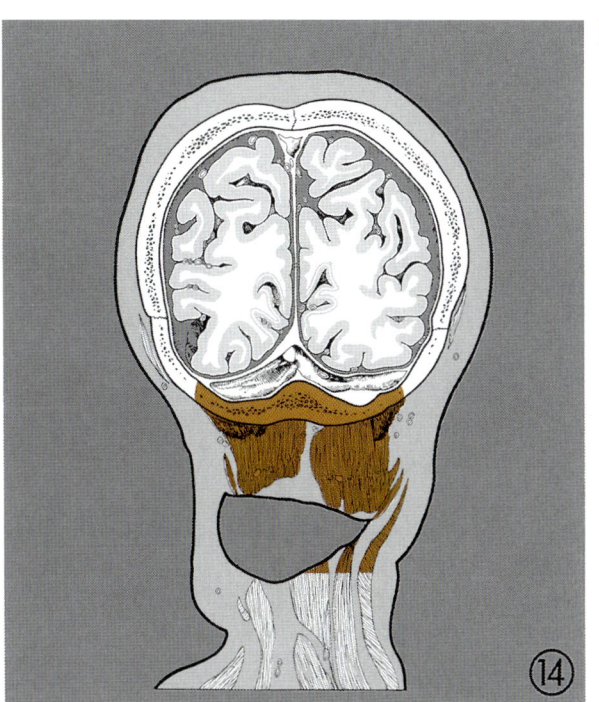

▮ Bones and muscles of craniocervical junction

216   3   Topography of the Facial Skeleton and its Cavities in Multiplanar Parallel Slices

■ Nasal cavity and paranasal sinuses
■ Oral cavity
■ Pharynx
■ Bones and muscles of craniocervical junction
■ Orbit
■ Parapharyngeal space

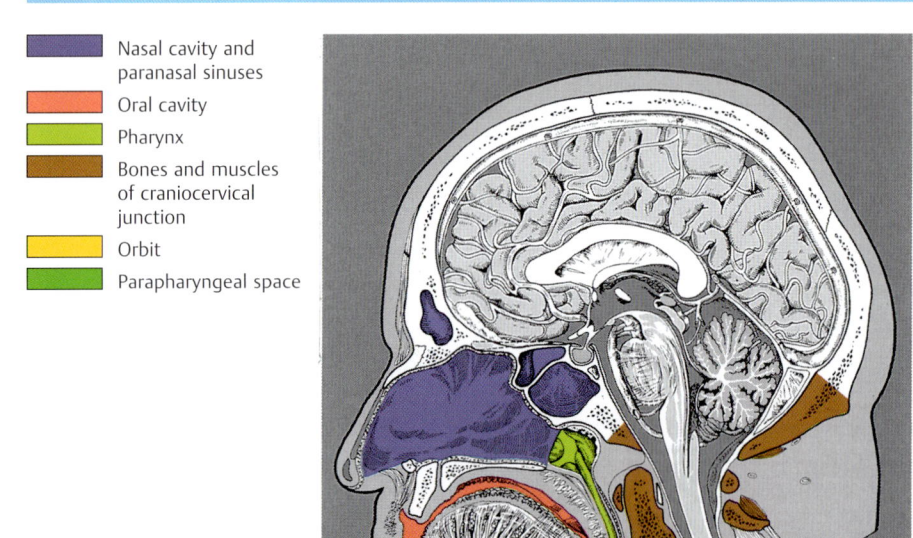

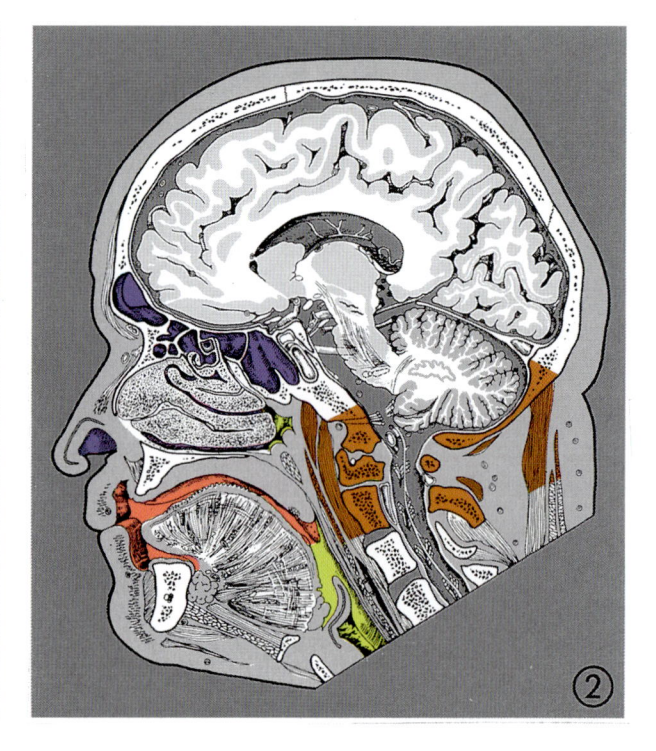

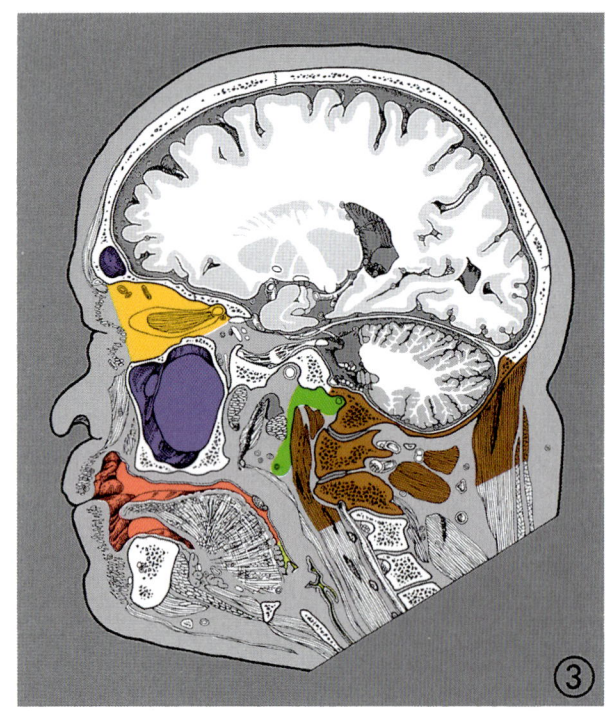

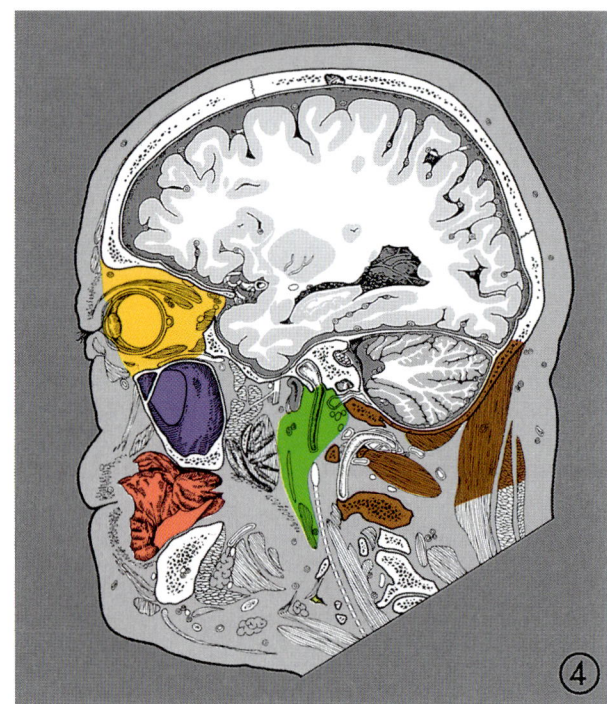

Fig. 80 Sagittal serial illustrations showing the compartments of the facial skeleton and the craniocervical junction. The encircled number indicates the number of the respective slice (Figs. 29, 30a,b, 31).

3.2 Nasal Cavity and Paranasal Sinuses

▬	Orbit
▬	Paranasal sinus
▬	Oral cavity
▬	Parapharyngeal space
▬	Bones and muscles of craniocervical junction

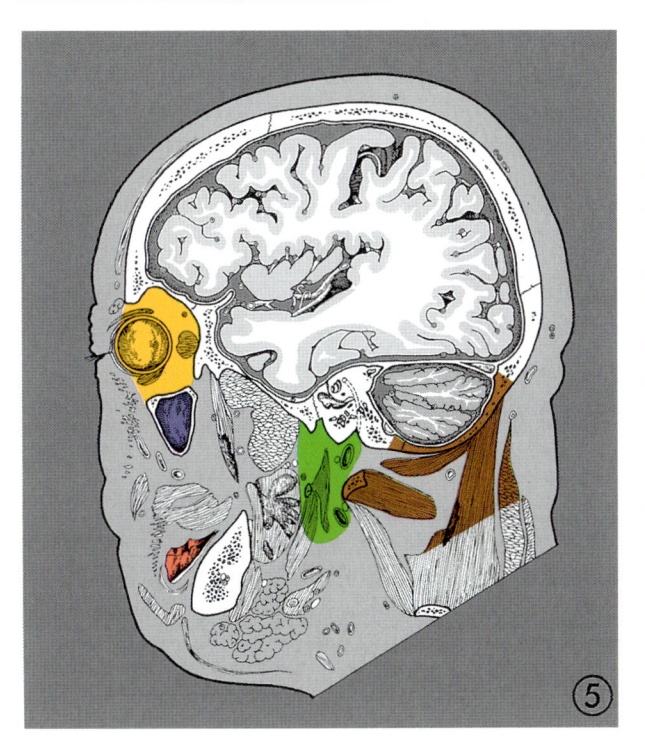

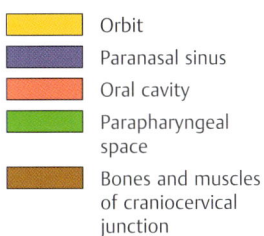

The lateral wall of the nasal cavity is enlarged by three nasal conchae projecting medially, each running above a nasal meatus. The superior nasal meatus is short, averaging less than 2 cm in length (265). Into it drain the posterior ethmoidal cells. The **middle nasal meatus** is connected with the frontal sinus, the anterior and middle ethmoidal cells, and the maxillary sinus via the **semilunar hiatus** (Figs. 4a.12, 5a.13). In Figure 33a.32 the middle nasal concha is partly cut tangentially, so that the anterior and upper portion of the semilunar hiatus (Fig. 33a.28) is visible. The lower posterior portion, which is covered by the middle nasal concha, is indicated by a dotted line. The nasolacrimal duct (Fig. 71a.2), through which the tears are conducted into the nasal cavity, drains into the **inferior nasal meatus**.

The topography of the nasal cavities and the paranasal sinuses can be deduced by comparison of a coronal and sagittal series (Figs. 79, 80). The variability of these cavities between different individuals is quite marked.

The ethmoidal cells and the maxillary sinus have been described above with their corresponding bones. The sphenoidal and the frontal are paired sinuses.

All the paranasal sinuses can be of clinical significance as the site of infectious or neoplastic lesions or trauma. Ultrasound, CT, MRI, and endoscopy compete in elucidating the diagnosis.

The **sphenoidal sinus** is usually in the body of the sphenoid. In 12% of cases the sphenoidal sinus extends only as far as a perpendicular drawn through the tuberculum sellae (presellar type); in 84% it surrounds the pituitary fossa (sellar type); and in 4% it is located outside the body of the sphenoid (265). In the coronal series a sphenoidal sinus of the sellar type can be seen (Figs. 2a.12, 7a.19, 8a.23, 9a.34, 10a.40). The sphenoidal sinus drains into the sphenoethmoidal recess, above the superior concha (375). The septum that separates the two sphenoidal sinuses is often asymmetrical (Fig. 7a.19). The roof of the sphenoidal sinus is very closely related to the optic nerve (Fig. 7a.13). Familiarity with the sphenoidal sinus is of particular importance in the transsphenoidal approach for operations on the pituitary gland. In 4% of cases portions of the optic canal are formed only by the sheath of the optic nerve and the mucous membrane of the sinus. The optic nerve may, therefore, very easily be damaged in the transsphenoidal approach to the pituitary (265).

The **frontal sinus** is particularly variable and often asymmetrical (Fig. 30a.3). The left frontal sinus is cut in the anterior part of the frontal bone in the right half of the head (Fig. 32a.13). Its anterior wall forms the bony supraciliary arch, which shows individual variations. The floor of the frontal sinus is separated from the orbit by a thin layer of bone.

Vessels of the Nasal Cavity

The walls of the nasal cavities are supplied by branches from the maxillary and ophthalmic arteries. The **maxillary artery** gives off the sphenopalatine artery, which runs out of the pterygopalatine fossa, through the sphenopalatine foramen underneath the nasal mucous membrane, and supplies the posterior part of the lateral and medial walls of the nasal cavity.

The **ophthalmic artery** gives off the anterior ethmoidal artery, which makes a detour through the cranial cavity and only then enters the nasal cavity. This complicated course probably arose as a result of the late phylogenetic development of a complete bony encapsulated orbital cavity, in association with the marked development of the neocortex in the mammals. The anterior ethmoidal artery leaves the orbital cavity through the anterior ethmoidal foramen, runs into the anterior cranial fossa, then through the cribriform plate into the anterior part of the nasal cavity, where it divides to supply its medial and lateral walls.

The veins from the nasal mucous membrane drain into the veins of the orbit, the pterygoid venous plexus, and facial veins.

The lymphatic vessels of the nasal mucous membrane run to the lymph nodes at the angle of the jaw and behind the pharynx.

Nerves of the Nasal Cavity

In the nasal mucous membrane one can distinguish between the ciliated epithelium of the respiratory area and the **olfactory epithelium**, which is thicker and has a slightly brown tinge. The olfactory epithelium consists of four fields, each about 8 mm in diameter, in the central part of the superior concha and the corresponding area of the nasal septum lying opposite. Histologically, the olfactory epithelium contains bipolar neurons. Their receptor endings are numerous cilia in the epithelial surface. The central axons of these neurons collectively constitute the **olfactory nerve**. These fibers of the first cranial nerve run through the cribriform plate of the ethmoid into the cranial cavity and terminate in the olfactory bulb.

The sensory nerves of the nasal cavity are branches of the ophthalmic and maxillary nerves. The terminal branches of these nerves contain the viscerosecretory (autonomic) fibers to the mucous glands in the nasal mucous membrane.

The **ophthalmic nerve** gives off the nasociliary nerve, from which the anterior ethmoidal nerve follows the anterior ethmoidal artery in its indirect course through the anterior cranial fossa to supply the anterior nasal mucous membrane.

Branches of the **maxillary nerve** supply the posterior part of the nasal mucous membrane on the medial and lateral sides.

The parasympathetic preganglionic nerve fibers for the glands of the nasal mucous membrane run in the greater petrosal nerve to the pterygopalatine ganglion (Fig. 151.10). The postganglionic fibers mingle in the pterygopalatine fossa with the sensory fibers.

The sympathetic postganglionic fibers run with the arterial branches to the pterygopalatine fossa as well and then continue with the sensory fibers to the glands of the nasal mucous membrane.

3.3 Orbit

(Figs. 79, 80)

The **orbit** contains the globe of the eye. It is the receptor organ of the visual system (Chap. 6.6). The eyeball is protected by the following structures (57):
- Bony walls of the orbit
- Eyelids
- Conjunctiva
- Lacrimal apparatus.

The fascial sheath (capsule of Tenon) surrounds the eyeball as a joint capsule might surround a globe.

The extraocular muscles are able to rotate the eyeball with the greatest precision. The optic nerves extend backward from the eyeballs as far as the partial crossing of the optic nerves in the optic chiasm.

The orbital cavity has the shape of a hollow four-sided pyramid. Its base is directed outward and its apex is at the optic canal, the exit point of the optic nerve. The apex of the pyramid is directed backward and medially. The conical shape of the orbit can be deduced from the colored areas in the coronal slices (Fig. 79).

The **four walls of the orbit** can best be seen in the coronal slices (Figs. 4c.9, orbital roof, and 4c.22, orbital floor). Moving posteriorly the walls change into a well-rounded cross-section (Fig. 20.3). In the optic canal the optic nerve and the ophthalmic artery are closely related (Figs. 7a.13, 7c.9).

The anterior pole of the eyeball is at a plane that runs between the upper and lower borders of the orbit. Forward displacements of the eyeball arise as a result of space-occupying retrobulbar lesions in the orbit. Edema, hematomas, inflammatory lesions, and tumors can push the eyeball forward if the bony walls of the orbit do not give way. As the inferior wall of the orbit is thin, a blunt compression injury, such as a blow with a fist, can lead to a fracture of the floor of the orbit and the orbital contents being forced into the maxillary sinus (Figs. 4a.19, 5a.19) (blow-out fracture).

Various openings connect the orbital cavity with:
- The middle cranial fossa, through the **optic canal** (Fig. 21.3) for the optic nerve and the ophthalmic artery, and through the **superior orbital fissure** (Fig. 21.5) for the oculomotor, trochlear, trigeminal (first division), and abducent nerves and the superior ophthalmic vein
- The infratemporal fossa and the pterygopalatine fossa, through the inferior orbital fissure, for the zygomatic nerve and inferior ophthalmic vein.

- The nasal cavity, through the **nasolacrimal canal** for the nasolacrimal duct
- The face, through the infraorbital canal (Figs. 18.10, 19.10) for the nerves and vessels of the same name (Figs. 4a.15, 4c.23, 5a.14, 5c.19)
- The anterior cranial fossa, through the anterior ethmoidal foramen for the vessels and nerves of the same name
- The posterior ethmoidal cells and the sphenoidal sinus, through the posterior ethmoidal foramen for the vessels and nerves of the same name.

Since the invention of the ophthalmoscope by Hermann von Helmholtz in 1850, ophthalmoscopic examination of the eyeball has maintained its importance to the present day. The advances in the new imaging techniques are most evident in the diagnosis of retrobulbar pathology, and therefore the retrobulbar space will be described in more topographic detail than the eyeball.

Eyelids and Lacrimal Apparatus

The eyelids and the lacrimal apparatus protect the cornea from drying, clouding, and/or ulceration. In the larger upper lid (Fig. 35a.15) and the smaller lower lid (Fig. 35a.24) are the lacrimal and palpebral parts of the **orbicularis oculi**. The lacrimal portion of this muscle arises from parts of the tear ducts. The orbital section of the orbicularis oculi (Fig. 4c.19) partly extends over the margin of the orbit. With its three parts this muscle surrounds the palpebral fissure like a ring. Its function is to close the lids and, with the lacrimal portion, to direct the tears into the nasal cavity. It is supplied by the facial nerve.

The **levator palpebrae superioris** (Figs. 4c.10, 5c.8, 6c.10, 35c.13, 36c.13) arises from the common tendinous ring of the eye muscle cone, runs forward to the upper part of the orbit, and is inserted into the connective tissue of the upper eyelid. Its function is to raise the upper lid. The nerve supply arises from the oculomotor nerve.

The **superior and inferior tarsal muscles** form a ring consisting of a thin layer of smooth muscle between striated muscles and the eyelids. The upper tarsal muscle arises from the levator palpebrae superioris and spreads out toward the tarsus (tough connective tissue) of the upper eyelid. The lower and weaker tarsal muscle takes its origin from the inferior rectus and is inserted into the tarsus of the lower lid. An increase in the tonus of the tarsal smooth muscles can widen the palpebral fissure. Innervation is by cervical sympathetic fibers. With a decrease in sympathetic tone (e.g. fatigue) the palpebral fissure narrows.

The sensory supply to the upper lid is from branches of the first division of the trigeminal nerve, and the lower lid from branches of its second division.

The conjunctiva covers the deep surface of the upper and lower eyelids as well as the sclera of the eyeball, as far as the margins of the cornea. Together, the parts of the conjunctiva cover a narrow cleft, the conjunctival sac, which is filled with tears.

The **lacrimal gland** is located behind the lateral part of the upper eyelid, close beneath the frontal bone (Figs. 4c.14, 36c.12). Its innervation consists of parasympathetic fibers from the facial nerve via the greater petrosal nerve—pterygopalatine ganglion—zygomatic nerve—lacrimal nerve, and sympathetic fibers from the cervical sympathetic trunk through the periarterial vascular plexus.

The lacrimal gland secretes the tears into the conjunctival sac. They are then transported by lid movements to the medial angle of the eye. The lacrimal ducts remove the tears with the help of the lacrimal portion of the orbicularis oculi, and they then drain through the lacrimal sac and the nasolacrimal duct into the inferior nasal meatus.

Fascial Sheath

The fascial sheath forms a sort of joint cavity in which the eyeball, as in a ball-and-socket joint, can rotate freely in the three main axes. Around the vertical axis that runs through the central point of the eyeball, the visual axis can be turned inward (adduction) or outward (abduction). Around the frontal axis the visual axis can be raised or lowered, and around the sagittal axis it can be rotated inward or outward. The function(s) of the extraocular muscles are decided by their positions and the final directions of pull in relation to the individual main axes. The fascial sheath consists of a firm connective tissue sheath which is attached to the sclera only at the point of entry of the optic nerve and at the corneoscleral junction (limbus corneae). The tendons of the extraocular muscles run through slits in this fascial sheath before they attach to the eyeball.

Extraocular Muscles

The extraocular muscles are situated in the orbital fat. They rotate the eyeball. Five of these muscles and also the levator palpebrae superior arise from the common tendinous ring. This encircles the opening of the optic canal containing the optic nerve and the ophthalmic artery and the medial part of the superior orbital fissure containing the oculomotor, nasociliary, and abducens nerves. In the coronal slices the extraocular muscles are easily recognized because the positional relationships, superior–inferior and medial–lateral, are quite clearly defined (Fig. 81).

The **superior rectus** (Figs. 4c.13, 5c.10, 6c.11, 6d.8, 35c.17, 77a.6) runs forward obliquely, forming an angle of 25° to the sagittal visual axis. Its effective terminal attachment lies medial to the adduction and abduction axes when the visual axis is directed straight forward. It acts as an elevator and its auxiliary functions are adduction and internal rotation. With abduction of the eye by 25° the final direction of pull of the muscle is displaced to the adduction and abduction axis, so that in this position the muscle is a pure elevator. Nerve supply: oculomotor nerve.

The **inferior rectus** (Figs. 4c.20, 5c.18, 6c.19, 6d.15, 35c.21, 74a.9) runs foward obliquely beneath the eyeball forming an angle of 25° to the sagittal visual axis. Its final direction of pull resembles that of the rectus superior above, when the visual axis is directed straight forward. Its main function is to direct the eye downward and its auxiliary functions are adduction and external rotation. Nerve supply: oculomotor nerve.

The **medial rectus** (Figs. 4c.15, 5c.14, 6b.14, 6c.15, 6d.14, 34c.16, 50b.4, 50d.4, 75a.8) runs medial to the eyeball. Its final direction of pull lies medial to the adduction and abduction axes, runs through the frontal main axis of eye elevation and depression, and in the same direction as the rotation axis. The muscle is, therefore, a pure adductor. Nerve supply: oculomotor nerve.

The **lateral rectus** (Figs. 5c.15, 6c.17, 6d.13, 35c.18, 36c.15, 50b.6, 75a.10, 76c.4, 76d.4) lies lateral to the eyeball. Its effective terminal attachment is found lateral to the axes of adduction and abduction in all positions of the globe. The muscle moves the eye laterally (pure abductor). Nerve supply: abducens nerve.

The **superior oblique** (Figs. 4c.12, 5c.9, 6c.12, 6d.11, 77a.5) first runs forward to the upper medial wall of the orbit. Its tendon then runs through a cartilaginous half-ring, the trochlea (pulley), and turns back at an angle of 55°; it then runs medial to the adduction and abduction axes to the posterior lateral quadrant of the eyeball. Its main function is to depress the eye, as its effective terminal attachment pulls anteriorly. In addition it abducts and rotates the eye internally. The internal rotation gets stronger the further the eye is already abducted. Nerve supply: trochlear nerve.

The **inferior oblique** (Figs. 4c.21, 35c.20, 36c.18, 73a.4) takes its origin near the floor of the orbit close to the entrance of the nasolacrimal duct. It runs backward obliquely and forms an angle of about 50° with the visual axis. Its tendon is inserted into the posterior and lateral quadrant. Its final direction of pull lies medial to the adduction and abduction axes. Its function is to elevate the visual axis, as well as abduction and outward rotation of the eyeball. Nerve supply: oculomotor nerve.

Clinical notes about disturbances of function of the ocular muscles are to be found in the chapter on the oculomotor systems (Chap. 6.8.3).

Arteries of the Orbit

The **ophthalmic artery** is the main artery of the orbit. This vessel is a branch of the internal carotid artery and leaves the middle cranial fossa through the optic canal. It enters the orbit through the common tendinous ring. It usually crosses the optic nerve and lies laterally (Fig. 6c.16), running forward above the superior oblique (Fig. 5c.12). The branches of the ophthalmic artery supply the contents of the orbit and take part in the blood supply of the eyelids, the mucous membrane of the ethmoid and sphenoidal sinuses, as well as the face and scalp regions. In the orbit it usually anastomoses with branches of the middle meningeal artery. In 4% of cases the main supply for the ophthalmic artery comes from the middle meningeal artery (265). Larger anastomoses from the terminal branches of the ophthalmic artery are found at the medial canthus of the eye with the facial artery, and in the temporal region with branches of the superficial temporal artery of the external carotid artery. These arterial anastomoses between the branches of the internal and external carotid arteries are of clinical significance. With stenoses or occlusions of the internal carotid artery, the blood supply can often be maintained by such anastomoses. The direction of flow in the ophthalmic artery can be determined by Doppler sonography (15, 183a, 374a, 488).

Branches of the Ophthalmic Artery:
- The central artery of the retina runs into the optic nerve. An occlusion of this artery, only 0.2 mm wide, leads to blindness.
- Further branches from the ophthalmic artery supply the choroid layer of the eyeball, the lacrimal gland, the ethmoidal cells and sphenoidal sinus, the medial canthus, and the forehead.
- The anterior ethmoidal artery has already been mentioned in the description of the nasal cavity. This artery courses through the foramen of the same name, reaches the anterior cranial fossa and there gives off the anterior meningeal artery. The anterior ethmoidal artery then passes through the lamina cribrosa into the anterior part of the nasal cavity.

The **veins of the orbit** almost always run separately from the arteries and most are wider in caliber. The superior ophthalmic vein (Figs. 5c.11, 6c.9, 7c.10) drains blood from the eyeball, upper part of the orbit, upper eyelid, and ethmoidal cells. It anastomoses with the facial vein and, through the superior orbital fissure, with the cavernous sinus. As neither the superior ophthalmic nor the facial vein has valves, blood from the orbital cavity drains not only forward to the face, but also posteriorly to the cavernous sinus. It is from this latter route, especially with furuncles or purulent infections of the face, that the danger of meningitis or thrombophlebitis of a dural sinus exists. The inferior ophthalmic vein runs along the floor of the orbit and drains into the superior ophthalmic vein, or through the inferior orbital fissure into the pterygoid venous plexus.

3.3 Orbit 221

- Oculomotor nerve
- Trochlear nerve
- Abducens nerve
- Motor root of trigeminal nerve
- Facial nerve
- Hypoglossal nerve
- Cervical spinal nerves

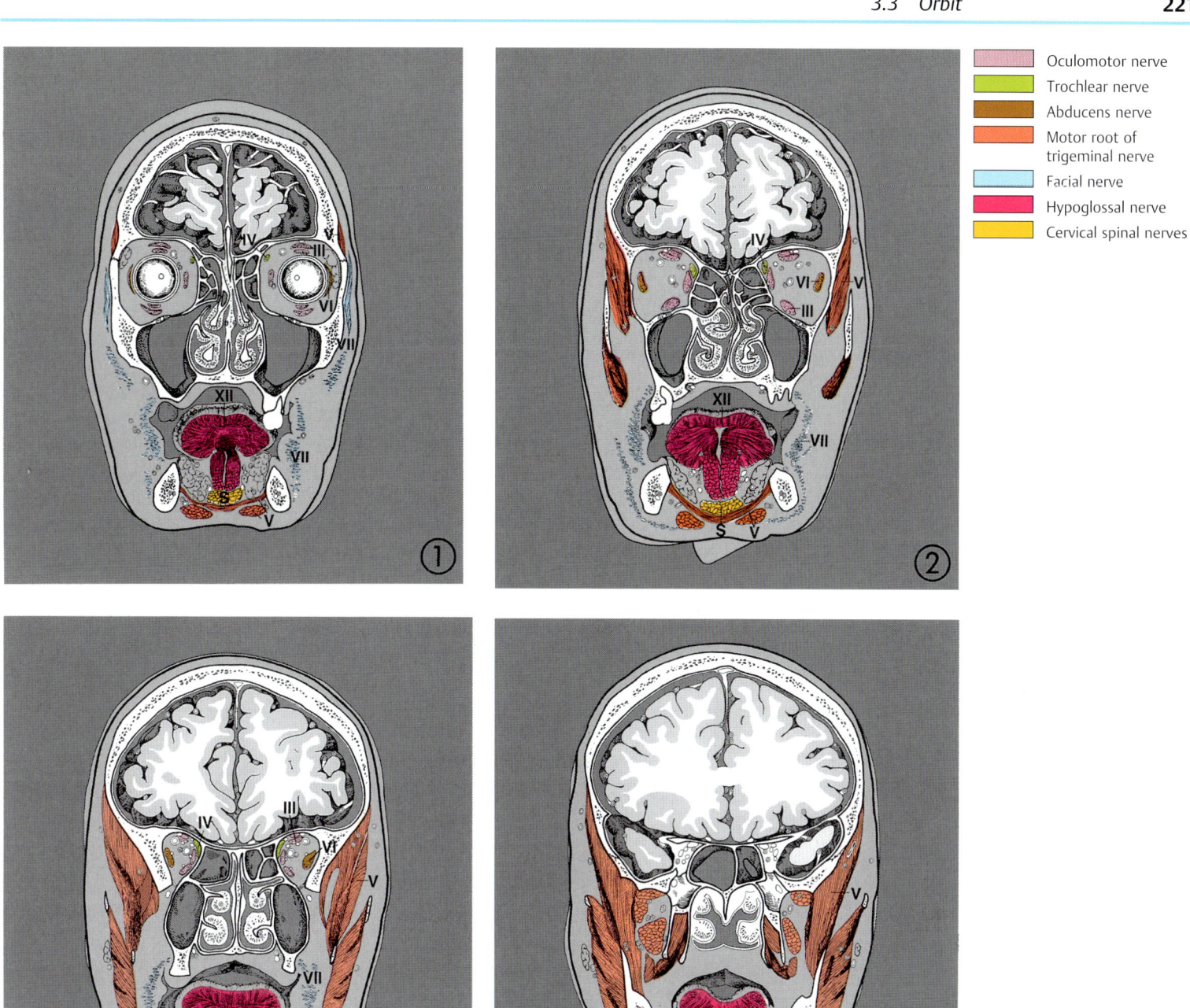

Fig. 81 Coronal serial illustrations of the groups of muscles that are innervated by cranial nerves (III, IV, V, VI, VII, IX, X, XI, XII) and/or spinal nerves (S). The encircled numbers (1–4) show the number of the respective slice (Figs. 1a, 2a,b, 3).

222 3 Topography of the Facial Skeleton and its Cavities in Multiplanar Parallel Slices

- Motor root of trigeminal nerve
- Glossopharyngeal nerve
- Vagus nerve
- Hypoglossal nerve
- Cervical spinal nerves
- Facial nerve
- Accessory nerve and cervical spinal nerves

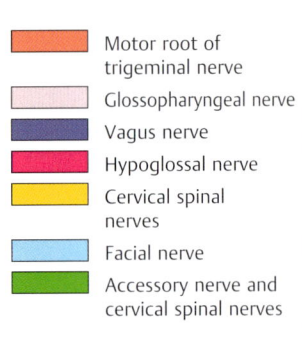

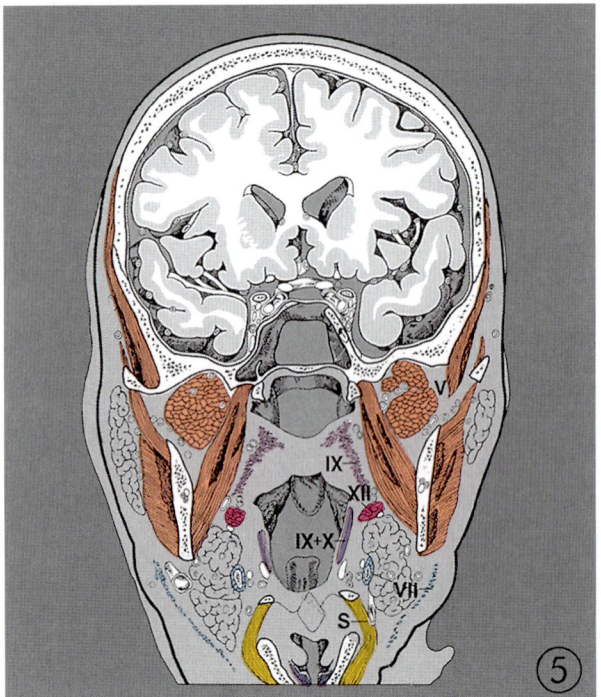

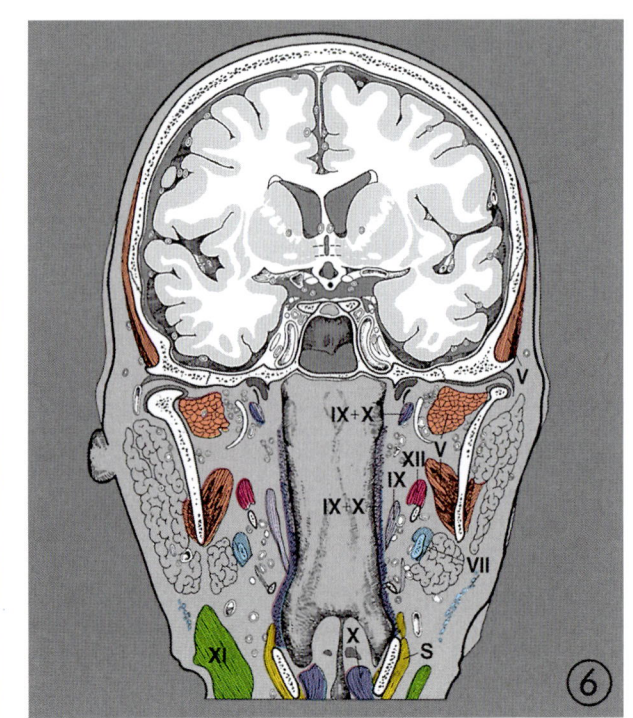

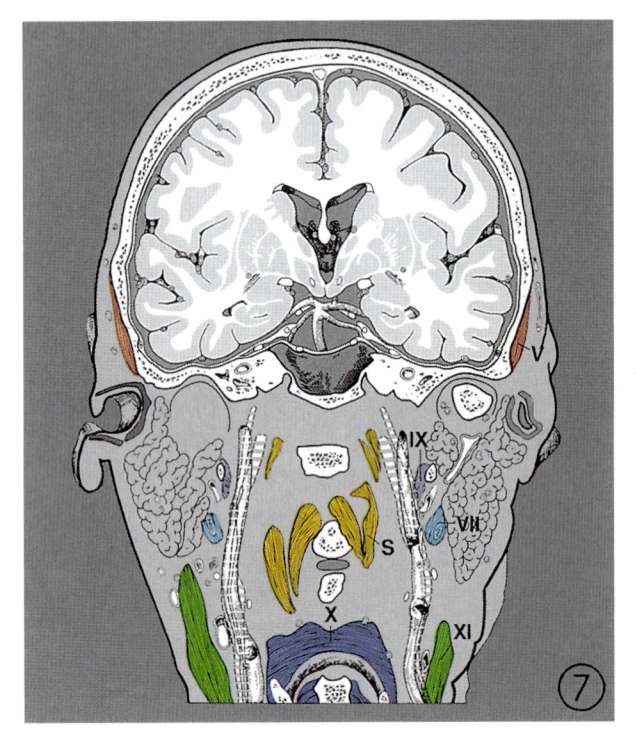

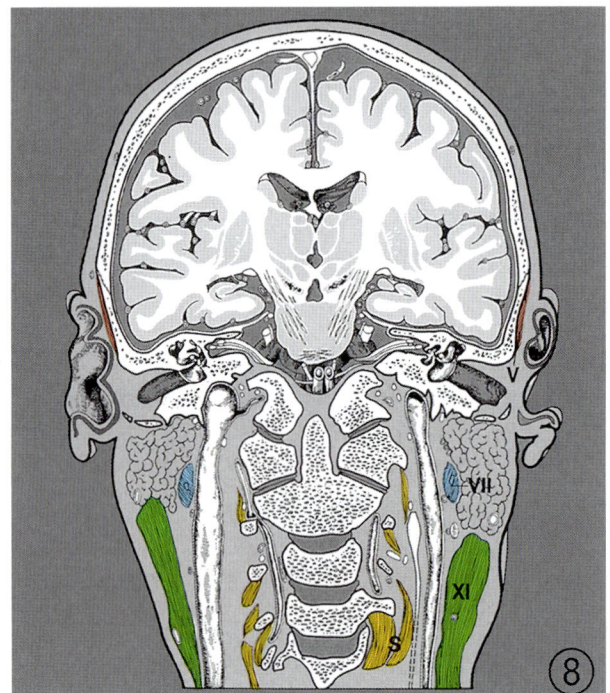

Fig. **81** Coronal serial illustrations of the groups of muscles that are innervated by cranial nerves (III, IV, V, VI, VII, IX, X, XI, XII) and/or spinal nerves (S). The encircled numbers (5–8) show the number of the respective slice (Figs. 1a, 2a,b, 3).

3.3 Orbit 223

Motor root of trigeminal nerve
Accessory nerve and cervical spinal nerves
Facial nerve
Cervical spinal nerves

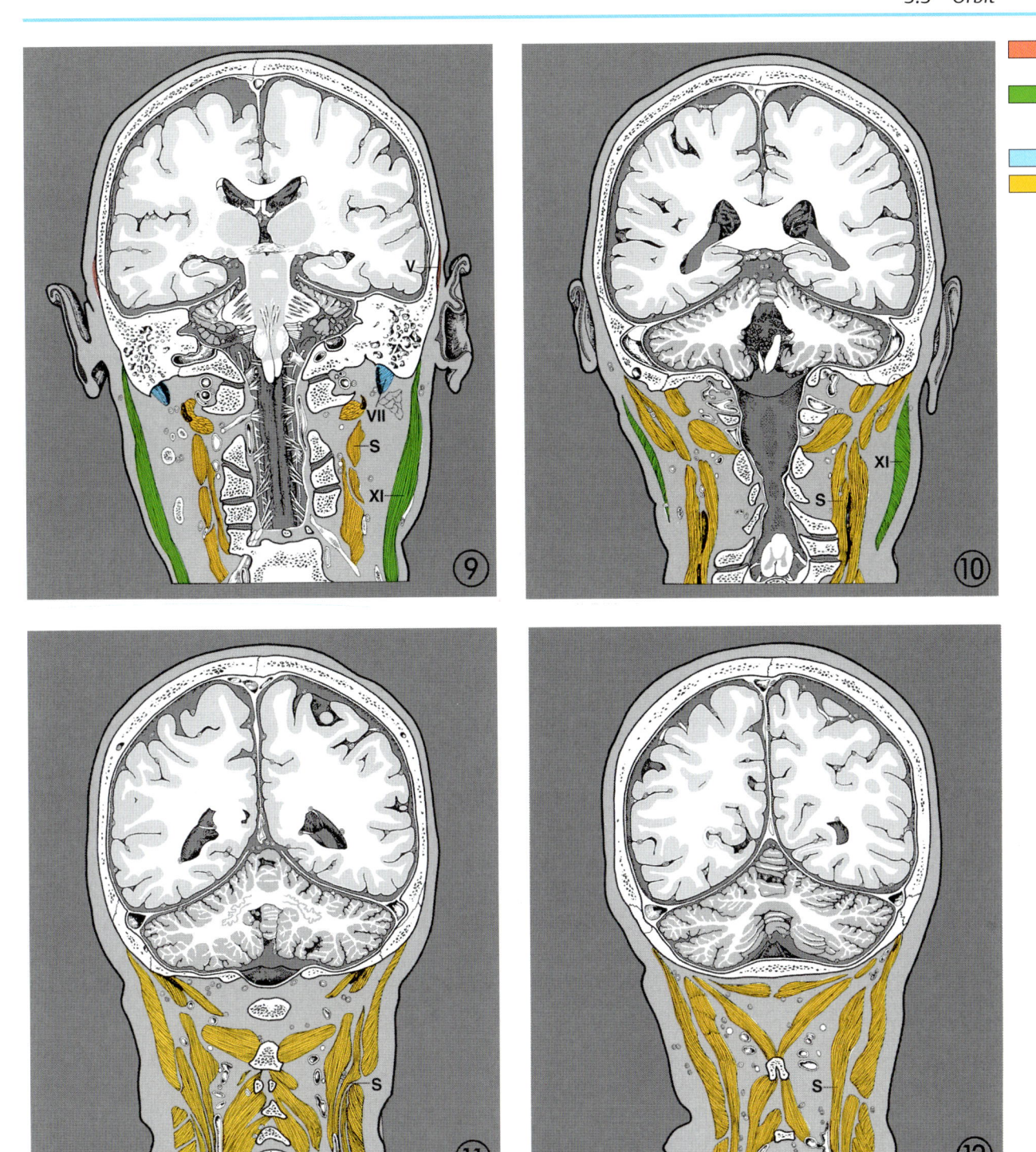

Fig. 81 Coronal serial illustrations of the groups of muscles that are innervated by cranial nerves (III, IV, V, VI, VII, IX, X, XI, XII) and/or spinal nerves (S). The encircled numbers (9–12) show the number of the respective slice (Figs. 1a, 2a,b, 3).

224   3 *Topography of the Facial Skeleton and its Cavities in Multiplanar Parallel Slices*

■ Facial nerve
■ Accessory nerve and cervical spinal nerves
■ Cervical spinal nerves

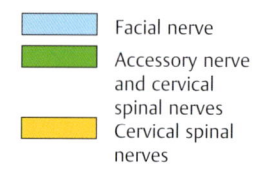

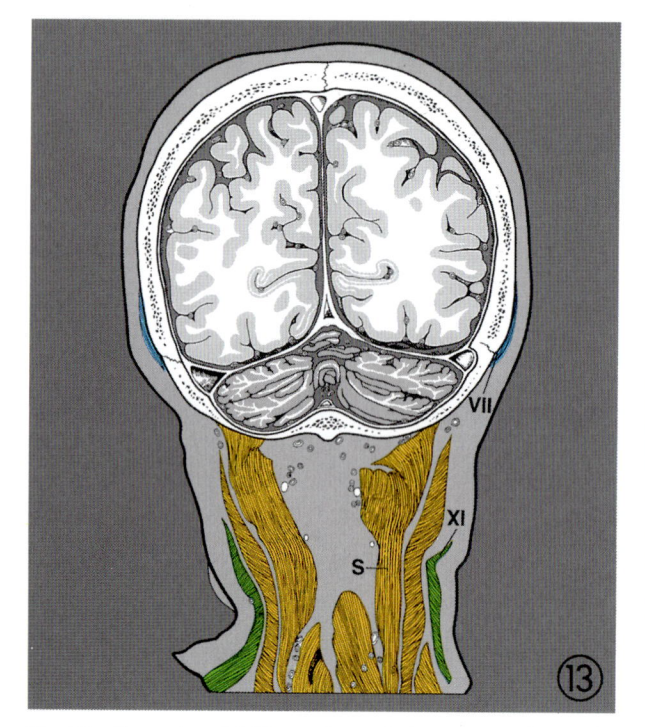

Fig. **81** Coronal serial illustrations of the groups of muscles that are innervated by cranial nerves (III, IV, V, VI, VII, IX, X, XI, XII) and/or spinal nerves (S). The encircled numbers (13–14) show the number of the respective slice (Figs. 1a, 2a,b, 3).

■ Facial nerve
■ Hypoglossal nerve
■ Cervical spinal nerves
■ Motor root of trigeminal nerve
■ Glossopharyngeal nerve
■ Vagus nerve
■ Accessory nerve and cervical spinal nerves

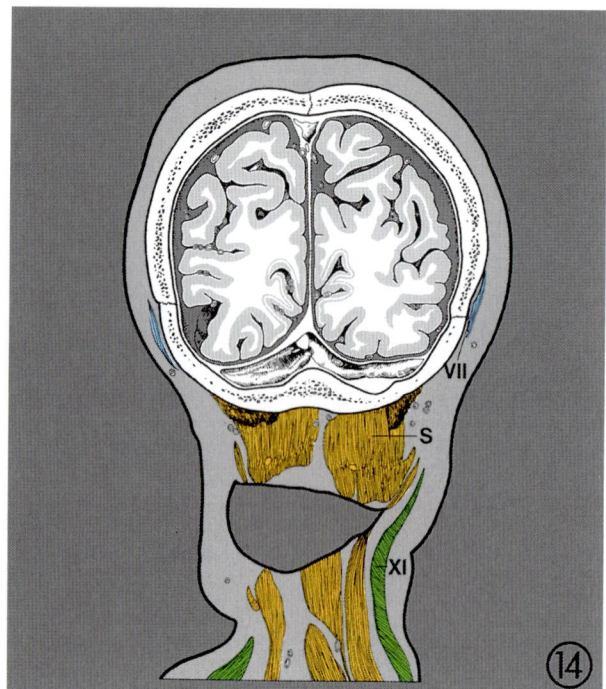

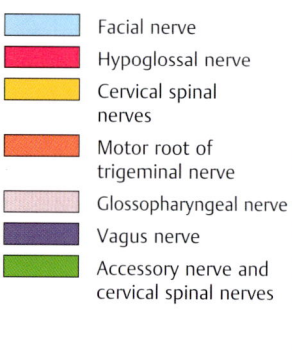

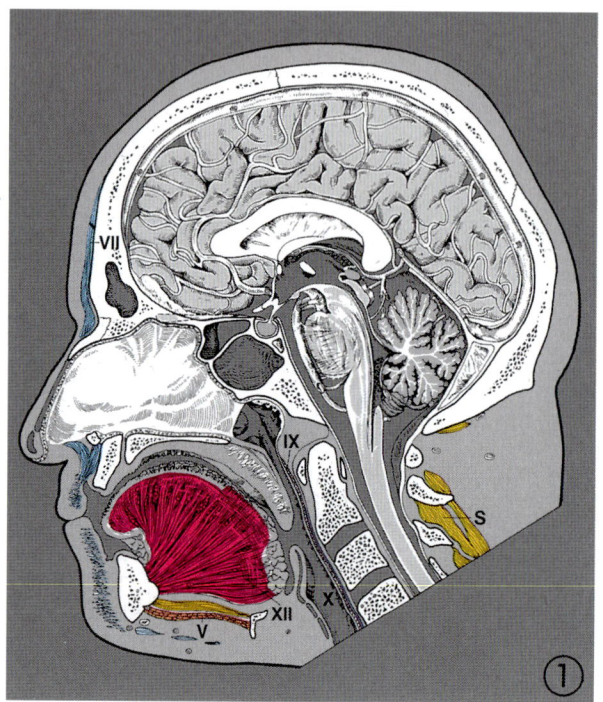

Fig. **82** Sagittal serial illustrations of the groups of muscles that are innervated by cranial nerves (III, IV, V, VI, VII, IX, X, XI, XII) and/or spinal nerves (S). The encircled numbers (1–2) show the number of the respective slice (Figs. 29, 30a,b, 31).

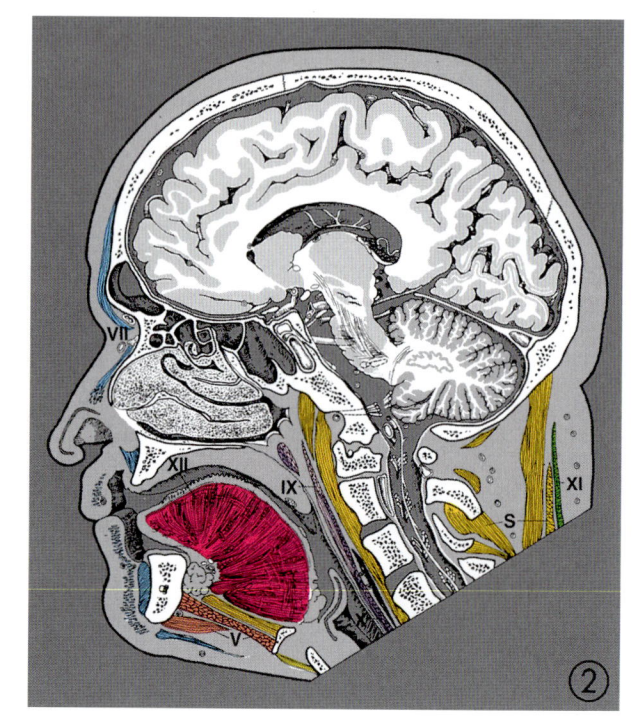

3.3 Orbit   225

Oculomotor nerve
Abducens nerve
Motor root of trigeminal nerve
Facial nerve
Glossopharyngeal nerve
Vagus nerve
Hypoglossal nerve
Cervical spinal nerves
Accessory nerve and cervical spinal nerves

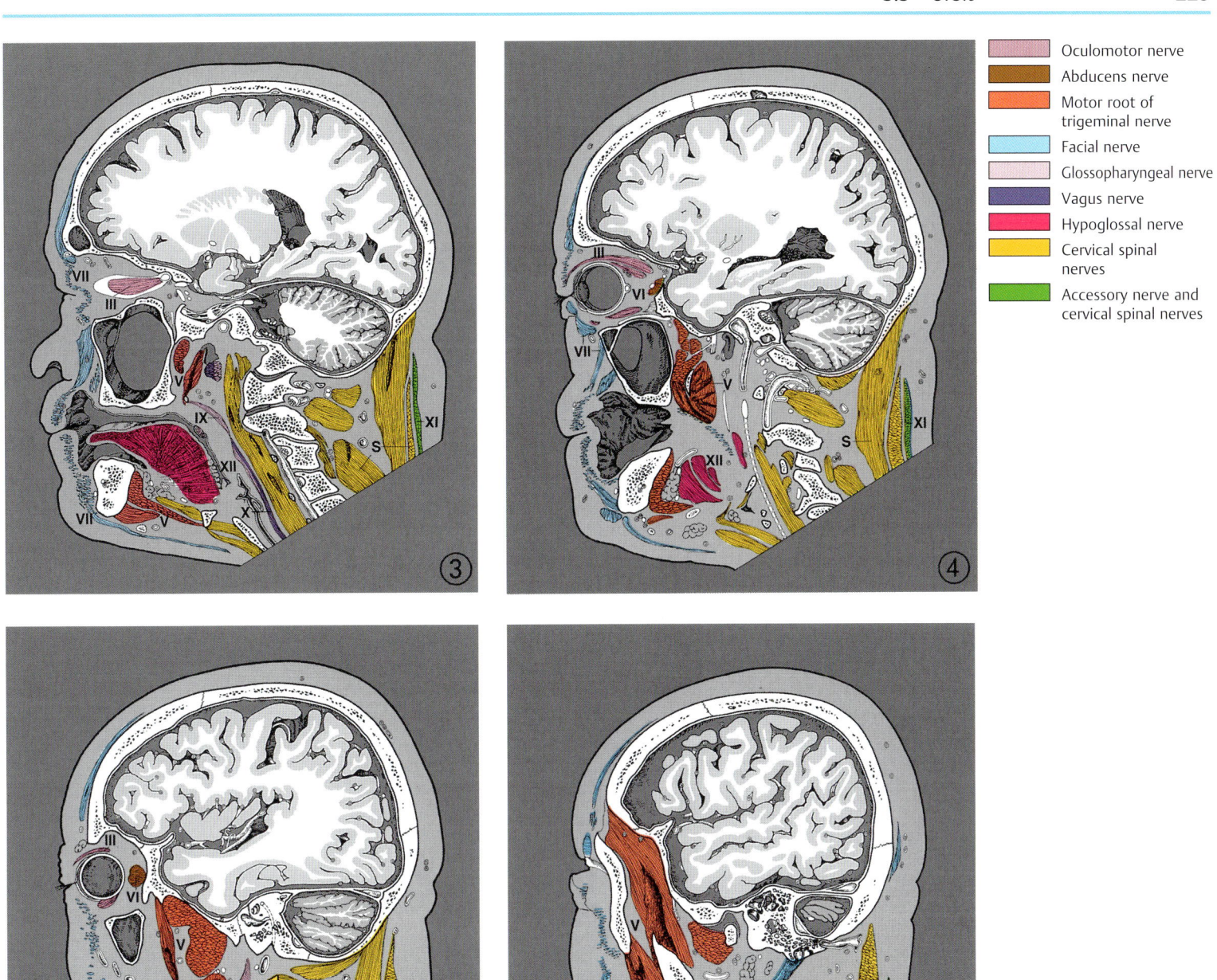

Fig. 82 Sagittal serial illustrations of the groups of muscles that are innervated by cranial nerves (III, IV, V, VI, VII, IX, X, XI, XII) and/or spinal nerves (S). The encircled numbers (3–6) show the number of the respective slice (Figs. 29, 30a,b, 31).

Nerves of the Orbit

The branches of the **ophthalmic nerve** arising from the trigeminal nerve give a sensory supply to the eyeball, mainly to the cornea and the conjunctiva, but also to the lacrimal gland, upper lid, the skin of the forehead and medial canthus, the mucous membrane of the ethmoidal cells and sphenoidal sinus, as well as the anterior part of the nasal mucous membrane and the skin of the bridge of the nose.

As a rule the ophthalmic nerve divides before the superior orbital fissure into its four main branches:
- Tentorial nerve, which courses backward to the tentorium cerebelli.
- Lacrimal nerve, which runs over the lateralis rectus to the lacrimal gland.
- Frontal nerve (Fig. 6a.12), which lies on the levator palpebrae superioris and then divides into branches for the forehead (including the supraorbital nerve [Figs. 4a.6, 5a.8], a pressure point for V/1 above the orbit).
- Nasociliary nerve (Figs. 5a.9, 6a.13), which lies within the muscle cone and gives branches to the eyeball, the mucous membrane of the ethmoidal cells and sphenoidal sinus and the anterior nasal cavity, and finally branches to the medial canthus and the skin over the bridge of the nose.

The motor nerve supply to the six extraocular muscles and the levator palpebrae superioris comes from the third, fourth, and sixth cranial nerves as already described. In addition, the third cranial nerve transmits parasympathetic impulses to the ciliary ganglion, where they are relayed to postganglionic fibers innervating intrinsic muscles of the eye, namely the sphincter pupillae and the ciliary muscle.

The **oculomotor nerve** (Fig. 7a.15) enters the orbit through the superior orbital fissure and the common tendinous ring, then divides into a superior division for the superior rectus and the levator palpebrae superioris, and a larger inferior division (Fig. 6a.17) that supplies the medial rectus and inferior rectus and the inferior oblique. In addition this inferior branch gives off a branch to the ciliary ganglion (Fig. 151.9). This parasympathetic ganglion is, on average, 3 mm long and is situated 18 mm behind the eyeball (265).

The **trochlear nerve** (Figs. 7a.14, 6a.10) runs through the superior orbital fissure and above the common tendinous ring. The trochlear nerve thus lies outside and above the muscle cone and supplies the superior oblique.

The **abducens nerve** (Figs. 7a.18, 6a.15) runs through the superior orbital fissure and the common tendinous ring to supply the rectus lateralis.

The infraorbital nerve runs on or beneath the floor of the orbit (Figs. 4a.15, 5a.14, 6a.20, 35a.25) without supplying any of its contents.

Eyeball

The eyeball (Figs. 4a.11, 35a.17, 36a.14, 48a.1, 49a.1, 50a.1, 75a.4) is almost spherical in shape, with a diameter of 24 mm. Anteriorly the eyeball is covered by the translucent cornea. The axis of the globe runs through the anterior and posterior poles. Just medial to the posterior pole the optic nerve leaves the eyeball. This point of exit corresponds within the eyeball to the optic disc (Fig. 4a.8), which is the region where the axons of the retinal ganglion cells converge to form the optic nerve. The fovea centralis of the retina (Fig. 4a.9), the area of most perfect vision, is located lateral to the optic disc. The optic axis runs through the fovea centralis and through the point of maximal convexity of the lens and the cornea. The equator of the globe is the maximum diameter of the eyeball in a frontal plane.

The **wall of the eyeball** has three layers:
- The external layer comprises the opaque sclera and the transparent cornea.
- The middle layer is the vascular layer consisting of the choroid, the ciliary body, and the iris. Within the iris are the sphincter pupillae and dilator pupillae.
- The inner layer is the retina, comprising an optic part containing the rods and/or cones (visual receptor cells) and a nonvisual retina (devoid of receptor cells).

In the eyeball there are two chambers, the anterior chamber in front of the iris and the posterior chamber behind it. The posterior chamber borders on the vitreous body

The **lens** (Figs. 35a.16, 75a.2) is supported by the zonular fibers. Lens, zonular fibers, ciliary body, and iris form the accommodation mechanism for near and far vision. In the process of accommodation, contraction and dilatation of the pupils by the sphincter and dilator are coordinated. Further details about the eyeball can be found in other publications (203, 265).

Optic Nerve

The **optic nerve** (Figs. 5a.11, 6a.16, 6b.10, 7a.13, 34a.20, 35a.18, 49a.2, 50a.5) begins at the lamina cribrosa of the sclera. Its average intraorbital length is 3 cm (265) and it is surrounded by a firm dural layer as well as by arachnoid and pia mater. The slightly sinuous course of the optic nerve in the orbit facilitates the free movement of the eyeball. In the optic canal the sheath of the optic nerve is closely attached to the bony walls. The optic canal can be demonstrated radiologically in a special projection devised by Rhese. For the solution of various clinical problems associated with lesions of the optic nerve, CT and MRI are important diagnostic aids.

3.4 Oral Cavity
(Figs. 79, 80)

The mouth or **oral cavity** (Figs. 4a.21, 5a.23, 6a.27, 7a.25, 32a.44, 33a.41, 34a.35, 35a.35) begins at the slitlike space bounded by the lips and ends at the isthmus of the fauces (Fig. 8a.30). The two rows of teeth and the alveolar margins covered by the gums divide the cavity of the mouth into the oral vestibule, a narrow space between the lips or cheeks and the teeth, and the oral cavity proper or mouth proper.

Inspection and palpation of oral lesions, and occasionally the biopsy of a tumor, will often be sufficient to arrive at a diagnosis. For planning and control of treatment modern imaging methods may be advisable in order to assess accurately the extent and nature of a tumorous growth as well as its malignancy. For example, such information is essential for a surgeon who has to decide whether a pathologic process requires a partial or a total glossectomy.

In this chapter and the following chapters, therefore, the topographic relationships of the oral cavity, particularly to its neighboring areas such as the infratemporal fossa (deep lateral facial region) and the oropharynx, will be emphasized. For the systematic descriptions of the oral cavity the reader should consult special references (408, 492).

Roof of the Mouth
The roof of the mouth is formed in its anterior two-thirds by the hard palate and in the posterior one-third by the soft palate.

The **hard palate** (Figs. 2a.30, 4c.25, 5c.24, 6c.23, 18.16, 19.15, 20.15, 33c.28, 39.20) is also the floor of the nasal cavity. Through the incisive canal (Figs. 32c.34, 38.32) a branch of the sphenopalatine artery and a branch of the nasopalatine nerve run from the nasal cavity into the mouth.

The **soft palate** (Figs. 7c.21, 8c.25) is the mobile portion (velum palatinum) that extends posteriorly to reach the unpaired conical process, the uvula (Figs. 8c.29, 32a.46). The muscles of the soft palate, namely the tensor veli palatini (Figs. 7c.22, 34c.31) and the levator veli palatini, function respectively as its tensor and elevator.

Floor of the Mouth
The floor of the mouth is muscular. It consists of the mylohyoid, geniohyoid, and digastric, which are all, either directly or indirectly, connected to the hyoid bone.

The **mylohyoid** (Figs. 4c.37, 5c.38, 6c.39, 7c.30, 32c.46, 33c.43, 34c.46, 35c.46) forms with its fellow of the opposite side a muscular floor for the oral cavity. It arises from the mylohyoid line of the mandible. Nerve supply: mylohyoid nerve of the mandibular nerve (V/3).

The **geniohyoid** (Figs. 4c.34, 5c.37, 6c.38, 32c.45, 33c.42, 34c.47) lies above the medial part of the mylohyoid. Nerve supply: second cervical nerves.

The anterior belly of the **digastric** arises from the inner surface of the mandible and lies beneath the mylohyoid (Figs. 4c.38, 5c.39, 6c.37, 33c.44, 34c.45). The digastric has the digastric tendon (Figs. 7c.34, 8c.37, 35c.47) that leads into the posterior belly. Nerve supply: mylohyoid nerve of the mandibular nerve (V/3).

The posterior belly of the digastric (Figs. 9c.39, 10c.32, 11c.32, 12c.26, 36c.46, 37c.37) arises from the mastoid process of the temporal bone (Fig. 12c.23). Nerve supply: facial nerve.

Tongue
The **tongue** (lingua) lies on the floor of the mouth. In the coronal sections (Figs. 4a.22, 5a.24, 6a.28, 7a.26) the tongue is seen between the sides of the mandible and appears mushroom- or "block"-shaped. In sagittal sections (Figs. 32a.47, 33a.43, 34a.37) the tip, body, and base of the tongue can be identified. The tongue is a muscular organ covered with mucous membrane. On the dorsum of the tongue a shallow furrow, the sulcus terminalis, divides the body (anterior) from the base (posterior). Immediately in front of the sulcus are the vallate papillae.

The tongue is very mobile. Its extrinsic muscles are the genioglossus, hyoglossus, and styloglossus. These muscles arise from the inner aspect of the mandible, hyoid bone, and styloid process and are able to move the tongue along their directions of pull.

The intrinsic muscles of the tongue are able to change its shape. They consist of vertical, longitudinal, and transverse muscles that interweave in the three dimensions of space. The nerve supply is via the hypoglossal nerve, which reaches the tongue from the floor of the mouth (Figs. 7a.29, 6a.31, 5a.26, 4a.23, 34a.33, 33a.47).

> *Clinical Notes*
> A **peripheral paresis** of the hypoglossal nerve results in wrinkling of the surface of the tongue and in a diminution of its muscle bulk. In a unilateral lesion of the hypoglossal nerve the tongue deviates to the affected side on protrusion.

Isthmus of Fauces
The isthmus of fauces (Fig. 8a.30) connects the oral cavity with the oropharynx. Two palatal folds containing muscle fibers, the palatoglossal and the palatopharyngeal arches are able to narrow the food passage, like curtains. Within these folds are the muscles of the same name. They spread out into the soft palate. During nasal breathing these muscles, together with the muscles of the uvula, close off the oral cavity.

The **palatoglossus** and **palatopharyngeus** surround the palatine tonsil. In the heads of the coronal series (Fig. 8a.28) and the sagittal series (Fig. 33a.42) the tonsil is small, as a result of atrophy in old age.

Vessels of the Oral Cavity
The walls of the oral cavity have a rich blood supply from branches of the external carotid artery having many anastomoses. The lingual artery runs above the hyoid bone (Fig. 8c.36) and supplies the tongue. The submental artery (Figs. 7c.31, 6c.35, 5c.35, 4c.36), a branch of the facial artery, runs to the floor of the mouth. The roof of the mouth is also well supplied by branches from the facial, maxillary, and ascending pharyngeal arteries.

Venous drainage from the walls of the oral cavity takes place through tributaries of the internal jugular vein.

Regional lymph pathways from the tongue and the palate drain to the submandibular and to the deep cervical lymph nodes.

Afferent Nerves of the Oral Cavity
The **lingual nerve**, a branch of the mandibular nerve (Figs. 5a.25, 6a.29, 7a.27, 8a.29, 33a.44, 34a.40, 35a.38), is the sensory nerve to the mucous membrane of the tip and anterior part of the tongue, the glossopharyngeal nerve to the area of the sulcus terminalis, and the **vagus nerve** to the base of the tongue. The nerve of taste for the anterior two-thirds of the tongue is the **chorda tympani** (Fig. 151.17), a branch of the facial nerve. The taste buds of the vallate papillae are supplied from the glossopharyngeal nerve, and those buds in the base of the tongue by the vagus nerve.

The roof of the mouth receives its sensory supply from branches of the maxillary nerve (V/2).

3.5 Masticatory Apparatus

Temporomandibular joint
In the temporomandibular joint the head of the mandible articulates with the articular surface of the mandibular fossa and the articular tubercle (Figs. 9c.21, 37c.17, 37c.16, 43.7). Between the head of the mandible and the articular surface of the temporal bone there is an articular cartilage named the articular disc (Figs. 9c.22, 37c.18). The articular surface of the mandibular fossa is much larger than the head of the mandible. This coupled with a slack joint capsule means that the heads of the mandible are very mobile. As the mouth is opened the heads of the mandible glide forward on their articular cartilages onto their articular tubercles. It is a combination of a hinge and gliding movement. During mastication the mandible can perform unilateral rotation movements around a vertical axis, alternating between the two sides.

Muscles of Mastication
Four masticatory muscles arise from the side and base of the skull and insert into the lower jaw, as follows
- Temporalis
- Masseter
- Medial pterygoid
- Lateral pterygoid.

The **temporalis** (Figs. 4c.6, 5c.16, 6c.18, 7c.15, 8c.18, 9c.15, 10c.15, 36c.23, 37c.10) is a fan-shaped muscle that arises in the temporal fossa. Its fibers converge for insertion into the coronoid process of the mandible (Figs. 2a.21, 6c.25, 7c.23, 37c.22). Within the muscle there is a supplementary tendon with a bipennate attachment of muscle fibers, which thus show a complicated fiber pattern in the sections. It is a powerful muscle for biting.

The **masseter** (Figs. 5c.25, 6c.27, 7c.26, 8c.28, 9c.37, 37c.29) arises from the zygomatic arch (Figs. 2a.15, 6c.21, 7c.14, 8c.20) and inserts into the lateral aspect of the ramus of the mandible (Figs. 7c.27, 8c.31, 9c.30). It works in cooperation with the temporalis and the medial pterygoid.

The **medial pterygoid** arises from the pterygoid fossa of the sphenoid (Fig. 7c.19). It is inserted into the medial surface of the ramus of the mandible (Figs. 8c.31, 9c.30) and forms, with the masseter, a muscular sling.

The **lateral pterygoid** has two origins (Fig. 7c.18). The upper head arises from the under surface of the greater wing of the sphenoid, the lower head from the lateral pterygoid plate. Both portions run together almost horizontally and are, therefore, cut transversely in the coronal series (Figs. 8c.22, 9c.27). The muscle runs slightly obliquely from medial to lateral, hence it is cut obliquely in the sagittal series (Figs. 35c.32, 36c.25, 37c.23). The muscle is inserted into the neck of the mandible and pulls the corresponding ramus of the mandible obliquely forward and inward. With unilateral contraction it leads to masticatory movements and with bilateral contraction assists in opening the mouth by pulling forward the condyle of the mandible and the articular disc.

The motor supply to these four muscles is from branches of the mandibular nerve (V/3). Their topography can be clearly seen in the coronal slices (Fig. 81).

Apart from these masticatory muscles in the narrower sense, the muscles of the lips, the cheeks, and the tongue cooperate in the act of chewing.

3.6 Lateral Facial Region

The lateral facial region includes the space which extends from the zygomatic arch above (Figs. 2a.15, 6c.21, 7c.14, 8c.20) and reaches the angle of the mandible below (Fig. 2a.35). Anteriorly the lateral facial region continues toward the cheeks without any sharp boundary, and posteriorly it includes the auricle and the external acoustic meatus (Figs. 11c.19, 11c.24). The ramus of the mandible (Figs. 7c.27, 8c.31, 9c.30) divides the space into superficial and deep lateral facial regions.

Superficial Lateral Facial Region
The superficial lateral facial region contains the masseter (Figs. 6c.27, 7c.26, 8c.28), a powerful muscle of mastication. Anterior to this muscle is the fat pad of Bichat and posterior to it the **parotid gland** (Figs. 9c.34, 10c.30). A small portion of the parotid gland lies superficial to the masseter (Fig. 8c.24). The parotid duct (from this upper part of the gland) drains into the vestibule of the mouth. The parotid is enclosed in a capsule formed from the cervical fascia. It contains the gland, a plexus formed by the facial nerve, branches of the auriculotemporal nerve, a section of the external carotid artery, the retromandibular vein, and lymph nodes.

The **external ear** comprises the auricle (pinna) (Fig. 11c.19) and the **external acoustic meatus** (Fig. 11c.24). In adults the external acoustic meatus is about 36 mm long. The medial two-thirds of the meatus is within the temporal bone, the lateral third is reinforced with cartilage and is mainly behind the the articular head of the mandible (Fig. 10c.22). The tympanic membrane (eardrum) (Fig. 11c.23) is a thin membrane separating the external acoustic meatus from the tympanic cavity (Fig. 11c.22).

Deep Lateral Facial Region
The main space of the deep lateral facial region is taken up by the infratemporal fossa. The lateral wall of the infratemporal fossa, the ramus of the mandible, has already been mentioned. Its medial wall is formed by the lateral pterygoid plate (Figs. 7c.17, 21.17). The infratemporal fossa extends backward and medially without any partition to the parapharyngeal space, the border between these two spaces being formed by the medial surfaces of the lateral and medial pterygoid (Figs. 9c.27, 9c.31). Anteriorly the infratemporal fossa extends forward as far as the posterior wall of the maxillary sinus (Fig. 6a.22). This border area lies within the third coronal slice (Fig. 6c). More posteriorly where the ramus of the mandible is absent, the infratemporal fossa continues into the superficial lateral facial region. The roof of the infratemporal fossa is formed by the lower surface of the greater wing of the sphenoid containing the foramen ovale (Fig. 41.12). In addition the infratemporal fossa continues superolaterally into the temporal fossa. The lower part of the temporalis is found in this area (Fig. 37c.10).

Vessels in the Lateral Facial Region
The **external carotid artery** runs vertically through the parotid gland. In the coronal series this section of the artery is located within the sixth slice and is, therefore, not visible on the surface of the section (Fig. 9c). At the level of the temporomandibular joint the external carotid artery bifurcates into its two terminal branches, the superficial temporal and the maxillary arteries. The maxillary artery runs medially from the neck of the mandible into the infratemporal fossa. It generally lies lateral to the lateral pterygoid (Fig. 36c.24). In Figures 9c.28 and 8c.21 of the coronal series the artery is found on the medial side of the lateral pterygoid. The artery runs into the pterygopalatine fossa (Fig. 34c.21) and there divides into its terminal branches. The maxillary artery supplies the muscles of mastication and most of the mucous membrane of the nasal and oral cavities, the teeth, the roof of the mouth, and the greater part of the dura mater and the bones of the skull.

In the infratemporal fossa the veins form the pterygoid venous plexus (Fig. 9c.25), an extensive network that drains through the maxillary veins into the retromandibular vein. The lymphatic vessels drain into deep cervical and retropharyngeal lymph nodes.

Nerves in the Lateral Facial Region
The **facial nerve** (Fig. 11a.44) leaves the skull through the stylomastoid foramen (Fig. 11c.28). A small branch is given off to the posterior belly of the digastric. The main nerve runs through the parotid gland where it divides into separate branches that supply the muscles of facial expression.

The **mandibular nerve** (Fig. 35a.29) runs through the foramen ovale to the infratemporal fossa. Immediately below the base of the skull it has on its medial surface the otic ganglion (Fig. 151.12). The mandibular nerve is the motor supply to the muscles of mastication and of the floor of the mouth. It is the sensory nerve to the floor of the mouth, to the mucous membrane of the tongue in its anterior two-thirds, and also to the skin over the lower jaw.

The mandibular nerve (Figs. 9a.36, 35a.29) divides in the upper part of the infratemporal fossa into:
- Branches to the muscles of mastication
- The buccal nerve to the mucous membrane and skin over the lower jaw
- The inferior alveolar nerve to the teeth in the lower jaw. It enters the mandibular foramen (Figs. 37a.19, 37c.31) and runs through the mandibular canal (Figs. 4a.24, 5a.27, 6a.30, 7a.28, 8a.27, 33a.46, 34a.39, 35a.37, 36a.24). Its terminal branch emerges through the mental foramen and supplies the skin of the chin and the lower lip.
- The lingual nerve (Figs. 5a.25, 6a.29, 7a.27, 8a.29) for the lingual mucous membrane. In the infratemporal fossa it is joined posteriorly by the chorda tympani which carries the preganglionic parasympathetic fibers to the submandibular ganglion and also contains taste fibers for the tongue.

4 Topography of the Pharynx and Craniocervical Junction in Multiplanar Parallel Slices

The craniocervical junction is the border area between the head and neck. From a systematic point of view the pharynx is part of the neck. In clinical practice, lesions of the nasal cavity spread easily into the nasopharynx (the nasal part of the nasopharynx), or from the nasopharynx into the nasal cavity. Anatomically and pathologically the oral cavity is closely related to the oropharynx. Therefore, in this chapter the topography of the pharynx will be discussed first of all, particularly in its clinical relationships with the oral and nasal cavities. The description of the region of the craniocervical junction—extending from the dorsal surface of the base of the skull (level of the mastoid processes to the external occipital protuberance), down to the second cervical vertebra (265)—will follow.

4.1 Pharynx and Parapharyngeal Space
(Figs. 79, 80)

The **pharynx** is a 12–15 cm long fibromuscular tube that extends from the base of the skull to the commencement of the esophagus at the level of the cricoid cartilage. It lies in front of the cervical spine and reaches the level of the sixth cervical vertebra. Flexion and extension movements of the cervical spine can influence the appearance of the pharynx in tomographs. In the coronal series the posterior wall of the pharynx is located almost coronally (Figs. 9c.29, 9c.35). In the sagittal series it runs obliquely to the coronal plane (Fig. 32a.48).

Whereas the posterior wall is closed, the anterior wall has three openings for the air and food passages. The pharynx is thus correspondingly divided into:
- **Nasopharynx** (the nasal part of the pharynx). This upper part communicates with the nasal cavities through the choanae.
- **Oropharynx** (the oral part of the pharynx). This middle level opens anteriorly into the oral cavity through the isthmus of fauces.
- **Laryngopharynx** (the laryngeal part of the pharynx). From this lower level (hypopharynx) the aditus laryngis leads into the larynx.

For examination of the nasopharynx and the oropharynx, median and paramedian slices are suitable (Fig. 80). In these planes the retropharyngeal space can also be evaluated quite well.

Nasopharynx
The nasopharynx (Figs. 8a.25, 9c.29, 32a.42) shows its functional similarity to the nasal cavity through the same type of mucous membrane, a ciliated epithelium. The roof of the nasopharynx forms the outer aspect of the base of the skull, in the area between the pharyngeal tubercle of the occipital bone, the apex of the temporal bone, and a small portion of the lower surface of the sphenoid. Located on the posterior wall is an unpaired mass of lymphoid tissue known as the pharyngeal tonsil. In the head of a 70-year-old man the pharyngeal tonsil is small and atrophic (Fig. 32a.39).

On the lateral wall of the nasopharynx, in the posterior prolongation of the inferior nasal concha, there is the pharyngeal opening of the **pharyngotympanic tube** (Eustachian tube) (Fig. 33c.24). The upper and posterior border of this opening is raised by the pharyngeal end of the cartilage of the tube. Elevation of the mucous membrane at the lower border of the tubal opening is produced by the levator veli palatini. The mucous membrane at the tubal opening contains lymphoreticular connective tissue, the tubal tonsil. This is all part of the ring of lymphoid tissue that surrounds the pharyngeal opening. If this is pathologically enlarged it can cause imflammatory changes (quinsy) that may obstruct the pharyngotympanic tube and block ventilation of the tympanic cavity.

Oropharynx
The oropharynx (Figs. 9c.35, 32a.48, 33a.45) is the space behind the root of the tongue, the paired palatopharyngeal arches and the uvula. Radiologists (470) define the oropharynx as the portion extending from the level of the hard palate to the hyoid bone.

Laryngopharynx
The lowest part of the pharynx (hypopharynx) starts opposite the opening of the larynx and extends downward as far as the entrance to the esophagus. The posterior wall of the larynx bulges into the lumen of the pharynx.

Muscles of the Pharyngeal Wall
The muscles of the pharyngeal wall comprise:
- Constrictor of the pharynx
- Slender elevators of the pharynx, namely the palatopharyngeus and the stylopharyngeus.

The topography of these thin muscles of the pharyngeal wall can best be understood by comparison of a coronal and sagittal series (Figs. 81, 82).

The superior, middle, and inferior **constrictor of the pharynx** arises from the skull, the hyoid bone, and the larynx, and the fibers run dorsally and upward to meet in the midline raphe on the posterior wall of the pharynx. Therefore, when the superior constrictor of the pharynx contracts it simultaneously pulls the hyoid bone and the larynx upward. The superior bulges like a torus (ring) into the lumen of the pharynx (Passavant's torus), which acts as an area of resistance against the soft palate closing off the nasal cavity. Nerve supply: glossopharyngeal and vagus.

The **stylopharyngeus and salpingopharyngeus** contract and raise the walls of the pharynx. Both pharyngeal elevators are inserted into the thyroid cartilage. Nerve supply: glossopharyngeal.

Parapharyngeal Space
The parapharyngeal (lateral pharyngeal) space is a space allowing movement of the pharynx in particular. It lies in the transitional area between head and neck, lateral and dorsolateral to the pharynx. Laterally this space is bounded by the lateral and medial pterygoid and the fascial capsule of the parotid gland. Medially the space reaches the wall of the pharynx. Cranially it extends up to the triangular area on the base of the skull which includes the openings for the internal carotid arteries, the jugular foramen and the hypoglossal canal. In a caudal direction the parapharyngeal space extends into the connective tissue layer of the carotid triangle. The styloid process with the stylopharyngeus, styloglossus, and stylohyoid project into the parapharyngeal space dividing the space into an anterior and a posterior compartment. The anterior compartment contains fatty tissue in which run small vessels including the ascending pharyngeal artery. All of the following run in the posterior compartment: the internal carotid artery (Figs. 10c.23, 35c.35); the internal jugular vein (Figs. 11c.37, 36c.32); the glossopharyngeal nerve (Figs. 11a.42, 35a.31); the vagus (Figs. 10a.42, 35a.30), accessory (Figs. 11a.45, 35a.32), and hypoglossal nerves (Figs. 11a.43, 35a.33). In the coronal slices the parapharyngeal space is easily identified and is usually bilaterally symmetrical (Fig. 79). Any departure from this symmetry suggests a space-occupying lesion. In the T1-weighted MR images the space can be recognized by its fatty tissue, between the muscles of mastication and the constrictors of the pharynx (470). The retropharyngeal space is the cleft between the posterior wall of the pharynx and the prevertebral layer in front of the cervical vertebrae.

Vessels of the Pharyngeal Wall
The ascending pharyngeal artery supplies the wall of the pharynx. There are numerous anastomoses with branches from the superior and inferior thyroid and lingual arteries.

The venous drainage takes place through the pharyngeal plexus, which lies dorsal to the constrictor of the pharynx.

The lymph drainage from the pharyngeal wall runs through the retropharyngeal lymph nodes and then through the deep cervical lymph nodes.

Nerves of the Pharyngeal Wall
The afferent and efferent nerves of the pharyngeal wall are provided by the glossopharyngeal and vagus nerves and the sympathetic trunk. They are pathways of such vital reflexes as the swallowing and the protective reflexes. Afferent and efferent pathways of the swallowing reflex are coordinated in the medulla oblongata.

4.2 Craniocervical Junction
(Figs. 79, 80)

The craniocervical junction includes the dorsally and caudally situated portion of the base of the skull from the level of the external occipital protuberance (Figs. 32c.30, 38.19, 45a.20, 51c.26, 65.19) to the pharyngeal tubercle (Figs. 32c.32, 38.22) of the occipital bone, the first two cervical vertebrae (Figs. 2a.28, 2a.32, 2a.34), and the attached musculature. Laterally the region extends to the mastoid processes (Figs. 2a.23, 12c.23, 26.8, 30a.19, 37c.24, 43.14, 45a.24, 48c.17, 62.14). The occipital bone, atlas, and axis form the joints of the head, a functional unit consisting of a chain of bones capable of free movement in three directions. The musculature takes the form of a virtual cone around the cranial end of the vertebral column, reaching up to the skull. This muscular cone consists dorsally and laterally of the superficial and deep neck muscles; two prevertebral muscles are found ventrally. The individual state of contraction of the muscles in the three spatial axes can cause variable images of the craniocervical junction, and thus complicate the interpretation of CT and MR scans in this region. The median and paramedian slices facilitate anatomic orientation (Fig. 80).

Bones of the Craniocervical Junction
The main bones of the craniocervical junction are:
- Occipital bone
- Atlas
- Axis.

The **occipital bone** is bowl-shaped, with the foramen magnum placed eccentrically (Figs. 2a.26, 14c.13, 26.9, 27.8, 38.23, 48c.20). The lambdoid suture (Fig. 38.4) reaches above the upper limit of the craniocervical junction, the external occipital protuberance (Fig. 38.19). The paired occipital condyles (Figs. 11c.26, 25.13, 30a.16, 34c.27, 40.22) are located anterolateral to the foramen magnum (Fig. 25.11) and form the convex articular surface for the atlanto-occipital joint.

The **atlas** (Figs. 2a.28, 2a.32, 30a.20) is almost ring-shaped. It has a delicate anterior arch (Figs. 10c.26, 24.12, 32c.35, 38.29) and a posterior arch (Figs. 13c.24, 27.9, 32c.38, 38.30), as well as two lateral masses (Figs. 11c.31, 12c.28, 25.17, 26.11, 34c.35, 40.26, 47a.17). On the upper surfaces of the lateral masses there are two concave articular surfaces for the condyles of the occipital bone (Figs. 12c.24, 26.10, 34c.30, 40.23). The lower surfaces of the lateral masses are almost flat for the lateral atlantoaxial joints (Figs. 11c.34, 25.19, 34c.40, 40.27). On the posteriorly directed inner aspect of the anterior arch of the atlas (Fig. 38.29) there is a smooth facet for the median atlantoaxial articulation (Fig. 38.28). On the posterior arch of the atlas there is a groove for the vertebral artery (Fig. 12b.29, 12d.29, 13c.21) and its accompanying veins. In the coronal series the atlas usually stands out because it is broader than the adjoining cervical vertebrae (Fig. 25.18).

The second cervical vertebra, the **axis** (Fig. 2a.34), has as its typical feature the strong toothlike process, the dens (Figs. 2a.29, 11c.30, 25.16, 32c.36, 38.31, 61.12). The dens projects upward into the ring of the atlas and forms the axis of a pivot joint. It articulates with the facet on the inner aspect of the anterior arch of the atlas in the median atlantoaxial joint (Fig. 38.28).

Head Joints

The articular attachments between the occipital bone, the atlas, and the axis are known as the head joints. They include:
- Atlanto-occipital joints
- Atlantoaxial joints.

The **atlanto-occipital joints** are the articulations between the atlas and the occipital bone (Figs. 12c.24, 34c.30). They are two ellipsoid joints between the paired occipital condyles and the paired articular surfaces on the upper surface of the atlas. The movements performed at this joint are, around a frontal axis, flexion and extension (nodding movements) and, around a sagittal axis, lateral movements to either side. Powerful ligaments between the occipital bone and the atlas reinforce these two joints.

The **median atlantoaxial joint** consists of two articular surfaces on the dens of axis and, respectively, a joint surface on the anterior arch of atlas and on the transverse ligament of the atlas. In a median section the two joints between the anterior arch of atlas (Fig. 32c.35) and the dens of axis (Fig. 32c.36) and between the dens of axis and the transverse ligament of atlas (Fig. 32c.37) can be easily identified. The axis of this pivot joint runs longitudinally through the dens of axis. These two median joints cooperate with the two lateral atlantoaxial joints.

The **lateral atlantoaxial joints** (Figs. 11c.34, 25.19, 34c.40, 40.27) are formed by the almost flat, paired joint surfaces on the lower aspect of the atlas and the corresponding paired facets on the upper surface of the axis. These two joints have a loose capsule so that rotatory movements of about 25° are possible.

Muscle Cone of the Craniocervical Junction

The group of muscles located immediately around the cervical vertebrae almost form a cone as they run up to the base of the skull. The muscles that lie dorsal and lateral to the cervical spine are powerful and numerous and are called the nuchal muscles. They are arranged into superficial and deep nuchal muscles and can pull the head backward, as well as rotate it right and left around the long axis of the dens. The anterior group of the muscle cone is located on the ventral aspect of the cervical spine, especially the two flexors of the cervical spine, the longus capitis and the rectus capitis anterior.

Muscles of the Neck

The most superficially positioned muscle at the back of the neck is the descending part of the **trapezius** (Figs. 16c.20, 17c.15, 33c.33, 34c.39, 35c.45, 36c.41, 37c.36). Its main origin is from the spinous processes of the cervical vertebrae and from the external occipital protuberance (Fig. 32c.30). It is inserted into the clavicle and scapula. The trapezius is supplied by the accessory nerve (motor) and by ventral branches from the cervical spinal nerves (proprioceptive). The muscles that lie deeper than the trapezius and dorsal to the vertebral column are the various components of the erector spinae. They are supplied by the posterior rami of the spinal nerves. In the different layers, from the outside inward, are the following muscles:
- Splenius capitis
- Semispinalis capitis and longissimus capitis
- Deep short nuchal muscles.

The **splenius capitis** (Figs. 14c.19, 15c.21, 16c.18, 33c.38, 34c.38, 35c.44, 36c.40, 37c.35) is flat and four-sided. It arises from the spinous processes of the third cervical to the third thoracic vertebrae and is inserted into the mastoid process. The splenius cervicis is related caudally to the splenius capitis.

The **semispinalis capitis** (Figs. 16c.17, 17c.12, 33c.32, 34c.37, 35c.39, 36c.39) arises from the transverse processes of the third cervical to the sixth thoracic vertebrae. It is inserted into the posterior aspect of the occipital bone, lateral to the external occipital protuberance.

The **longissimus capitis** lies lateral to the semispinalis capitis. It arises from the transverse processes of the third cervical to the third thoracic vertebrae and is inserted into the mastoid process.

The deep, short nuchal muscles lie close to the bones between the axis and occipital bone. They

cooperate in the finer movements of the head. There are four paired deep nuchal muscles:
- Rectus capitis posterior minor
- Rectus capitis posterior major
- Obliquus capitis superior
- Obliquus capitis inferior.

The **rectus capitis posterior minor** (Figs. 14c.15, 15c.19) arises from a small tubercle on the posterior arch of atlas and runs up to the outer aspect of the occipital bone about 1 cm dorsal to the posterior margin of the foramen magnum.

The **rectus capitis posterior major** (Fig. 15c.20) arises from the spinous process of the axis (Figs. 2a.36, 15c.22) and is inserted laterally alongside its small fellow muscle into the outer surface of the occipital bone.

The **obliquus capitis superior** (Figs. 13c.22, 14c.16) arises from the transverse process of the atlas (Figs. 25.18, 30a.21) and is inserted laterally to the attachment of the rectus capitis posterior major on the outer surface of the occipital bone, about 2 cm lateral to the border of the foramen magnum.

The **obliquus capitis inferior** (Figs. 13c.26, 14c.20, 34c.42, 35c.41) takes its origin from the spinous process of the axis (Figs. 2a.36, 14c.21) and is inserted into the transverse process of the atlas (Figs. 25.18, 30a.21, 36c.34).

The **levator scapulae** lies almost lateral to the cervical spine, takes its origin from the transverse processes of the upper cervical vertebrae, and is inserted into the scapula. It belongs to the muscles of the shoulder girdle and is provided by the dorsal scapular nerve, a ventral branch of the cervical spinal nerves.

Anterior Part of the Muscle Cone

The two muscles in the anterior part of the muscle cone are prevertebral. The longus capitis (Fig. 33c.30) arises from the transverse processes of the third to the sixth cervical vertebrae and is inserted into the base of the occipital bone. The short rectus capitis anterior arises from the transverse process of the atlas and takes a similar course to the longus capitis.

Blood Vessels of the Craniocervical Junction

The dorsal region of the craniocervical junction is supplied by three vessels with multiple anastomoses:
- Occipital artery
- Vertebral artery
- Deep cervical artery.

The **occipital artery** is a branch of the external carotid artery and runs medially along the posterior belly of the digastric (Figs. 11c.35, 12c.25) and on the medial aspect of the mastoid process, ending in the posterior part of the scalp (Figs. 13c.25, 14c.18, 15c.18, 16c.16, 17c.11).

The **vertebral artery** arises as the first branch of the subclavian artery, enters the foramen in the transverse process of the sixth cervical vertebra and runs cranially through the foramina transversaria of the cervical vertebrae. The artery emerges beside the lateral mass of the atlas and then turns medially (Fig. 12b.29, 12d.29, 13c.21). In this part of its course it gives off branches to the deep cervical musculature. The further course of the vertebral artery through the atlanto-occipital membrane into the cranial cavity will be described with the arteries of the brain (Chap. 5.4).

The small deep cervical artery arises from the subclavian artery and runs between the last cervical vertebra and the transverse process of the first thoracic vertebra into the deep posterior neck where it supplies the local musculature.

The venous drainage of the neck takes place through superficial veins into the external jugular vein and through two deep veins, the vertebral and the deep cervical veins, into the **brachiocephalic vein**. The veins anastomose with the occipital vein and the suboccipital venous plexus (Figs. 13c.23, 14c.22, 15c.23). This venous network is connected to the confluence of sinuses (Figs. 97a.14, 97b.14, 32b.29, 32d.29, 17c.8) and the sigmoid sinus (Figs. 97a.16, 97b.10, 12c.19, 13c.16, 36c.30, 37c.21) through emissary veins.

Nerves of the Craniocervical Junction

The muscles of the craniocervical junction are innervated by:
- Accessory nerve
- Dorsal branches from cervical spinal nerves
- Ventral branches from cervical spinal nerves.

The corresponding muscles and groups of muscles are topographically arranged, which can be clearly seen in the coronal series (Fig. 81). The trapezius, provided by the **accessory nerve** and the ventral branches of the upper spinal nerves, lies in the most superficial and dorsal position. The dorsal branches of the spinal nerves run to the various subdivisions of the erector spinae. The dorsal branch of the first cervical spinal nerve is the suboccipital nerve. It is mainly a motor nerve and provides deep muscles of the neck, namely the rectus capitis minor and major, obliquus capitis superior and inferior, and longissimus capitis and the semispinalis capitis. The large dorsal branch of the second cervical nerve, the **greater occipital nerve** (Figs. 13a.29, 14a.20, 15a.22, 16a.17, 17a.12) is mainly sensory. Its branches supply the skin over the posterior part of the head.

> *Clinical Significance of the Craniocervical Junction*
> The clinical significance of the craniocervical junction extends from fractures, dislocations, congenital abnormalities to cisternal punctures. **Fractures** and **dislocations** are most often the result of a traffic accident with a whiplash injury, or a head-

first dive into shallow water. In most cases the first two cervical vertebrae are fractured. The posterior arch of the atlas is more frequently fractured than the anterior. A fracture of the dens of axis is the most frequent injury of the second cervical vertebra (265). If no serious dislocation between the first and second cervical vertebrae occurs there may be no neurologic deficits. The fracture may only be discovered later through a pseudoarthrosis. Luxations can occur as the result of hyperextension of the cervical spine with tearing of the transverse ligament of the atlas (Fig. 32c.37). The dens of axis (Fig. 32c.36) can be displaced backward and compress the spinal cord (Fig. 12b.28, 32a.45, 32b.40, 32d.40) causing paraplegia. Subluxations are seen in severe rheumatoid arthritis and atlantoaxial dislocation with rupture of the ligaments (5, 471a).

Atlas assimilations, basilar impression, and the Chiari malformation (synonym Arnold–Chiari malformation) occur as **congenital malformations** at the craniocervical junction (66a, 185, 471a). In **atlas assimilation** the atlas is fused with the occipital bone and the foramen magnum is reduced in size and often deformed. The first mobile cervical vertebra is the axis. The dens may be displaced backward and impair circulation in the vertebral artery as well as circulation of the cerebrospinal fluid (CSF). Ischemia of the medulla oblongata and hydrocephalus may result.

Basilar impression can produce similar symptoms. It is characterized by changes in the foramen magnum and the upper cervical vertebrae. In the **Chiari malformation** the cerebellar tonsils are tongue-shaped and also displaced into the spinal canal. The medulla oblongata is deformed and also displaced caudally. These changes can be easily demonstrated in median and paramedian MR images. A neurosurgical decompression of the medulla oblongata and restoration of the circulation of the CSF may be indicated (129a, 195, 253, 367, 374a). Characteristics of the **Dandy-Walker malformation** include hypoplasia of the vermis of the cerebellum and grotesque ballooning of the fourth ventricle. Furthermore, trabecular dysplasia, other cerebral and many extracerebral deformations may occur.

If there is clinical evidence of malformations or anomalies, MRI can clarify the individual pathology and reduce the risks of a cisternal puncture, which nowadays is seldom required.

4.3 Blood Vessels in the Head and Neck

The large vascular bundle between the trunk and the head runs upward in the neck. The component vessels are:
- Common carotid artery
- Internal jugular vein
- A network of lymphatic vessels merging to form the jugular trunk that drains into the jugulosubclavian junction.

The vagus nerve also runs in this neurovascular sheath. The neurovascular bundle follows a course close behind the sternoclavicular joint, up to the middle ear. The bundle leaves the thoracic inlet, runs medially to the sternocleidomastoid, and then enters the carotid triangle. Above the thyroid cartilage the internal carotid artery continues the course of the common carotid artery into the parapharyngeal space (Chap. 4.1).

Arteries in the Head and Neck

In two-thirds of cases, the **common carotid artery** (Figs. 10c.38, 37c.44) divides at the level of the fourth cervical vertebra into the external carotid artery (Figs. 10c.33, 37c.33) and the internal carotid artery (Figs. 10c.23, 37c.41). In the remainder the artery divides either at the level of the third or fifth, rarely at the level of the second or sixth cervical vertebra (267).

The **internal carotid artery** (Fig. 35c.35) runs into the carotid canal at the base of the skull, without giving off branches in this part of its course. Its further course will be described with the cerebral arteries (Chap. 5.4).

The **external carotid artery** divides in the carotid triangle into branches for organs in the neck, the face, and the scalp:
- anteriorly
  - Superior thyroid artery
  - Lingual artery
  - Facial artery
  - Maxillary artery
- medially
  - Ascending pharyngeal artery
- dorsally
  - Occipital artery
- superiorly
  - Superficial temporal artery.

The **superior thyroid artery** descends in the neck to the thyroid gland. The lingual artery (Figs. 9c.41, 8c.36, 36c.45) is given off in the carotid triangle in the neck and runs to the tip of the tongue. See description in the chapter on the mouth (Chap. 3.4).

The **facial artery** (Figs. 9c.36, 8c.33, 36c.44, 37c.40) also branches off the external carotid artery in the carotid triangle. It first runs toward the mandible, then, at the anterior border of the masseter, crosses the lower border of the mandible and runs into the face. The facial artery anastomoses at the medial canthus with terminal branches of the ophthalmic, supratrochlear, and supraorbital arteries.

The **maxillary artery** (Figs. 9c.28, 8c.21, 7c.16, 36c.24, 37c.26) supplies the deeper regions of the face (Chap. 3.6).

The small ascending pharyngeal artery runs in the parapharyngeal space toward the base of the skull. The **occipital artery** runs dorsally into the region of the craniocervical junction (Chap. 4.3).

The **superficial temporal artery** (Figs. 6c.13, 7c.12) runs over the zygomatic bone into the temporal region and, like the facial artery, anastomoses with the supratrochlear and the supraorbital arteries.

Clinical Notes

In a healthy individual the blood pressure in the branches of the internal carotid artery is higher than in those of the external carotid. As a result, the blood flows from the cranial cavity through the ophthalmic artery into the branches of the facial and superficial temporal arteries. If uncompensated stenosis or occlusion of the internal carotid artery exists, this physiologic flow (intracranially to extracranially) diminishes and may even be reversed. The speed and direction of flow can be measured by means of noninvasive **Doppler sonography**. The finding of a reversal of the direction of circulation allows the diagnosis of a stenosis or occlusion of the internal carotid artery to be made with 98 % certainty (15, 183a, 488).

Veins in the Head and Neck

The diploic veins are thin-walled veins in the cancellous bone of the calvaria. They communicate via emissary veins (Fig. 37c.25) with the sinuses of the dura mater and with the veins of the scalp. The blood from the soft tissues of the head is collected in the:
- Facial vein
- Pterygoid venous plexus
- Retromandibular vein
- External jugular vein.

These veins drain into the internal jugular or the subclavian vein.

The **facial vein** collects the blood from the superficial facial area. It starts at the medial canthus and runs obliquely across the cheek and the lower jaw. The pterygoid venous plexus (Fig. 9c.25) is a network of veins in the deep facial region (Chap. 3.6). It drains into the facial and retromandibular veins and connects with the cavernous sinus. The retromandibular vein collects the blood from the temporal region, runs in front of the external acoustic meatus behind the mandible and through the parotid gland in the direction of the internal jugular vein. The external jugular vein receives blood mainly from the nuchal region.

The **internal jugular vein** drains the blood from the venous sinuses of the cranial cavity. It is usually larger on the right side than on the left. In the brainstem series this difference is very marked (Figs. 70a.16, 70a.19). The internal jugular vein starts at the jugular foramen (Fig. 25.6). It lies (Figs. 11c.37, 35c.30) dorsal to the internal carotid artery (Figs. 10c.23, 35c.35). In the neurovascular sheath the internal jugular vein lies lateral to the common carotid artery. Behind the sternoclavicular joint the internal jugular vein joins the subclavian vein, forming the brachiocephalic vein.

5 Topography of the Neurocranium and its Intracranial Spaces and Structures in Multiplanar Parallel Slices

5.1 Neurocranium

The neurocranium comprises the skull bones that enclose the brain, namely the:
- Occipital bone
- Sphenoid
- Temporal bones
- Frontal bone
- Ethmoid
- Parietal bones.

Occipital Bone

The occipital bone encloses the greater part of the posterior cranial fossa. It is divided into four parts that surround the foramen magnum (Figs. 26.9, 27.8, 38.23): basilar part, two lateral parts, and squamous part.

The basilar part forms the anterior border of the foramen magnum. At age 16 to 18 years it fuses with the sphenoid to form the clivus, which is an important guideline structure for neuroimaging (Fig. 32c.28). Posterior to the clivus are the pons and the medulla oblongata (Figs. 32a.28, 32a.36, 32b.31, 32b.34).

The two lateral parts are joined to the temporal bones. On their lower surface the occipital condyles, lateral to the foramen magnum, bulge downward for articulation with the atlas. Above the occipital condyles are the exit foramina for the twelfth cranial nerves, the hypoglossal canals (Figs. 33a.36, 39.15, 48d.10).

The squamous part is almost triangular in shape. In the median section it seems to be bent and is divided into an upper and a lower part. At this border a prominence exists, the external occipital protuberance (inion) (Figs. 32c.30, 38.19). On the inner aspect of the squamous part the internal occipital protuberance lies opposite to the external one (Figs. 32c.27, 38.15). This is the site of the confluence of sinuses, where the superior sagittal sinus and the straight sinus drain into the transverse sinus. The dura of the transverse sinus is the beginning of the tentorium of cerebellum and hence forms the important topographic and neurosurgical boundary between the infratentorial and supratentorial spaces.

Sphenoid

The sphenoid forms the central part of the base of the skull. Comparison with a wasp aids in visualizing the different parts of the isolated sphenoid: The body of the sphenoid forms the unpaired middle portion from which two pairs of wings project laterally, the lesser wings and below these the greater wings.

Between each pair of wings there is a cleft, the superior orbital fissure (Figs. 20.4, 21.5, 30a.7, 34c.17, 50c.6). From the body of the wasp two paired "legs" hang downward, the pterygoid processes, each with a medial and a lateral pterygoid plate (Figs. 7c.20, 7c.17, 21.18, 21.17).

The **body of the sphenoid** is more or less cubical in shape and contains the sphenoidal sinus, which has already been described as a paranasal space (Chap. 3.2). The cerebral surface of the body of the sphenoid is related via the sphenoethmoidal suture to the cribriform plate of the ethmoid. Posteriorly the sella turcica, "Turkish saddle," forms a deep depression, the hypophysial fossa, for the pituitary gland (hypophysis). The hypophysial fossa is bounded anteriorly by the tuberculum sellae and posteriorly by the dorsum sellae (Figs. 38.11, 65.11). From each side of the dorsum sellae a posterior clinoid process (Fig. 65.10) projects upward.

The **lesser wing** of the sphenoid arises on each side of the body with two roots surrounding the optic canal (Figs. 21.3, 65.6). The lesser wings form the boundary between the anterior and middle cranial fossae. The posterior and medial angle of the lesser wing projects medially and anteriorly as the anterior clinoid process (Figs. 2a.5, 8c.12, 45a.8, 65.7).

The **greater wing** of the sphenoid arises on each side from the posterior part of the body. The medial portion of the greater wing is pierced by two nerve openings, anteriorly by the foramen rotundum for the maxillary nerve and posteriorly by the foramen ovale for the mandibular nerve. Lateral and posterior to the foramen ovale is the foramen spinosum for the middle meningeal artery. The greater wing is related anteriorly to the maxilla at the pterygopalatine fossa, and to the orbit, forming part of its lateral wall. The temporal portion of the greater wing is directed laterally and forms a small part of the lateral wall of the skull in the temporal fossa.

The **pterygoid process** is attached by two roots, between which the pterygoid canal (Fig. 21.12) runs, and continues downward into the lateral wall of the choana. The pterygoid canal continues into the pterygopalatine fossa. The pterygoid process is divided into medial and lateral pterygoid plates enclosing a longitudinal groove, the pterygoid fossa (Fig. 21.16). The lower end of the medial pterygoid plate curves laterally into a hooklike pterygoid hamulus (Figs. 20.16, 34c.34), around which passes the tendon of the tensor veli palatini. The lateral pterygoid plate is rounded at its lower border.

Temporal Bone
The paired temporal bone forms part of the base of the skull and part of its side wall. It contains the inner ear, the middle ear, and a portion of the external acoustic meatus. The temporal bone provides a protective covering for the facial and vestibulocochlear nerves, and for branches of the glossopharyngeal and vagus nerves. It carries the articular facet for the temporomandibular joint. The temporal bone consists of four parts:
- The petrous part contains the inner ear and forms part of the skull base.
- The tympanic part forms the floor, anterior, and lateral walls of the bony external acoustic meatus.
- The squamous part joins with the occipital, parietal, and sphenoid to form the lateral wall of the cranial cavity. On its lower surface the squamous part articulates with the head of the mandible.
- The styloid process.

The petrous part is roughly pyramidal in shape. Its apex is directed forward and medially and its base posteriorly and laterally. The superior margin (Figs. 24.3, 30a.10), disposed at an angle of approximately 55° with the midline when viewed from above, forms the boundary between the posterior and middle cranial fossae. It has a groove for the superior petrosal sinus; the groove divides the posterior surface, which faces the cerebellum, from the anterior surface, which faces the temporal lobe.

The medial portion of the **petrous part** consists of ivory-hard bony tissue, which is particularly responsible for the dense bony artifacts in the CT scans. The lateral portion forms commonly the mastoid process which is pneumatized from the tympanic cavity and contains the mastoid cells (Figs. 25.10, 43.13, 49c.20).

In the center of the posterior aspect of the pyramid is the **internal acoustic meatus** (Figs. 11b.23, 11c.20, 25.4, 35b.14, 35c.23, 41.9, 64.12), through which run the facial and vestibulocochlear nerves, together with the arteries and veins to the labyrinth. In the center of the anterior aspect of the pyramid is a small elevation, the arcuate eminence (Figs. 25.3, 42.6) formed by the anterior semicircular canal (Figs. 11b.24, 50b.18, 50c.17, 65.12). The area just lateral to the arcuate eminence is the roof of the tympanic cavity (tegmen tympani). In the medial part of the anterior surface are two small openings through which pass the parasympathetic fibers from the seventh and ninth cranial nerves (Chap. 6.14). The shallow trigeminal impression for the trigeminal ganglion is located close to the apex of the petrous part.

The inferior surface of the pyramid forms part of the external surface of the base of the skull. It forms the floor of the tympanic cavity and the bony portion of the musculotubal canal. In the center of the inferior surface is the beginning of the carotid canal. Anterior and lateral to this is the opening of the bony part of the pharyngotympanic (Eustachian) tube (Chap. 4.1).

Contents of the Petrous Part
Within the petrous part is the **labyrinth** containing the sensory receptors for the vestibular and auditory systems (Chaps. 6.4 and 6.5), the tympanic cavity, and the bony part of the pharyngotympanic tube. In the tympanic cavity are the auditory ossicles, the malleus (hammer), incus (anvil), and stapes (stirrup).

The **facial canal** begins at the outer end of the internal acoustic meatus and runs forward and laterally as far as the angle (genu) where the sensory geniculate ganglion of the facial nerve is located. At this site the parasympathetic fibers leave the trunk of the facial nerve. At the genu the facial nerve bends at an acute angle laterally and posteriorly. It runs in or on the medial wall of the tympanic cavity. In over 50% of cases the connective tissue of the facial nerve directly borders the mucous membrane of the tympanic cavity, so that pathologic lesions in the tympanic cavity can easily affect the facial nerve (260). Beneath the lateral semicircular canal the facial canal curves inferiorly and ends at the outer base of the skull at the stylomastoid foramen, between the mastoid process and the styloid process (237, 450). The facial nerve occupies the facial canal (Figs. 25.7, 36c.28, 42.11, 49c.18), which is about 20 mm long and 2 mm wide.

In the newborn the tympanic portion of the temporal bone consists only of a bony tympanic ring, which is open superiorly to receive attachment of the tympanic membrane. In the postnatal period it develops anteriorly, inferiorly, and posteriorly to form the bony part of the external acoustic meatus. The bony acoustic meatus is closed from above by the temporal squamous part.

The squamous part of the temporal bone consists of the true squama and a basal part from which the zygomatic process projects forward. The zygomatic process of the temporal bone together with the temporal process of the zygomatic bone forms the zygomatic arch (Figs. 2a.15, 7c.14, 8c.20, 21.14, 48c.7). The mandibular fossa is located on the inferior surface of the basal part, forming the articular surface for the temporomandibular joint (Figs. 9c.21, 23.8, 37c.17, 43.7).

The styloid process projects downward and forward (Figs. 24.11, 30a.17, 42.14).

Frontal Bone
The frontal bone encloses the cranial cavity anteriorly, forms the greater part of the roofs of the orbits, and borders on the upper portion of the nasal cavity. The frontal bone is divided into:
- Squamous part
- Orbital parts
- Nasal part.

The squamous part is connected via the coronal suture to the parietal bone and via the sphenofrontal suture to the greater wing of the sphenoid.

The orbital part is vaulted into the cranial cavity and forms the roof of the orbital cavity. The orbital parts border the cribriform plate of the ethmoid medially.

The unpaired nasal part joins together the two orbital parts of the frontal bone.

Ethmoid

The contribution of the ethmoid comprises the crista galli and cribriform plates in the interval between the orbital plates of the frontal bone.

Parietal Bone

The paired parietal bones, between the occipital and frontal bones, form a large part of the roof and the side walls of the skull (Figs. 2a.2, 10c.4, 24.1, 32c.3, 38.2, 45a.2, 54c.14). The bone has four borders:

- The upper border forms the sagittal suture in the median plane together with the parietal bone from the other side (Fig. 59c.9).
- The anterior border meets the frontal bone at the coronal suture (Figs. 32c.1, 33c.1, 38.1, 39.1, 57c.6).
- The posterior border meets the occipital bone at the lambdoid suture (Figs. 32c.10, 33c.8, 38.4, 39.4, 54c.25).
- The lower border forms the squamous suture with the squamous part of the temporal bone and the sphenoparietal suture with the greater wing of the sphenoid.

5.2 Cranial Cavity

(Figs. 4–17, 32–37, 47–60)

Located inside a rigid capsule, the cranial cavity is a hollow space with an average volume of 1550 ml in males and 1425 ml in females. This cavity houses the brain with its nerves and vessels, which is submerged in a liquid medium, the cerebrospinal fluid (CSF). Rigid sheets of dura mater divide the cranial cavity into compartments. The tentorium of cerebellum (Figs. 13a.17, 15a.17, 32a.21, 33a.21, 51a.19, 52a.40, 53a.40) divides the cranial cavity into an infratentorial and a supratentorial space.

Infratentorial Space

The floor of the infratentorial space or compartment is the posterior cranial fossa. Its roof is shaped like a shallow-pitched tent by the **tentorium of cerebellum**. The brainstem emerges through a large oval opening called the **tentorial notch** (incisura). A fluid jacket, the ambient cistern, is found here (Chap. 5.3). The foramen magnum is the other large opening of the infratentorial compartment (Figs. 2a.26, 14c.13, 27.8, 38.23, 48c.20). It can be oval or almost circular in shape, usually giving the appearance of two differently sized semicircles placed together. The area of the foramen magnum averages 8 cm^2, ranging from 5–10 cm^2. In cases of extreme cerebral edema, the brainstem and the cerebellum are pushed into a more caudal position. As a result, a pressure cone may develop in the inferior surface of the cerebellum and may cause tonsillar herniation.

Supratentorial Space

The supratentorial space is partially divided by the sickle-shaped **falx cerebri** (Figs. 4a.3, 10a.3, 17a.4, 52a.3, 55a.3, 57a.14). Fluid jackets, namely the interhemispheric cistern and the pericallosal cistern, protect the structures between the cerebral hemispheres. The subdivision of the cranial cavity into separate compartments by the fibrous sheets of dura mater determines the possibility and direction of a major displacement of the individual brain structures in the event of an increase in intracranial pressure. An increase in volume of the cerebrum in the supratentorial compartment may strangulate the brainstem, giving rise to a **midbrain syndrome**. Furthermore, a displacement in one hemisphere may bend the falx cerebri toward the opposite side. Awareness of possible movements such as these can be essential for diagnosis and/or surgical intervention. When planning a neurosurgical procedure, the position of the blood vessels and venous sinuses in the tentorium and falx cerebri must be taken into consideration in order to avoid unnecessary hemorrhagic complications (Chaps. 5.4 and 5.5).

In the frontal series the topography of the cranial cavity is clearly demonstrated through the superiorly located skullcap, the lateral walls, and the base of the skull (Figs. 4–17). In the sagittal series the structures of the infratentorial and supratentorial spaces can be differentiated especially well (Figs. 32–37).

As seen in the parallel canthomeatal planes (from the lateral corner of the eyelid to the external acoustic meatus), the serial cross-sections of the bones at the skull base and craniocervical junction appear as more complicated images when compared to those of the skullcap. Depending on the shape of the head, the **superior portion of the skull** appears in cross-sections as a bony, more or less oval ring (Figs. 52–60).

In sections through the craniocervical junction, CT scans show great variability when upper cervical vertebrae or intervertebral spaces are cut (Fig. 47a). The first cervical vertebra, the atlas, is characterized by the anterior and posterior arches, an absent vertebral body, and laterally positioned foramina transversaria through which the vertebral arteries ascend. These structures are better visualized in the radiograph of the 1 cm-thick section (Fig. 61). The second cervical vertebra, the axis, is easily identified by its toothlike process, the dens.

In Figure 48c, the sectioning plane lies at a slight angle to the foramen magnum, dissecting anteriorly the basal portion of the occipital bone and anteriolaterally the hypoglossal canal. The posterior part of the sectioning plane is located in a inferior position close to the foramen magnum (Fig. 62).

Cranial Fossae

The topography of the posterior, middle, and anterior cranial fossae is best clarified on the skull itself. "Hands-on" examination of a dry skull reveals the spatial relationships of these structures most easily. Studying illustrations of the internal cranial base in anatomic atlases may give an incorrect idea of the arrangement of these fossae. In an atlas, they frequently appear to lie on the same horizontal plane whereas, in reality, the fossae are in the form of **three terraces**, each set about 2.5 cm above or below the other (264). The floor of the middle cranial fossa (Fig. 45a.16) lies approximately in Reid's base plane (lower border of the orbit to the center of the external acoustic canal) (136). The floor of the posterior fossa is about 2.5 cm lower and the anterior fossa 2.5 cm higher than the middle cranial fossa. The sagittal series oriented in the coordinate system shows the topographic relation of the cranial fossae to Reid's base line most clearly in the slice where the middle cranial fossa has its deepest depression. This applies to the fourth sagittal slice and particularly to its radiograph (Figs. 41.4, 41.8, 41.15).

Knowledge of such simple spatial relationships is very useful when examining cross-sectional images made in parallel canthomeatal planes. On average, the canthomeatal plane is tilted about 19° to Reid's base line (264). The canthomeatal plane lies within the head slice (Fig. 49a). The sectioning plane lies in the inferior third of the posterior cranial fossa and extends along the floor of the middle fossa. The anterior fossa lies superior to the sectioning plane, and hence is not shown in the illustrations. The radiograph of this slice shows the jugular foramen in the posterior fossa and the foramina spinosum, ovale, and rotundum in the middle cranial fossa (Fig. 63). In the next slice (Figs. 50c and 64), the skull encloses the posterior and middle cranial fossae in the form of two forceps. The opening of the internal acoustic meatus is found in the posterior cranial fossa (Fig. 50c.15).

The **superior orbital fissure** (Figs. 50c.6, 64.7) connects the middle cranial fossa with the orbit (Fig. 50c.4). In the middle of Figure 50c the dorsum sellae has been partially dissected (Fig. 50c.11). The cribriform plate is shown as a part of the anterior cranial fossa. Resting on the cribriform plate is the olfactory bulb (Fig. 50a.3).

In the fifth slice, the sectioning plane dissects the tentorium of cerebellum (Fig. 51c.17). The infratentorial compartment appears to decrease gradually in size in the subsequent cranial slices until the ridge of the tentorium is reached. The radiograph of this slice shows the **optic canal** (Fig. 65.6) that forms a connection between the orbit and the middle cranial fossa. The roof of the orbit can be seen in the anterior cranial fossa (Figs. 51c.4, 65.3).

In the subsequent slice (Figs. 52c, 66) and in all further slices, the bony outline of the skull appears as an oval ring. The infratentorial compartment forms a smaller portion of these illustrations than the supratentorial compartment. The border between the two compartments is marked by the tentorium of cerebellum (Fig. 52c.17).

5.3 Cerebrospinal-Fluid-Containing Spaces (Figs. 83–87)

Subarachnoid Space

The brain is suspended in its protective jacket of cerebrospinal fluid (CSF) of an almost identical specific gravity. CSF is present throughout the ventricular system and the subarachnoid space. The cranial subarachnoid space, which lies between the pia mater and the more externally located arachnoid mater, holds 25–50 ml of CSF (264). The arachnoid mater is applied to the dura mater, a tough fibrous membrane. Due to the alcohol–formalin fixation, the subarachnoid spaces of our anatomic preparations are artificially enlarged.

Cisterns
(Figs. 83a, 84, 85, 86a, 87)

Expansions of the CSF-containing subarachnoid spaces are referred to as cisterns.

The **posterior cerebellomedullary cistern** (cisterna magna) fills the space between the medulla oblongata, the roof of the fourth ventricle, and the inferior surface of the cerebellum. It is approximately 3 cm wide and in the sagittal plane is up to 2 cm deep. In the median plane indentations are present, as the cistern follows the highly variable surface of the falx cerebelli. This is the cistern entered during **cisternal puncture**.

The **posterior** and **anterior basal cisterns** (Figs. 83a.12, 86a.12, 83a.9, 86a.9) are enlarged chambers of the subarachnoid space. They lie between the lower surface of the brain and the skull base and extend from the foramen magnum to the crista galli in the anterior cranial fossa. The posterior and anterior basal cisterns are separated by the dorsum sellae (264).

The **pontine cistern** is located between the clivus and the pons.

The **cerebellopontine cistern** occupies the cerebellopontine angle. The lateral recess of the fourth ventricle discharges CSF into this chamber through the lateral aperture (of Luschka), identifiable by "Bochdalek's bouquet," a protrusion of the choroid plexus of the fourth ventricle through this aperture. The flocculus (H X) of the cerebellum extends laterally into this chamber.

The **superior cerebellar cistern** is found between the tentorium and the superior surface of the cerebellum.

240 5 Topography of the Neurocranium and its Intracranial Spaces and Structures in Multiplanar Parallel Slices

1 Pericallosal cistern
2 Cistern of transverse cerebral fissure
3 Cistern of lamina terminalis
4 Pineal gland
5 Interpeduncular cistern
6 Ambient cistern
7 Quadrigeminal cistern (cistern of great cerebral vein)
8 Superior cerebellar cistern
9 Anterior basal cistern (dotted line)
10 Chiasmatic cistern
11 Pontine cistern
12 Posterior basal cistern (dashed line)
13 Cisterna magna (posterior cerebellomedullary cistern)
14 Spinal subarachnoid space

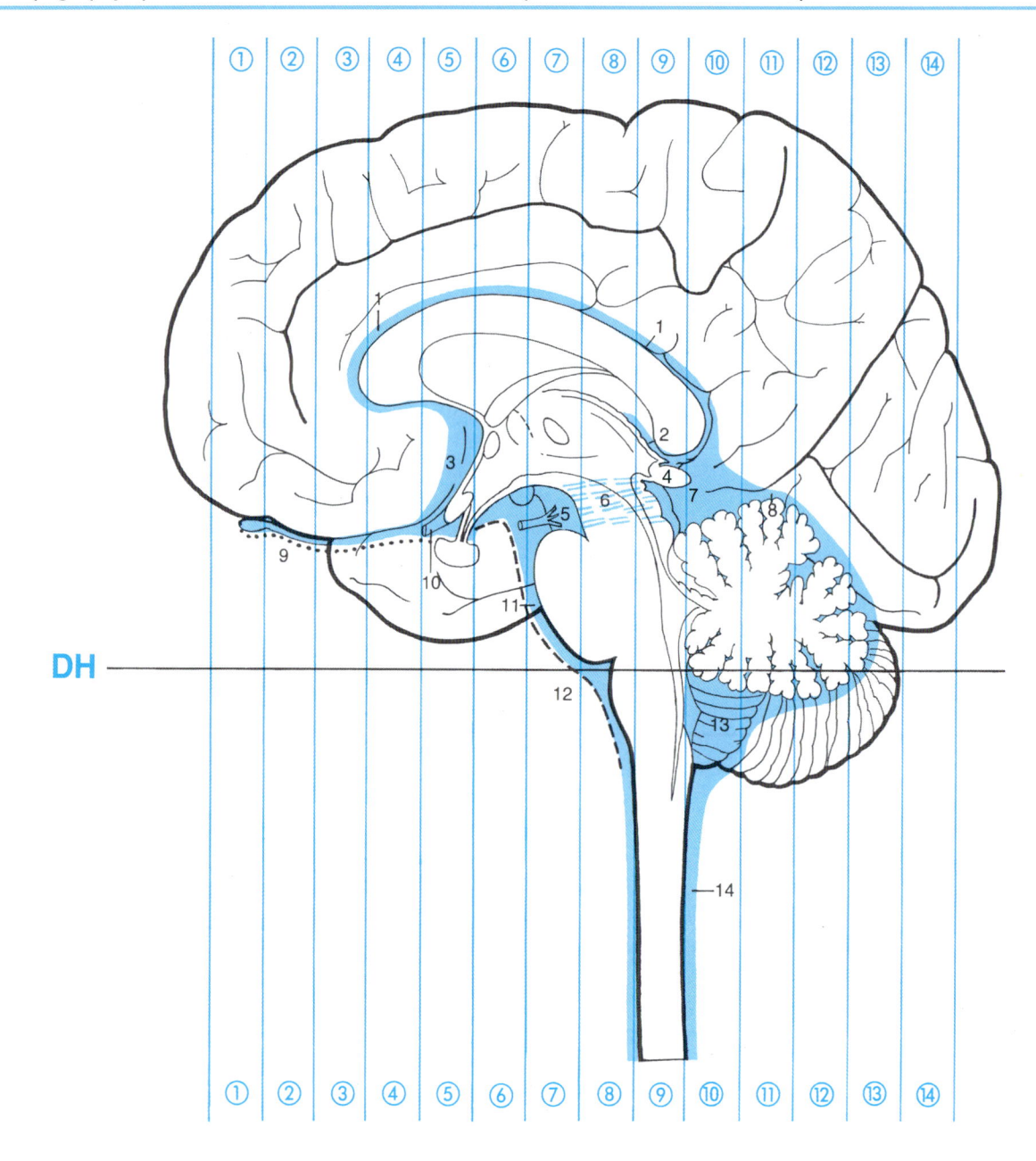

Fig. **83a** Medial view of the external CSF spaces in the cranial cavity and vertebral canal of the coronally cut brain. The ambient cistern encloses the cerebral peduncle. The cistern is, therefore, indicated with a blue dashed line.

5.3 Cerebrospinal-Fluid-Containing Spaces   241

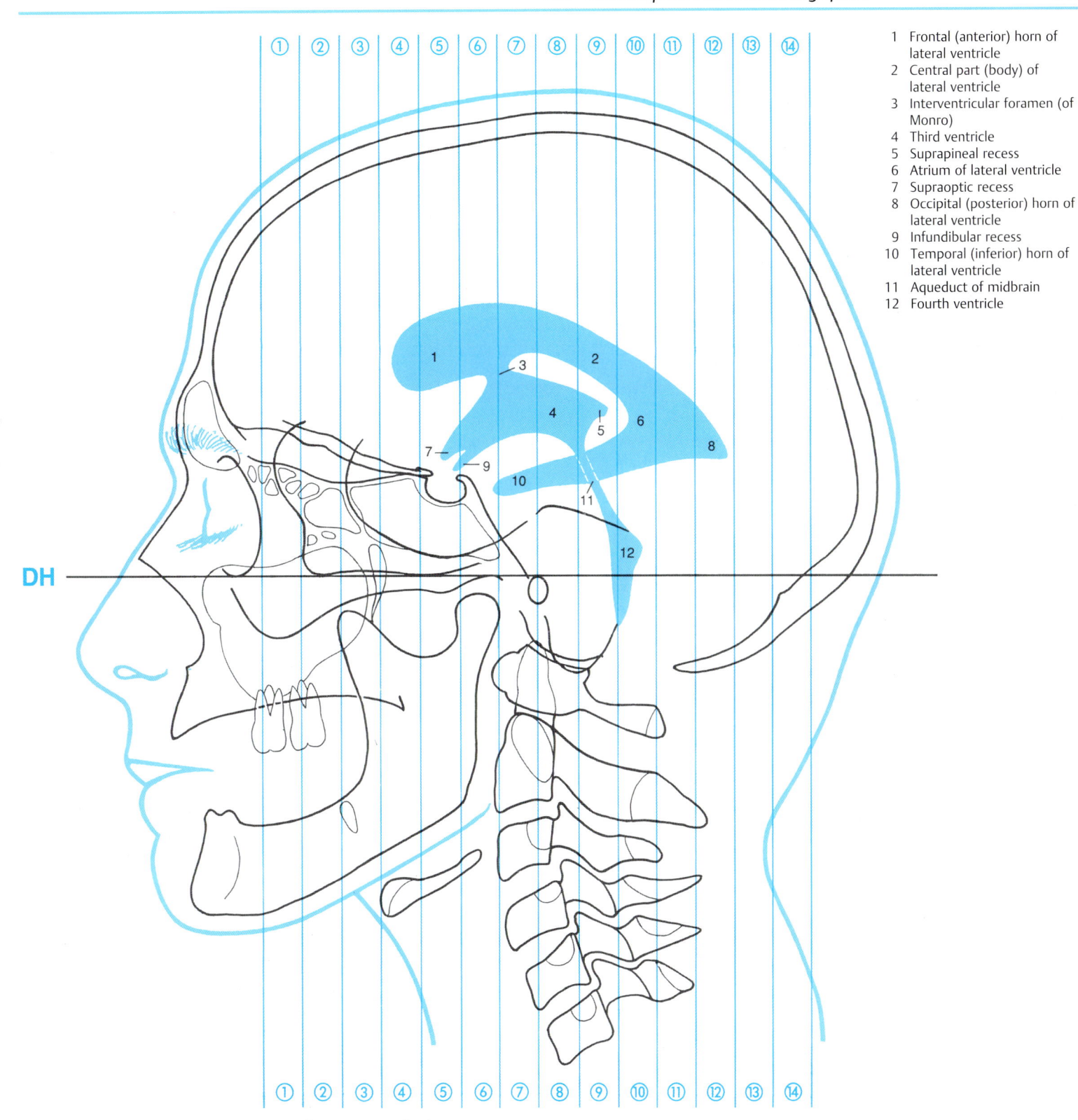

1 Frontal (anterior) horn of lateral ventricle
2 Central part (body) of lateral ventricle
3 Interventricular foramen (of Monro)
4 Third ventricle
5 Suprapineal recess
6 Atrium of lateral ventricle
7 Supraoptic recess
8 Occipital (posterior) horn of lateral ventricle
9 Infundibular recess
10 Temporal (inferior) horn of lateral ventricle
11 Aqueduct of midbrain
12 Fourth ventricle

Fig. 83b Lateral view of the ventricular system of the coronally cut head (Figs. 1, 2a,b, 3).
DH Reid's base line

The **interpeduncular cistern** is the anterior portion of the posterior basal cistern. It contains the third cranial nerve, the terminal bifurcation of the basilar artery (Fig. 51c.14), namely the origin of the superior cerebellar arteries and the posterior cerebral arteries (Fig. 51c.13).

The **ambient cistern** (Fig. 52b.18) encloses the lateral surfaces of the cerebral peduncles and forms a fluid jacket around the tentorial notch (incisura) beside the sharp edge of the tentorium of cerebellum. The ambient cistern courses in a posterior direction to the quadrigeminal cistern and continues in an anterior direction to the cistern of vallecula cerebri. Furthermore, the ambient cistern is connected with the unpaired pericallosal cistern and the paired interhemispheric cisterns (Figs. 7d.2, 16d.4). The ambient cistern contains the trochlear nerve and three blood vessels, namely the posterior cerebral artery, the superior cerebellar artery, and the basal vein (of Rosenthal).

The **quadrigeminal cistern** (Figs. 52b.20, 52d.20) consists of the CSF space posterior to the tectal plate (quadrigeminal lamina). The quadrigeminal cistern and the cistern of great cerebral vein were assessed as synonyms by the Federative Committee on Anatomical Terminology since these two cisterns describe a similar space between the quadrigeminal lamina and the great cerebral vein.

The **trigeminal cistern** opens into the cerebellopontine cistern (Figs. 50d.13, 73c.9, 73d.9). The flat appendix of the trigeminal cistern (Figs. 74b.7, 87.5) lies on the petrous part of the temporal bone and sphenoid in the middle cranial fossa and houses the root of the fifth cranial nerve (Fig. 74b.8) together with the trigeminal (Gasserian) ganglion.

The **anterior basal cistern** reaches from the dorsum sellae to the anterior limit of the anterior cranial fossa. This cistern borders on the mammillary bodies, infundibulum, optic chiasm, optic tracts, olfactory bulbs and tracts, and the base of the frontal lobes. One part of this cistern is the **chiasmatic cistern** that encloses the optic chiasm. Posteriorly, the anterior basal cistern is related to the interpeduncular cistern (Figs. 11b.17, 11d.17, 52b.11, 52d.11). The medial part of the anterior basal cistern and the interpeduncular cistern are conjointly named the **suprasellar cistern** (pentagonal cistern) (Fig. 87.9); this contains the cerebral arterial circle (circle of Willis) and its central branches.

The anterior basal cistern is linked laterally to the cistern of lateral cerebral fossa by the cistern of the vallecula cerebri. The **cistern of vallecula cerebri** (Figs. 51d.8, 78c.3, 78d.3, 87.8) is the CSF-filled space between the posterior edge of the lesser wing of the sphenoid and the anterior perforated substance containing the first segment of the middle cerebral artery.

The **cistern of lateral cerebral fossa** (Sylvian fissure) (Figs. 11b.11, 36b.9, 53d.16, 84.5, 85.36, 87.13) forms the space between the insula and the opercular portions of the frontal, parietal, and temporal lobes (38). Therefore, this space is also referred to as the insular cistern. Branches of the middle cerebral artery, the insular arteries, are found here.

The **cistern of transverse fissure** (Figs. 84.20, 85.5, 86a.2) is a fluid accumulation located in the fissure between the corpus callosum and the roof of the third ventricle including the thalamus. This space lies between the telencephalon and diencephalon. The cistern of the transverse fissure extends anteriorly toward the interventricular foramen (of Monro) (Fig. 54a.22). This cistern is 2.5 cm long in sagittal direction and has a transverse diameter of 4 cm. It contains the internal cerebral veins (Fig. 54c.12) and portions of the posterior medial and posterior lateral choroidal arteries (Figs. 54c.17, 54c.16).

The cistern of transverse fissure is in continuity with the quadrigeminal, pericallosal, and interhemispheric cisterns. The pericallosal cistern (Figs. 83a.1, 85.2) is the unpaired CSF-filled space between the corpus callosum and the inferior free edge of the falx cerebri. The **interhemispheric cisterns** (Figs. 7d.2, 16d.4, 84.1) are the paired spaces between the falx cerebri and the medial surface of the cerebral hemisphere on each side. The cistern of lamina terminalis (Figs. 84.6, 86a.4, 87.12) connects the chiasmatic cistern (Figs. 83a.10, 84.7, 85.13) with the pericallosal cistern enclosing the corpus callosum.

Ventricles
(Figs. 83b, 84, 85, 86b, 87)

The internal CSF-containing spaces are the four ventricles with their connections. The Volume and shape of these spaces vary greatly, even among healthy individuals. The average ventricular volume of an extracranially fixed adult brain is approximately 20 ml, ranging from 7 to 57 ml (233, 271). According to CT examinations of healthy brains, the volume lies between 15 and 46 ml, the average being 31 ml (52).

Fourth Ventricle

The fourth ventricle (Figs. 2b.38, 13b.19, 32a.32, 32b.32, 71a.20, 73b.29) is shaped like a small tent, its floor being the rhomboid fossa and the roof being the two medullary vela, the cerebellar peduncles, and the cerebellum. The superior part of the roof is formed by the superior medullary velum and the inferior portion by the inferior medullary velum. The choroid plexus of the fourth ventricle is attached to the inferior medullary velum suspended in a sheet of connective tissue.

Three openings release CSF from the ventricle into the subarachnoid space: the median aperture (of Magendie) on the midline at the obex (Figs. 32a.40, 32b.35, 70b.29, 70d.9) at the inferior margin of the fourth ventricle, and the paired lateral apertures (of Luschka) laterally beside the medulla oblongata (Figs. 72b.21, 72c.6).

5.3 Cerebrospinal-Fluid-Containing Spaces

1. Interhemispheric cistern
2. Anterior basal cistern
3. Pericallosal cistern
4. Frontal (anterior) horn of lateral ventricle
5. Cistern of lateral cerebral fossa (cistern of Sylvian fissure)
6. Cistern of lamina terminalis
7. Chiasmatic cistern
8. Third ventricle
9. Infundibular recess
10. Cistern of vallecula cerebri
11. Trigeminal cistern

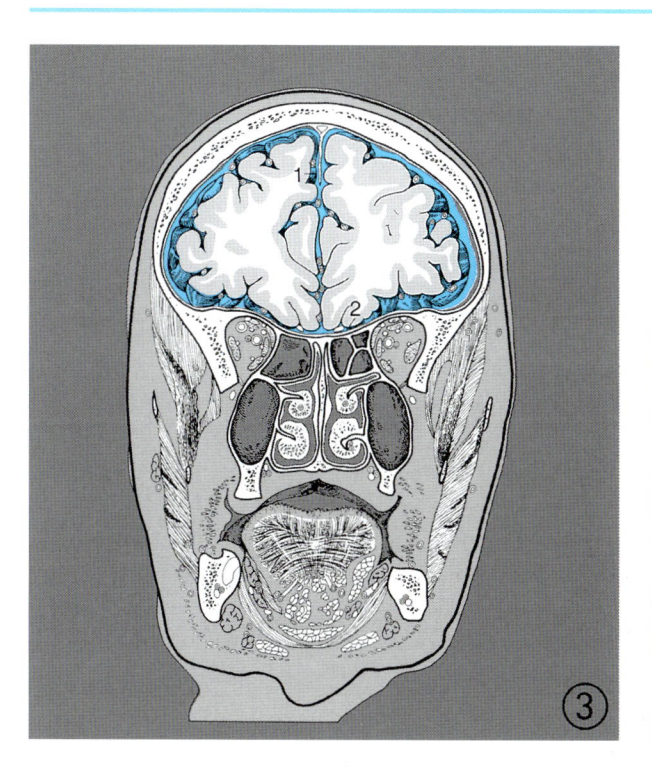

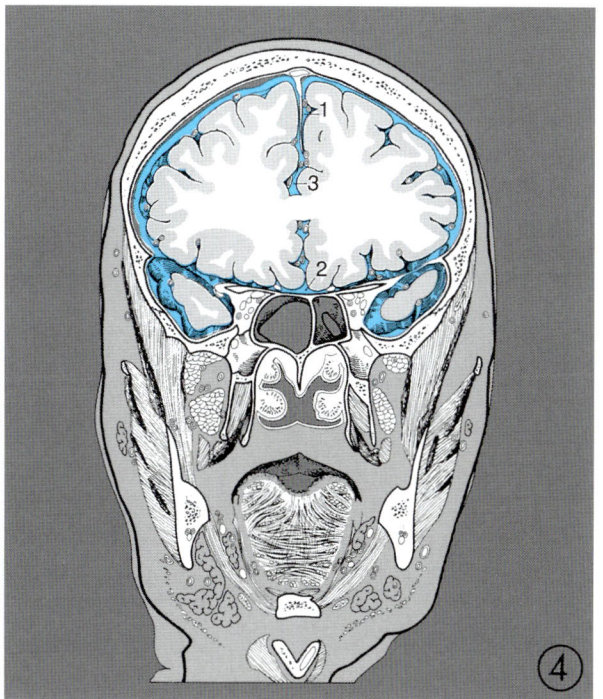

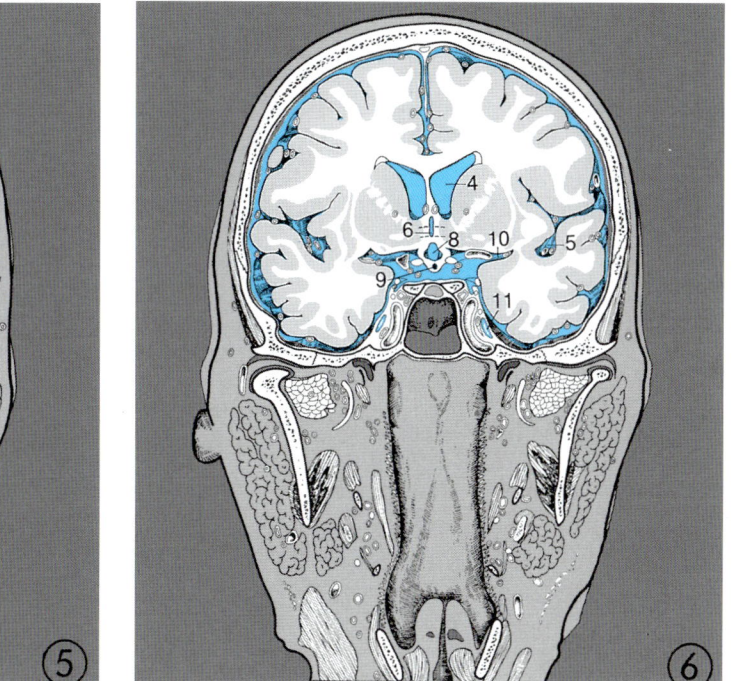

Fig. 84 Coronal serial illustrations of the CSF spaces in the cranial cavity and in the vertebral canal. The encircled numbers (3–6) show the number of the respective slice (Figs. 1, 2a,b, 3).

5 Topography of the Neurocranium and its Intracranial Spaces and Structures in Multiplanar Parallel Slices

1 Interhemispheric cistern
3 Pericallosal cistern
4 Frontal (anterior) horn of lateral ventricle
5 Cistern of lateral cerebral fossa (cistern of Sylvian fissure)
8 Third ventricle
11 Trigeminal cistern
12 Interventricular foramen (of Monro)
13 Ambient cistern
14 Temporal (inferior) horn of lateral ventricle
15 Pontine cistern
16 Lateral ventricle
17 Interpeduncular cistern
18 Cerebellopontine cistern
19 Central part (body) of lateral ventricle
20 Cistern of transverse cerebral fissure
21 Suprapineal recess
22 Aqueduct of midbrain
23 Posterior basal cistern
24 Spinal subarachnoid space
25 Atrium of lateral ventricle
26 Quadrigeminal cistern (cistern of great cerebral vein)
27 Roof of fourth ventricle
28 Cisterna magna (posterior cerebellomedullary cistern)

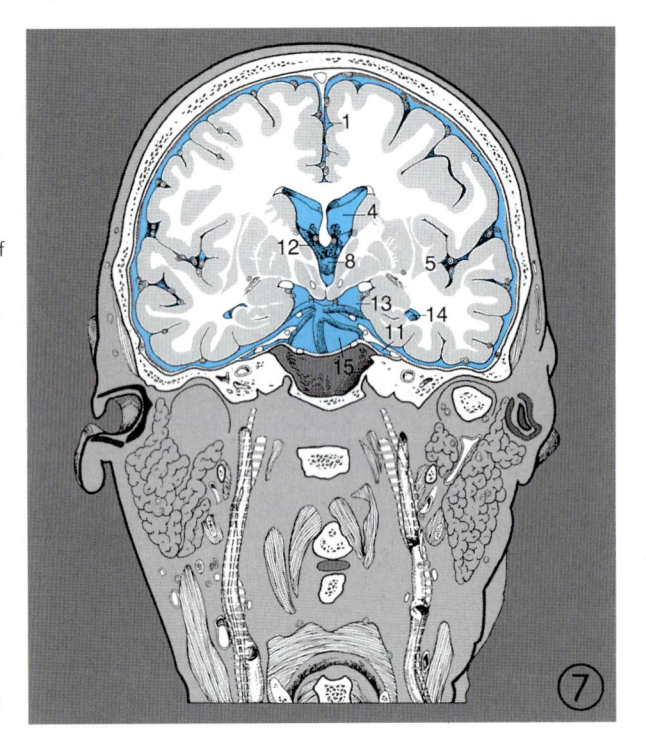

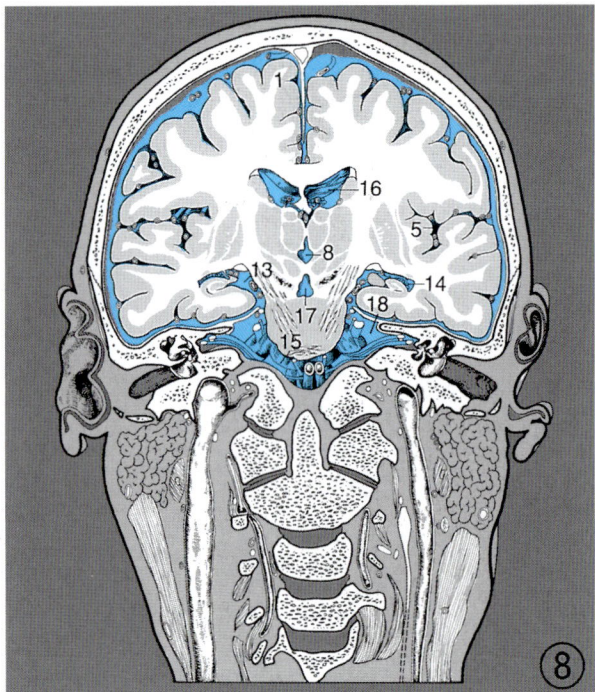

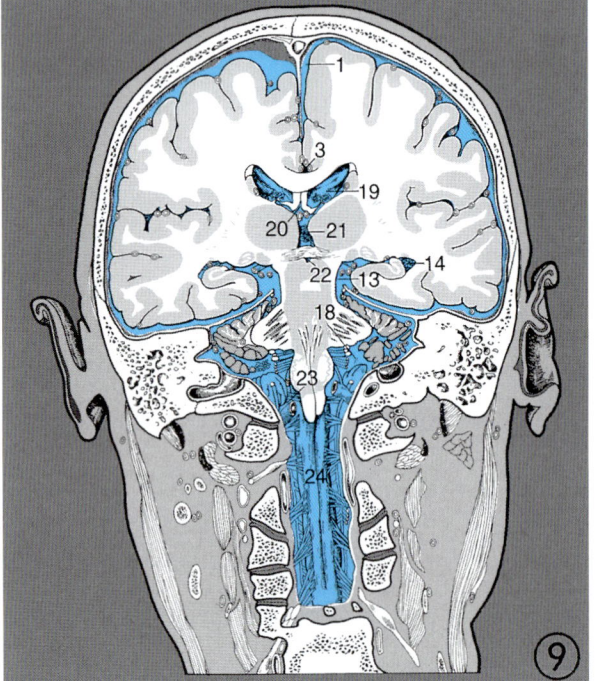

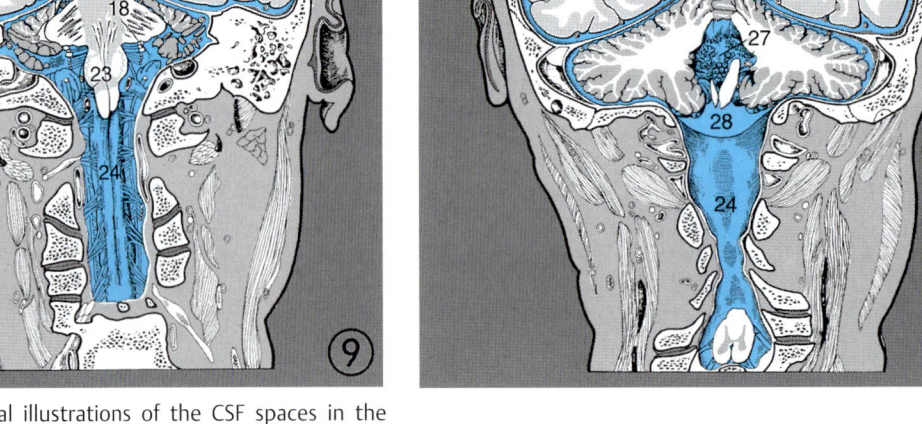

Fig. 84 Coronal serial illustrations of the CSF spaces in the cranial cavity and in the vertebral canal. The encircled numbers (7–14) show the number of the respective slice (Figs. 1, 2a,b, 3).

5.3 Cerebrospinal-Fluid-Containing Spaces 245

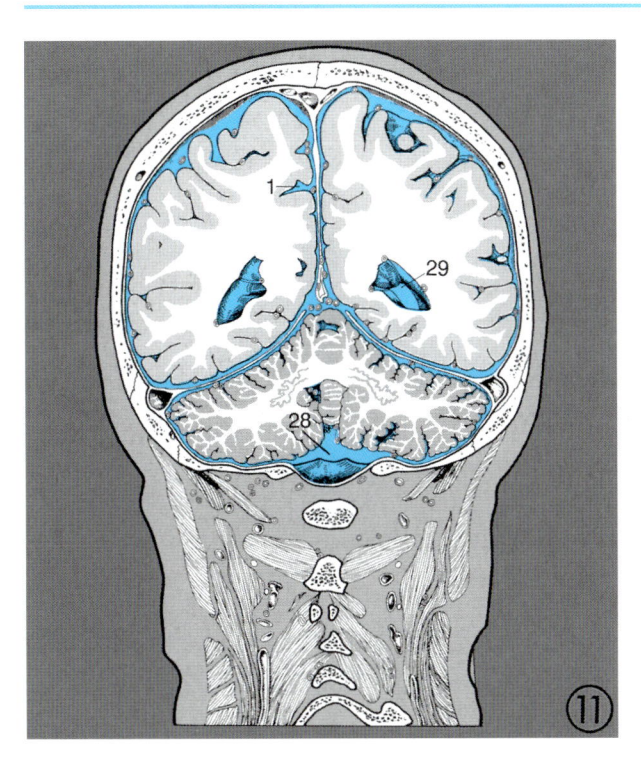

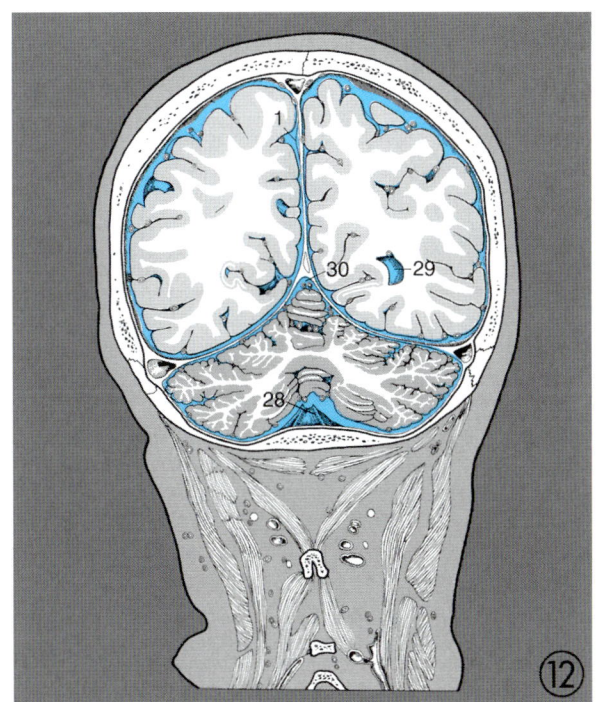

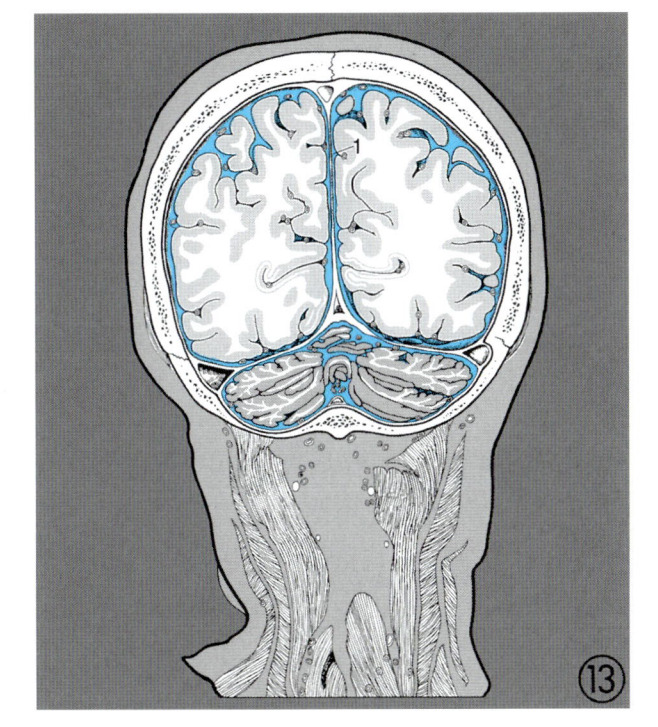

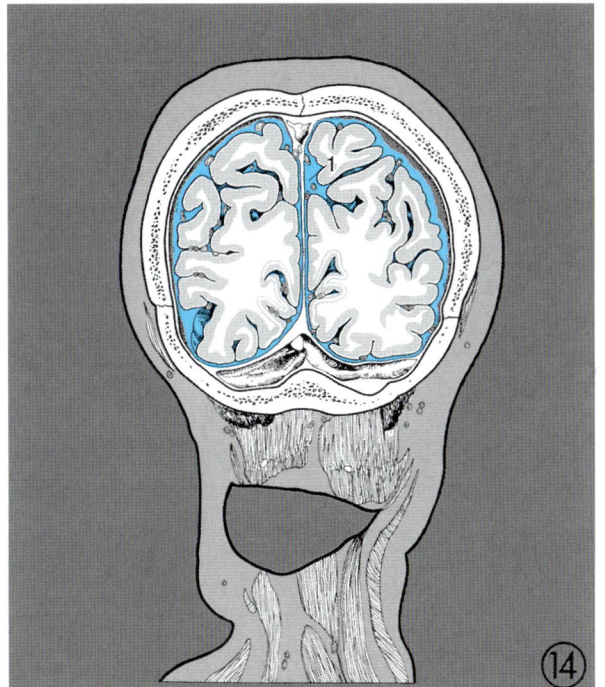

1 Interhemispheric cistern
28 Cisterna magna (posterior cerebellomedullary cistern)
29 Occipital (posterior) horn of lateral ventricle
30 Superior cerebellar cistern

246　　5　Topography of the Neurocranium and its Intracranial Spaces and Structures in Multiplanar Parallel Slices

1　Interhemispheric cistern
2　Pericallosal cistern
3　Interventricular foramen (of Monro)
4　Choroid plexus of third ventricle
5　Cistern of transverse cerebral fissure
6　Suprapineal recess
7　Pineal gland
8　Quadrigeminal cistern (cistern of great cerebral vein)
9　Cistern of lamina terminalis
10　Supraoptic recess
11　Infundibular recess
12　Third ventricle
13　Chiasmatic cistern
14　Interpeduncular cistern
15　Aqueduct of midbrain
16　Superior cerebellar cistern
17　Pontine cistern
18　Fourth ventricle
19　Choroid plexus of fourth ventricle
20　Posterior basal cistern
21　Central canal
22　Cisterna magna (posterior cerebellomedullary cistern)
23　Spinal subarachnoid space
24　Central part (body) of lateral ventricle
25　Frontal (anterior) horn of lateral ventricle
26　Anterior basal cistern
27　Ambient cistern
28　Lateral ventricle
29　Choroid plexus of lateral ventricle
30　Cistern of vallecula cerebri
31　Occipital (posterior) horn
32　Trigeminal cistern
33　Cerebellopontine cistern
34　Atrium of lateral ventricle
35　Temporal (inferior) horn of lateral ventricle

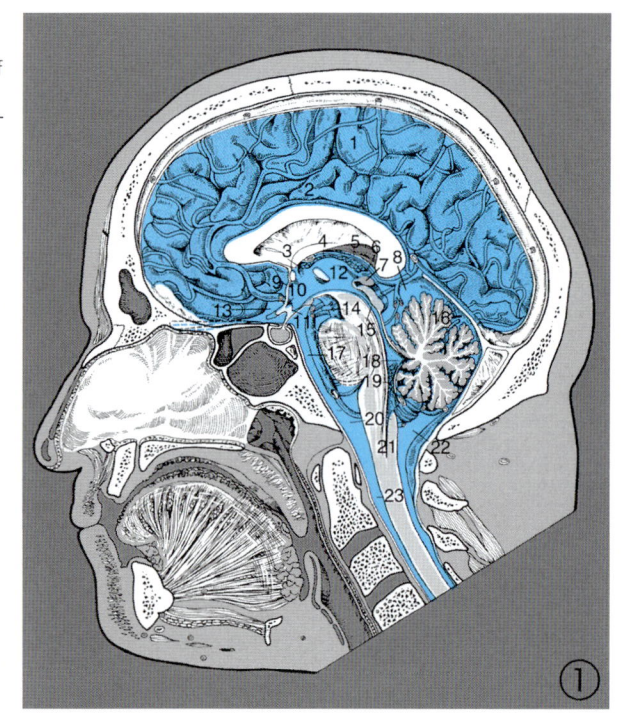

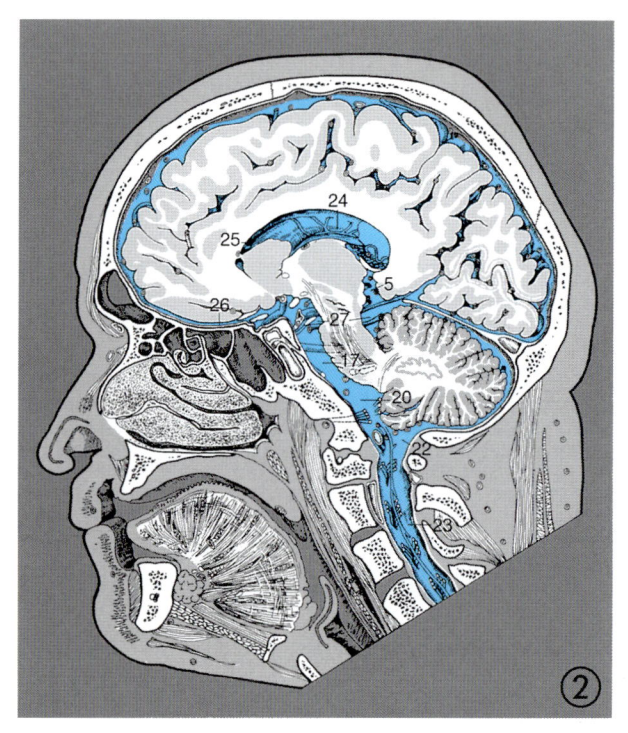

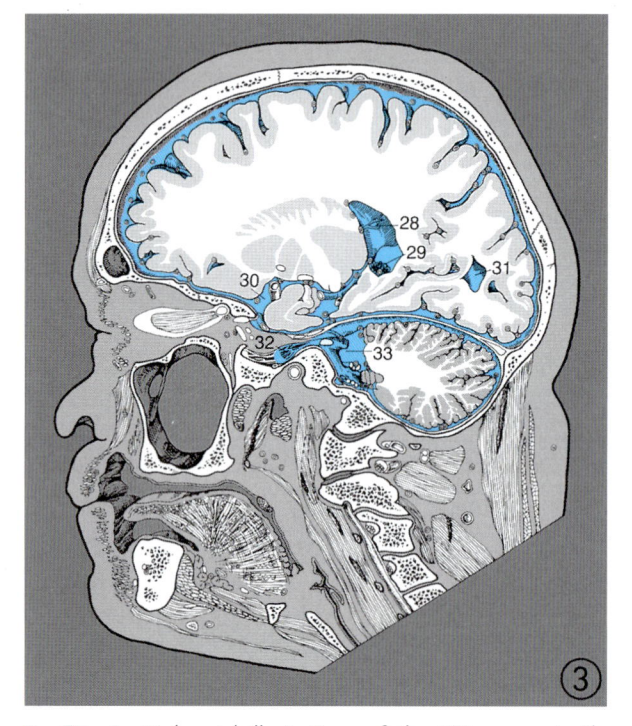

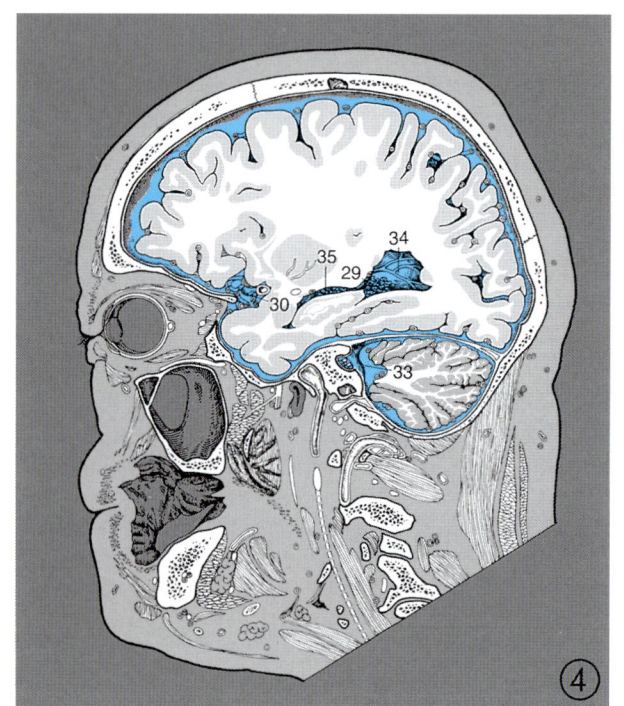

Fig. 85 Sagittal serial illustrations of the CSF spaces in the cranial cavity and in the vertebral canal. The encircled number (1–5) shows the number of the respective slice (Figs. 29, 30a,b, 31).

5.3 Cerebrospinal-Fluid-Containing Spaces

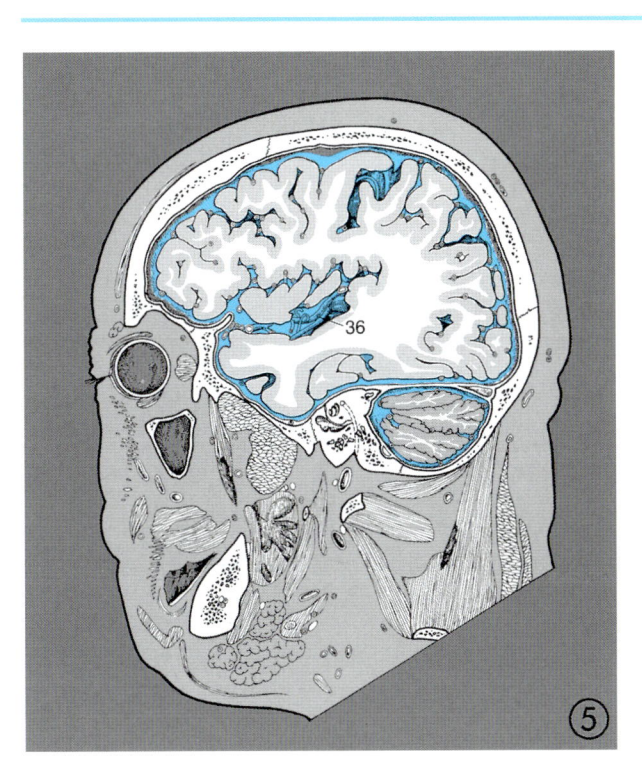

36 Cistern of lateral cerebral fossa (cistern of Sylvian fissure)

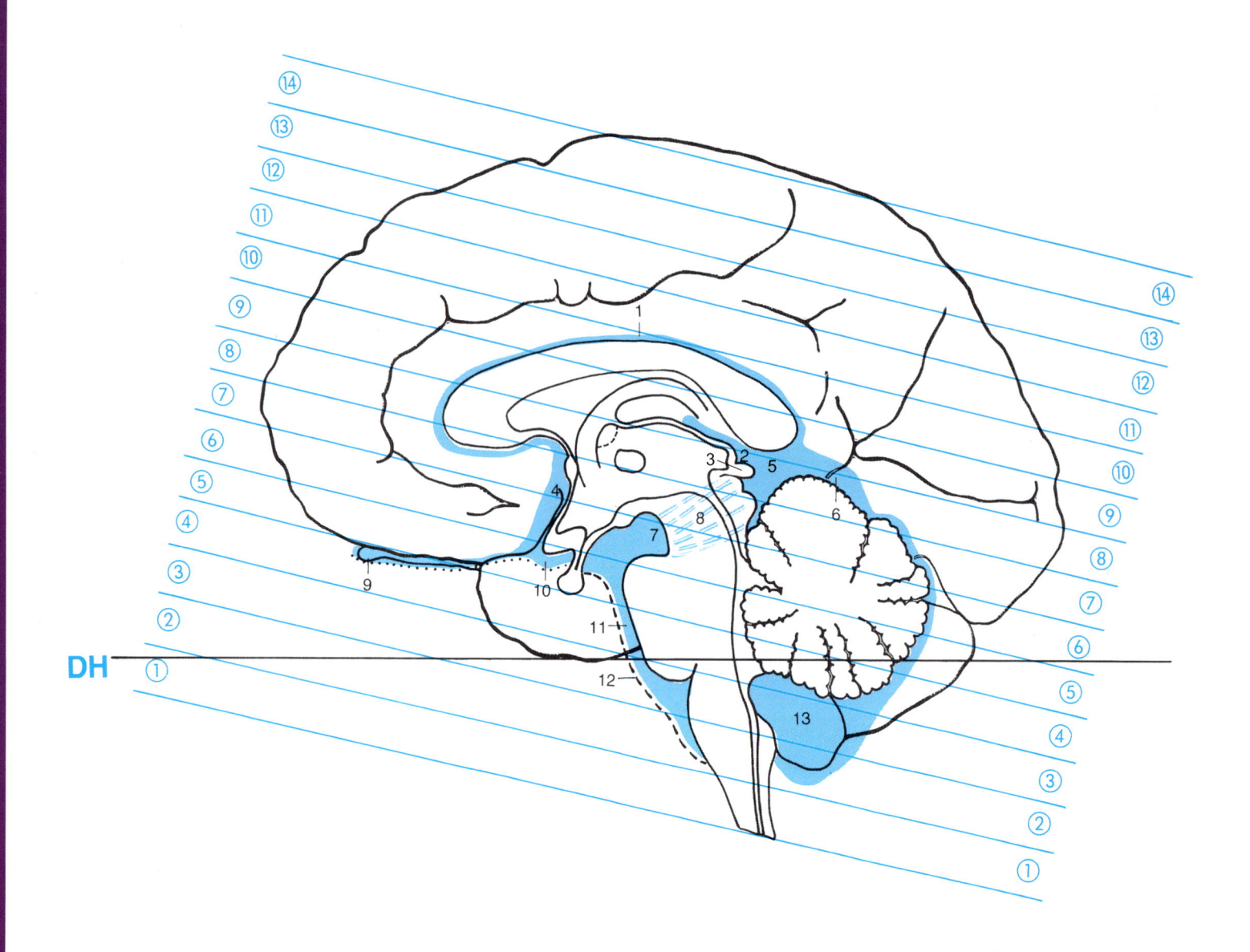

248   5 Topography of the Neurocranium and its Intracranial Spaces and Structures in Multiplanar Parallel Slices

Fig. **86a** Medial view of the external CSF spaces of the canthomeatal series. The ambient cistern encloses the cerebral peduncle laterally. This cistern is, therefore, indicated with a blue dashed line.

1 Pericallosal cistern
2 Cistern of transverse cerebral fissure
3 Pineal gland
4 Cistern of lamina terminalis
5 Quadrigeminal cistern (cistern of great cerebral vein)
6 Superior cerebellar cistern
7 Interpeduncular cistern
8 Ambient cistern
9 Anterior basal cistern (dotted line)
10 Chiasmatic cistern
11 Pontine cistern
12 Posterior basal cistern (black dashed line)
13 Cisterna magna (posterior cerebellomedullary cistern)

5.3 Cerebrospinal-Fluid-Containing Spaces 249

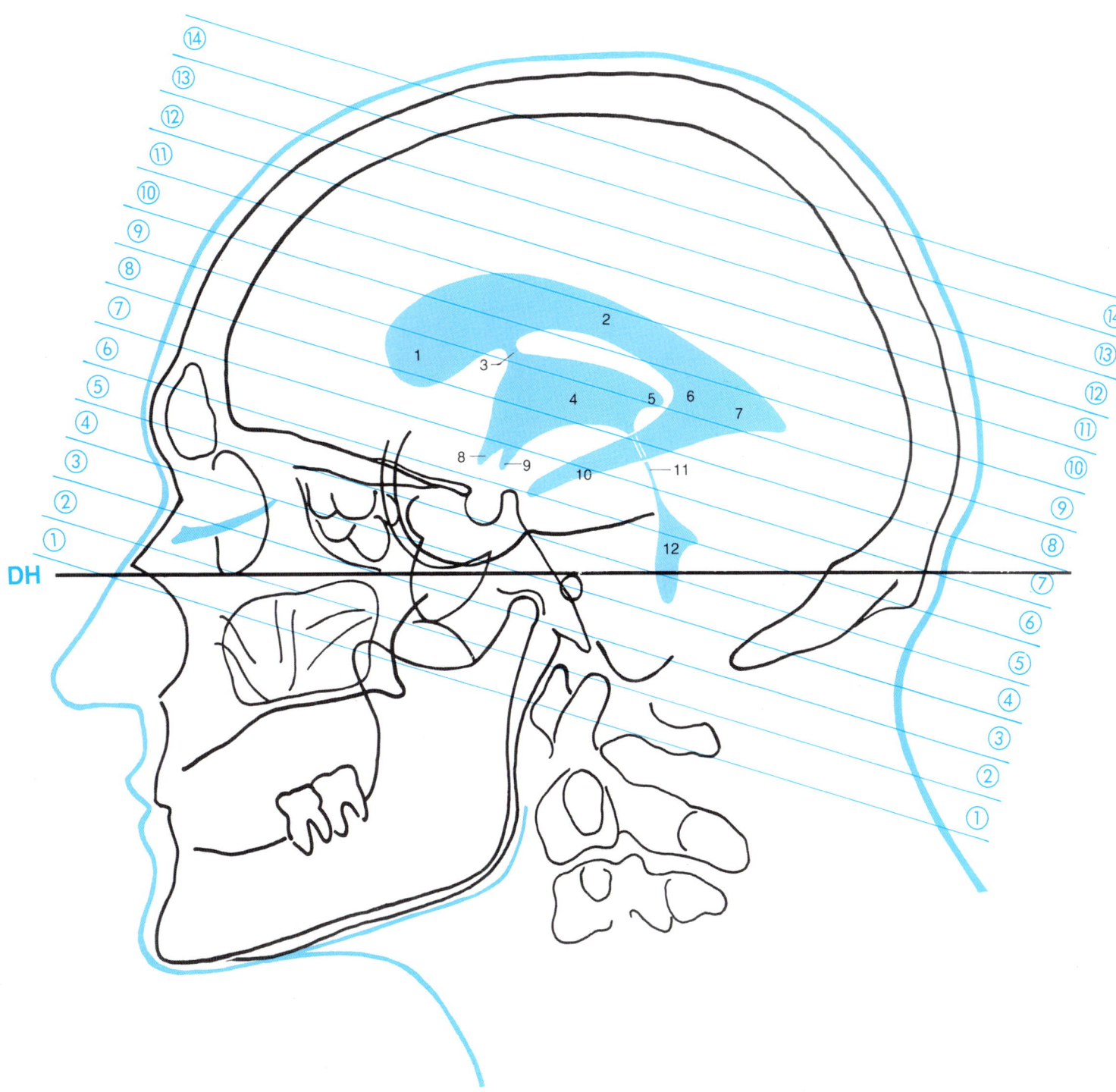

Fig. **86b** Lateral view of the ventricular system derived from a radiograph of the head of the canthomeatal series (Figs. 44, 45a,b, 46).
DH Reid's base line

1 Frontal (anterior) horn of lateral ventricle
2 Central part (body) of lateral ventricle
3 Interventricular foramen (of Monro)
4 Third ventricle
5 Suprapineal recess
6 Atrium of lateral ventricle
7 Occipital (posterior) horn of lateral ventricle
8 Supraoptic recess
9 Infundibular recess
10 Temporal (inferior) horn of lateral ventricle
11 Aqueduct of midbrain
12 Fourth ventricle

1 Posterior basal cistern
2 Cisterna magna (posterior cerebellomedullary cistern)
3 Anterior basal cistern
4 Pontine cistern
5 Trigeminal cistern
6 Cerebellopontine cistern
7 Fourth ventricle
8 Cistern of vallecula cerebri
9 Suprasellar cistern
10 Lateral ventricle

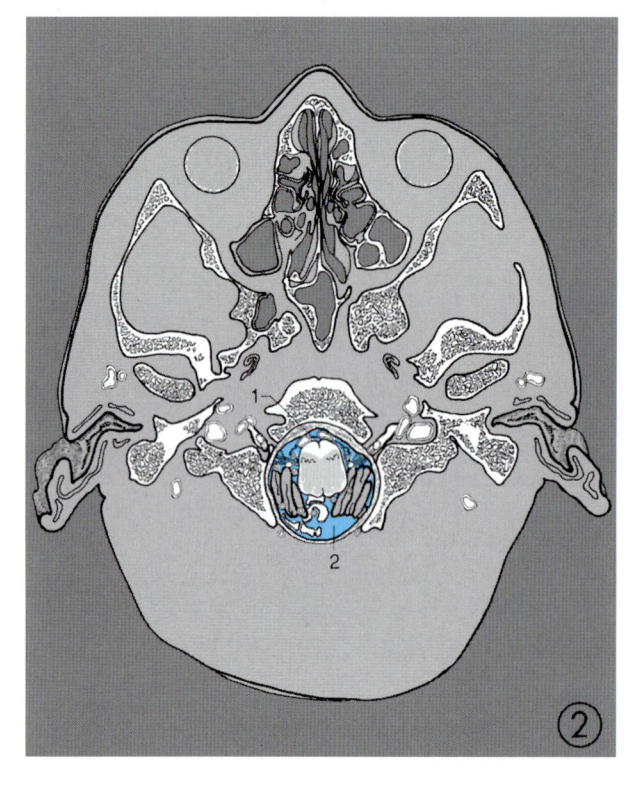

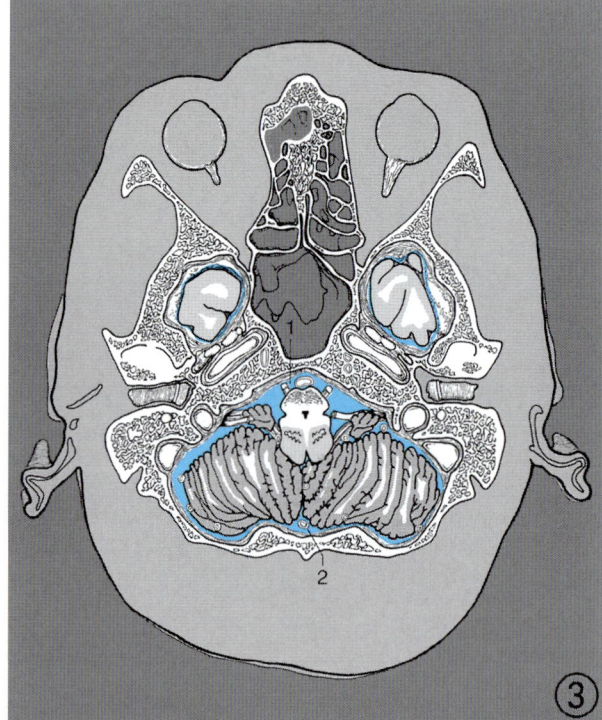

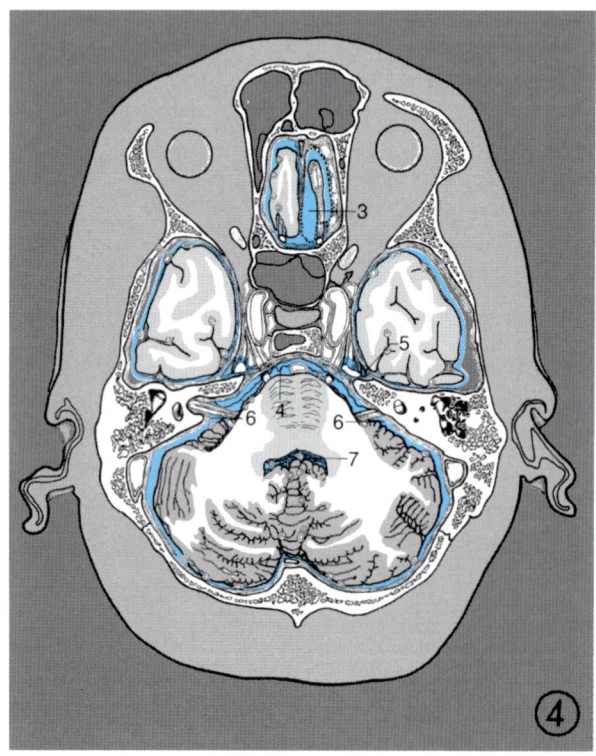

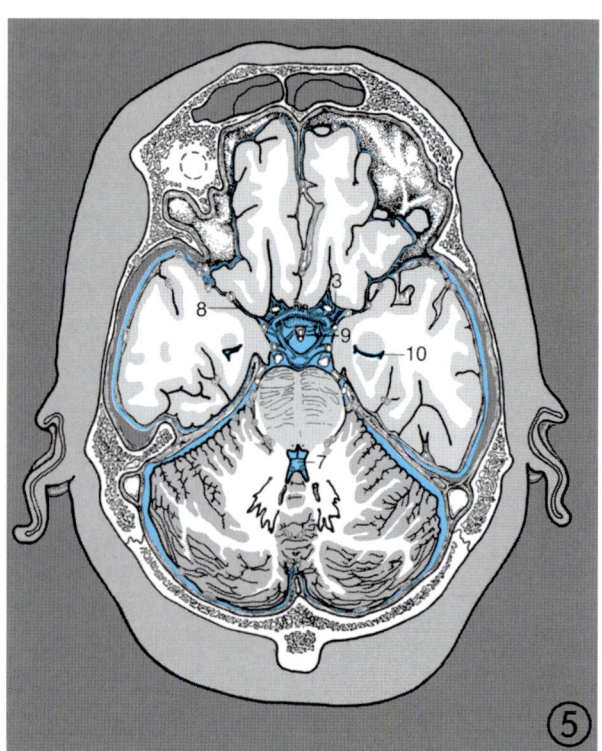

Fig. 87 Canthomeatally oriented serial illustrations of the intracranial CSF spaces. The encircled numbers (2–9) indicate the number of the respective slice (Figs. 44, 45a,b, 46, 86a,b).

5.3 Cerebrospinal-Fluid-Containing Spaces

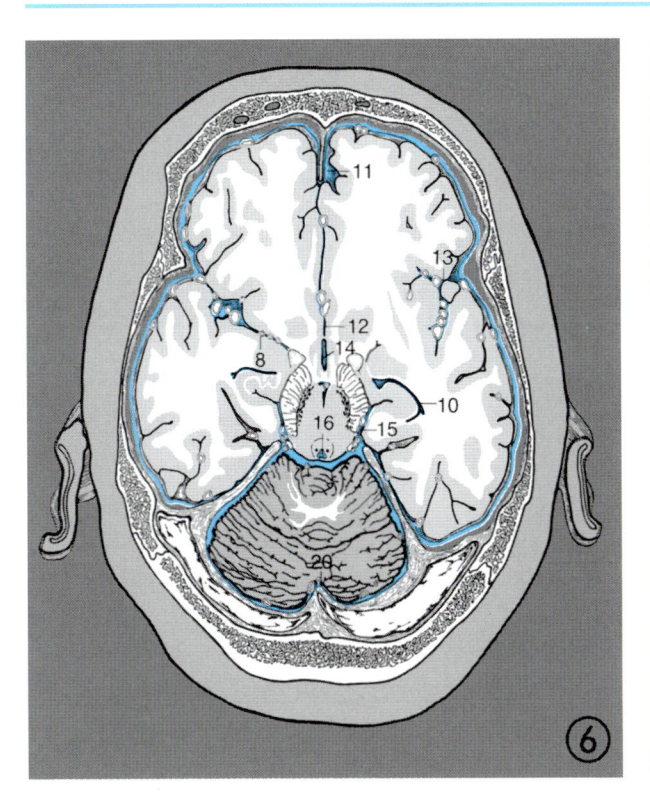

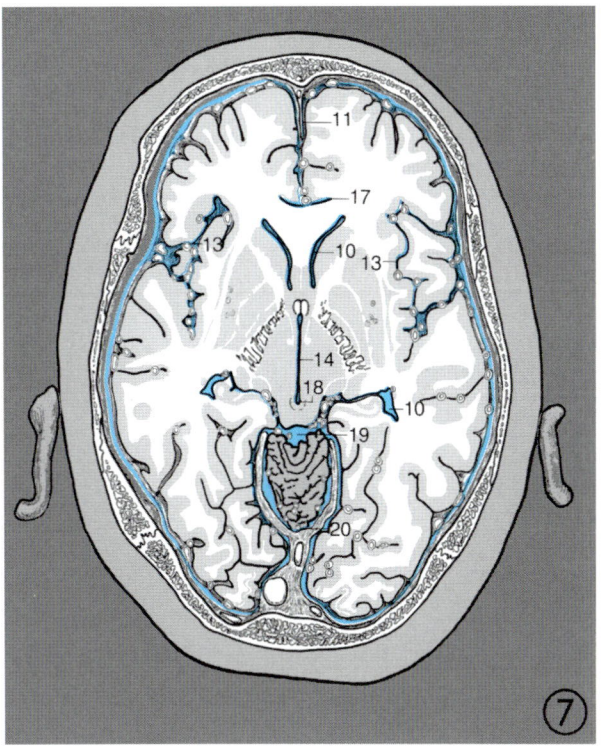

8 Cistern of vallecula cerebri
10 Lateral ventricle
11 Interhemispheric cistern
12 Cistern of lamina terminalis
13 Cistern of lateral cerebral fossa (cistern of Sylvian fissure)
14 Third ventricle
15 Ambient cistern
16 Transition of aqueduct into the fourth ventricle
17 Pericallosal cistern
18 Aqueduct of midbrain
19 Quadrigeminal cistern (cistern of great cerebral vein)
20 Superior cerebellar cistern

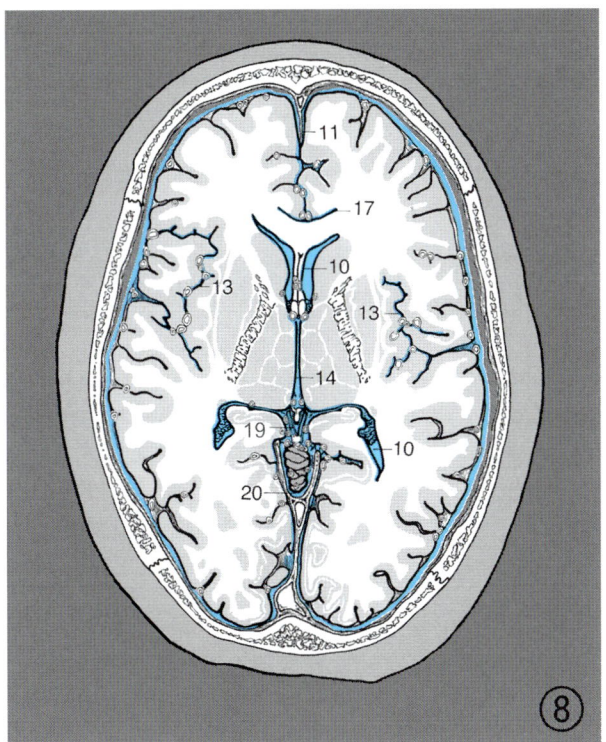

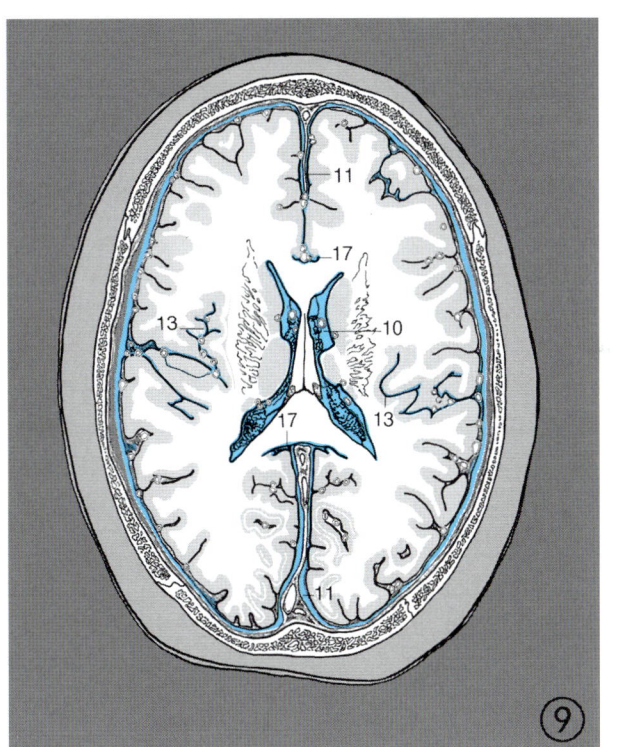

10 Lateral ventricle
11 Interhemispheric cistern
17 Pericallosal cistern

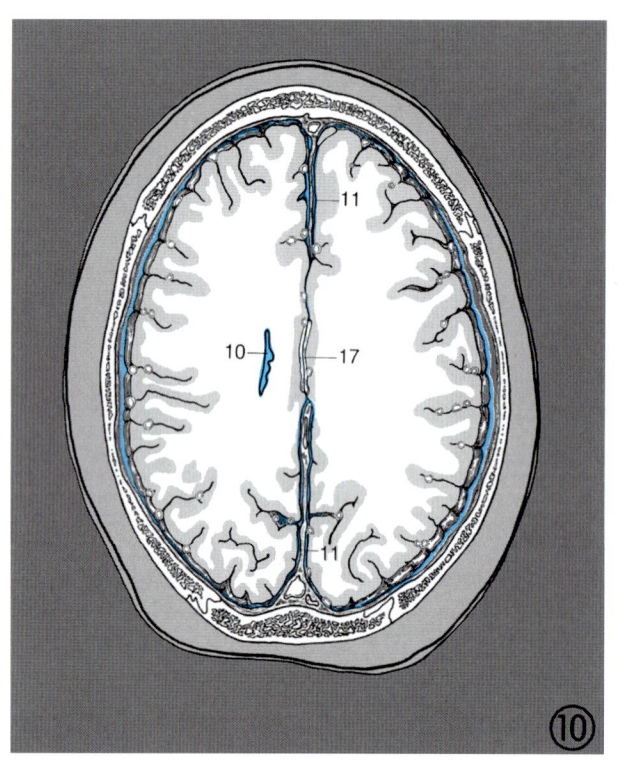

Fig. 87 Canthomeatally oriented serial illustrations of the intracranial CSF spaces. The encircled numbers (10–11) indicate the number of the respective slice (Figs. 44, 45a,b, 46, 86a,b).

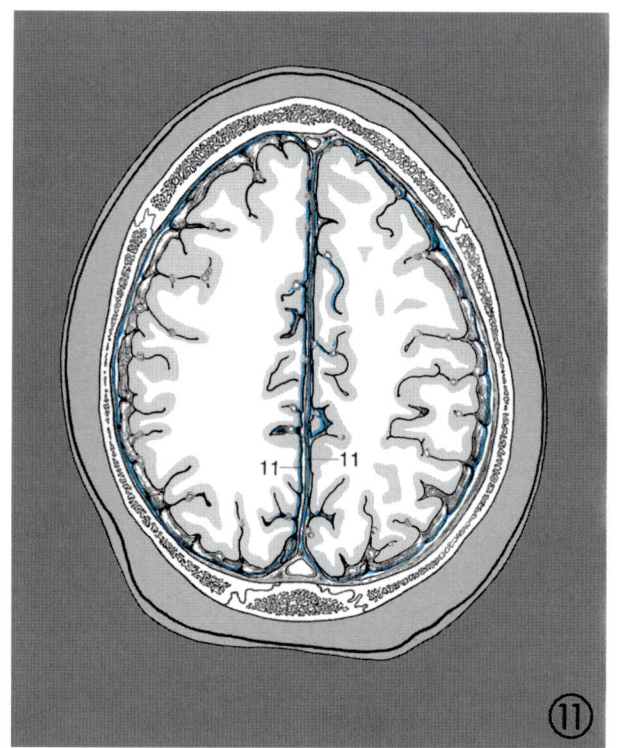

Aqueduct of Midbrain
The aqueduct (approximately 15 mm long) is located in the midbrain (Figs. 2b.30, 12a.23, 32b.22, 52a.33, 52d.17, 53c.17, 85.15). It curves slightly anteriorly, connecting the third ventricle with the fourth.

Third Ventricle
The third ventricle is an unpaired slit-shaped cavity in the median plane. Its walls are formed from its posterior to basal region by the epithalamus (Chap. 5.7.4), thalamus, and hypothalamus. In 75% of brains an interthalamic adhesion (intermediate mass) can be demonstrated between the right and left thalamus. The lamina terminalis forms the anterior boundary of the third ventricle (Figs. 2b.17, 32a.14, 52a.16). In the area near the hypothalamic sulcus, a groove for the anterior commissure can be found. Near the hypothalamus, two additional diverticula can be seen: the supraoptic recess (Fig. 86b.8), leading toward the optic chiasm, and the infundibular recess (Figs. 9a.26, 85.11, 86b.9) directed toward the pituitary stalk.

The choroid plexus appears as a canopy in the third ventricle above the **interventricular foramen (of Monro)**. Connected to the choroid plexus is a thin ependymal lining, the tela choroidea. It stretches between the medullary striae of the thalamus (a tract on the medial margin of the thalamus) and forms a diverticulum above the pineal gland, the suprapineal recess (Fig. 83b.5). A few millimeters below the suprapineal recess is a small niche, the pineal recess. Located anterior to the pineal and below the suprapineal recess is the habenular commissure. The posterior commissure is found underneath the pineal recess, below which the aqueduct leaves the third ventricle (262).

Lateral Ventricles
The two lateral ventricles take the form of two ram's-horn-shaped cavities in the telencephalon. They are linked to each other and to the third ventricle by the interventricular foramina (of Monro). In accordance with the four lobes of the telencephalon, the lateral ventricle is divided into four parts:
1. Frontal or anterior horn, located in the frontal lobe (Figs. 9a.9, 9b.7, 54a.8, 54d.5, 85.25)
2. Central part or body, located in the parietal lobe (Figs. 12a.7, 12b.8, 55c.13, 85.24)
3. Occipital or posterior horn, located in the occipital lobe (Figs. 14a.6, 14b.6, 85.31)
4. Temporal or inferior horn, located in the temporal lobe (Figs. 11a.24, 11b.19, 35a.14, 35d.8, 52a.31).

The **frontal horn** forms the anterior pole of the lateral ventricle and reaches the interventricular foramen (of Monro) (Figs. 2b.11, 10a.13, 54a.22, 54d.13, 83b.3, 85.3). The frontal horn is bordered medially by the septum pellucidum and laterally by the head of the caudate nucleus. The radiation of the corpus callosum forms its roof.

The **central part** of the lateral ventricle is narrow due to the protruding thalamus. The floor of the central part is formed by a narrow strip of ependyma on the superior surface of the thalamus (lamina affixa) and laterally by the body of the caudate nucleus. The roof consists of the corpus callosum. The choroid plexus extends through the interventricular foramen from the medial side into the central part. The central part reaches the splenium of the corpus callosum where it bifurcates into the occipital and temporal horns. The junction of the occipital horn, the temporal horn, and the central part of the lateral ventricle is referred to as the **atrium of lateral ventricle** (Figs. 54b.26, 83b.6, 84.25, 85.34, 86b.6). The collateral trigone is a triangular area at the beginning of the temporal horn that lies in close topographic relationship to the deep collateral sulcus.

The **occipital horn** is covered by a radiation of the corpus callosum, the major (occipital) forceps. An inward curvature on the medial wall of the occipital horn, the calcarine spur, is caused by the calcarine sulcus.

The **temporal horn** deviates from the collateral trigone in a small curve in a laterobasal direction. Located on its roof is the tail of caudate nucleus. The amygdaloid body (amygdala) (Figs. 9b.20, 10a.27, 35a.21, 51a.12, 51b.11, 52a.21) is found at the tip of the temporal horn. The choroid plexus enters the temporal horn on the medial side and extends to the fimbria of hippocampus. Mediobasally, the temporal horn is bordered by the hippocampus (Figs. 10a.30, 10d.22, 35a.22, 35b.9, 52a.24, 52b.16) with its alveus protruding into the horn (Fig. 52a.23).

Clinical Notes
Despite the large interindividual and very variable width and configuration of the ventricle system and the CSF-containing cisterns, these spaces are of significance for the detection and assessment of pathologic intracranial processes. Asymmetries of the lateral ventricles, deformation of a ventricle wall or several ventricles, variable width of the outer and inner fluid spaces, or disproportion of the width of the supratentorial positioned ventricle with the size of the fourth ventricle give the examiner an indication of the clinical findings and aid with the topical and functional diagnostic orientation: obstructive hydrocephalus, malresorptive hydrocephalus, hypersecretory hydrocephalus, external and internal hydrocephalus, hydrocephalus e vacuo. Further references (17, 129a, 185, 253, 374a, 375, 403, 409, 471b, 502).

5.4 Arteries of the Brain and their Vascular Territories (Figs. 88–96)

The blood vessels of the brain are only inadequately demonstrated in routine CT and MR scans, so that in dealing with particular problems cerebral **CT angiography (CTA)** or **MR angiography (MRA)** may still be necessary. This is true for vascular disorders, for the differential diagnosis of tumors, and for operation planning. Some specific cases require **cerebral angiography**. CT and MRI depict the pathologic changes caused by vascular disorders and any lesions developing in the brain such as edema, infarction, hemorrhage, or hydrocephalus. Therefore, very often the topographic anatomy of the cerebral arteries derived from the angiographic anteroposterior and lateral projections has to be correlated three-dimensionally with results from the new imaging techniques. For this reason, we have compared the diagrams of angiograms and their most common arterial variations with the arteries as shown in the brain sections.

Occlusions of major brain arteries—basilar and middle cerebral arteries—may be seen on CT studies by hyperdensity in the vascular lumen and with MRI by the absence of blood flow. **Occlusions of the middle-sized brain arteries** are seen in CT only some hours later, shown by hypodense areas and in some cases by a faint cortex–medullary border in the arterial supply area. Intracranial hemorrhages are seen immediately in CT. Special MR sequences are required in imaging to detect intracranial hemorrhages during the first few hours. In cerebral ischemia MRI has a greater sensitivity than CT because the brain infarct can be diagnosed earlier and the brainstem and cerebellum are better visualized. The extension and size of the hypodensity in CT, the abnormal signal in MRI as correlate of the edema and infarct, are determined not only by the size of the occluded vessels, but also by the available **collateral circulation**. Aneurysms are only shown in CT if their diameter is above 5–10 mm. In these cases, as well as for diagnosing angiomas, it is usually necessary to inject contrast medium. With precontrast MRI, angiomas are shown by a flow phenomenon.

Over the past few decades, a number of thorough studies showing the **variability of the arteries** of the brain have been completed (111, 145, 157, 238, 264, 265, 474). Clinicians, however, have only partially adopted the international anatomic nomenclature and, as a result, synonyms are often used in publications. For this reason, in addition to the Terminologia Anatomica, synonyms are included in parentheses in this text.

Many of the anatomic **names for the arteries** of the brain are more than 100 years old. In many instances, a single conspicuous topographic feature was chosen as the basis for these names (29). For example, "cerebellar" arteries, which branch on the cerebellum, send important circumferential branches to parts of the medulla oblongata, pons, and midbrain. As a result, proximal occlusion of a cerebellar artery may lead to dysfunction in one or more of these four divisions of the brain.

Vertebral Artery

The vertebral artery (Fig. 88.1) emerges from the atlas through the transverse foramen and runs initially in a dorsal direction before turning into the groove for this artery on the atlas (Fig. 47a.24). In this way, a "reserve loop" of the artery is formed, allowing for free movement of the head. This portion of the vertebral artery can be seen in the lateral view of an angiogram as the V3 segment.

The vertebral artery extends diagonally from its groove, through the atlanto-occipital membrane, the dura mater, and the arachnoid mater. At this last point the atlanto-occipital sinus is attached to the ampulloglomerular organ, most likely a receptor apparatus for vascular reflexes. The vertebral artery continues in an arch and finally reaches the medulla oblongata (Figs. 11c.25, 12c.21, 32c.31, 48c.15). The intracranial portion of the artery is referred to as the V4 segment. The **junction** of the left and right vertebral arteries, forming the basilar artery, is located at the inferior edge of the pons in two-thirds of cases. In the remaining third, this junction is found anteriorly on the superior portion of the medulla oblongata. In the V4 segment the right or the left vertebral artery may be somewhat wider than its fellow, or may take the form of a loop (Figs. 70c.6, 70d.6, 71c.4, 71d.4).

Angiographic examination of the **vertebral artery** can demonstrate branches, namely the anterior spinal artery and the posterior inferior cerebellar artery (PICA). Just before the junction with its fellow, the vertebral artery gives off the **anterior spinal artery** that runs in a mediocaudal direction. In 77% of cases, the right and left arteries form an unpaired median anterior spinal artery approximately 2–3 cm from their origin (264). In 20% of cases the anterior spinal artery is unilaterally absent, and in about 13% the paired branches do not join. Paramedian branches arise from the anterior spinal artery and extend toward the medulla oblongata.

The **posterior inferior cerebellar artery (PICA)** (Figs. 12c.20, 33c.25, 48c.18) generally arises intracranially from the vertebral artery, but in 18% of cases it arises extracranially caudal to the foramen magnum. In about 10% of all patients examined, the PICA arises not from the vertebral artery but from the basilar artery. The PICA is unilaterally absent in 10% of cases. A bilateral absence is recorded in only 2% of cases (264). This cerebellar artery takes a highly variable route along the lateral edge of the medulla oblongata (238, 264). The PICA sends fine branches into the anterolateral and lateral, and partially the posterior, territories of the medulla oblongata, where the nucleus ambiguus and other structures including the central sympathetic pathway, the spinal tract of the trigeminal nerve, and the spinothalamic tract are located (Figs. 69b.24, 69b.28, 70b.17, 70b.31, 71b.16, 72b.17). The PICA continues and occasionally forms loops on or around the cerebellar tonsil. In 18% of cases, the PICA lies caudal to the foramen magnum (238), so low caudal localization does not necessarily indicate brain edema complicated by a downward shift of the tonsil of cerebellum. One branch of this cerebellar artery extends into the choroid plexus of the fourth ventricle. The last portion of the PICA is located on the inferior surface of the cerebellum and branches into two directions: one branch supplies the inferior surface of the vermis and the other the inferior surface of the cerebellar hemisphere including a small part of the dentate nucleus.

Basilar Artery

The basilar artery is formed by the union of the vertebral arteries. Located in the basilar sulcus of the pons, the basilar artery runs superiorly through the pontine cistern and into the interpeduncular cistern (Figs. 10c.17, 32b.25, 32c.25, 49c.11, 50b.12, 50c.12, 51c.14). It is 15 to 40 mm long, averaging 32 mm. In 51% of cases the superior end of the basilar artery has been found to lie at the level of the dorsum sellae, in 30% above it, and in 19% below it (238). The artery forms a right or left concave arch in 10% of cases. This arch is usually combined with a wider contralateral vertebral artery and is assumed therefore to be the result of existing hemodynamic factors (178). This curved course is not to be confused with a pathologic displacement due to a space-occupying process.

Branches of the basilar artery are:
- Pontine arteries (these fine branches are not cut in our sections and hence are not included in the illustrations)
- Anterior inferior cerebellar artery (AICA) (Figs. 32c.29, 49c.15, 50c.18)
- Superior cerebellar artery (Figs. 10c.18, 32c.22, 51c.16)
- Posterior cerebral artery (Figs. 10c.13, 32c.21, 51c.13).

The **pontine arteries**, in most cases about eight, arise almost at right angles from the basilar artery. Their medial branches supply the anteromedial, their lateral branches the anterolateral and partially the lateral territories of the pons. Generally the pontine arteries are not seen in angiograms.

The **anterior inferior cerebellar artery (AICA)** has been found to originate in 52% of cases from the inferior third of the basilar artery. In 46% of cases it arises from the middle third and in 2% from the upper third of the basilar artery. Exceptionally, the AICA arises from the vertebral artery. In 10% of cases there is a duplication of the AICA on one side, in approximately 1% of cases it is unilaterally absent, and only

5.4 Arteries of the Brain and their Vascular Territories

1. Vertebral artery
2. Variation of posterior inferior cerebellar artery (PICA)
3. Posterior inferior cerebellar artery (PICA)
4. Basilar artery
5. Anterior inferior cerebellar artery (AICA)
6. Superior cerebellar artery
7. Origin of posterior cerebral artery
8. Posterior communicating artery
9. Internal carotid artery

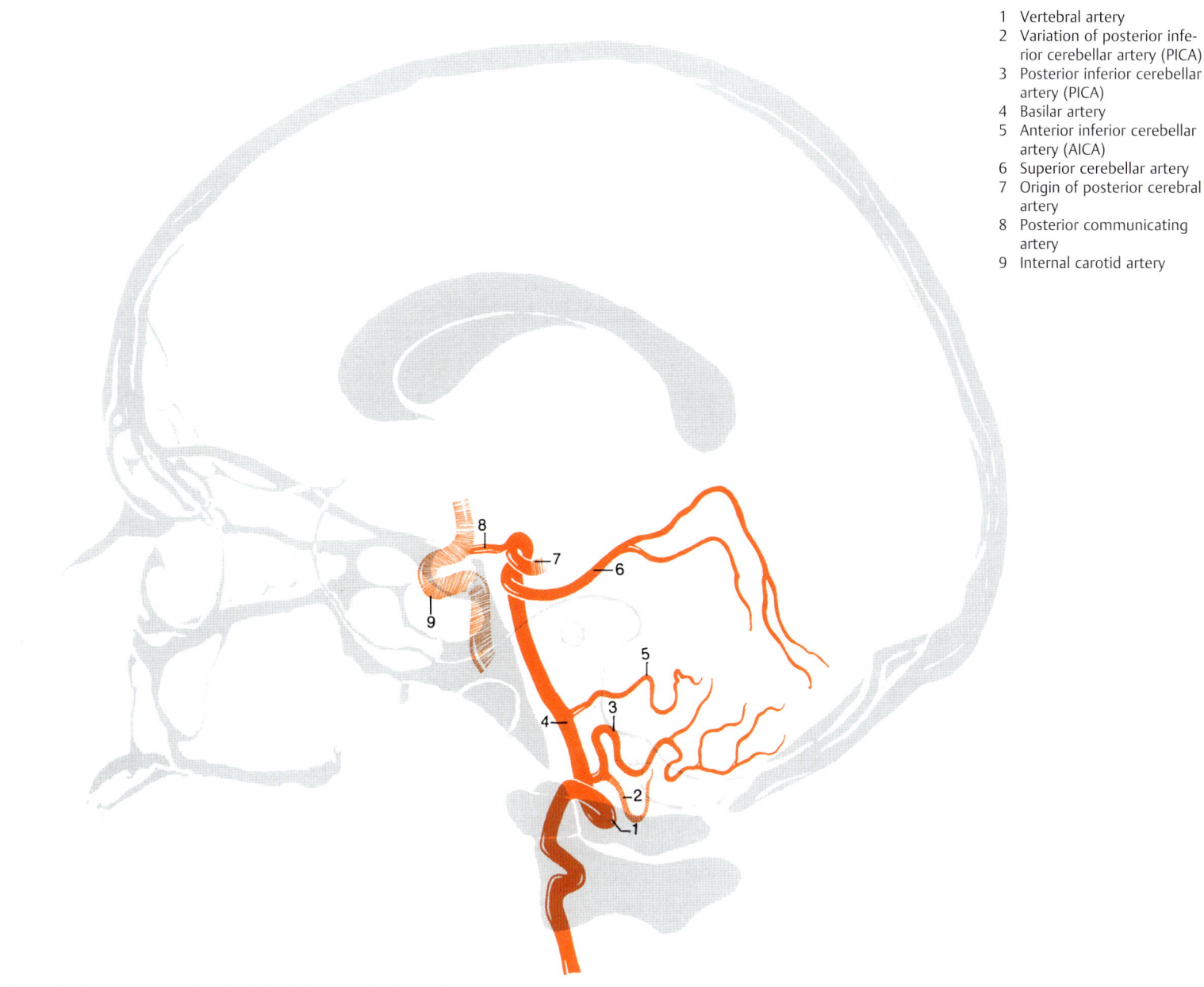

Fig. 88 Lateral view of the infratentorial arterial tree with its connection to the internal carotid artery. According to (238).

rarely is it bilaterally absent. The first part of the AICA usually extends lateroinferiorly over the pons and gives off a few fine branches. It then continues as a loop from which, in approximately 70% of cases, the labyrinthine artery arises. In the remaining instances, the labyrinthine artery emerges directly from the basilar artery. The AICA either crosses the flocculus (H X) or encircles and supplies it with fine branches. From this floccular portion of the artery, additional fine branches extend into the medulla oblongata and the middle cerebellar peduncle of the pons. The hemispheric branches of the AICA supply the inferior surface of the cerebellum as well as the choroid plexus of the fourth ventricle.

The **superior cerebellar artery** is the most form-constant cerebellar artery. It arises from the basilar artery just before its terminal bifurcation. In about 4% of cases, this cerebellar artery arises from the posterior cerebral artery (265). In about 10% of cases, the superior cerebellar artery is duplicated on both sides. The superior cerebellar artery gives off fine branches to the posterior territory of the pons, the superior cerebellar peduncle, and partly to the posterior territory of the midbrain. Wider branches reach the superior surface of the cerebellum. The cerebellar arteries of each side are commonly joined through anastomoses.

In the case of an aplasia of a cerebellar artery, the group of cerebellar arteries has the ability of partial or complete compensation. With an aplasia of the PICA, for instance, the AICA and the superior cerebellar artery take over the blood supply to the inferior surface of the cerebellum. In 60% of cases, one PICA can independently supply the inferior surface of the cerebellum. The PICA is supplemented in 26% of cases by the AICA and in 3% by the superior cerebellar artery. The superior surface of the cerebellum, on the other hand, is supplied in 67% of cases by the superior cerebellar artery. The AICA and the PICA supplement the superior cerebellar artery (264).

Posterior Cerebral Artery

The posterior cerebral arteries (Figs. 89a.6, 10c.13, 32c.21, 33d.15, 51c.13, 52b.15, 91d.16) arise, in 90% of cases, as the terminal bifurcation of the basilar artery and reach into the interpeduncular cistern between the cerebral peduncles and the clivus. In the other 10% a **fetal type** is present, in which the posterior cerebral artery forms an extension of the posterior communicating artery. In this instance, the posterior cerebral artery is, in fact, a branch of the internal carotid artery. The portion of the posterior cerebral artery between the basilar and the posterior communicating artery is referred to as the **precommunicating part** of the posterior cerebral artery. It ranges from 3 to 9 mm in length, averaging 6 mm. The midbrain and diencephalon are partially supplied by small penetrating branches of the precommunicating part (collicular artery, posteromedial and posterolateral central arteries; Fig. 89a.7). These fine arterial branches are seldom visible in angiograms (265).

The **postcommunicating part** of the posterior cerebral artery arches around the midbrain and lies in the ambient cistern. Small penetrating arteries (posterolateral central arteries; Fig. 89a.7) of the postcommunicating part of the posterior cerebral artery supply the tectum of the midbrain, posterior parts of the thalamus, and the pineal gland. The posterior medial and posterior lateral choroidal arteries arise at the beginning of the postcommunicating part of the posterior cerebral artery (Fig. 52c.14). They run between the quadrigeminal plate and the parahippocampal gyrus and supply the choroid plexus of the third and lateral ventricles. In addition, fine branches run to the quadrigeminal plate, pineal gland, and to other portions of the diencephalon. Several branches reach the lateral and medial geniculate bodies, the posterior side of the thalamus, and the parahippocampal gyrus. Between one and four hemispheric branches of the posterior cerebral artery supply the parahippocampal gyrus, the hippocampal formation, and parts of the splenium of the corpus callosum. In patients with cerebral edema the tentorium of cerebellum may strangulate branches of the parahippocampal arteries because of transtentorial herniation. As a result, the sector (of Sommer) of the hippocampal formation usually degenerates. Additional hemispheric branches of the parahippocampal arteries run toward the inferior side of the temporal lobe.

Underneath the pulvinar thalami and above the tentorium of cerebellum, the posterior cerebral artery divides into two hemispheric branches: the **medial occipital artery** (Figs. 12c.13, 33c.16, 52c.12, 53c.15, 54c.21) and the **lateral occipital artery** (Figs. 12c.15, 34c.15, 52c.13, 53c.18). The division of the posterior cerebral artery into two approximately equal-sized main branches generally takes place at the most lateral point of the cerebral peduncles. This division is usually a bifurcation, sometimes a trifurcation, and only occasionally a quadrifurcation (265).

The **lateral occipital artery** reaches over the posterior section of the parahippocampal gyrus supplying the inferior surface of the occipital lobe. The **medial occipital artery** runs beneath the splenium of the corpus callosum and crosses the isthmus of the cingulate gyrus (152). The artery divides into its terminal branches, namely the parieto-occipital and calcarine arteries. The parieto-occipital artery (Figs. 15c.7, 32c.14, 55c.21, 56c.16) runs, for the most part, in the sulcus of the same name and supplies the cuneus and precuneus. The **calcarine artery** (Figs. 15c.11, 32c.15, 54c.22, 55c.23) lies on or in the calcarine sulcus. It arises only occasionally from the lateral occipital artery. The primary visual cortex is completely supplied by the calcarine artery in only 25% of all cases (433). In the remainder, the visual cortex is partially supplied by neighboring arteries. Vascular occlusions of the calcarine artery can give rise to a homonymous hemianopia. The macula can be spared if a neighboring artery sufficiently supplies the portion of the striate area that lies at the posterior margin and has a point-to-point connection with the macula lutea.

Arterial Territories of the Brainstem and Cerebellum (Fig. 89b)

Despite all the **anastomoses** between brain arteries so far described (238), the sudden occlusion of a large artery will lead to ischemic brain infarction. Usually the supply through neighboring collaterals does not suffice. Arterial territories can be defined.

The clinical symptoms of an arterial occlusion depend on the neurofunctional systems that are affected. Knowledge of the topography of arterial territories and neurofunctional systems is necessary, therefore, for the evaluation of neurovascular disorders.

The arteries supplying the **brainstem** consist mainly of thin branches that lead directly from the larger arteries to supply mostly four territories (111, 456). The arteries of the brainstem vascularize:
- anteromedial,
- anterolateral,
- lateral,
- posterior territories.

The posterior territory is absent in the upper third of the medulla oblongata and the lower two-thirds of the pons.

The borders of these territories are variable and not identical to those of the neurofunctional systems. Long nuclei and wide fiber paths often lie in the region of two neighboring arterial territories. For example, the medial lemniscus system (Figs. 69b.29, 69b.30, 73b.17, 77b.23, 113) courses from the medulla

5.4 Arteries of the Brain and their Vascular Territories

1 Vertebral artery
2 Origin of posterior inferior cerebellar artery (PICA)
3 Basilar artery
4 Origin of anterior inferior cerebellar artery (AICA)
5 Origin of superior cerebellar artery
6 Posterior cerebral artery
7 Posteromedial and posterolateral central arteries
8 Posterior medial and posterior lateral choroidal arteries
9 Medial occipital artery
10 Parieto-occipital artery
11 Calcarine artery
12 Lateral occipital artery
13 Temporal arteries
14 Posterior communicating artery
15 Internal carotid artery

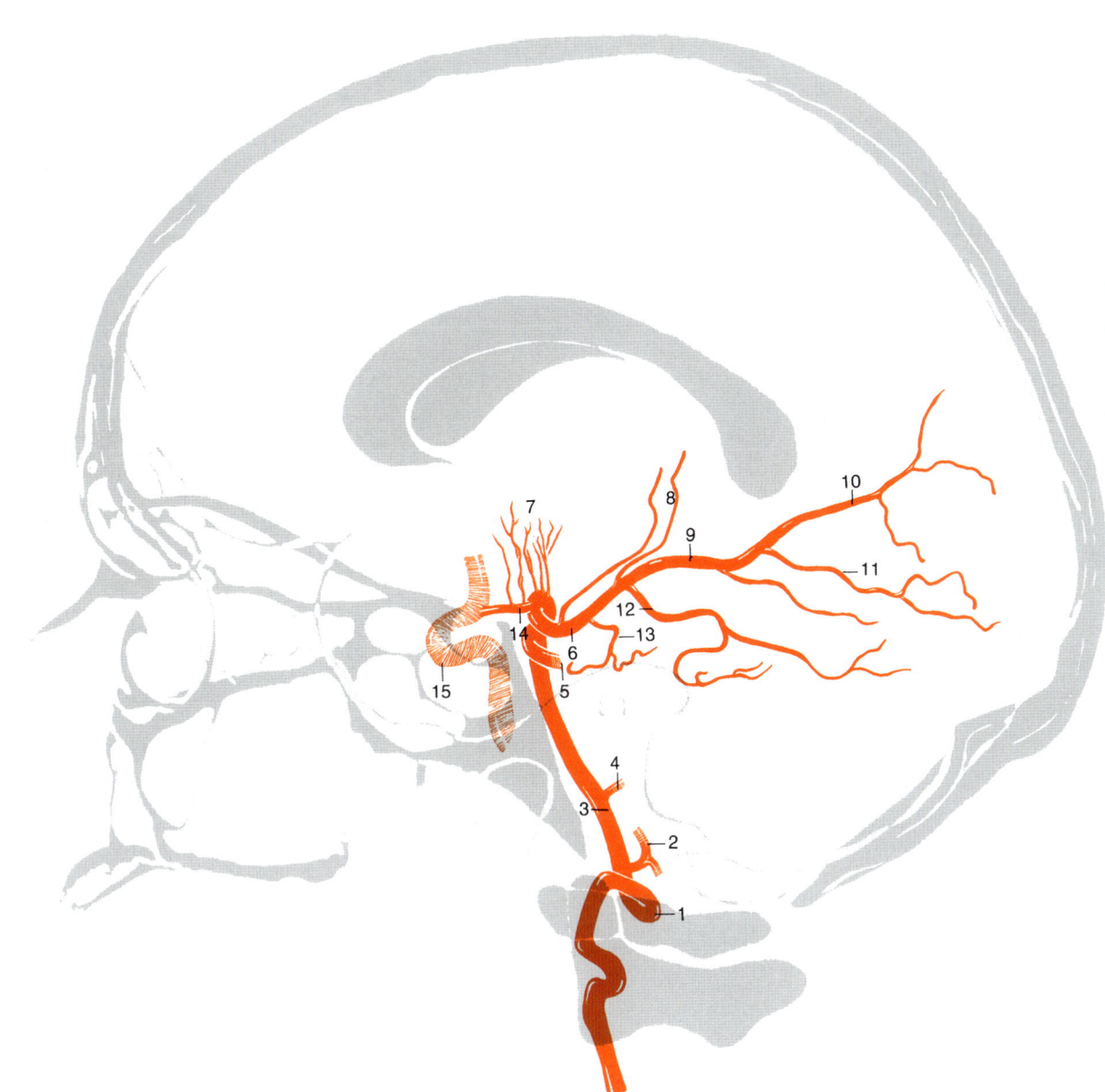

Fig. 89a Lateral view of the posterior cerebral artery. According to (238).

oblongata to the midbrain through a posterior, lateral, anterolateral, and anteromedial territory and, finally, through pairs of territories (anteromedial and lateral, anterolateral and lateral). Following color injection in the arteries of the brainstem, a marked difference can be seen between both sides of these territories, also between the left and right halves of the same brainstem (111).

Arterial Territories of the Medulla Oblongata
The medulla oblongata is for the most part supplied by the branches from the anterior spinal artery, the vertebral artery, the PICA, and the two posterior spinal arteries. Thin branches of the basilar artery and the AICA vascularize a small lateral part of the medulla oblongata close to the pontomedullar junction.

Thin branches of the anterior spinal artery penetrate the surface of the anterior median fissure and branch out into the **anteromedial territory** of both sides. In the upper quarter of the medulla oblongata the branches of the vertebral artery also supply the anteromedial territory. This territory contains the medial part of the corticospinal fibers (Figs. 69b.21, 70b.12, 71b.10, 72b.9), a large part of the medial lemniscus (Figs. 70b.14, 71b.13, 72b.11), the medial longitudinal fasciculus (Figs. 69b.22, 70b.19, 71b.20, 72b.16), most of the hypoglossal nucleus (Figs. 70b.24, 71b.25), and the prepositus nucleus (Fig. 72b.22).

The **anterolateral territory** is vascularized by branches of the anterior spinal artery, the vertebral artery, and the PICA. This territory comprises the lateral part of the corticospinal fibers (Figs. 69b.21, 70b.12, 71b.10, 72b.9), a small part of the medial lemniscus, medial parts of the inferior olivary nucleus (Figs. 70b.16, 71b.14, 72b.14), and the reticular formation.

258   5 Topography of the Neurocranium and its Intracranial Spaces and Structures in Multiplanar Parallel Slices

Arterial territories of the medulla oblongata: penetrating arteries of
- anteromedial: Anterior spinal artery
- anterolateral: Anterior spinal artery, Vertebral artery, Posterior inferior cerebellar artery (PICA)
- lateral: Posterior inferior cerebellar artery (PICA)
- posterior: Posterior spinal artery

Arterial territories of the cerebellum
- Lateral branch of posterior inferior cerebellar artery (PICA)
- Medial branch of posterior inferior cerebellar artery (PICA)

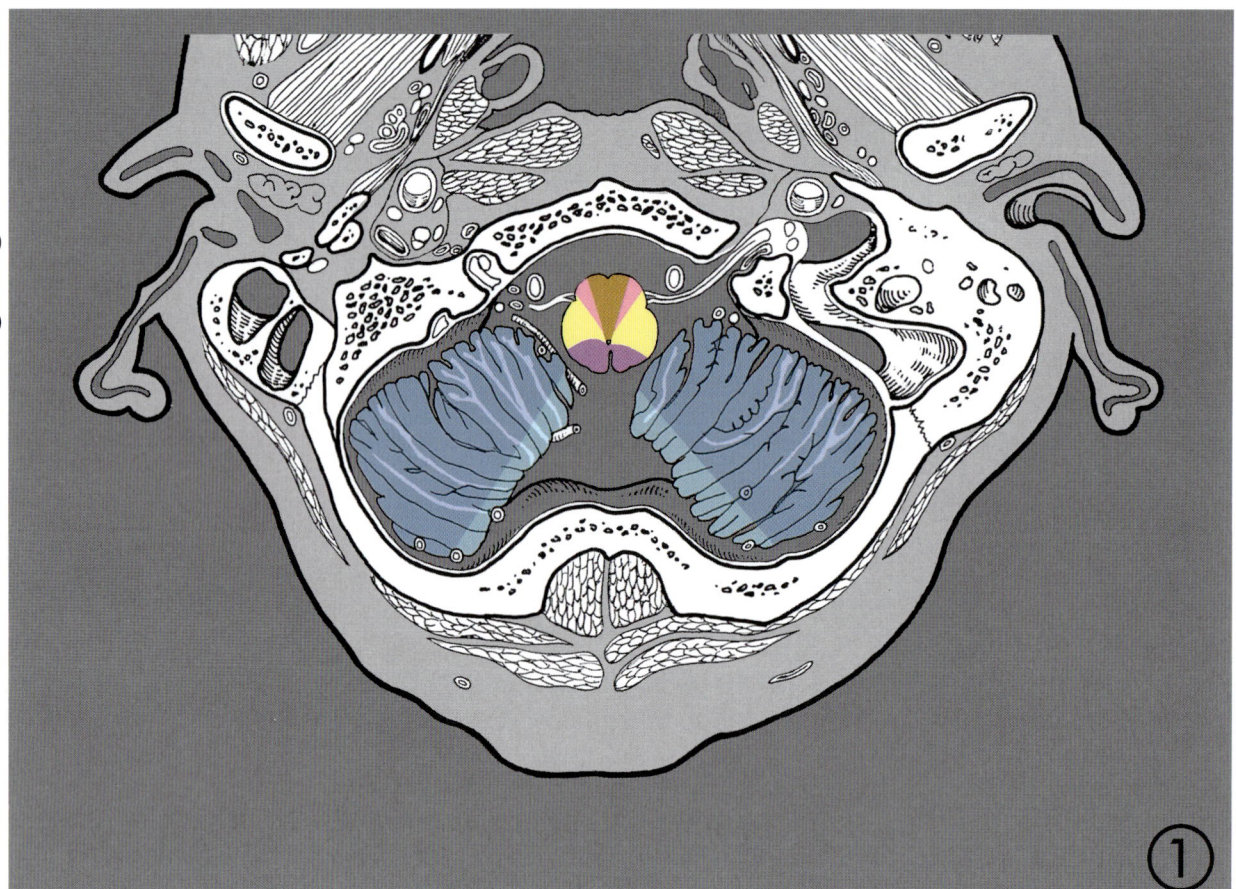

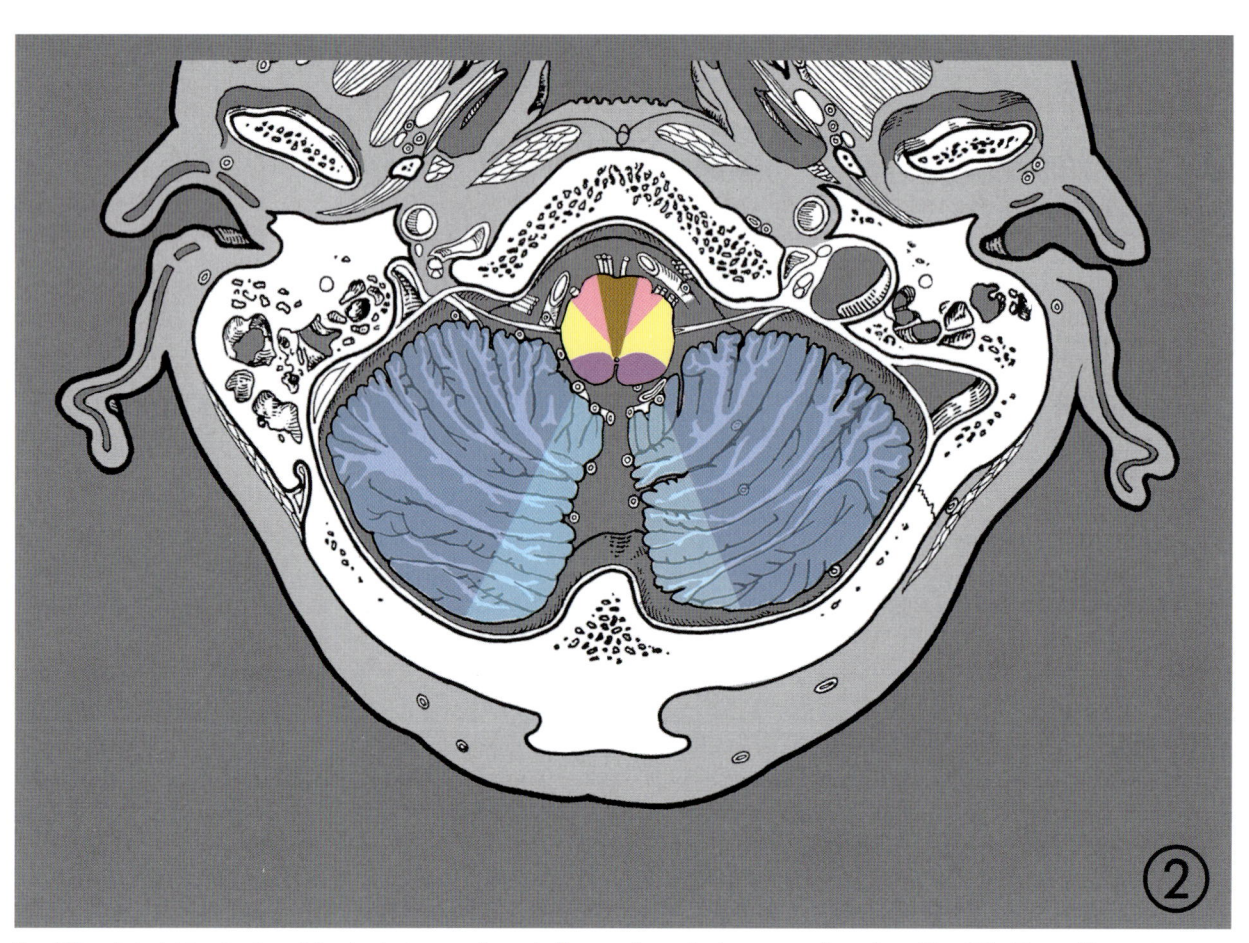

Fig. **89b** Arterial territories of the brainstem and cerebellum. These serial slices were cut vertically to the median plane and Meynert's axis. The encircled numbers (1, 2) indicate the number of the respective slice (Fig. 67). These illustrations are details of Figs. 69a and 70a. According to (111, 456).

5.4 Arteries of the Brain and their Vascular Territories 259

Arterial territories of the medulla oblongata: penetrating arteries of

- anteromedial: Anterior spinal artery
- anterolateral: Anterior spinal artery, posterior inferior cerebellar artery (PICA)
- lateral: Posterior inferior cerebellar artery (PICA)
- posterior: Posterior inferior cerebellar artery (PICA)

Arterial territories of the cerebellum

- Lateral branch of posterior inferior cerebellar artery (PICA)
- medial branch of posterior inferior cerebellar artery (PICA)

③

Arterial territories of the medulla oblongata: penetrating arteries of

- anteromedial: Anterior spinal artery, Vertebral artery
- anterolateral: Anterior spinal artery, Vertebral artery, Posterior inferior cerebellar artery (PICA)
- lateral: Vertebral artery

Arterial territories of the cerebellum

- Anterior inferior cerebellar artery (AICA)
- Lateral branch of posterior inferior cerebellar artery (PICA)
- Medial branch of posterior inferior cerebellar artery (PICA)

④

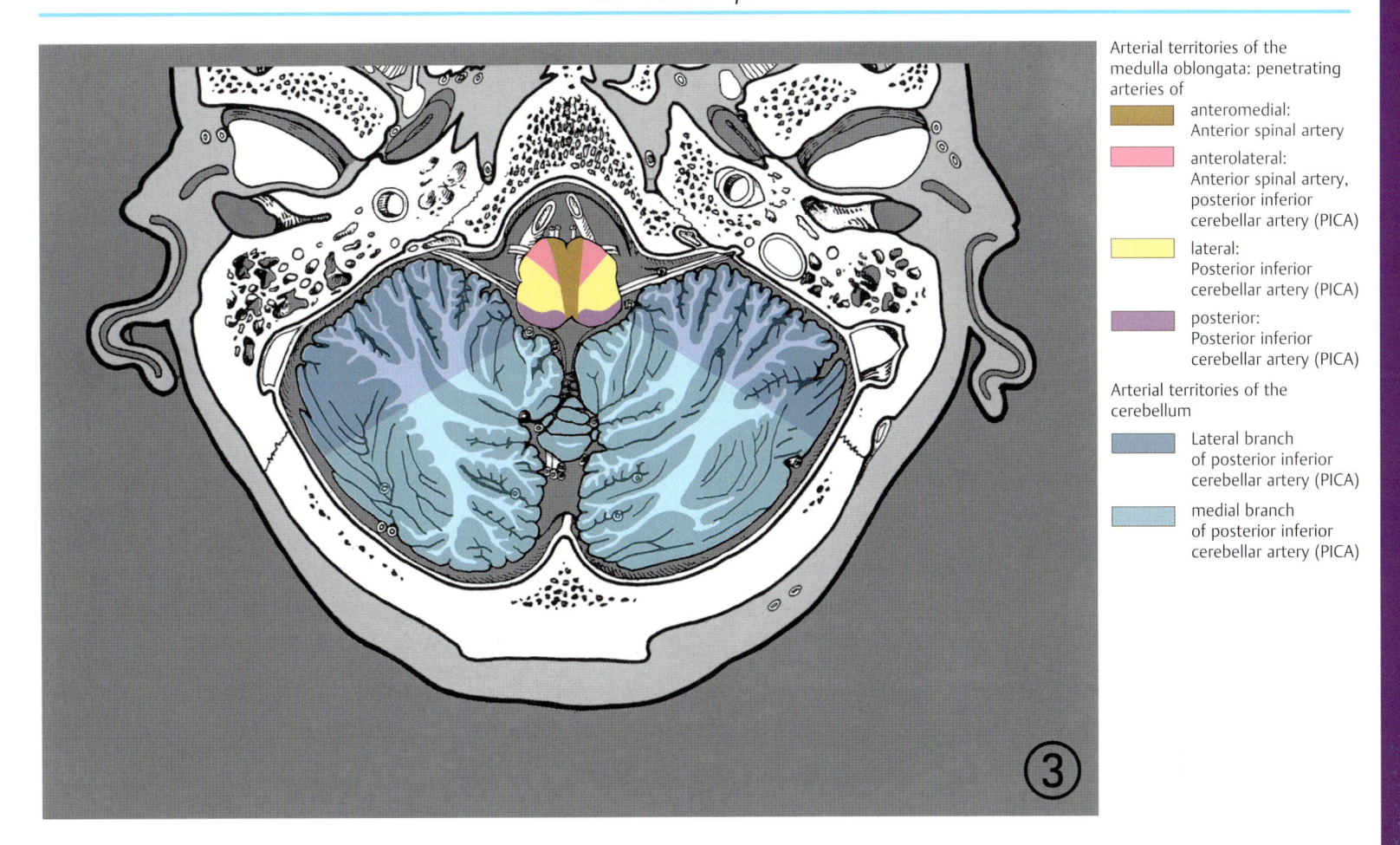

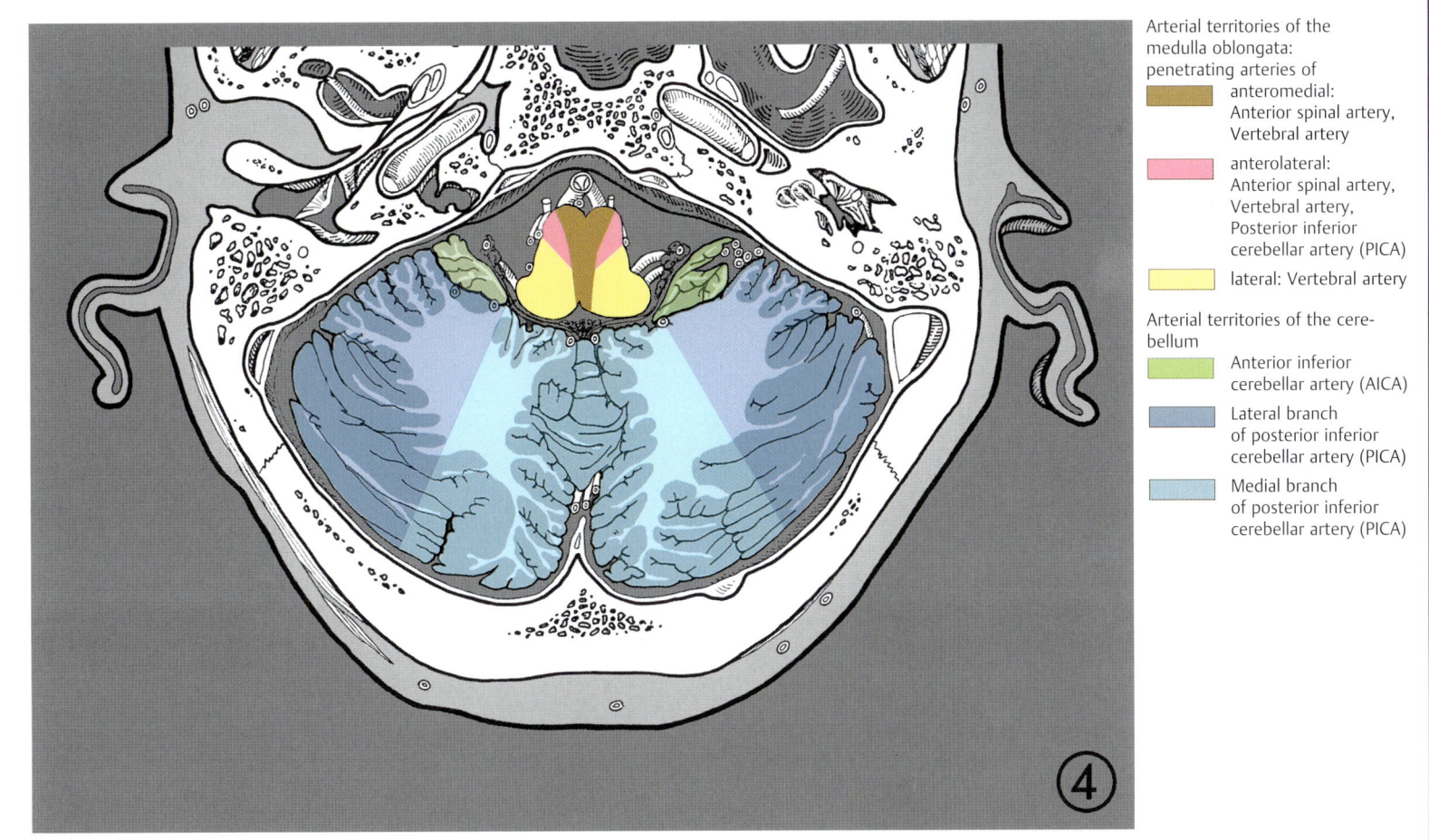

Fig. **89b** Arterial territories of the brainstem and cerebellum. These serial slices were cut vertically to the median plane and Meynert's axis. The encircled numbers (3, 4) indicate the number of the respective slice (Fig. 67). These illustrations are details of Figs. 71a and 72a. According to (111, 456).

260 5 Topography of the Neurocranium and its Intracranial Spaces and Structures in Multiplanar Parallel Slices

Arterial territories of the pons: penetrating arteries of

- anteromedial: Medial pontine arteries of the basilar artery
- anterolateral: Lateral pontine arteries of the basilar artery
- lateral: Lateral pontine arteries of the basilar artery, anterior inferior cerebellar artery (AICA)

Arterial territories of the cerebellum

- Anterior inferior cerebellar artery (AICA)
- Lateral branch of superior cerebellar artery
- Medial branch of superior cerebellar artery
- Medial branch of posterior inferior cerebellar artery (PICA)

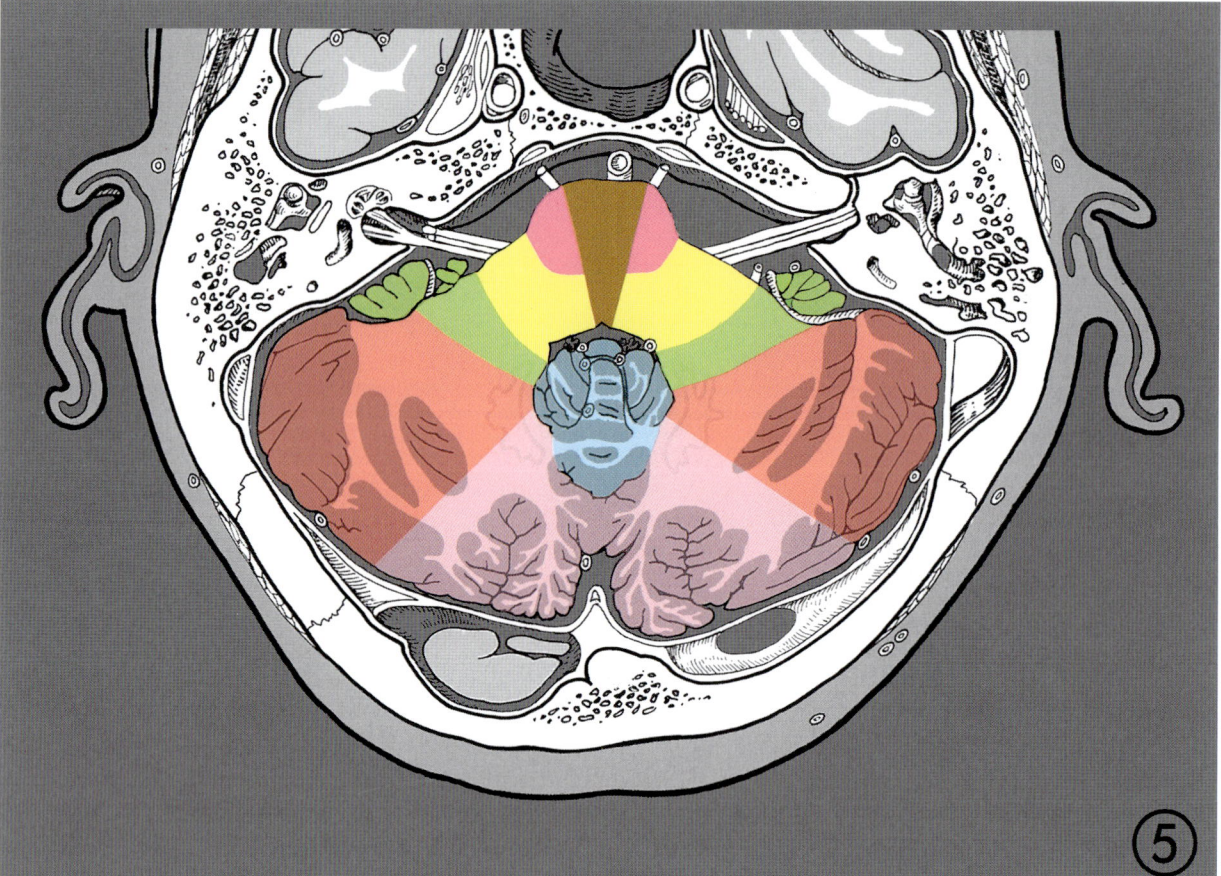

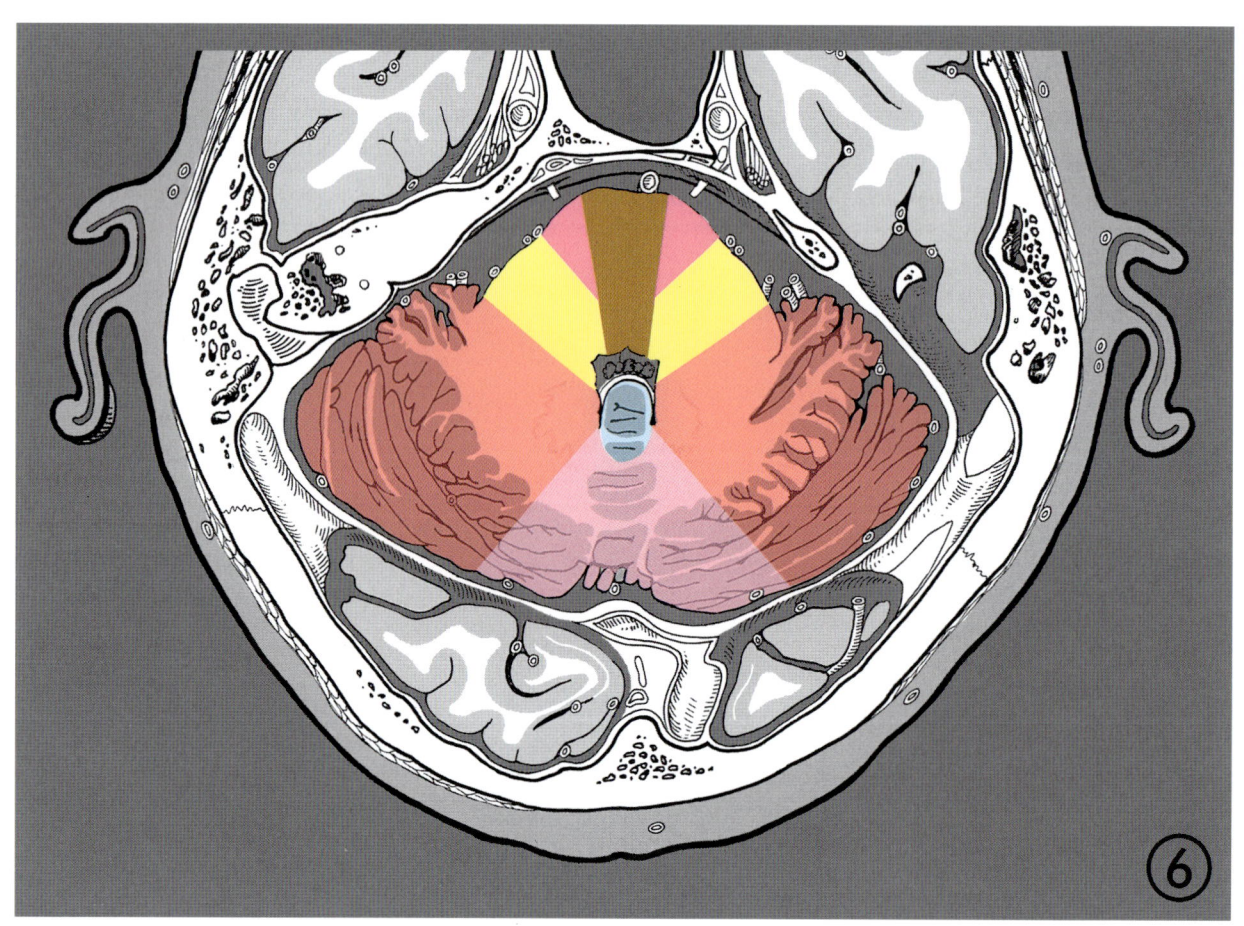

Fig. **89b** Arterial territories of the inferior portion of the pons and cerebellum. These serial slices were cut vertically to the median plane and Meynert's axis. The encircled numbers (5, 6) indicate the number of the respective slice (Fig. 67). These illustrations are details of Figs. 73a and 74a. According to (111, 456).

5.4 Arteries of the Brain and their Vascular Territories

Arterial territories of the pons: penetrating arteries of
- anteromedial: Medial pontine arteries of the basilar artery, Descending branches of posteromedial central arteries of posterior cerebral artery from the interpeduncular fossa
- anterolateral: Lateral pontine arteries of the basilar artery
- lateral: Lateral pontine arteries of the basilar artery
- posterior: Superior cerebellar artery

Arterial territories of the cerebellum
- Lateral branch of superior cerebellar artery
- Medial branch of superior cerebellar artery

⑦

Arterial territories of the pons: penetrating arteries of
- anteromedial: Medial pontine arteries of the basilar artery, Descending branches of posteromedial central arteries of posterior cerebral artery from the interpeduncular fossa
- anterolateral: Lateral pontine arteries of the basilar artery
- lateral: Superior cerebellar artery
- posterior: Superior cerebellar artery

Arterial territories of the cerebellum
- Lateral branch of superior cerebellar artery
- Medial branch of superior cerebellar artery

⑧

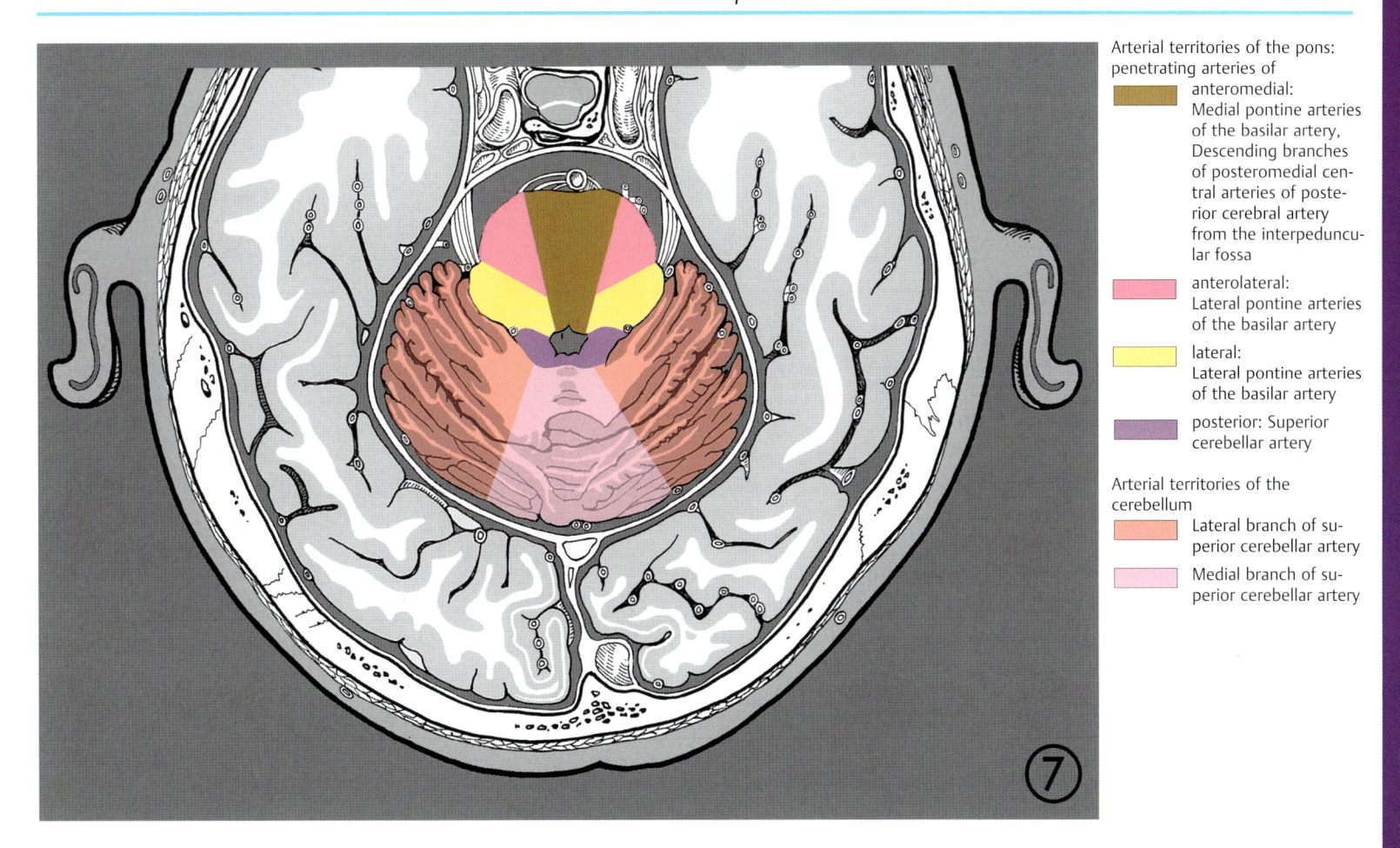

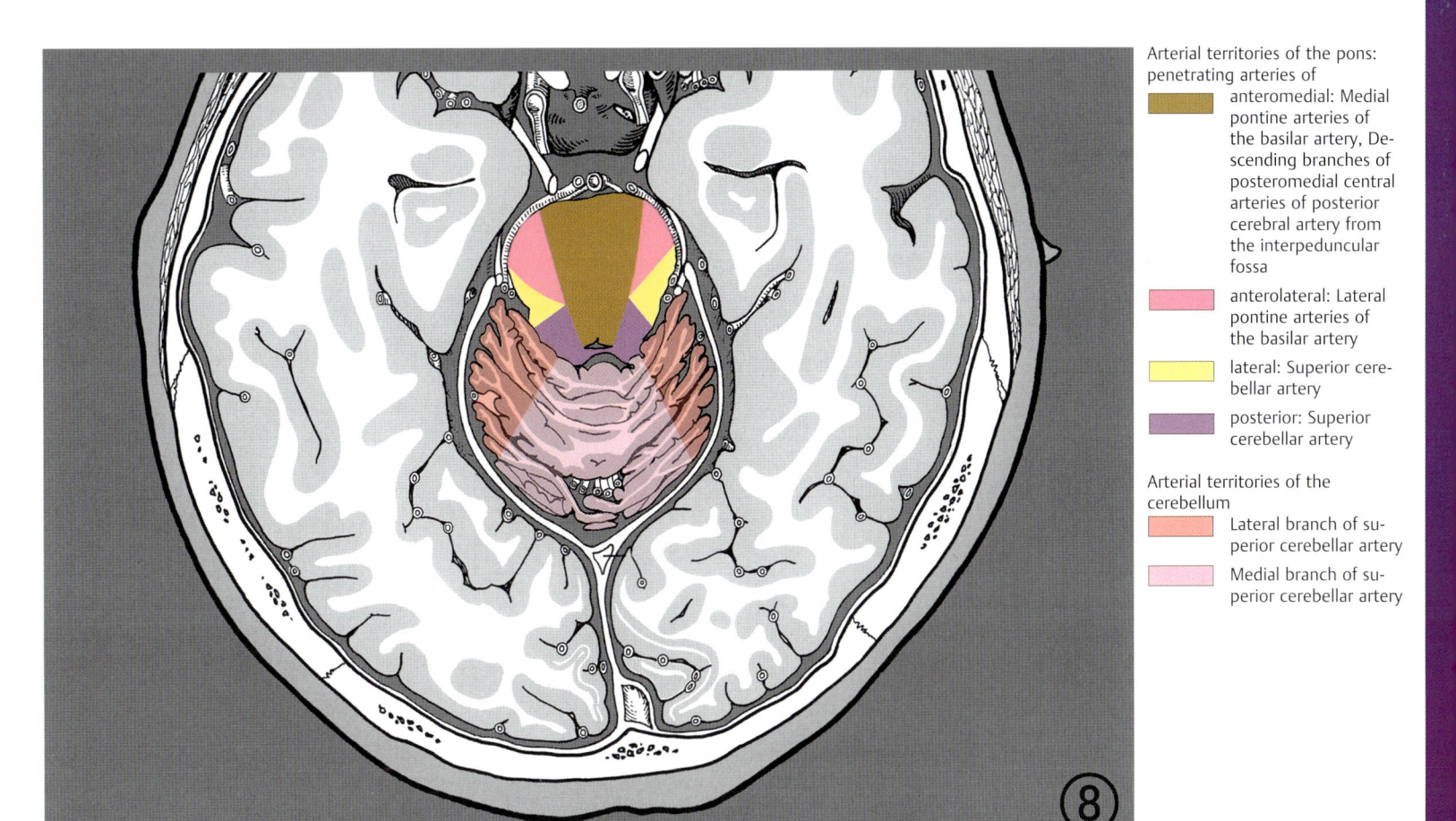

Fig. **89b** Arterial territories of the superior portion of the pons and cerebellum. These serial slices were cut vertically to the median plane and Meynert's axis. The encircled numbers (7, 8) indicate the number of the respective slice (Fig. 67). These illustrations are details of Figs. 75a and 76a. According to (111, 456).

262   5   Topography of the Neurocranium and its Intracranial Spaces and Structures in Multiplanar Parallel Slices

Arterial territories of the midbrain: penetrating arteries of
- anteromedial: Posteromedial central arteries of posterior cerebral artery
- anterolateral: Collicular artery and posterior medial choroidal arteries of posterior cerebral artery
- lateral: Collicular artery of posterior cerebral artery
- posterior: Collicular artery of posterior cerebral artery and superior cerebellar artery

Arterial territories of the cerebellum
- Lateral branch of superior cerebellar artery
- Medial branch of superior cerebellar artery

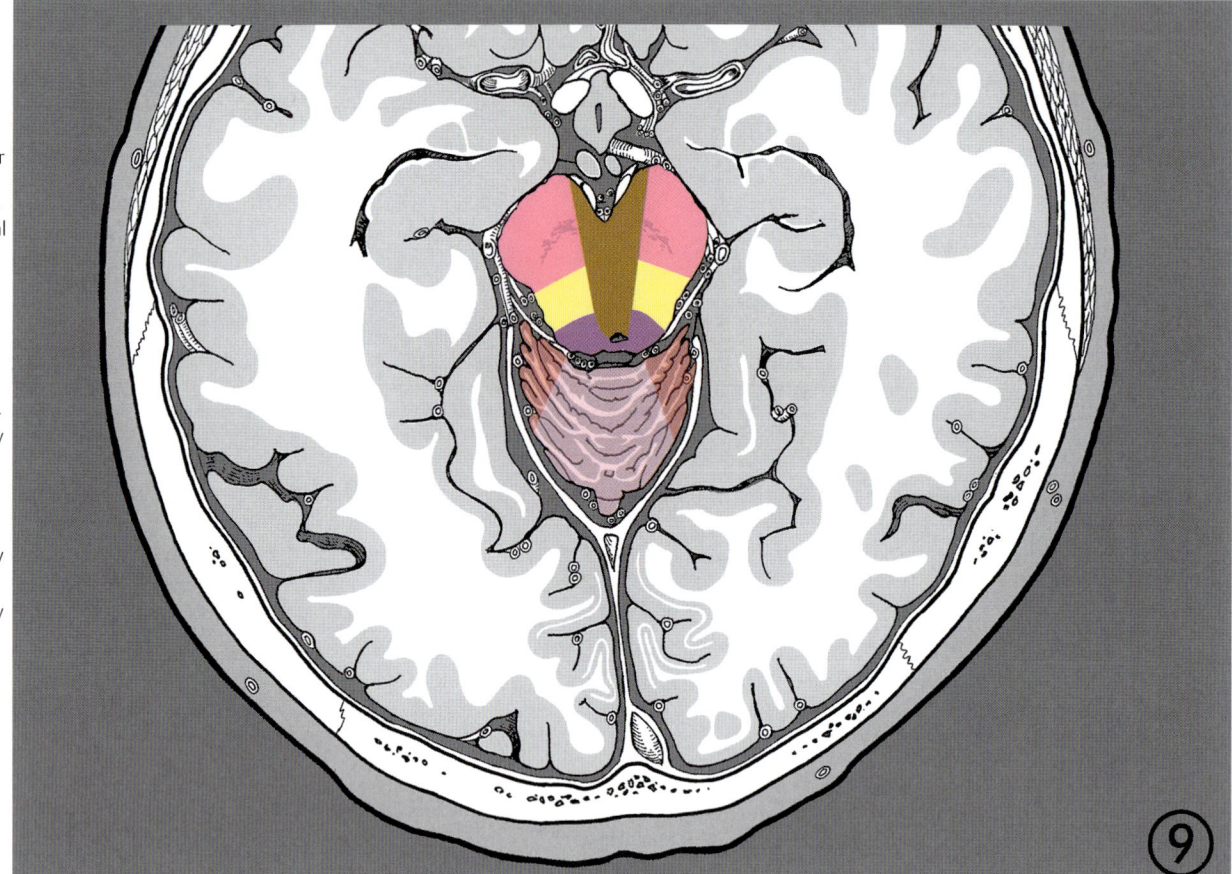

Arterial territories of the midbrain: penetrating arteries of
- anteromedial: Posteromedial central arteries of posterior cerebral artery
- anterolateral: Collicular artery, Posterior medial choroidal arteries of posterior cerebral artery and anterior choroidal artery
- lateral: Collicular artery and posterior medial choroidal arteries of posterior cerebral artery
- posterior: Collicular artery and posterior medial choroidal arteries of posterior cerebral artery

Arterial territories of the cerebellum
- Medial branch of superior cerebellar artery

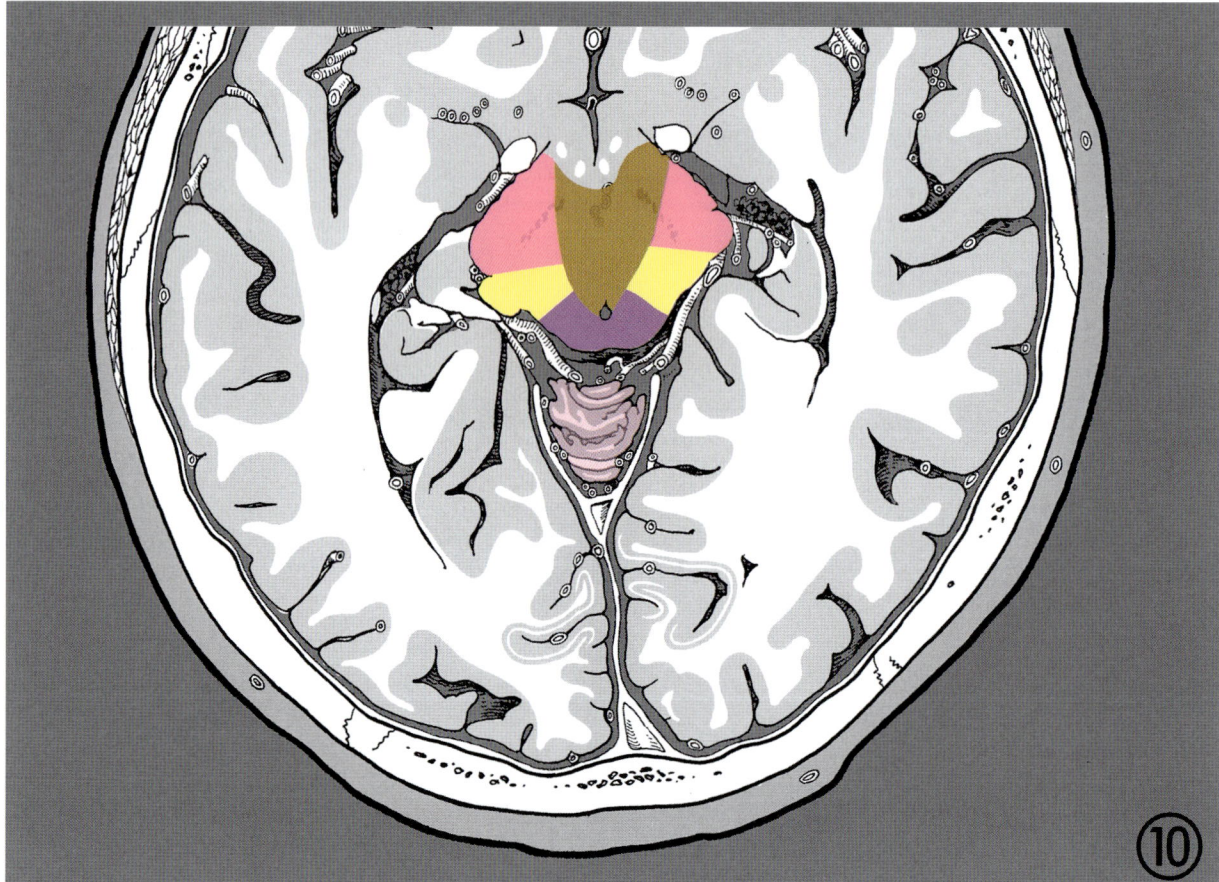

Fig. **89b** Arterial territories of the midbrain and cerebellum. These serial slices were cut vertically to the median plane and Meynert's axis. The encircled numbers (9, 10) indicate the number of the respective slice (Fig. 67). These illustrations are details of Figs. 77a and 78a. According to (111, 456).

The **lateral territory** is supplied by the penetrating branches of the PICA and the vertebral artery. This territory is made up of the spinothalamic tract (Figs. 70b.17, 71b.17), the anterior spinocerebellar tract (Figs. 70b.21, 71b.21), a small part of the hypoglossal nucleus and posterior nucleus of the vagus nerve, a part of the solitary nucleus, the lateral part of the inferior olive, in addition to the roots of the glossopharyngeal and vagus nerves. In the lateral territory of the superior portion of the medulla oblongata are the posterior and anterior cochlear nuclei (Fig. 72b.26) and the medial and inferior vestibular nuclei (Fig. 72b.24).

The **posterior territory** is vascularized mainly by the posterior spinal artery. In the inferior portion of the medulla oblongata (closed part with the central canal) are the gracile and cuneate nuclei, the solitary nucleus, and the posterior nucleus of the vagus nerve. In the middle portion of the medulla oblongata are the area postrema, also the posterior nucleus of the vagus nerve and the solitary nucleus. There is no posterior territory on either side of the superior portion of the medulla oblongata.

Arterial Territories of the Pons

The pons is mainly vascularized by branches of the basilar artery, the AICA, and the superior cerebellar artery. In the lower and mid portion of the pons, containing the wide part of the floor of the fourth ventricle, there are three territories on each side: anteromedial, anterolateral, and lateral. There is also a posterior territory in the superior portion of the pons.

The **anteromedial territory** is supplied by the medial pontine arteries of the basilar artery, which penetrates mainly the surface of the basilar sulcus. In a cross-section the anteromedial territory appears as a paramedian strip from the basilar sulcus to the floor of the fourth ventricle. This territory is made up of medial parts of the corticospinal tract (Figs. 73b.11, 74b.11, 75b.9) and the medial lemniscus (Figs. 73b.17, 74b.18, 75b.16) and extends into the lower pons to the abducens nucleus. In the inferior portion of the pons the territory close to the ventricle is supplied by small arteries that penetrate the foramen cecum before ascending further. In the superior portion of the pons narrow arteries descend through the interpeduncular fossa to reach the anteromedial territory close to the ventricle. Should these arteries be able to function during an anteromedial infarct, the anteromedial infarct will not reach the floor of the fourth ventricle (111).

The **anterolateral territory** is connected laterally to the anteromedial territory and is confined to the basal part of the pons without reaching the tegmentum of the pons. The anterolateral territory contains the lateral part of the corticospinal tract.

The **lateral territory** varies considerably in size and form. In the inferior and middle portions of the pons it is large, and in the upper portion small or absent. It is made up of the lateral part of the anterior and tegmental pons. Here can be seen the root fibers of the trigeminal nerve (Fig. 75b.13), parts of the motor and principal sensory nuclei of the trigeminal nerve (Figs. 74b.24, 74b.25) and the lateral lemniscus, the superior olivary nucleus (Fig. 73b.19), and the facial nucleus (Fig. 73b.21).

The **posterior territory** in the superior portion of the pons is made up of parts of the superior cerebellar peduncle, the mesencephalic nucleus of the trigeminal nerve (Fig. 75b.24), and the cerulean nucleus.

Arterial Territories of the Midbrain

Branches from the initial stage (precommunicating part) of the posterior cerebral artery supply mainly the midbrain. The anterior choroidal artery and narrow branches of the superior cerebellar artery are also involved (111). The posteromedial central arteries penetrate the interpeduncular fossa and supply the **anteromedial territory**. The oculomotor nucleus (Fig. 78b.20), trochlear nucleus (Fig. 77b.27), the red nucleus (Fig. 78b.16), and medial parts of the substantia nigra (Figs. 77b.21, 78b.15) are found here.

The **anterolateral territory** receives the flow from the longer branches of the posterior cerebral artery, namely, the collicular artery and the posterior medial choroidal arteries. In this territory are the cerebral crus with the corticospinal tract (Figs. 77b.17, 78b.12), large parts of the substantia nigra (Figs. 77b.21, 78b.15), and parts of the medial lemniscus (Fig. 77b.23).

The **lateral territory** is supplied by the collicular artery and in the superior portion of the midbrain by the anterior choroidal artery. This territory contains parts of the medial lemniscus (Figs. 77b.23, 78b.22).

The **posterior territory** is supplied mainly by the collicular artery and the superior cerebellar artery. This area corresponds to the tectal plate with its inferior and superior colliculi (Figs. 77b.34, 78b.31).

Arterial Territories of the Cerebellum

The cerebellum is supplied by three long arteries:
- PICA (Fig. 88.3)
- AICA (Fig. 88.5)
- superior cerebellar artery (Fig. 88.6).

As mentioned above, the arterial cerebellar supply demonstrates a high variability. Also, right–left asymmetries are not infrequent. Therefore the territories marked in color can only be used as a rough guide (Fig. 89b).

The **posterior inferior cerebellar artery (PICA)** is divided into a medial and a lateral branch and supplies the inferior part of the vermis and the inferior and posterior surfaces of the cerebellar hemispheres.

The **anterior inferior cerebellar artery (AICA)** flows through the middle cerebellar peduncle, the flocculus (H X), the posterior quadrangular lobule (H VI), and the superior and inferior semilunar lobule

1 Internal carotid artery
2 Branches of middle cerebral artery
3 Anterior cerebral artery
4 Medial frontobasal artery
5 Callosomarginal artery
6 Polar frontal artery
7 Anteromedial frontal artery
8 Intermediomedial frontal artery
9 Pericallosal artery
10 Posteromedial frontal artery
11 Paracentral artery
12 Superior precuneal artery
13 Inferior precuneal artery

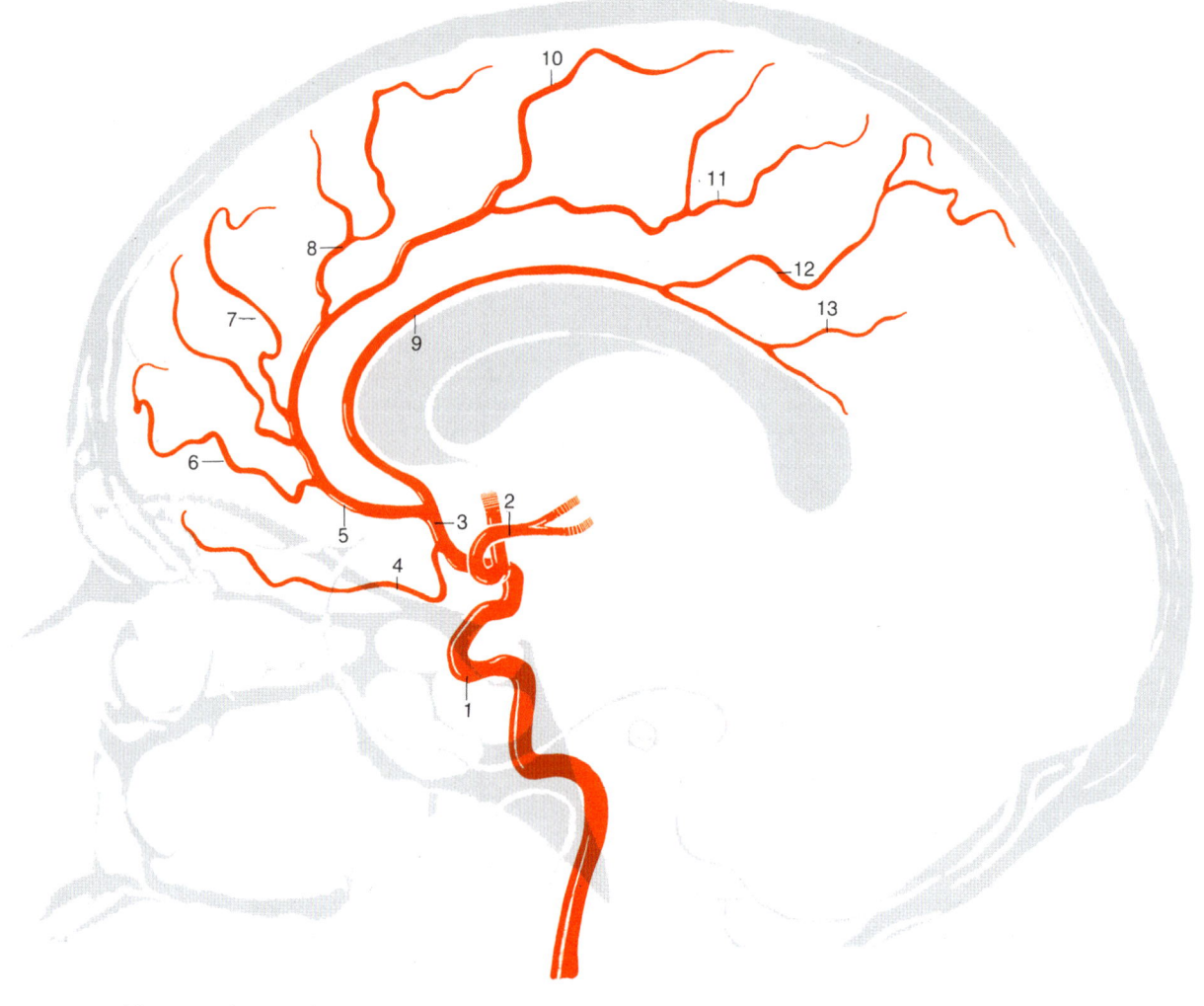

Figs. **90a** and **b** Lateral view of two main variations of the anterior cerebral artery; a) secondary branches originate from the callosomarginal artery, a main branch of the anterior cerebral artery; b) secondary branches arise directly from the anterior cerebral artery. According to (238).

(H VII A). The great reciprocal variability of the PICA and AICA has already been referred to above. In the case that an artery has a smaller territory, then the other arteries take over the supply of a larger area.

The **superior cerebellar artery** is the most consistent of the three cerebellar arteries. This artery consists of a medial and a lateral branch and vascularizes the upper half of the cerebellar hemisphere, the upper cerebellar vermis, and mainly the dentate nucleus. All three cerebellar arteries are involved in the supply of the brainstem.

Clinical Notes
A unilateral lesion of the medial territory causes the syndrome of "crossed" paralyses. The motoneurons of the hypoglossal nucleus on the side of the lesion are affected, and a paralysis of the ipsilateral muscles of the tongue results. The pyramidal tract is interrupted prior to the pyramidal decussation (crossing) and, therefore, a contralateral hemiparesis results.

A unilateral lesion of the lateral territory of the medulla oblongata causes Wallenberg's syndrome with "crossed" disorders of pain and temperature sensation mostly caused by an occlusion of the vertebral artery or PICA (471b). As the spinal nucleus of the trigeminal nerve is affected, pain and temperature sensations from the ipsilateral side of the face are lost. An interruption of the spinothalamic tract (above the decussation) results in a disorder of pain and temperature transmission in the contralateral arm, trunk, and leg. Infarction in the vestibular system causes vertigo, vomiting, and nausea. A lesion of the ninth and tenth cranial nerves may result in dysphagia and hoarseness (paralysis of pharyngeal and laryngeal muscles). Horner's syndrome is usually found in an ipsilateral position. Cerebellar infarcts are not as consistently distributed as cerebral, due to the variable nature of the arterial supply of the cerebellum (403).

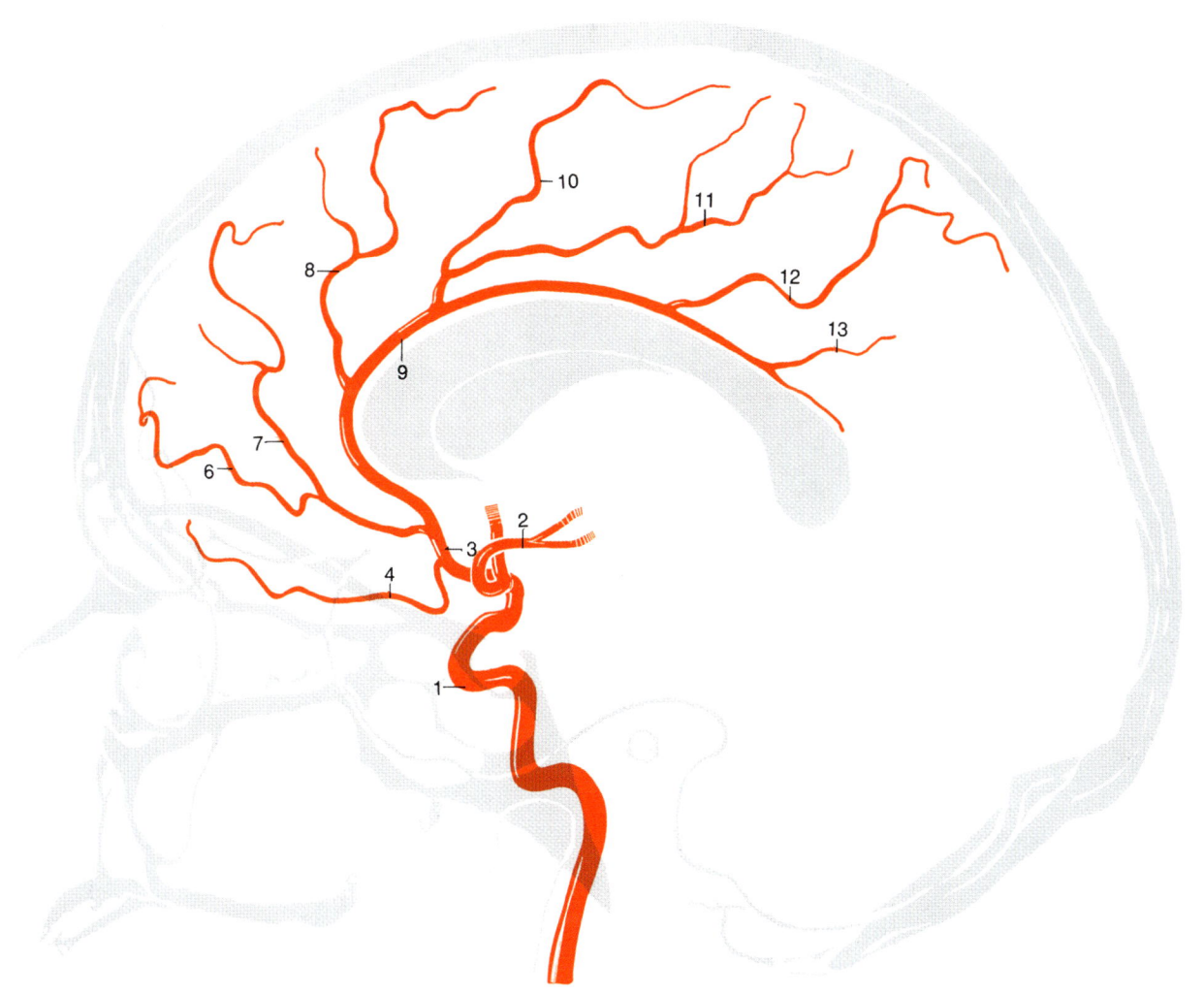

5.4 Arteries of the Brain and their Vascular Territories

1 Internal carotid artery
2 Branches of middle cerebral artery
3 Anterior cerebral artery
4 Medial frontobasal artery
6 Polar frontal artery
7 Anteromedial frontal artery
8 Intermediomedial frontal artery
9 Pericallosal artery
10 Posteromedial frontal artery
11 Paracentral artery
12 Superior precuneal artery
13 Inferior precuneal artery

Internal Carotid Artery

The internal carotid artery (Figs. 90.1, 10c.23, 34c.23, 48c.12, 49c.9) enters the skull base through the carotid canal in the petrous part of the temporal bone. The artery runs vertically at first, then bends sharply in an anteromedial direction. It ascends a short distance almost in an anterior and again in a vertical direction (C5 segment) in the cavernous sinus (Figs. 9c.17, 33c.17, 33d.18, 50c.10, 50c.9). In its next path, the internal carotid artery turns anteriorly and lies lateral to the pituitary gland (C4 segment). It curves backward below the anterior clinoid process. The frontally directed convex arch forms the carotid genu (C3 segment, carotid knee). In some recent publications the intracavernous section of the internal carotid artery has been referred to as the juxtasellar segment (238). Passing through the dura mater and the arachnoid mater (C2 segment), the internal carotid artery enters the subarachnoid space in a posterior direction. This subarachnoid part of the artery averages 13 mm in length, ranging from 8 to 18 mm (265). The next section reaches the point of its terminal bifurcation (C1 segment) into the anterior cerebral artery (Figs. 8c.10, 8d.14, 32c.20, 51c.10) and the middle cerebral artery (Figs. 8d.13, 9c.9, 34c.13, 51c.11). Direct branches of the internal carotid artery supply the optic chiasm, the pituitary stalk, the anterior lobe of the pituitary gland, as well as small portions of the hypothalamus, the genu of the internal capsule, and occasionally the globus pallidus and anterior portions of the thalamus (264).

The **posterior communicating artery** (Fig. 51c.12) arises from the internal carotid artery in the region between the sella turcica and the tuber cinereum of the diencephalon. It runs occipitally along the upper edge of the tentorium. In 1% of cases, the posterior communicating artery is absent. In 10% of cases, a **fetal type** is present in which the posterior communicating artery has such a large lumen that the posterior cerebral artery receives the principal portion of its blood from the internal carotid artery through the posterior communicating artery (265). Branches of the posterior communicating artery supply the optic chiasm, portions of the optic tract, the mammillary body, the tuber cinereum, additional portions of the hypothalamus, the anterior portion of the thalamus between the interthalamic adhesion and the interventricular foramen (of Monro), the cerebral peduncles, and the tail of the caudate nucleus.

1 Internal carotid artery
2 Middle cerebral artery
3 Origin of anterior cerebral artery
4 Lateral frontobasal artery
5 Insular arteries
6 Prefrontal arteries
7 Artery of precentral sulcus
8 Artery of central sulcus
9 Anterior parietal artery
10 Posterior parietal artery
11 Angular artery
12 Temporo-occipital artery
13 Posterior temporal artery
14 Middle temporal artery
15 Anterior temporal artery
16 Polar temporal artery

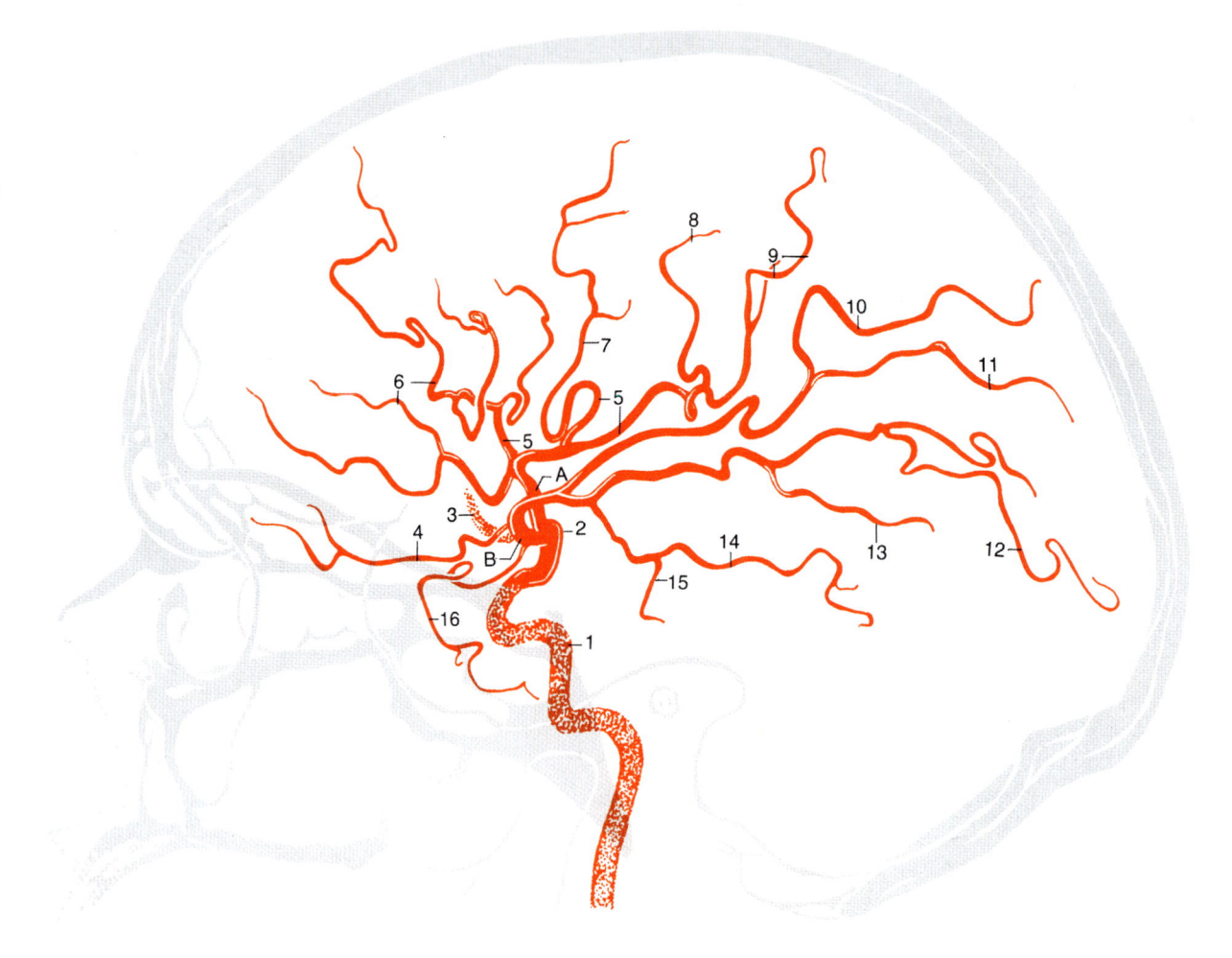

Figs. **91a** and **b** Lateral view of two variants of the middle cerebral artery; a) with a bifurcation A,B; b) with a trifurcation A,B,C. According to (238).

The **anterior choroidal artery** almost always arises from the internal carotid artery distal to the posterior communicating artery and about 3 mm proximal to the bifurcation of the internal carotid artery (265). Exceptionally, the anterior choroidal artery arises from the posterior communicating artery. Approximately 25 mm long, the anterior choroidal artery extends between the optic tract and the parahippocampal gyrus, enters the interpeduncular cistern, and runs through the ambient cistern to the tip of the temporal horn of the lateral ventricle into the choroid plexus. Additionally, it supplies parts of the telencephalon, diencephalon, and midbrain. Fine branches of the anterior choroidal artery reach the uncus of the parahippocampal gyrus, the amygdaloid body, the internal portion of the globus pallidus, as well as the posterior limb of the internal capsule in which the corticonuclear and corticospinal tracts are located.

Anterior Cerebral Artery

The anterior cerebral artery (Figs. 90.3, 7c.5, 7d.10, 32c.20, 32d.11, 51c.10, 52c.6, 53c.5, 54c.7) arises with the middle cerebral artery from the terminal bifurcation of the internal carotid artery. This bifurcation lies in the cleft between the optic chiasm and the anterior pole of the temporal lobe in the region of the anterior clinoid process. Aplasia of the anterior cerebral artery is observed in less than 1 % of cases (265). The anterior cerebral artery curves anteromedially and thereafter is located above the optic nerve. The initial precommunicating part (A1 segment) of the anterior cerebral artery averages 14 mm in length (265) and reaches the anterior communicating artery. The second postcommunicating part (A2 segment) begins distal to its connection with the anterior communicating artery (Fig. 32c.18).

Several short central (medial lenticulostriate) arteries (36) arise from the **precommunicating part** of the anterior cerebral artery and penetrate the anterior perforated substance. The long central artery (Heubner's recurrent artery) arises mostly from the postcommunicating part. In only 10 % of cases does it arise from the precommunicating part (264). This penetrating artery and the anteriomedial central (medial lenticulostriate) arteries supply deep structures of the forebrain: lamina terminalis, anterior commissure, anterior parts of the hypothalamus, occasionally the anterior tubercle of the thalamus, the anterior limb and genu of the in-

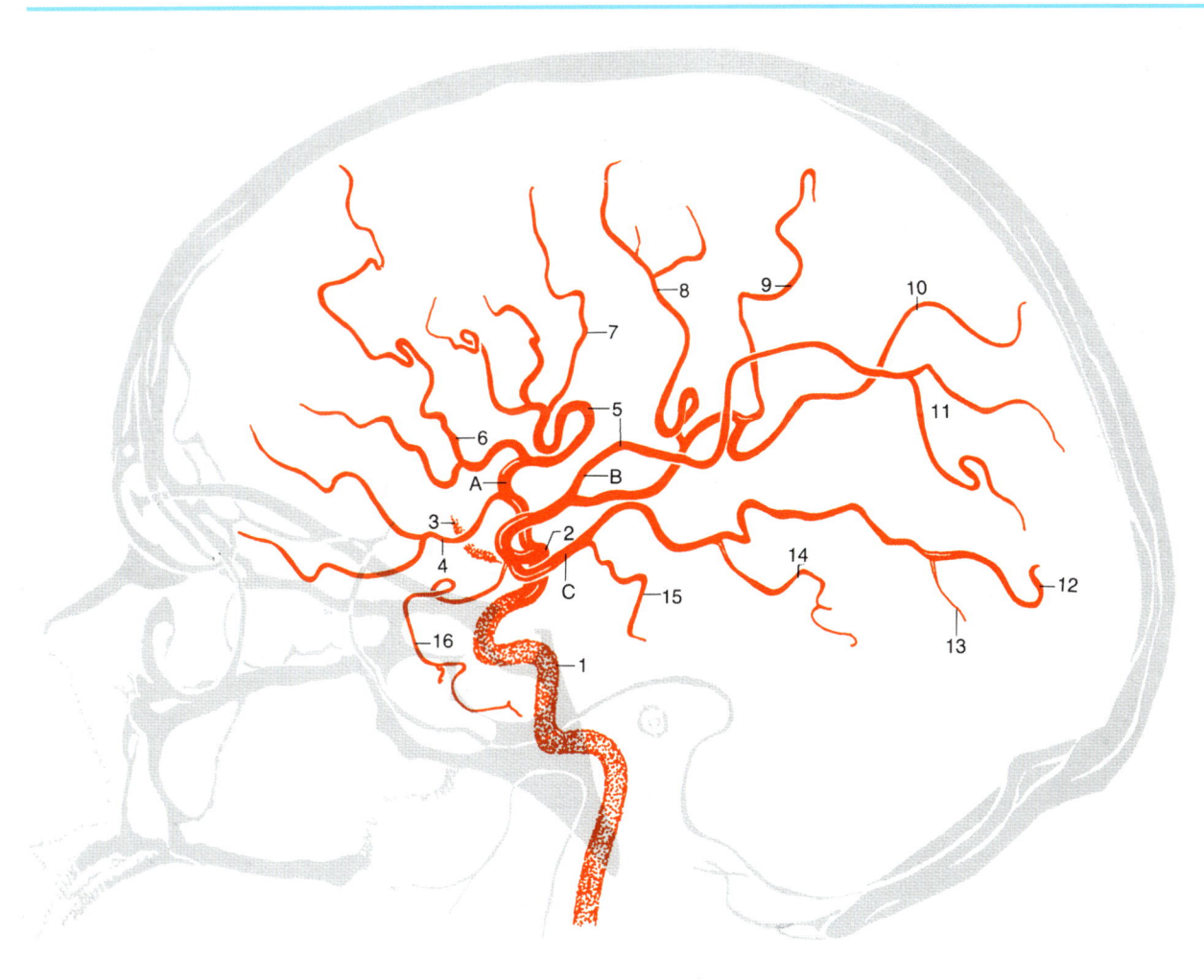

5.4 *Arteries of the Brain and their Vascular Territories*

1 Internal carotid artery
2 Middle cerebral artery
3 Origin of anterior cerebral artery
4 Lateral frontobasal artery
5 Insular arteries
6 Prefrontal arteries
7 Artery of precentral sulcus
8 Artery of central sulcus
9 Anterior parietal artery
10 Posterior parietal artery
11 Angular artery
12 Temporo-occipital artery
13 Posterior temporal artery
14 Middle temporal artery
15 Anterior temporal artery
16 Polar temporal artery

ternal capsule, anterior portion of the globus pallidus, and anteroinferior part of the head of the caudate nucleus.

Terminal branches from the **postcommunicating part** of the anterior cerebral artery extend into the cerebral cortex and the adjacent white matter. The medial frontobasal artery (Figs. 6c.8, 32c.19, 51c.5, 90a.4) arises near the subcallosal area and supplies the medial portion of the orbital forebrain. The polar frontal artery (Fig. 52c.3) extends diagonally in an oblique anterior direction toward the frontal pole. This artery is used as a point of reference in the interpretation of angiograms. The horizontally running terminal part of the anterior cerebral artery is known as the pericallosal artery (Figs. 7b.7, 7c.4, 7d.7, 32b.3, 32c.9, 55c.8, 56c.10) (381).

Further branching of the anterior cerebral artery generally takes one of two forms (238):

1. A principal branch of the anterior cerebral artery, the **callosomarginal artery** (Figs. 54c.5, 55c.6, 56c.7, 57c.7, 91d.5), lies in the cingulate sulcus and gives off branches (Fig. 90a.5).

2. The branches may arise directly from the anterior cerebral artery or from the pericallosal artery (Fig. 90b.9).

The **terminal** (formerly cortical) **arteries** of the anterior cerebral artery supply the medial surface of the frontal and parietal lobes almost as far as the parieto-occipital sulcus. The additional region supplied by the anterior cerebral artery is a longitudinal, 2–3-cm-wide territory overlapping the superior margin of the hemisphere including the superior frontal gyrus, the anterior portion of the middle frontal gyrus, the portions of the precentral and postcentral gyri near the superior margin, and a part of the superior parietal lobule. Additionally, the corpus callosum, with the exception of the splenium, is supplied by the anterior cerebral artery (150).

The **anterior communicating artery** (Figs. 32c.18, 51c.9, 91d.3) forms a connection, about 3 mm in length, between the right and left anterior cerebral arteries. It is located above the optic chiasm at the level of the anterior clinoid process. Fine branches supply the optic chiasm, the infundibulum, and the preoptic area of the hypothalamus.

Middle Cerebral Artery

The middle cerebral artery (Figs. 91a.2, 8b.13, 8d.13, 9c.9, 34c.13, 35d.7, 51c.11) is a continuation of the internal carotid artery running from its medial point of

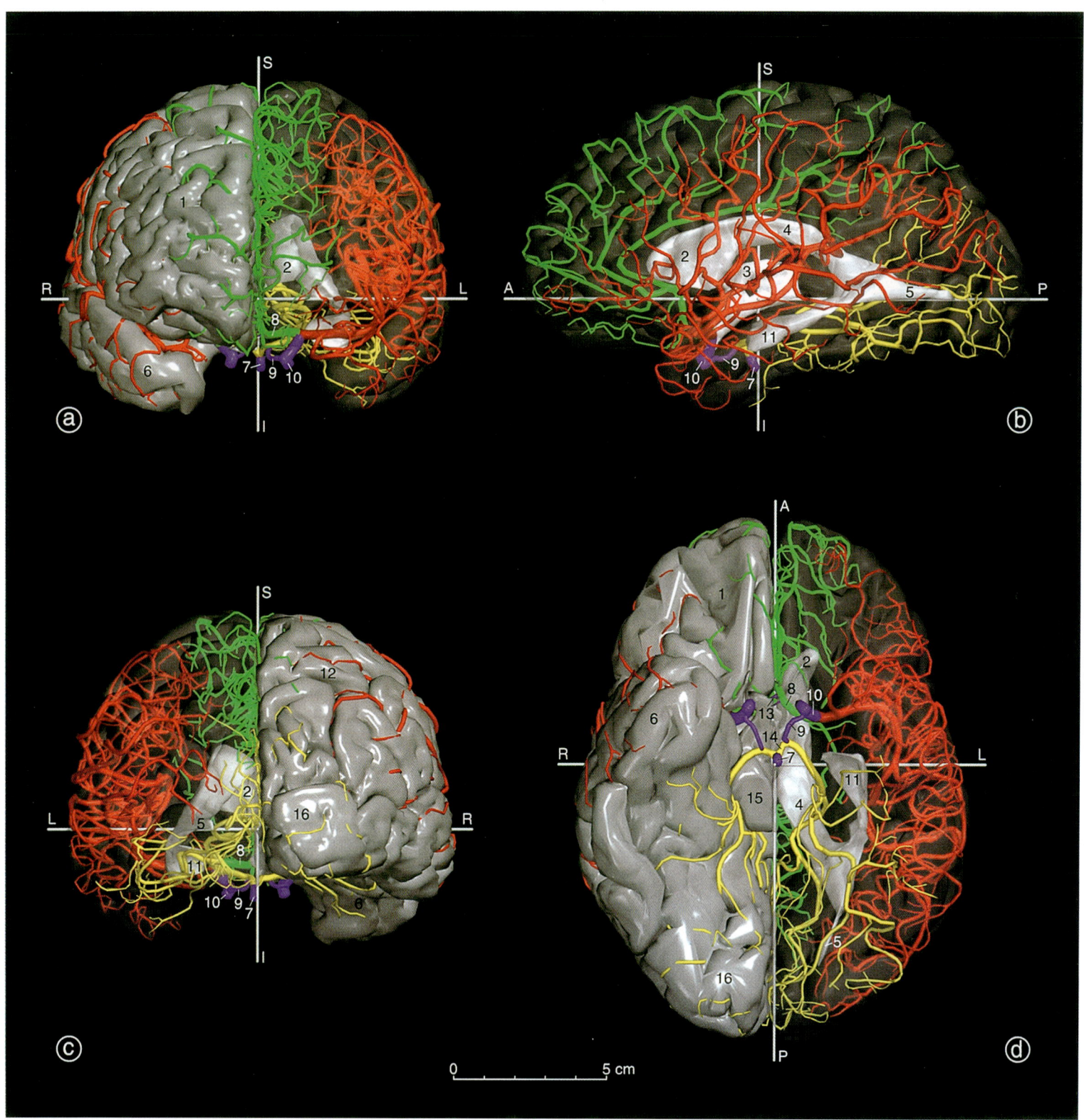

268   5   Topography of the Neurocranium and its Intracranial Spaces and Structures in Multiplanar Parallel Slices

Fig. 91c Computer-generated images of the circle of Willis and the anterior cerebral artery (green), the middle cerebral artery (red), and the posterior cerebral artery (yellow) within the bicommissural coordinate system. The left cerebral hemisphere is shown as transparent. The left lateral ventricle, the third ventricle, and the right cerebral hemisphere are shown as nontransparent. In the right hemisphere only those parts of the cerebral arteries are visible running on the surface. According to (149, 243, 244).

ⓐ Anterior view
ⓑ Lateral view of the left cerebral hemisphere only
ⓒ Posterior view
ⓓ Inferior view

1 Frontal lobe ⓐⓓ
2 Frontal (anterior) horn of lateral ventricle
3 Third ventricle ⓑ
4 Central part (body) of lateral ventricle ⓑⓓ
5 Occipital (posterior) horn of lateral ventricle ⓑⓒⓓ
6 Temporal lobe ⓐⓒⓓ
7 Terminal part of basilar artery
8 Precommunicating part of anterior cerebral artery ⓐ ⓒⓓ
9 Posterior communicating artery
10 Terminal part of internal carotid artery
11 Temporal (inferior) horn of lateral ventricle ⓑⓒⓓ
12 Parietal lobe ⓒ
13 Anterior communicating artery ⓓ
14 Precommunicating part of posterior cerebral artery ⓓ
15 Midbrain ⓓ
16 Occipital lobe ⓒⓓ

A   ANTERIOR
P   POSTERIOR
R   RIGHT
L   LEFT
S   SUPERIOR
I   INFERIOR

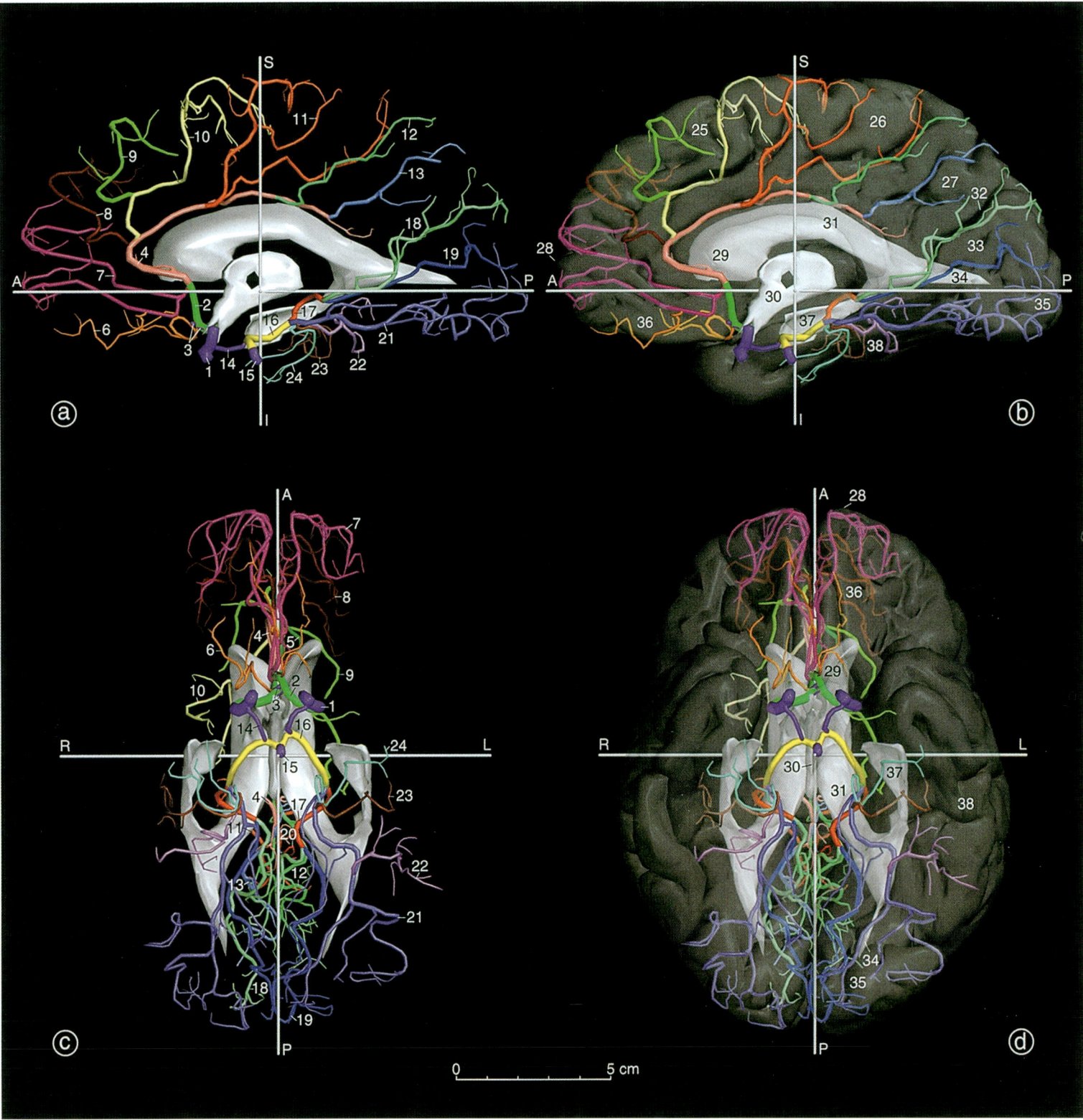

5.4 Arteries of the Brain and their Vascular Territories

Fig. 91d Computer-generated images of the circle of Willis, the anterior cerebral artery with its terminal branches, and the posterior cerebral artery with its terminal branches within the bicommissural coordinate system. According to (149, 243, 244).

ⓐ Medial view of the arteries of the right side with the right lateral ventricle and the third ventricle
ⓑ as ⓐ, also indicating the transparent right cerebral hemisphere
ⓒ Inferior view of both arteries with the lateral ventricles and the third ventricle
ⓓ as ⓒ, also indicating the transparent cerebrum

1 Terminal part of internal carotid artery (dark violet) ⓐⓒ
2 Anterior cerebral artery (green) ⓐⓒ
3 Anterior communicating artery (dark violet) ⓐⓒ
4 Pericallosal artery (pink) ⓐⓒ
5 Callosomarginal artery (dark green), only present in left hemisphere ⓒ
6 Medial frontobasal artery (ocher) ⓐⓒ
7 Polar frontal artery (red-violet) ⓐⓒ
8 Anteromedial frontal artery (brown) ⓐⓒ
9 Intermediomedial frontal artery (light green) ⓐⓒ
10 Posteromedial frontal artery (yellow-green) ⓐⓒ
11 Paracentral artery (light orange) ⓐⓒ
12 Superior precuneal artery (blue-green) ⓐⓒ
13 Inferior precuneal artery (light blue) ⓐⓒ
14 Posterior communicating artery (dark violet) ⓐⓒ
15 Terminal part of basilar artery (dark violet) ⓐⓒ
16 Posterior cerebral artery (yellow) ⓐⓒ
17 Medial occipital artery (orange) ⓐⓒ
18 Parieto-occipital artery (light turquoise) ⓐⓒ
19 Calcarine artery (blue) ⓐⓒ
20 Posterior pericallosal artery (red), only present in left hemisphere ⓒ
21 Lateral occipital artery (mauve) ⓐⓒ
22 Posterior inferior temporal artery (light violet) ⓐⓒ
23 Middle inferior temporal artery (light brown) ⓐⓒ
24 Anterior inferior temporal artery (turquoise) ⓐⓒ
25 Medial frontal gyrus ⓑ
26 Paracentral lobule ⓑ
27 Precuneus ⓑ
28 Pole of frontal lobe ⓑⓓ
29 Frontal (anterior) horn of lateral ventricle ⓑⓓ
30 Third ventricle ⓑⓓ
31 Central part (body) of lateral ventricle ⓑⓓ
32 Parieto-occipital sulcus ⓑ
33 Cuneus ⓑ
34 Occipital (posterior) horn of lateral ventricle ⓑⓓ
35 Occipital lobe ⓑⓓ
36 Medial orbital part of frontal lobe ⓑⓓ
37 Temporal (inferior) horn of lateral ventricle ⓑⓓ
38 Temporal lobe ⓑⓓ
A ANTERIOR
P POSTERIOR
R RIGHT
L LEFT
S SUPERIOR
I INFERIOR

- Terminal branches of anterior cerebral artery
- Terminal branches of middle cerebral artery
- Terminal branches of posterior cerebral artery
- Anterior choroidal artery

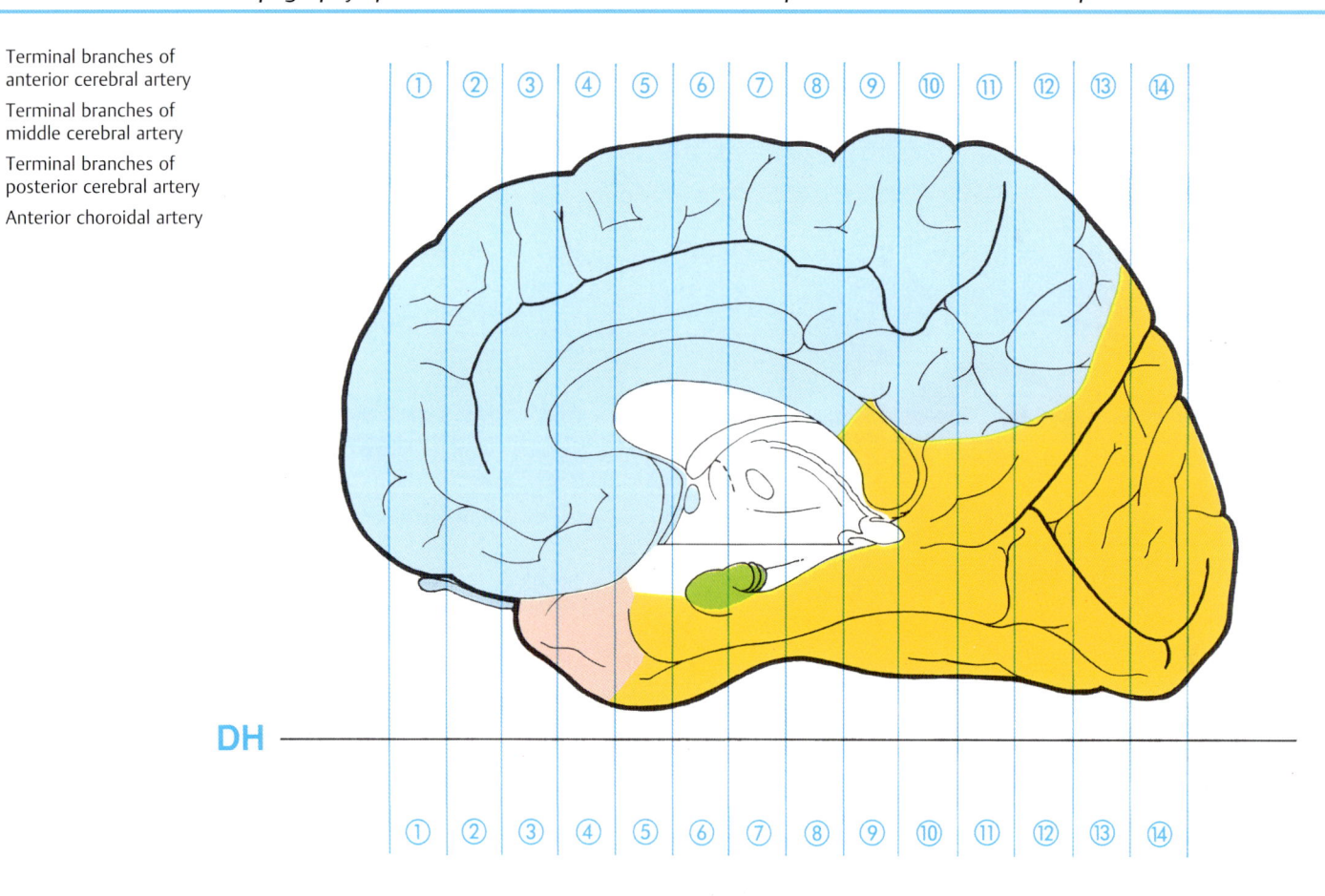

Fig. **92a** Medial view of the coronally cut cerebrum showing the vascular territories of the terminal branches of the anterior, middle, and posterior cerebral arteries and the anterior choroidal artery. The encircled number indicates the number of the respective slice (Figs. 1, 2a,b, 3).
DH Reid's base line

origin deep into the cistern of the lateral cerebral fossa. The initial or sphenoid part (M1 segment) of the middle cerebral artery is located just below the anterior perforated substance. Here 3 to 13 thin arteries, the anterolateral central (formerly lateral lenticulostriate) arteries, branch off mainly to supply deeper telencephalic and diencephalic structures: the genu and posterior limb of the internal capsule, the majority of the putamen and caudate nucleus, and part of the globus pallidus. Prior to its division into two or more branches, the middle cerebral artery averages 16 mm (5–24 mm) in length. Aplasia of the middle cerebral artery is reported rarely and was seen only in about 0.3% of cases (265). In the region between the anterior perforated substance and the insula, the middle cerebral artery divides into its hemispheric branches as a **bifurcation** in 20% of cases (Fig. 91a), as a trifurcation in about 50% (Fig. 91b), and only seldom forms a quadrifurcation or quintafurcation (265). The **insular arteries** (insular part, M2 segment) (Figs. 8c.9, 36c.9, 52c.7, 53c.6, 54c.9, 55c.10) ascend in an oblique manner and lie on the insula. They run around the frontal, parietal, and temporal opercula. During evolution the neocortex pushed the opercula over the insula together with these arteries (438, 439). The arteries are enclosed by the opercula of the insula (M3 segment) and assume the shape of a candelabra. The concave portion of the curve in the ascending arteries is directed upward. Likewise, in descending arteries of the temporal operculum the concave portion of the candelabra is directed downward. The segments of the insular arteries lie on the surface of the cerebrum (M4 and M5 segments). The terminal branches are named according to the terminal territory that they supply (151).

The lateral frontobasal artery (Figs. 6c.6, 35c.10, 91a.4) supplies the inferior frontal gyrus and partially the orbital gyri. The prefrontal artery (Figs. 6c.4, 35c.4, 55c.5, 56c.5) lies on the triangular part of the operculum and branches on the external surface of the frontal lobe. The artery of precentral sulcus (prerolandic artery) (Figs. 9c.6, 35c.2, 54c.8, 55c.9) lies to some extent in the precentral sulcus and supplies the middle frontal gyrus and the basilar part of the precentral gyrus. The artery of central sulcus (Rolandic artery) (Figs. 10c.7, 35c.6, 55c.14, 56c.9) assists in supplying the precentral and postcentral gyri as well as the adjacent areas. The anterior and posterior parietal arteries supply the anterior and posterior parts of the parietal lobe. The **angular artery** (Figs. 12c.9, 35c.8, 55c.19, 56c.15) runs partially in the superior temporal sulcus in the direction of the angular gyrus and can be seen as the terminal branch of the middle cerebral artery. The temporo-occipital artery runs on the su-

5.4 Arteries of the Brain and their Vascular Territories

☐ Terminal branches of anterior cerebral artery
☐ Terminal branches of middle cerebral artery
☐ Terminal branches of posterior cerebral artery

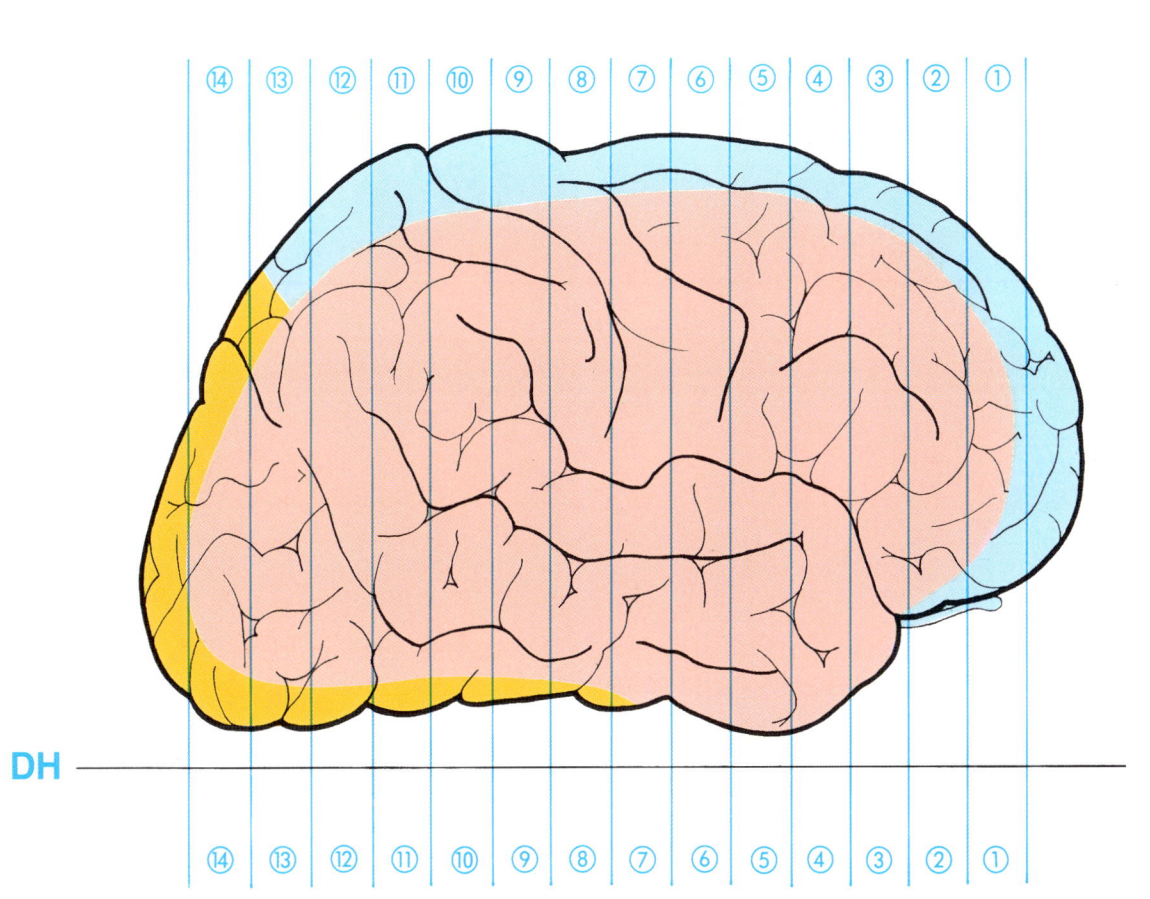

Fig. 92b Lateral view of the coronally cut cerebrum demonstrating the vascular territories of the terminal branches of the anterior, middle, and posterior cerebral arteries. The encircled number indicates the number of the respective slice (Figs. 1, 2a,b, 3).
DH Reid's base line

perior temporal gyrus to the occipital lobe. There are four temporal arteries that descend along the surface of the temporal lobe (Figs. 91a,b.13, 91a,b.14, 91a,b.15, 91a,b.16).

Circle of Willis

In all but 4% of cases, the circle of Willis forms a vascular ring joining the blood flow systems of basilar and internal carotid arteries. The circle can act as an adaptive distributor during variations in the blood supply of one of the arteries. In about 2% of cases, the left or right posterior communicating artery is absent (264). Hemodynamically speaking, connections between the large cerebral arteries are not sufficient in about 50% of cases (8). The preferred localization of arteriosclerosis in the cerebral arterial circle can further impair its compensational functions. In adults a complete ligation of one internal carotid artery generally results in neurologic deficits. The compensating function of the circle of Willis as a distributor of the blood stream is confirmed by the fact that brain infarcts are significantly more frequent in patients with a congenitally incomplete circle than in those with a complete circle.

Anastomoses of Cerebral Arteries

Most cerebral arteries have arterial interconnections (anastomoses) that can partially supply neighboring brain areas. An insufficient blood supply to the brain through the internal carotid and vertebral arteries can (within limits) be compensated for by anastomoses from the facial and superficial temporal arteries with the ophthalmic artery and a **reversal of the direction of flow** of the ophthalmic artery into the internal carotid artery (Chap. 3.3). Furthermore, leptomeningeal anastomoses between the three main cerebral arteries and the three cerebellar arteries exist. Across the midline blood can be supplied to the contralateral hemisphere through the pericallosal artery or the callosomarginal artery. Generally, arterial anastomoses are present also between the anterior choroidal artery and the posterior choroidal artery.

Arterial Territories of the Forebrain
(Figs. 92–96)
Basically two main arterial territories can be distinguished:
- Central territories located in the diencephalon, caudate nucleus, putamen, and the internal capsule
- Terminal territories located in the cerebral cortex and the white matter situated directly beneath it. The synonym "cortical territories" describes these territories incompletely.

272   5   Topography of the Neurocranium and its Intracranial Spaces and Structures in Multiplanar Parallel Slices

Terminal branches of anterior cerebral artery
Terminal branches of middle cerebral artery

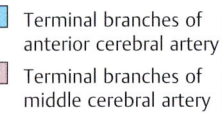

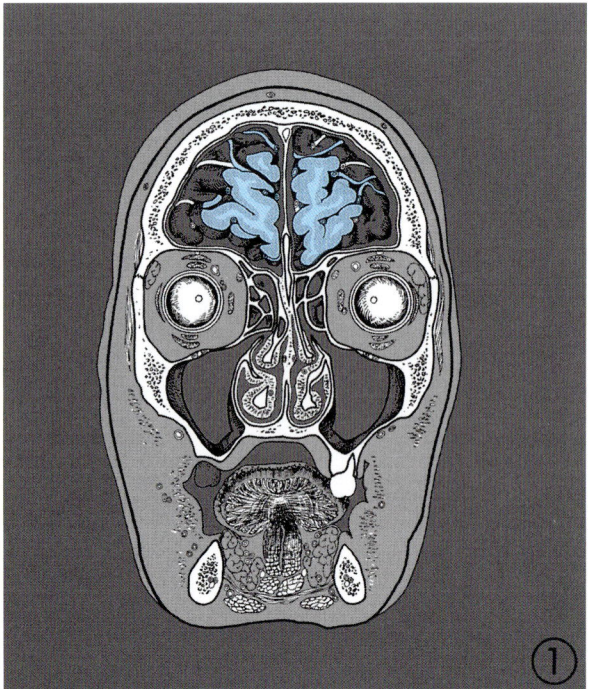

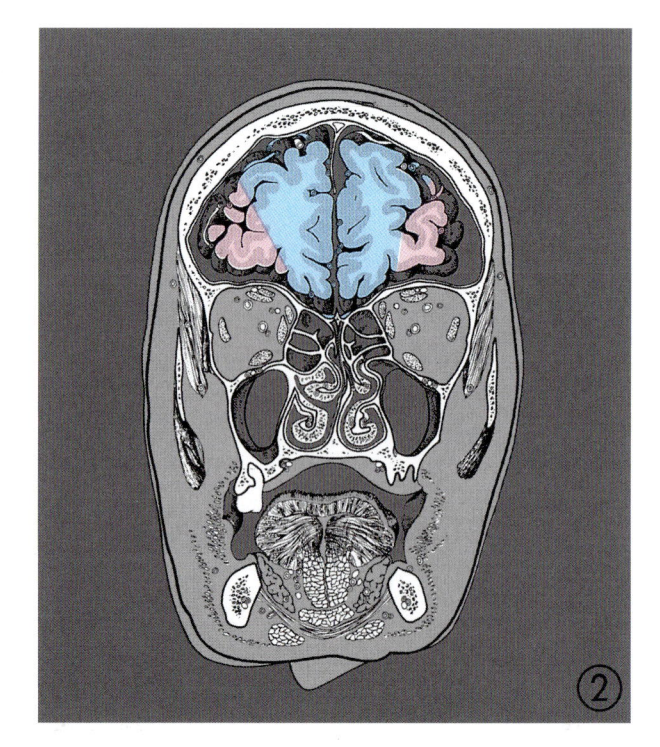

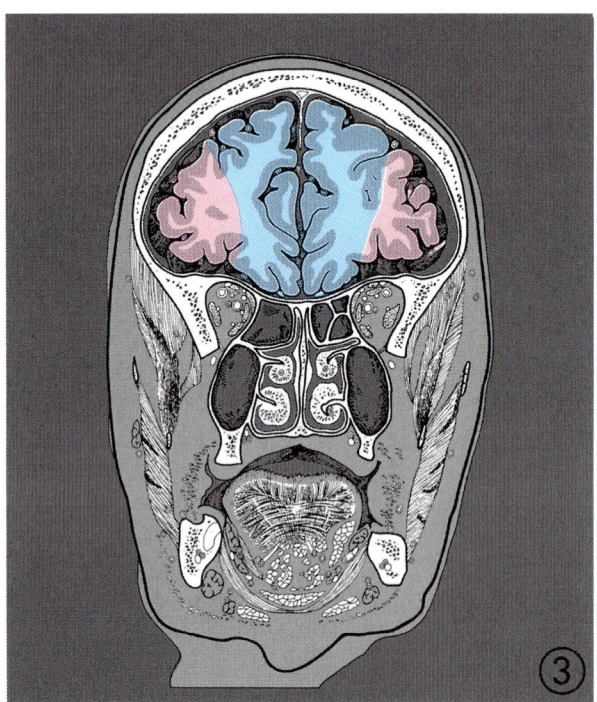

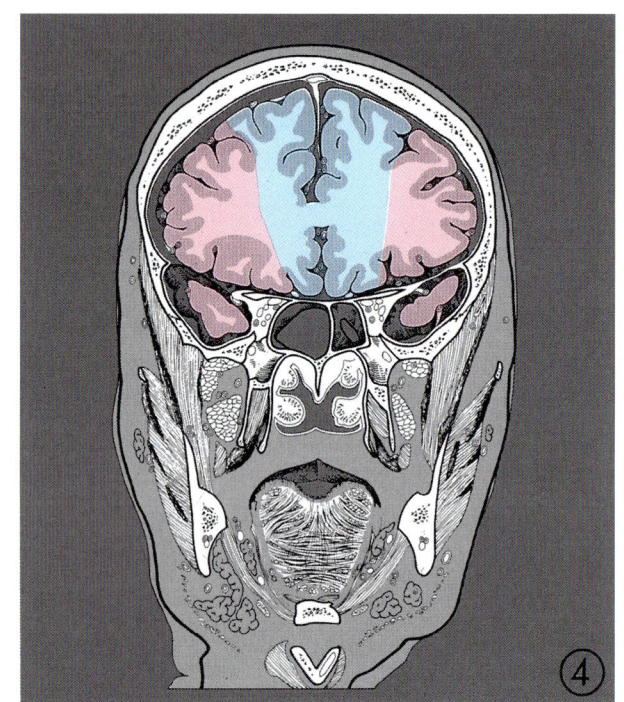

Fig. 93 Coronal serial illustrations showing the vascular territories of the terminal and penetrating (central) branches of the anterior, middle, and posterior cerebral arteries, and the anterior choroidal artery. The encircled numbers (1–8) indicate the number of the respective slice (Figs. 1, 2a,b, 3, 92a,b). According to (29, 35, 36, 89, 179).

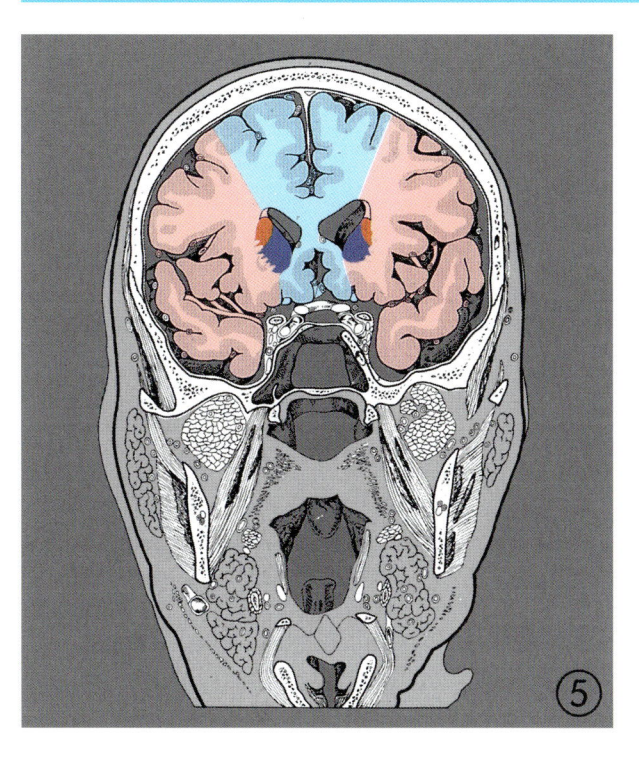

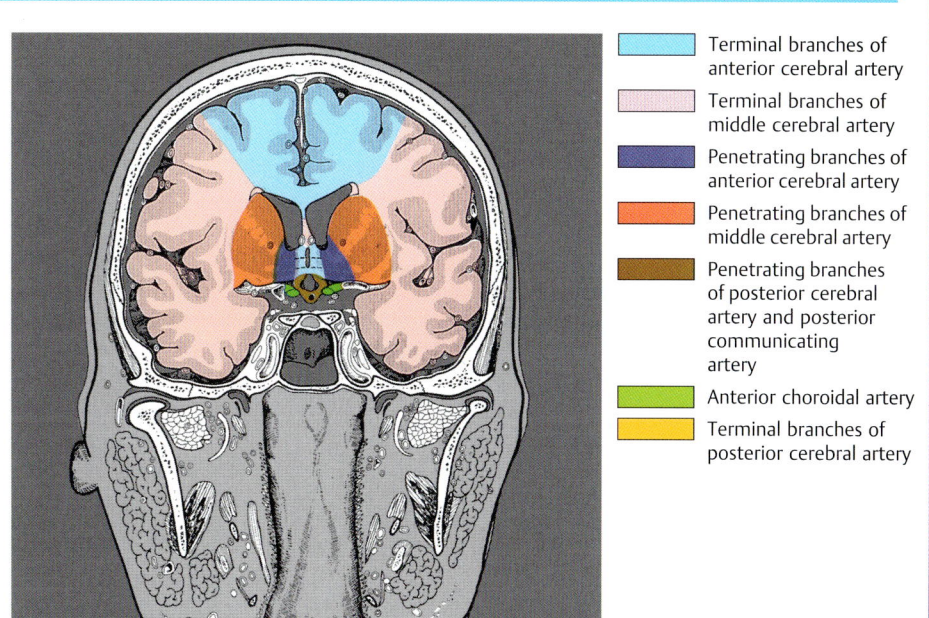

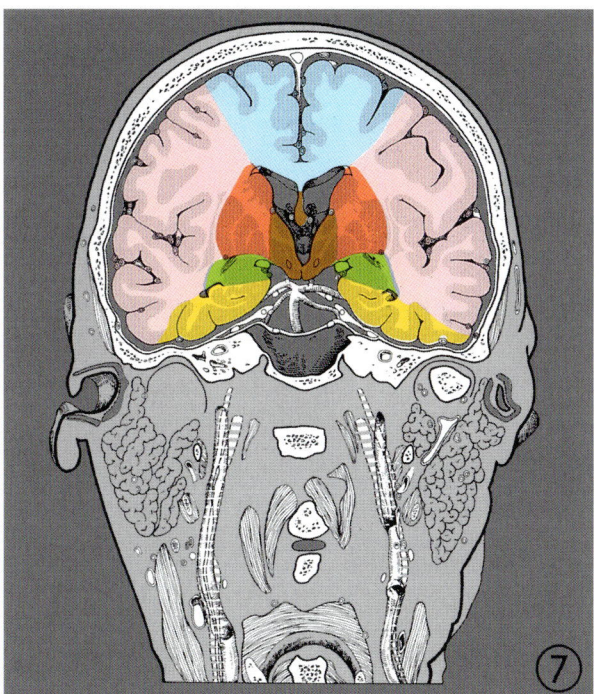

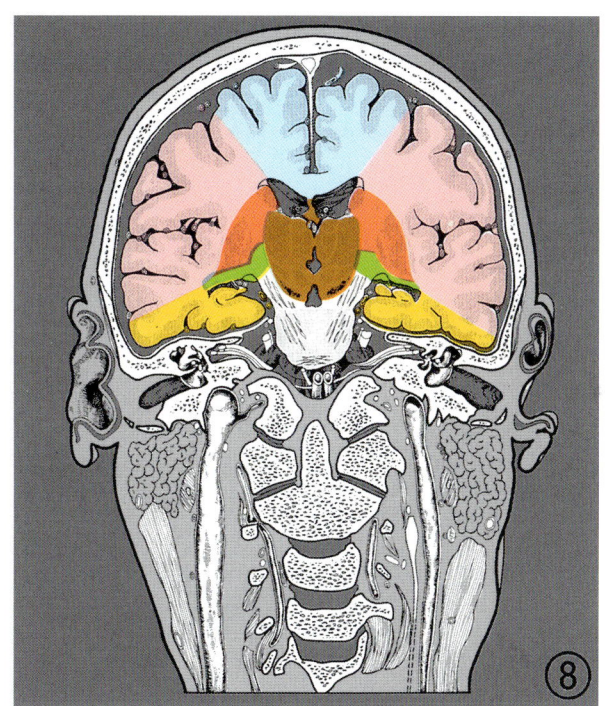

5.4 Arteries of the Brain and their Vascular Territories

■ (light blue)	Terminal branches of anterior cerebral artery
■ (pink)	Terminal branches of middle cerebral artery
■ (dark blue)	Penetrating branches of anterior cerebral artery
■ (orange)	Penetrating branches of middle cerebral artery
■ (brown)	Penetrating branches of posterior cerebral artery and posterior communicating artery
■ (green)	Anterior choroidal artery
■ (yellow)	Terminal branches of posterior cerebral artery

273

274   5   Topography of the Neurocranium and its Intracranial Spaces and Structures in Multiplanar Parallel Slices

- Terminal branches of anterior cerebral artery
- Terminal branches of middle cerebral artery
- Terminal branches of posterior cerebral artery
- Penetrating branches of middle cerebral artery
- Penetrating branches of posterior cerebral artery

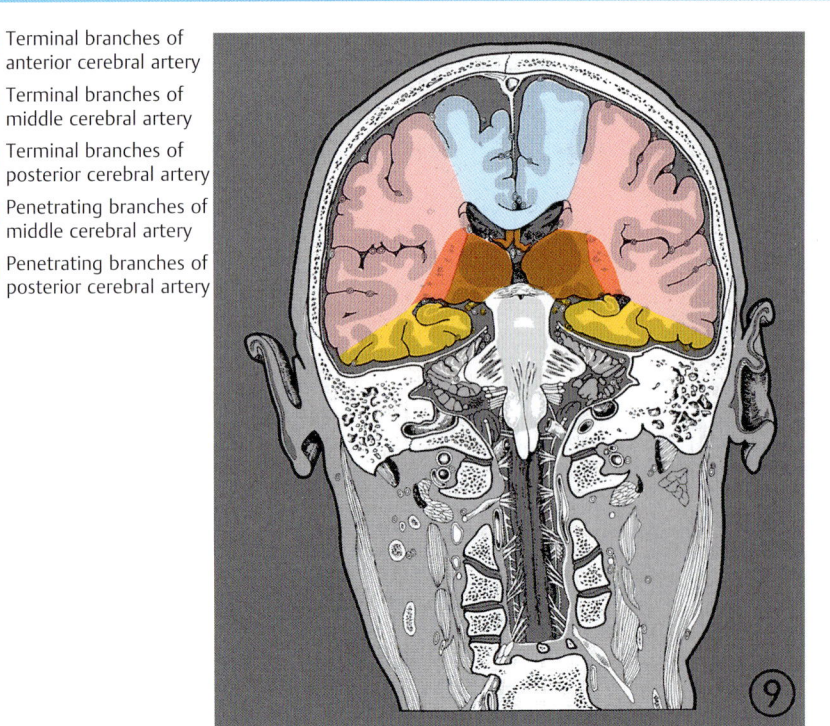

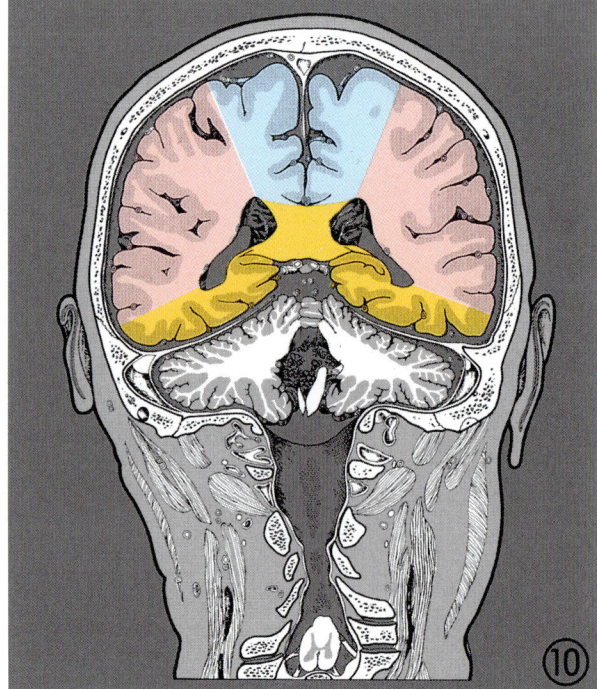

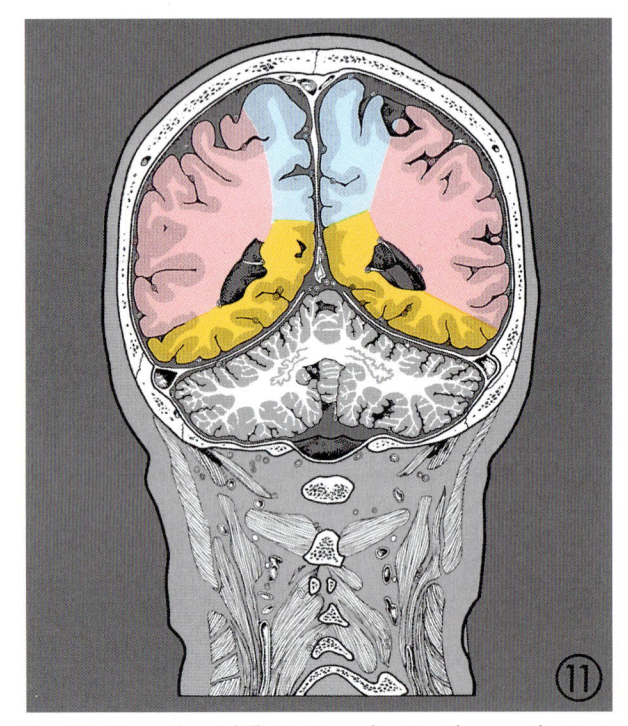

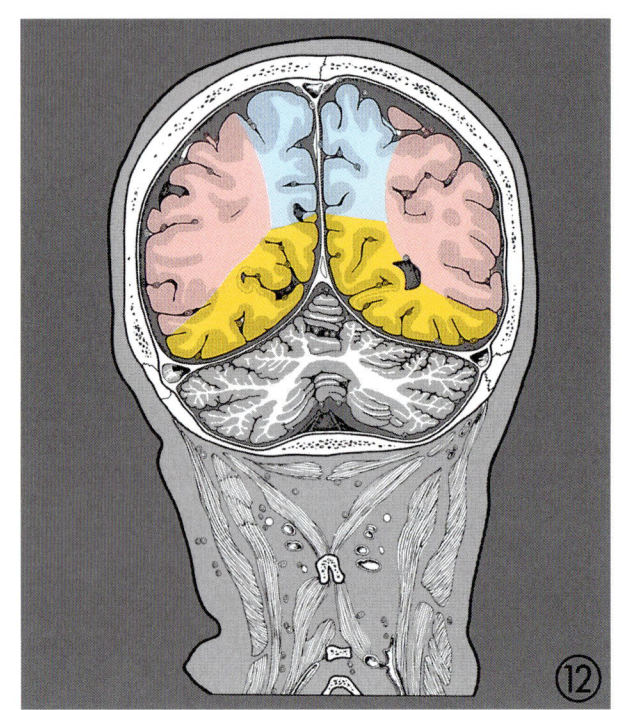

Fig. 93 Coronal serial illustrations showing the vascular territories of the terminal and penetrating (central) branches of the anterior, middle, and posterior cerebral arteries and the anterior choroidal artery. The encircled numbers (9–14) indicate the number of the respective slice (Figs. 1, 2a,b, 3, 92a,b). According to (29, 35, 36, 89, 179).

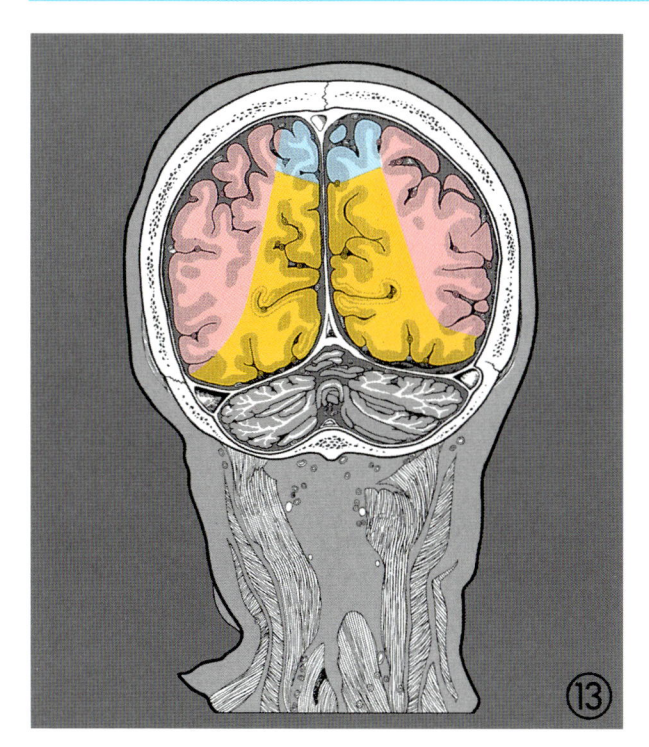

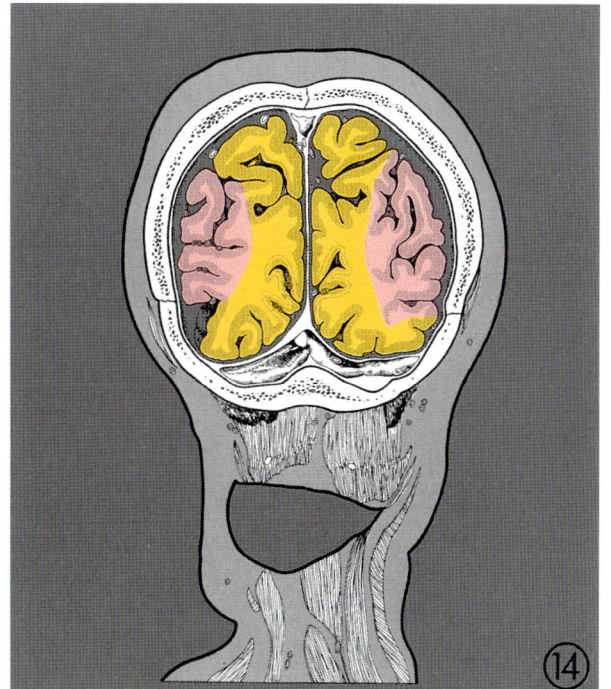

5.4 Arteries of the Brain and their Vascular Territories

☐ Terminal branches of anterior cerebral artery
☐ Terminal branches of middle cerebral artery
☐ Terminal branches of posterior cerebral artery

Central Territories

The central territories of the forebrain are supplied by **"penetrating" arteries**. They are end arteries and in the case of a lesion hypoperfusion results. Penetrating arteries are:

- The penetrating branches of the anterior cerebral artery include the **long central artery** (distal medial striate artery, Heubner's recurrent artery) and **anteromedial central arteries** (medial lenticulostriate arteries [35]) (Fig. 77b.4). Reaching the forebrain through the anterior perforated substance they supply the anteroinferior part of the caudate nucleus and putamen, and the anteroinferior part of the internal capsule (35).
- The **anterolateral central** (lateral lenticulostriate) **arteries** (Fig. 77b.5) are branches of the middle cerebral artery and penetrate basal parts of the forebrain to supply the innominate substance, the lateral part of the anterior commissure, most of the putamen, the lateral portion of the globus pallidus, the superior half of the internal capsule and adjacent corona radiata, and the body and head (except the anteroinferior part) of the caudate nucleus (36).
- The **posteromedial and posterolateral central arteries** are the penetrating branches of the posterior cerebral artery and branches from the circle of Willis. They reach the basal and posterior diencephalic areas and supply the thalamus, metathalamus, hypothalamus, and subthalamic nucleus.

Clinical Notes
Occlusion of a penetrating artery produces a small, well-circumscribed infarct. If only the pyramidal tract is affected, a contralateral paresis without sensory disturbances will develop. Infarcts in the ventral posterior nucleus of the thalamus produce "pure hemisensory loss."

Terminal Territories

The terminal territories of the cerebral hemispheres are supplied by the anterior, middle, and posterior cerebral arteries and of the anterior choroidal artery (29, 35, 36, 89, 179). These territories are demonstrated in Figures 92–96. The borders of these four territories are independent of the boundaries of the telencephalic lobes (Figs. 104–108a).

276 5 Topography of the Neurocranium and its Intracranial Spaces and Structures in Multiplanar Parallel Slices

- Terminal branches of anterior cerebral artery
- Terminal branches of middle cerebral artery
- Terminal branches of posterior cerebral artery
- Penetrating branches of anterior cerebral artery
- Penetrating branches of middle cerebral artery
- Penetrating branches of posterior cerebral artery and posterior communicating artery
- Anterior choroidal artery

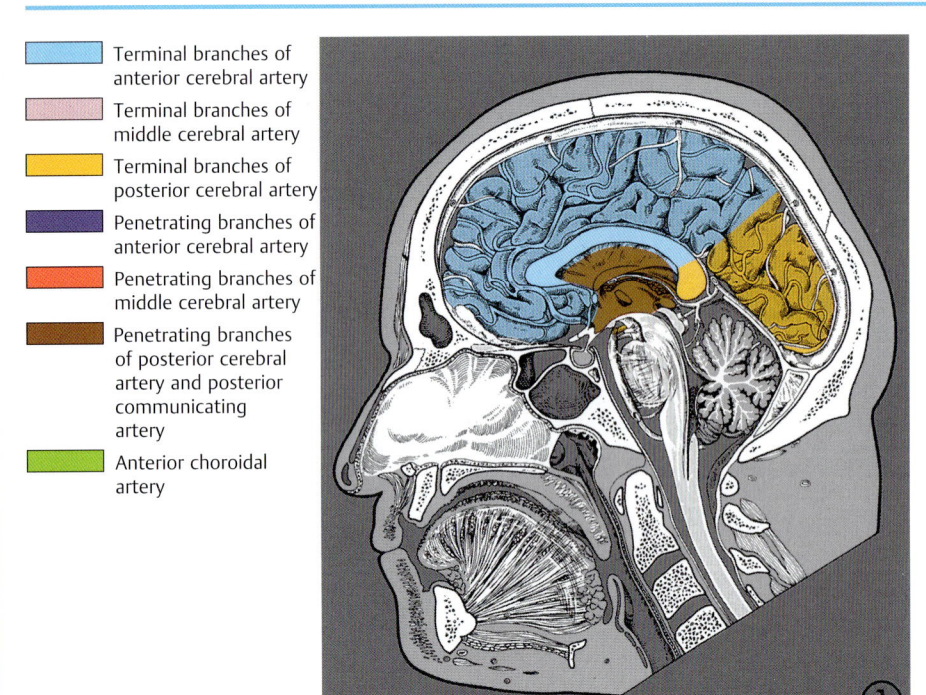

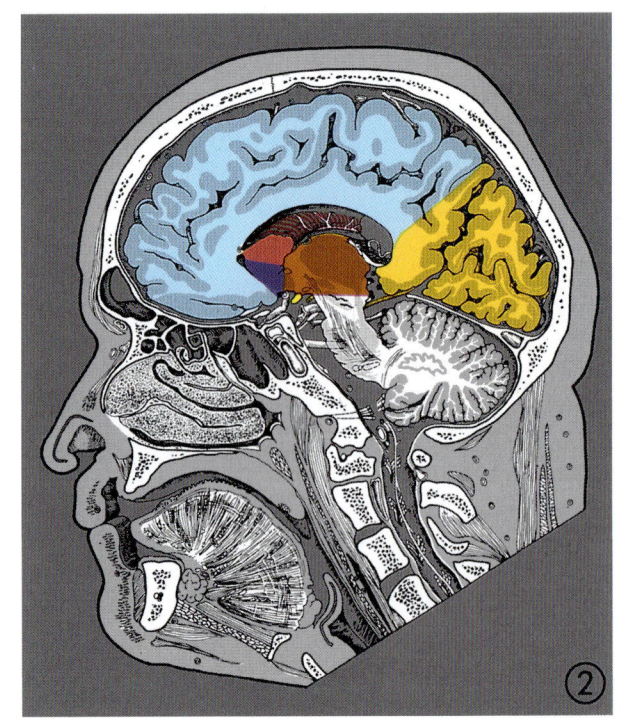

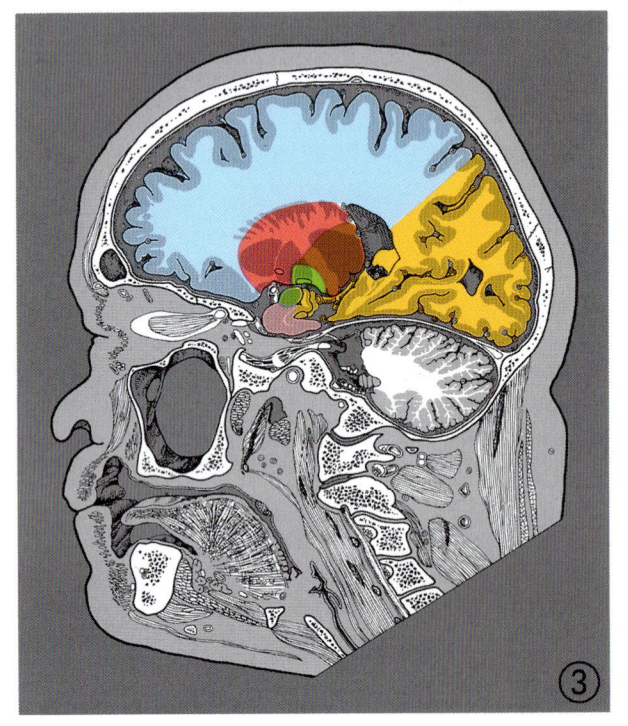

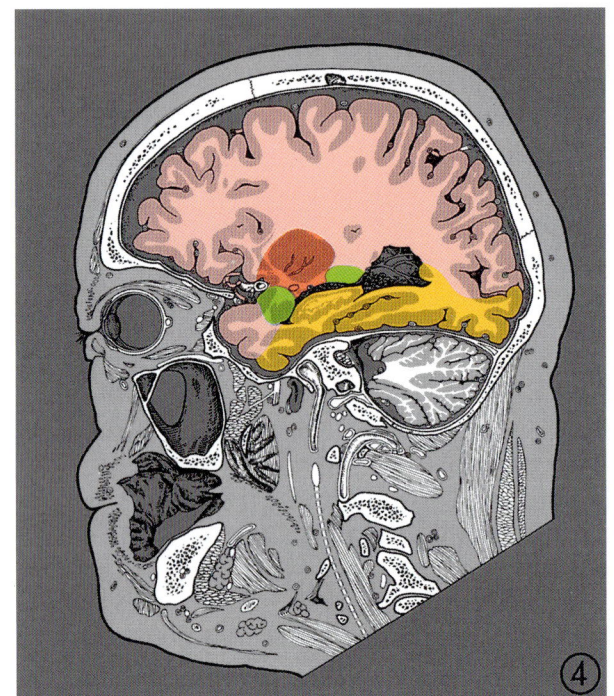

Fig. 94 Sagittal serial illustrations showing the vascular territories of the terminal and penetrating (central) branches of the anterior, middle, and posterior cerebral arteries and the anterior choroidal artery. The encircled number (1–6) indicates the number of the respective slice (Figs. 29, 30a,b, 31). According to (29, 35, 36, 89, 179).

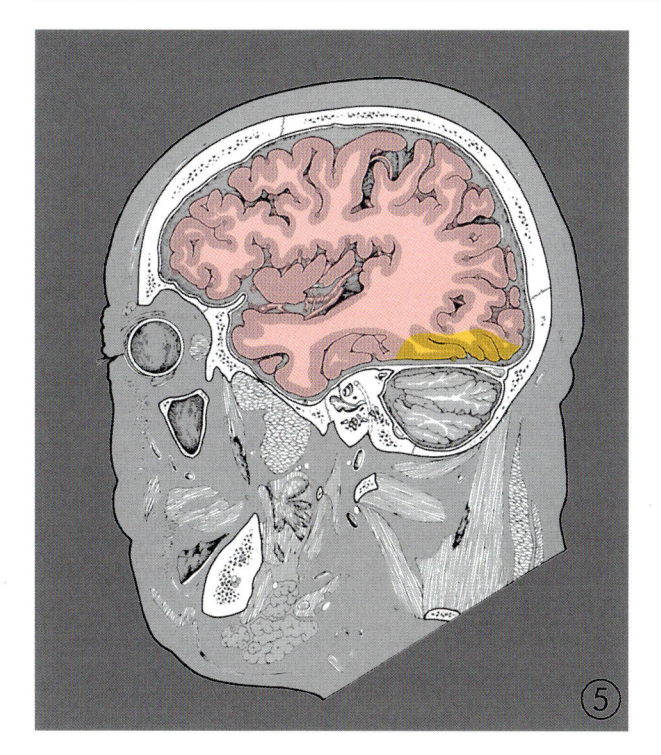

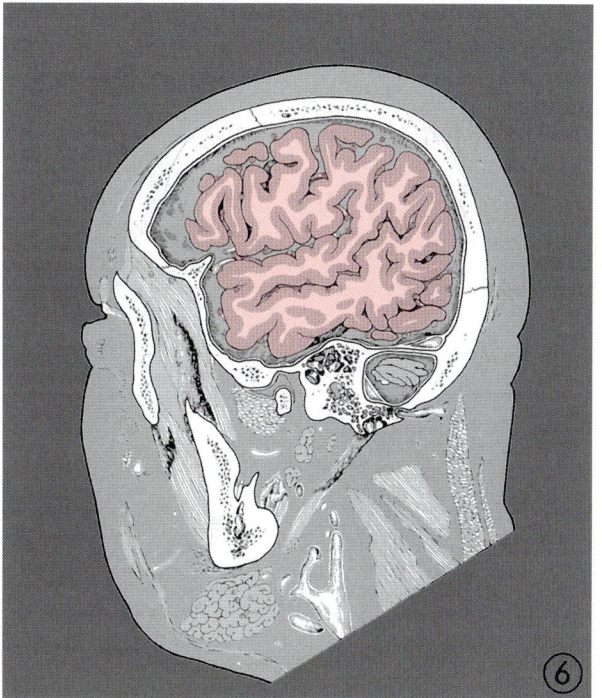

Terminal branches of middle cerebral artery

Terminal branches of posterior cerebral artery

Terminal Territories of the Anterior Cerebral Artery

The anterior cerebral artery supplies the anterior three-quarters of the medial surface of the cerebral hemisphere as far as the level of the parieto-occipital sulcus. Furthermore, it supplies the anterior four-fifths of the corpus callosum with the exception of the splenium. Additional small branches supply a 2–3-cm-wide strip along the convexity of the hemisphere along the superior margin. This area includes the superior frontal gyrus, the parts of the pre- and postcentral gyri close to the superior margin, as well as the upper parietal gyri. These vascular territories of the cortex and adjacent white matter contain the primary motor and sensory areas for the contralateral leg.

Clinical Notes
Occlusions of the terminal branches of the anterior cerebral artery cause a contralateral weakness and sensory loss in the leg.

Terminal Territories of the Middle Cerebral Artery

The terminal branches of the middle cerebral artery supply the insula, frontal, parietal, and temporal opercula and an oval territory around the lateral sulcus (Sylvian fissure) (Figs. 93, 94, 96). This territory includes the lower part of the precentral and postcentral gyri close to the central sulcus and, therefore, the primary motor and sensory areas of the trunk, arm, and head. Furthermore, the middle cerebral artery supplies the white matter beneath the parietal and temporal cortical areas. The upper part of the optic radiation (geniculocalcarine tract) is located in the parietal white matter and the lower part in the temporal white matter. In the dominant hemisphere the frontal operculum holds Broca's area and the superior temporal gyrus in the temporal operculum includes Wernicke's area.

Clinical Notes
Terminal infarcts in the territory of the middle cerebral artery cause contralateral weakness and sensory disturbances of the trunk, arm, and head, as well as contralateral inferior quadrantanopia (interruption of the parietal optic radiation) or contralateral superior quadrantanopia (interruption of the temporal optic radiation). If the language areas in the dominant hemisphere are affected, Broca's aphasia or Wernicke's aphasia may result (Chap. 6.10). When opercular damage is widespread in the dominant hemisphere, a severe language disturbance of a mixed type (global aphasia [59]) results.

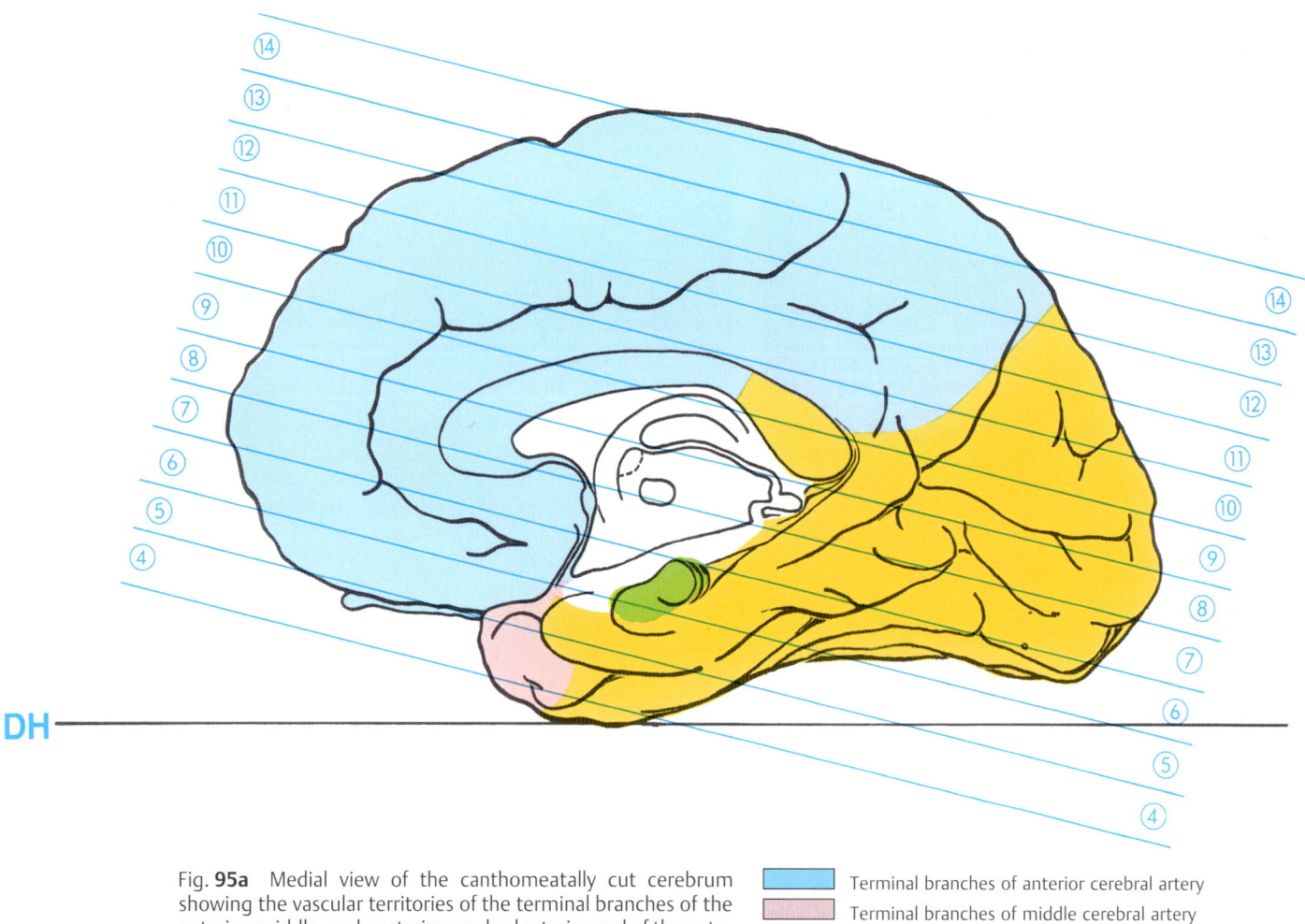

Fig. 95a Medial view of the canthomeatally cut cerebrum showing the vascular territories of the terminal branches of the anterior, middle, and posterior cerebral arteries and of the anterior choroidal artery. The encircled number indicates the number of the respective slice. According to (29, 35, 36, 89, 179). DH Reid's base line

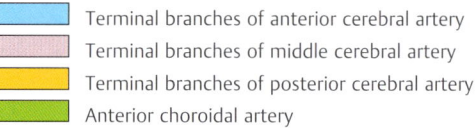

- Terminal branches of anterior cerebral artery
- Terminal branches of middle cerebral artery
- Terminal branches of posterior cerebral artery
- Anterior choroidal artery

Terminal Territories of the Posterior Cerebral Artery

On the medial surface of the hemisphere, the terminal branches of the posterior cerebral artery supply the inferior temporal lobe and large parts of the occipital lobe, especially the primary visual cortex (Figs. 92a, 95a). At the convexity of the hemispheres a small strip of the occipital and temporal lobes is supplied by them as well (Figs. 92b, 95b). The posterior cerebral artery also supplies the splenium of the corpus callosum.

Clinical Notes
An occlusion of the posterior cerebral artery causes a contralateral homonymous hemianopia. A lesion of the splenium leads to the disconnection of the primary visual cortex with the language areas. These patients may develop reading problems (alexia due to disconnection).

In Figures 92–96 the arterial territories of cerebral arteries are demonstrated in coronal, sagittal, and canthomeatal series according to references (35, 36, 59, 89, 179, 238, 264, 374a, 474). They are simplified and an average size was chosen; individual variations have to be taken into account. The extent of an infarct depends on the respective collateral supply.

Border zone infarcts constitute a special type of circulatory impairment. These occur in the border areas between the anterior, middle, and posterior cerebral territories, if two (less commonly three) of these arteries have an insufficient circulation.

For the assessment of regional cerebral circulation, perfusion CT, perfusion MRI, and emission computed tomography (Chap. 2.3) are suitable procedures. Intracranial arteries can be shown by the noninvasive MRA (Chap. 2.2) and CTA (Chap. 2.1). With this method vascular anomalies, dislocation of vessels, and pathologic patterns of the blood flow can be demonstrated.

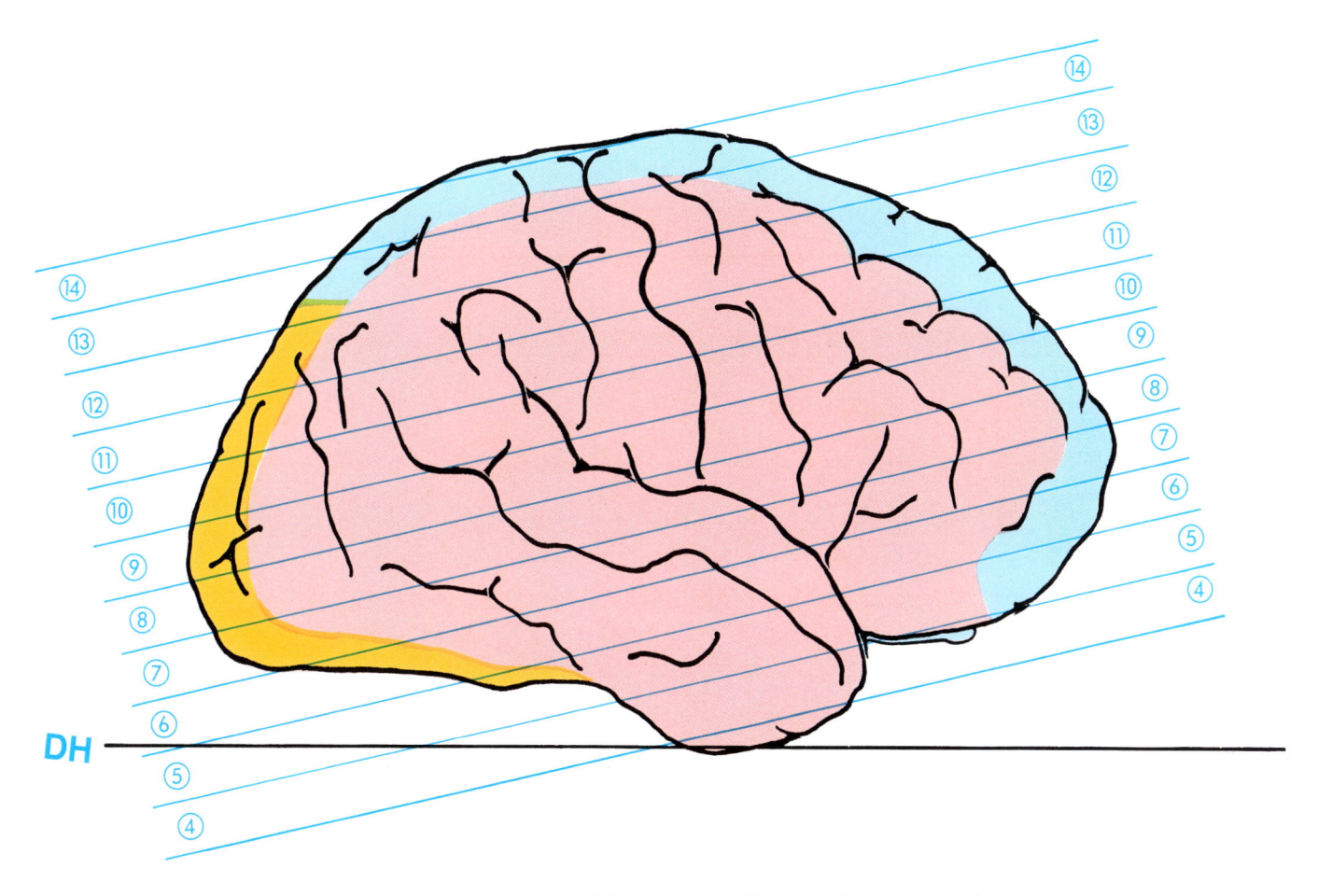

5.4 Arteries of the Brain and their Vascular Territories

Fig. 95b Lateral view of the canthomeatally cut cerebrum showing the vascular territories of the terminal branches of the anterior, middle, and posterior cerebral arteries. The encircled number indicates the number of the respective slice. According to (29, 35, 36, 89, 179).
DH Reid's base line

- Terminal branches of anterior cerebral artery
- Terminal branches of middle cerebral artery
- Terminal branches of posterior cerebral artery

280   5   Topography of the Neurocranium and its Intracranial Spaces and Structures in Multiplanar Parallel Slices

- Terminal branches of anterior cerebral artery
- Terminal branches of middle cerebral artery
- Terminal branches of posterior cerebral artery
- Penetrating branches of anterior cerebral artery
- Penetrating branches of middle cerebral artery
- Penetrating branches of posterior cerebral artery and posterior communicating artery
- Anterior choroidal artery

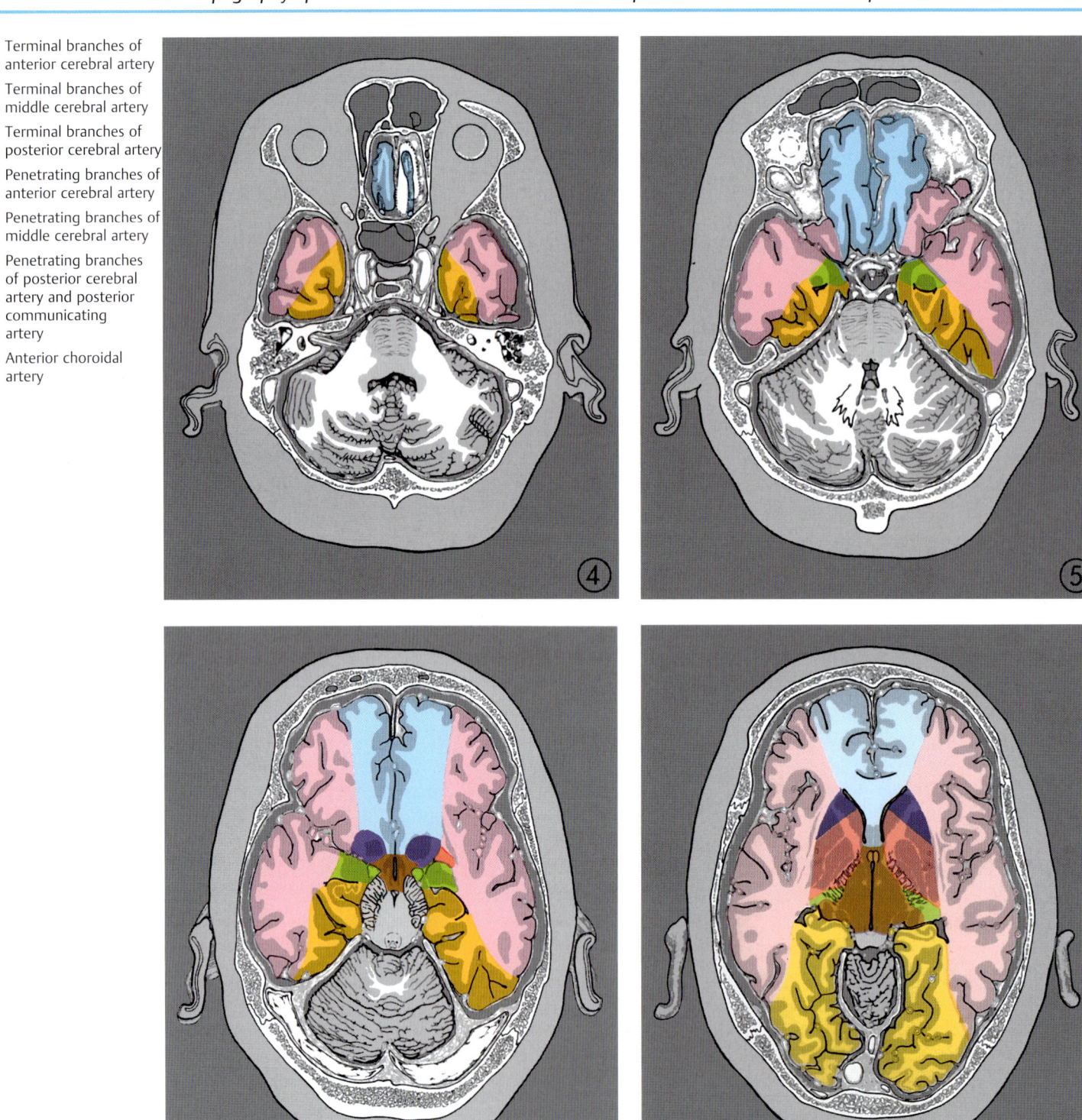

Fig. 96 Canthomeatally oriented serial illustrations showing the vascular territories of the terminal and penetrating (central) branches of the anterior, middle, and posterior cerebral arteries and the anterior choroidal artery. The encircled numbers (4–11) indicate the number of the respective slice (Figs. 44, 45a,b, 46). According to (29, 35, 36, 89, 179).

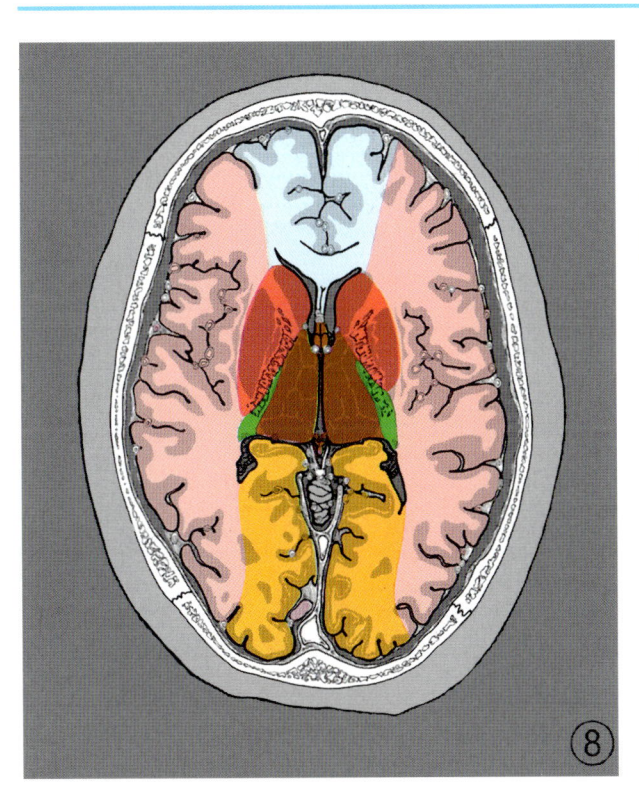

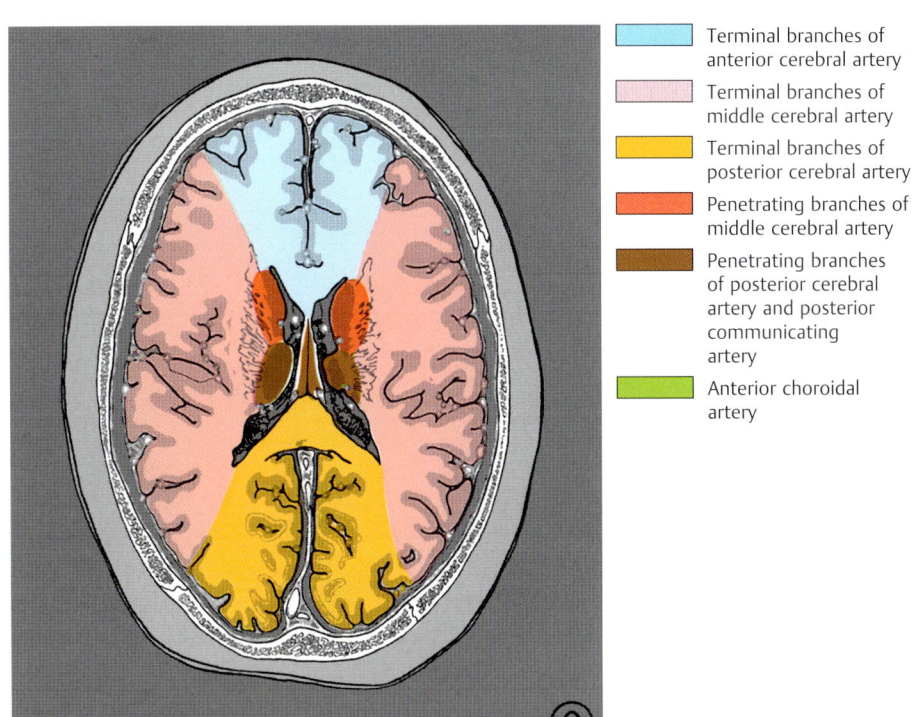

5.4 Arteries of the Brain and their Vascular Territories 281

	Terminal branches of anterior cerebral artery
	Terminal branches of middle cerebral artery
	Terminal branches of posterior cerebral artery
	Penetrating branches of middle cerebral artery
	Penetrating branches of posterior cerebral artery and posterior communicating artery
	Anterior choroidal artery

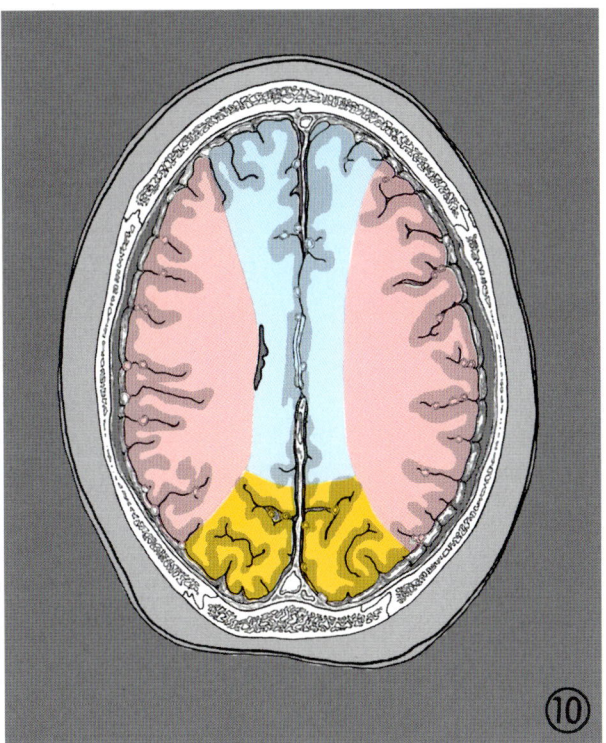

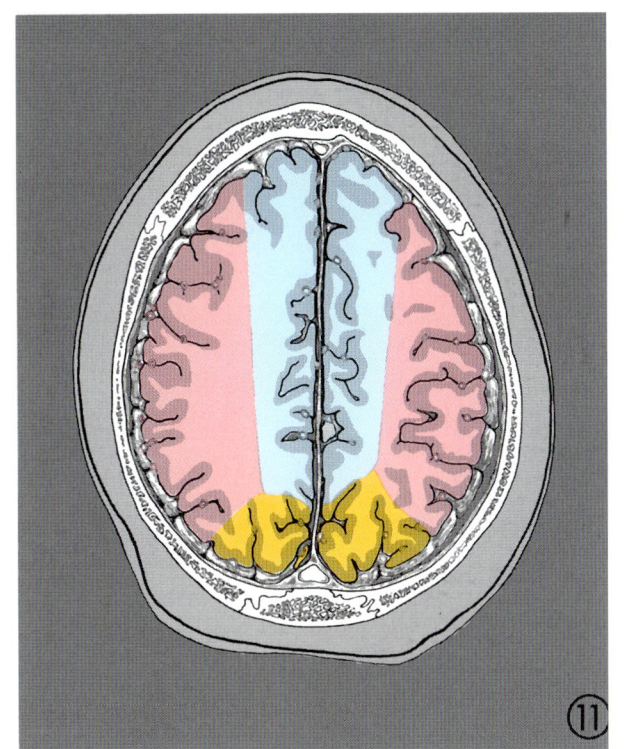

282   5   *Topography of the Neurocranium and its Intracranial Spaces and Structures in Multiplanar Parallel Slices*

☐ Terminal branches of anterior cerebral artery
☐ Terminal branches of middle cerebral artery
☐ Terminal branches of posterior cerebral artery

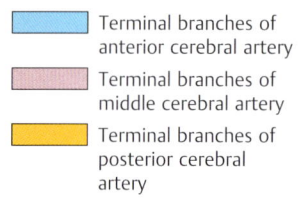

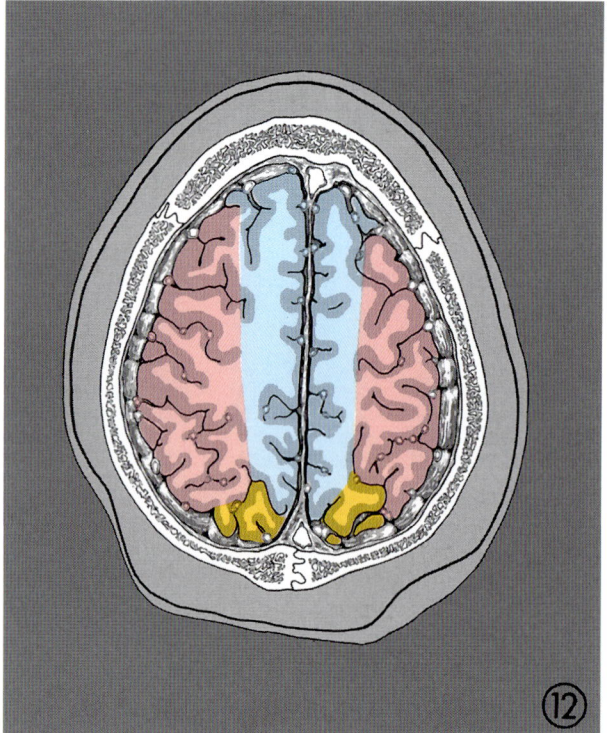

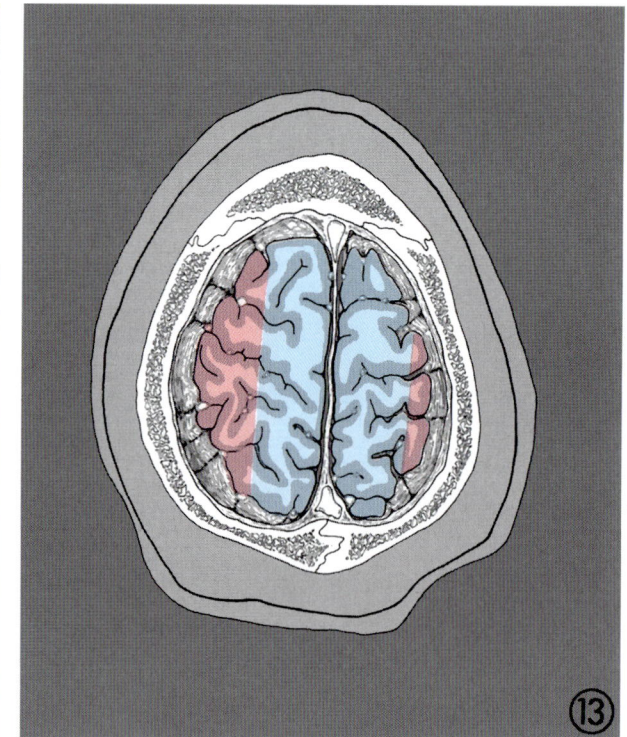

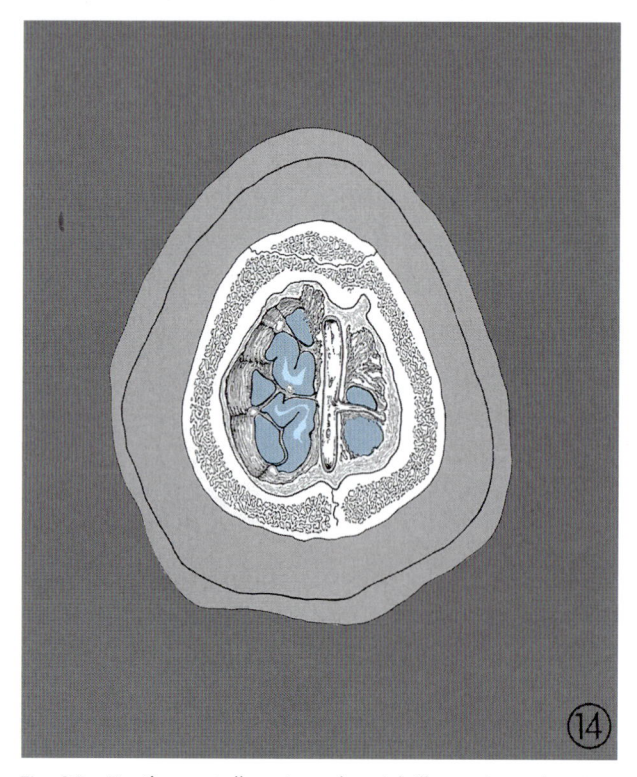

Fig. **96** Canthomeatally oriented serial illustrations showing the vascular territories of the terminal and penetrating (central) branches of the anterior, middle, and posterior cerebral arteries. The encircled numbers (12–14) indicate the number of the respective slice (Figs. 44, 45a,b, 46). According to (29, 35, 36, 89, 179).

5.5 Veins of the Brain

(Figs. 97a,b, 4c–17c, 32c–37c, 47a, 48c–60c)

In the human body numerous veins run along common vascular routes parallel to their corresponding arteries. The veins of the brain, however, run **spatially independent of the arteries of the brain**. In addition, these veins also show a greater variability than the arteries. Nevertheless, the topography of veins can be described by a general scheme. The topography of the deep intracerebral veins, as shown in angiograms, is of particular diagnostic importance. In the venous phase of the angiogram space-occupying lesions can be recognized by the displacement of the deep cranial veins. The superficial arteries of the brain may appear normal in such angiographic images.

The veins and sinuses can be used to some extent as guideline structures in CT and MRI (Chap. 2.5.5). Pathologic changes or displacements are frequently discrete or not visible at all. Dislocations of the medial structures are often more clearly identified by changes of the ventricular system than by displacement of the veins.

The veins of the brain contain no valves and form a tubular network with many anastomoses. The principal venous drainage occurs via the venous sinuses through the **internal jugular vein** (Figs. 11c.37, 48c.13, 49c.17). The internal jugular vein leaves the skull through the jugular foramen (Figs. 25.6, 35c.30, 49c.16, 63.16). Other veins can take over the drainage of the internal jugular veins. The internal vertebral venous plexus can drain blood from a basilar venous plexus located on the clivus. The **cavernous sinus** may drain through the ophthalmic veins into the facial vein. Cerebral blood can be drained via the veins passing through the foramen ovale into the pterygoid venous plexus, via veins located in the carotid canal (not indicated in Fig. 97a), and via emissary veins.

The telencephalon and diencephalon are drained by two groups of veins:

- **Superficial veins** drain blood mainly from the cortical areas.
- **Deep veins** receive most of their blood from the white matter and the nuclear regions located there. In a few instances, these deep veins also drain cortical regions. Blood from the tributaries of the deep veins is collected in a cascading manner in the great cerebral vein (of Galen) (Figs. 97a.10, 32c.13, 54c.19, 55c.20). This large vein usually joins the inferior sagittal sinus (Fig. 97a.11) at its junction with the straight sinus (Figs. 97a.13, 14c.7, 32c.23) (264).

Superficial Veins of the Brain

The superficial cerebral veins include the superior cerebral veins (Figs. 54c.3, 55c.3, 56c.3, 57c.3, 58c.4), inferior cerebral veins, and superficial middle cerebral veins (Figs. 52c.5, 53c.9). The superior cerebral veins, known simply as the superficial cerebral veins, ascend in an arch along the curvature of the cerebral hemisphere to join the superior sagittal sinus (Figs. 4c.1, 9b.1, 9c.1, 17c.1, 32c.2, 54c.2, 60c.5). The veins close to the sinus break through the arachnoid mater and fasten their adventitia to the tough connective tissue of the dura mater. These veins are referred to as "bridging veins" (Fig. 32b.1, 53c.3). They are easily subjected to mechanical injury and can be the source of a subdural hematoma (164).

The superficial cerebral veins are divided into prefrontal, frontal, parietal, and occipital veins. The inferior cerebral veins descend from the external surfaces of the frontal, temporal, and occipital lobes. The frontal veins generally flow into the superficial middle cerebral vein. The temporal and occipital veins flow directly into the transverse sinus (Figs. 14c.11, 14d.13, 17c.9, 33c.22, 37c.14, 52c.19) or indirectly via the posterior anastomotic veins. The superficial middle cerebral vein originates on the lateral wall of the cerebral hemisphere above the lateral sulcus. It may join the cavernous sinus (Figs. 8c.15, 9c.13, 33c.21, 50c.9), sphenoparietal sinus, paracavernous sinus into the veins of the foramen ovale, superior petrosal sinus (Figs. 51c.19, 75b.7), or sigmoid sinus (Figs. 12c.19, 13c.16, 36c.30, 49c.19, 50c.20, 50d.22, 51b.19, 51c.20).

Deep Veins of the Brain

The great cerebral vein (of Galen), which is approximately 1 cm long, collects the blood of the deep cerebral veins. It originates at the junction of both internal cerebral veins (Figs. 12c.10, 13c.10, 32c.12, 54c.12), curves around the posterior surface of the splenium of the corpus callosum, and usually terminates by draining into the junction of the inferior sagittal sinus and the straight sinus. At this point the cerebral falx meets the ridge of the tentorium of cerebellum.

The **internal cerebral vein** is the confluence of the anterior vein of the septum pellucidum (Fig. 54c.11), superior thalamostriate vein (also known as the terminal vein) (Figs. 10c.8, 12c.8, 55c.11), and the superior choroid vein (Fig. 55c.12). The entry of the anterior vein of the septum pellucidum into the superior thalamostriate vein can be observed in lateral projections of the brain. This junction is referred to as the venous angle. It is usually located at the level of the interventricular foramen. Dislocation of the venous angle indicates an intracranial displacement, especially in the median plane. The superior thalamostriate vein lies in about 50% of cases between the caudate nucleus and the thalamus. It may change its course in an occipital direction before it reaches the interventricular foramen. In this case, the confluence of the anterior vein of the septum pellucidum and the superior thalamostriate vein at the venous angle is located several millimeters occipital to the interventricular foramen (264).

The internal cerebral vein runs posteriorly inside the cistern of the transverse fissure (cistern of velum

Superficial veins of cortical regions and their sinuses:

1. Superior cerebral veins
2. Superior sagittal sinus
3. Superficial middle cerebral vein
4. Cavernous sinus
5. Inferior petrosal sinus

Deep veins of central and nuclear regions and their sinuses:

6. Anterior vein of septum pellucidum
7. Superior thalamostriate (terminal) vein
8. Venous angle
9. Internal cerebral vein
10. Great cerebral vein (of Galen)
11. Inferior sagittal sinus
12. Basal vein (of Rosenthal)
13. Straight sinus
14. Confluence of sinuses
15. Transverse sinus
16. Sigmoid sinus
17. Internal jugular vein

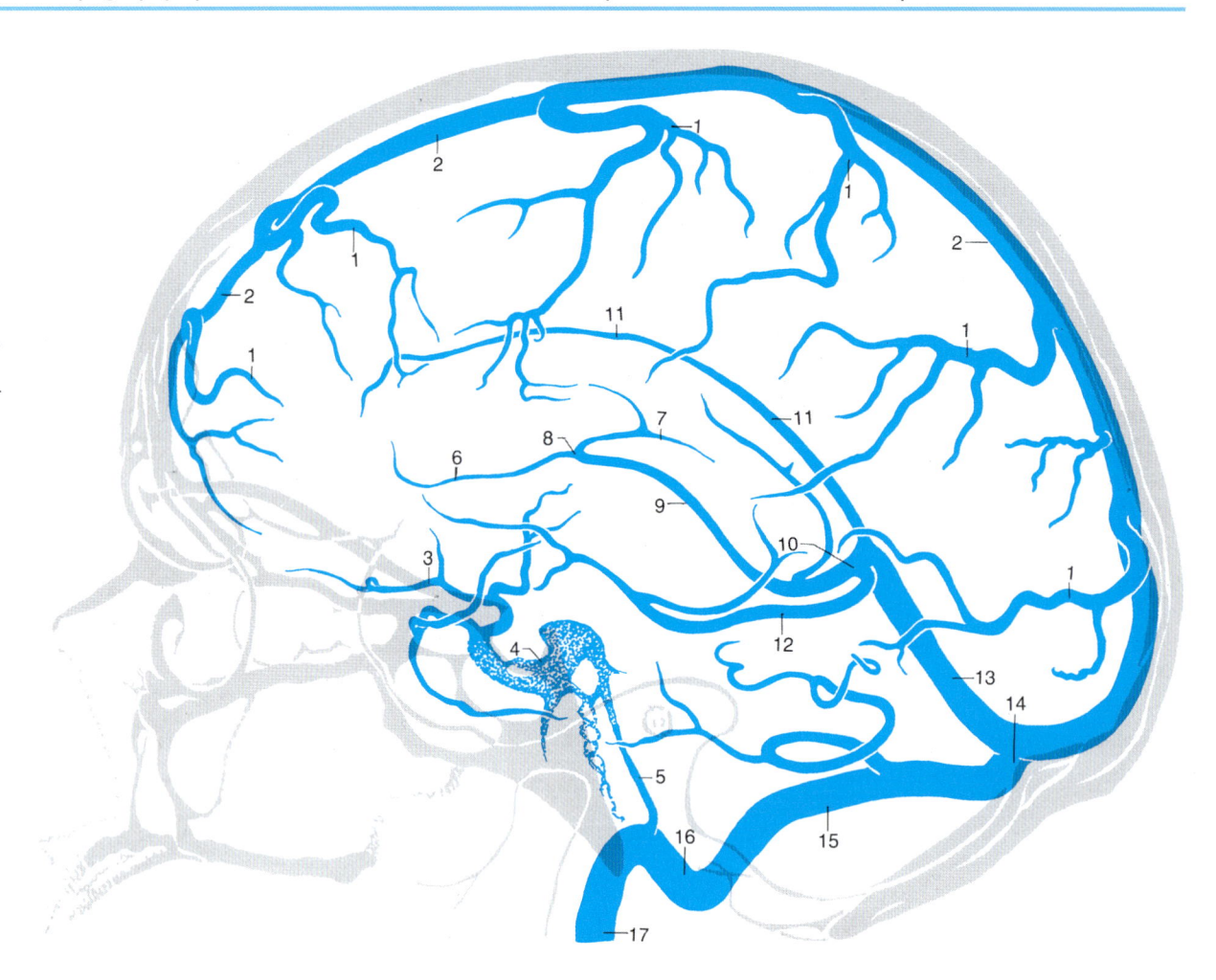

Fig. **97a** Lateral view of the head illustrating the cerebral veins and sinuses. The sequence of the numbers takes into account both the areas drained by the veins and the direction of blood flow. According to (238).

interpositum) in a slightly wavelike manner. Approximately 3.5 cm posterior to the interventricular foramen, the right and left internal cerebral veins join to form the great cerebral vein. Dislocation of an internal cerebral vein visible in angiograms indicates a supratentorial displacement of a cerebral hemisphere.

The **basal vein** (of Rosenthal) (Figs. 8c.11, 12c.14, 51c.15, 52c.15, 53c.19) is formed by various confluences: the anterior cerebral vein, the inferior central veins, and the deep cerebral vein of the anterior perforated substance. These veins receive blood from the basal and medial parts of the frontal lobe, the basal ganglia, and the insula. The basal vein runs occipitally along the optic tract between the cerebral peduncle and the diencephalon. The vein ascends posteriorly around the cerebral peduncle in the ambient cistern. In addition to the above-mentioned drainage of the frontal and insular parts of the telencephalon, the initial basilar segment of the basal vein receives blood from the pole of the temporal lobe and the hippocampus, as well as from portions of the midbrain and diencephalon. The second lateroposterior segment of the basal vein is located between the cerebral peduncle and its variable junction with the internal cerebral vein, the great cerebral vein, or the straight sinus. The second segment receives venous blood from the cerebral peduncle, the tectum, the geniculate bodies, the body and splenium of the corpus callosum, the medial surface of the occipital lobe, and portions of the cerebellum.

The unpaired vessels, namely the great cerebral vein and the straight sinus, collect blood from the paired internal cerebral veins and the basal veins. These veins drain the large regions of the white matter of the telencephalon, diencephalon, striatum, midbrain, pons, cerebellum, and medial and basal regions of the frontal, temporal, and occipital surfaces of the telencephalon.

The straight sinus unites with the **superior sagittal sinus** at the **confluence of sinuses** (Figs. 17c.8,

5.5 Veins of the Brain

1. Sphenoparietal sinus
2. Anterior intercavernous sinus
3. Cavernous sinus
4. Posterior intercavernous sinus
5. Basilar plexus
6. Venous plexus of foramen ovale
7. Superior petrosal sinus
8. Inferior petrosal sinus
9. Internal jugular vein (running inferiorly)
10. Sigmoid sinus
11. Transverse sinus
12. Occipital sinus
13. Superior sagittal sinus
14. Confluence of sinuses

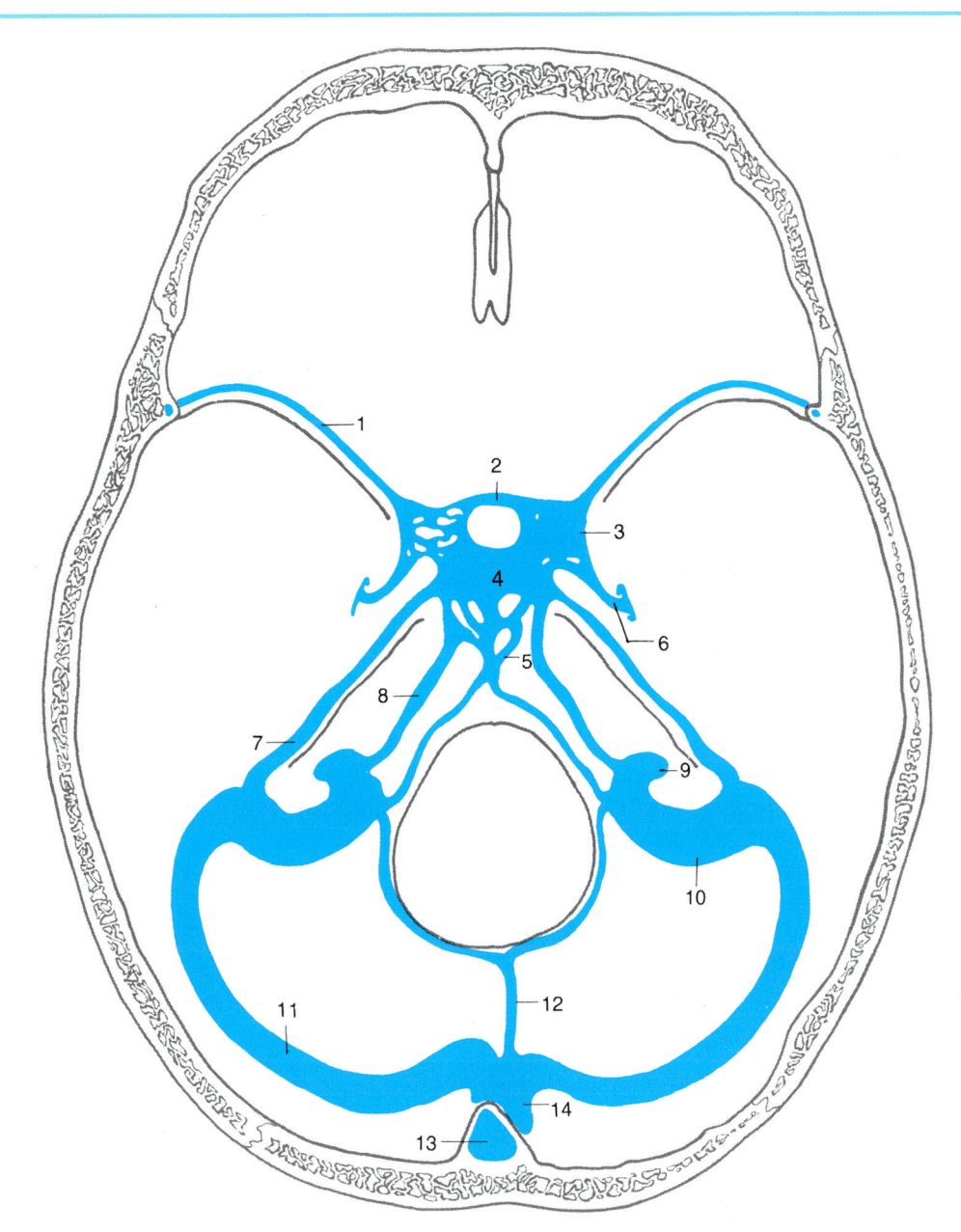

Fig. **97b** Illustration of the basal sinuses. According to (238).

32b.29, 32c.26, 32d.29, 53c.25) to form the transverse sinus. From there the venous blood flows via the sigmoid sinus into the internal jugular vein.

Blood generally drains from the midbrain through the great cerebral vein. Furthermore, small veins originating in the upper anterior portion of the cerebellum flow into the great cerebral vein. The large veins of the cerebellum run through the subarachnoid space independent of the arteries and join various blood vessels of the posterior cranial fossa. The petrosal vein drains the lower anterior portions of the cerebellum and of the pons. This vein flows into the superior petrosal sinus. The remaining cerebellar veins drain into the straight sinus, the confluence of sinuses, and occasionally into the transverse sinus. Venous drainage of the pons and the medulla oblongata varies greatly, taking place through tributaries of the basal vein, the transverse sinus, the inferior and superior petrosal sinuses, the occipital sinus, or the internal vertebral venous plexus.

Clinical Notes

Cerebral venous and dural sinus thrombosis are divided clinically into bland and septic categories and functional–anatomically into deep and superficial venous vascular illnesses. Untypical complaints and a multitude of different symptoms make diagnosis difficult. Imaging using specific blood-sensitive MR sequences and MRA are diagnostic aids featuring the highest degree of accuracy (403, 468). A DSA is necessary in the case of an indecisive diagnosis with MRI. Primary examinations usually include a CT (198), important for obtaining a differential diagnosis of the brain veins and dural sinus thrombosis, which may not be gained by clinical signs and symptoms only. Suspect findings on neuroimaging may include extremely narrow ventricles and/or external fluid spaces, also symmetrical bilateral hypodensity or hemorrhage with atypical localization. Thrombosis of the cerebral veins and dural sinuses constitute the most frequent wrong diagnosis (198).

5.6 Cranial Nerves

(Figs. 68, 81, 82, 114, 119, 122, 126)

The cranial nerves emerge from the base of the brain and pass through the subarachnoid space before penetrating the dura mater and leaving through the foramina in the skull base. The second cranial nerve is the only one retaining its sheath of dura mater outside the cranial cavity. Cranial nerves XII through VII leave via foramina in the posterior cranial fossa. Cranial nerves VI through II leave via foramina in the middle cranial fossa. The first cranial nerve passes through the cribriform plate, thus emerging from the anterior cranial fossa.

> *Clinical Notes*
> T2-weighted MR images with FLAIR sequences are more suitable for MRI for localization of the exit positions of the cranial nerves (508).

Twelfth Cranial Nerve

The twelfth cranial or **hypoglossal nerve** (Figs. 3.34, 11a.43, 12a.40, 33a.36, 33a.47, 48a.5) appears as 12 to 16 rootlets sprouting out of the medulla oblongata between the pyramid and inferior olive. These rootlets join to form several bundles that, as a rule, lie posterior to the vertebral artery and extend as far as the hypoglossal canal of the occipital bone. The hypoglossal nerve innervates the muscles of the tongue.

Eleventh Cranial Nerve

The eleventh cranial or **accessory nerve** (Figs. 3.37, 12a.39, 30b.26, 49a.10, 70b.22) has two roots: the spinal and the cranial roots. The fibers of the spinal root (Figs. 3.39, 33a.38, 47a.23, 48a.6, 49a.11) arise from the C1 through C6 (maximal C7, minimal C3) segments of the spinal cord. They emerge from the lateral side of the spinal cord, extend cranially, and pass through the foramen magnum to the posterior cranial fossa. The fibers of the cranial root arise as three to six rootlets on the lateral side of the medulla oblongata. Both roots join up with the ninth and tenth cranial nerves just proximal to the dural opening above the jugular foramen. These three nerves IX, X, and XI leave through the medial part of the jugular foramen. The spinal root of the accessory nerve together with direct branches of the cervical plexus innervate the ipsilateral sternocleidomastoid and trapezoid. The cranial root assists in the motor innervation of the pharynx and partially innervates the muscles of the soft palate and the larynx.

Tenth Cranial Nerve

The tenth cranial or **vagus nerve** (Figs. 3.33, 11a.42, 12a.36, 30b.23, 33a.34, 49a.9, 71c.7, 71d.7) emerges from the lateral edge of the medulla oblongata by 10 to 18 fine rootlets. It stretches about 1.5 cm within a cistern to the dural opening above the jugular foramen (264). It conveys sensory information from a small area in the external acoustic meatus and the sensory taste buds in the pharynx. It also carries visceral afferent information from the mucous membranes of the thoracic and abdominal viscera. The vagus nerve provides the intrinsic laryngeal muscles and the caudal portion of the pharyngeal constrictor except the stylopharyngeus. It is the parasympathetic nerve of the thoracic viscera, the upper abdominal organs, and intestinal tract down to the splenic fissure.

Ninth Cranial Nerve

The ninth cranial or **glossopharyngeal nerve** (Figs. 3.33, 11a.42, 12a.36, 30b.22, 33a.34, 49a.9) has some morphologic similarities with the vagus nerve. These similarities include a lateral exit from the medulla oblongata and a passage through the jugular foramen. Likewise, the glossopharyngeal nerve provides the primary visceral regions including the mucosa of the palate and pharynx, the taste buds on the posterior third of the tongue, as well as the parasympathetic innervation of the parotid gland and the cranial portion of the pharyngeal muscles including the stylopharyngeus.

Eighth Cranial Nerve

The eighth cranial or **vestibulocochlear nerve** (Figs. 3.30, 11a.40, 12a.35, 30b.20, 34a.30, 50a.15, 50d.14) is a combination of two pathways: one serves the vestibular system, the other the auditory system. Following the direction of the afferent fibers, the nerve passes through the internal acoustic meatus and enters the medulla oblongata at the lateral edge near the border with the pons. The intracisternal portion of the vestibulocochlear nerve is approximately 1.4 cm long (264).

Seventh Cranial Nerve

The seventh cranial or **facial nerve** arises together with the intermediate nerve (of Wrisberg) (Figs. 3.28, 11a.39, 11a.44, 12a.34, 30b.17, 34a.29, 50a.14, 50d.14) from the lateral wall between the pons and medulla oblongata. The intermediate nerve is an extremely thin bundle that runs in an inferior position parallel to the main part of the seventh cranial nerve. The seventh cranial nerve lies superior to the vestibulocochlear nerve in the internal acoustic meatus. The facial nerve measures approximately 1.6 cm from its origin to the internal acoustic meatus (264). The **intermediate nerve** contains sensory nerve fibers from the taste buds on the anterior two-thirds of the tongue, and parasympathetic fibers for the lacrimal glands, the nasopharyngeal, sublingual, and submandibular glands. The facial nerve is principally motor and innervates the muscles of facial expression, the stapedius, and the posterior belly of the digastric. In one out of three cases, the anterior inferior cerebellar artery (AICA) forms a loop in the direct vicinity of the facial nerve.

This vascular loop may compress the facial nerve resulting in a hemifacial spasm (211, 371, 398).

Sixth, Fourth, and Third Cranial Nerves

The abducens nerve (VI), trochlear nerve (IV), and oculomotor nerve (III) innervate the extraocular muscles. The **abducens nerve** (Figs. 3.32, 10a.34, 11a.41, 30b.18, 32a.35, 33a.31, 49a.5, 72b.8) emerges in 94% of cases from the fissure between the pons and the medulla oblongata and in 6% of cases just above this fissure from the lower portion of the pons (508). It passes through the pontine cistern and pierces the dura mater (Figs. 50a.11, 74b.9) at the clivus mediobasal to the tip of the petrous part of the temporal bone. The intracisternal portion of the abducens nerve is 1.5 cm long (264). It continues through the venous basilar plexus and enters the lateral wall of the cavernous sinus. It then leaves the middle cranial fossa through the superior orbital fissure and innervates the lateral rectus. A complete lesion of the abducens nerve leads to an ipsilateral strabismus: the affected eye is strongly adducted.

The **trochlear nerve** (Figs. 12a.25, 51a.16, 76b.14, 77b.24) is the only cranial nerve that emerges from the posterior side of the brainstem. The trochlear nerve originates from the midbrain just inferior to the inferior colliculus of the tectum. It traverses the ambient cistern around the midbrain and pierces the dura mater where the tentorial notch attaches to the posterior clinoid process. On most occasions the nerve enters the dura about 1 cm inferior to the posterior clinoid process. The trochlear nerve runs along the roof of the cavernous sinus, passing through the superior orbital fissure into the orbit. It innervates the superior oblique, which rotates the eye downward and laterally. A lesion of the trochlear nerve allows the antagonist muscles to rotate the eye upward and medially.

The **oculomotor nerve** (Figs. 2b.29, 9a.27, 10a.31, 30b.13, 32a.16, 33a.23, 51a.11, 76b.7, 77b.13, 77d.8) is the largest of the three nerves for the extraocular muscles. It innervates the remaining four extraocular muscles and the levator palpebrae superioris. In addition, the oculomotor nerve carries parasympathetic fibers for the sphincter pupillae and the ciliary muscles. The oculomotor nerve emerges from the interpeduncular fossa, passes through the similarly named cistern, and runs between the superior cerebellar artery and the posterior cerebral artery toward the cavernous sinus. There it runs in the lateral wall of the cavernous sinus and leaves the middle cranial fossa through the superior orbital fissure.

Fifth Cranial Nerve

The fifth cranial or **trigeminal nerve** (Figs. 10a.37, 11a.38, 30b.16, 33a.26, 34a.25, 50a.10, 74c.7, 74d.7, 75b.11) arises from the lateral edge of the pons (77). It emerges from the posterior cranial fossa and reaches the trigeminal cave in the middle cranial fossa. This flat dural pouch (Meckel's cave) is lined with the arachnoid mater. The trigeminal ganglion (formerly Gasserian or semilunar ganglion) (Figs. 9a.31, 34a.28, 73b.3) is found here and contains unipolar neurons for the sensory root of the trigeminal nerve. Beyond the ganglion, the trigeminal nerve divides into three large branches: the ophthalmic, maxillary, and mandibular nerves. These branches emerge from the middle cranial fossa through the superior orbital fissure (Fig. 64.7), the foramen rotundum (Fig. 63.5), and foramen ovale (Fig. 63.8), respectively. For the most part, the trigeminal nerve transmits afferent signals from the skin of the face, the conjunctiva and cornea, the mucosa of the nasal and oral cavities, and the teeth. The afferent fibers from the muscle spindles of the muscles of mastication are interconnected in a special way in the trigeminal system (Chap. 6.1.3).

The motor fibers of the trigeminal nerve lie in the medial portion of the nerve and project toward the mandibular nerve. The motor fibers innervate the muscles of mastication, the tensor tympani, and the majority of the muscles of the floor of the mouth.

The most common situation, according to neurosurgical findings, shows that the superior cerebellar artery can compress the trigeminal nerve and may cause trigeminal neuralgia (210, 212, 398).

Second Cranial Nerve

The second cranial or **optic nerve** (Figs. 2b.26, 7a.13, 7d.14, 8a.17, 32a.23, 33a.18, 49a.2, 50a.5, 50b.5, 76a.14, 77b.2) enters the middle cranial fossa through the optic canal (77). The topography of the optic nerve is described further in visual system (Chap. 6.6).

First Cranial Nerve

The first cranial or **olfactory nerve** projects through the cribriform plate into the anterior cranial fossa. It is described in detail in olfactory system (Chap. 6.7).

Syndromes of the Cranial Nerves

The topography of the cranial nerves, in relation to each other and to structures at the skull base as well as to blood vessels and to different parts of the human brain, is of considerable clinical relevance. Lesions that simultaneously affect several cranial nerves can aid in locating an injury in relation to the course of these nerves. This may be the case with an inflammation or a tumor at the skull base or of the brain itself. **Garcin's syndrome** is characterized by a lesion of all 12 cranial nerves on one side of the skull base. In many cases isolated cranial nerves are spared.

The **jugular foramen syndrome** includes: disorders of the glossopharyngeal nerve with sensory impairment, frequent pain indicating glossopharyngeal neuralgia, paresis of the soft palate, a lesion of the vagus nerve with vocal cord palsy, and unilateral paralysis of the accessory and hypoglossal nerves. Such signs, together with concurrent pressure on the medulla oblongata and a resultant contralateral hemiparesis, are referred to as **Vernet's syndrome**.

The **cerebellopontine angle syndrome** is a disorder of the fifth, seventh, and eighth cranial nerves often caused by a schwannoma of the eighth cranial nerve. Sensory impairment (including loss of the corneal reflex) and/or pain in the facial region, peripheral facial paresis, and unilateral acoustic and vestibular defects are to be expected. In advanced cases, cerebellar involvement may cause ipsilateral ataxia and nystagmus. Occasionally paresis of the abducens nerve may be found.

Gradenigo's syndrome or syndrome of the apex of the petrous part of the temporal bone is marked by unilateral paresis of the abducens nerve and by disorders of the trigeminal nerve with sensory impairment or facial pain, especially in the forehead. Larger lesions may also cause peripheral facial paralysis.

The **cavernous sinus syndrome** involves a disorder of the three ocular nerves, namely the third, fourth, and sixth cranial nerves, as well as the trigeminal nerve.

If, in addition to the three ocular cranial nerves, only the first trigeminal division is affected, a **syndrome of the superior orbital fissure** is present. Additional presence of unilateral headaches, especially in the temporal region, and a nonpulsating exophthalmos indicate a **syndrome of the sphenoid wing**. The cause is frequently a meningioma in this region.

A disorder of the third, fourth, sixth, and first division of the fifth (ophthalmic nerve) cranial nerves with involvement of the optic nerve is referred to as the **orbital apex syndrome**. Frequently, the primary symptom is an increasing optic atrophy with corresponding visual impairment.

The **olfactory groove syndrome** presents first with unilateral and eventually with bilateral anosmia. The lesion may also affect the optic nerve, thereby leading to blindness. Large space-occupying lesions, such as meningiomas, are frequently marked by a frontal lobe syndrome with corresponding psychopathologic findings.

In the initial stages, lesions responsible for the cranial nerve syndromes located in the region of the skull base are difficult to demonstrate in the CT because the lesions are closely related to the base of the skull. Enhancement, CT scans of reduced thickness, other projections, special bone examinations (high-resolution technique), and intrathecal contrast medium are necessary for better portrayal. Frequently MRI leads to earlier demonstration of pathologic lesions. Thinner MR scans and occasionally i.v. administration of contrast medium are also necessary at times. For early detection of basal cerebral lesions MRI is more suitable than CT. The use of both procedures can improve the diagnostic accuracy (Chap. 2.6).

5.7 Subdivisions of the Brain
(Figs. 98–103)

The brain can be divided into two basic parts:
1. Brainstem together with the cerebellum
2. Forebrain or prosencephalon.

According to Terminologia Anatomica the medulla oblongata, pons, and midbrain are collectively called the brainstem. The cerebellum is connected to the brainstem by three paired cerebellar peduncles. The forebrain is further divided into the diencephalon and telencephalon. The longitudinal axis of the brainstem (**Meynert's axis**) and the longitudinal axis of the forebrain (Forel's axis) lie, as mentioned in the introduction (Chap. 1.1), at an approximate 110–120° angle to one another. The axis of the brainstem lies approximately at the floor of the fourth ventricle. Forel's axis extends from the frontal to the occipital pole of the telencephalon. The angle between the two axes as measured in brains fixed extracranially usually differs from the angle measured in living patients (Chap. 1.3).

5.7.1 Medulla Oblongata and Pons
(Figs. 98–103)

The **medulla oblongata** is a small subdivision of the brain. Its volume is about 7 ml and its basilar surface between the spinal cord and pons is approximately 2 to 2.5 cm long. The area of the cross-section through its inferior portion is on average 1 cm^2.

External Features

On the anterior side of the medulla the anterior median fissure continues into the spinal cord. A longitudinal column rises on the medulla oblongata along both sides of the fissure. This paired elevation is called the pyramid (Figs. 48b.8, 69c.7). The pyramidal pathway (Chap. 6.8.1) crosses deep within the fissure.

The paired inferior olive-shaped bodies lateral to the pyramids are referred to as inferior olives. The inferior olive contains the inferior olivary nucleus. Nuclear regions of the posterior funiculi form small elevations on the posterior side of the medulla oblongata. These are called the tubercles of the gracile nucleus (of Goll) and cuneate nucleus (of Burdach).

Further posterior parts of the medulla are visible upon removal of the cerebellum along the peduncles (Fig. 68). The fourth ventricle can now be opened. The floor of the fourth ventricle is formed by the rhomboid fossa. At its inferior tip the fourth ventricle connects with the central canal of the spinal cord (Figs. 32a.43, 69c.9). A small transverse fold, the obex (Figs. 32a.40, 32b.35, 67.37, 70b.29, 70c.9), forms the inferior boundary of the rhomboid fossa. At the level of the obex the medulla oblongata can be divided into (302):
- Inferior or **closed portion**
- Superior or **open portion**.

5.7 Subdivisions of the Brain

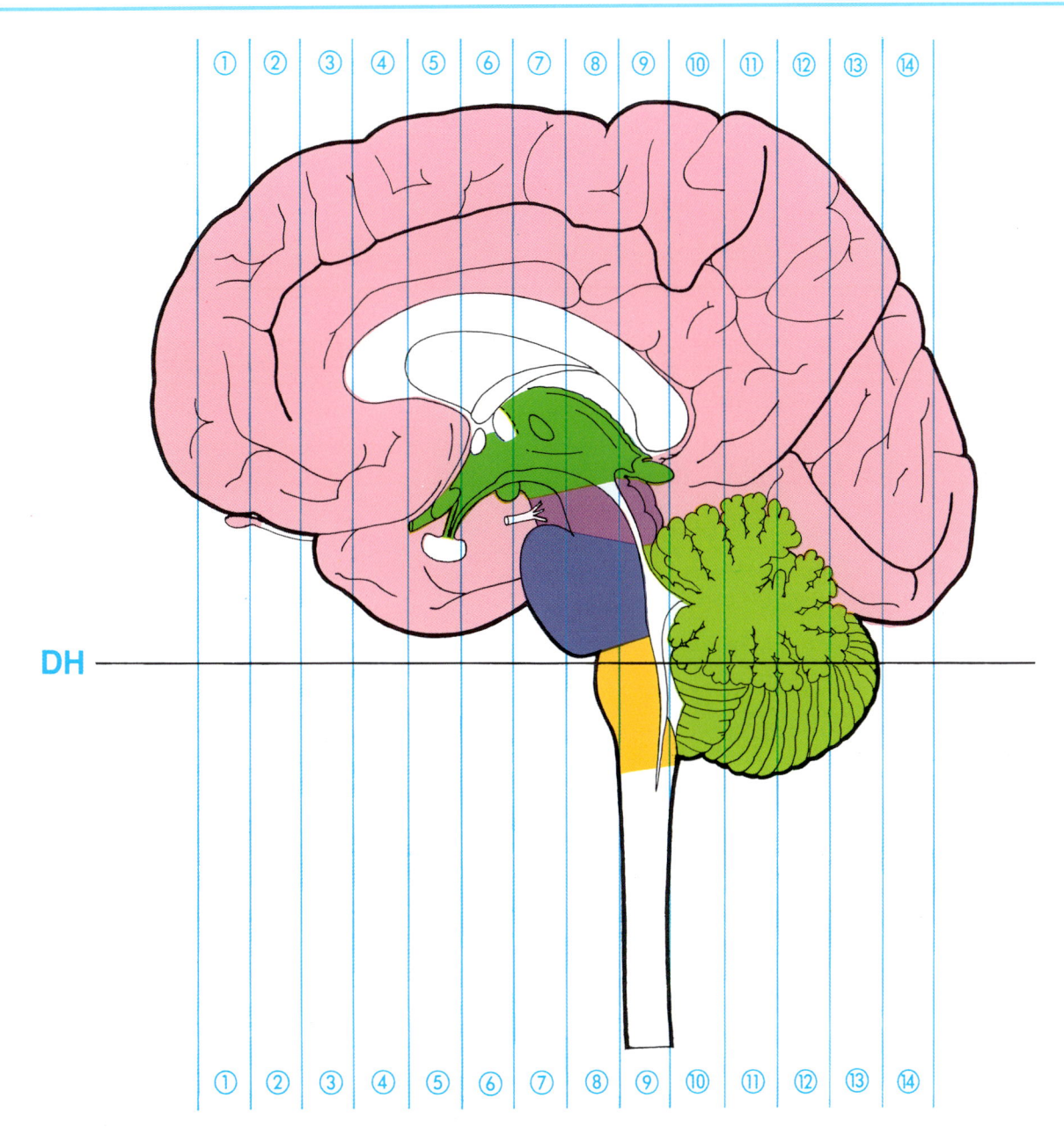

Fig. 98 Medial view of the subdivisions of the coronally cut brain (Fig. 2b). The corpus callosum, anterior commissure, fornix, olfactory tract, pituitary gland, and the oculomotor nerve are portrayed in white (Chap. 8).
DH Reid's base line

- Cortex of telencephalon
- Diencephalon
- Midbrain
- Pons
- Cerebellum
- Medulla oblongata

290 5 Topography of the Neurocranium and its Intracranial Spaces and Structures in Multiplanar Parallel Slices

Cortex of telencephalon

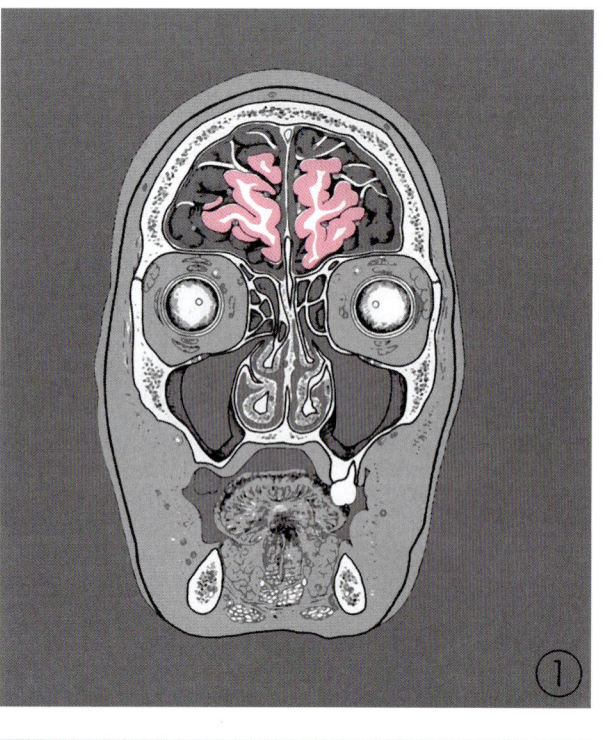

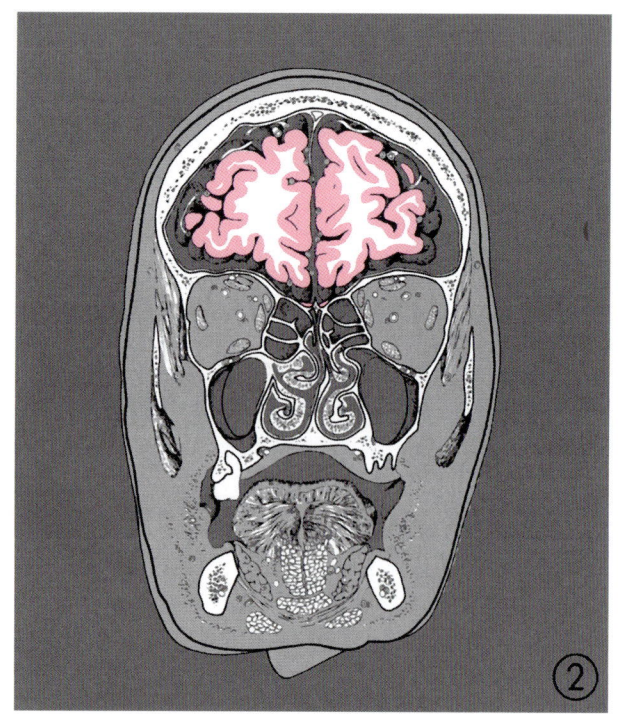

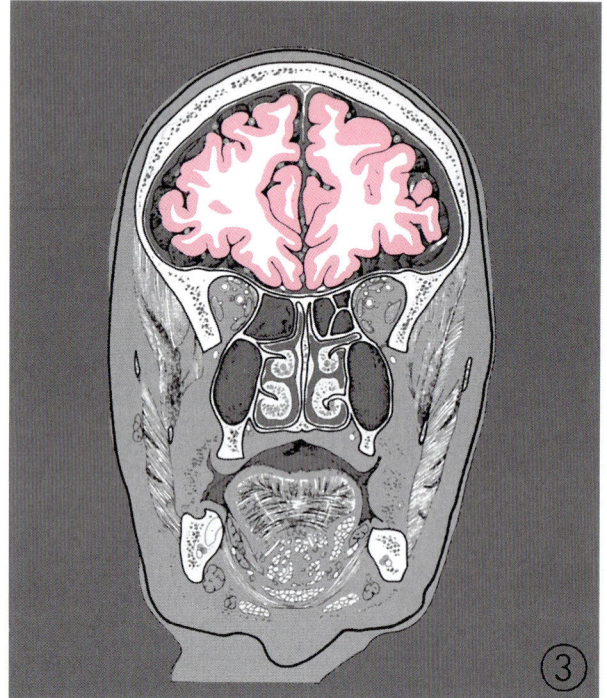

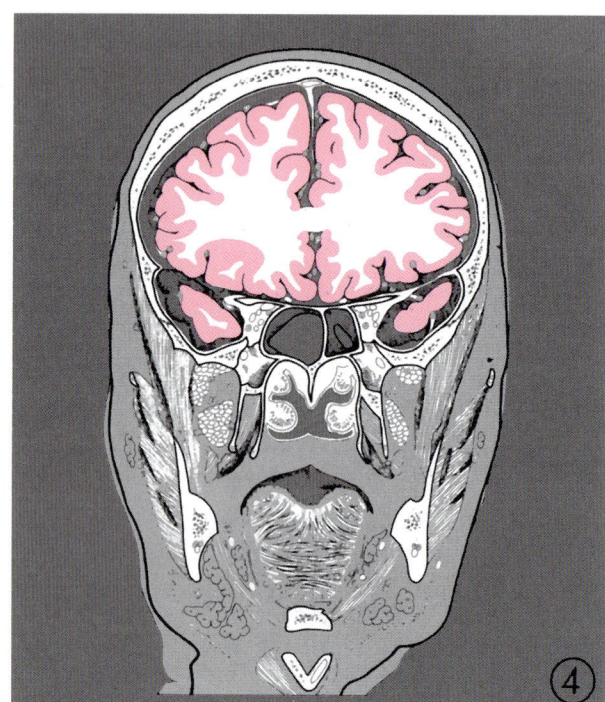

Fig. **99** Coronal serial illustrations of the subdivisions of the brain. The encircled numbers (1–8) indicate the number of the respective slice (Figs. 1, 2a,b, 3).

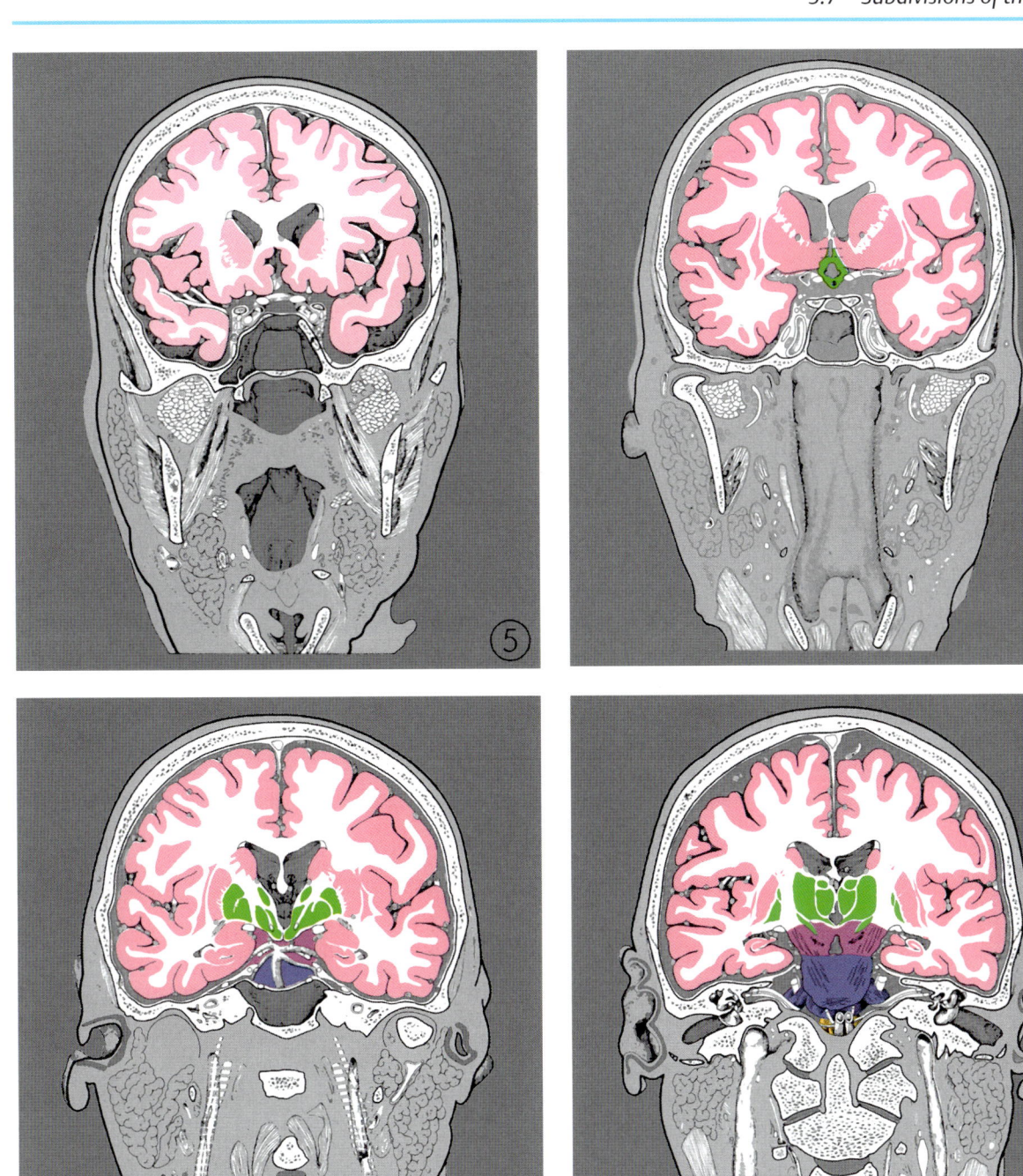

5.7 Subdivisions of the Brain   291

	Cortex and basal ganglia of telencephalon
	Diencephalon
	Midbrain
	Pons
	Medulla oblongata

292   5   Topography of the Neurocranium and its Intracranial Spaces and Structures in Multiplanar Parallel Slices

- Cortex and basal ganglia of telencephalon
- Diencephalon
- Midbrain
- Cerebellum
- Pons
- Medulla oblongata

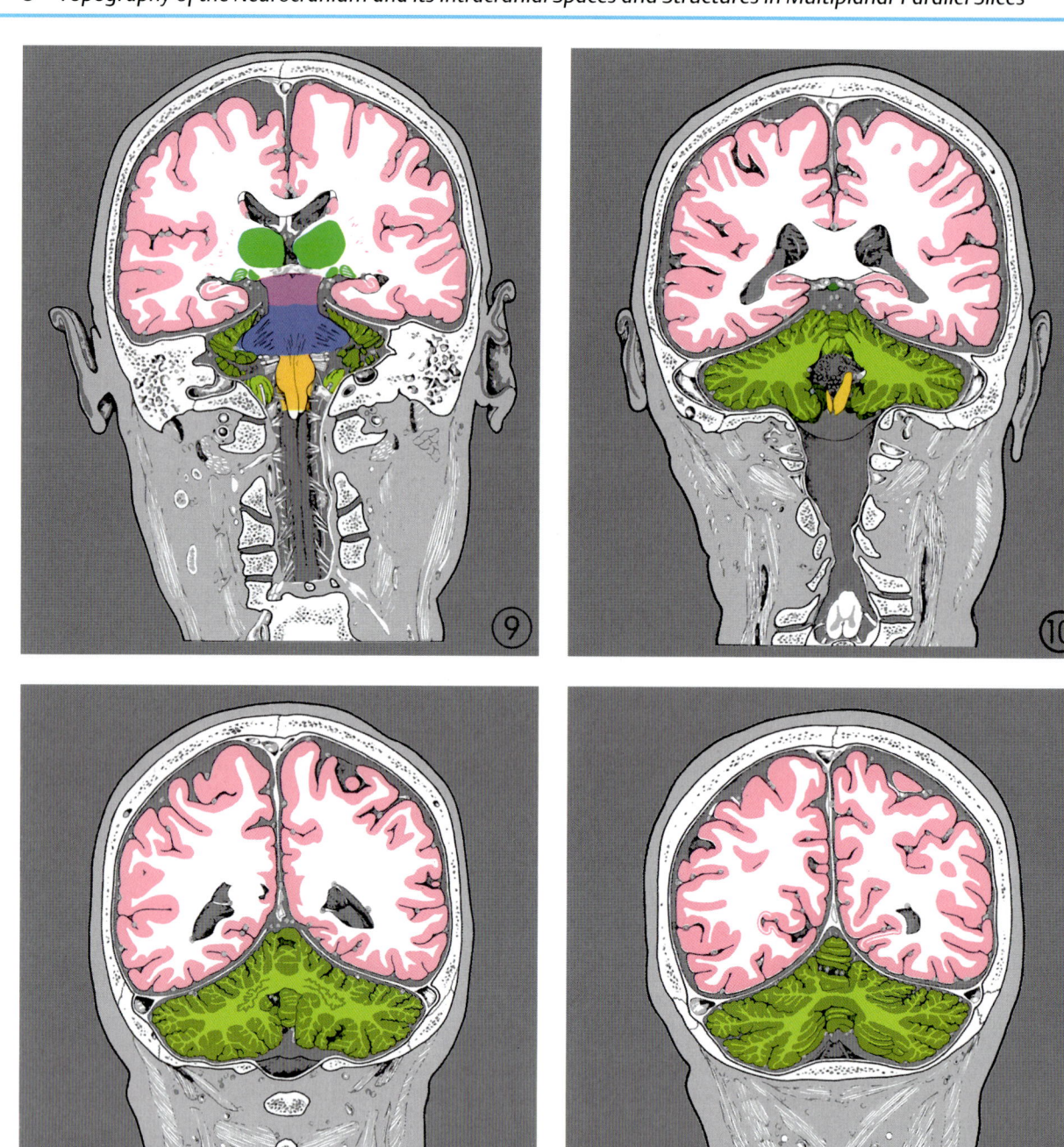

Fig. **99** Coronal serial illustrations of the subdivisions of the brain. The encircled numbers (9–14) indicate the number of the respective slice (Figs. 1, 2a,b, 3).

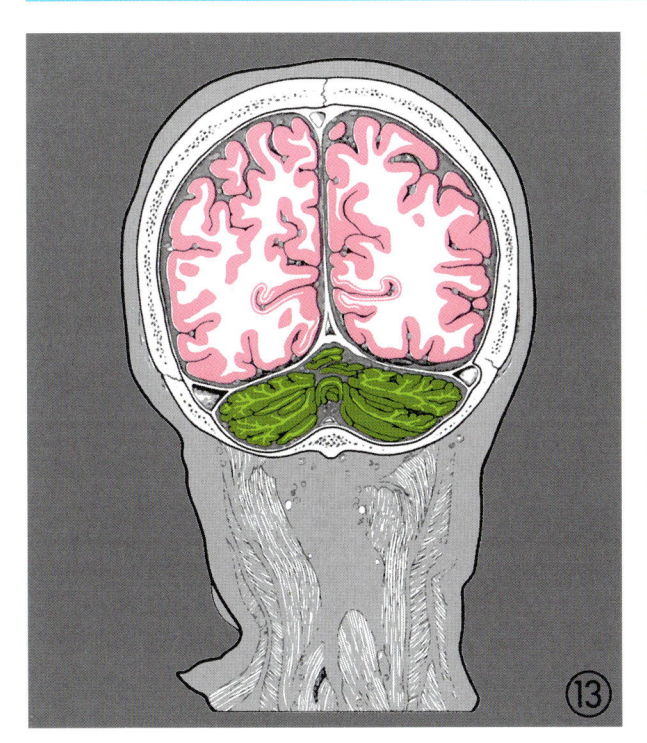

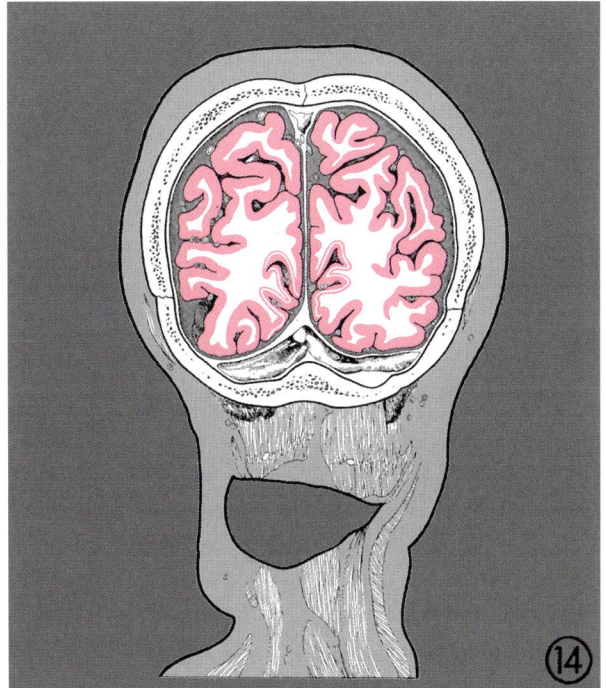

In a transverse section the closed portion of the medulla appears pear-shaped (Fig. 69b). The pyramids (Fig. 69b.19) are located paramedian to the anterior median fissure (Fig. 69b.20). Posterior to the central canal (Fig. 69b.26) the gracile and cuneate nuclei bulge outward (Figs. 69b.30, 69b.29).

In the open portion of the medulla oblongata the floor of the rhomboid fossa can be identified posteriorly (Figs. 71a.19, 72b.23). Because the inferior olivary nuclei bulge outward (Fig. 71b.14), the lateral walls of this section of the medulla oblongata are biconcave. Between the closed and the open portion of the medulla oblongata a transitional area exists at the level of the obex (Fig. 70b).

The twelfth cranial nerve leaves the medulla oblongata as 12–16 rootlets, between the pyramid and the inferior olive (Figs. 69b.17, 70b.9, 70b.15, 71b.7), while the branchial nerves IX, X, and XI leave the lateral wall of the medulla oblongata posterior to the inferior olives (Figs. 70b.22, 71b.18). The eighth and seventh cranial nerves originate laterally in the area of transition between the medulla oblongata and pons (Figs. 72b.20, 73b.12, shown by dotted lines). The sixth cranial nerve emerges anteriorly out the fold between the medulla oblongata and the pons (Figs. 3.32, 11a.41, 32a.35, 49a.5, 72b.8).

When viewed from anteriorly, the **pons** is almost twice as wide as the superior portion of the medulla oblongata. The superior border of the pons is formed by the cerebral peduncle of the midbrain. Both middle cerebellar peduncles arise from the lateral part of the pons (Fig. 144a.14). The median sulcus (Fig. 71b.24) of the rhomboid fossa continues from the medulla oblongata to the pons.

The pons can be divided into (302):
- Inferior (lower) portion
- Middle portion
- Superior (upper) portion.

The **inferior portion of the pons** extends from the boundary of the medulla oblongata to a level below the entry point of the trigeminal nerve. The floor of the rhomboid fossa forms the posterior wall. It narrows toward the aqueduct. In the lower portion of the pons the fourth ventricle shows the paired posterior recesses (Fig. 73b.31) that surround the nodule of the vermis (X) laterally (Figs. 32b.33, 73b.30, 73c.11, 73d.11). Lateral to the middle cerebral peduncle (Fig. 73b.24) the flocculus (H X) can be found in the cerebellopontine cistern (Figs. 49b.18, 72c.5, 73b.23). On account of its elliptical shape and the partial volume effect produced, the flocculus (H X) can be mistaken for a tumor (302).

The **middle portion of the pons** is characterized by the exit zone of the trigeminal nerve (Fig. 75b.11), which can be shown in CT and MR scans. The fifth cranial nerve runs from the cerebellopontine cistern (Figs. 50d.13, 73d.9, 75b.12) into the trigeminal cistern in the middle cranial fossa.

The **superior portion of the pons** is characterized by the paired superior cerebellar peduncles (Fig. 76b.21), which are found posteriorly and interrupt the continuity of the adjoining cisterns. Between the superior cerebellar peduncles lies the narrow portion of the fourth ventricle.

Internal Organization
All three portions of the pons are divided in the axial slices into an anterior and a posterior part. Its **anterior part**, the pons in a restricted sense, contains relay nuclei, the pontine nuclei (Figs. 73b.10, 74b.14, 75b.10, 76b.12), in which the corticopontine fibers terminate. The fibers from the pontine nuclei form the typical pontocerebellar fibers that run into the cerebellum.

The **posterior part of the pons** is the **tegmentum**, which merges inferiorly into the tegmentum of the medulla oblongata.

The **fifth through twelfth cranial nerve nuclei** are arranged in a topographic pattern in the tegmentum of the medulla oblongata and pons (Fig. 68). In the floor of the rhomboid fossa the afferent cranial nerve nuclei lie laterally and the efferent nuclei are located medially. The afferent or sensory nuclei are separated from the efferent nuclei by a weakly developed groove. Two afferent nerves and their sensory nuclei can be seen on the left in Figure 68. On the right the efferent nuclei are illustrated together with the efferent nerves. The sensory nuclei belong to the trigeminal (Chap. 6.1.3), vestibular (Chap. 6.4), auditory (Chap. 6.5), and gustatory (Chap. 6.2) systems.

The **afferent nucleus** for the pain and temperature pathways from the ipsilateral side of the face is the caudal part of the spinal nucleus of trigeminal nerve (Figs. 69b.28, 70b.31), which extends from the obex of the medulla oblongata (Fig. 32a.40) to the second cervical segment of the spinal cord. The mechanoreceptor signals of the trigeminal nerve are conveyed principally to the principal sensory nucleus of trigeminal nerve in the middle portion of the pons (Figs. 68.3, 74b.25). Mainly signals from the muscle spindles of the masticatory muscles reach the mesencephalic nucleus of trigeminal nerve (Figs. 68.2, 74b.29, 75b.24, 76b.24, 77b.31, 78b.28). This nucleus extends from the middle portion of the pons upward as far as the midbrain. The vestibular nuclei extend from the superior portion of the medulla oblongata almost to the center of the pons (Figs. 68.6, 72b.24, 73b.26, 74b.30). The sensory nuclei for the auditory nerve, the cochlear nuclei (Figs. 68.7, 72b.26), are located in the superior portion of the medulla oblongata near to the lateral openings of the fourth ventricle. The sensory nucleus for the taste fibers, the solitary nucleus (Figs. 68.8, 70b.23, 71b.23), extends from the transitional area between the closed and open portions of the medulla oblongata almost to the cranial limit of the medulla.

The motor neurons of the twelfth, eleventh, tenth, ninth, seventh, sixth, and fifth cranial nerves and the visceroefferent nerve cells of the tenth, ninth, and seventh cranial nerves are located in the **efferent nuclei**:

The hypoglossal nucleus (Figs. 68.19, 70b.24, 71b.25) consists of a cell column 10 mm long, which extends from the inferior part of the rhomboid fossa to the closed portion of the medulla oblongata. Its axons leave the medulla oblongata anterolaterally from the groove between the pyramid and inferior olive and innervate the muscles of the tongue.

The nucleus ambiguus (Figs. 68.17, 70b.20, 71b.16, 72b.17) is 16 mm long and lies immediately posterior to the inferior olivary nucleus in the medulla oblongata. Its motor fibers run in the ninth, tenth, and eleventh cranial nerves and innervate the muscles of the pharynx (in part), the larynx, and the esophagus.

The facial nucleus (Figs. 68.15, 73b.21, 74b.23) is 4 mm long (in the direction of Meynert's axis) and lies in the inferior portion of the pons anterior to the abducens nucleus. Its fibers loop around the abducens nucleus and form the genu of the facial nerve (Figs. 68.13, 74b.27). The neurons of the facial nerve provide the muscles of facial expression, the stapedius, and the stylohyoid.

The motor nucleus of trigeminal nerve (Figs. 68.12, 74b.24) is about 4 mm long, lies in the middle portion of the pons, and forms with its axons the motor root of the trigeminal nerve. These nerve fibers provide the muscles of mastication, muscles of the floor of the mouth, and the tensor tympani.

The following nuclei belong to the **visceroefferent nuclei**:
- Posterior (dorsal) nucleus of vagus nerve (Figs. 68.18, 70b.25, 71b.26). The nucleus is found mainly in the inferior part of the rhomboid fossa. Its fibers form the parasympathetic portion of the vagus nerve and innervate the organs of the respiratory and digestive tracts. The posterior nucleus of the vagus nerve is also the afferent nucleus for the fibers from the ninth and tenth cranial nerves.
- Inferior salivatory nucleus (Figs. 68.16. 151.4). This small nucleus is located in the superior portion of the medulla oblongata. Its neurons provide parasympathetic innervation to the parotid gland.
- Superior salivatory nucleus (Figs. 68.16, 151.3). This nucleus is located in the inferior portion of the pons. Its parasympathetic secretory fibers innervate the lacrimal, submandibular, and sublingual glands, as well as the glands of the nasal and oral mucous membrane.

Reticular Formation
The reticular formation is a loose network of large and small nerve cells situated in the medulla oblongata and the pons. It can be divided into three loosely demarcated longitudinal zones (188):
- Median and paramedian zone
- Medial zone
- Lateral zone.

The **median and paramedian zone** contains the nuclei of the raphe (numbered B1–B8 from inferior to superior), in which serotonin and other neurotransmitters have been identified. These nuclei of

5.7 Subdivisions of the Brain   295

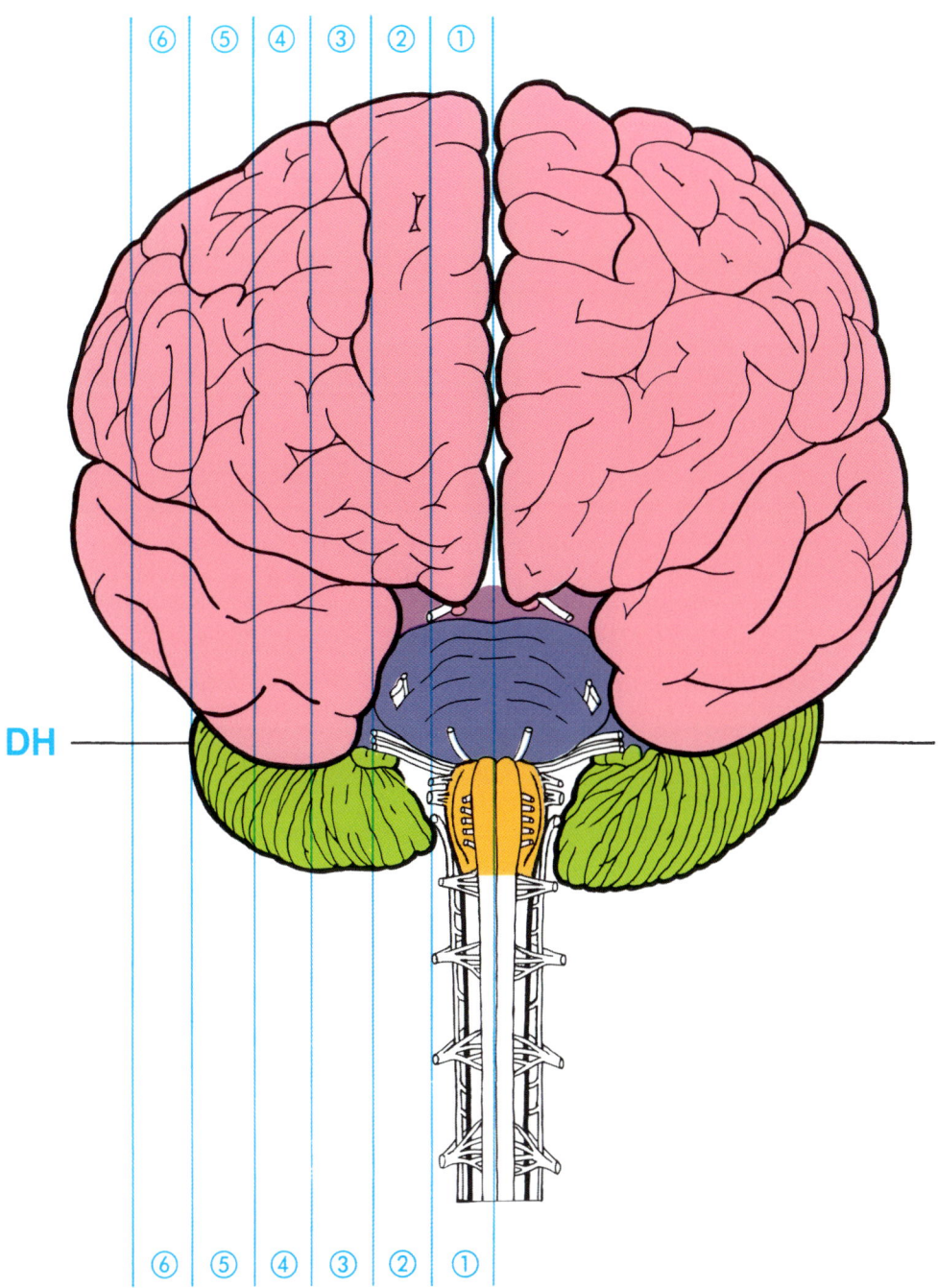

Fig. 100 Coronal view of the subdivisions of the sagittally cut brain and the medulla spinalis. The sagittal slices were fitted together and numbered as shown in Fig. 30b (Chap. 8).
DH Reid's base line

- Cortex of telencephalon
- Midbrain
- Pons
- Cerebellum
- Medulla oblongata

the raphe (simplified) belong to the serotoninergic nerve cells (Chap. 7.2). The pontine visual center, the **p**aramedian **p**ontine **r**eticular **f**ormation (PPRF), is located in the middle portion of the pons (Figs. 75b.15, 76b.19).

The **medial zone** contains many large nerve cells, the axons of which have long ascending and descending branches with many synaptic connections.

The **lateral zone** comprises predominantly small nerve cells with presumed associative functions. The reticular formation consists of polysynaptic nerve cells that are connected to afferent and efferent pathways and to the autonomic systems. Stimulation of the reticular formation in animals causes an arousal reaction from sleep. Regulatory regions for circulation and respiration are also located in the reticular formation.

Inferior Olivary System
The inferior olivary nucleus (Figs. 12a.38, 70b.16, 71b.14, 72b.14) with its two accessory olivary nuclei is the most striking nuclear group in the open portion of

296   5   Topography of the Neurocranium and its Intracranial Spaces and Structures in Multiplanar Parallel Slices

- Cortex and basal ganglia of telencephalon
- Diencephalon
- Midbrain
- Pons
- Cerebellum
- Medulla oblongata

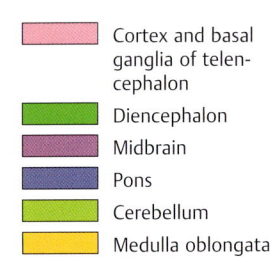

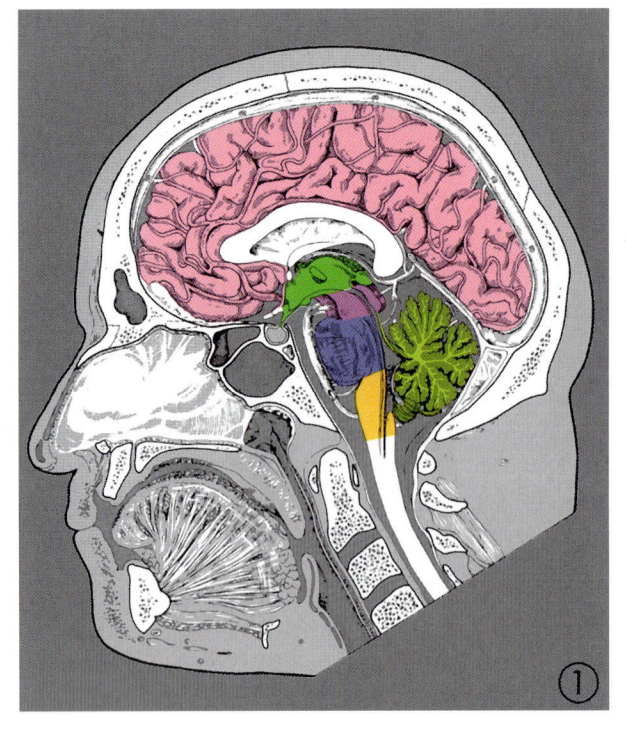

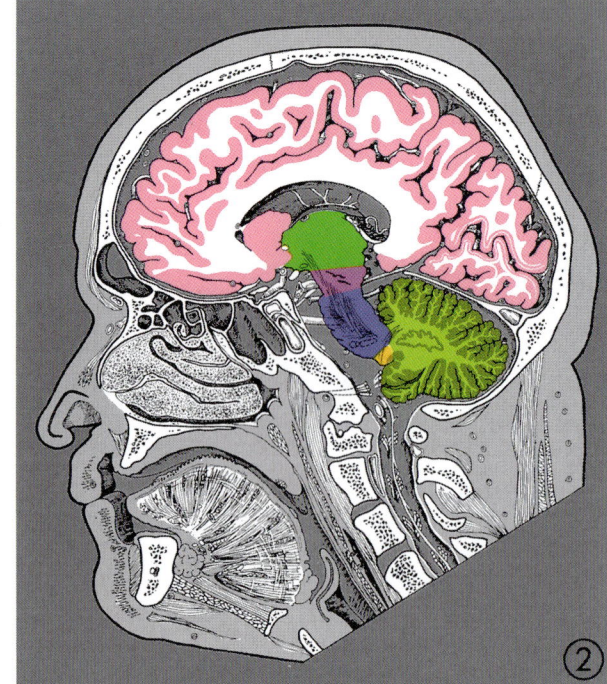

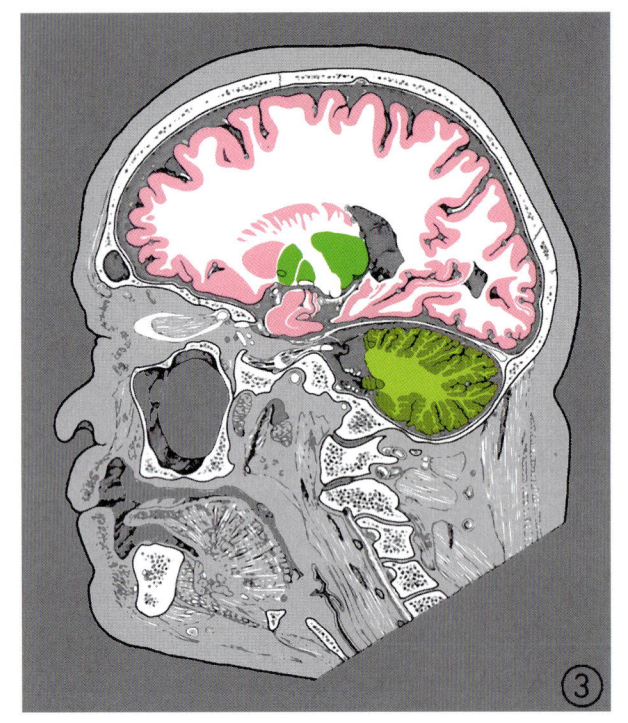

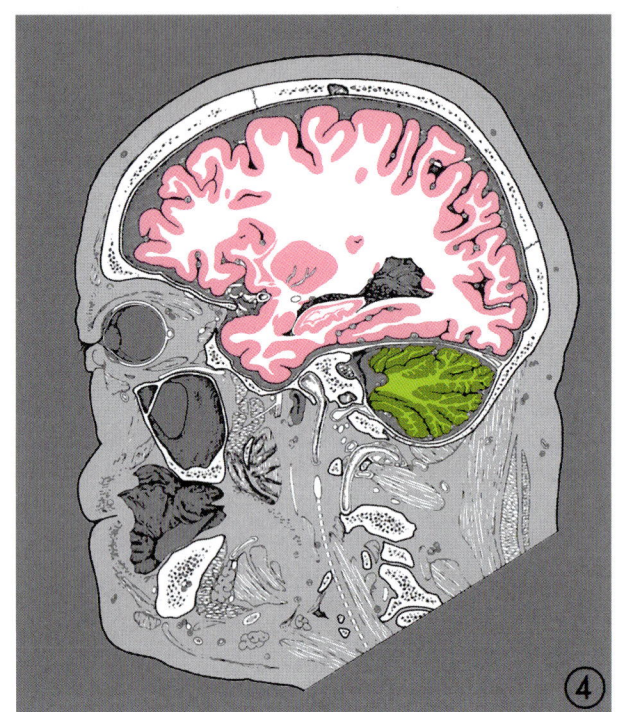

Fig. 101 Sagittal serial illustrations of the subdivisions of the brain. The corpus callosum, anterior commissure, and fornix are portrayed in white. The encircled number (1–6) indicates the number of the respective slice (Figs. 29, 30a,b, 31).

	▢ Cortex of telencephalon
	▢ Cerebellum

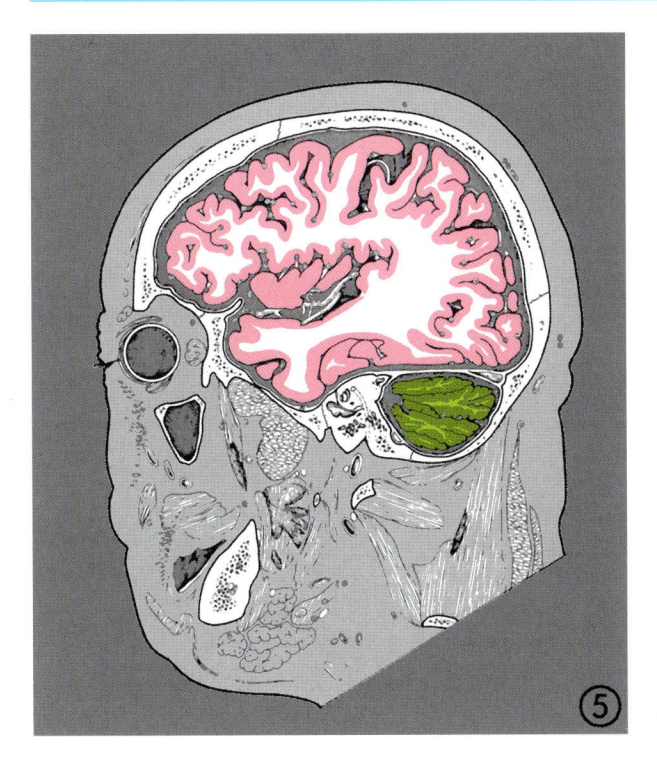

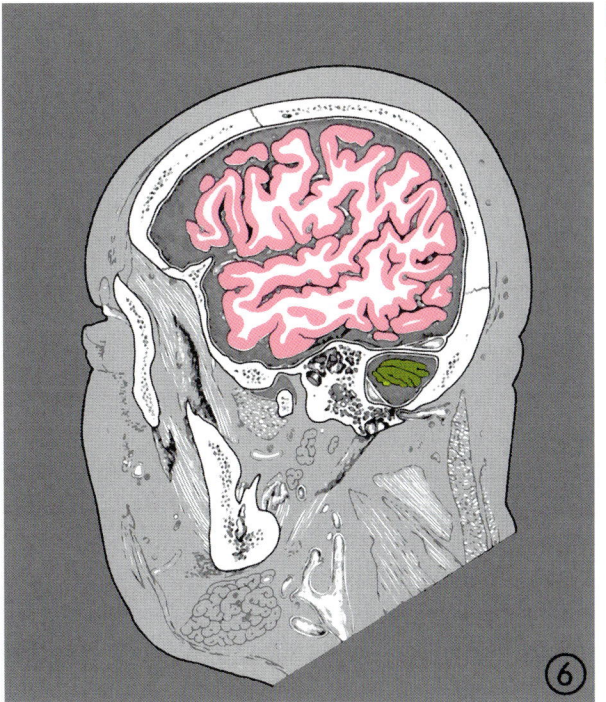

⑤

⑥

the medulla oblongata. The 15-mm-long inferior olivary nucleus extends into the superior part of the closed portion of the medulla oblongata. The inferior olivary nucleus can be compared to a sack with many folds, its opening pointing medially. The inferior olivary nuclei are relay centers for connections with the cerebellum. They receive signals from the spinal cord, midbrain, and from an accessory pathway in the motor cortex and basal ganglia of the telencephalon. As a whole, the olivary system is a relay station of the cerebellum.

Chemically Identifiable Neurons

Using histochemical techniques for transmitter identification, the following nerve cell groups can be demonstrated in the medulla oblongata and pons, predominantly in the reticular formation:

- Noradrenergic cell groups (A1–A7). Because of its neuromelanin content the most striking group (A6) is the cerulean nucleus in the locus ceruleus (Figs. 75b.22, 76b.23).
- Adrenergic cell groups in the superior portion of the medulla oblongata.
- Serotoninergic cell groups (B1–B9).
- Cholinergic cell groups.
- Neuropeptide-containing cells.

These groups will be described in detail in Chapter 7.

Pathways

Pathways ascending from the anterolateral (Chap. 6.1.1), medial lemniscus (Chap. 6.1.2), trigeminal (Chap. 6.1.3), gustatory (Chap. 6.2), vestibular (Chap. 6.4), and auditory (Chap. 6.5) systems, as well as pathways descending from the motor (Chap. 6.8) and cerebellar (Chap. 6.9) systems, pass through the medulla oblongata and pons. In canthomeatal parallel planes the medulla oblongata and pons are cut diagonally—at a slight angle to the plane perpendicular to Meynert's axis—so that the resulting sectioning planes lie anteriorly in a more superior position and posteriorly in a more inferior position than the transverse sections of conventional neuroanatomy books (55, 85, 219, 247, 285, 332, 350, 370, 380, 408, 492). Typical of this phenomenon is the sectioning plane of the third slice (Fig. 49a), which is located at the border region between the pons and medulla oblongata. In Figure 49a.6 the anterior part of the pons is cut. The medulla oblongata follows underneath the pons, the posterior part being cut almost at the end of the rhomboid fossa. Lying between the pons and medulla oblongata, a blind canal (known as the foramen cecum) indicates the superior end of the anterior median fissure of the medulla oblongata. The medulla oblongata (Fig. 48a) and the pons (Figs. 50a.13, 51a.18) can also be seen.

Clinical Notes

Lesions of the medulla oblongata and pons frequently affect the cranial nerve nuclei and their connections with one another as well as their connections with the spinal cord, cerebellum, and cerebrum. The afferent and efferent pathways between the cerebrum, or, more specifically, between the efferent nuclei and spinal cord, are affected simultaneously. Small foci lead to ipsilateral disorders of the inferior cranial nerves and to contralateral paresis of the extremities and/or sensory impairment. Clinically recognizable symptoms usually suffice to localize the damage and identify the type of brainstem syndrome. The different syndromes are seldom described with any consistency and clinically rarely present in their pure form. One of the most common syndromes is **Wal-**

lenberg's syndrome showing acute symptoms like rotatory vertigo, nausea, vomiting, and hoarseness. Examination reveals nystagmus, ipsilateral Horner's syndrome, trigeminal disorder, palatal and pharyngeal paresis, and hemiataxia of the extremities. A dissociated sensory loss (for pain and temperature) of the extremities and trunk exists contralaterally.

Extensive lesions of the medulla oblongata and the pons cause **bulbar palsy** with tetraplegia. Most of the small lesions in the inferior brainstem are rarely shown in the CT because of the bony artifacts. For the demonstration of ischemic lesions, multiple sclerosis foci, and small brainstem tumors, MRI is the method of choice. Only fresh hemorrhages can be overlooked or misinterpreted where no appropriate specific sequences are used.

5.7.2 Midbrain
(Figs. 98–103)

The midbrain (mesencephalon) is a small subdivision of the brain with a volume of about 10 ml. The base of the midbrain is approximately 1.5 cm long. At the tectum it has a length of 2 cm.

Posterior Surface

The posterior surface of the midbrain is formed by the tectal (quadrigeminal) plate. The superior colliculi (Figs. 2b.21, 32a.18, 78b.31, 78c.12) are broader and higher than the inferior colliculi (Figs. 2b.31, 32a.19, 52d.19, 77b.34, 77c.14, 77d.14). Immediately below the inferior colliculi the trochlear nerve (IV) emerges as the only cranial nerve from the posterior surface of the brainstem. It turns anteriorly and runs through the orbit to the superior oblique.

Anterior Surface

On the anterior surface the paired cerebral peduncles, the cerebral crura (Figs. 77a.14, 77c.10, 77d.10, 78b.9), bulge forward enclosing the interpeduncular fossa (Fig. 77b.14) and partially enclosing the interpeduncular cistern (Figs. 77c.9, 77d.9). The oculomotor nerve (III) (Figs. 77b.13, 77d.8) emerges from this fossa and supplies extraocular and intrinsic ocular muscles.

Internal Organization

The midbrain can be divided into three levels, which are oriented in the transverse plane around the aqueduct. The roof of the midbrain is called the tectal plate. The tegmentum lies in the middle of the midbrain. The basal portion of the midbrain is formed by the cerebral crus. The aqueduct ascends in a concave curve between the fourth and third ventricles. Transverse sections through the midbrain, which are cut perpendicular to the aqueduct, cannot, therefore, be parallel to each other. Histologic serial sections through a block of midbrain tissue can be made against either the superior or inferior transverse plane of the aqueduct. For this reason, transverse serial sections through the midbrain vary greatly (55, 85, 219, 247, 285, 332, 350, 370, 408, 492). After CT and anatomic studies it was recommended to examine the midbrain in an approximately infraorbitomeatal parallel plane (37). Furthermore, CT examination of the interpeduncular cistern, ambient cistern, and quadrigeminal cistern, along with their contents, is recommended in the infraorbitomeatal plane rather than in the canthomeatal plane. The particular advantage of MRI for the clinical assessment of the midbrain is that it allows the brain structures and the cisterns to be displayed free of artifacts. The sagittal MR scans in addition to the axial views improve topical orientation.

The **tectum of midbrain** (Fig. 32b.21) is a thin plate marked by four roundish elevations. The inferior colliculi are relay stations for the auditory system. The superior colliculi, on the other hand, serve as a visual reflex center. From here, the short tectobulbar tract and long tectospinal tract descend to motor neurons in the brainstem and spinal cord.

The **tegmentum of midbrain** contains the motor nuclei of the third and fourth cranial nerves (Figs. 68.9, 68.10, 68.11, 77b.27, 78b.20) (77). The medial and most superiorly located parasympathetic accessory nucleus of oculomotor nerve (Edinger–Westphal) (Fig. 151.2) innervates the sphincter pupillae (miosis) and the ciliary muscle (accommodation). The root fibers of the third cranial nerve project basally through the red nucleus and emerge at the interpeduncular fossa. The motor nucleus of the fourth cranial nerve lies inferior to the oculomotor nucleus. The root fibers of the trochlear nerve extend posteriorly, cross over, and leave the tectum inferior to the inferior colliculi (Figs. 68, 77b.33). Posterolateral to these motor nuclei lies the mesencephalic nucleus of the trigeminal nerve (Chap. 6.1.3).

The reticular formation constitutes the framework of the tegmentum. Structure and function of the reticular formation have been described in connection with the medulla oblongata and pons (Chap. 5.7.1). The red nucleus is considered a part of the basal ganglia (Chap. 6.8.2) and is located in the tegmentum of the midbrain. It has the shape of a short ellipsoid, which is surrounded by a capsule of longitudinally running fibers (Fig. 78b.16). Inferiorly the red nucleus borders on the superior cerebellar peduncle. Anteriorly the red nucleus is separated from the subthalamic nucleus by an almost 2-mm-thick layer of fibers. The main part of the red nucleus consists of small cells (parvocellular); only an inferior cap of about 1 mm contains large nerve cells (magnocellular). This last part contains fewer than 300 cells.

The characteristic black color of the substantia nigra, a plate of nerve cells located in the **cerebral**

5.7 Subdivisions of the Brain   299

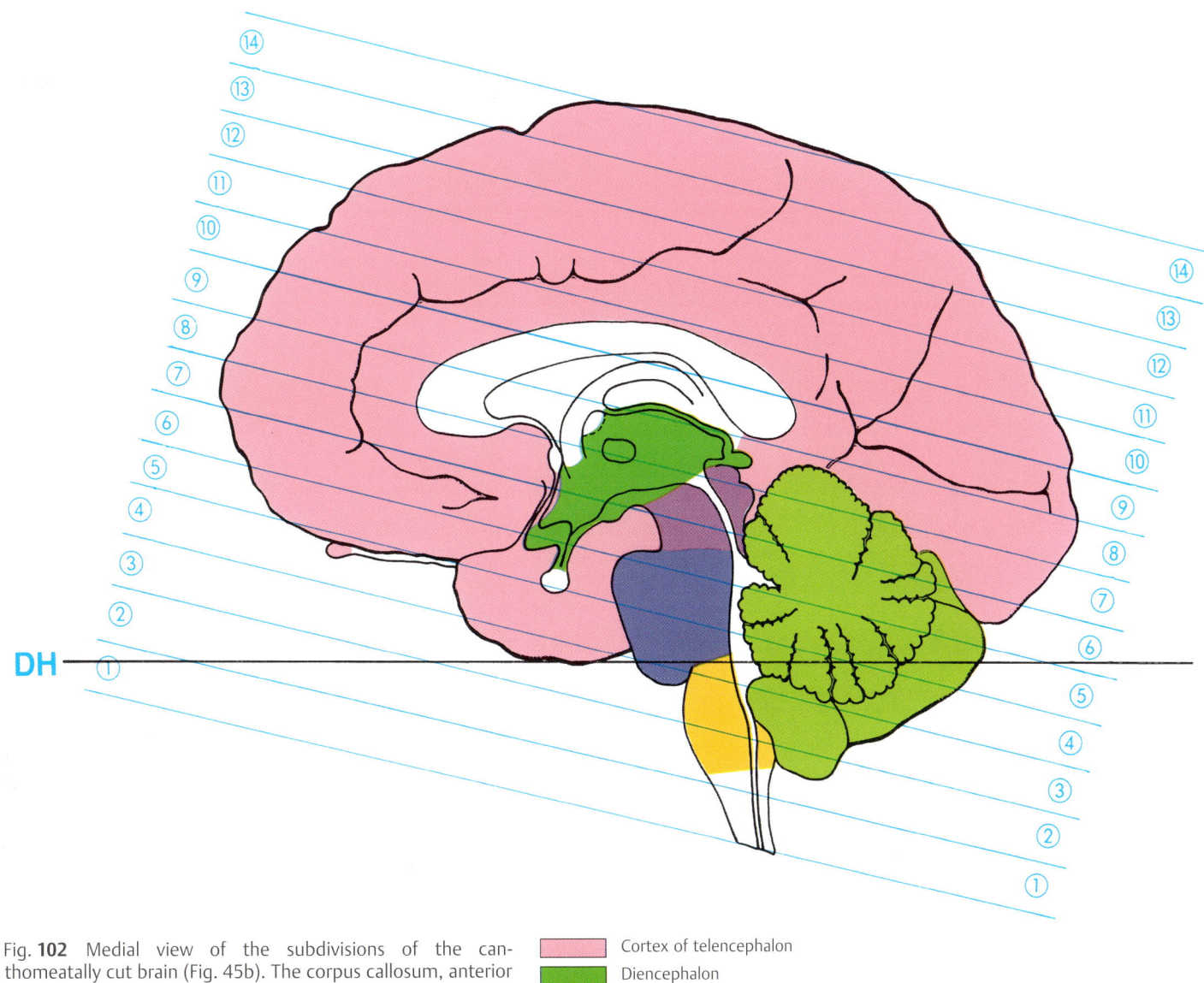

Fig. **102** Medial view of the subdivisions of the canthomeatally cut brain (Fig. 45b). The corpus callosum, anterior commissure, fornix, olfactory tract, and pituitary gland are portrayed in white (Chap. 8).
DH Reid's base line

- Cortex of telencephalon
- Diencephalon
- Midbrain
- Pons
- Cerebellum
- Medulla oblongata

300   5   Topography of the Neurocranium and its Intracranial Spaces and Structures in Multiplanar Parallel Slices

- Medulla oblongata
- Pons
- Cerebellum
- Diencephalon
- Cortex and basal ganglia of telencephalon

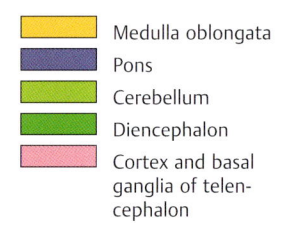

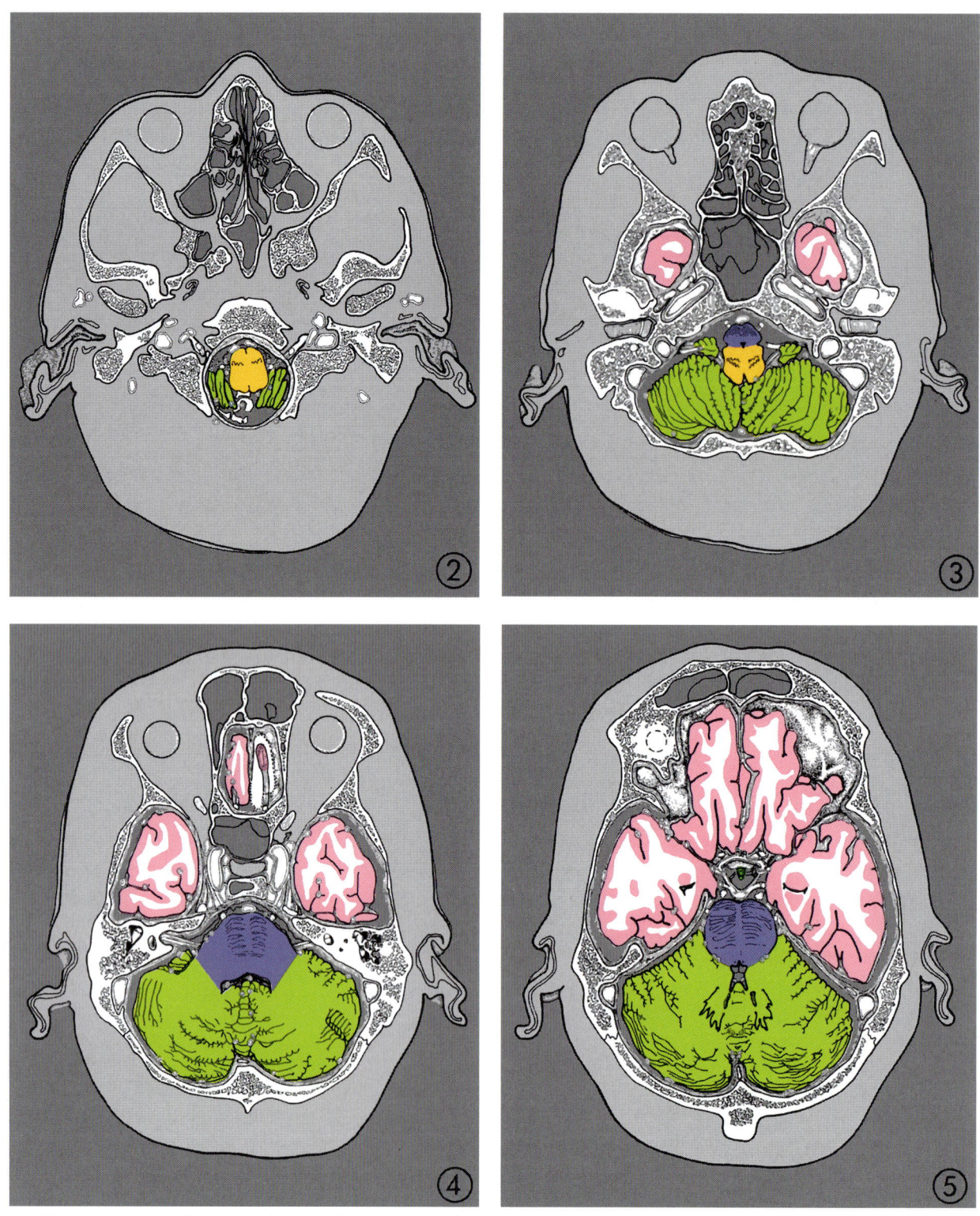

Fig. 103 Canthomeatally oriented serial illustrations of the subdivisions of the brain. The encircled numbers (2–9) indicate the number of the respective slice (Figs. 44, 45a,b, 46).

5.7 Subdivisions of the Brain 301

- Cerebellum
- Midbrain
- Diencephalon
- Cortex and basal ganglia of telencephalon

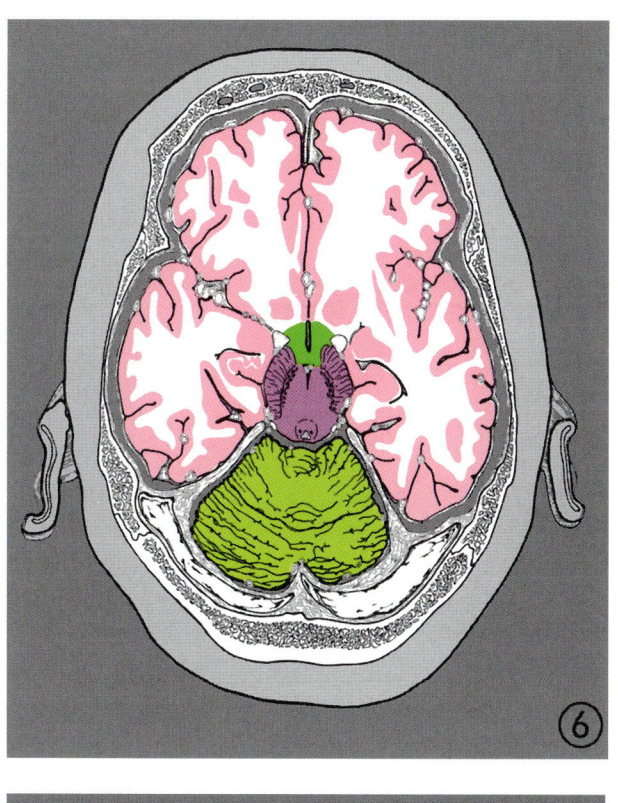

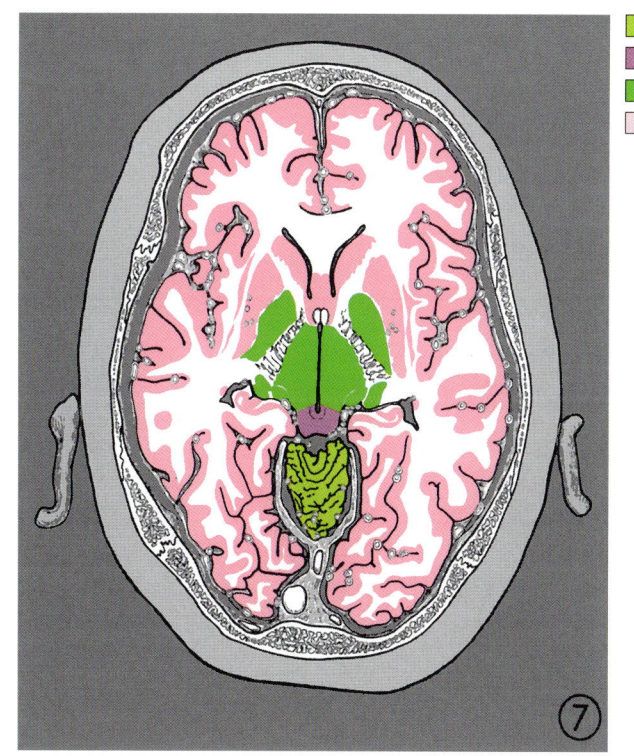

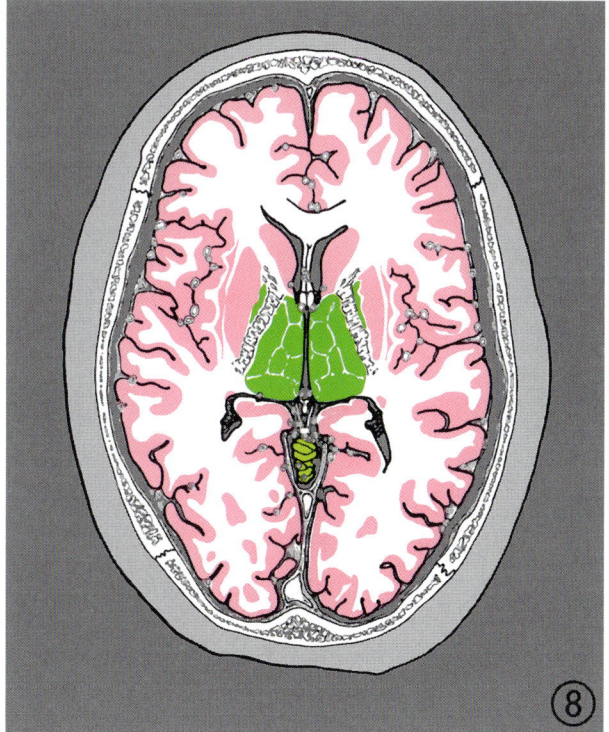

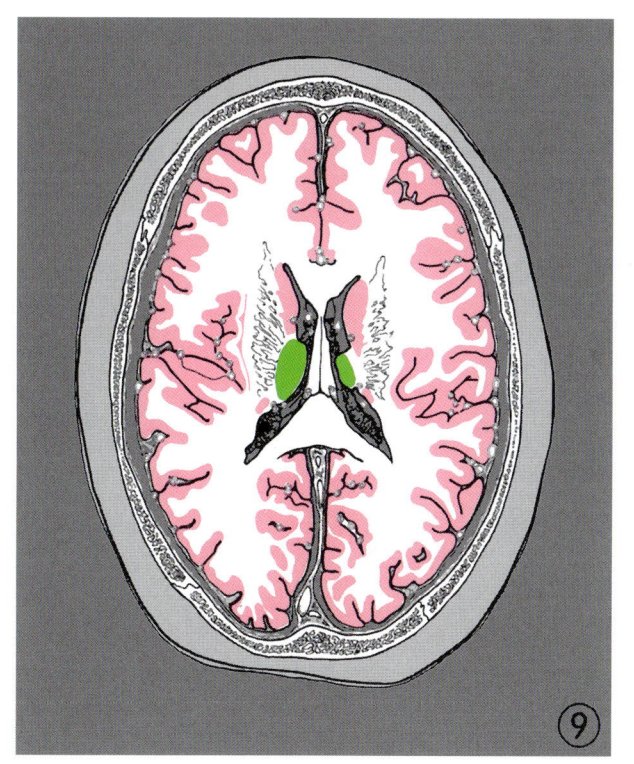

5   Topography of the Neurocranium and its Intracranial Spaces and Structures in Multiplanar Parallel Slices

☐ Cortex of telencephalon

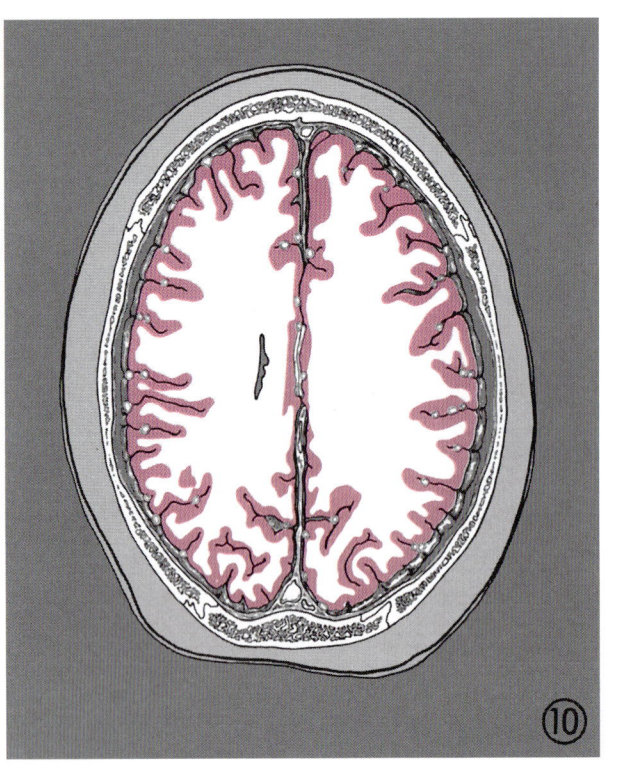

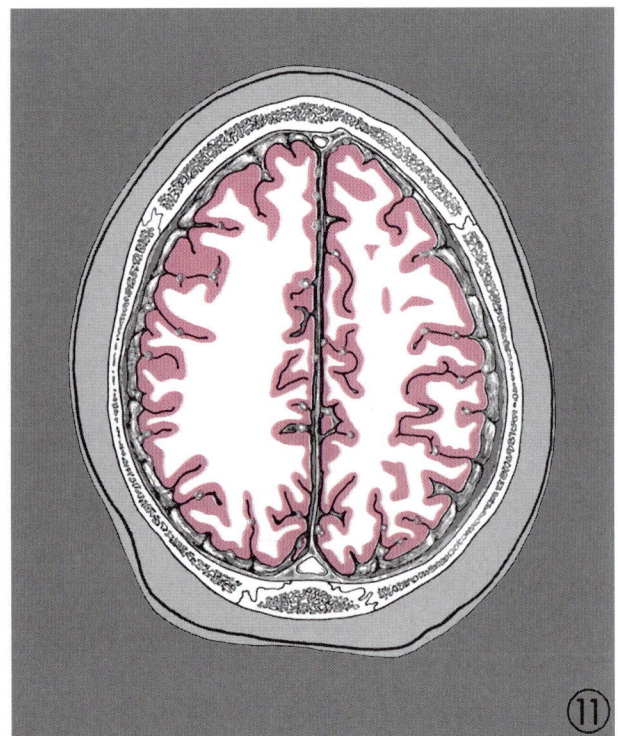

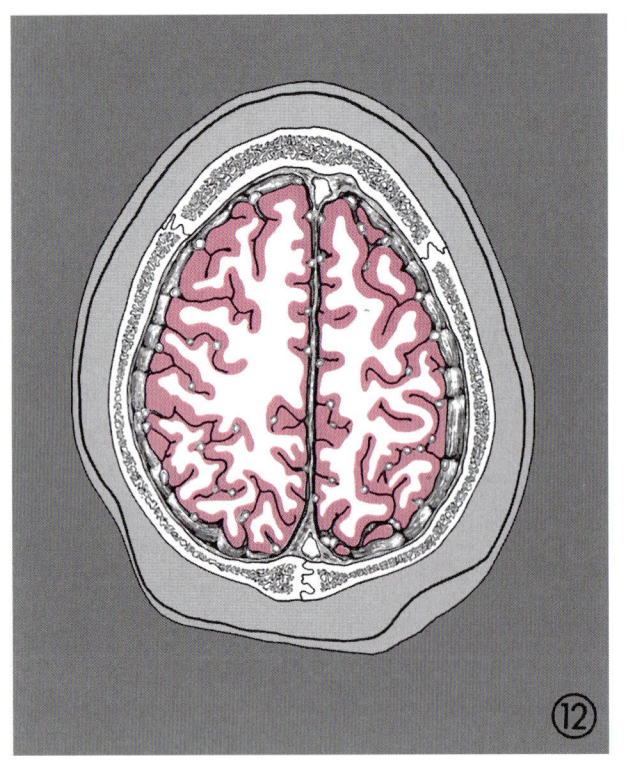

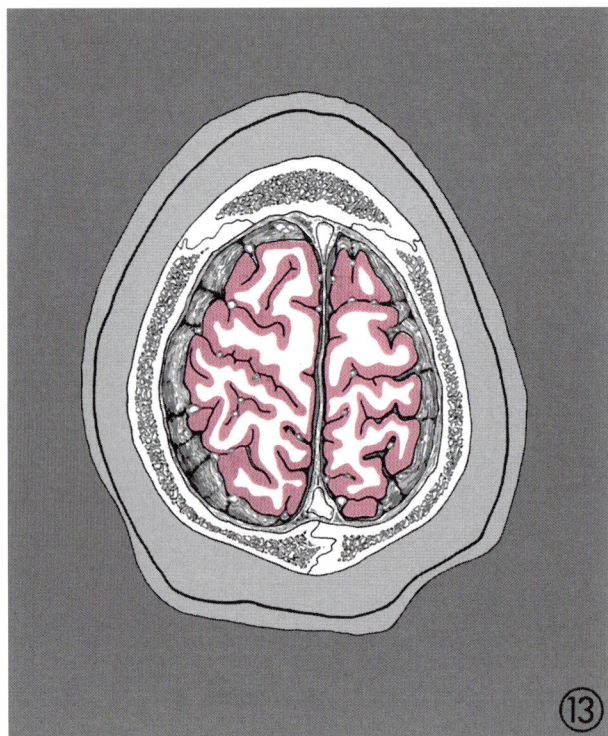

Fig. 103 Canthomeatally oriented serial illustrations of the subdivisions of the brain. The encircled numbers (10–14) indicate the number of the respective slice (Figs. 44, 45a,b, 46).

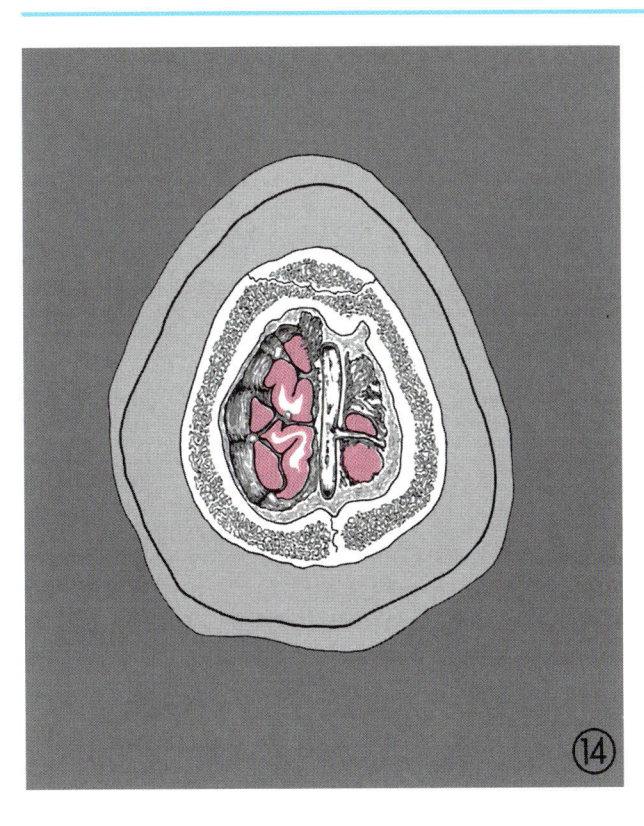

peduncle of the midbrain (Figs. 52a.29, 77b.21, 78b.15), is due to the high concentration of neuromelanin in its nerve cells. The axons of these dopaminergic neurons (A9) project into the striatum. These nigrostriatal neurons are described in Chapter 7.1.1. The **cerebral crus** lies on the basal side of the cerebral peduncle and contains only descending pathways from the neocortex. These pathways as seen in medial to lateral direction are:

- Frontopontine tract (Figs. 77b.15, 78b.10)
- Motor cranial nerve pathway or corticonuclear tract (Figs. 77b.16, 78b.11)
- Pyramidal pathway or corticospinal tract (Figs. 77b.17, 78b.12)
- Occipitopontine and temporopontine tracts (Figs. 77b.18, 78b.13).

The frontopontine, occipitopontine, and temporopontine tracts are part of the cerebellar system (Chap. 6.9). The corticonuclear and corticospinal tracts are part of the pyramidal system (Chap. 6.8.1). The ascending pathways run through the tegmentum. The medial lemniscus (Chap. 6.1.2) lies posterolateral to the red nucleus (Figs. 78b.22, 78b.16). The fibers of the anterolateral and trigeminal systems lie close to the medial lemniscus. Located further posteriorly is the lateral lemniscus (Fig. 77b.30) that projects to the inferior colliculus (Fig. 77b.34). These are part of the auditory system (Chap. 6.5).

> *Clinical Notes*
> Mesencephalic dysfunctions are characterized by paralysis of vertical gaze, paresis of the eye muscles controlled by the third and fourth cranial nerves, and by ataxia and, occasionally, tremor. Injuries to the reticular formation and rostral mesencephalic structures, as well as to those structures localized in the border region between the midbrain and diencephalon, can cause akinetic mutism. Such dysfunctions often develop posttraumatically.

5.7.3 Cerebellum
(Figs. 98–103, 142, 143)

External Features
The cerebellum is divided into a narrow median part, the **vermis**, and **two hemispheres**. The **primary fissure** (Figs. 32a.26, 32b.26, 52a.41, 67.20, 74a.17, 75a.18, 76a.20) separates the anterior lobe of the cerebellum from the posterior lobe. The lobes and lobules of the cerebellum are best identified from the median (midline) plane because the vaulted surface of the primary fissure runs only approximately vertically in the median plane and obliquely in the paramedian planes. The vermis (not the hemispheres) shows the typical pattern of the arbor vitae with the deep cleft of the primary fissure between the culmen (IV and V) and the declive (VI) (Figs. 142.1, 142.2,

Table 1 Parts of the vermis, lobules, and lobes of the cerebellum with the numeric and alphanumeric abbreviations according to Larsell (122, 268)

Vermis of cerebellum (I–X)	Hemisphere of cerebellum (H II–H X)	Lobes of cerebellum
Lingula (I)		Anterior lobe of cerebellum
Central lobule (II, III)	Wing of central lobule (H II, H III)	
Culmen (IV, V)	Anterior quadrangular lobule (H IV, H V)	
Primary fissure		
Declive (VI)	Posterior quadrangular lobule (H VI)	Posterior lobe of cerebellum
Folium of vermis (VII A)	Superior and inferior semilunar lobules (H VII A)	
Tuber of vermis (VII B)	Gracile lobule (H VII B)	
Pyramis of vermis (VIII)	Biventral lobule (H VIII)	
Uvula of vermis (IX)	Tonsil of cerebellum (H IX)	
Posterolateral fissure		
Nodule of vermis (X)	Flocculus (H X)	Flocculonodular lobe

142.3). The anterior lobe is positioned in the upper canthomeatal plane (Fig. 143). The sagittal series reveals that large parts of the posterior lobe lie below the anterior lobe (Fig. 142).

The flocculus (H X) (Figs. 49a.12, 49b.18, 72a.14, 72c.5, 73b.23, 142.11) and the nodules of vermis (X) (Figs. 67.29, 73b.30, 73d.11, 74b.32, 142.8) form the flocculonodular lobe. The posterolateral fissure separates the flocculonodular lobe from the posterior lobe (Table 1).

The cerebellum is connected to the brainstem on each side by **three cerebellar peduncles**:
- Inferior cerebellar peduncle (Fig. 144a.13) with the medulla oblongata
- Middle cerebellar peduncle (Fig. 144a.14) with the pons
- Superior cerebellar peduncle (Fig. 144a.6) with the midbrain.

The functions and somatotopy of the lobules of the cerebellum have been examined using PET and fMRI and individual functions related to these lobules coordinated. The lobules were assigned historical names that gave no indication of their functions or development. Larsell suggested a clear **alphanumerical nomenclature** for the cerebellum (268), which was accepted as an alternative in 1998 by the Federative Committee on Anatomical Terminology. The parts of the vermis are numbered in a topologic order using roman numerals. In the mid section of the right half of the cerebellum (Fig. 32a), most of the component parts of the vermis with these numbers are shown in brackets and printed clockwise on this side. The letter H has been placed in front of the corresponding parts of the hemisphere, for example wing of central lobule (H II, H III) or flocculus (H X). In Table 1 the names with alphanumerical abbreviations have been listed. These abbreviations are used for PET and fMRI examinations (412).

Internal Organization

The cerebellum has a thin cortex of gray matter (approximately 1 mm thick). In the white matter, from lateral to medial, lie the following paired cerebellar nuclei: dentate, anterior interpositus (emboliform), posterior interpositus (globose), and fastigial nuclei. The afferent and efferent cerebellar pathways are described in cerebellar systems (Chap. 6.9).

Topography

The cerebellum fills most of the infratentorial space. On average the cerebellum has a volume of 150 ml in males and 135 ml in females (390, 482). The relatively large portion of the infratentorial space occupied by the cerebellum compared to that occupied by the medulla oblongata and pons is clearly evident in Figures 99, 101, and 103.

The tonsils (H IX) of the cerebellum reach furthest into the posterior cranial fossa and are thereby its most inferior portion (Figs. 48a.9, 48b.14, 48d.14). The posterior lobe is located superior to the tonsils. The flocculus (H X) (Figs. 49a.12, 49b.18, 72c.5, 72d.5, 73b.23) lies in the cerebellopontine cistern (Figs. 73b.16, 73c.9, 73d.9, 87.6). As seen in canthomeatal serial illustrations, the anterior lobe is also the most superior (Figs. 52a.38, 52a.39, 53a.41, 54a.41, 142, 143).

Clinical Notes

Cerebellar lesions are characterized by dyssynergias (disturbances of muscular coordination with ataxia), postural anomalies, hypotonia (decreased muscle tone), and disturbances of equilibrium and speech. Lesions of the vermis and flocculus resulting in impairment of the transmission of vestibular signals cause equilibrium disorders as well as truncal ataxia. Lesions of the lateral zone of the cerebellar hemisphere (Chap. 6.9) cause an ipsilateral impairment of movement in the extremities with ataxia, intention tremor, and dysdiadochokinesia. A frequent additional cerebellar symptom is nystagmus.
Bony artifacts can reduce the diagnostic accuracy of the CT images. This accounts for the superiority of MRI in this region, which is still further increased by the possibility of imaging sagittal and coronal scans (Chiari malformation: Chap. 4.2 Craniocervical Junction).

5.7.4 Diencephalon and Pituitary Gland
(Figs. 98–103)

External Features
The diencephalon encircles the third ventricle and is bordered by the midbrain and telencephalon. It consists of nuclear regions traversed by fiber bundles.

As mentioned earlier, the shift of the longitudinal axis of the forebrain (Forel's axis) during evolution of the neuronal systems of the neocortex forced the nuclear regions of the human diencephalon into new topographic positions. Many of these diencephalic nuclear regions were first described in lower mammals in which the neocortex is not as highly developed. The names given to the nuclear diencephalic regions in comparative anatomy did not change in human neuroanatomy. Thus, when referring to the positions of the subnuclei of the human diencephalon, directional descriptions like "ventral" and "dorsal" are only correct in relation to Forel's axis and do not correspond to the long axis of the human body. This inconsistency in the nomenclature is especially obvious in the illustrations of the forebrain made in the canthomeatal parallel planes, as in serial sections of the whole head the anatomic position can be easily identified by the frontal (anterior) and occipital (posterior) part of the skull.

Arranged in an inferior to superior sequence, the illustrations of the diencephalon first show only the hypothalamus and its infundibulum (Figs. 51a.9, 77d.6) in the canthomeatal series. In the next illustration, the hypothalamus (Fig. 52a.17) and telencephalic lamina terminalis are visible (Fig. 52a.16). The subsequent illustrations depict the hypothalamus (Fig. 53a.22), thalamic parts (Fig. 53a.30), metathalamus (Figs. 53a.31, 53a.32), and globus pallidus (Figs. 53a.14, 53a.15). The next parallel plane, the subnuclei of the thalamus with the habenular nuclei (Figs. 54a.23–28), and the globus pallidus (Fig. 54a.18) are seen in Figure 54. The last and most superior section of the series shows only the thalamus (Fig. 55a.18).

Internal Organization
With occasional exceptions, the diencephalon is divided in an inferior to superior direction into the following parts:
- Hypothalamus
- Subthalamus
- Metathalamus
- Thalamus
- Epithalamus

Hypothalamus
The hypothalamus forms the base of the diencephalon (Figs. 52a.17, 53a.22, 67.11, 77b.9, 78b.5). It surrounds the funnel-shaped inferior portion of the **third ventricle** that extends inferiorly into the infundibular recess. The infundibulum connects the hypothalamus with the pituitary gland. The hypothalamus borders anteriorly on the lamina terminalis (Figs. 2b.17, 32a.14, 52a.16, 78b.3) and the **anterior commissure** (Figs. 32a.8, 32b.12, 53b.12). The optic chiasm is located basal to the hypothalamus (Figs. 2b.20, 8a.16, 8b.15, 8d.15, 32a.24, 32b.18, 45b.29, 51a.8, 67.14, 77b.3). Posterior to the infundibulum lie the tuber cinereum and mammillary bodies (Figs. 2b.22, 10a.25, 32a.15, 32b.19, 45b.22, 67.18, 77b.10). The hypothalamic sulcus forms the border on the wall of the third ventricle between the hypothalamus and thalamus. The hypothalamus laterally reaches the subthalamic nucleus.

Morphologically and functionally, the hypothalamus is closely **connected with the pituitary gland** or hypophysis. The axonal fibers of the neurosecretory cells in the hypothalamus project through the infundibulum into the neurohypophysis or posterior lobe of the pituitary gland. These neurosecretory cells produce the neurohypophysial hormones oxytocin and vasopressin (ADH, antidiuretic hormone). Damage to this hypothalamic–neurohypophysial system results in diabetes insipidus. The adenohypophysis or anterior lobe of the pituitary gland is connected to the hypothalamus through the hypophysial portal system. The hypothalamic–infundibular system produces substances that either trigger the release of hormones in the anterior lobe of the pituitary gland (releasing factors [RF]—liberins), or inhibit the secretion of hypophysial hormones (inhibiting factors [IF]—statins). This system is partly controlled by the tuberoinfundibular dopaminergic system (Chap. 7.1.1).

The hypothalamus can be divided according to its content of myelinated nerve fibers into:
- Weakly myelinated hypothalamus
- Strongly myelinated hypothalamus.

The nerve cells of the hypothalamic–neurohypophysial system and the hypothalamic–infundibular system and nonhypophysial nerve cells are part of the weakly myelinated hypothalamus. The nonhypophysial nerve cells are located, for the most part, in the lateral regions of the hypothalamus and control autonomic activities such as regulation of body temperature, food and water intake, sleep, and emotional behavior. The nuclear groups in the mammillary body are part of the strongly myelinated hypothalamus. Morphologically and functionally, these groups are closely related to the limbic system (Chap. 6.11).

Subthalamus
The subthalamus is located in the lateral portion of the diencephalon but does not come into contact with the wall of the third ventricle. The subthalamic nucleus, the globus pallidus, and the zona incerta are parts of the subthalamus. The subthalamic nucleus lies posterior to the mammillary body and post-

eromedial to the posterior limb of the internal capsule deep in the seventh slice of the canthomeatal series (Fig. 138.7). The **subthalamic nucleus** is shaped like a biconvex lens and can be seen macroscopically (Figs. 11a.22, 33a.15). Located in the vicinity of the subthalamic nucleus but lateral to the internal capsule is the **globus pallidus** (Figs. 9b.11, 9d.11, 11a.23, 11a.15, 34a.8, 34a.14, 53a.14, 53a.15, 53b.13, 53d.13). Laterally the globus pallidus is separated from the putamen by a thin layer of fibers, the lateral medullary lamina. Inferiorly the globus pallidus borders on the innominate substance and on olfactory areas. The globus pallidus is considered part of the basal ganglia and is involved in motor activities (Chap. 6.8.2). The zona incerta is a continuation of the reticular formation of the midbrain. It consists of a thin layer of cells located above the subthalamic nucleus. It borders on two medullated fiber laminae (Forel's fields H1 and H2).

Metathalamus
The metathalamus consists of the **medial** and **lateral geniculate bodies** (Figs. 12a.18, 12a.19, 34a.15, 53a.31, 53a.32) that are located posterior to the thalamus. The medial geniculate body is a relay nucleus for the auditory system (Chap. 6.5), while the lateral geniculate body is a relay center for the visual system (Chap. 6.6).

Thalamus
The thalamus is a somewhat egg-shaped aggregate of numerous nuclear regions. The tip of this "egg" is directed toward the interventricular foramen (of Monro) (Figs. 2b.11, 10a.13, 54a.22, 83b.3). The medial surface of the thalamus borders on the third ventricle. Its lateral surface contacts the posterior limb of internal capsule (Figs. 11a.15, 54a.20, 54d.20). The posterior portion of the thalamus is the pulvinar (Figs. 12b.13, 54a.28). The interthalamic adhesion (intermediate mass) (Figs. 2b.13, 32a.9, 45b.15), a narrow bridge of glial cells, usually connects the thalami of both sides. A narrow portion of the superior side of the thalamus develops embryonally into the floor of the central part of lateral ventricle. This area is called the lamina affixa and would appear in Figure 55a.18 just above the visible portion of the thalamus. Lateral and superior to the thalamus lies the caudate nucleus (Figs. 11a.9, 12a.9, 34a.5, 34b.5, 34d.5, 55a.12, 55a.22). The superior thalamostriate vein (Figs. 11c.9, 12c.8, 55c.11) and the stria terminalis run in the groove between these two nuclear regions.

The **medullary laminae** divide the nuclear complexes of the thalamus into several groups. In the anterior portion of the thalamus two laminae separate the **anterior nuclei** (Figs. 10a.14, 54a.23). These nuclei are, for the most part, relay stations of the limbic system (Chap. 6.11). Medially, an internal lamina forms the border of the **medial nuclei** (Figs. 11a.13, 54a.24). They have corticopetal and corticofugal connections with the frontal lobe of the telencephalon.

Of the many lateral nuclei of the thalamus, only those which are of special importance to the neurofunctional systems will be described. In general, the thalamic nuclei have both thalamocortical and corticothalamic fibers, although often only one projectional system may be mentioned. Stereotactic surgery can be performed on several of the relay nuclei. The ventral lateral nucleus (Figs. 11a.14, 54a.25) is connected with area 4 (located anterior to the central sulcus in the frontal lobe). The frontal portion of the ventral lateral nuclei contains afferent fibers from the globus pallidus, while the occipital portion contains afferent fibers from the cerebellum. The **ventral posterolateral nucleus** (Figs. 34a.9, 53a.30) is a relay nucleus for the anterolateral and the medial lemniscus systems. In its immediate vicinity lies the **ventral posteromedial nucleus** (Figs. 114.3, 115.17, 116.11). This nucleus provides a similar relay center to its neighboring nucleus for the trigeminal system with a somatotopic projection into the postcentral gyrus (Chap. 6.1.3). The ventral posterolateral and posteromedial nuclei belong to the specific nuclei of the thalamus. They have point-to-point connections with the body periphery and specific areas of the cerebral cortex.

The mode of connection of these specific nuclei is different from that of the nonspecific nuclei that project diffusely into large areas of the telencephalon. The intralaminar nuclei, as described in Chapter 6.3 (ascending reticular system), belong to these nonspecific nuclei. The **pulvinar** transmits both auditory and optic signals and projects into association cortical areas of the telencephalon.

Epithalamus
The epithalamus is composed of structures located on and around the roof of the third ventricle. These structures include the choroid plexus of the third ventricle, the stria medullaris of the thalamus, the habenular nuclei (Figs. 54a.27, 147.11), and the **pineal gland** (formerly pineal body) (Figs. 2b.19, 13a.14, 32a.12, 32b.16, 54b.22, 54c.18, 54d.22). Just anterior to the superior colliculi lies the **posterior commissure** (Figs. 2b.18, 12a.17, 32a.11, 32b.15, 45b.18) that joins nuclear groups of the midbrain. The pineal gland, which has an average length of slightly less than 1 cm, lies on the tectum and is attached to the roof of the diencephalon. In about 10% of school children examined, acervulus (brain sand) is found in the pineal gland. CT scans reveal the presence of pineal gland calcifications in more than 50% of examined individuals above age 25 (497). These calcifications are a CT guideline structure indicating the position of the pineal gland.

Clinical Notes
Diencephalic lesions result in characteristic dysfunctions that, in certain cases, enable a topical assessment after clinical examination. A "central" dysregulation of body temperature and/or dis-

orders of fluid balance, for instance, indicates hypothalamic or, more specifically, hypothalamic–neurohypophysial dysfunction. Other symptoms indicating hypothalamic dysfunction are severe impairments of sympathetic/parasympathetic regulatory functions.

The **subthalamus** is in close contact with the basal ganglia via the globus pallidus. A lesion in this region results in contralateral hemiballism. A vascular disorder is the most frequent cause.

Depending on the anatomic location, **thalamic dysfunctions** may take on many forms. The thalamus is not only a subcortical collection point for exteroceptive and proprioceptive impulses (110), but also an important integration and coordination center for afferent impulses and their affective influences. Lesions cause contralateral disorders of both exteroceptive sensitivity, especially thermal sense and proprioceptive sensitivity. Patients develop hemiataxia and involuntary movements as well as choreoathetoid movements. Contralateral spontaneous pain and hyperpathia may arise. Thalamic disorders can often be traced to vascular causes. Tumors seldom cause a complete thalamic syndrome.

A unilateral lesion of the **medial geniculate body** usually remains undetected because of the bilateral nature of the auditory pathway. A unilateral injury of **the lateral geniculate body**, on the other hand, leads to a contralateral visual field defect up to a homonymous contralateral hemianopia.

Pituitary Gland
(Figs. 8b.17, 9c.14, 32a.27, 32b.24)

The pituitary gland or hypophysis is an endocrine organ. It is connected anatomically and functionally with the hypothalamus. The pituitary gland weighs on average 0.7 g and is bean-shaped. It is situated in the hypophysial fossa of the body of the sphenoid and is separated superiorly from the cranial cavity by a layer of dura, the diaphragma sellae. The infundibular stalk runs through a small opening in the diaphragma sellae.

Subdivisions
The pituitary gland is divided into:
- Adenohypophysis, anterior lobe (Fig. 75b.2)
- Neurohypophysis, posterior lobe (Fig. 75b.5).

The **adenohypophysis** or anterior lobe is divided into distal, tuberal, and intermediate portions. The distal part is the largest section of the adenohypophysis. The tuberal portion surrounds the pituitary stalk. The intermediate portion borders on the neurohypophysis.

The adenohypophysis controls the activity of the other endocrine glands through glandotropic hormones. In the adenohypophysis the following cells have been identified by electron microscopy and by immunohistochemical methods for the listed hormones (in parentheses):
- Somatotropic cells (growth hormone (GH) = STH)
- Thyrotropic cells (thyrotropic hormone = TSH)
- Mammotropic cells (prolactin = PRL)
- Corticotropic cells (adrenocorticotropic hormone = ACTH)
- Gonadotropic cells (follicular stimulating hormone = FSH, luteinizing hormone = LH).

In the intermediate lobe melanotropin and lipotropin are produced by endocrine cells.

The **neurohypophysis** is divided into:
- Infundibulum, infundibular stalk
- Posterior lobe of the pituitary gland.

No hormones are produced in the neurohypophysis. It is an area for the storage and release of hormones that are transported to the neurohypophysis via axons from nerve cells of the hypothalamus.

The following arteries supply the pituitary gland:
- Superior hypophysial arteries from the internal carotid artery
- Inferior hypophysial arteries from the circle of Willis.

Parts of both vessels reach the pituitary gland directly and other parts form capillary plexuses around the stalk. From here the blood reaches one or two veins (portal veins) that run to the adenohypophysis and there (once again) form capillaries (**portal circulation of the pituitary gland**). The regulatory hypothalamic neurohormones are transported by these infundibular vessels to the adenohypophysis, their effector site.

5.7.5 Telencephalon
(Figs. 102–108)

The telencephalon is the largest subdivision of the brain (more than 80% of total brain weight, average volume above 1000 ml). The supratentorial space is predominantly filled with telencephalic structures. The telencephalon covers great parts of the diencephalon. The telencephalon is separated from the cerebellum by a deep transverse furrow, the transverse cerebral fissure where the tentorium of cerebellum is located.

External Features
The telencephalon consists of two hemispheres. The **longitudinal cerebral** (interhemispheric) **fissure** separates the two hemispheres in the median plane down to the corpus callosum. Between the hemispheres is a dural septum, the falx cerebri (Figs. 4a.3, 4b.3, 10a.3, 17a.4, 52a.3, 55a.3, 55d.3, 57a.14). The medial surface of each hemisphere merges into the lateral surface at the superior margin. The lateral surface of the human telencephalon is formed entirely

- Frontal lobe
- Parietal lobe
- Occipital lobe
- Temporal lobe

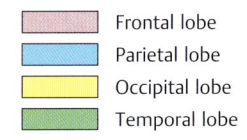

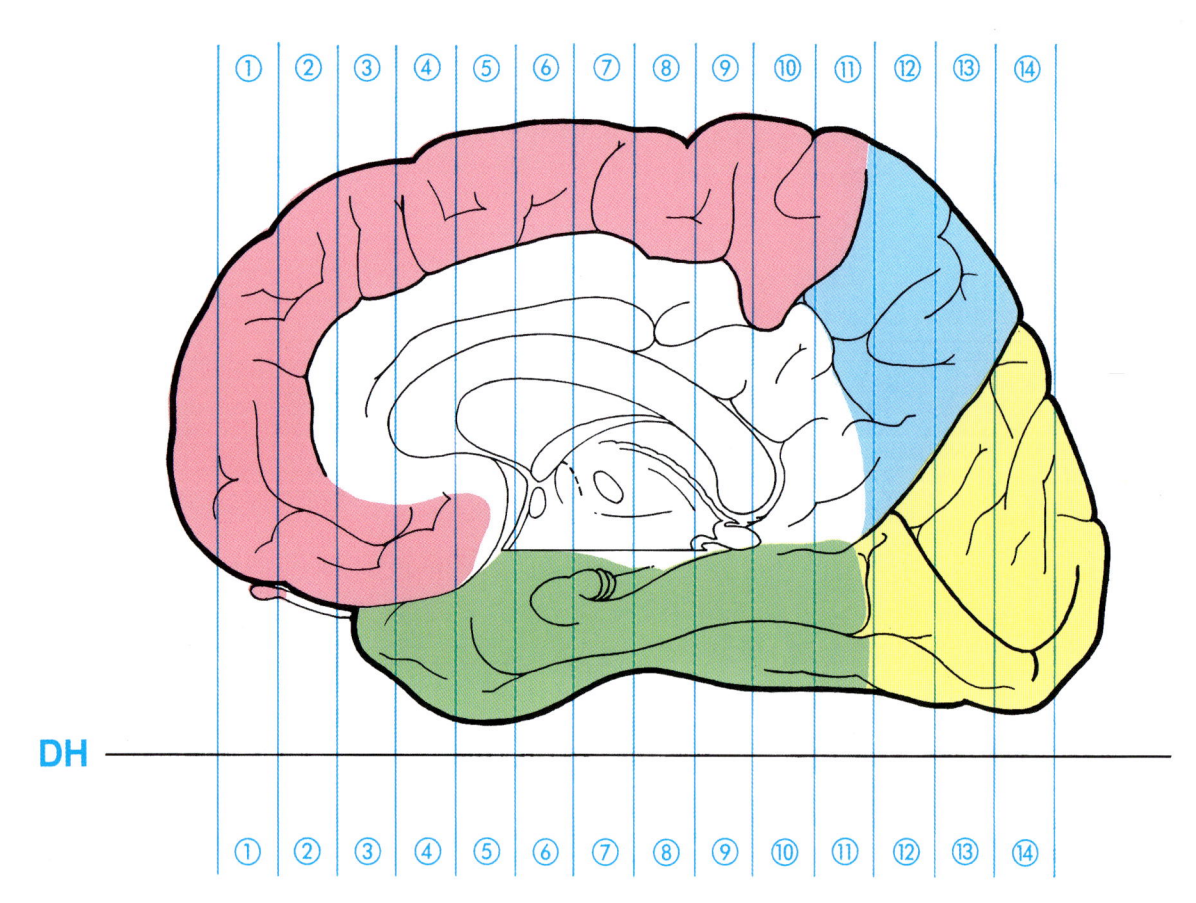

Fig. **104a** Medial view of the coronally cut cerebrum indicating the boundaries of the frontal, parietal, occipital, and temporal lobes. The cingulate gyrus, the paraterminal gyrus, and the subcallosal area are not included in the above-mentioned lobes (Chap. 8).
DH Reid's base line

by the neocortex. During evolution, its surface area increased through the development of convolutions or gyri and furrows or sulci. Each hemisphere is divided into four lobes and an insula. The olfactory bulb and tract are located underneath the frontal lobe. They belong to the olfactory system (Chap. 6.7).

Internal Organization

The telencephalon consists of gray and white matter. The **gray matter,** which contains nerve cells, can be divided into:
- Telencephalic nuclei
- Cerebral cortex.

The **white matter** consists of nerve fibers that transmit afferent and efferent signals and facilitate information processing between the different regions of the telencephalon. Each hemisphere includes a lateral ventricle that communicates with the third ventricle through the interventricular foramen (of Monro).

Telencephalic Nuclei

The nuclei of the telencephalon border on the lateral ventricles. These nuclei have been divided by the ascending and descending neencephalic pathways into the following formations:

- Caudate nucleus (Figs. 8a.9, 10a.9, 12a.20, 33a.7, 34a.5, 35a.11, 53a.16, 53a.33, 54a.34, 55a.22, 55b.8, 55d.8)
- Putamen (Figs. 9a.14, 9b.12, 9d.12, 11a.16, 34a.7, 34b.10, 34d.10, 35a.10, 53a.13, 54a.17)
- Claustrum (Figs. 9a.16, 10a.22, 10b.17, 35a.9, 52a.13, 54a.15, 55a.13)
- Amygdaloid body (Figs. 9b.20, 9d.20, 10a.27, 35a.21, 51a.12, 51b.11, 52a.21)
- Septal nuclei (formerly septal verum) (Fig. 53a.20).

During evolution of the neocortex, the **caudate nucleus** assumed the shape of a comma, with a head and an arched tail contoured along the wall of the lateral ventricle. The head is a relatively large bulging protuberance on the lateral wall of the frontal horn of the lateral ventricle. It continues occipitally along this wall as the body of the caudate nucleus, turning anteriorly in the roof of the lateral ventricle, where it forms the tail of the caudate nucleus. This tail tapers to the tip of the temporal horn. Neencephalic pathways separate the caudate nucleus from the putamen, with the exception of those parts located in the anterobasal region (floor of the striatum, Fig. 52a.12). The striatum includes caudate nucleus, putamen, and nucleus accumbens. The nucleus accumbens verges

5.7 Subdivisions of the Brain   309

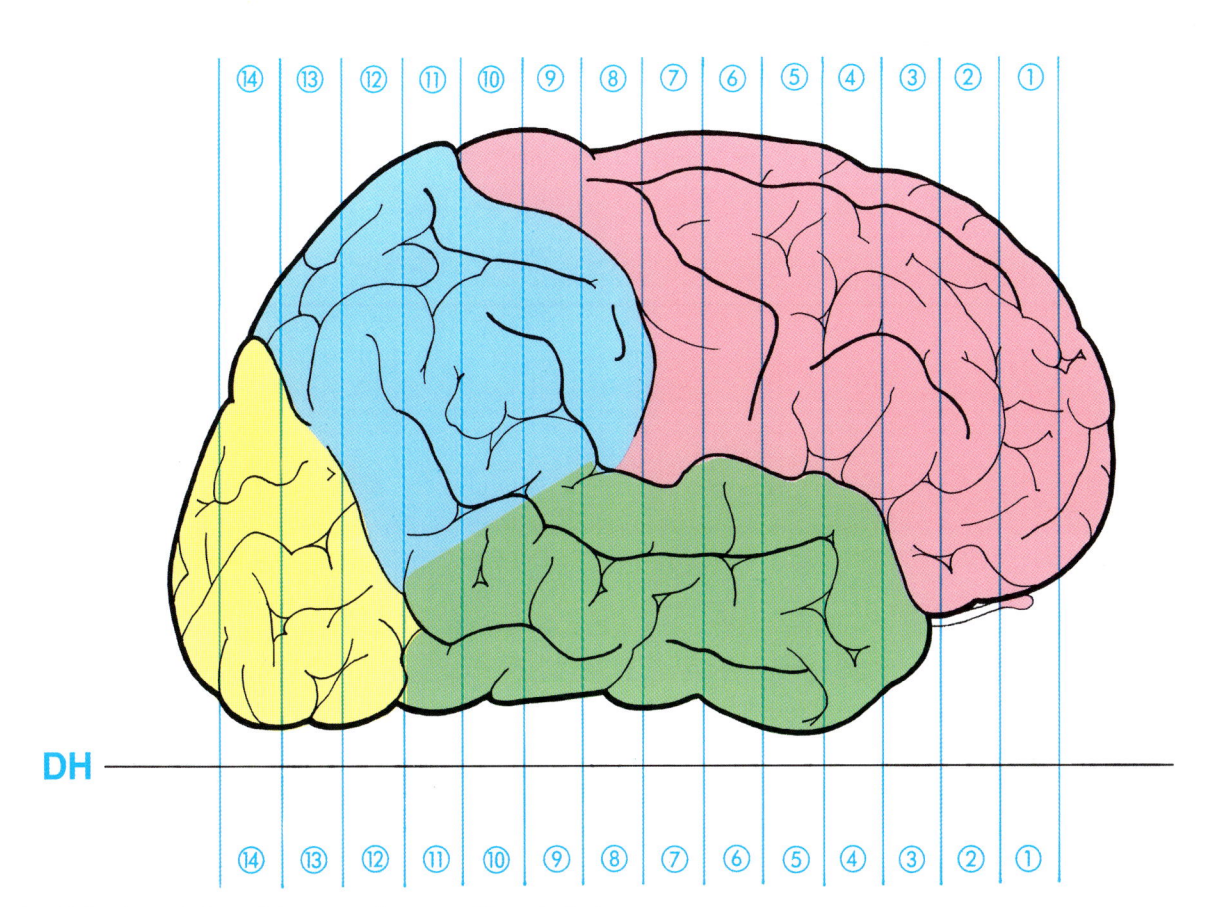

Fig. **104b** Lateral view of the coronally cut cerebrum indicating the boundaries of the frontal, parietal, occipital, and temporal lobes (Chap. 8).
DH Reid's base line

towards the septum pellucidum, therefore its full name is nucleus accumbens septi pellucidi. It is located on the floor of the striatum (Figs. 52a.12, 138.1). Stimulation of the nucleus accumbens induces an intense sense of well-being comparable to that experience by intake of addictive drugs, such as heroin (127). As the nerve cells of the three nuclei are similar in form, they are referred to as **striatum**. The striatum has an important motor function (Chap. 6.8.2).

The **putamen** is a shell-shaped structure located medial to the external capsule. The globus pallidus of the diencephalon lies inside the concave portion of the putamen. Topographically, the putamen and globus pallidus form the lentiform nucleus. The nerve cells of these two nuclear regions, however, differ substantially.

The **claustrum** lies as a small platelike structure lateral to the putamen and is bordered on opposite sides by the external and extreme capsules.

The **amygdaloid body** (amygdala) is located in a medial position at the tip of the temporal horn of the lateral ventricle. One part of the amygdaloid body belongs to the olfactory system (Chap. 6.7), the other part to the limbic system (Chap. 6.11).

The **septal nuclei** (formerly precommissural septum) is a nuclear region located anterior to the anterior commissure and to the column of the fornix. It is described further in Chapter 6.11 as part of the limbic system.

Cerebral Lobes

The brain mantle or pallium consists of the cerebral cortex and the white matter beneath it and encloses the lateral ventricles. The cerebral cortex is divided into four lobes and the insula, which has been covered by the opercula during evolution of the neocortex (Figs. 104–108a):

- Frontal lobe
- Parietal lobe
- Occipital lobe
- Temporal lobe
- Insula or island (of Reil).

The individual lobes are only partially separated by sulci (342). Located on the lateral surface of each hemisphere, the **central sulcus** (Figs. 3.4, 11a.4, 12a.4, 12b.4, 31.9, 36a.4, 36b.3, 54a.29, 56a.7, 58b.9, 59a.4, 59d.9) separates the frontal lobe from the parietal lobe. The central sulcus does not run in a straight line but as two arches from the superior margin in the direction of the lateral sulcus. The upper arch borders the "knob" demonstrating a protrusion in a posterior direction and a concavity in an anterior direction (458, 495, 507). The "knob" contains the hand area. The course of the central sulcus is shown clearly in the 3D illustrations (Fig. 108b). With help of a PC, red–blue spectacles, and a CD-ROM (243), the different

310   5 Topography of the Neurocranium and its Intracranial Spaces and Structures in Multiplanar Parallel Slices

Cortex of frontal lobe

Cortex of temporal lobe

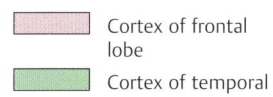

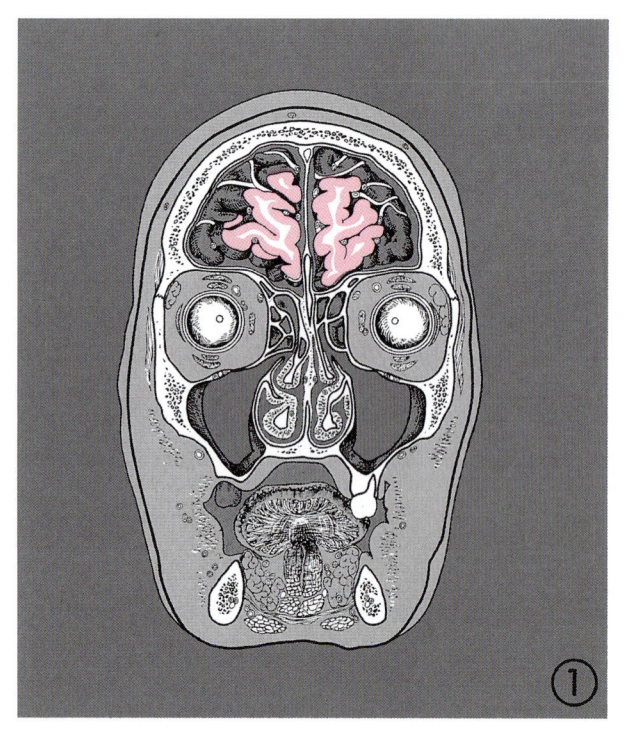

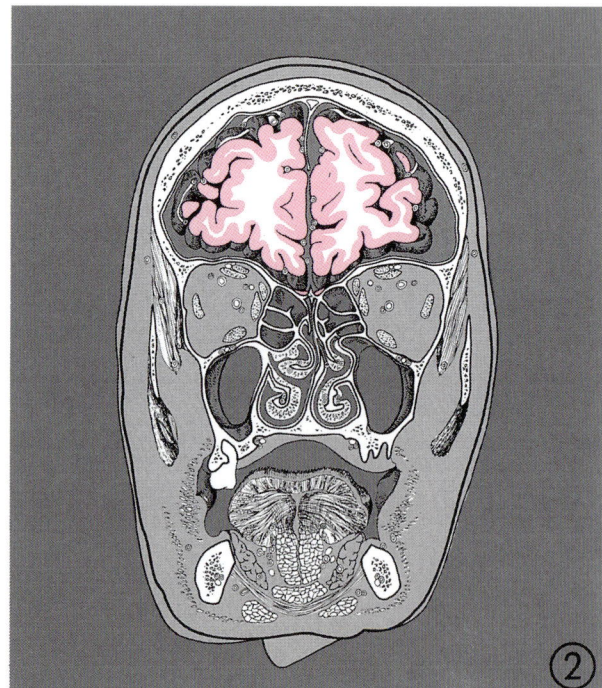

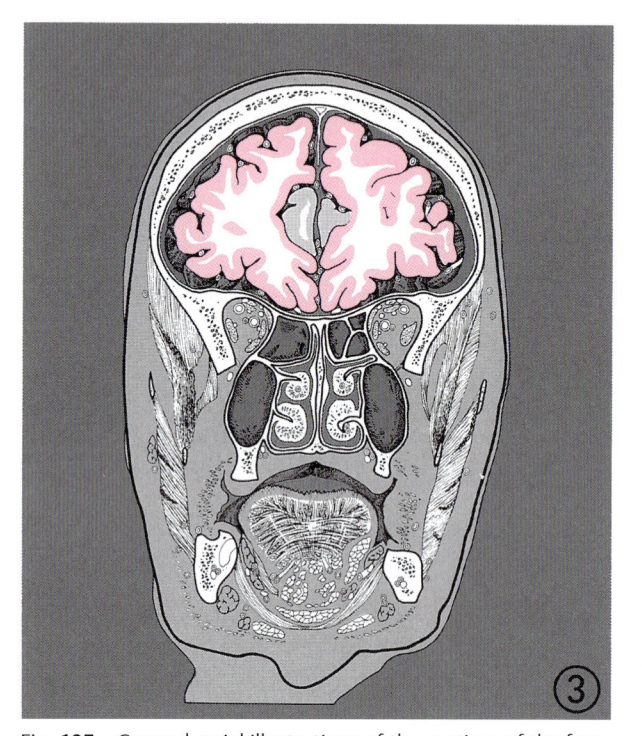

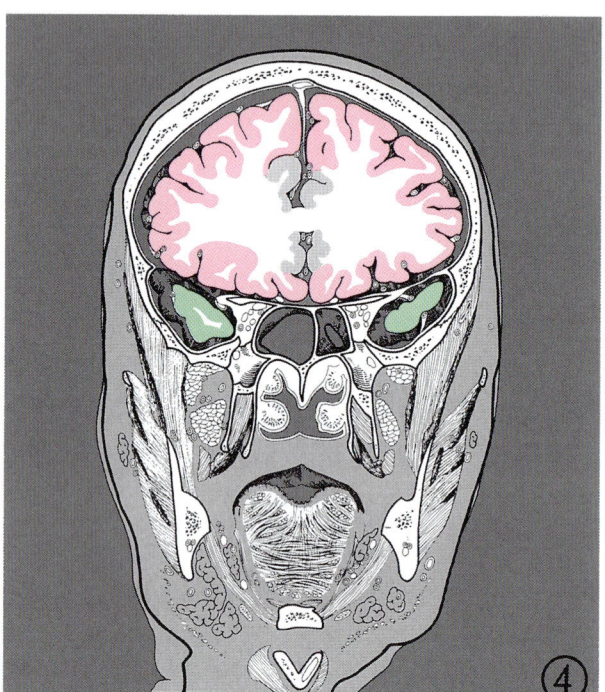

Fig. 105 Coronal serial illustrations of the cortices of the frontal, parietal, occipital, and temporal lobes. The cortices of the insula, cingulate gyrus, subcallosal area, and paraterminal gyrus are not included in the above-mentioned lobes. The encircled numbers (1–8) indicate the number of the respective slice.

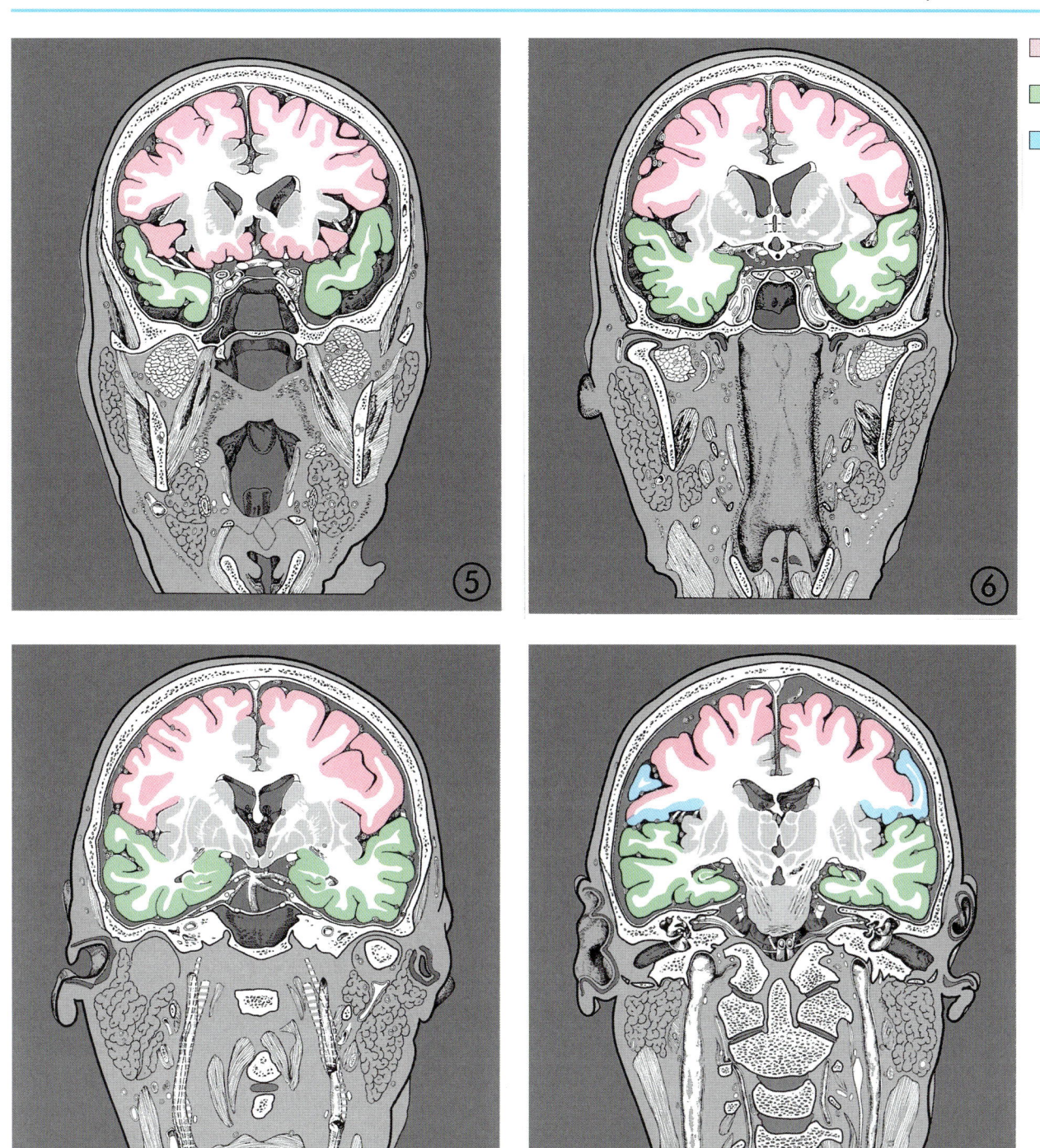

5.7 Subdivisions of the Brain

Cortex of frontal lobe

Cortex of temporal lobe

Cortex of parietal lobe

- Cortex of frontal lobe
- Cortex of parietal lobe
- Cortex of temporal lobe
- Cortex of occipital lobe

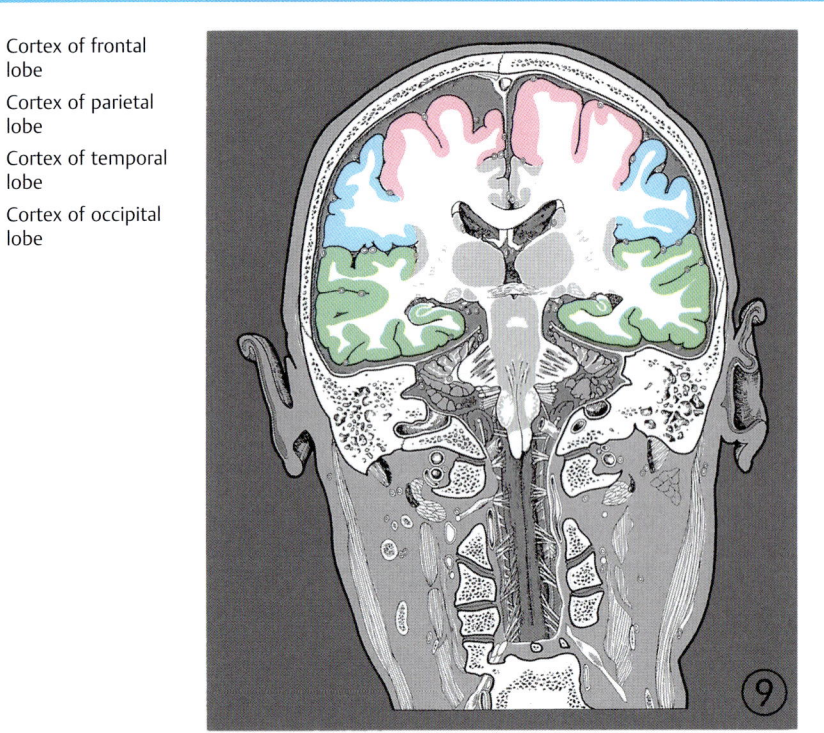

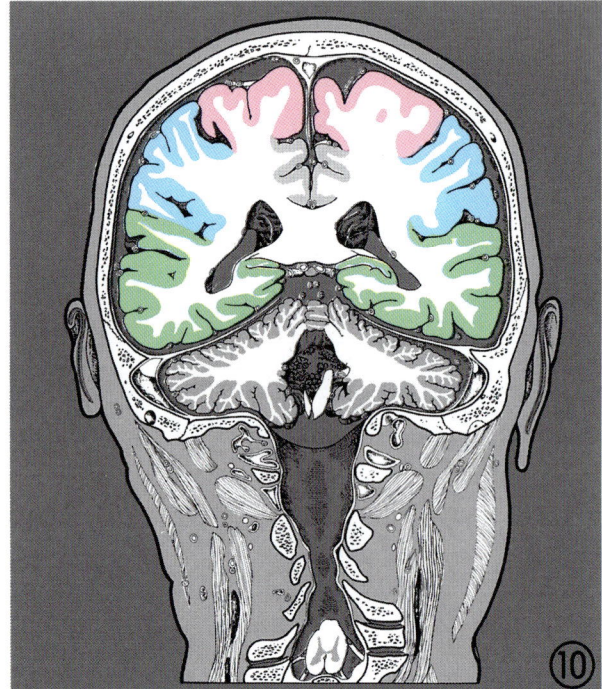

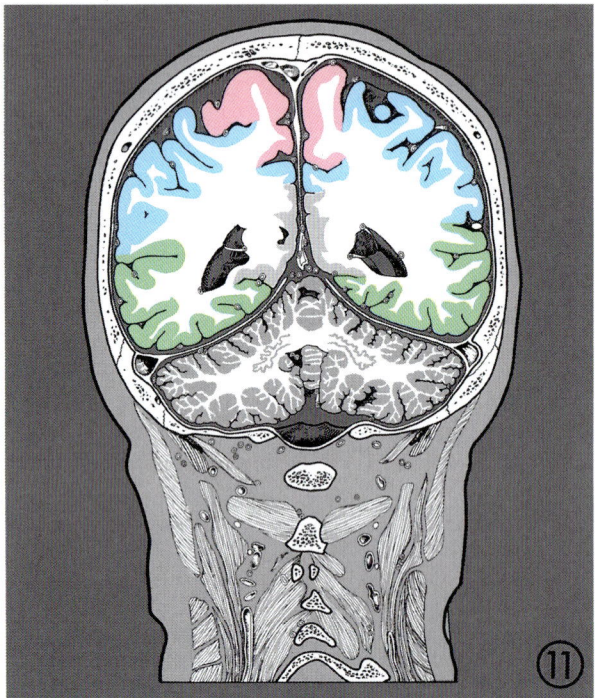

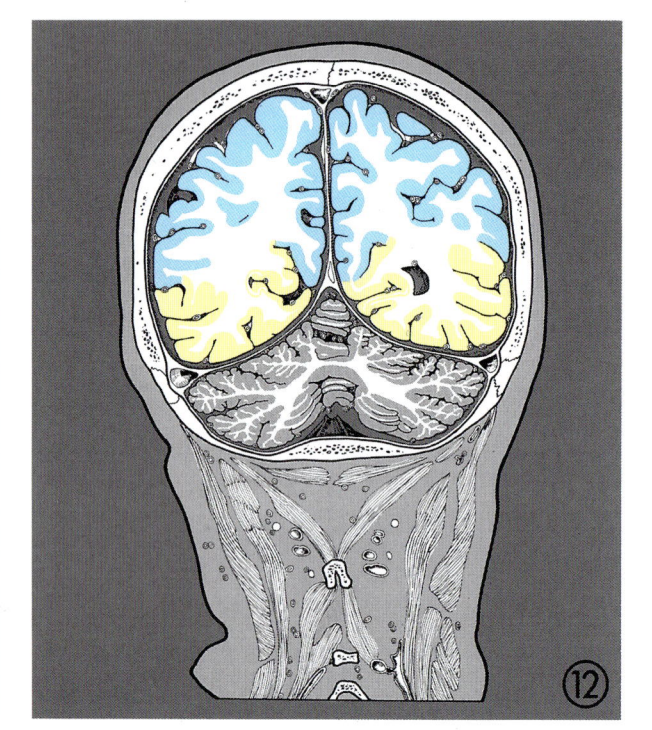

Fig. 105 Coronal serial illustrations of the cortices of the frontal, parietal, occipital, and temporal lobes. The cortices of the insula, cingulate gyrus, subcallosal area, and paraterminal gyrus are not included in the above-mentioned lobes. The encircled numbers (9–14) indicate the number of the respective slice.

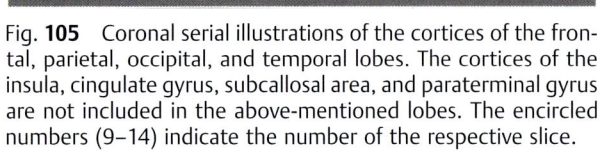

angles of inclination of the central sulcus can be recognized leading to the mid plane and the bicommissural plane.

Clinical Notes
In CT and, less frequently, MR images, this variable angle of inclination produces an irregular partial volume effect, resulting in an indistinct illustration of the central sulcus and therefore making identification difficult.

The criteria for detecting the **central sulcus** are
- Localization of the "knob" (229) (see above).
- Differences in the cortical thickness of the precentral and postcentral gyri. In regions where the central sulcus lies approximately vertical to the layers of the MR image, the cortex of the precentral gyrus is wider than that of the postcentral gyrus. The lateral walls of the central sulcus showed the cortical thickness of the precentral gyrus to be on average 2.7 mm and the postcentral gyrus 1.8 mm (508).

5.7 Subdivisions of the Brain

Cortex of parietal lobe
Cortex of occipital lobe

- The superior frontal sulcus ends usually in the precentral sulcus, which courses directly anterior to the central sulcus. Here the axial illustrations are seen most clearly.
- The bracket signs. In axial CT and MR images the marginal branch of the cingulate sulcus close to the superior margin of the cerebrum appears to form a "bracket" to the central sulcus. The medial end of the central sulcus reaches this "bracket region" in around 95% percent of cases compared to the postcentral sulcus in only 3% of cases (508).

The **lateral sulcus** (Sylvian fissure) (Figs. 8a.11, 10a.18, 10b.15, 13a.8, 36a.8, 37b.8, 37d.8, 52a.7, 53a.25, 53b.8, 53d.8, 54a.12) forms the boundary between the temporal lobe and the frontal lobe and reaches deep into the brain toward the insula. For a short distance it also separates the temporal and parietal lobes. On the medial surface of each hemisphere, the **parietooccipital sulcus** (Figs. 2b.6, 15a.6, 15b.4, 16b.5, 17a.3, 32a.2, 32b.4, 33a.6, 55a.25, 55b.21, 56d.15, 57a.12) divides the parietal and occipital lobes. In the posterolateral region of the lateral surface of each hemisphere, there are no clear boundaries between the parietal, occipital, and temporal lobes.

Frontal Lobe

The lateral surface of the frontal lobe shows three arched gyri only partially separated by sulci:
- Superior frontal gyrus (Figs. 3.1, 4a.2, 5b.4, 8a.1, 11a.1, 30b.4, 33a.3, 33b.4, 52a.1, 55a.1, 55b.2, 59a.1, 59d.4)
- Middle frontal gyrus (Figs. 3.8, 4a.4, 8a.3, 8b.4, 10a.2, 10d.3, 30b.3, 35a.1, 36b.1, 52a.4, 55a.2, 58a.2, 58b.6, 58d.6)
- Inferior frontal gyrus (Figs. 3.13, 5a.6, 8a.6, 9b.9, 30b.6, 31.5, 36a.7, 36b.5, 52a.5, 55a.7).

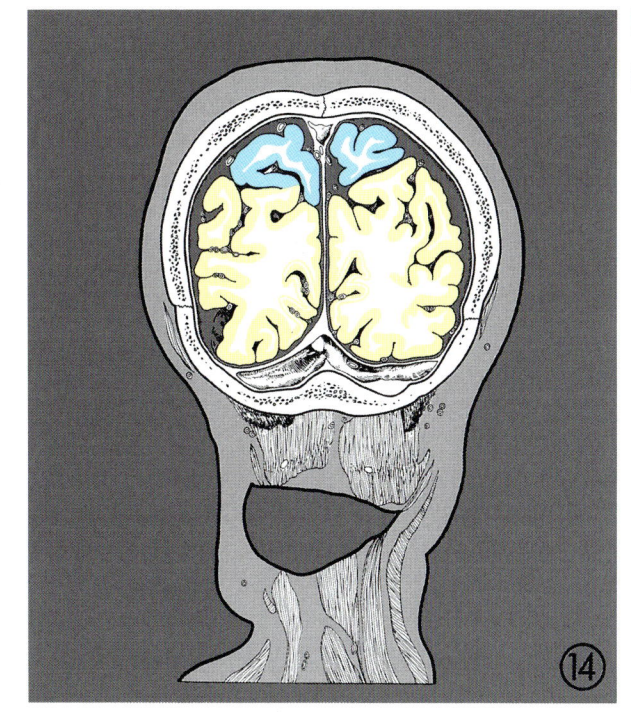

The inferior frontal gyrus is further divided by two branches of the lateral sulcus (Sylvian fissure). In the sagittal MR and CT images, which lie close to the surface of the inferior frontal gyrus, a skew M-shaped cortical band can be determined at the lateral sulcus. The vertically ascending ramus of the lateral sulcus borders the opercular part and the triangular part of the inferior frontal gyrus. The V-form of the letter M can be found at the triangular part. The anterior ramus of the lateral sulcus divides the triangular part from the orbital part of the inferior frontal gyrus (508).

The portion of the inferior frontal gyrus located posterior to the ascending ramus is called the **frontal operculum**. In more than 95% of all individuals, Broca's area (motor language area) is located in this region of the left hemisphere (Chap. 6.10). All three frontal gyri terminate at the **precentral sulcus** (Figs. 3.7, 31.8, 36a.2, 37a.5, 56a.5, 56b.5, 56d.5, 58a.3, 58d.7, 59a.2). Located between the precentral and central sulci is a motor region, the **precentral gyrus** (Figs. 3.10, 10a.5, 10b.5, 11a.3, 14a.1, 31.10, 33a.1, 33b.2, 34a.2, 34d.5, 54a.11, 59a.3, 59d.7). The precentral gyrus runs across the lateral aspect of the cerebral hemisphere, not vertically to Reid's base line, but obliquely from anteroinferiorly to posterosuperiorly toward the superior margin of the hemisphere. In the **frontopetal type** of hemisphere the precentral gyrus (Fig. 46.3) runs more steeply, in the occipitopetal type less steeply to Reid's base line (Fig. 3 DH) (136, 260). Therefore, in the brain of the coronal series the precentral gyrus reaches relatively far occipitally at the superior margin of the hemisphere. Situated on the medial surface of each hemisphere, the paracentral lobule is a portion of this motor region. The medial frontal gyrus lies also on the medial surface of each hemisphere (Fig. 91d.25). Above the roof of the orbit in the anterior cranial fossa lie variable convolutions

314   5 Topography of the Neurocranium and its Intracranial Spaces and Structures in Multiplanar Parallel Slices

- Cortex of frontal lobe
- Cortex of parietal lobe
- Cortex of occipital lobe
- Cortex of temporal lobe

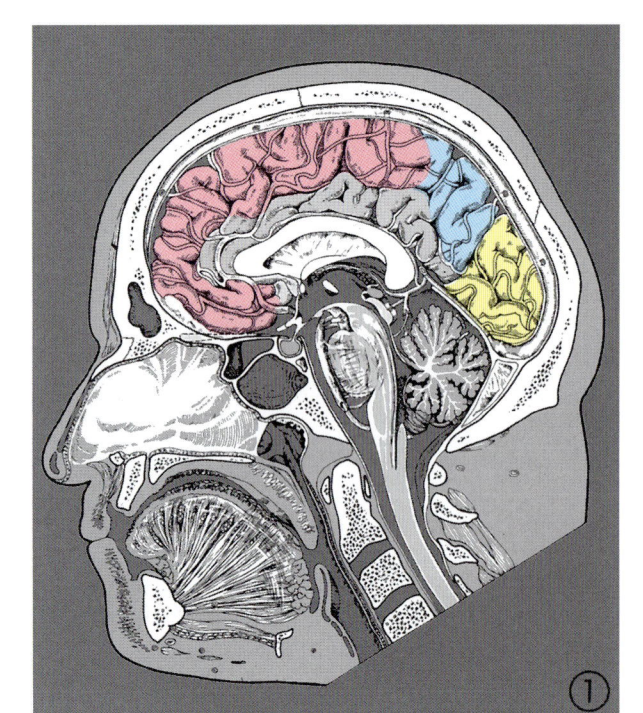

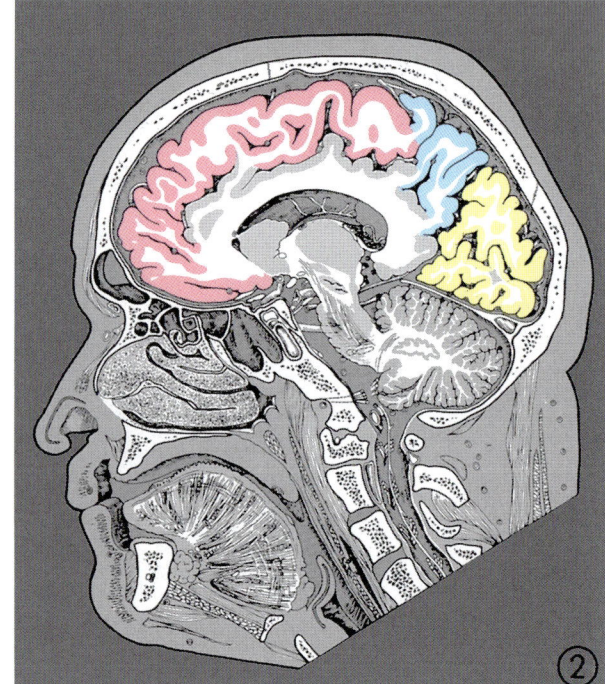

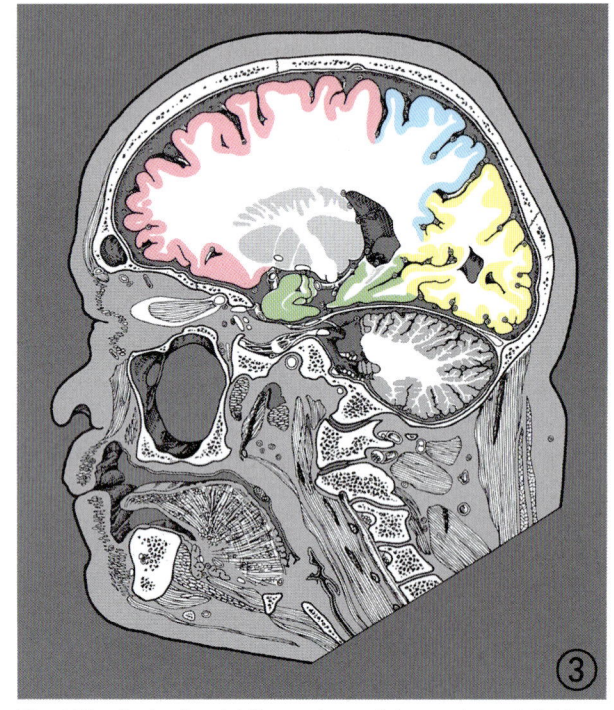

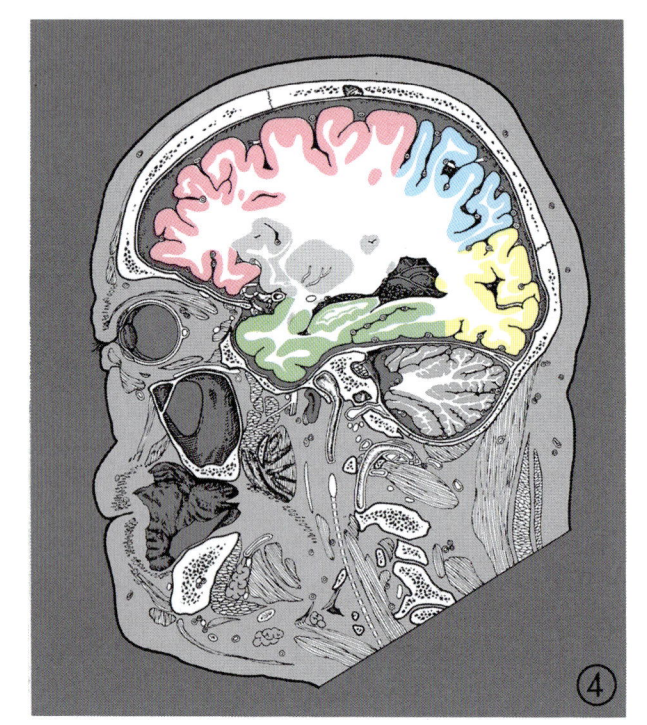

Fig. **106** Sagittal serial illustrations of the cortices of the frontal, parietal, occipital, and temporal lobes. The cortices of the insula, cingulate gyrus, subcallosal area, and paraterminal gyrus are not included in the above-mentioned lobes. The encircled number (1–6) indicates the number of the respective slice (Figs. 29, 30a,b, 31).

5.7 Subdivisions of the Brain

	Cortex of frontal lobe
	Cortex of parietal lobe
	Cortex of occipital lobe
	Cortex of temporal lobe

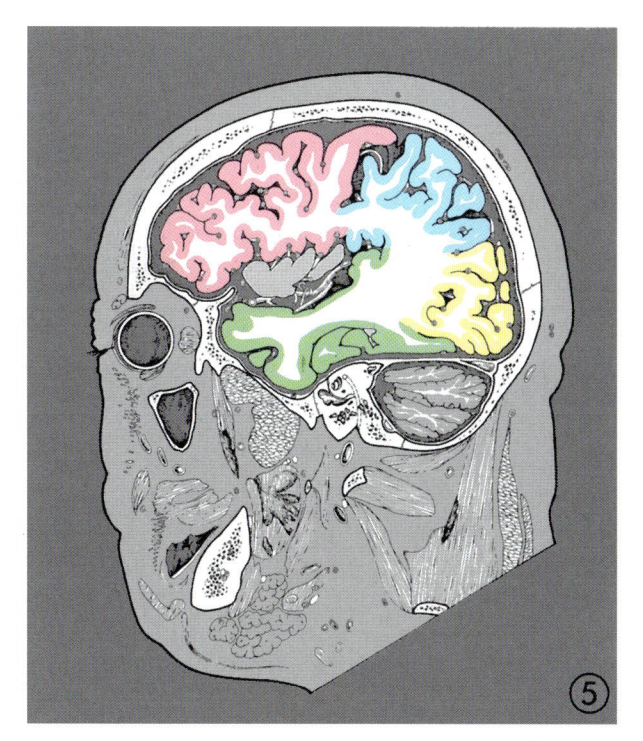

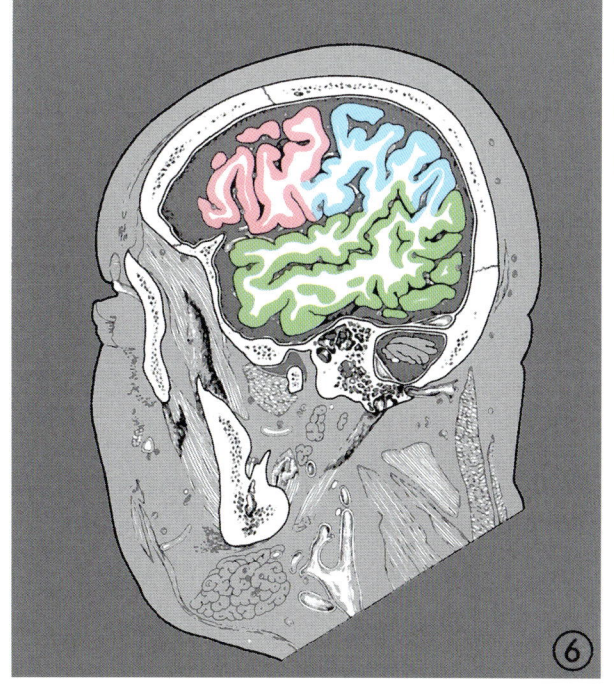

of the frontal lobe known as the orbital gyri (Figs. 5a.5, 6a.8, 6b.6, 51a.2). The straight gyrus (Figs. 5a.7, 8a.14, 50a.2, 51a.3) is bordered laterally by the olfactory sulcus.

Parietal Lobe
The **postcentral gyrus** (Figs. 3.3, 11a.7, 13a.5, 13b.4, 31.12, 33a.2, 33b.3, 34a.3, 37a.4, 55a.15, 59a.5, 59b.10, 59d.10) of the parietal lobe borders on the central sulcus. The postcentral sulcus runs posterior to the postcentral gyrus, partitioning off the superior parietal lobule (Figs. 3.6, 15a.1, 15b.2, 31.15, 58a.9, 58b.14, 58d.14, 59a.9). The **supramarginal gyrus** (Figs. 3.9, 12a.6, 13a.7, 31.11, 36a.6, 37a.6, 37b.5, 46.9, 56a.13, 56b.13, 57a.9) and the **angular gyrus** (Figs. 3.11, 15a.5, 16a.4, 31.14, 35a.4, 36a.9, 46.11, 56a.15, 57a.10) are considered as portions of the parietal lobe. The supramarginal gyrus forms a concave convolution around the posterior end of the lateral sulcus (Sylvian fissure). The angular gyrus curves around the occipital end of the superior temporal sulcus. The precuneus (Figs. 2b.4, 15a.4, 17a.1, 33a.4, 45b.2, 56a.16, 57a.11, 58a.11), located on the medial surface of each hemisphere, extends from the marginal branch of the cingulate sulcus to the parieto-occipital sulcus, and is considered part of the parietal lobe.

Occipital Lobe
The **occipital gyri** (Figs. 3.18, 16a.8, 17a.5, 17b.4, 31.17, 33a.12, 35a.7, 36a.17, 36b.12, 53a.45, 53b.28, 53d.28, 56a.19, 56b.16, 56d.16) are somewhat irregularly shaped convolutions located on the lateral surface of the occipital lobe. Lying on the inferior surface of the occipital lobe and facing the tentorium of cerebellum are the lateral occipitotemporal gyrus (Figs. 15a.15, 15b.9, 15d.9, 16a.13, 16b.10, 17a.11, 53a.42) and the medial occipitotemporal gyrus (Figs. 15a.14, 15b.8, 16a.12, 16b.9, 17a.10, 34a.19, 35a.23, 53a.44). Half of these gyri belong to the occipital lobe, half to the temporal lobe. The cuneus (Figs. 2b.16, 16a.7, 17a.6, 45b.12, 55a.26, 56a.20, 57a.15) lies on the medial side of the occipital lobe between the parieto-occipital (Fig. 33a.6) and calcarine sulci. The area on each side of the **calcarine sulcus** (Figs. 2b.23, 15a.12, 15b.6, 15d.6, 16a.9, 17a.8, 17b.5, 32b.17, 32d.17, 33a.16, 45b.20, 54a.44, 126.17) belongs to the primary visual cortex.

Temporal Lobe
The temporal lobe has three temporal gyri (Fig. 46):
- Superior temporal gyrus (Figs. 3.19, 8a.13, 8b.12, 11a.20, 14a.8, 30b.8, 37a.10, 37b.7, 37d.7, 46.20, 52a.10, 52b.5, 52d.5, 54b.15, 55a.20)
- Middle temporal gyrus (Figs. 3.23, 8a.20, 8b.16, 11a.27, 14a.9, 30b.10, 37a.15, 37b.9, 37d.9, 46.25, 52a.22, 52b.10, 52d.10, 54a.38)
- Inferior temporal gyrus (Figs. 3.26, 9a.32, 9b.23, 14a.14, 36a.19, 36b.13, 36d.13, 37a.16, 50a.8, 50b.9, 51a.17, 52a.32).

These temporal gyri cross the parallel lines of the Reid's base line at an acute angle (Fig. 46). They are separated by the superior and inferior temporal sulci. Lying in the lateral sulcus between the superior temporal gyrus and the posterior edge of the insula are the **transverse temporal gyri** (of Heschl). As a rule there are two transverse gyri on the right side and only one on the left side (139, 140). They run obliquely to the median plane from anterolaterally to posteromedially. They are more easily recognized in the coronal slices (Figs. 11a.18, 11b.13, 12a.10, 12a.11, 12a.14, 12b.14) and in the sagittal slices (Figs. 36a.11, 36a.12, 36b.8, 37a.11, 37a.12) than in the canthomeatal slices (Figs. 54a.32, 54d.21, 55a.21, 55b.15, 55d.15). In the coronal MR images, the transverse

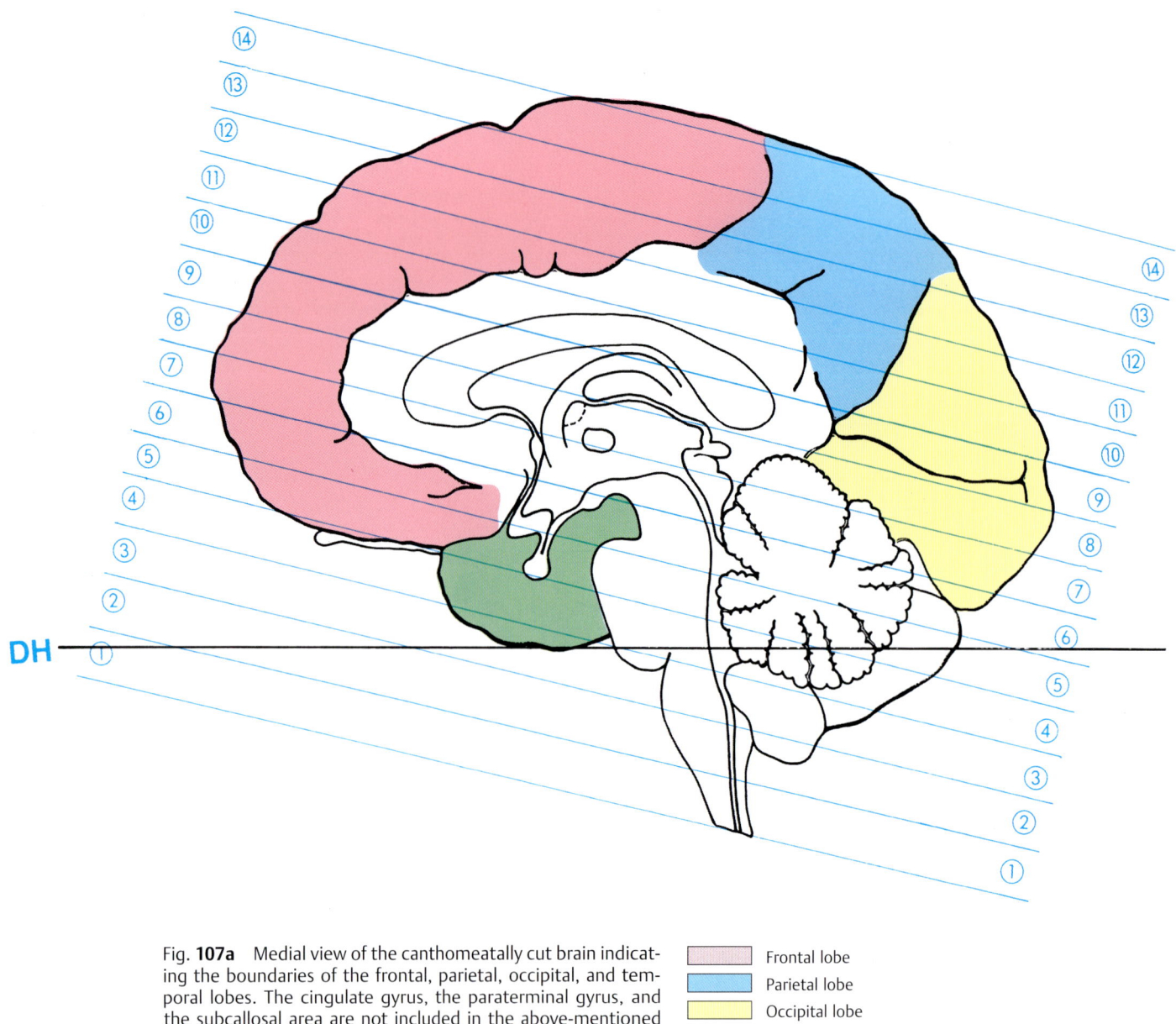

Fig. **107a** Medial view of the canthomeatally cut brain indicating the boundaries of the frontal, parietal, occipital, and temporal lobes. The cingulate gyrus, the paraterminal gyrus, and the subcallosal area are not included in the above-mentioned lobes (Chap. 8).
DH Reid's base line

- Frontal lobe
- Parietal lobe
- Occipital lobe
- Temporal lobe

temporal gyrus forms a protrusion in a superior direction. In the sagittal MR images, the transverse temporal gyrus can be recognized by its Omega form (Ω), also known as mushroom form. Sometimes the image takes on a heart form. In the axial layers the described oblique course taken by the transverse temporal gyrus from the median plane in an anterolateral direction is typical (508). The primary auditory cortex is located in the transverse temporal gyrus (of Heschl) or, if there are two transverse temporal gyri, to a large extent in the anterior transverse temporal gyrus. Posteriorly the transverse temporal gyrus adjoins the temporal plane (Fig. 37a.13), which is often larger on the left side than on the right (138, 140). This finding is thought to be related to the lateralization of language (140).

On the inferior side of the temporal lobe, the lateral and medial occipitotemporal gyri (mentioned above) border on the inferior temporal gyrus. Further medial lies the **parahippocampal gyrus** (Figs. 9a.29, 10a.36, 10b.23, 12a.26, 12b.21, 12d.21, 51a.15, 52a.27, 53a.37) with the uncus of the parahippocampal gyrus (Figs. 34a.17, 52a.25). These portions of the temporal lobe belong to the phylogenetically older divisions of the brain. Buried deep in the temporal lobe, the **hippocampus** (113) borders on the temporal horn of the lateral ventricle (Figs. 10a.30, 10b.22, 10d.22, 11a.31, 11b.18, 13a.15, 35a.22, 35b.9, 35d.9, 52a.24, 53a.36, 53b.24, 54a.37). Together with rudimentary cortical structures on the corpus callosum and a small convolution frontal to the corpus callosum, the hippocampus serves as the internal boundary of the **limbic system** (Chap. 6.11). The parahippocampal gyrus, the part of the cingulate gyrus near the corpus callosum (Figs. 2b.3, 6a.5, 6b.4, 9a.5, 9b.4, 13a.6, 32b.2, 32d.2, 33a.5, 45b.4, 53a.4, 55b.4, 56a.8, 56b.10, 147.1), and the subcallosal area (Figs. 52a.11, 147.6) surround the corpus callosum and form the external boundary of the limbic system. This outer ring of gyri courses at the medial side of the cerebral hemispheres and is

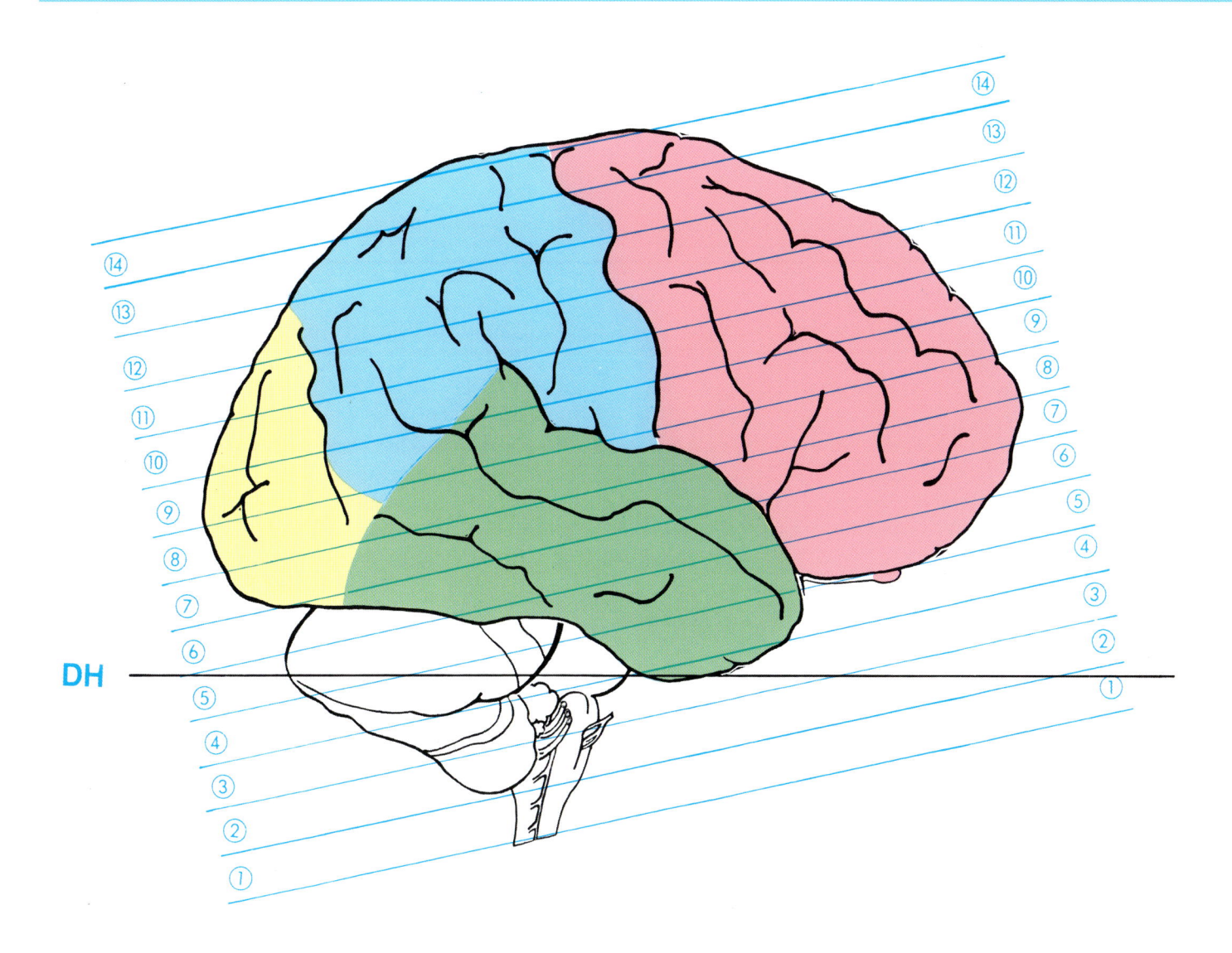

5.7 Subdivisions of the Brain

Fig. **107b** Lateral view of the canthomeatally cut brain indicating the boundaries of the frontal, parietal, occipital, and temporal lobes (Chap. 8).

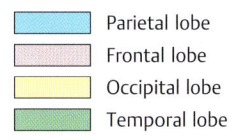

- Parietal lobe
- Frontal lobe
- Occipital lobe
- Temporal lobe

called the **limbic lobe**. It borders the other cerebral lobes (Figs. 104a, 107a).

Insula
The insula lies deep in the lateral sulcus (Figs. 8a.10, 9a.18, 9b.13, 10a.17, 36a.10, 36b.7, 52a.14, 53a.9, 53b.9, 53d.9, 54a.13, 55a.14, 55b.11). It is covered by the frontal, parietal, and temporal portions of the neencephalon. The corresponding gyri are referred to as the frontal, parietal, and temporal opercula. The insula contains visceral areas.

When observed from an inferior to superior direction, the parallel canthomeatal planes initially show the basal surface of the temporal lobe lying in the middle cranial fossa (Fig. 108a, third slice). In the fourth slice, one centimeter higher, the sectioning plane cuts through the recess in the anterior cranial fossa, the cribriform plate. The olfactory bulb and tract, as well as basal portions of the frontal lobe, are located in this recess. The cross-sectional areas of the frontal and temporal lobes increase in the fifth and sixth slices. At the level of the lateral ventricle, the occipital and parietal lobes appear. In the ninth slice, the frontal, parietal, temporal, and occipital lobes interdigitate. The temporal lobe does not extend into the supraventricular area. The two most superior slices contain parts of the frontal and parietal lobes only.

Organization of the Cerebral Cortex
The cerebral cortex is a 2 to 5 mm thick layer of gray matter averaging 600 ml in males and 540 ml in females. This sex-based volume difference is statistically significant.

On the basis of phylogenetic and ontogenetic studies of the development of the telencephalon, the cerebral cortex can be divided into:
- Paleocortex
- Archicortex
- Neocortex.

318 5 Topography of the Neurocranium and its Intracranial Spaces and Structures in Multiplanar Parallel Slices

- Cortex of temporal lobe
- Cortex of frontal lobe
- Cortex of occipital lobe

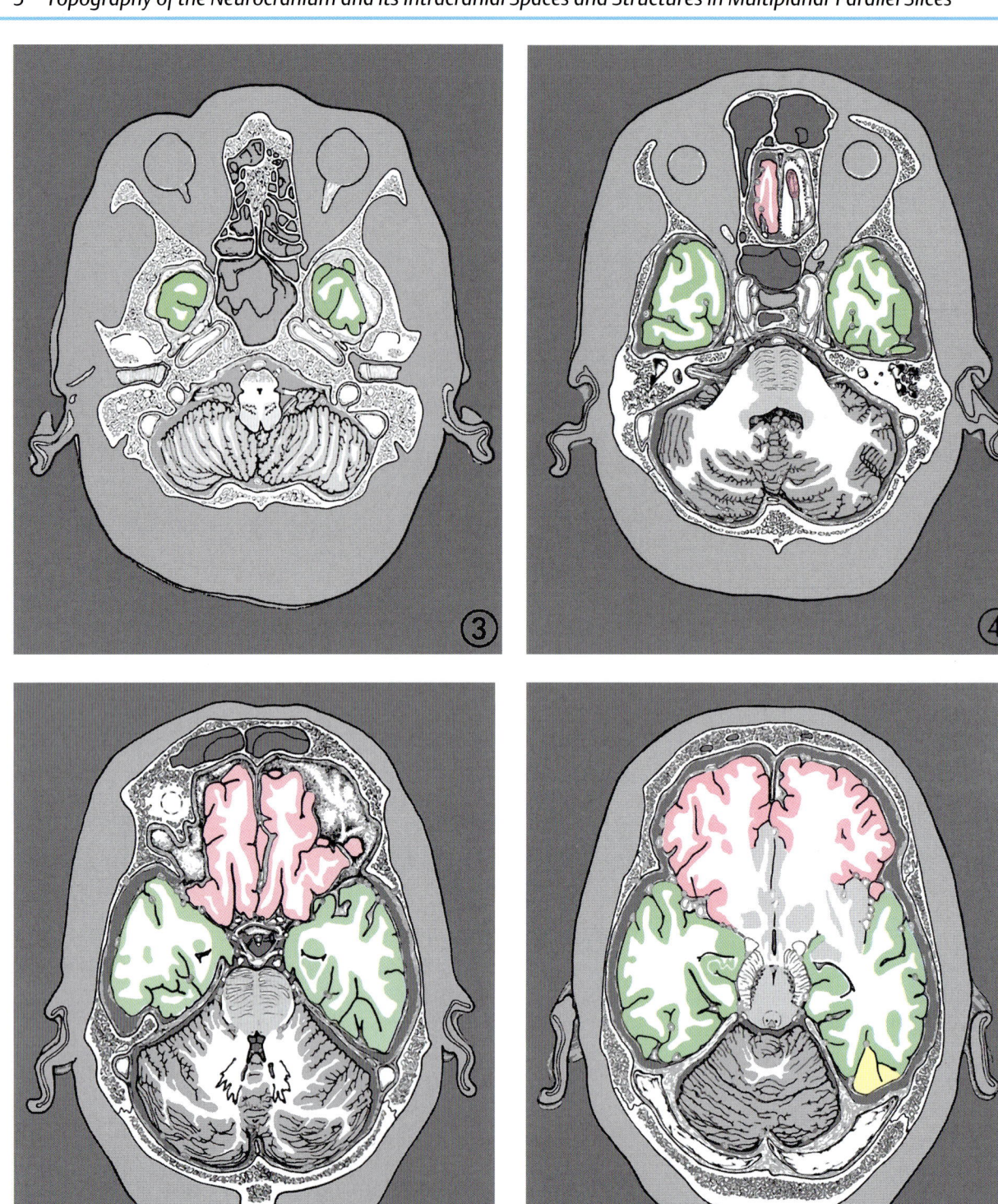

Fig. **108a** Canthomeatally oriented serial illustrations of the cortices of the frontal, parietal, occipital, and temporal lobes. The cortices of the insula, cingulate gyrus, subcallosal area, and paraterminal gyrus are only shaded in gray. The encircled numbers (3–10) indicate the number of the respective slice (Figs. 44, 45a,b, 46).

5.7 Subdivisions of the Brain

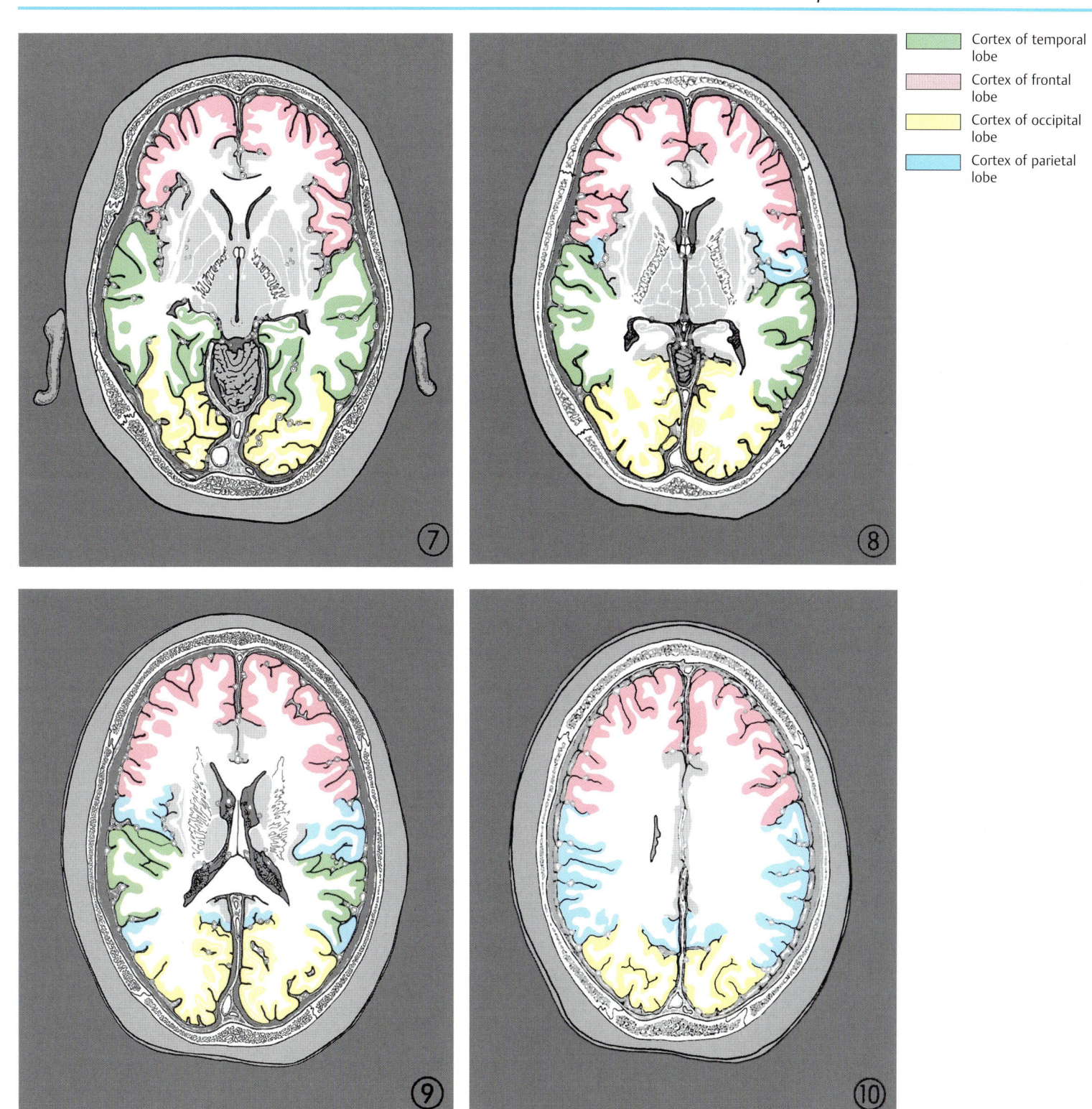

	Cortex of temporal lobe
	Cortex of frontal lobe
	Cortex of occipital lobe
	Cortex of parietal lobe

Cortex of frontal lobe
Cortex of occipital lobe
Cortex of parietal lobe

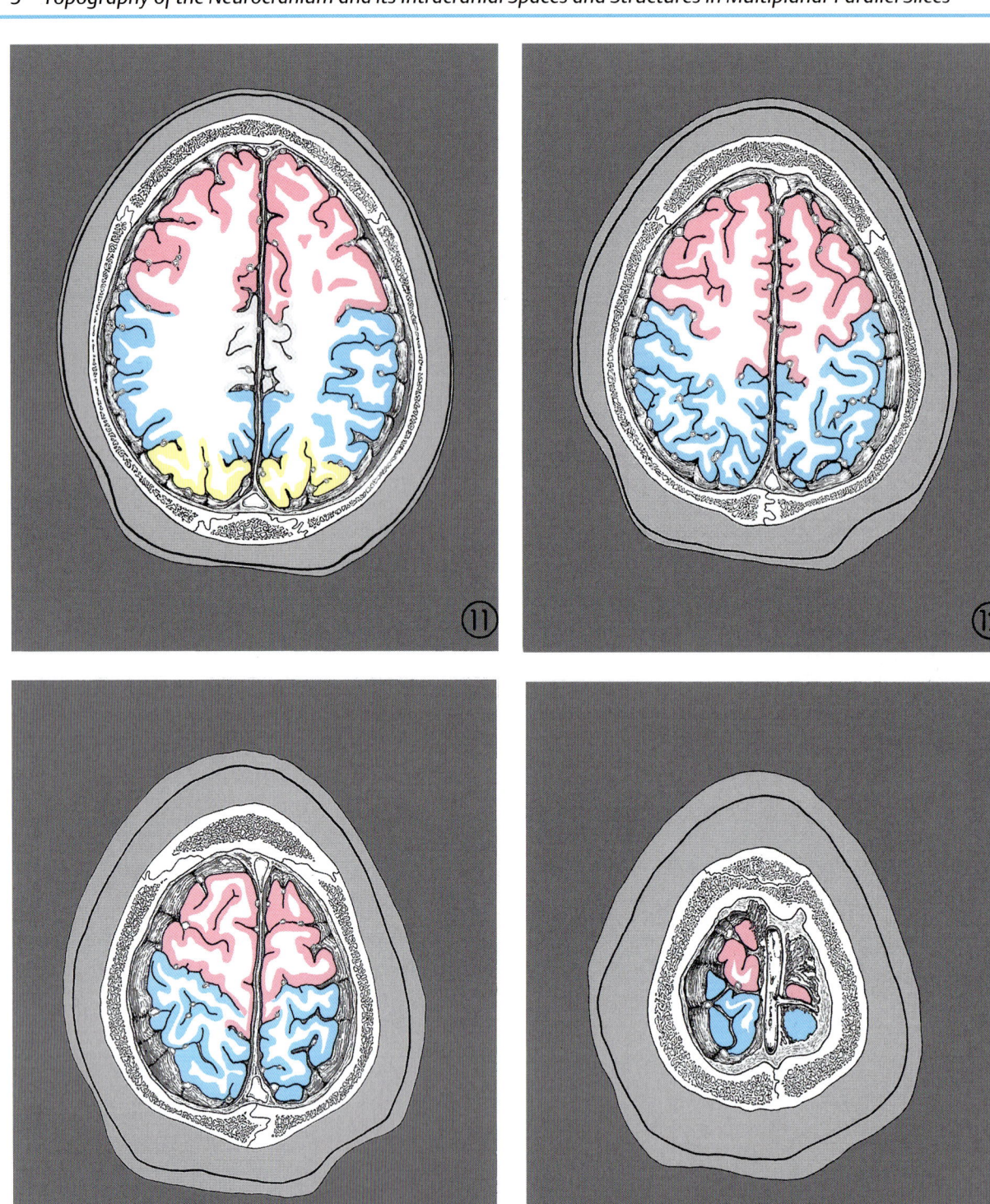

Fig. **108a** Canthomeatally oriented serial illustrations of the cortices of the frontal, parietal, occipital, and temporal lobes. The cortices of the insula, cingulate gyrus, subcallosal area, and paraterminal gyrus only are shaded in gray. The encircled numbers (11–14) indicate the number of the respective slice (Figs. 44, 45a,b, 46).

5.7 Subdivisions of the Brain   321

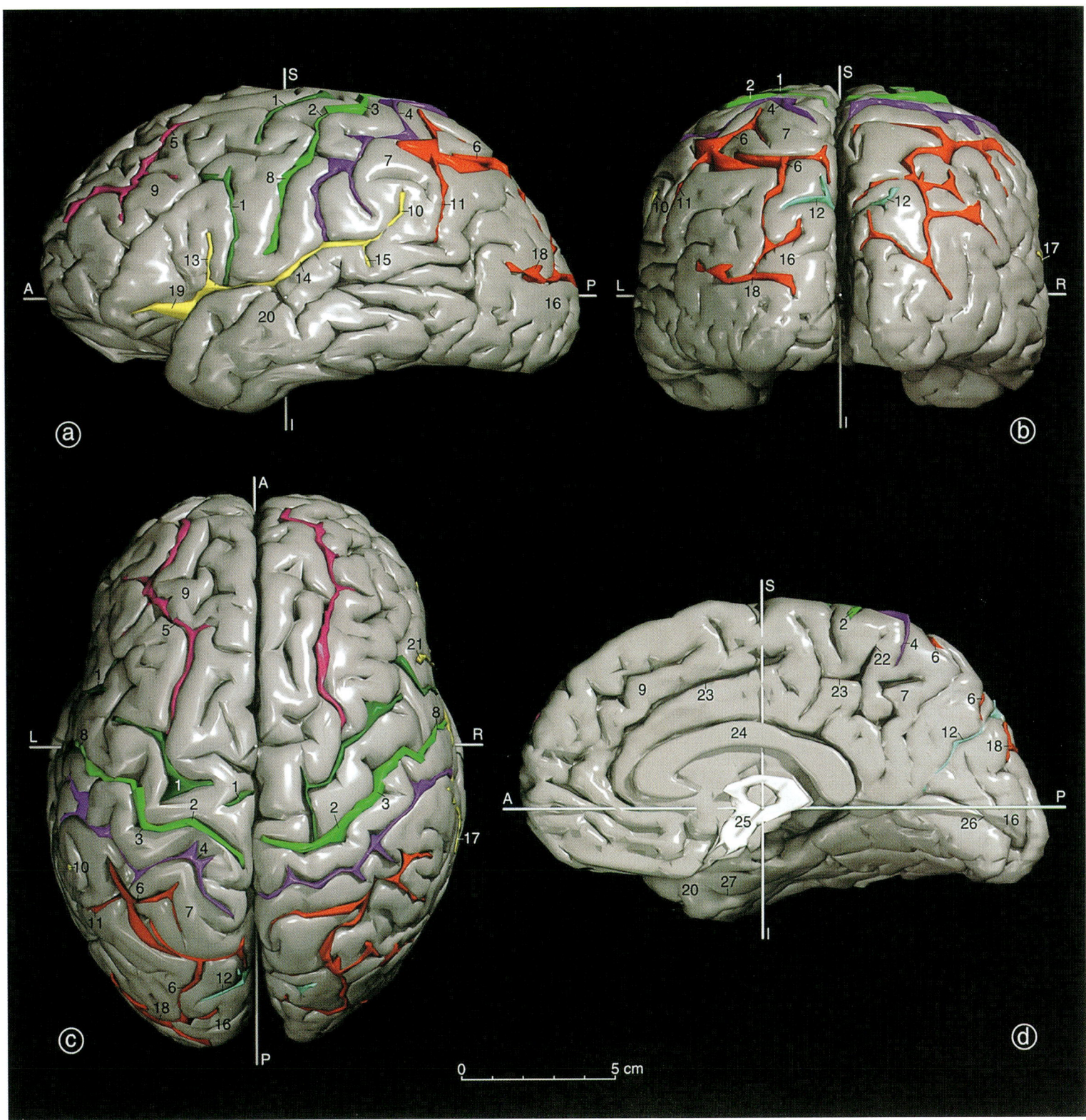

Fig. **108b** Computer-generated images of seven sulci with a nontransparent representation of the brain within the bicommissural coordinate system. According to (243, 244).

ⓐ Lateral view of the left cerebral hemisphere
ⓑ Posterior view
ⓒ Superior view
ⓓ Medial view of the right cerebral hemisphere

1 Precentral sulcus ⓐⓑⓒ
2 Central sulcus
3 Superior genu of central sulcus ⓐⓒ
4 Postcentral sulcus
5 Superior frontal sulcus ⓐⓒ
6 Intraparietal sulcus
7 Parietal lobe
8 Inferior genu of central sulcus ⓐⓒ
9 Frontal lobe ⓐⓒⓓ
10 Posterior ascending ramus of lateral sulcus ⓐⓑⓒ
11 Primary intermediate sulcus ⓐⓑⓒ
12 Parieto-occipital sulcus ⓑⓒⓓ
13 Ascending ramus of lateral sulcus ⓐ
14 Posterior ramus of lateral sulcus ⓐ
15 Posterior descending ramus of lateral sulcus ⓐ
16 Occipital lobe
17 Lateral sulcus (Sylvian fissure) ⓑⓒ
18 Transverse occipital sulcus
19 Anterior ramus of lateral sulcus ⓐ
20 Temporal lobe ⓐⓓ
21 Diagonal sulcus ⓒ
22 Marginal branch of cingulate sulcus ⓓ
23 Cingulate sulcus ⓓ
24 Corpus callosum ⓓ
25 Third ventricle ⓓ
26 Calcarine sulcus ⓓ
27 Rhinal sulcus ⓓ

A ANTERIOR
P POSTERIOR
R RIGHT
L LEFT
S SUPERIOR
I INFERIOR

The **paleocortex** is a phylogenetically old part of the cerebral cortex, the olfactory cortex. It was shifted to the mediobasal side of the temporal lobe through the great development of the neocortex. The paleocortex can be found if the lateral bundle of the olfactory tract (lateral olfactory stria) is followed to the medial surface of the temporal lobe. Here there are two small bulging areas about the size of a millet seed. They are covered by the prepiriform cortex and periamygdaloid cortex, which belong to the paleocortex and to the olfactory system (Chap. 6.7).

The **archicortex** also consists of a phylogenetically old cerebral cortex that was located originally on the medial side of the hemisphere. Through the marked development of the neocortex the greater part of the archicortex, such as the dentate gyrus, hippocampus, and subiculum, was forced into the interior of the temporal lobe.

More than 90% of the human cerebral cortex is **neocortex**. During the process of phylogenesis it extended almost completely over the surface of the telencephalon and hence covered phylogenetically older neocortical areas such as the insula.

As a result of cytoarchitectonic, myeloarchitectonic, glioarchitectonic, angioarchitectonic, chemoarchitectonic, and pigmentarchitectonic investigations, the cerebral cortex can be divided into:
- Isocortex
- Allocortex
- Mesocortex.

The isocortical area of the cerebral cortex is organized principally in six layers of cells. The isocortex corresponds largely to the neocortex (439).

The allocortex consists mostly of three or four layers. The paleocortex and archicortex are parts of the allocortex.

The mesocortex is a transitional cortex that developed between the isocortex and the allocortex during their evolution. The structure of the mesocortex stands between the typical six-layered isocortex and the three- or four-layered allocortex.

The mesocortex consists of:
- Peripaleocortex
- Periarchicortex

(these are grouped together as Periallocortex)
- Proisocortex.

The peripaleocortex is very small in the human and surrounds the paleocortex. The periarchicortex surrounds the corpus callosum like a bow and consists of the following parts: paraterminal gyrus, the part of the cingulate gyrus close to the corpus callosum, fasciolar gyrus, and the entorhinal cortex. These regions belong to the limbic system (Chap. 6.11).

The proisocortex lies on the edge of the isocortex and developed during evolution at the border between the isocortex and periallocortex.

Information gained from morphologic, physiologic, and clinical investigations indicates the following division of the **isocortex**:
- Primary cortical areas
- Association areas
- Supplementary areas.

The **primary cortical areas** have afferent and efferent topical connections with the periphery. Basically, these are marked by point-to-point connections between the periphery and the cortex or vice versa. The anterolateral, medial lemniscus, and trigeminal systems project into the postcentral gyrus, into Brodmann's areas 3, 1, 2 (Figs. 3.3, 11a.7, 13a.5, 31.12, 33a.2, 34a.3, 37a.4, 55a.15, 59a.5). These cytoarchitectonic areas form three vertical bands arranged 3, 1, 2 from frontal to occipital in the postcentral gyrus. Their somatotopic organization is described in sensory systems (Chap. 6.1). The primary cortical area of the gustatory system is located in the parietal operculum and in an area on the edge of the insula (Chap. 6.2). The vestibular system has connections with parietal cortical areas around the intraparietal sulcus and insular cortex. The primary cortical area of the auditory system is about 1.5 cm in diameter. It is located deep in the lateral sulcus in the anterior transverse temporal gyrus (of Heschl) in the temporal lobe (Figs. 12a.11, 36a.11, 37a.11). Cytoarchitectonically this area corresponds to Brodmann's area 41. The primary visual cortical areas of both hemispheres have a volume of 12 ml. They can be recognized macroscopically by occipital stripe (stria of Gennari) located in the occipital lobe in the upper and lower lips of the calcarine sulcus (Figs. 54a.44, 126.17, 127.10, 127.9, 128.4, 128.5). There is a precise point-to-point projection from the photoreceptors of the retina to the ocular dominance columns of the primary visual cortex (Chap. 6.6).

The primary motor area or motor cortex is located in the frontal lobe and, for the most part, in and around the precentral gyrus (Figs. 3.10, 10a.5, 14a.1, 31.10, 33a.1, 34a.2, 54a.11, 59a.3). This location corresponds cytoarchitectonically to Brodmann's area 4. The premotor cortex comprises the area 6. It is six times larger than the primary motor cortex. Additional motor neurons arise from Brodmann's sensory areas 3, 1, 2 and their neighboring parietal area 5 (102, 270). The somatotopic pattern of the motor cortex is described in Chapter 6.8.1 (pyramidal system).

During evolution of the neocortex, the cortical **association areas** developed between the primary areas in a mosaic pattern. This development is especially evident in primate brains. The association cortex is connected with other cortical areas or subcortical nuclei but not with motor neurons or sensory receptors in point-to-point relation. The cortical association areas have predominantly gnostic functions. Included among the association areas are the Broca's area located in the opercular and triangular parts of the inferior frontal gyrus and Wernicke's area located in the superior temporal gyrus (374a) (Chap. 6.10).

The **supplementary areas** lie at the border between the primary cortex and phylogenetically older regions of the brain:
- The supplementary somatic sensory area (SII) lies on the medial surface of the parietal operculum between the primary somatosensory cortex and insula (400).
- The supplementary auditory area is located between the primary auditory cortex and insula.
- The supplementary visual area lies on the medial surface of the hemisphere between the visual cortex and periarchicortex (400).
- The supplementary motor area is a part of Brodmann's area 6 and extends onto the medial surface of each hemisphere between Brodmann's area 4 and the paralimbic transitional cortex of the isocortex or proisocortex (46, 356).

The topical arrangement of the supplementary areas with the periphery is less developed than that of the primary areas. Nevertheless, a supplementary area can partially compensate the loss of the corresponding primary area.

White Matter

The white matter underlying the cerebral cortex is formed by the many fibers of the various pathways that connect the cortical areas with each other or with other regions of the central nervous system (CNS). These connecting pathways include:
- Association fibers
- Commissural fibers
- Projection fibers.

The **association** (intrahemispheric) **fibers** are short or long axons that interconnect the cortical areas of one cerebral hemisphere. The short arcuate fibers lie directly beneath the cerebral cortex and appear as small connecting arches between adjacent gyri. The long association fibers interconnect the gyri of the individual cerebral lobes. The cingulum (Figs. 56a.9, 56b.11, 147.2) is a fiber bundle located in the white matter of the cingulate gyrus. It arches around the corpus callosum from the frontal lobe to the temporal lobe and belongs to the Papez circuit (Chap. 6.11).

The **commissural** (interhemispheric) **fibers** interconnect the corresponding cortical areas of the two hemispheres. The **anterior commissure** lies within the seventh section of the canthomeatal series and is seen in the median view of the brain (Fig. 45b.14). It connects the paleocortex (olfactory cortex) of one hemisphere with its counterpart in the contralateral hemisphere (Chap. 6.7). In addition, the anterior commissure contains fibers that connect small neocortical areas of the frontal and temporal lobes with their counterparts. The **corpus callosum** is a large transverse connection between both sides of the neocortex. The divisions of the corpus callosum, the genu, trunk, and splenium, are depicted from frontal to occipital in the median view of the brain (Figs. 32a.3, 32a.6, 32b.5, 32b.8, 45b.5, 45b.8, 45b.11).

The parallel canthomeatal illustrations show the genu of the corpus callosum (Figs. 53a.6, 53d.5), a portion of the trunk (Fig. 55a.8), and the splenium (Figs. 55a.23, 55b.17). Two groups of U-shaped fibers emerge from the corpus. The minor (frontal) forceps (Fig. 55a.6) passes from the genu into the frontal lobes. The major (occipital) forceps (Fig. 55a.24) extends from the splenium into the occipital and temporal lobes.

The posterior commissure (Figs. 2b.18, 12a.17, 32a.11, 32b.15, 45b.18) is not a commissural fiber bundle of the telencephalon. It connects nuclear areas in the tegmentum of the midbrain.

The **projection fibers** form afferent and efferent connections between the cerebral cortex and subcortical centers of the brain and spinal cord. The projection fibers of the telencephalon include the terminal fibers of the sensory (Chap. 6.1), gustatory (Chap. 6.2), vestibular (Chap. 6.4), auditory (Chap. 6.5), visual (Chap. 6.6), and olfactory (Chap. 6.7) systems. They also include the initial parts of pyramidal and oculomotor pathways (Chap. 6.8). The limbic system has many synaptic contacts via projection fibers with the diencephalon (Chap. 6.11).

During evolution, the **neencephalic projection fibers** formed a crown of radiating fibers called the corona radiata (Fig. 55a.16). These projection fibers form the internal capsule. Lying in the diencephalic–telencephalic area, the internal capsule appears in the parallel canthomeatal planes as a fan-shaped band of fibers bent outward to form two limbs. The tip of the obtuse angle between these two limbs points in a medial direction. The **internal capsule** forms the medial border of the lentiform nucleus, a collective term for the globus pallidus and putamen. The internal capsule can be divided into an anterior limb, a genu, and a posterior limb. The anterior limb lies between the head of the caudate nucleus and the lentiform nucleus. The genu of the internal capsule lies between the anterior and posterior limbs at the level of the interventricular foramen of Monro. The posterior limb is located between the thalamus and the lentiform nucleus (Figs. 53a.19, 54a.20, 54d.20). The efferent projection fibers lie in the posterior limb of the internal capsule. The acoustic and visual radiations run from the metathalamus behind the internal capsule to the primary auditory and primary visual cortex (Chaps. 6.5 and 6.6). The projection fibers from the thalamus branch off in fan-shaped bundles that extend into the anterior and posterior limbs. A small number of the projection fibers form the **external capsule** (Figs. 53a.12, 54a.16), which is located between the putamen and claustrum. The fibers from the internal and external capsules converge in the cerebral crus of the midbrain (Figs. 52a.28, 77a.14, 77c.10, 78b.9, 78c.8). **Projection fibers of the hippocampal formation** extend via the fimbria of the hippocampus and the fornix mainly to the hypothalamus (Figs. 13a.13, 12a.12, 11a.12, 10a.25, 10b.10, 32b.7, 55a.19, 55b.12, 55d.12, 54a.21, 53a.21). The semioval center is the white matter of the telencephalon above the corpus callosum (Figs. 56a.14, 56d.12, 57a.8, 57b.11, 58a.7). In cross-sectional images, the white matter of one hemisphere above the corpus callosum appears semioval in shape. This semioval center consists of association, commissural, and projection fibers.

> *Clinical Notes*
>
> Depending on their relationship to neurofunctional systems in the individual lobes, telencephalic lesions will cause characteristic clinical symptoms enabling a preliminary topical diagnosis.
>
> A lesion in the motor cortex of the **frontal lobe** may take the form of a patterned convulsion (Jacksonian motor seizure) that begins, at least initially, with a tonic contraction of the fingers of one hand, one side of the face, or one foot, and spreads to other muscles on the same side of the body. An acute lesion of the primary motor cortex in the posterior part of the frontal lobe produces a contralateral flaccid hemiplegia with a positive Babinski sign without spasticity. Only later may the reflexes be accentuated. Fine voluntary movements involving the distal muscles of the extremities will remain impaired. Lesions of the premotor cortex lead to a slowing of movements. Widespread injuries cause apraxia. Defects in the opercular and triangular parts of the inferior frontal gyrus of the language-dominant hemisphere lead to Broca's aphasia. Injuries involving the middle region of the precentral sulcus may result in paralysis of the conjugate movement of the eyes; generally, the gaze will drift toward the side of the focus. Extensive lesions of the frontal lobe cause an organic psychosyndrome with lack of initiative, psychomotoric retardation, and emotional impairment. Frequently a dysbasia is also seen. The close topographic relation of the frontal lobe and the olfactory bulb and tract explains the appearance of anosmia following pathologic changes in the area of the anterior cranial fossa.
>
> Lesions in the postcentral gyrus of the **parietal lobe** lead to contralateral disturbances of peripheral sensitivity and spatial orientation. The perception of vibration and pain is seldom impaired. Abnormal stimulation of the parietal lobe may result in a sensory Jacksonian seizure. Characteristic symptoms for a parietal lobe syndrome are altered spatial and body orientation usually affecting the contralateral side, though very seldom this may occur bilaterally. In such cases, patients often forget activities such as putting a sock on the contralateral foot (dressing apraxia). Adolescents may develop muscle atrophy and skeletal hemiatrophy. An injury of the lower part of the parietal cortex in the hemisphere dominant for language causes alexia (127).
>
> Lesions of the **occipital lobe** that affect the optic radiation and/or the visual cortex are characterized by impairments of the corresponding portions of the contralateral visual field (homonymous hemianopia). Lesion of the occipital lobe may cause photopsy. Visual hallucinations arise with transient ischemia of the occipital pole and are frequently observed in connection with migraines (352). A complete bilateral loss of the primary visual cortex leads to cortical blindness.
>
> Pathologic changes in the **temporal lobe** can cause a wide variety of symptoms. Bilateral lesions of the transverse temporal gyri (of Heschl) cause cortical deafness. Unilateral lesions, however, may remain clinically unnoticed. Pathology in the superior temporal gyrus leads to Wernicke's aphasia. Bilateral lesions of the hippocampal formation lead to memory and learning impairments or even to a severe amnestic syndrome. Injuries to the posterior region of the temporal lobe may cause homonymous hemianopia or superior quadrantanopia. Pathologic lesions or foci of scars are frequently manifested by epileptic attacks (psychomotor epilepsy).
>
> The commissural fibers of the **corpus callosum** transmit information from one hemisphere to the other. Interruption of the corpus callosum leads to an "interhemispheric disconnection effect." Lesions of the anterior portion of the corpus callosum produce a unilateral apraxia. Furthermore, tumors in this region may cause the patient to become apathetic. A severe loss of drive may result in mutism. Interruption of the splenium of the corpus callosum causes impairment of the patient's verbal articulation of experiences perceived in reading material in the right half of the visual field, but material in the left half would be meaningless.

6 Neurofunctional Systems

The broad term neurofunctional system signifies a group of neurons that share a common pathway and transmit a specific afferent or efferent signal. Familiar neurofunctional systems are those serving visual, auditory, and voluntary motor functions. In this book descriptions are restricted to those systems that may easily be tested clinically and are known to be of diagnostic significance. A satisfactory description of these pathways must collate findings from the realms of neuroanatomy, neurophysiology, neuropathology, clinical neurology, neuroradiology, neurosurgery, psychiatry, and psychology, as well as from animal experiments and ontogenetic investigations.

In the prenatal period, the neurofunctional systems are not fully developed. It is also true that populations of embryonic nerve cells possess **plasticity**. The younger the brain, the greater the potential for compensation in the case of a lesion. For example, if a cerebellum fails to form for genetic or environmental reasons (agenesis), a different neuron population may almost totally take over the cerebellar function. Cases of inborn cerebellar hypoplasia have been described, yet no cerebellar symptoms were observed during the entire lifetime. Similar observations have been made in cases of inborn aplasia of the corpus callosum (469). Even infant brains can compensate for neurofunctional deficiencies much better than adult brains. A possible explanation for this compensation, especially in young individuals, could be the formation of new synapses among another group of neurons. It has been shown in mammals that more nerve cells are formed prenatally and develop perinatally than actually function in later life. The role of stem cells for the reorganization in both the infant and the adult brain is of great interest at present for neuroscience (374a, 435). Not all prenatal and perinatal lesions can be compensated for and, as a result, some perinatal lesions may cause serious functional disorders. Blindness resulting from a bilateral occipital cortex defect is one example. Our knowledge about localization of specific functions in neuron populations of the brain is mainly based on neurologic findings in children of school age and in adults.

The **positions of the neurofunctional systems** are presented in the serial illustrations of the slices, which are depicted in the atlas in Figures 4–17 (coronal series), 32–37 (sagittal series), 47–60 (canthomeatal series), and 69–78 (brainstem series).

The difficulties inherent in transferring neuroanatomic findings from the cadaver to the corresponding in vivo situation are reviewed critically in Chapter 1.3. This problem must be taken into consideration in the analysis of the neurofunctional systems. Only a few investigations concerning the individual variability of the neurofunctional systems have been published to date (65, 146, 249, 417, 479).

In spite of these limitations, hemianopia, ataxia, aphasia, and many other neurologic syndromes are diagnosed daily in clinical practice and are correlated with the probable site of the lesion. Our illustrations of the main neurofunctional pathways in the parallel coronal, sagittal, and axial planes should serve as an aid to diagnosis. We are convinced that the present knowledge of human neurofunctional pathways can be expanded by a scientific evaluation of the correlations observed between clinical, CT, MRI, fMRI, MEG, and PET findings (101, 131, 198, 311, 374a, 403, 440, 465).

6.1 General Sensory Systems

6.1.1 Anterolateral System
(Figs. 109, 110)

The anterolateral system receives its input from nociceptors (pain), thermoreceptors (heat, cold), and mechanoreceptors located in the legs, trunk, arms, and neck. The cell bodies of the first-order neurons are located in the **spinal ganglia** and their central axons terminate in the marginal cells and cells of the nucleus proprius of the dorsal gray horn of the spinal cord. From there, the second-order neurons extend cranially as the anterior and lateral spinothalamic tracts and as the spinoreticular tract. The spinothalamic tracts cross in the white commissure of the spinal cord and ascend contralaterally in the anterolateral funiculus.

The spinoreticular tract extends (partly ipsilaterally) as a polysynaptic pathway to the medial reticular nucleus of the brainstem and from there to the **intralaminar nuclei of the thalamus**. These thalamic neurons project widely throughout the cerebral cortex, notably into cortical areas of the cingulate gyrus and the prefrontal cortex.

The anterior and lateral spinothalamic tracts extend alongside the reticular formation in the medulla oblongata and pons. In the pons–midbrain region they join the medial lemniscus. Here a lesion involving only one pathway is unlikely. The spinothalamic tracts terminate in the **ventral posterolateral nucleus** of the thalamus. From there the axons of the third-order neurons extend as thalamoparietal fibers through the posterior limb of the internal capsule to the postcentral gyrus. Located in the **postcentral gyrus** is the somatic sensory projection field (Brodmann's areas 3, 1, 2). These somatic sensory cortical areas are organized somatotopically. The projection field for the contralateral leg is localized in a triangular region within the paracentral lobule on the medial surface of the hemisphere. On the convex brain curvature, the areas for the trunk, arm, and neck of the opposite side extend in the upper two-thirds of the postcentral gyrus between the superior margin and the lateral sulcus (Fig. 109.1). The axons of the third-order neurons also reach the supplementary somatic sensory area (SII) for pain located in the parietal operculum near the insula (Fig. 109.2). The pain is consciously localized in the primary and supplementary areas. Perception of location and intensity of pain depends upon the primary and supplementary areas. Perception of the aversive (repellent) quality of pain depends upon activity in the medial (spinoreticular) pathway terminating in the cingulate gyrus. Interruption of the spinothalamic tract results in pain and temperature perception disorders (221, 374a, 471b).

6.1.1 Anterolateral System   327

1 Postcentral gyrus
2 Parietal operculum near insula
3 Thalamoparietal fibers
4 Intralaminar nuclei of thalamus
5 Ventral posterolateral nucleus of thalamus
6 Medial reticular nucleus
7 Anterior and lateral spinothalamic tracts
8 Spinoreticular tract
9 Posterior (dorsal) root of spinal nerve
10 Spinal ganglion
11 White commissure of spinal cord

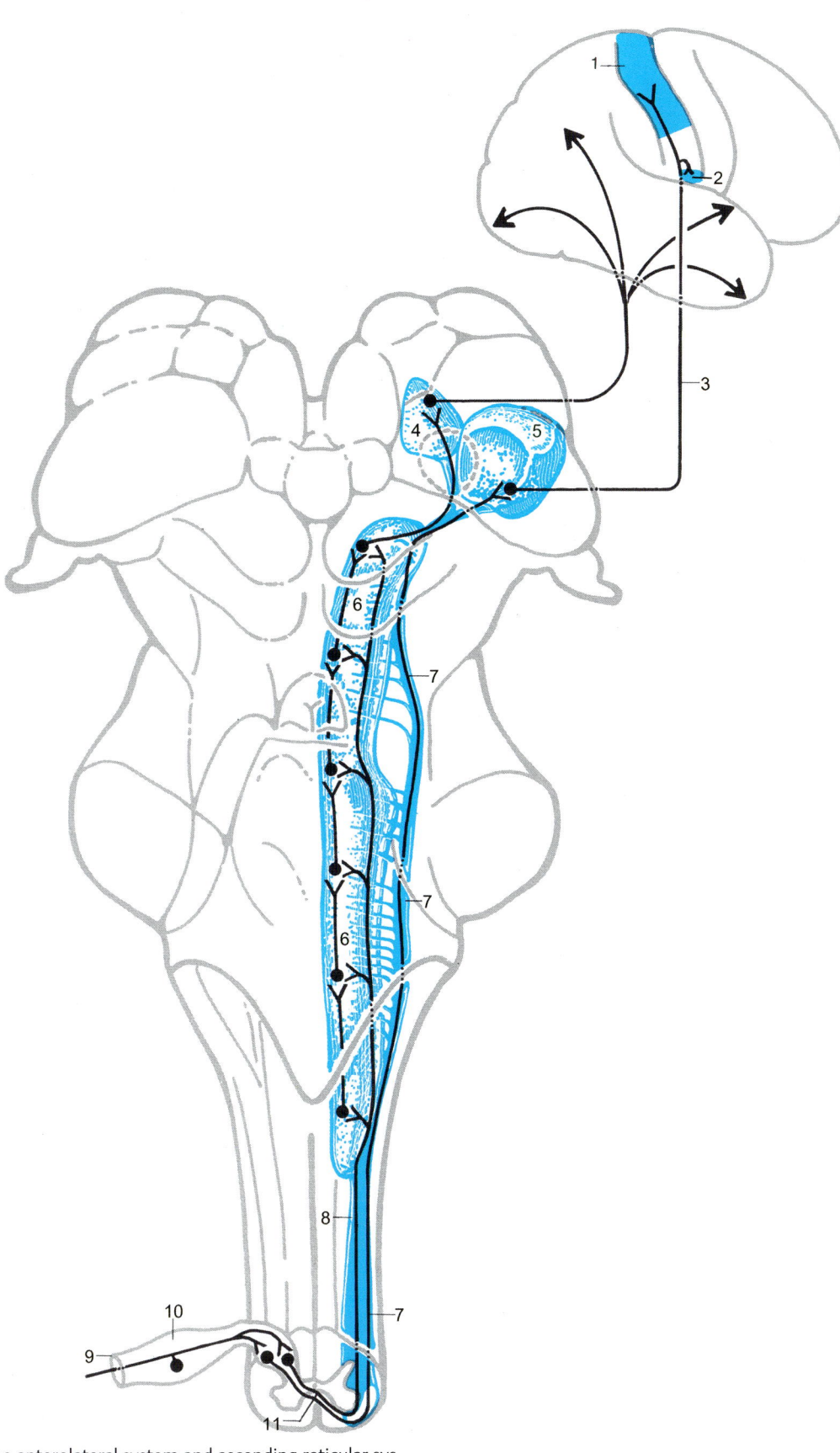

Fig. **109** The anterolateral system and ascending reticular system in the spinal cord, medulla oblongata, pons, midbrain, and diencephalon as seen from a posterior aspect, and in the cerebrum as seen from a lateral aspect. According to (332).

328 6 Neurofunctional Systems

1 Anterior and lateral spinothalamic tracts

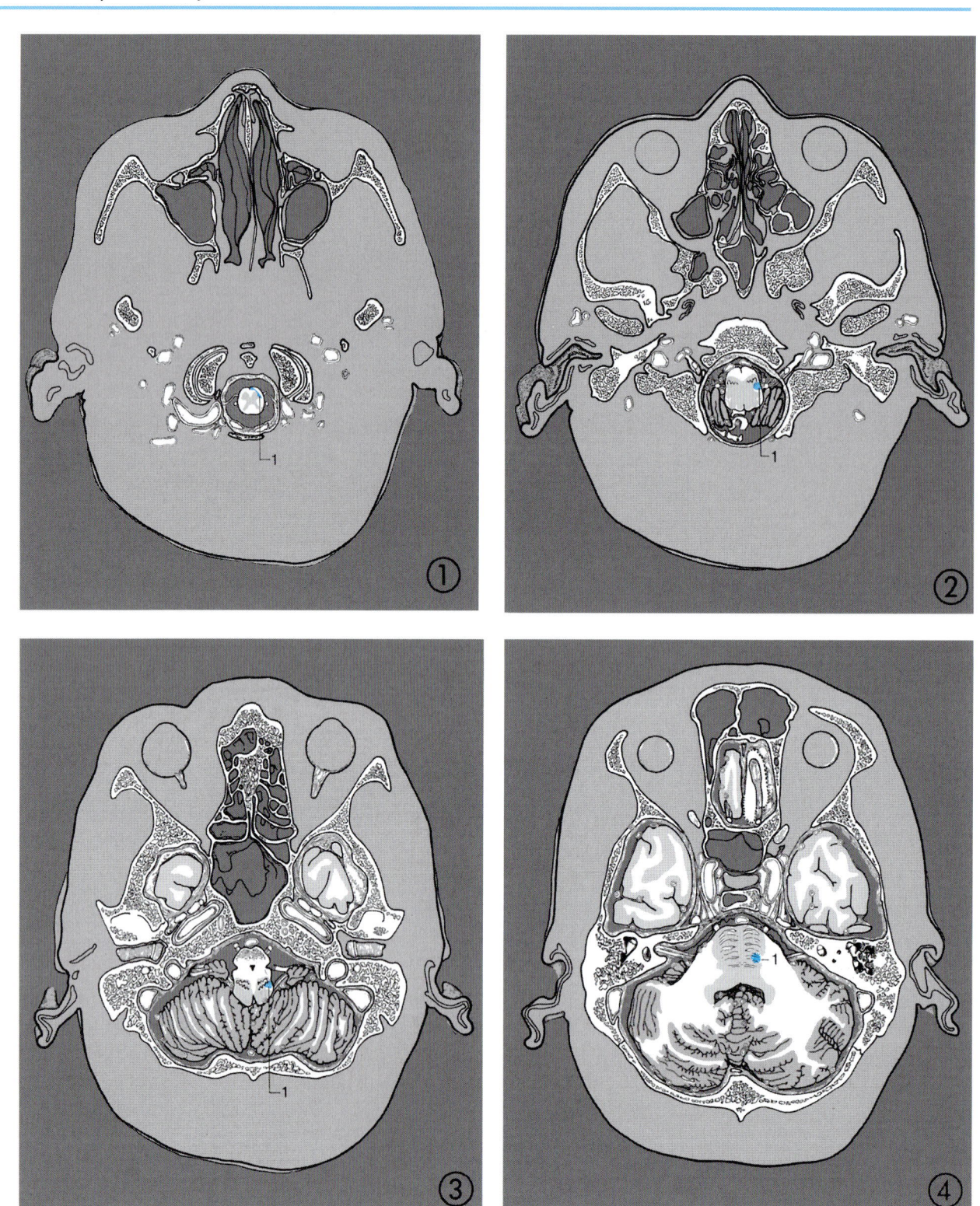

Fig. 110 Canthomeatally oriented serial illustrations of the anterolateral system. The encircled numbers (1–8) indicate the number of the respective slice (Figs. 44, 45a,b, 46).

6.1.1 *Anterolateral System*

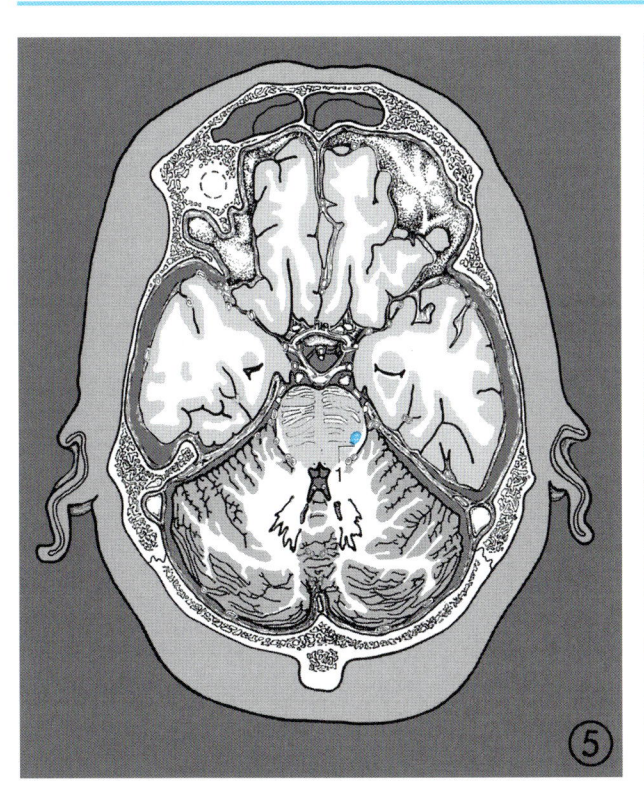

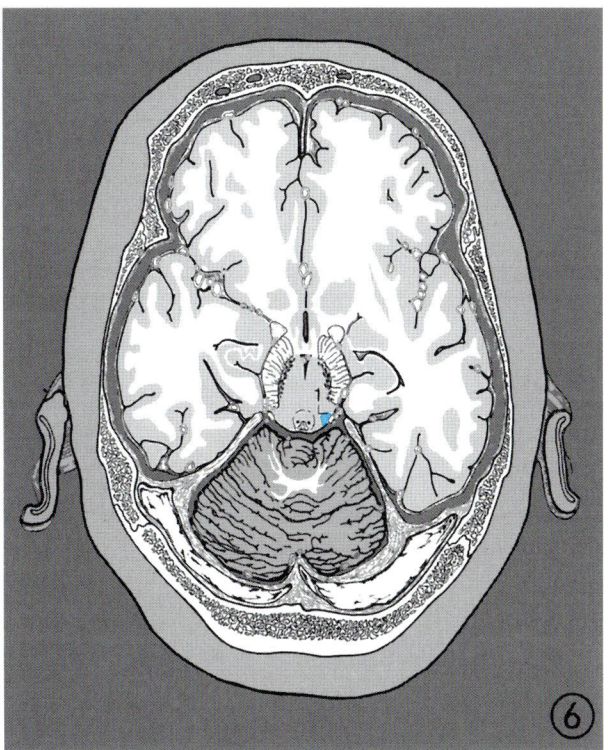

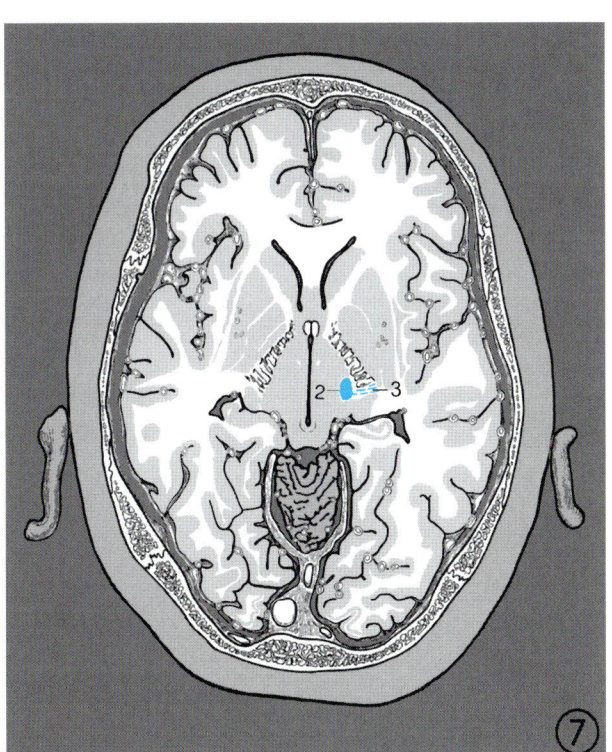

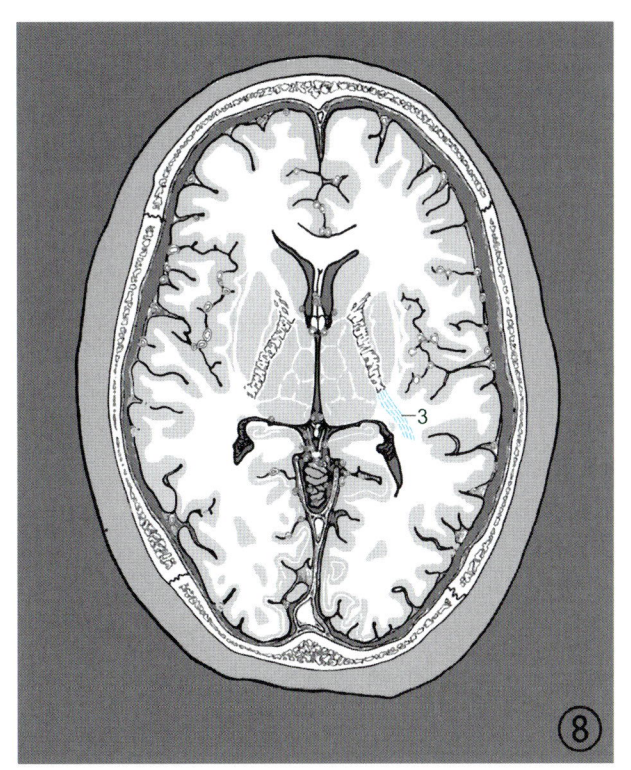

1 Anterior and lateral spinothalamic tracts
2 Ventral posterolateral nucleus of thalamus
3 Thalamoparietal fibers

330   6 Neurofunctional Systems

3 Thalamoparietal fibers
4 Postcentral gyrus

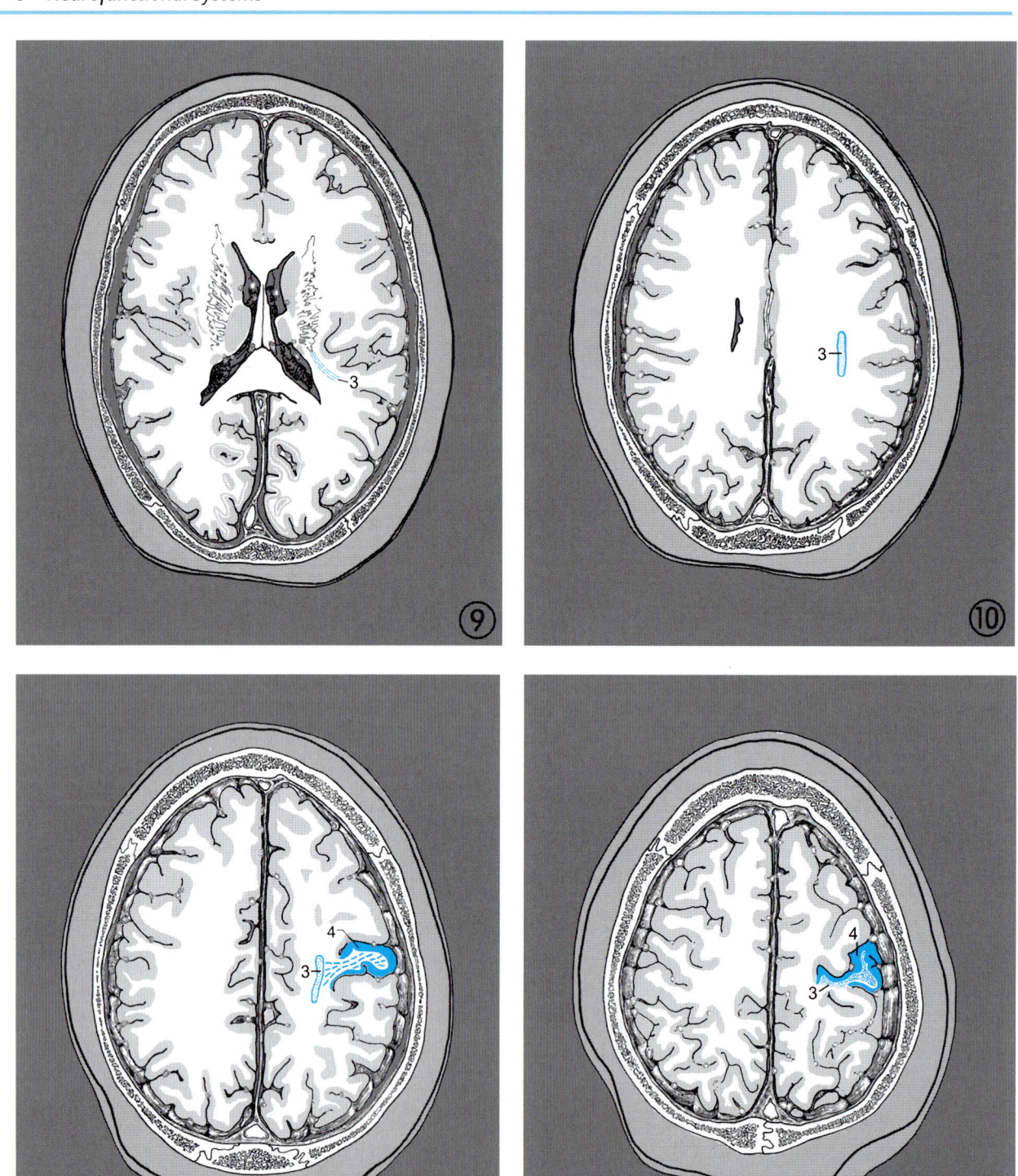

Fig. 110 Canthomeatally oriented serial illustrations of the anterolateral system. The encircled numbers (9–14) indicate the number of the respective slice (Figs. 44, 45a,b, 46).

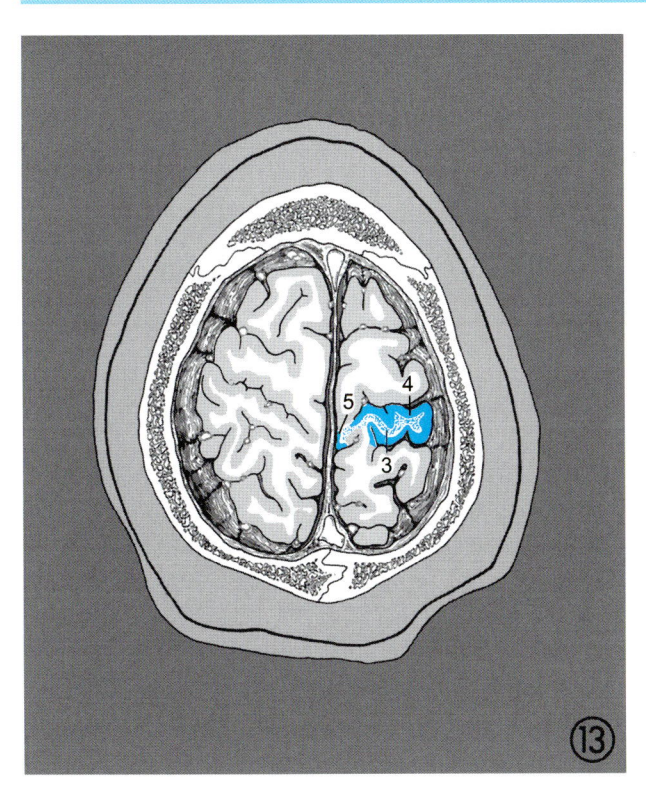

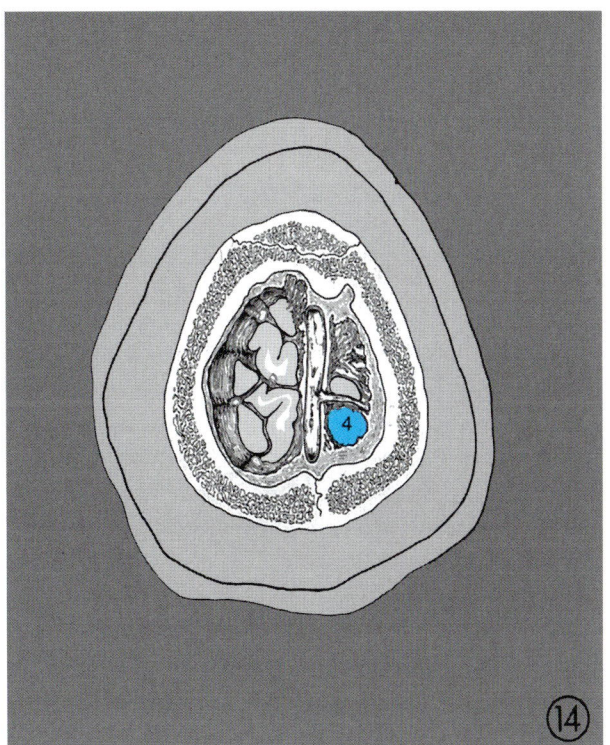

3 Thalamoparietal fibers
4 Postcentral gyrus
5 Primary somatic sensory cortex in paracentral lobule

6.1.2 Medial Lemniscus System
(Figs. 111–113)

The receptors of the medial lemniscus system (dorsal column–lemniscal pathway) are the mechanoreceptors in the skin, muscle spindles, tendon organs and the remaining stimulus transducers in the legs, trunk, arms, and neck. The cell bodies of the first-order neurons are located in the **spinal ganglia.** The axons of the unipolar nerve cells enter the posterior funiculus of the spinal cord and are organized somatotopically, that is, the pathways from each dermatome and myotome are organized in layers. Axons from the caudal half of the body run in the gracile fasciculus to the gracile nucleus. Those from the cranial half form the cuneate fasciculus, which runs alongside the gracile fasciculus and terminates in the cuneate nucleus. The two nuclei form two macroscopically visible protrusions on the posterior surface of the lower third of the medulla oblongata. The gracile tubercle is located on the medial aspect and on the lateral aspect the cuneate tubercle. From multipolar second-order neurons in these nuclei, axons cross to the opposite side as internal arcuate fibers and ascend to the thalamus as the **medial lemniscus**. In a cross-section through the upper medulla oblongata, the medial lemnisci appear as two fiber bundles facing one another across the median plane. In the pons, the medial lemniscus lies posterior to the pontine nuclei of the pontocerebellar pathways. In the midbrain, it occupies the lateral region of the tegmentum. At the midbrain–diencephalon junction it shifts in a lateral direction. In T2-weighted MR images of axial planes the medial lemniscus can be identified through its shape and its contrast to the surrounding structures (50, 97). It terminates in the ventral posterolateral nucleus of the thalamus.

The lateral border of the **ventral posterolateral nucleus** is demarcated by the triangular area (of Wernicke) (406, 479). It forms a groove on the inferior part of the lateral side of the thalamus. In axial MR images the ventral posterolateral nucleus can be identified by the posterior limb of the internal capsule, the pulvinar, and to some extent the triangular area (of Wernicke) (404) serving as a guideline structure. From the ventral posterolateral nucleus, the third-order neurons project as thalamoparietal fibers to the postcentral gyrus and paracentral lobule.

The **thalamoparietal fibers** are neither macroscopically nor microscopically identified in specimens of adult human brains. Therefore, they are demarcated and in comparison with histological brain sections of infants (postnatal age 2 to 6 months). The thalamoparietal fibers course diagonally upward through the posterior limb of the internal capsule posterior to the corticospinal fibers. Superior to the optic radiation, they run at the lateral edge of the corona radiata toward the postcentral gyrus and the paracentral lobule.

The anterior border of the primary somatic sensory cortex in the **postcentral gyrus** is formed through the floor of the central sulcus, even though the somatic sensory and motor regions seldom meet exactly at the floor of the sulcus (362). Accordingly the floor of the postcentral sulcus forms the posterior border. Inferior to the postcentral gyrus the primary somatic sensory cortex of the medial lemniscus system cannot be morphologically demarcated from the primary sensory cortex of the trigeminal system. Therefore, the demarcation of this border is based on physiological–experimental descriptions (499). The primary somatic sensory cortex of neurosurgical patients has been stimulated under local anesthesia by means of electrodes applied directly to the cerebral surface. Using these investigations as a guideline, the approximate distance from the superior margin of hemisphere to the lateral sulcus on the postcentral gyrus was measured using a form of tape measure (479). Approximately two-thirds of the postcentral gyrus belongs to the medial lemniscus system, one third to the trigeminal system. To identify the postcentral gyrus in MR images, the central sulcus can be used as a point of orientation since it is identified in the sagittal as well as in the axial planes (404) (Chap. 5.7.5).

A triangle is demarcated as the primary somatic sensory cortex on the medial side of the hemisphere in the **paracentral lobule**. Its form is similar to that shown in the illustrations of the brain by Brodmann (56). The triangle approximately 1 cm in height is demarcated on the medial side of the hemisphere within the paracentral lobule close to the postcentral gyrus at the superior margin. The base of the triangle is formed by the postcentral gyrus at the superior margin. The tip of the triangle indicates the middle of the corpus callosum. The marginal branch of the cingulate sulcus is used to identify the paracentral lobule in axial MR images (Chap. 5.7.5).

These cortical areas of the medial lemniscus system are, like the spinothalamic system, **somatotopically organized** (Chap. 6.1.1). The projection field from the contralateral leg is localized in the above-mentioned triangle within the paracentral lobule. The areas from the contralateral trunk, arm, and neck are located more laterally in the postcentral gyrus on the convex brain curvature. An interruption of the medial lemniscus system leads to an impairment of proprioceptive perception (vibration and position senses) and of exteroceptive perception (disturbances of two-point discrimination) (471b).

6.1.2 Medial Lemniscus System   333

1 Postcentral gyrus
2 Thalamoparietal fibers
3 Ventral posterolateral nucleus of thalamus
4 Medial lemniscus
5 Internal arcuate fibers
6 Cuneate nucleus (of Burdach)
7 Gracile nucleus (of Goll)
8 Cuneate fasciculus
9 Gracile fasciculus
10 Posterior (dorsal) root of spinal nerve
11 Spinal ganglion

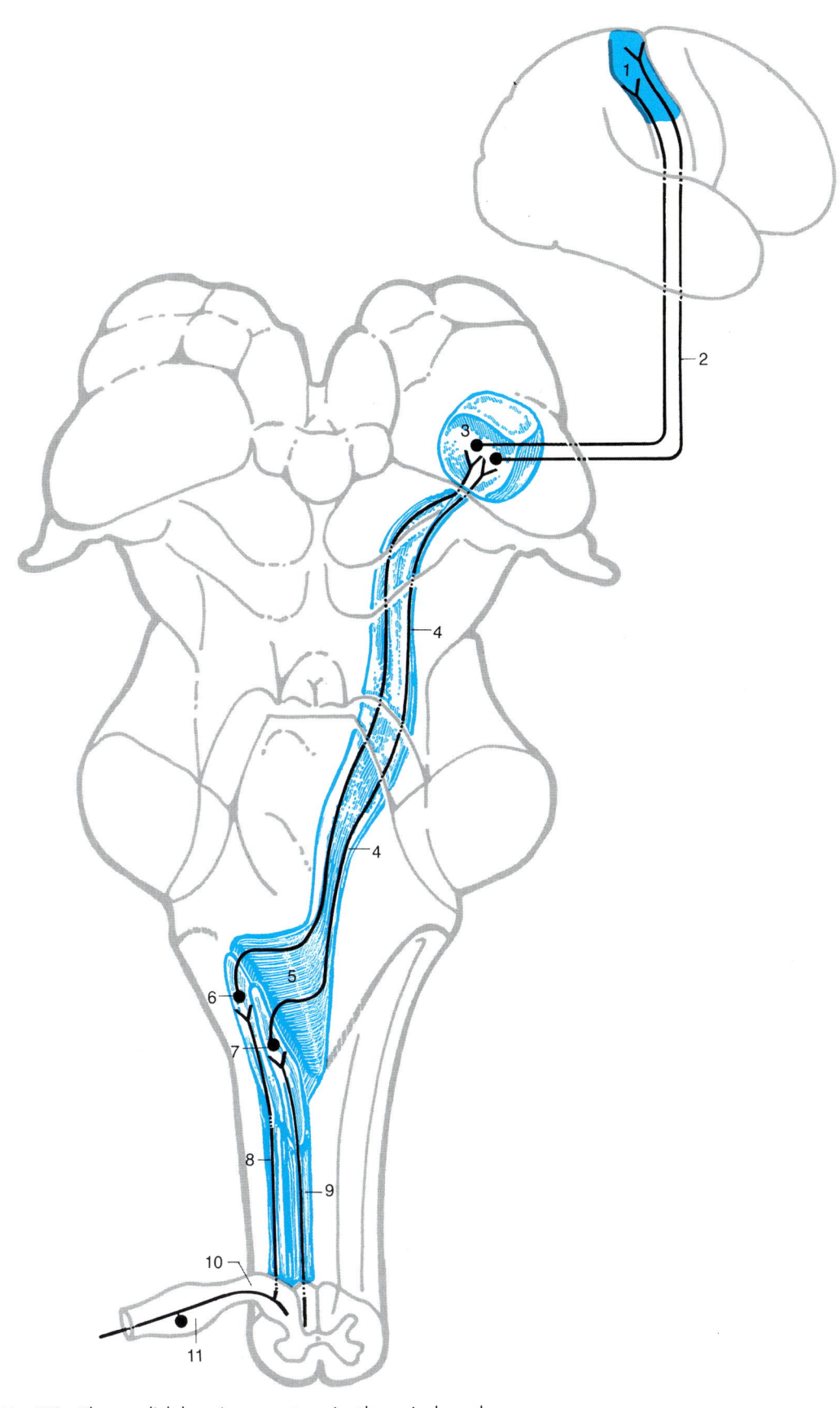

Fig. 111 The medial lemniscus system in the spinal cord, brainstem, and diencephalon (posterior view) and in the cerebrum (lateral view). According to (332).

334   6 Neurofunctional Systems

1 Thalamoparietal fibers (in the posterior part of the slice)
2 Ventral posterolateral nucleus of thalamus (in the posterior part of the slice)
3 Medial lemniscus (in the posterior part of the slice)
4 Postcentral gyrus
5 Thalamoparietal fibers
6 Medial lemniscus
7 Internal arcuate fibers
8 Cuneate nucleus (of Burdach) (in the posterior part of the slice)
9 Gracile nucleus (of Goll) (in the posterior part of the slice)
10 Gracile fasciculus (in the posterior part of the slice)
11 Cuneate fasciculus (in the posterior part of the slice)
12 Postcentral gyrus and primary somatic sensory cortex in paracentral lobule (within the slice)

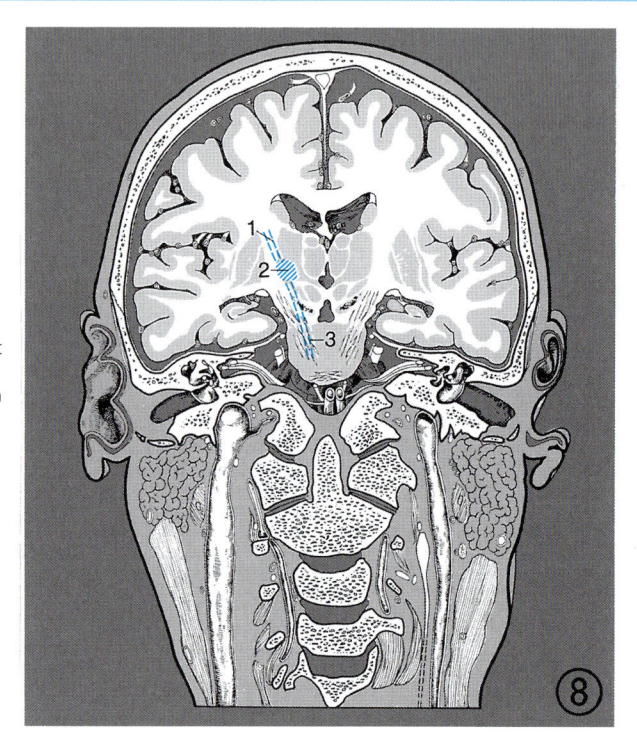

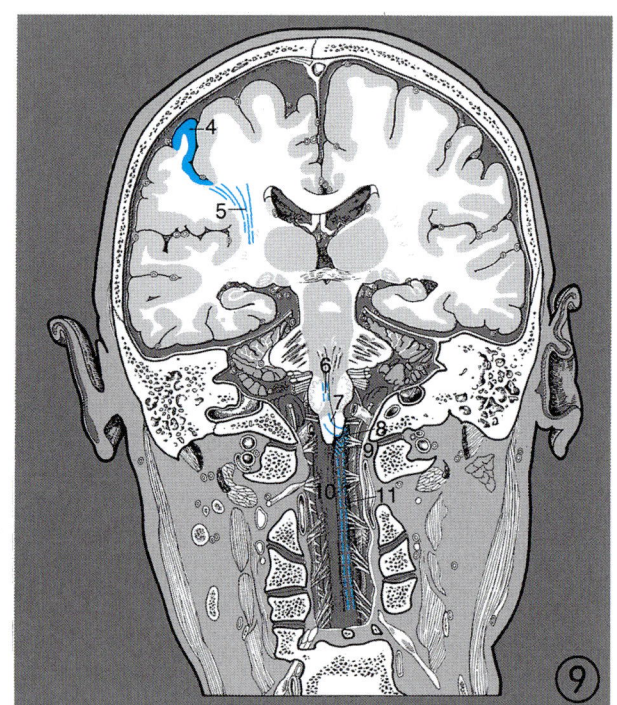

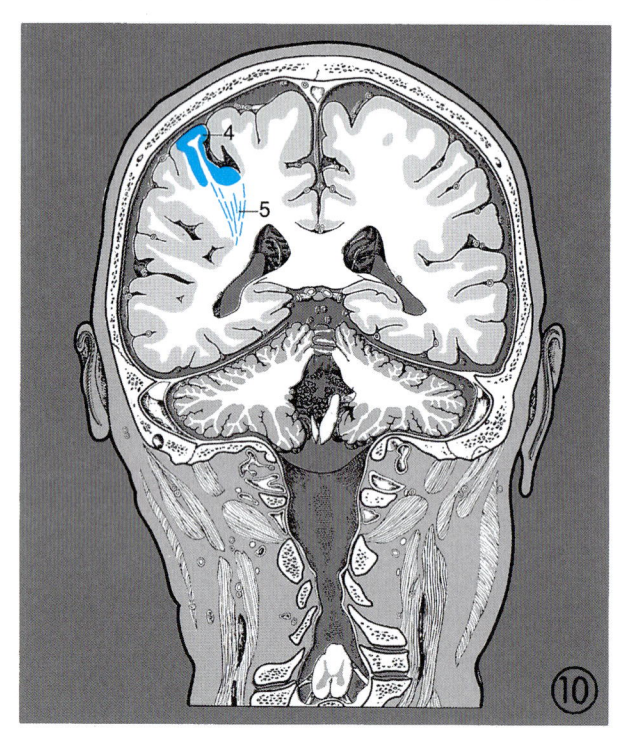

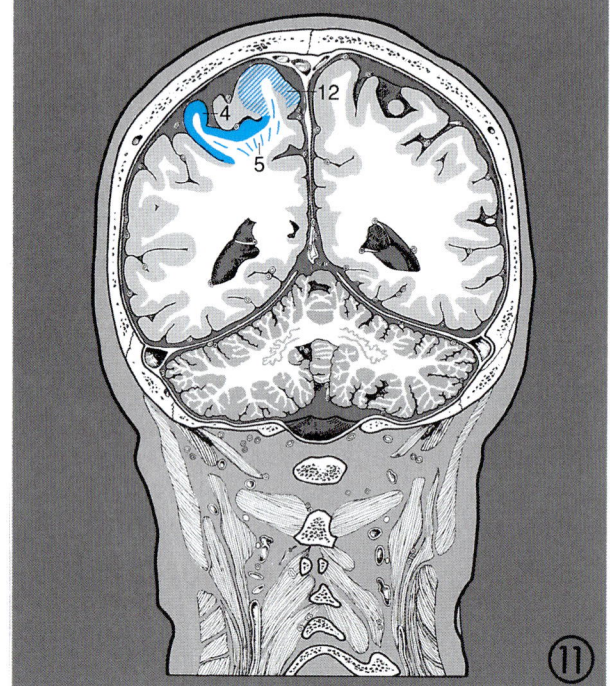

Fig. 112 Coronal serial illustrations of the medial lemniscus system. The encircled numbers (8–11) indicate the number of the respective slice (Figs. 1, 2a,b, 3).

6.1.2 Medial Lemniscus System

1 Cuneate fasciculus
2 Gracile fasciculus
3 Internal arcuate fibers
4 Cuneate nucleus (of Burdach)
5 Gracile nucleus (of Goll)
6 Medial lemniscus

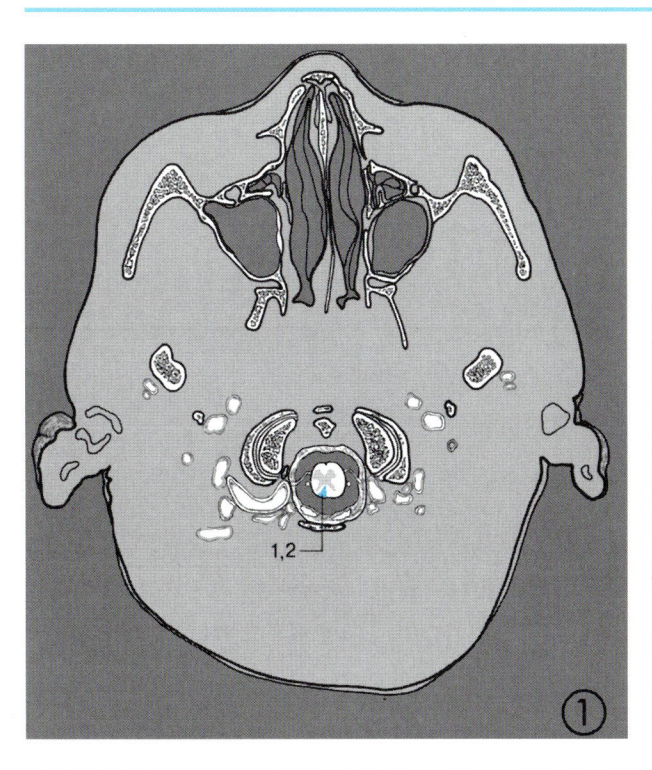

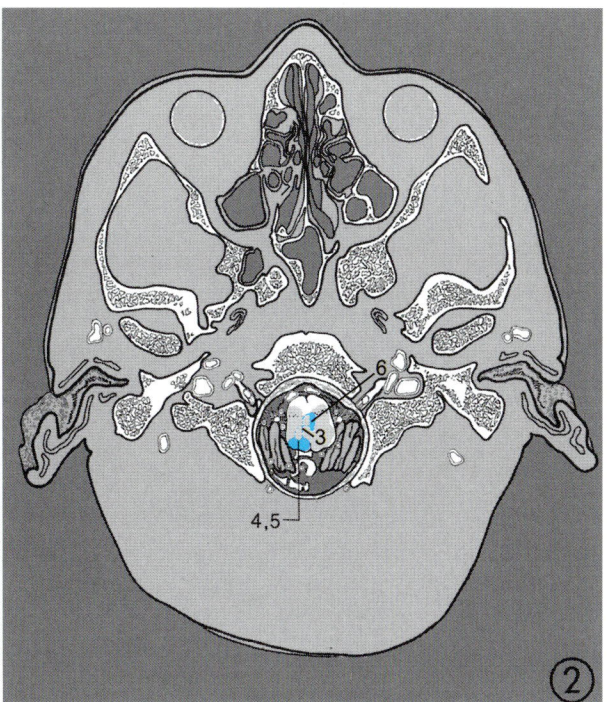

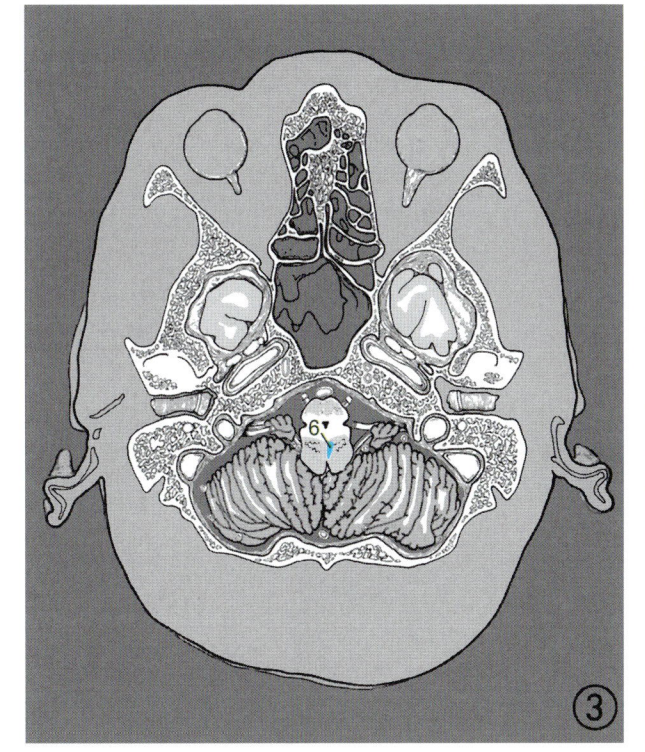

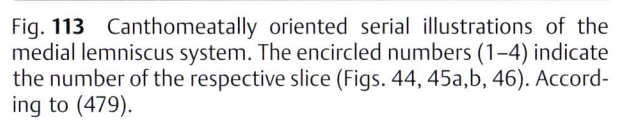

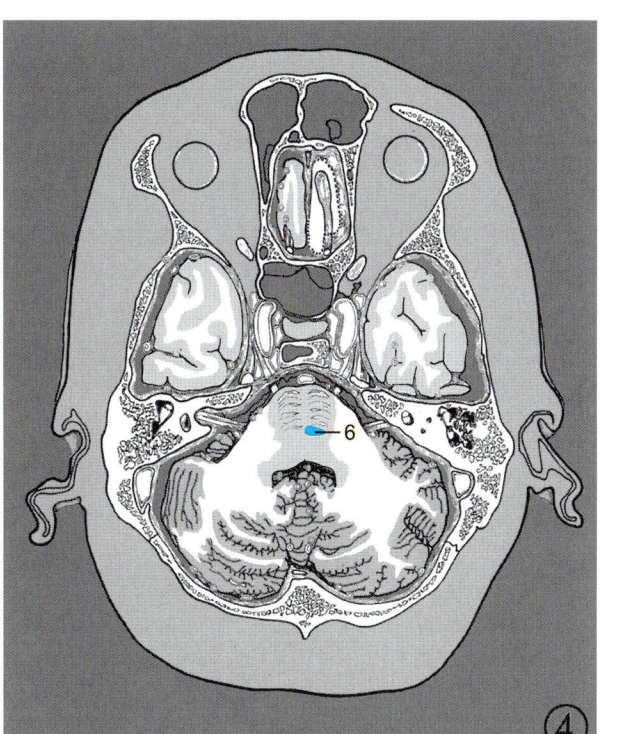

Fig. 113 Canthomeatally oriented serial illustrations of the medial lemniscus system. The encircled numbers (1–4) indicate the number of the respective slice (Figs. 44, 45a,b, 46). According to (479).

6 Medial lemniscus
7 Ventral posterolateral nucleus of thalamus
8 Thalamoparietal fibers

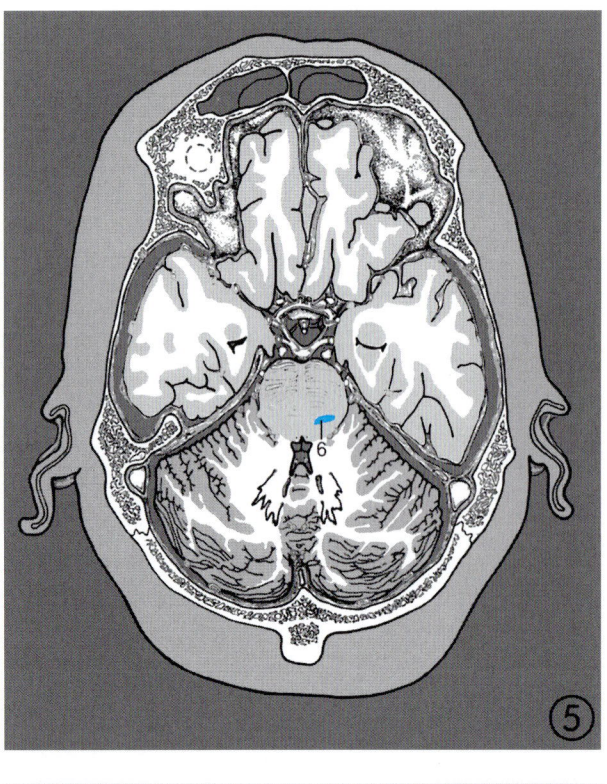

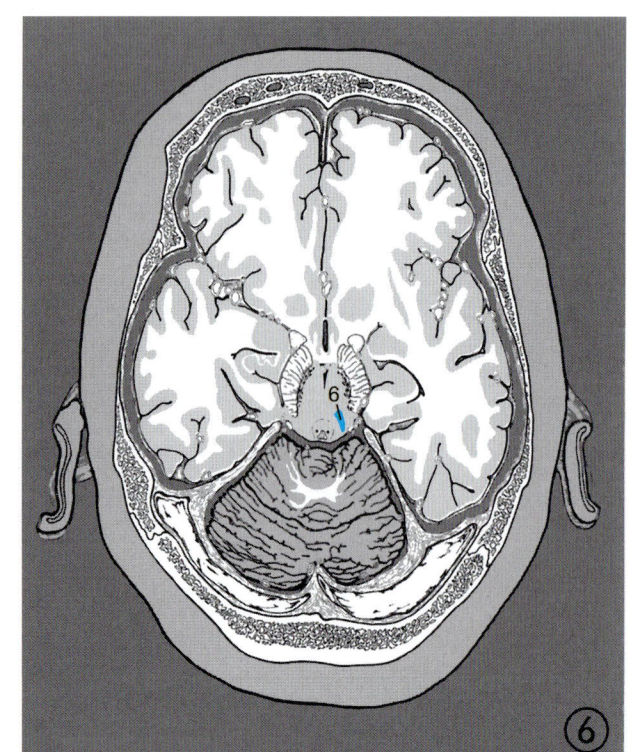

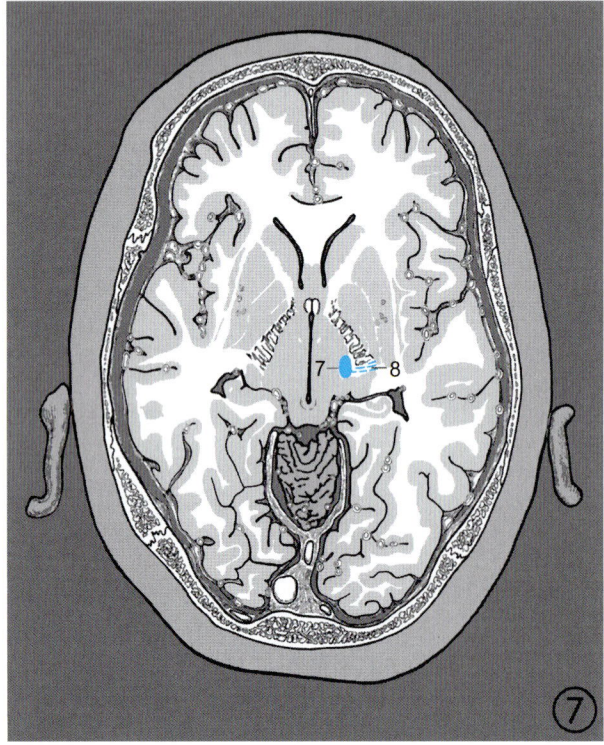

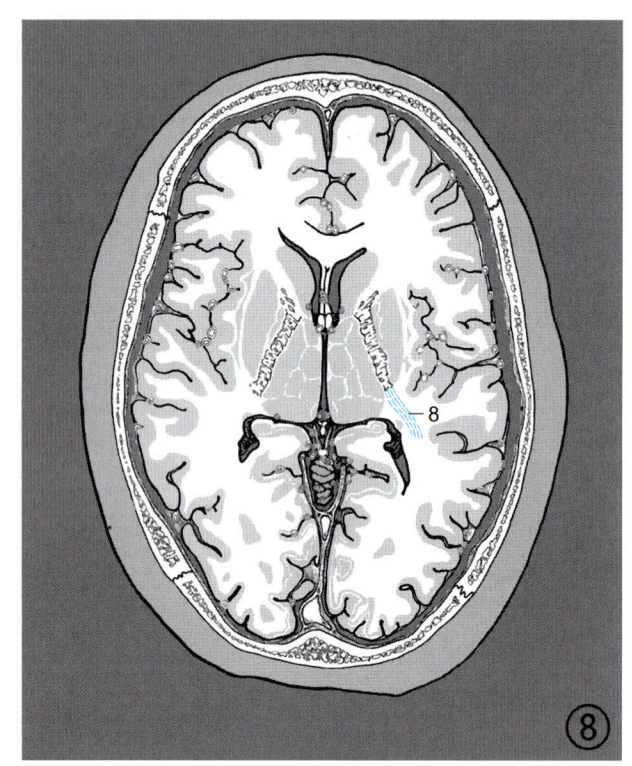

Fig. 113 Canthomeatally oriented serial illustrations of the medial lemniscus system. The encircled numbers (5–12) indicate the number of the respective slice (Figs. 44, 45a,b, 46). According to (479).

6.1.2 *Medial Lemniscus System* **337**

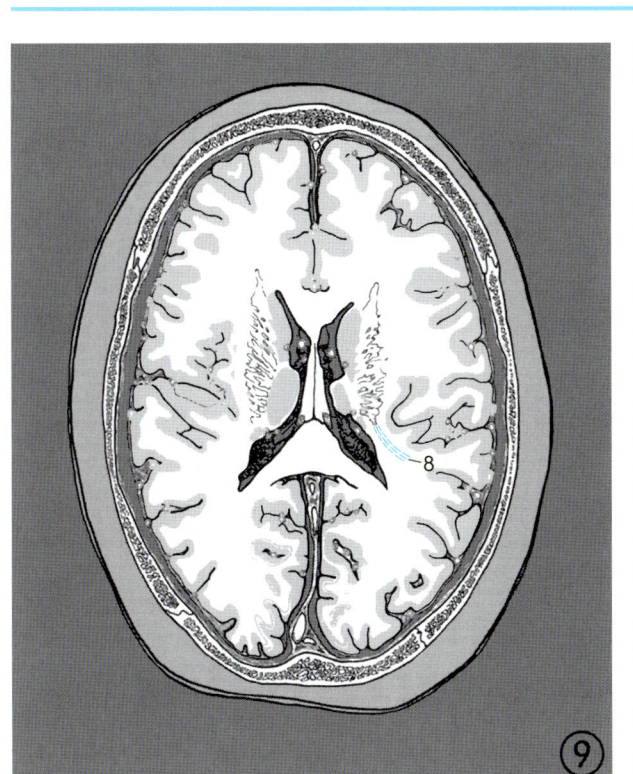

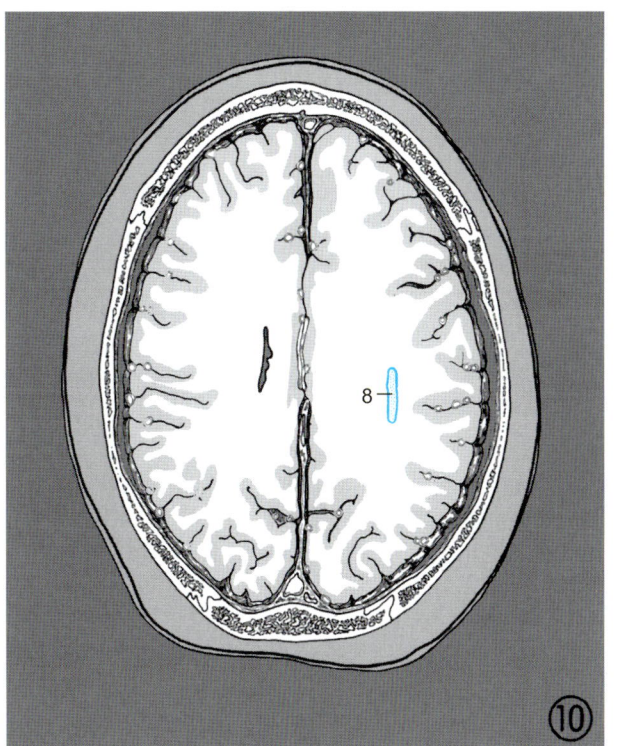

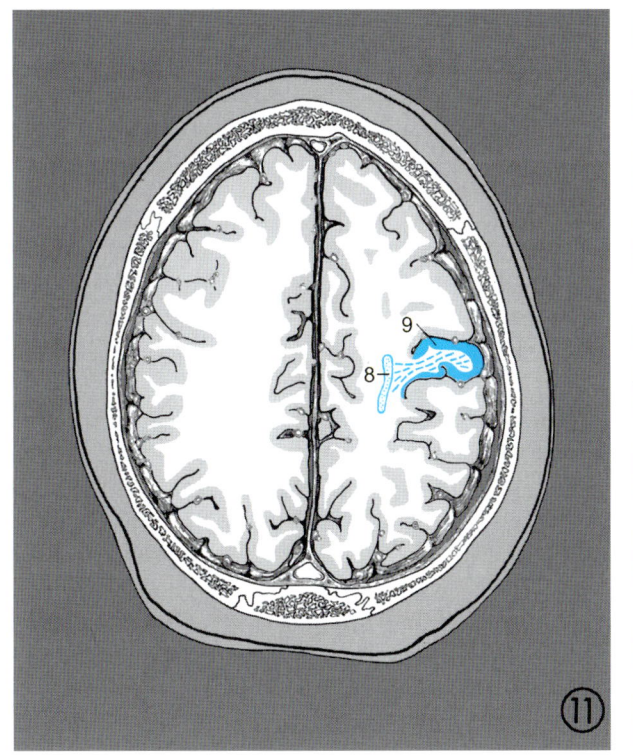

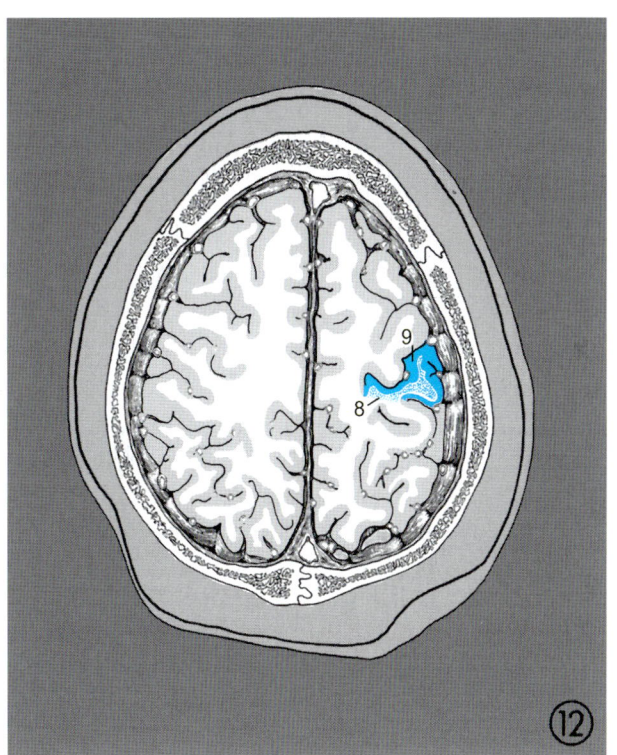

8 Thalamoparietal fibers
9 Postcentral gyrus

8   Thalamoparietal fibers
9   Postcentral gyrus
10 Primary somatic sensory cortex in paracentral lobule

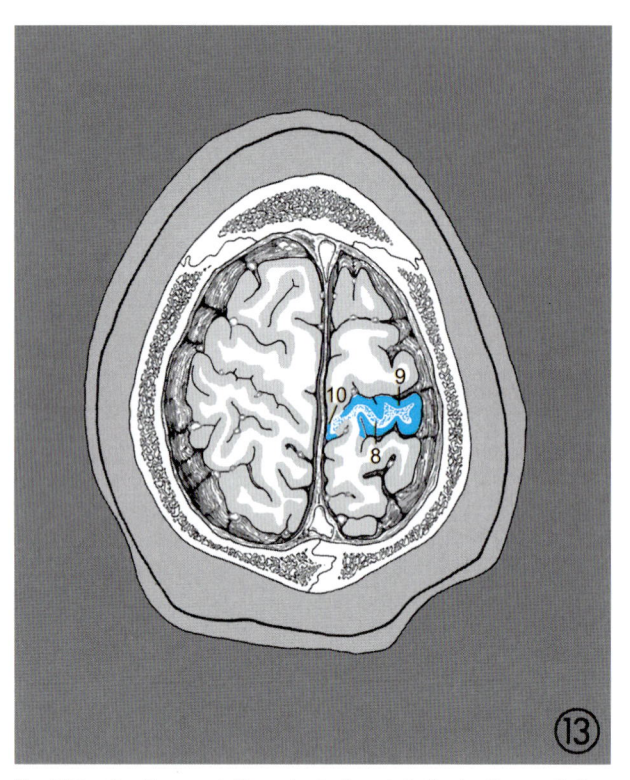

Fig. 113 Canthomeatally oriented serial illustrations of the medial lemniscus system. The encircled numbers (13–14) indicate the number of the respective slice (Figs. 44, 45a,b, 46). According to (479).

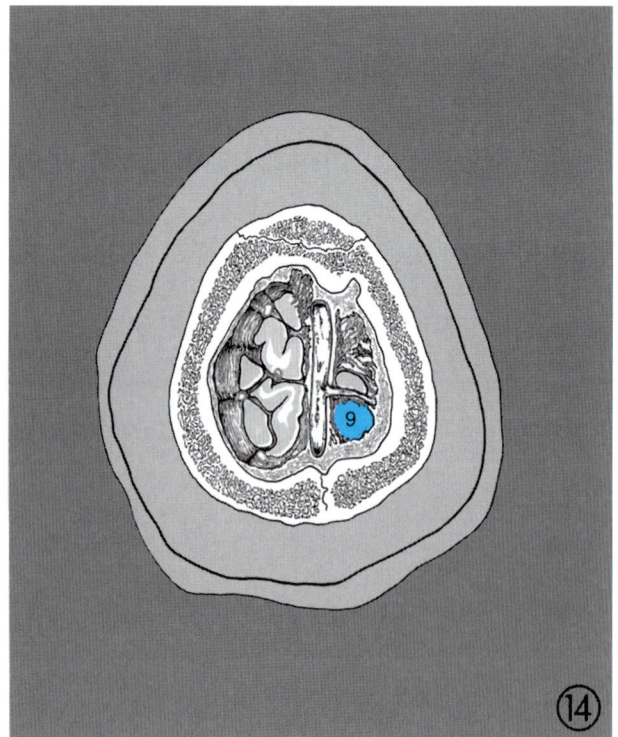

6.1.3 Trigeminal System
(Figs. 114–116)

The pain, cold, and heat receptors of the facial skin, as well as those of the mucous membranes of the nose with its paranasal sinuses, the oral cavity, and the teeth transmit their signals via branches of the trigeminal nerve to the unipolar nerve cells of the **trigeminal** (Gasserian) **ganglion**. The central axons of the trigeminal ganglion run to the pons and as the spinal tract of the trigeminal nerve through the pons to reach the caudal part of the **spinal nucleus of trigeminal nerve**. This nucleus consists of caudal, interpolar, and oral parts. The caudal part of the nucleus is located laterally in the medulla oblongata and extends from the obex down to the cervical spinal cord segment C2. It corresponds to the marginal cells and cells of the nucleus proprius in the dorsal gray horn of the spinal cord, which also transmit nociceptive and thermal signals. Arising from the second-order neurons of the caudal part of the spinal nucleus of the trigeminal nerve, axons cross in the medulla oblongata, ascend as the lateral trigeminothalamic tract, and synapse in the ventral posteromedial nucleus of the thalamus. The interpolar part (approximate length 11 mm) of the spinal nucleus is located in the medulla oblongata (4) and transmits nociceptive signals from the teeth (153, 484). The oral part (approximate length 14 mm) of the spinal nucleus is found in the lower portion of the pons. Fibers from the interpolar and oral parts of the spinal nucleus also cross to the anterior trigeminothalamic tract to reach the ventral posteromedial nucleus of the thalamus. The primary somatic sensory fields for these pathways are situated at the foot of the **postcentral gyrus** close to the lateral sulcus.

The mechanoreceptors of the facial skin, the eyes, and the nasal and oral cavities transmit their signals via branches of the trigeminal nerve to the unipolar nerve cells of the **trigeminal ganglion**. The central axons of this ganglion extend as the sensory root (formerly portio major) of the trigeminal nerve, mainly to the principal sensory (formerly main sensory) nucleus of the trigeminal nerve. The **principal sensory nucleus of trigeminal nerve** is located in the lateral part of the tegmentum of the pons at the height of entry of the trigeminal nerve. From the principal sensory nucleus the axons of the second-order neurons cross over to the opposite side and extend as trigeminothalamic fibers alongside the medial lemniscus to the ventral posteromedial nucleus of the thalamus. The uncrossed fibers coursing from the principal sensory nucleus to the ventral posteromedial nucleus are known as the Wallenberg tract or the posterior trigeminothalamic tract (417). This fiber pathway courses in a more posterior direction in the tegmentum of the pons and the midbrain than does the main pathway from the principal sensory nucleus. The ipsilateral and contralateral pathways are only joining just before reaching the **ventral post-**

6.1.3 Trigeminal System 339

1 Postcentral gyrus
2 Thalamoparietal fibers
3 Ventral posteromedial nucleus of thalamus
4 Trigeminal (Gasserian) ganglion
5 Sensory root of trigeminal nerve
6 Mesencephalic nucleus of trigeminal nerve
7 Trigeminal lemniscus
8 Posterior trigeminothalamic tract
9 Principal sensory nucleus of trigeminal nerve
10 Trigeminothalamic tract from principal sensory nucleus of trigeminal nerve
11 Anterior trigeminothalamic tract
12 Spinal nucleus of trigeminal nerve
13 Spinal tract of trigeminal nerve
14 Lateral trigeminothalamic tract

V Trigeminal nerve
VII Facial nerve
IX Glossopharyngeal nerve
X Vagus nerve

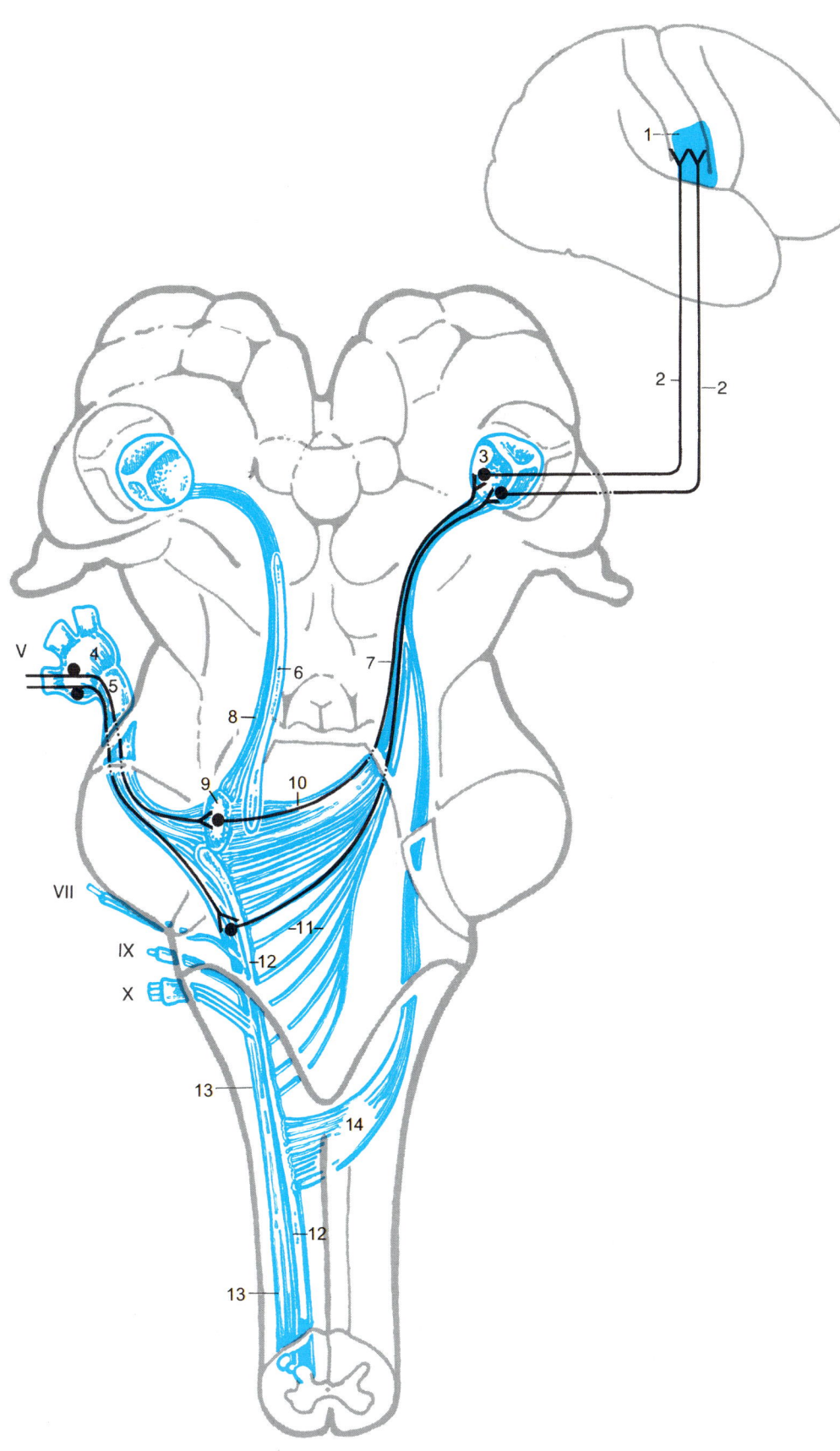

Fig. 114 The trigeminal system in the spinal cord, brainstem, and diencephalon (posterior view) and in the cerebrum (lateral view). Roman numerals indicate the cranial nerves. According to (332, 416).

340   6   Neurofunctional Systems

1 Supraorbital nerve
2 Infraorbital nerve
3 Inferior alveolar nerve
4 Nasociliary nerve
5 Greater palatine nerve
6 Lingual nerve
7 Frontal nerve
8 Palatine nerves
9 Ophthalmic nerve
10 Maxillary nerve

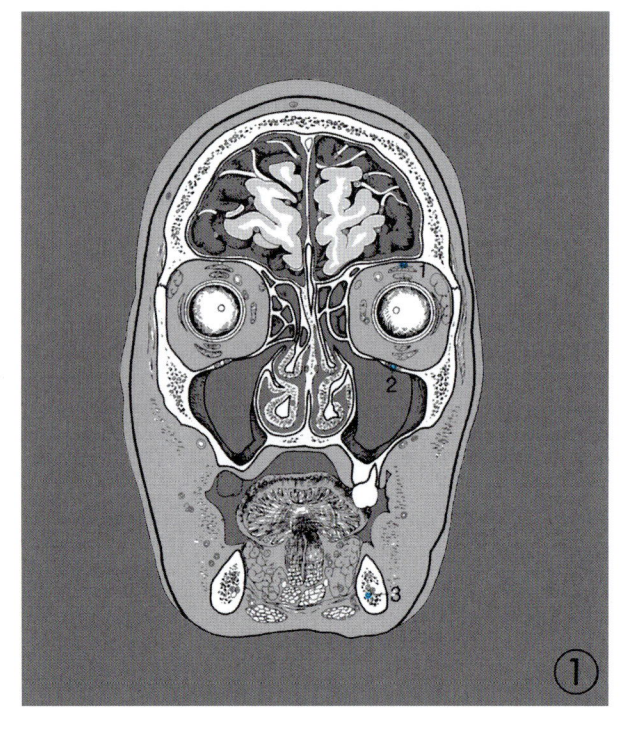

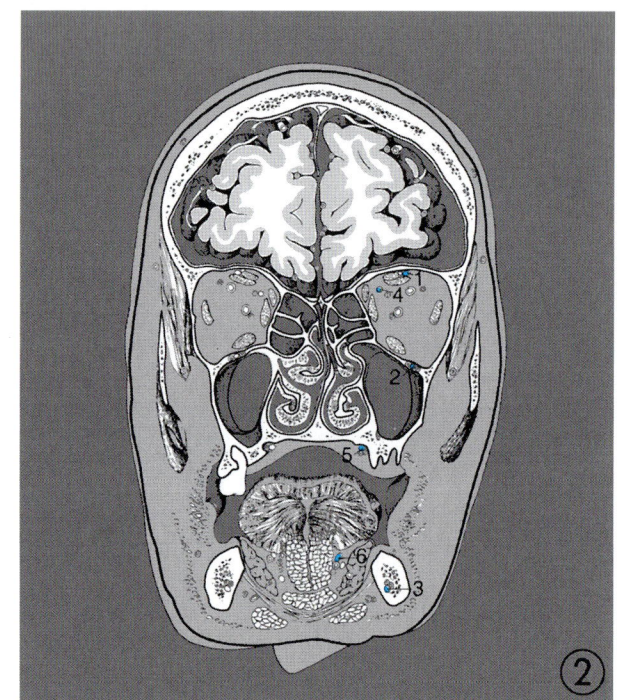

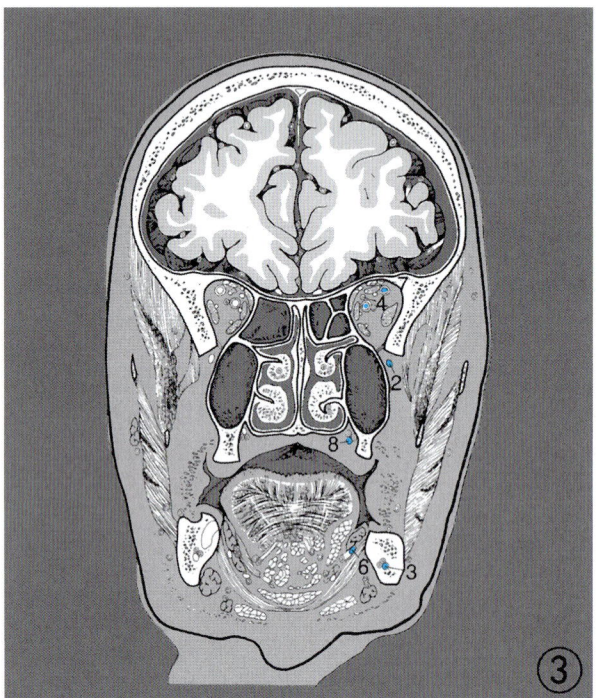

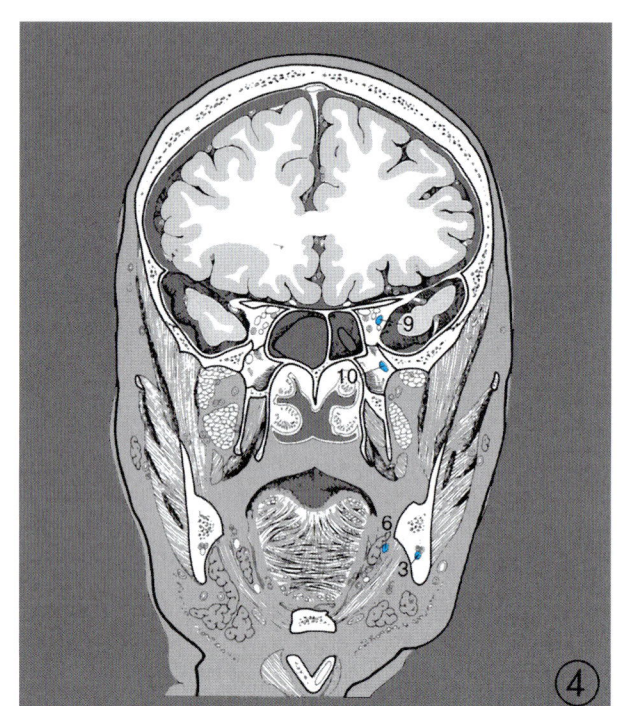

Fig. **115** Coronal serial illustrations of the peripheral and central trigeminal system. The encircled numbers (1–8) indicate the number of the slice (Figs. 1, 2a,b, 3). According to (295, 416).

6.1.3 Trigeminal System

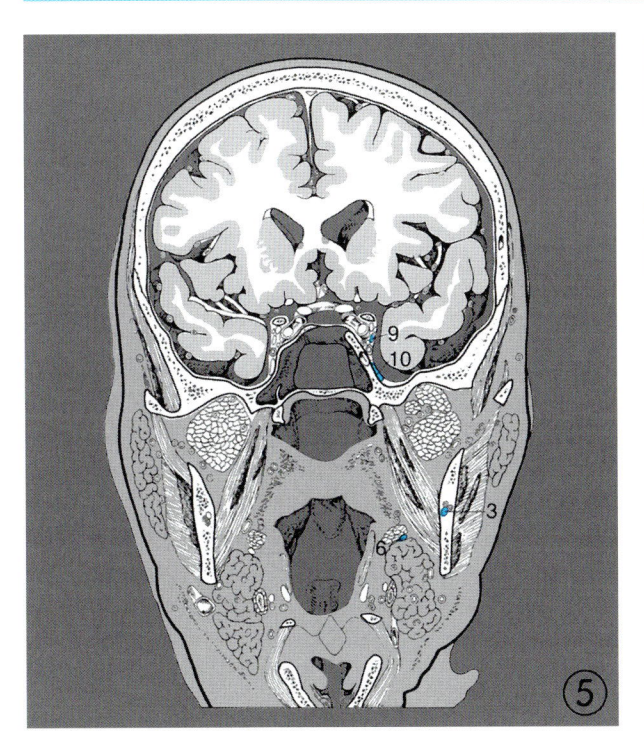

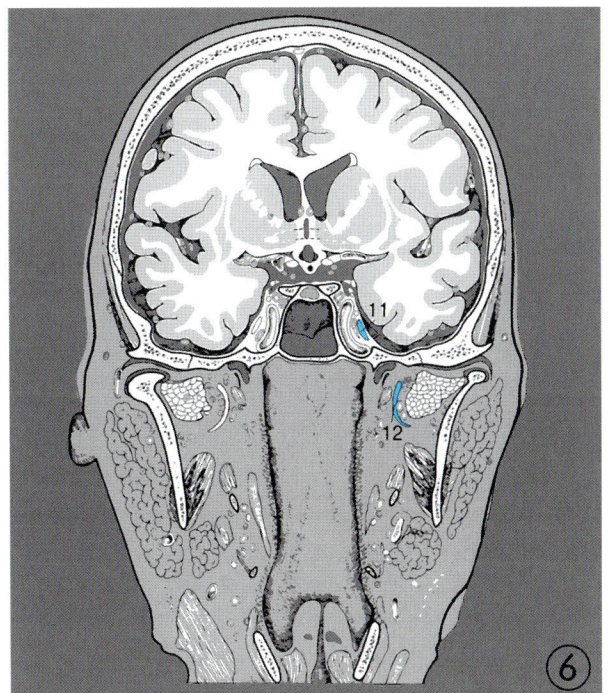

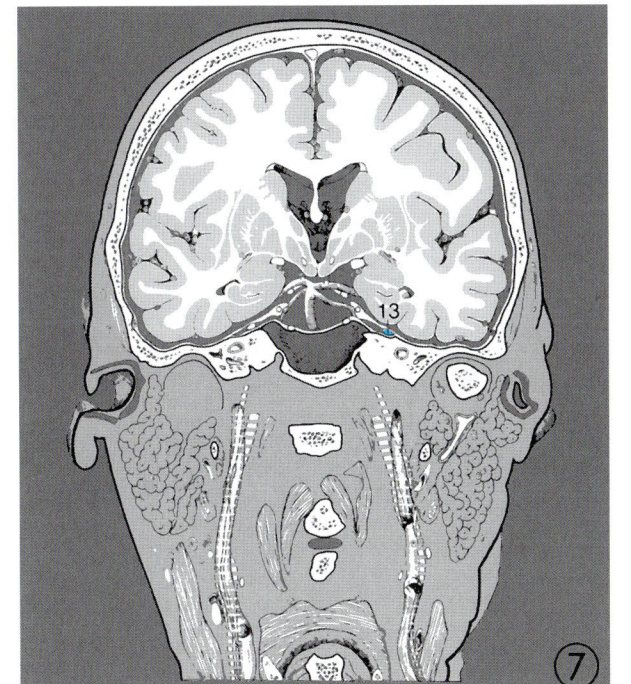

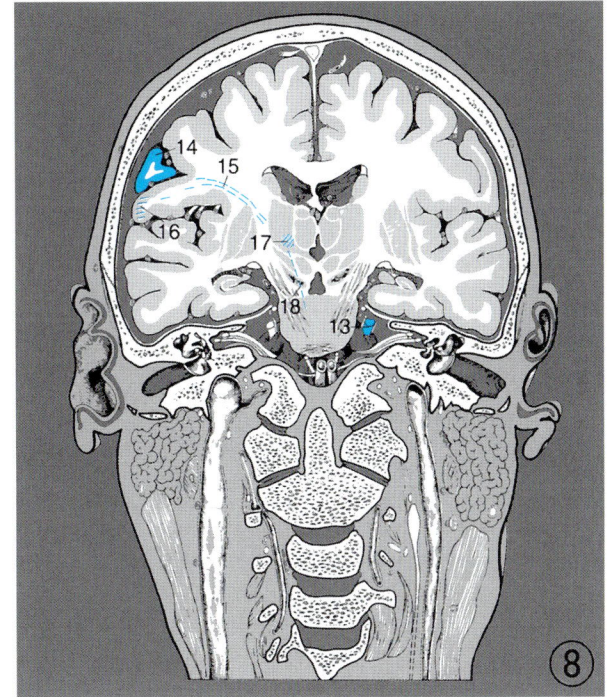

3 Inferior alveolar nerve
6 Lingual nerve
9 Ophthalmic nerve
10 Maxillary nerve
11 Trigeminal (Gasserian) ganglion
12 Mandibular nerve
13 Trigeminal nerve
14 Postcentral gyrus
15 Thalamoparietal fibers
16 Postcentral gyrus (within the slice)
17 Ventral posteromedial nucleus of thalamus (in the posterior part of the slice)
18 Trigeminal lemniscus (within the slice)

14 Postcentral gyrus
15 Thalamoparietal fibers
18 Trigeminal lemniscus (within the slice)
19 Principal sensory nucleus of trigeminal nerve (in the posterior part of the slice)
20 Spinal nucleus of trigeminal nerve (within the slice)
21 Lateral trigeminothalamic tract (within the slice)

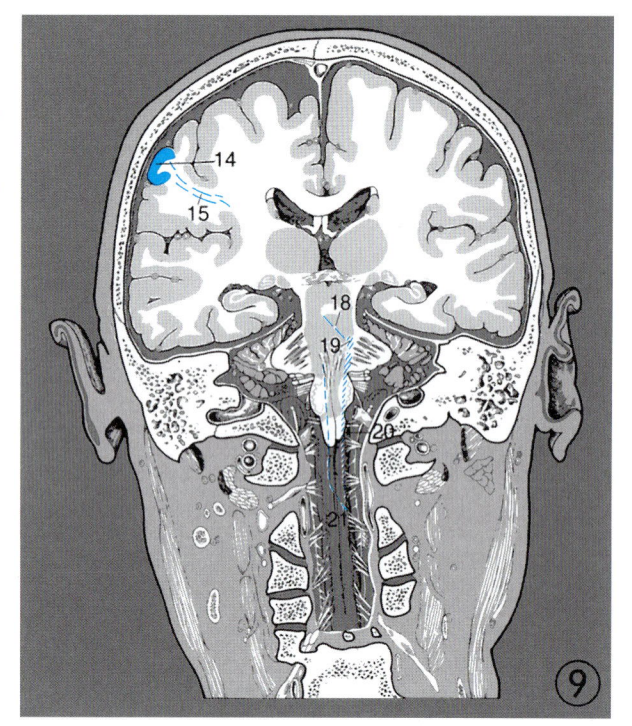

Fig. 115 Coronal serial illustrations of the peripheral and central trigeminal system. The encircled number (9) indicates the number of the respective slice (Figs. 1, 2a,b, 3). According to (295, 416).

6.1.4 Topography of Sensory Disorders

Clinical Notes

The separate courses of the anterolateral and medial lemniscus systems in the medulla oblongata explain the appearance of a **dissociated sensory disorder** as a result of an isolated lesion of the anterolateral system in the **medulla oblongata**. Small infarcts in the anterolateral system cause a contralateral loss of pain and temperature sensation with preservation of tactile sensivity. With an additional lesion of the primary trigeminal neurons and/or of the initial part of the secondary trigeminal neurons, ipsilateral sensory impairments may involve the face. This produces a **crossed impairment**, such as that of the Wallenberg's syndrome, caused by lesions in the lateral medulla oblongata.

A lesion of the medial lemniscus system impairs tactile discrimination, i.e. sensations of touch, position, and vibration. Lesions near the midline of the medulla oblongata may give rise to impairments on one or both sides of this sensory system. Due to the close proximity of both sensory systems further cranially, dissociated sensory disorders above the pons are rare. The same is true for the trigeminal system. Isolated pain and temperature sensory disorders arise only in connection with injuries of the upper cervical spinal cord and/or the medulla oblongata.

Foci in the posterior region of the **internal capsule** usually cause sensory disorders affecting the entire contralateral side of the body. This is due to the compact bundling of all sensory systems in this area. Increasing somatotopic fanning of the thalamoparietal pathways in the **semioval center**, as they extend toward the sensory cortex, results in isolated sensory disorders of individual (contralateral) parts of the body. Such disorders include the entire range of sensory qualities.

Objective measurement of functional disturbances of the sensory systems in their peripheral as well as their central parts is made possible through recording the somatosensory evoked potentials (SEP). Repeated electrical stimulation of a nerve allows a topical delineation if the typical patterns of the SEP components are recorded with surface electrodes over the spinal cord, the brainstem, and the primary somatic sensory field (80a, 167a, 288, 374a, 446).

eromedial nucleus. From this nucleus the third-order neurons project thalamoparietal fibers to the **lower third of the postcentral gyrus**. The pathway from the principal sensory nucleus transmits exteroceptive and proprioceptive sensory signals with the exception of pain and temperature modalities.

Figure 114 shows the lateral trigeminothalamic tract (pain and temperature signals), the anterior trigeminothalamic tract (pain and temperature signals), and the trigeminothalamic tract from the principal sensory nucleus (mechanosensibility) first meeting at the level of the pontomesencephalic transition, prior to simultaneously reaching the ventral posteromedial nucleus. The **trigeminal lemniscus** runs alongside to the medial lemniscus in the upper portion of the pons and the midbrain; thus these two fiber pathways can only be differentiated histologically after experimental marking in mammalian brains. According to these histologic findings the fibers of the trigeminal lemniscus are found in the common fiber bundle in a posterior position to those of the medial lemniscus.

The muscle spindle afferents of the masticatory muscles pass through unipolar nerve cells that are not located in the trigeminal ganglion but in the **mesencephalic nucleus of the trigeminal nerve** (located laterally in the floor of the rhomboid fossa of the pons and beside the periaqueductal gray substance of the midbrain). Their central axons give collaterals to the motor nucleus of the trigeminal nerve, thus providing a monosynaptic pathway for the masseter reflex elicited by a downward tap on the lower jaw.

6.1.3 Trigeminal System

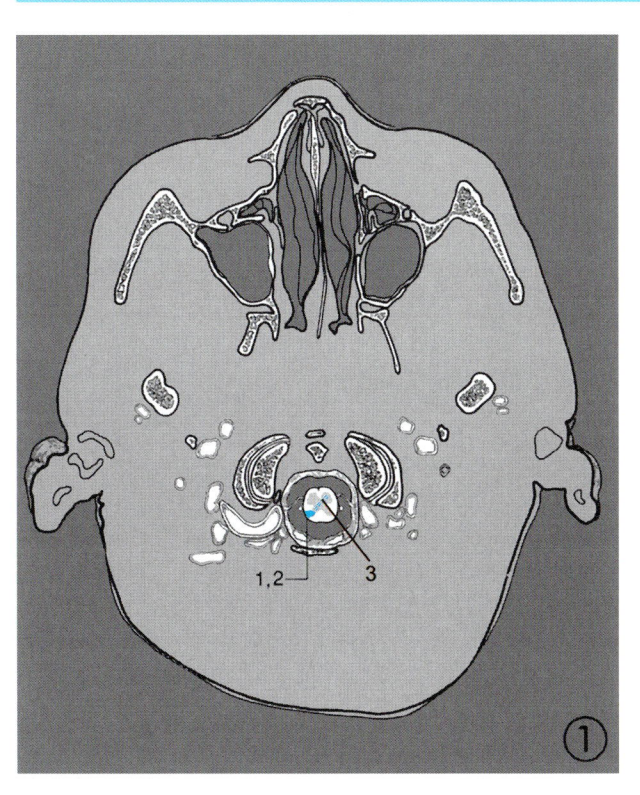

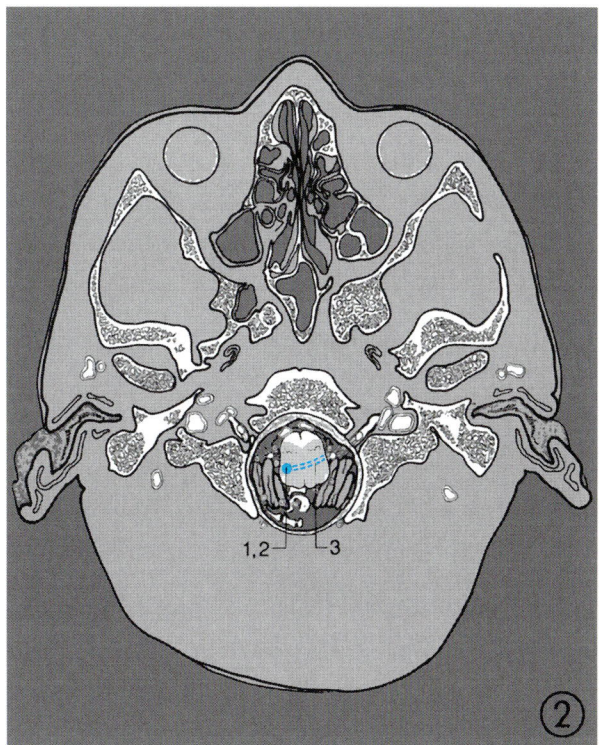

1 Spinal tract of trigeminal nerve
2 Spinal nucleus of trigeminal nerve
3 Lateral trigeminothalamic tract (within the slice)
4 Lateral trigeminothalamic tract
5 Trigeminal (Gasserian) ganglion
6 Principal sensory nucleus of trigeminal nerve
7 Trigeminothalamic tract from principal sensory nucleus of trigeminal nerve
8 Posterior trigeminothalamic tract

V   Trigeminal nerve
V/2 Maxillary nerve
V/3 Mandibular nerve

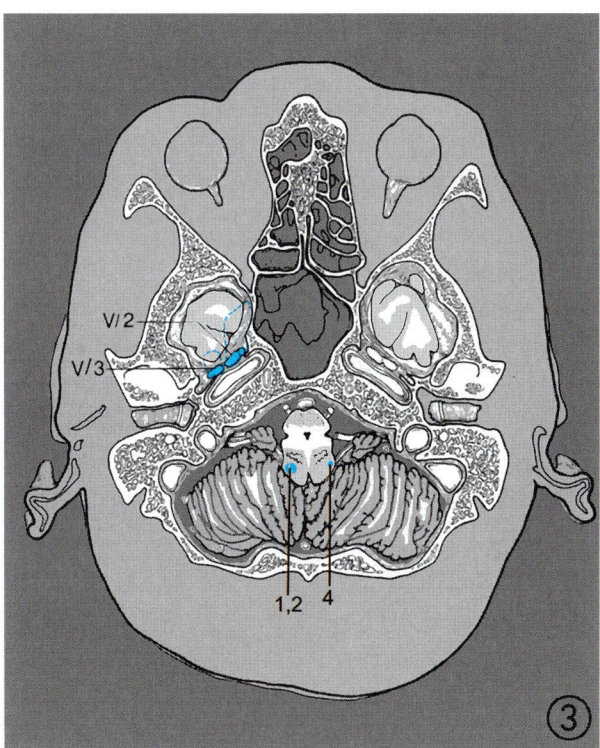

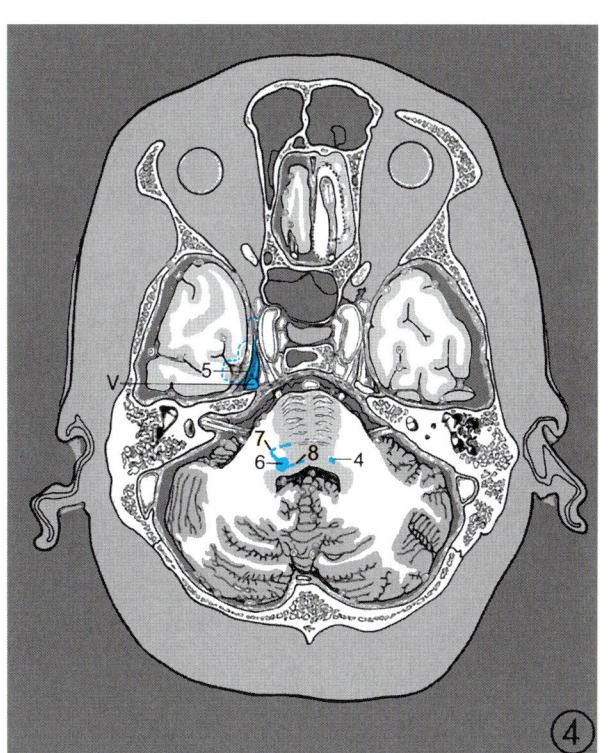

Fig. 116 Canthomeatally oriented serial illustrations of the central trigeminal system. The encircled numbers (1–4) indicate the number of the respective slice (Figs. 44, 45a,b, 46). According to (295, 416).

344 6 Neurofunctional Systems

4 Lateral trigeminothalamic tract
7 Trigeminothalamic tract from principal sensory nucleus of trigeminal nerve
8 Posterior trigeminothalamic tract
9 Trigeminal lemniscus
10 Mesencephalic nucleus of trigeminal nerve
11 Ventral posteromedial nucleus of thalamus
12 Thalamoparietal fibers
13 Postcentral gyrus

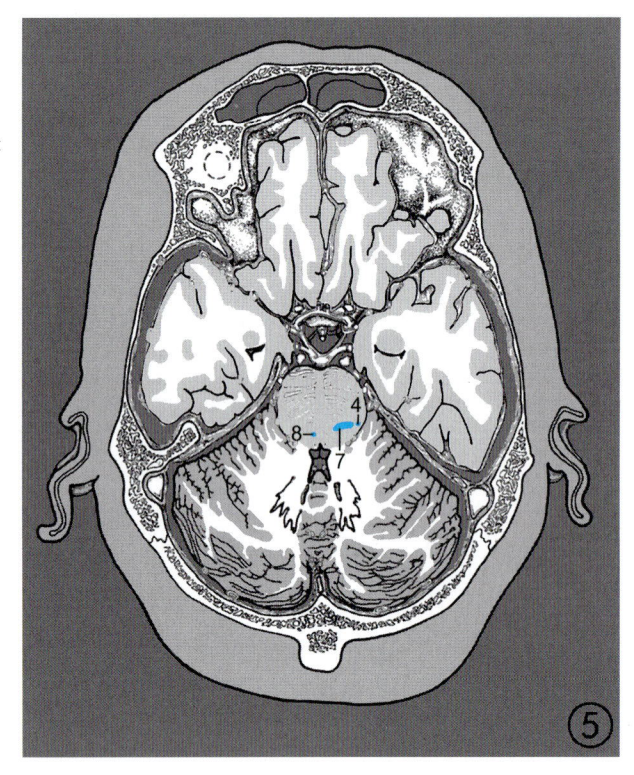

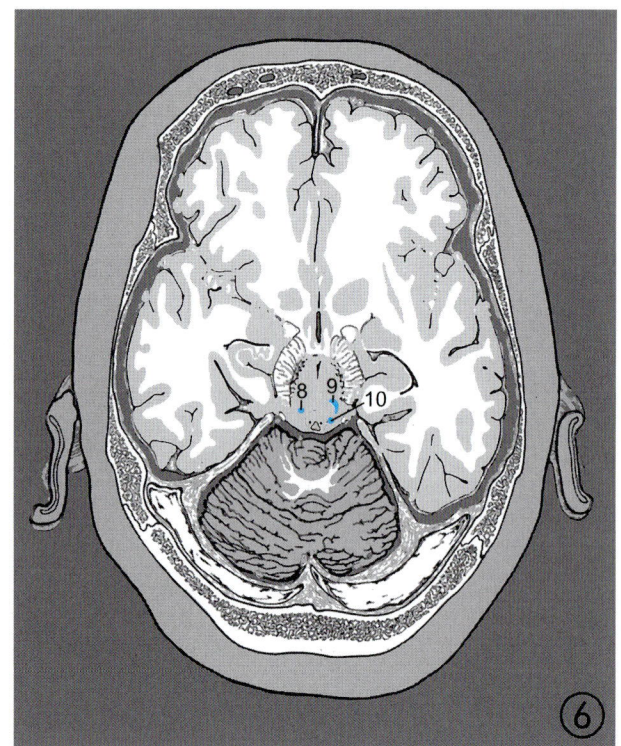

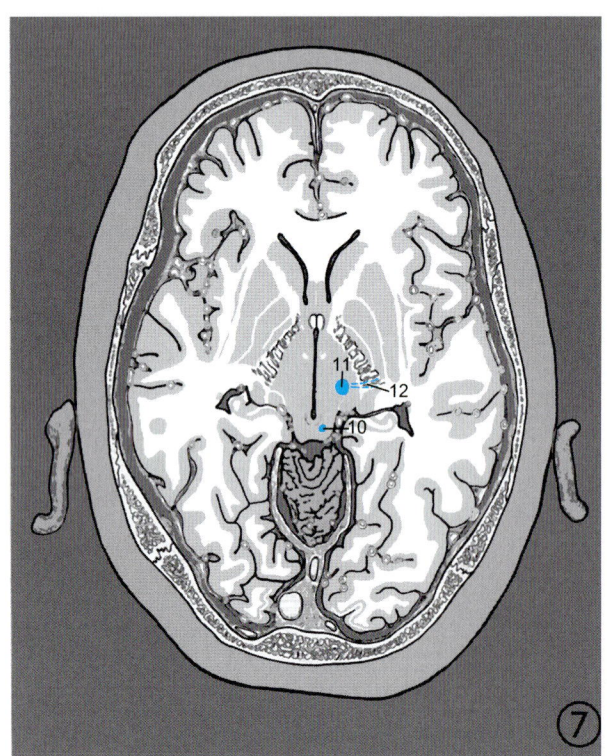

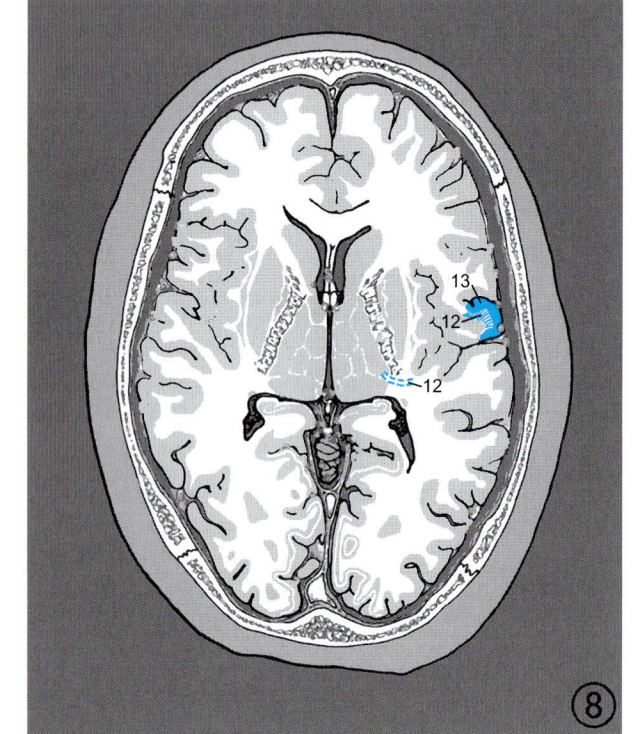

Fig. 116 Canthomeatally oriented serial illustrations of the central trigeminal system. The encircled numbers (5–10) indicate the number of the respective slice (Figs. 44, 45a,b, 46). According to (295, 416).

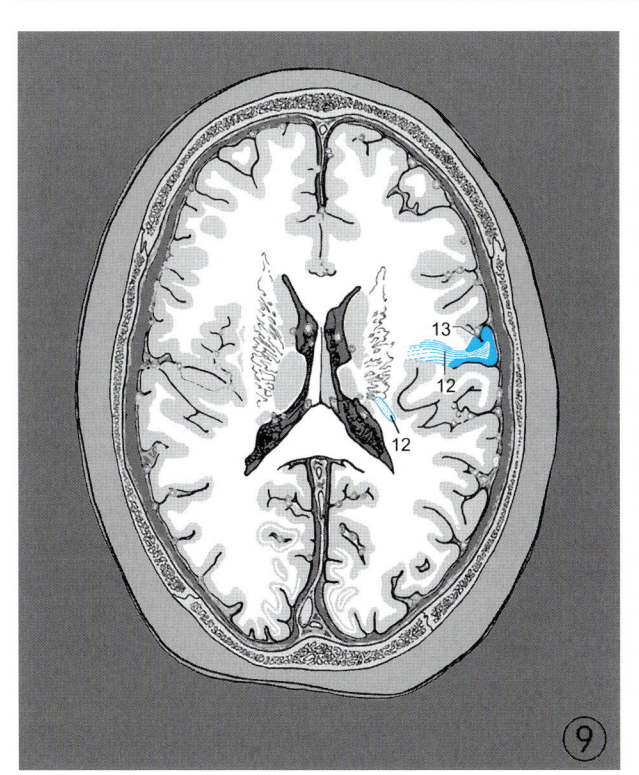

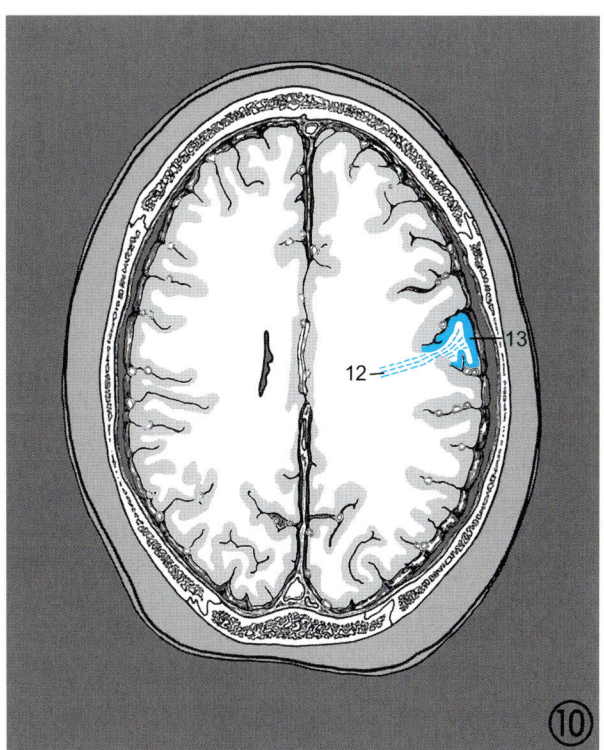

12 Thalamoparietal fibers
13 Postcentral gyrus

6.2 Gustatory System
(Figs. 117, 118)

The **facial, glossopharyngeal**, and **vagus nerves** receive gustatory signals from the taste buds of the tongue, palate, and epiglottis and transmit these signals to the medulla oblongata. The unipolar cell bodies of the first-order neurons are located in the ganglia of the seventh, ninth, and tenth cranial nerves, namely the **geniculate ganglion** and the **superior and inferior ganglia of IX and X**. Their central axons terminate in the gustatory part of the **solitary nucleus** and in its upward extension, the nucleus ovalis. The continuing pathway takes an ascending contralateral route similar to that of the trigeminal system close to the medial lemniscus and reaches the ventral posteromedial nucleus of the **thalamus**. The third-order neurons project from here to the parietal operculum and to an area on the edge of the insula (332, 374a).

Clinical Notes
Impairments of the sense of taste are predominantly accounted for by peripheral lesions of the taste buds or lesions of the seventh, ninth, and/or tenth cranial nerves and not by lesions in the aforementioned gustatory nuclei and cortical areas.

346   6 Neurofunctional Systems

1 Parietal operculum
2 Gustatory cortical area near insula
3 Ventral posteromedial nucleus of thalamus
4 Gustatory fibers in posterior (dorsal) trigeminothalamic tract
5 Nucleus ovalis
6 Pars gustatoria of solitary nucleus
VII Facial nerve
IX Glossopharyngeal nerve
X Vagus nerve

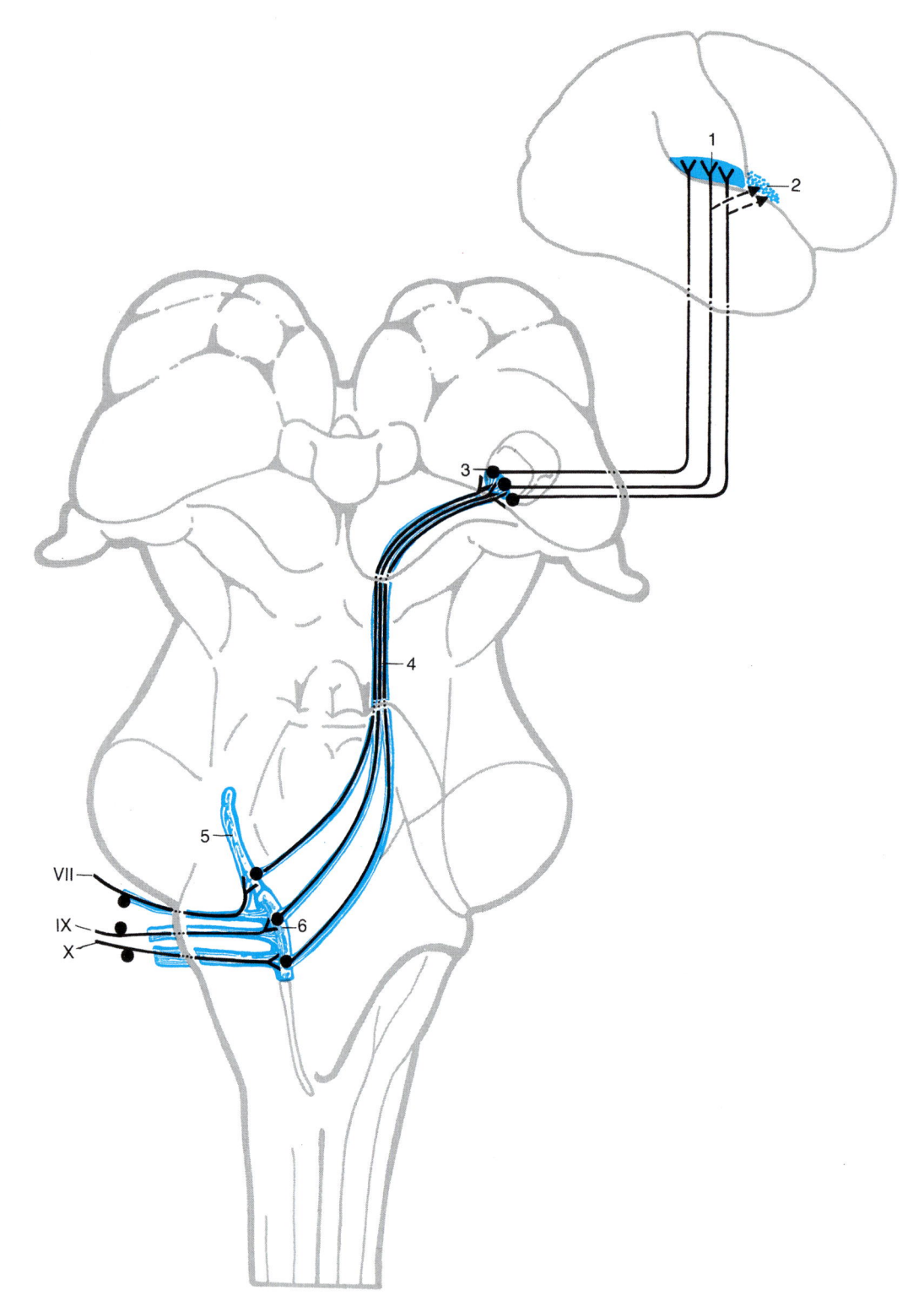

Fig. 117 The gustatory system in the brainstem and diencephalon (posterior view) and in the cerebrum (lateral view). Roman numerals indicate the facial, glossopharyngeal, and vagus nerves. According to (332).

6.2 Gustatory System

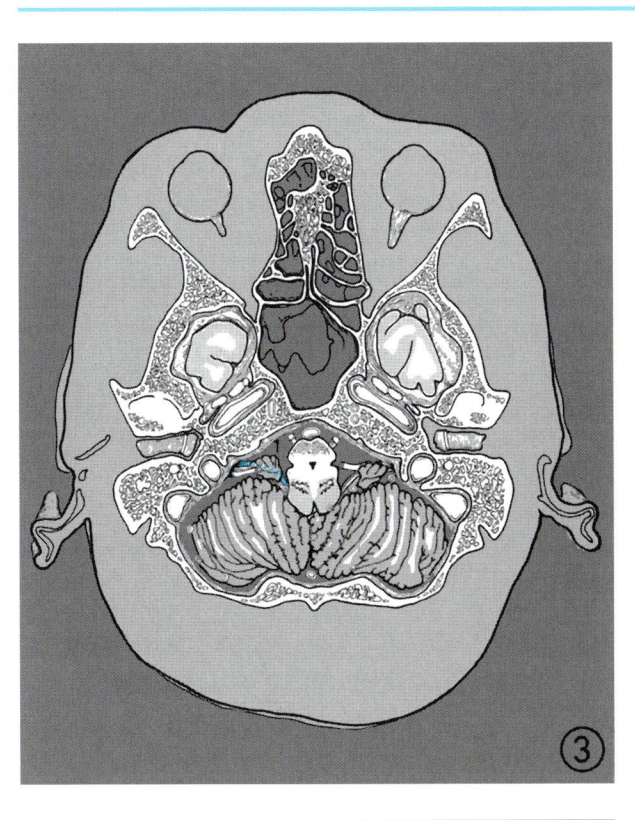

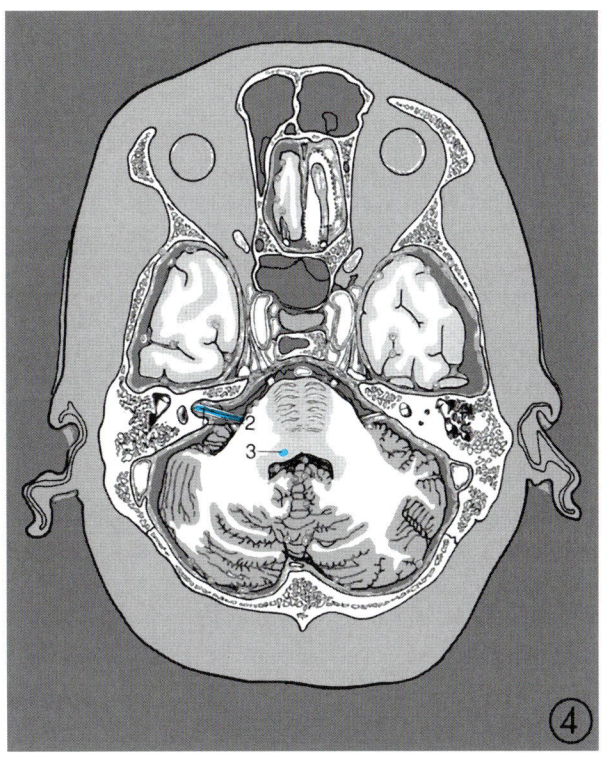

1 Glossopharyngeal nerve, vagus nerve
2 Facial nerve with chorda tympani
3 Solitary nucleus (within the slice)
4 Gustatory fibers in posterior (dorsal) trigeminothalamic tract

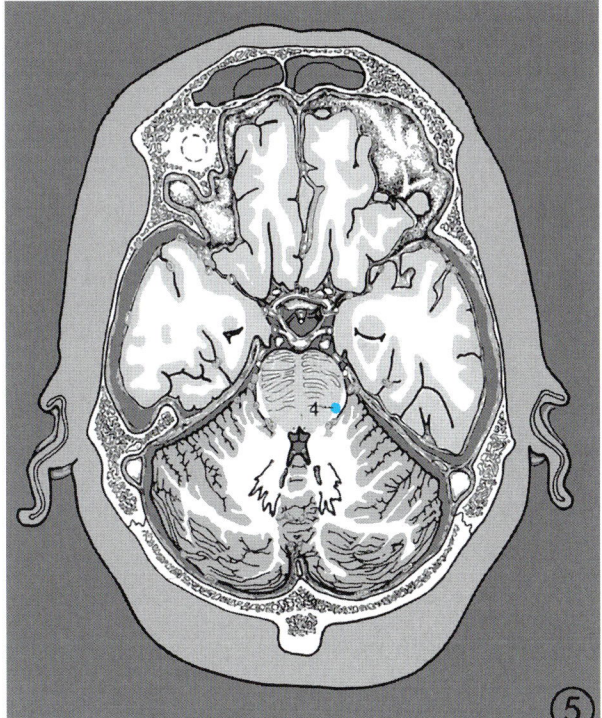

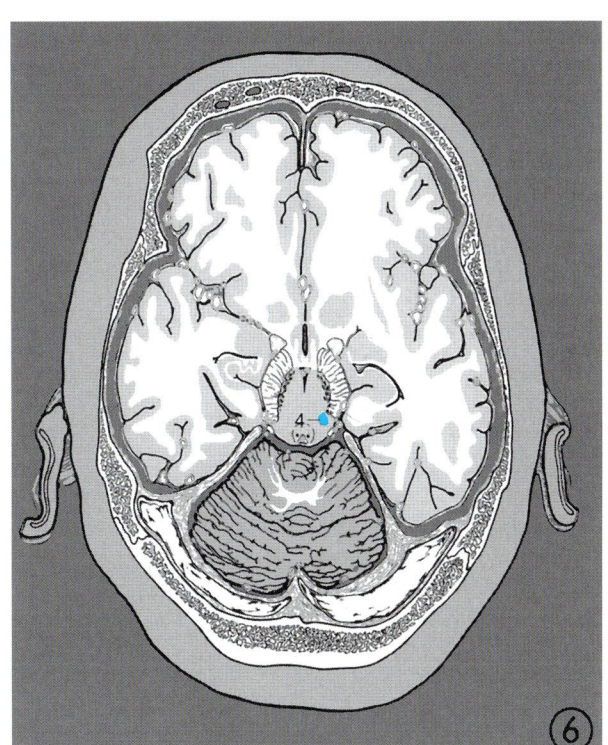

Fig. 118 Canthomeatally oriented serial illustrations of the gustatory system. The encircled numbers (3–6) indicate the number of the respective slice (Figs. 44, 45a,b, 46).

5 Ventral posteromedial nucleus of thalamus
6 Parietal operculum
7 Hypothetical fibers from thalamus to parietal operculum

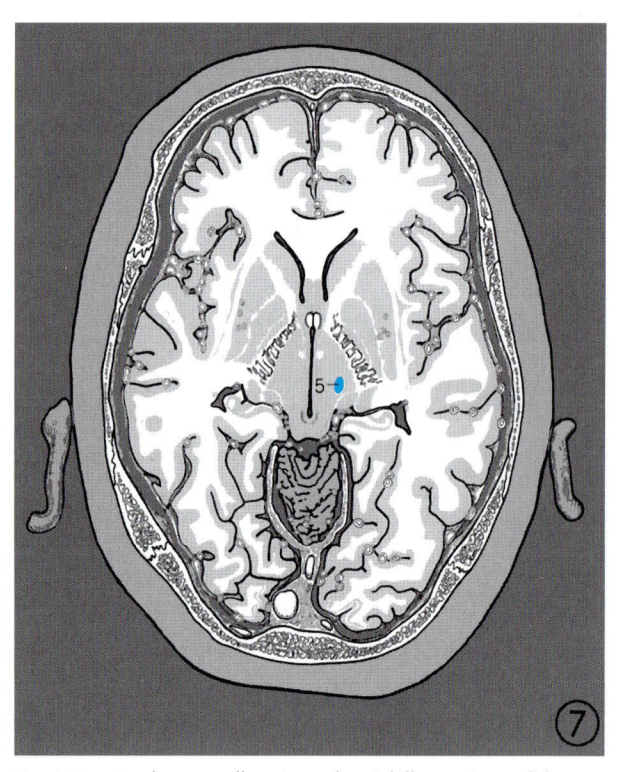

Fig. 118 Canthomeatally oriented serial illustrations of the gustatory system. The encircled numbers (7–8) indicate the number of the respective slice (Figs. 44, 45a,b, 46).

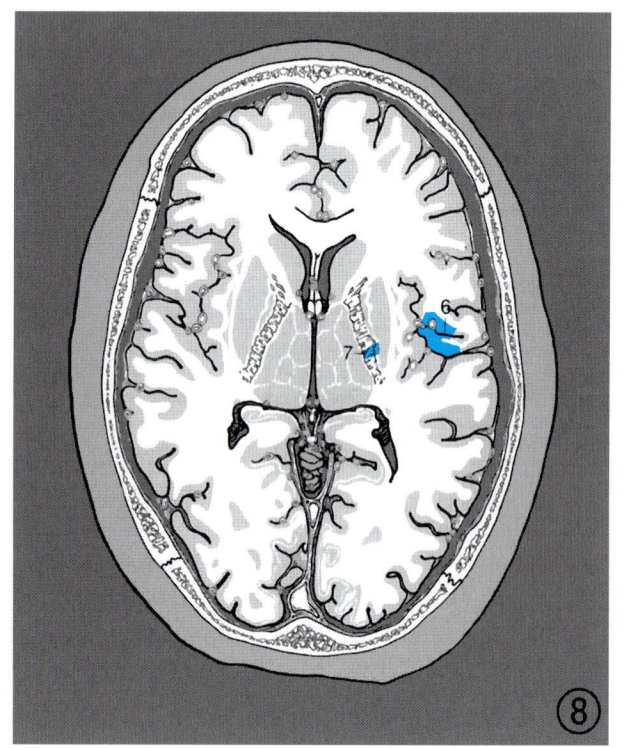

6.3 Ascending Reticular System
(Fig. 109)

The reticular formation consists of a network of organized nerve cells in the medial tegmentum of the **medulla oblongata, pons**, and **midbrain**. The cranial nerve nuclei, several relay nuclei, and the descending pathways surround the reticular formation. The medial lemniscus system passes through it. The reticular formation receives **afferent signals** from the **spinal cord** and from all **sensory cranial nerves**. These signals are relayed through the intralaminar nuclei of thalamus via widespread projections to the cerebral cortex. Due to its polysynaptic conduction of impulses and **extensive overlap**, the reticular formation forms a nonspecific system of neurons extending between the receptors and the cortical nerve cells. In contrast to this nonspecific system are specific processing systems, with a point-to-point relay between the signal-producing receptors and the nerve cells in the primary cortical areas. Examples of specific signal-processing systems include the medial lemniscus system and the visual pathway. The ascending reticular system projects into numerous subcortical centers, including the striatum, preoptic region, septal nuclei, and hypothalamus (45, 332). It should also be noted that the ascending reticular system is closely connected with the descending reticular system (55).

Clinical Notes
The complex connections of the reticular formation with the motor systems, limbic system, and other systems explain the difficulty in analyzing isolated functional disorders. The fiber system ascending from the reticular formation serves to activate the forebrain. Lesions of the reticular system may result in a disturbance of vigilance and disorders or total loss of consciousness (195, 374a, 471b, 513).

6.4 Vestibular System
(Figs. 119–121)

The receptor cells of the vestibular system are located in the **semicircular ducts** and in the **saccule** and **utricle**. The sensory cells of the semicircular ducts monitor angular acceleration of the head. The sensory cells in the saccule and utricle are in contact with small calcium carbonate crystals (otoliths) embedded in a gelatinous layer and emit signals registering the effect of linear acceleration on the head (i.e. gravitiy). In this way, information about rotation of the head or other movement of the head in space is relayed to the central nervous system (72).

The signals of angular and linear acceleration are transmitted by the neurons of the vestibular system. The perikarya of the first-order vestibular neurons are located in the internal acoustic meatus, in the **vestibular ganglion**. The peripheral axons of these bipolar cells make synaptic contact with the sensory cells of the semicircular ducts and those of the saccule and utricle. The central axons form the **vestibular nerve** (vestibular component of the eighth cranial nerve) that enters the brainstem at the cerebellopontine angle. The afferent fibers from the sensory cells of the semicircular ducts terminate primarily in the superior and medial vestibular nuclei; some branches extend directly to the flocculonodular lobe of the cerebellum. The afferent fibers triggered by the otoliths project mainly to the superior and inferior vestibular nuclei. Only a few of the primary vestibular afferent fibers from the saccule terminate in the large-celled lateral vestibular nucleus (of Deiters).

The **vestibular nuclei** receive afferent signals from the spinal cord, reticular formation, cerebellum, and cerebral cortex. Efferent connections from the lateral vestibular nucleus descend in the lateral vestibulospinal tract to the spinal cord. The remaining vestibular nuclei send their fibers via the medial longitudinal fasciculus to the motor neurons in the brainstem for the extraocular muscles and via the medial vestibulospinal tract to reach the spinal cord. These pathways form a compensatory system that stabilizes, in cases of external disturbances, the retinal image and posture of the head and trunk. Each movement of the head is followed by **vestibulo-ocular reflexes** that maintain the position of an image on the retina. In this way, constant visual orientation in space is achieved.

The vestibular system has numerous connections with the motor neurons of the eye, neck, trunk, arm, and leg muscles (vestibular reflexes).

There are a few recent reports on pathways between the vestibular system and the cerebral cortex. They are probably relayed in the small contralateral ventral intermediate nucleus of the thalamus (332) and further to a parietal cortical area around the intraparietal sulcus. The path courses further via the ventral posterolateral nucleus of the thalami to area 3 in the postcentral gyrus. This link is not demonstrated in Figures 119–121. Monkeys present further small vestibular cortical areas (area 7, parietoninsular and insular cortical areas) (73).

Clinical Notes
Vestibular system lesions result in **disturbances of equilibrium**. Acute vestibular lesions initially cause vertigo (a spinning sensation). Unilateral destruction of the vestibular system is compensated for after a period of several days or weeks, whereas bilateral lesions result in a permanently unsteady gait (110, 301, 318, 319, 471b). **Nystagmus** refers to a sequence of involuntary or reflex-released movements of both eyeballs with a slow and a rapid component that is released via the brainstem paths by saccade generators. Spontaneous nystagmus is always pathologic. A peripheral or a central lesion is to be suspected. Peripheral disorders affect the receptors in the semicircular ducts and/or the first-order vestibular neurons. Central disorders influence the second, third, and following sets of neurons of the vestibular system. Gaze-dependent nystagmus is observed as a result of lesions in the cerebellum, the brainstem, or oculomotor regions (276, 301). Fixation nystagmus can be identified by the pendular movement of the eyes upon fixation and is a congenital central disorder of the oculomotor system. Since different lesions may cause similar forms of nystagmus, the detection of a nystagmus alone is not sufficient for topical diagnosis. The nystagmus that occurs only in the abducting eye (**dissociated nystagmus**) is one of the few symptoms that can be attributed specifically to a lesion of the midline pontine tegmentum affecting the medial longitudinal fasciculus between the oculomotor and abducens nuclei. Rotatory and vertical nystagmus also indicate the presence of a central lesion.

350   6 Neurofunctional Systems

1 Parietal cortical area
2 Ventral intermediate nucleus of thalamus
3 Oculomotor nucleus
4 Trochlear nucleus
5 Vestibulothalamic tract
6 Cerebellum
7 Medial longitudinal fasciculus
8 Superior vestibular nucleus
9 Abducens nucleus
10 Vestibular nerve
11 Inferior vestibular nucleus
12 Medial vestibular nucleus
13 Lateral vestibular nucleus (of Deiters)
14 Lateral vestibulospinal tract
15 Medial vestibulospinal tract

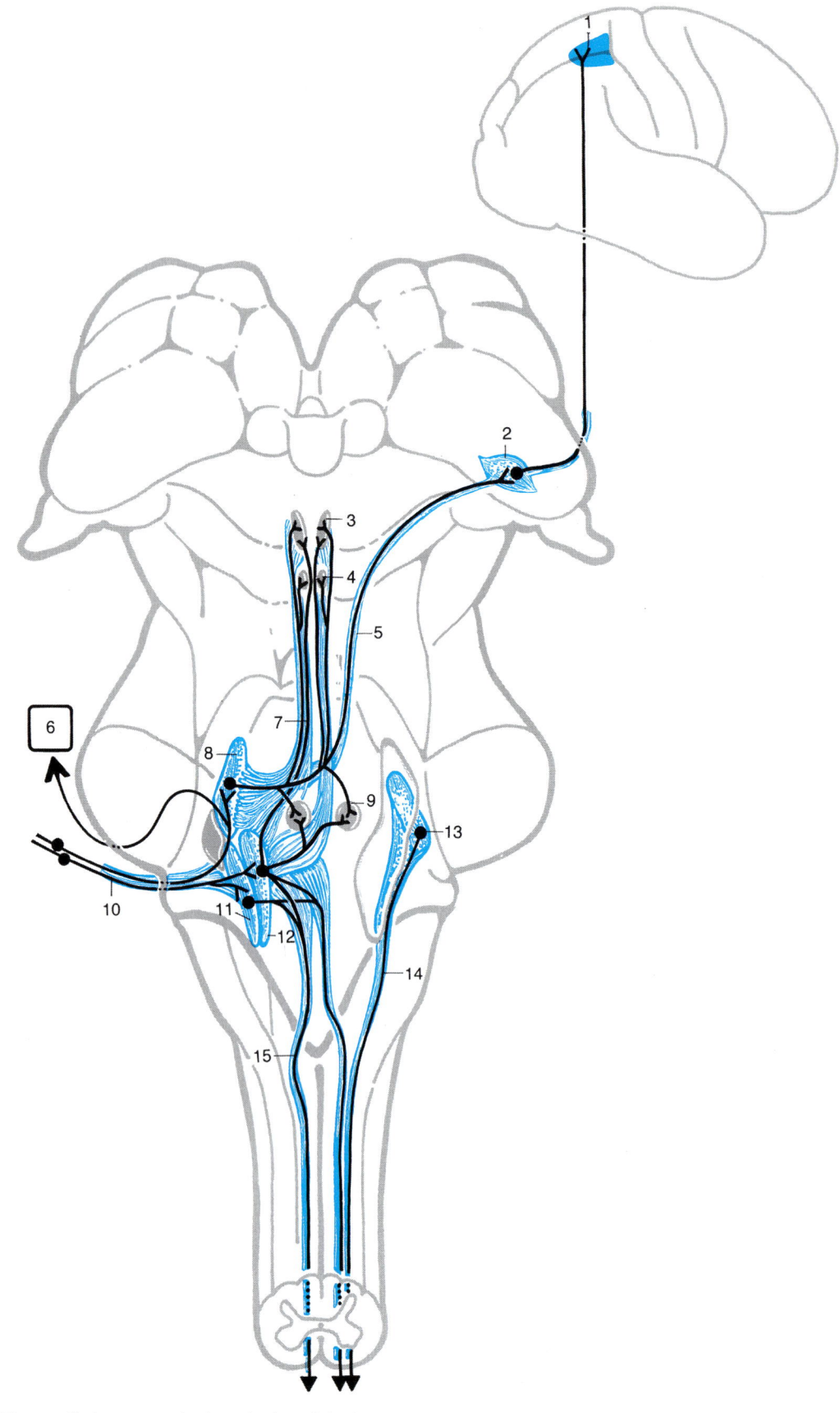

Fig. **119** The vestibular system in the spinal cord, brainstem, and diencephalon (posterior view), and in the cerebrum (lateral view). According to (332).

6.4 Vestibular System 351

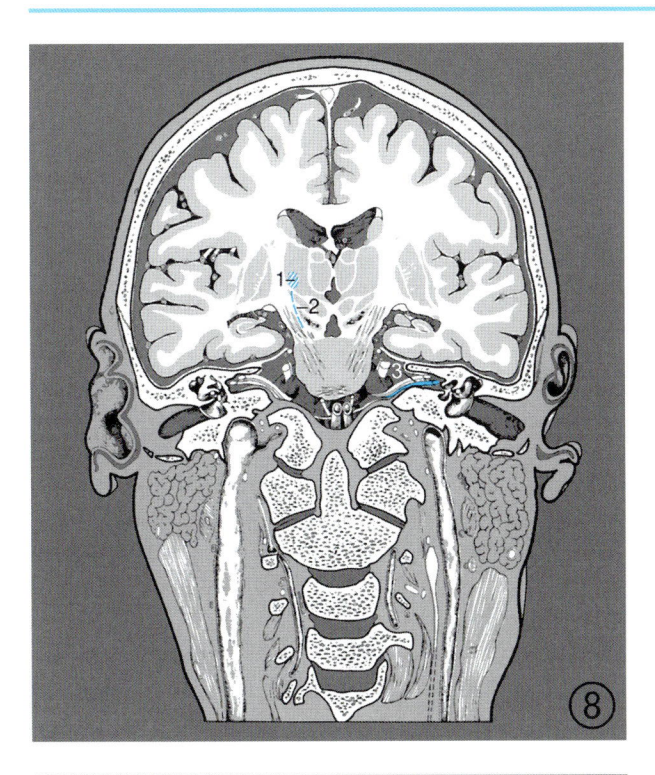

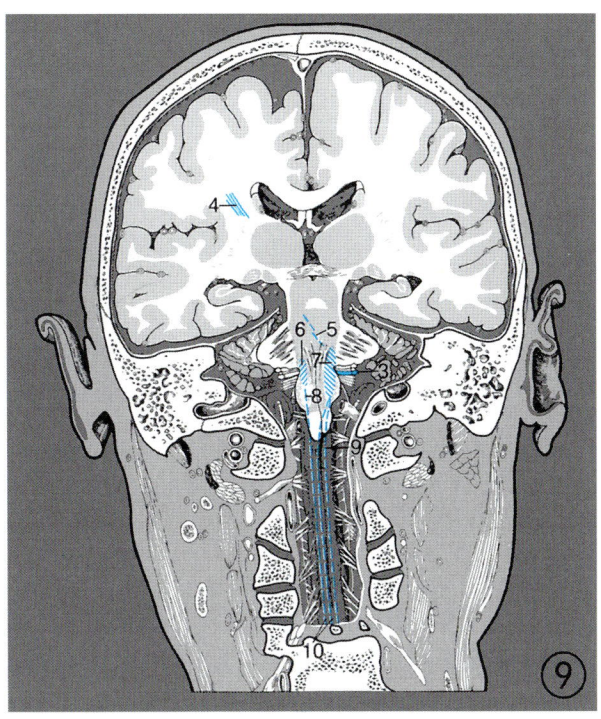

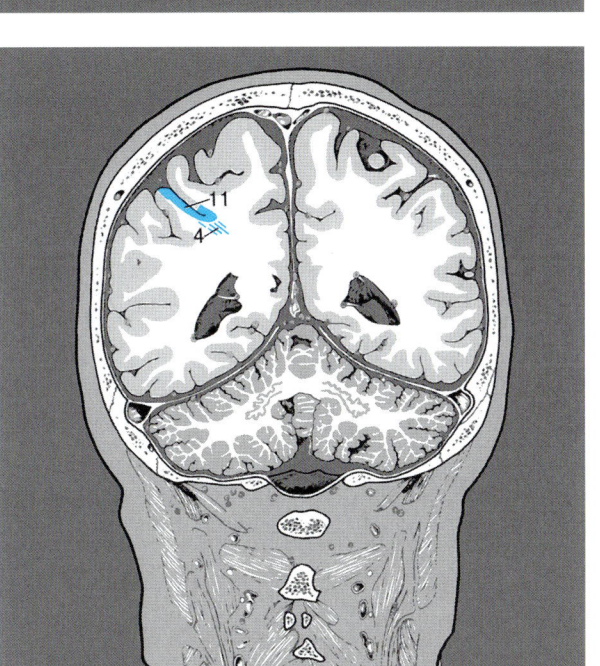

1 Ventral intermediate nucleus of thalamus (within the slice)
2 Vestibulothalamic tract (within the slice)
3 Vestibular nerve
4 Hypothetical fibers from thalamus to parietal cortical area
5 Vestibulothalamic tract
6 Lateral vestibular nucleus (of Deiters) (within the slice)
7 Vestibular nuclei (within the slice)
8 Lateral vestibulospinal tract (within the slice)
9 Medial vestibulospinal tract (within the slice)
10 Lateral and medial vestibulospinal tract (within the slice)
11 Parietal cortical area

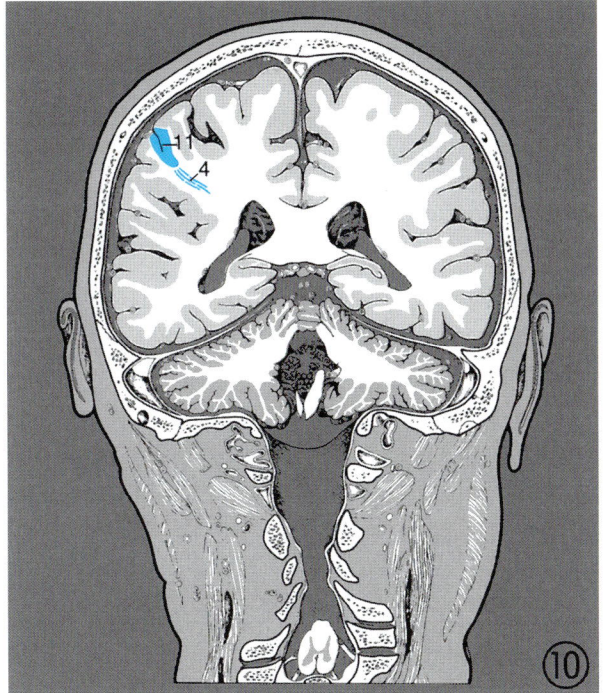

Fig. 120 Coronal serial illustrations of the vestibular system. The encircled number indicates the number of the respective slice (Figs. 1, 2a,b, 3).

352   6 Neurofunctional Systems

1 Medial vestibulospinal tract
2 Lateral vestibulospinal tract
3 Vestibular nerve
4 Vestibular nuclei
5 Lateral vestibular nucleus (of Deiters)

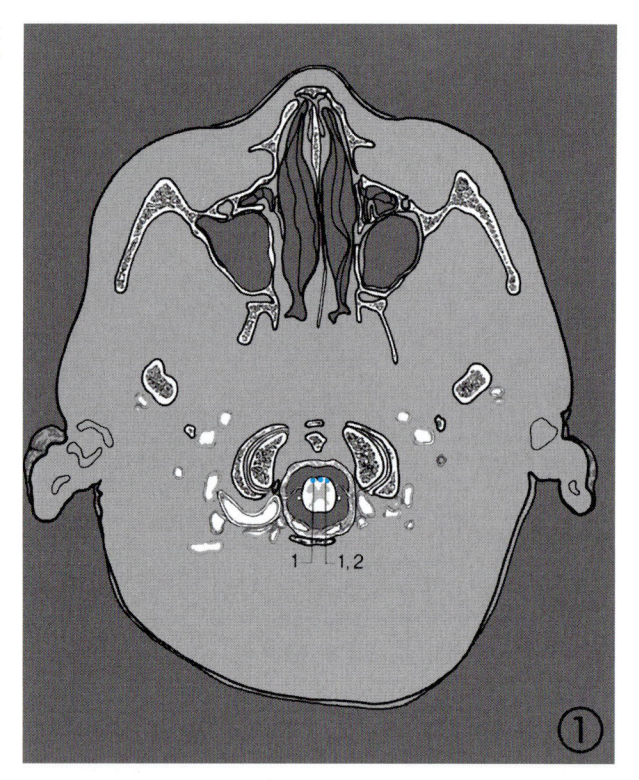

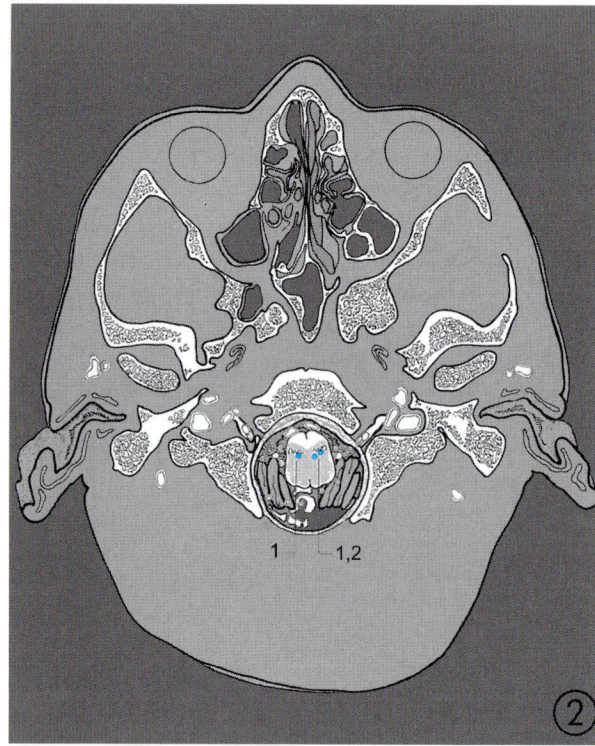

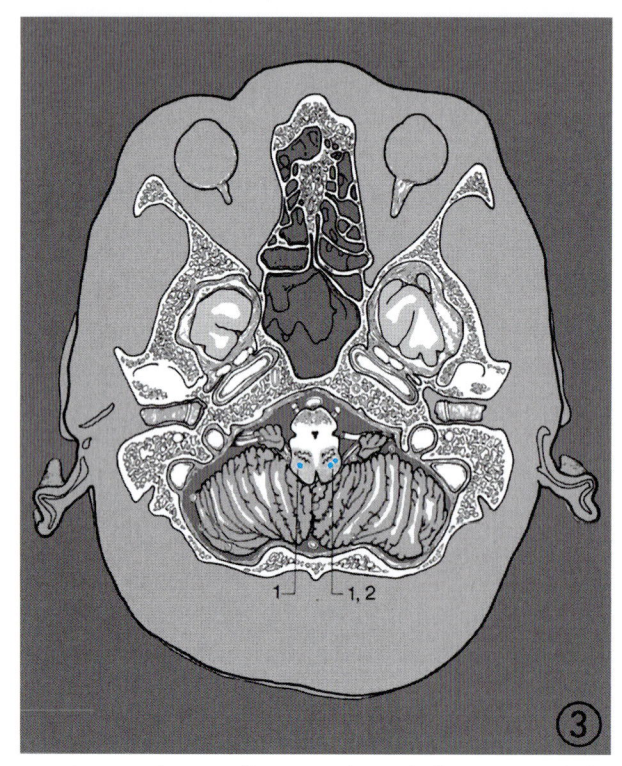

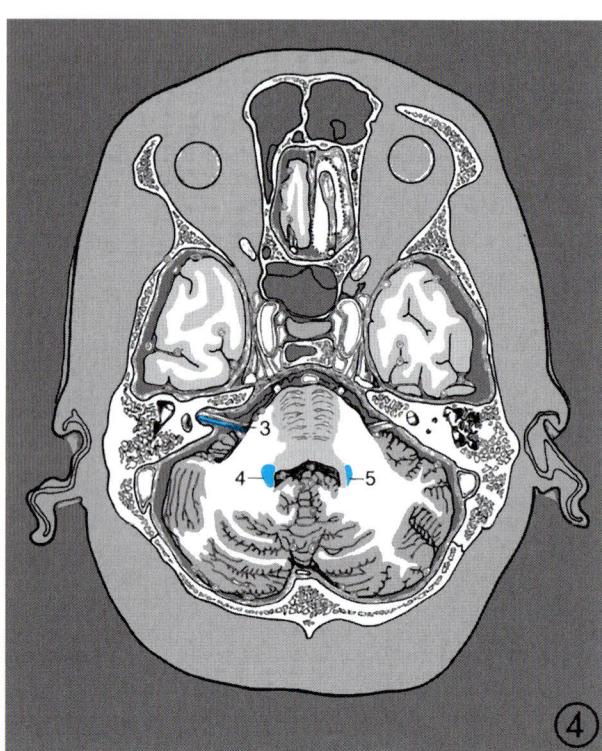

Fig. **121** Canthomeatally oriented serial illustrations of the vestibular system. The encircled numbers (1–8) indicate the number of the respective slice (Figs. 44, 45a,b, 46).

6.4 *Vestibular System* 353

6 Vestibulothalamic tract
7 Ventral intermediate nucleus of thalamus (within the slice)

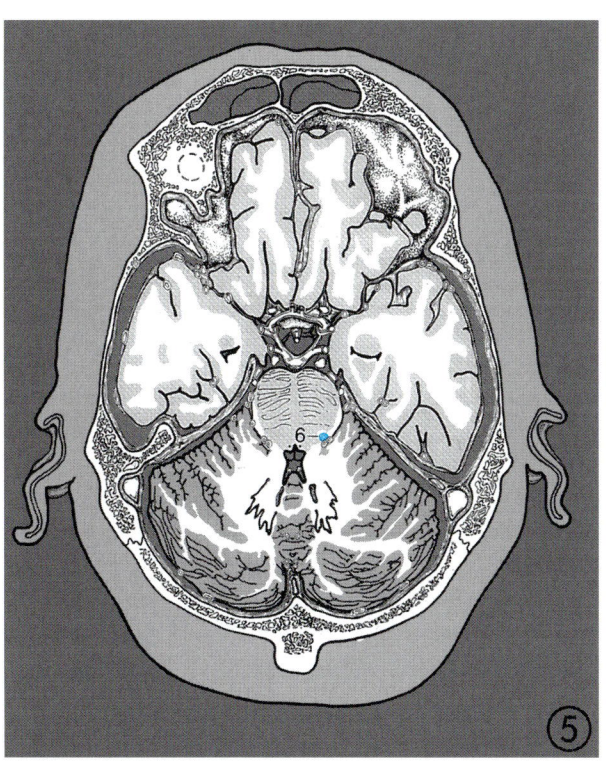

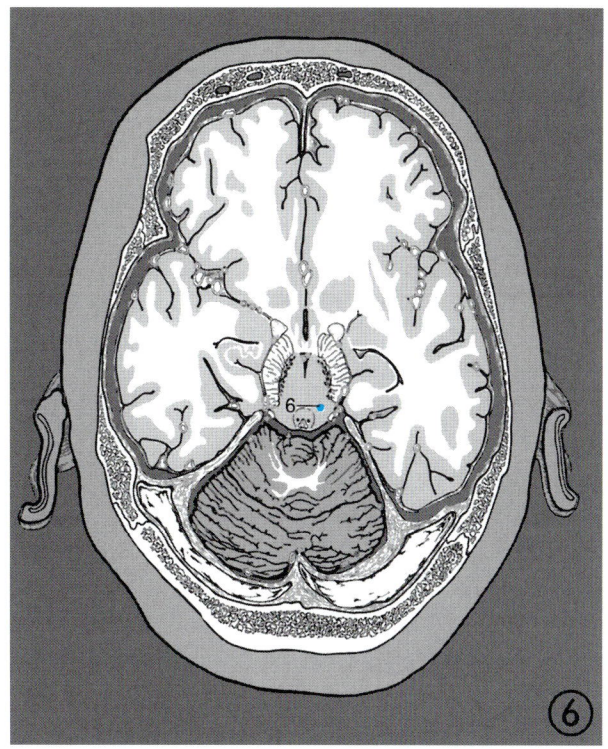

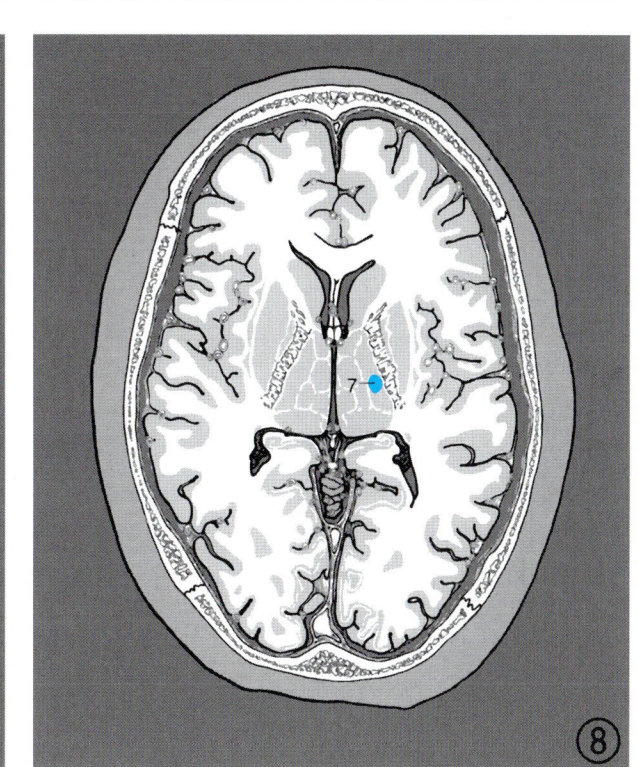

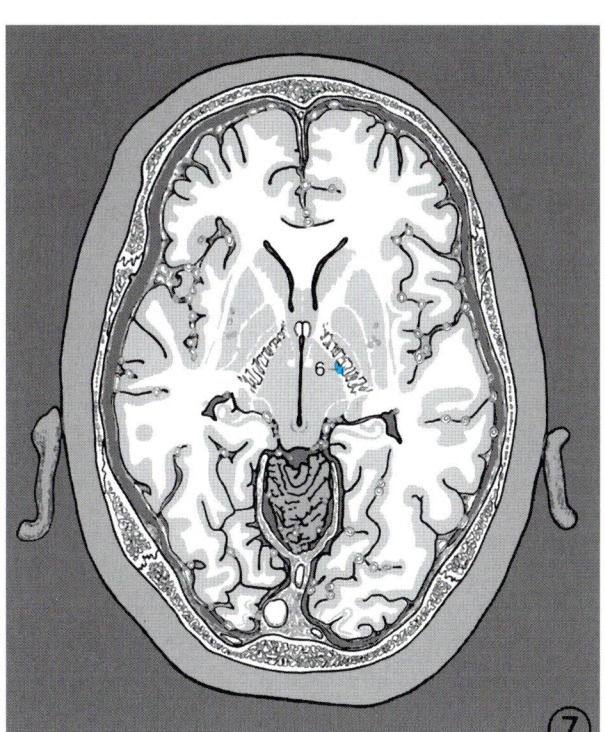

8 Hypothetical fibers from thalamus to parietal cortical area
9 Parietal cortical area

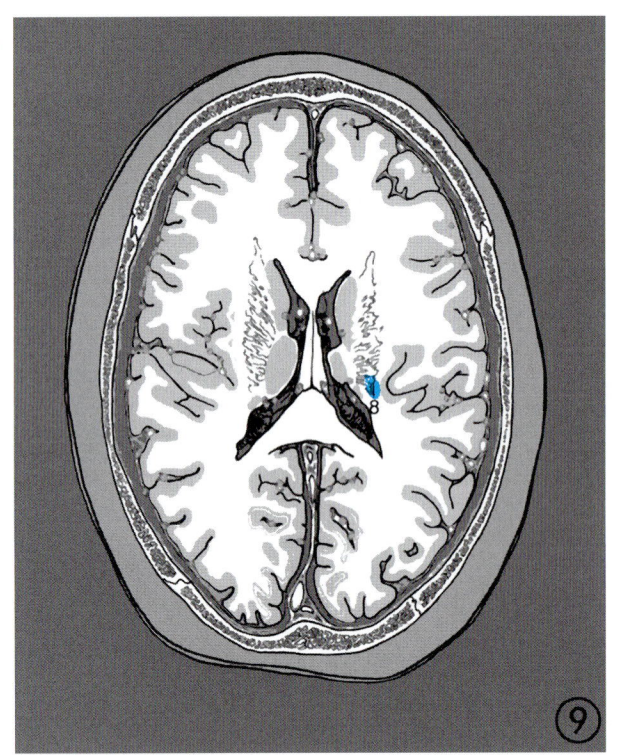

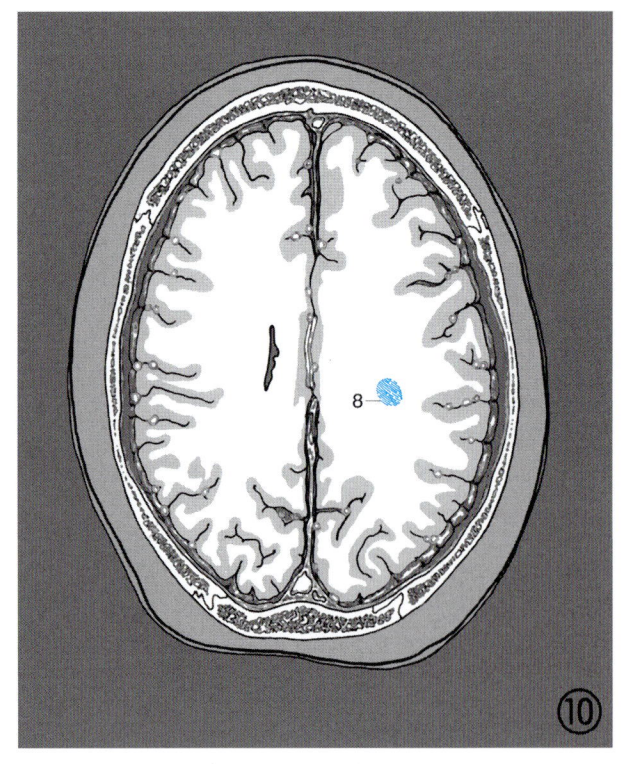

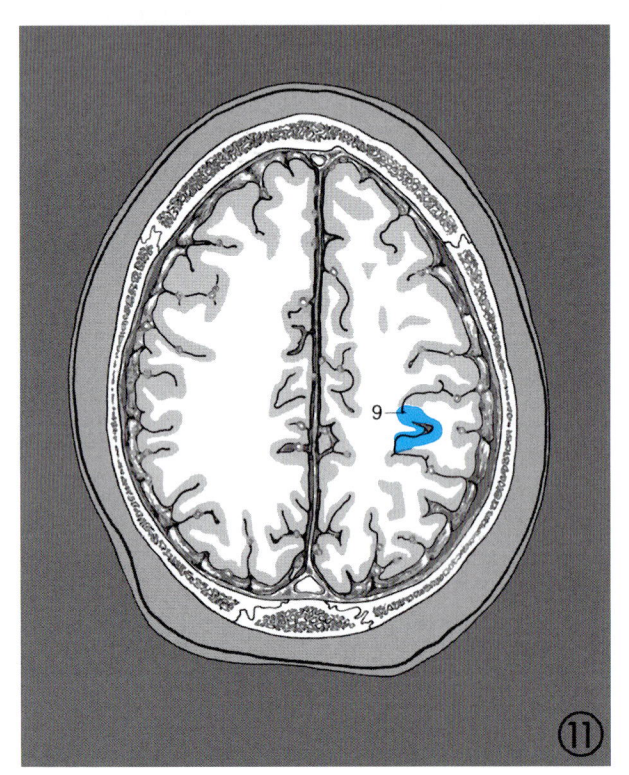

Fig. 121 Canthomeatally oriented serial illustrations of the vestibular system. The encircled numbers (9–11) indicate the number of the respective slice (Figs. 44, 45a,b, 46).

6.5 Auditory System
(Figs. 122–125)

Sound waves reach the tympanic membrane through the external acoustic meatus. The auditory ossicles mechanically amplify vibrations in the middle ear and transmit them onto the oval window. The resulting movements of the endolymph are received by the **hair cells of the spiral organ** (of Corti) in the inner ear and are transmitted to the chain of neurons in the auditory system. Anatomically speaking, retrocochlear hearing impairment is a lesion of this chain of neurons. The first-order neurons of this chain are formed in the cochlea by the bipolar nerve cells of the **spiral ganglion**. Their peripheral processes innervate the bases of the hair cells in the spiral organ of Corti. The central axons of the bipolar ganglion cells form the **cochlear nerve** (cochlear division of the eighth cranial nerve). The axons emerge near the opening of the internal acoustic meatus from the petrous part of the temporal bone and enter the medulla oblongata at the cerebellopontine angle. The central axons subsequently divide into two branches, one extending toward the posterior cochlear nucleus and the other toward the anterior cochlear nucleus. The second-order auditory neurons are located in these two nuclei.

- The axons of the **posterior cochlear nucleus** belong to the posterior part of the auditory pathway and pass along the floor of the rhomboid fossa just beneath the medullary striae of the fourth ventricle. They cross over to the opposite side and ascend in the **lateral lemniscus** to reach the **inferior colliculus**. Along the way, additional neurons may be interposed. The axons of the nerve cells of the inferior colliculus conduct the auditory signals by way of the brachium of the inferior colliculus to the **medial geniculate body**. The final neurons of this auditory chain extend from the medial geniculate body through the auditory radiation to the **primary auditory cortex** (area 41). The latter is located approximately in the **anterior transverse temporal gyrus** (of Heschl) on the superior bank of the temporal lobe. The anterior transverse temporal gyrus is hidden within the lateral sulcus and is only visible if the frontal and parietal opercula of the insula are removed.

- The anterior auditory pathway in the trapezoid body extends from the **anterior cochlear nucleus** to the **superior olivary nucleus** and the nuclei of the trapezoid body, crossing to the **opposite side** to join the **lateral lemniscus**. The pathway then continues in the same manner as the posterior part of the auditory pathway already described. A second portion of the anterior auditory pathway remains on the same side, ascending **ipsilaterally** through the above-mentioned auditory chain centers to the **primary auditory cortex** (area 41).

The ipsilateral and contralateral course of the auditory pathway enables highly specialized neurons to determine the time difference of a sound source located further from one ear than from the other. In this way the **direction of a sound source** can be localized by hearing alone. The second-order and higher auditory neurons are specialized to interpret the specific sound patterns. The second-order and higher neurons are able to filter out the useful sounds, for example, linguistic information from the background noise.

The **posterior and anterior cochlear nuclei** (Fig. 72b.26) are found in the medulla oblongata at the entry site of the vestibulocochlear nerve at the medullopontine junction (459). The cochlear nuclei are found close to the surface of the medulla oblongata at the level of the lateral aperture of the fourth ventricle (Fig. 72a.15). The cochlear nuclei are bordered anteromedially by the inferior cerebellar peduncle, which is used for indirect localization of the cochlear nuclei in MR images (14).

Only the anterior part of the auditory pathway is represented in Figures 123–125. This part courses through the **trapezoid body**. The fibers of the trapezoid body leave the cochlear nuclei at their anterior border. They run anteriorly in a gradual upward direction around the inferior cerebellar peduncle and continue to the ipsilateral and contralateral auditory complex consisting of the superior olivary nucleus and the nuclei of the trapezoid body. The fibers are situated posterior to the pontine nuclei in the inferior region of the pons and cross the anterior part of the medial lemniscus. In MR images the trapezoid body can be located directly and in topographic relation to the position of the medial lemniscus (14).

The **lateral lemniscus** (Figs. 74b.20, 75b.18, 76b.18) originates at the superior olivary nucleus and in the nuclei of the trapezoid body. It terminates in the inferior colliculus (Fig. 77b.34). Its length is about 25 mm. The auditory signals may be relayed through synapses in one or more nuclei of the lateral lemniscus. Our Figures 122–125 show no demarcation of these nuclei of the lateral lemniscus. The medial lemniscus runs upward in the lateral part of the tegmentum of the pons and lies in the transition between the pons and midbrain immediately beneath the posterolateral surface of the tegmentum pontis. Close to the inferior colliculus it borders on the lateral surface of the superior cerebellar peduncle. The lateral lemniscus enters the inferior colliculus anterolaterally. In axial T2-weighted MR images the position of the lateral lemniscus can be immediately determined by its contrast with the neighboring structures (97).

The **inferior colliculus** can be identified posterior to the aqueduct in the first sagittal slice by the inferior bulge of the tectal (quadrigeminal) plate (Fig. 32a.19). Because of its exposed position, the inferior colliculus can be clearly seen on sagittal, axial, and coronal MR images (14, 404).

The axons of the nerve cells of the inferior colliculus form the **brachium of inferior colliculus**. They collect together as a narrow band of fibers on the lateral side of the tegmentum of the midbrain. At the junction of the midbrain with the diencephalon the brachium of the inferior colliculus curves laterally over about 5 mm to enter the medial geniculate body on its posteromedial aspect.

The **medial geniculate body** is positioned lateral to the tegmentum of the midbrain in the junctional region of the diencephalon with midbrain. The anterior surface of the medial geniculate body borders on the internal capsule (Fig. 34a.15). The largest diameter of the medial geniculate body is around 8 to 9 mm and it has a vertical span of 5 to 6 mm.

It is made up of three parts:
- The largest nuclear area, the parvocellular, principal division receives purely auditory signals (217).
- The magnocellular medial division is posteromedial to the principal nucleus (312). Electrophysiological investigations indicate that it receives somatosensory, vestibular, and auditory afferents and is, therefore, multimodal (7, 312).
- The small triangular division is a nuclear area receiving visual and auditory signals.
  The fibers of the medial geniculate body leave as the acoustic radiation in an anterolateral direction (243, 244).

The **acoustic radiation** interconnects the medial geniculate body with the primary auditory cortex. This radiation was described in humans for the first time in connection with myelogenetic microscopic specimens of infant brains (360). Further details were given following later investigations (53, 247). The acoustic radiation ascends from the anterolateral border of the medial geniculate body, curving in a lateral direction. It lies above the optic tract and

356 6 Neurofunctional Systems

1 Optic chiasm
2 Temporal lobe
3 Third ventricle
4 Primary auditory cortex in transverse temporal gyrus (of Heschl)
5 Thalamus
6 Pineal gland
7 Lateral ventricle
8 Splenium of corpus callosum
9 Acoustic radiation
10 Medial geniculate body
11 Brachium of inferior colliculus
12 Inferior colliculus
13 Commissure of inferior colliculus
14 Nucleus of lateral lemniscus
15 Lateral lemniscus
16 Pons
17 Superior olivary nucleus
18 Bipolar nerve cells in spiral ganglion
19 Cochlear nerve
20 Anterior (ventral) cochlear nucleus
21 Trapezoid body
22 Nuclei of trapezoid body
23 Posterior (dorsal) cochlear nucleus
24 Posterior acoustic stria
25 Medulla oblongata

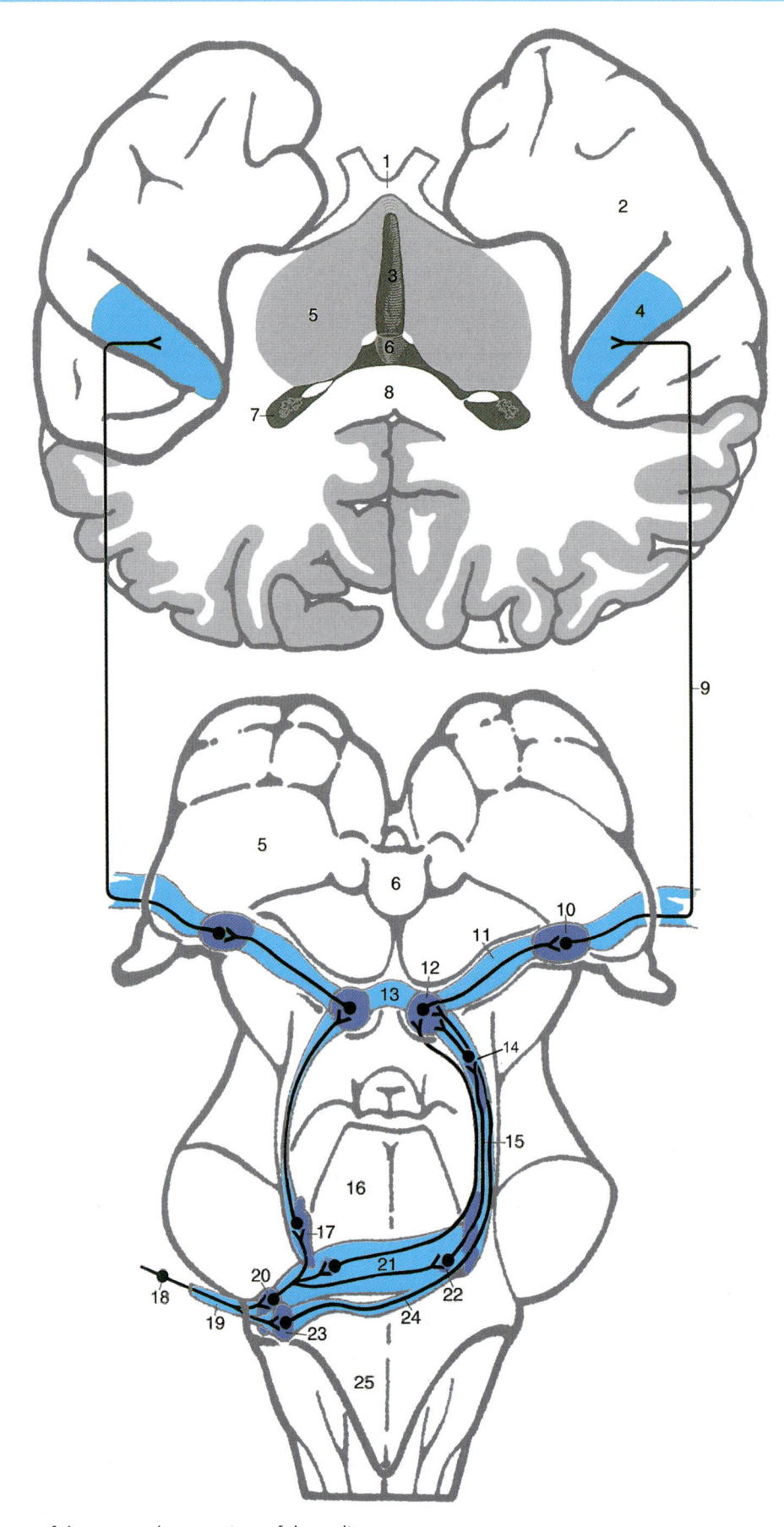

Fig. 122 Diagram of the neuronal connections of the auditory system in a posterior view of the brainstem and the diencephalon and in a superior view of both temporal lobes and the cut surface coursing just above the optic chiasm and through the middle of the splenium of the corpus callosum. This plane lies anteriorly approximately 20° below and posteriorly approximately 20° above the bicommissural plane. Modified according to (332).

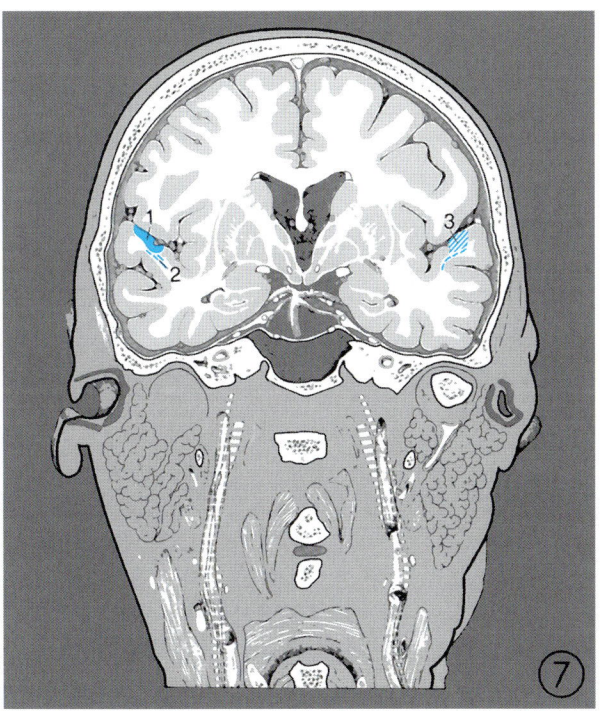

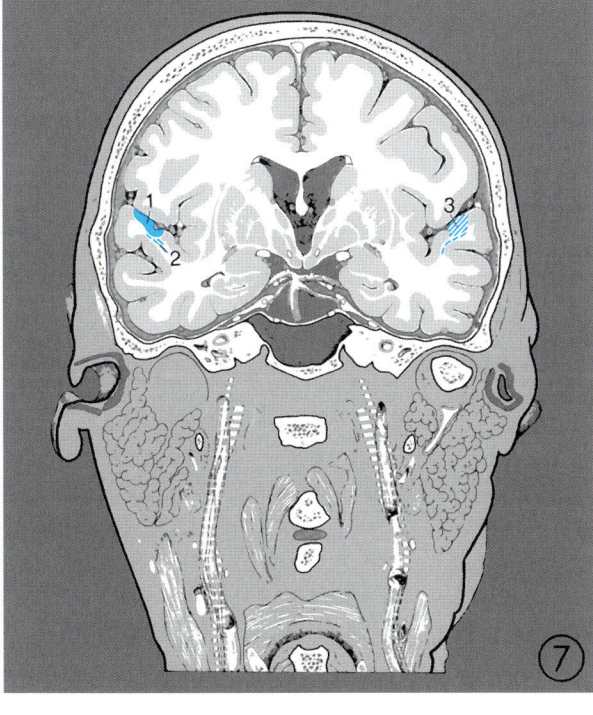

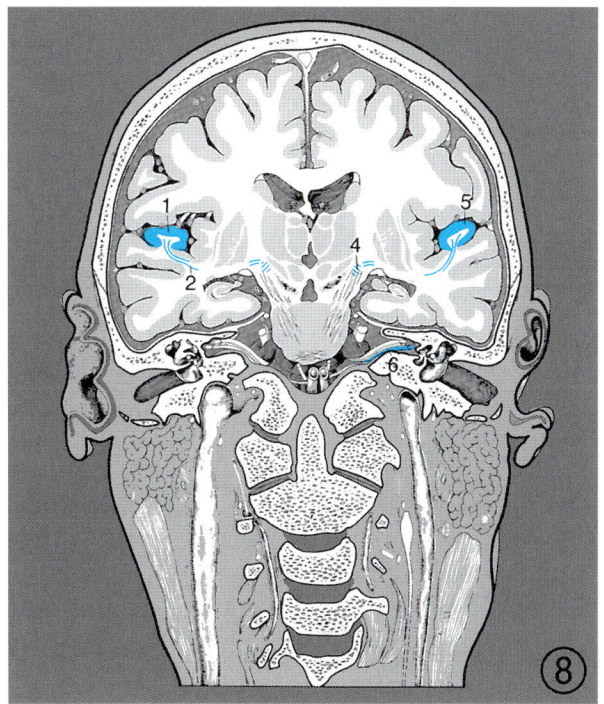

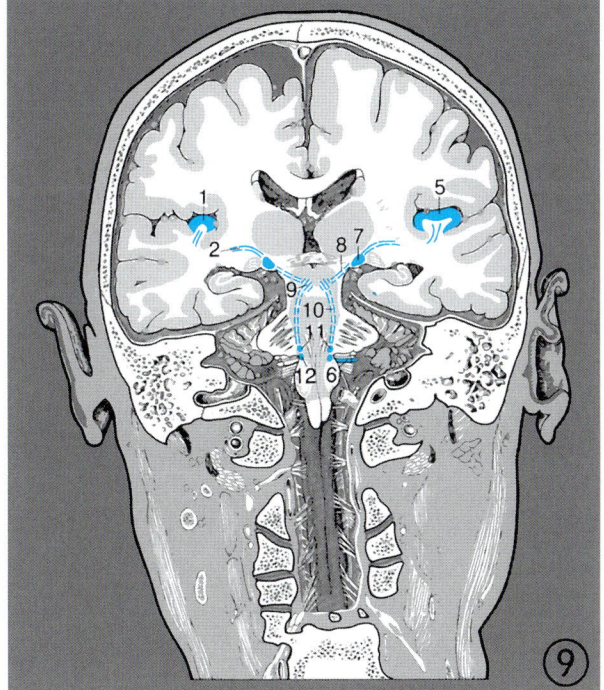

6.5 Auditory System

1 Anterior transverse temporal gyrus (of Heschl)
2 Acoustic radiation
3 Transverse temporal gyrus (of Heschl) (in the posterior part of the slice)
4 Medial geniculate body (in the posterior part of the slice)
5 Transverse temporal gyrus (of Heschl)
6 Cochlear nerve
7 Medial geniculate body
8 Brachium of inferior colliculus
9 Inferior colliculus (in the posterior part of the slice)
10 Lateral lemniscus (within the slice)
11 Superior olivary nucleus
12 Anterior (ventral) and posterior (dorsal) cochlear nuclei (within the slice)

Fig. 123 Coronal serial illustrations of the auditory system. The encircled number indicates the number of the respective slice (Figs. 1, 2a,b, 3). The ipsilateral and contralateral parts of the anterior auditory pathway are shown to emerge from the left cochlear nerve. Two transverse temporal gyri are present in the right hemisphere.

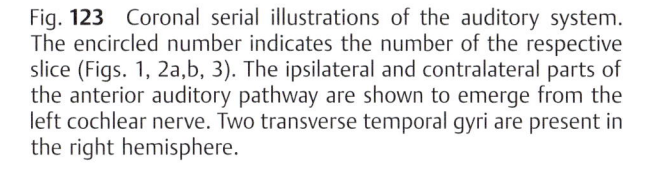

below the thalamoparietal fibers. As it projects anterolaterally, it passes over the lateral geniculate body and below the pulvinar. The acoustic radiation extends through the retrolentiform part behind the posterior limb of the internal capsule and then passes posterior to the lateral part of the globus pallidus, the putamen and the claustrum. Finally, the acoustic radiation curves in an anterior direction around the posterior border of the insular cortex and ascends into the white substance of the transverse temporal gyrus to reach the primary auditory cortex.

The **primary auditory cortex** is cytoarchitectonically cited as area 41 (514). Brodmann (56) localized area 41 in the region around the transverse temporal gyrus (of Heschl). Area 41 extends in an anterior direction over the transverse temporal gyrus. Area 42 forms an arc around area 41. Using pigmentoarchitectural methods the primary auditory cortex is indicated in the medial part of the gyrus of Heschl and a small bordering part of the temporal plane (46, 47, 465). Generally, two transverse temporal gyri are found on the right side (anterior and posterior transverse temporal gyri), and one gyrus on the left side (138, 139). The anterior transverse temporal gyrus is easily identified in axial, coronal, and sagittal MR images (14, 505, 508).

6 Neurofunctional Systems

1 Inferior colliculus
2 Lateral lemniscus (in the lateral part of the slice)
3 Trapezoid body
4 Medullary striae of fourth ventricle
5 Brachium of inferior colliculus
6 Lateral lemniscus
7 Superior olivary nucleus
8 Cochlear nerve (within the slice)
9 Posterior (dorsal) and anterior (ventral) cochlear nuclei (within the slice)
10 Acoustic radiation (in the lateral part of the slice)
11 Medial geniculate body
12 Cochlear nerve
13 Acoustic radiation (partially within the slice)

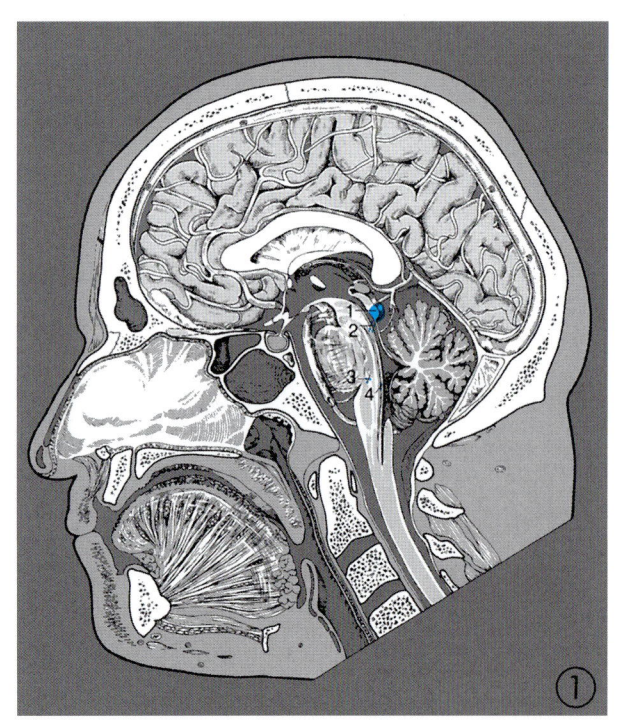

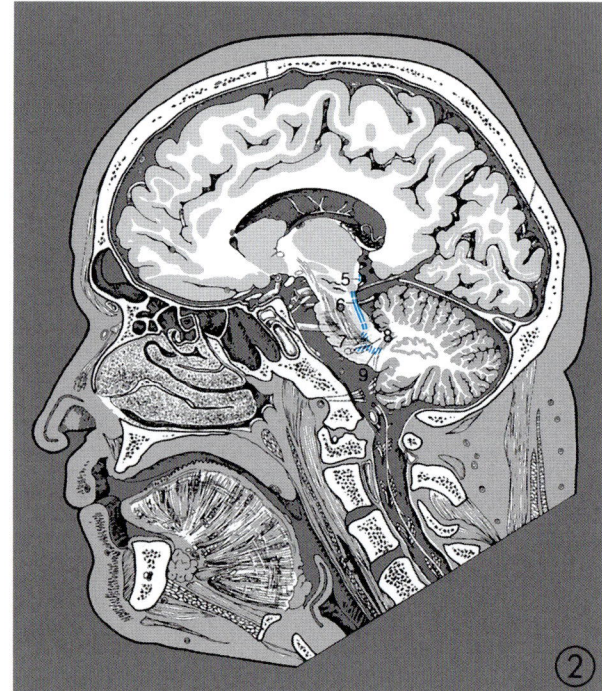

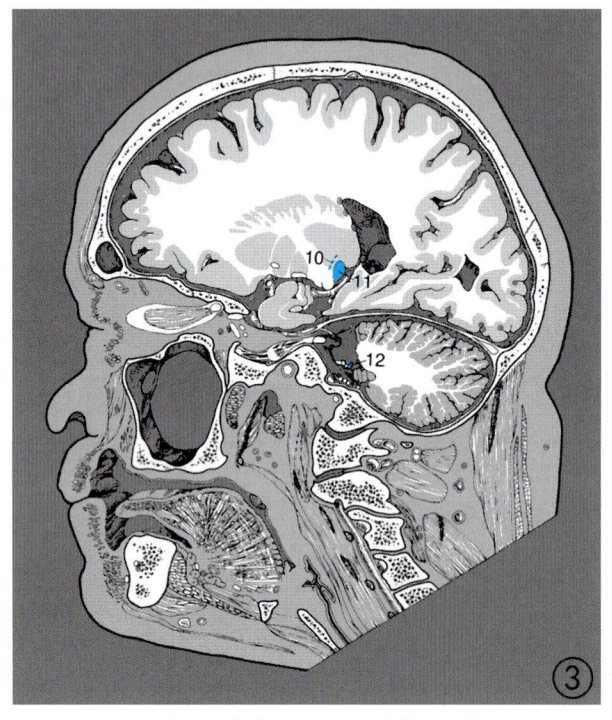

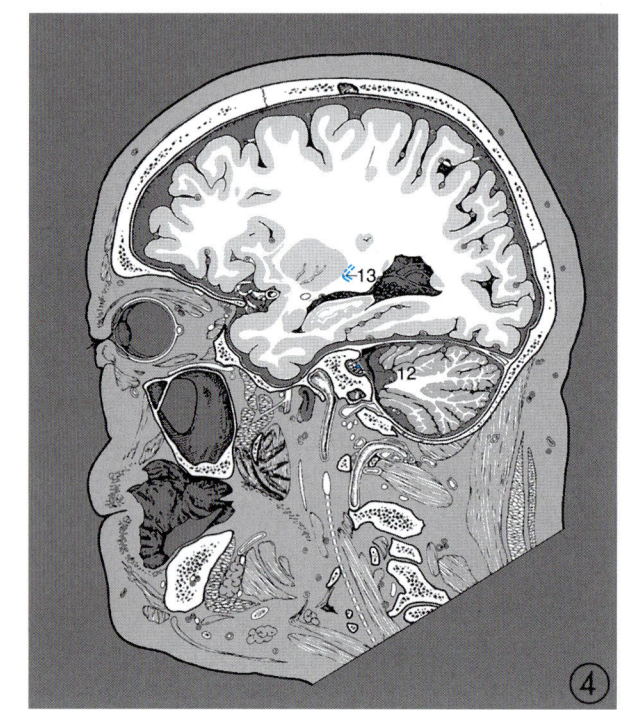

Fig. 124 Sagittal serial illustrations of the auditory system. The encircled number indicates the number of the respective slice (Figs. 29, 30a,b, 31).

Electrophysiological studies conducted on 20 patients with the help of auditory evoked potentials, showed that short latency evoked potentials were constant in the medial two-thirds of the anterior and posterior transverse temporal gyri (78, 283). The area surrounding the temporal plane and the superior temporal gyrus revealed evoked potentials with smaller amplitudes and long latencies.

The computer-generated images show that the auditory system compared to the medial lemniscus system and the visual system is the shortest pathway to its primary cortical area (243, 244).

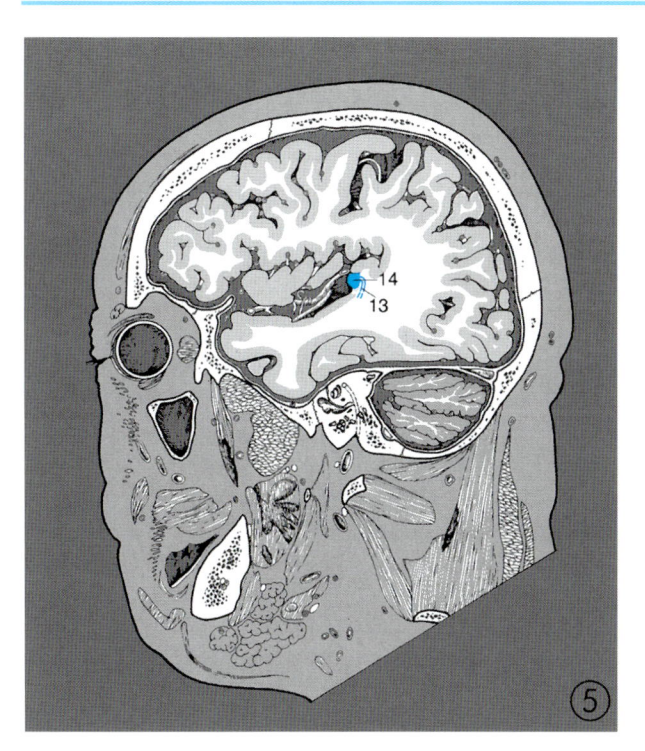

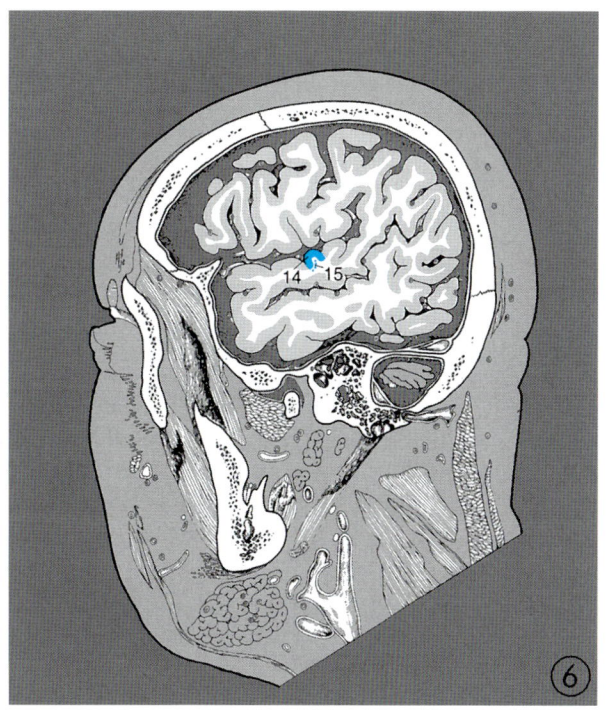

13 Acoustic radiation (partially within the slice)
14 Anterior transverse temporal gyrus (of Heschl)
15 Acoustic radiation

Clinical Notes
Several of the nuclei mentioned are not merely relay nuclei but also reflex centers, through which the nuclei of the trapezoid body are connected with the motor nuclei of the seventh cranial nerve. In this manner, a reflex arc is formed from the spiral organ of Corti to the stapedius. As a reflex response to high intensity tones, the muscle contracts and consequently dampens the transmission of sound waves from the tympanic membrane to the stapes. Loss of this reflex results in hyperacusis (excessive sensitivity to loud sounds). A similar reflex pathway controls the tensor tympani to reduce the loudness of one's own voice.

Additional reflex pathways extend from the inferior colliculus to the superior colliculus. These pathways modulate reflexes associated with eye and head movements caused by auditory stimuli. Furthermore, the neurons of the reticular formation are interconnected with the ascending portion of the auditory pathway.

A pathway from the auditory cortex and the inferior colliculi descends to the periolivary nuclei in the inferior portion of the pons. Originating in a subnucleus of the trapezoid body (periolivary nucleus), an efferent pathway (olivocochlear tract of Rasmussen) extends into the cochlea and terminates on the outer hair cells of the spiral organ (of Corti). This tract contains cholinergic and enkephalinergic fibers (Chaps. 7.4, 7.7.4). Experimentally, impulses arising in the auditory nerve can be suppressed by stimulation of this olivocochlear tract.

Clinical Notes
Clinically, middle ear, cochlear, and retrocochlear hearing impairments can be differentiated. Recognition of middle ear deafness involves a simple examination using a tuning fork. To distinguish a cochlear or retrocochlear hearing defect, audiometry and neurophysiologic tests such as the computerized auditory evoked potentials (AEP) or brainstem acoustic evoked potential (BAEP) (formerly brainstem electric response audiometry [BERA]) are utilized. The early acoustic evoked brainstem potentials have been differently described in the international nomenclature (301, 446). Recording of the AEP by surface electrodes after repeated acoustic stimuli enables localization of the lesions at various levels in the brainstem (80a, 167a, 288).

If an **acoustic schwannoma** or another space-occupying lesion is suspected in the cerebellopontine angle, together with central disturbances of hearing, then MRI is preferred. CT with thin slices and the use of i. v. contrast medium is the second choice of diagnostic technique.

1 Cochlear nerve
2 Cochlear nuclei (within the slice)
3 Trapezoid body (within the slice)
4 Lateral lemniscus
5 Medial geniculate body
6 Brachium of inferior colliculus
7 Inferior colliculus

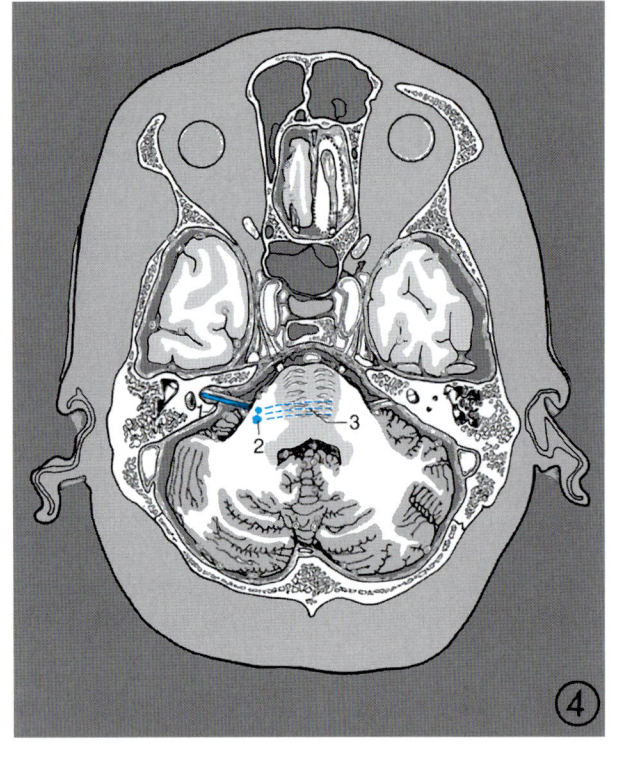

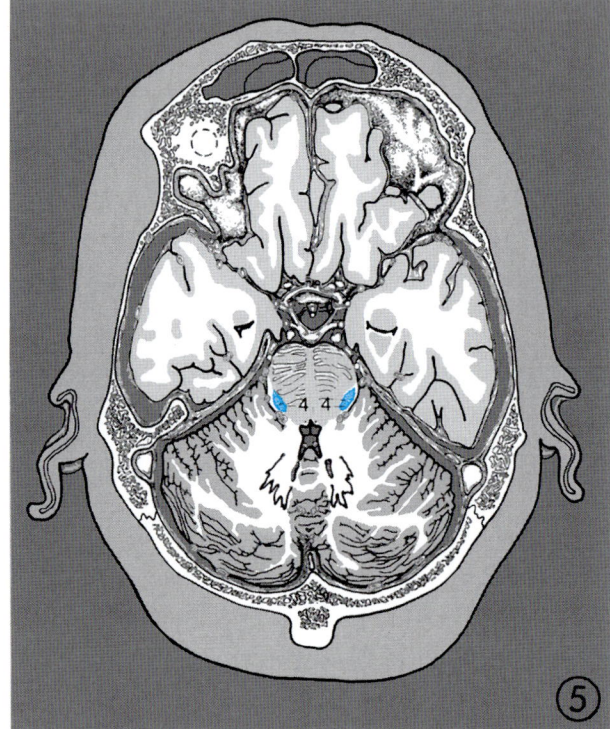

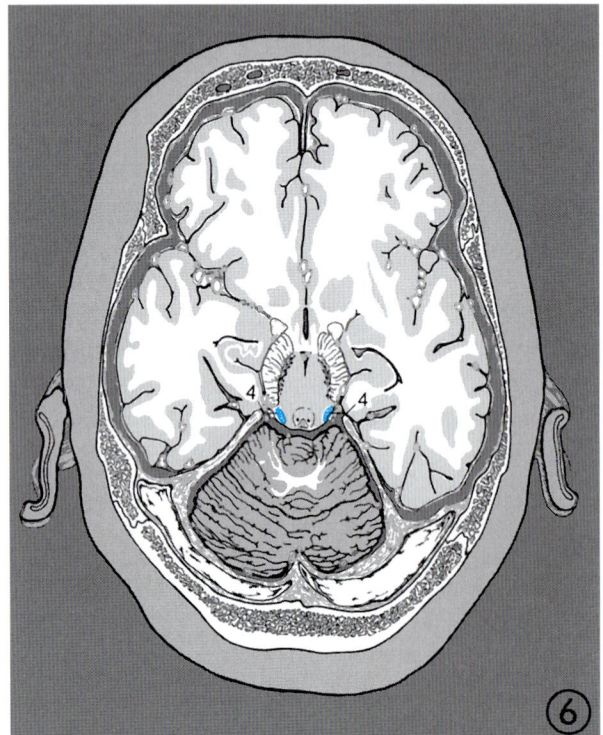

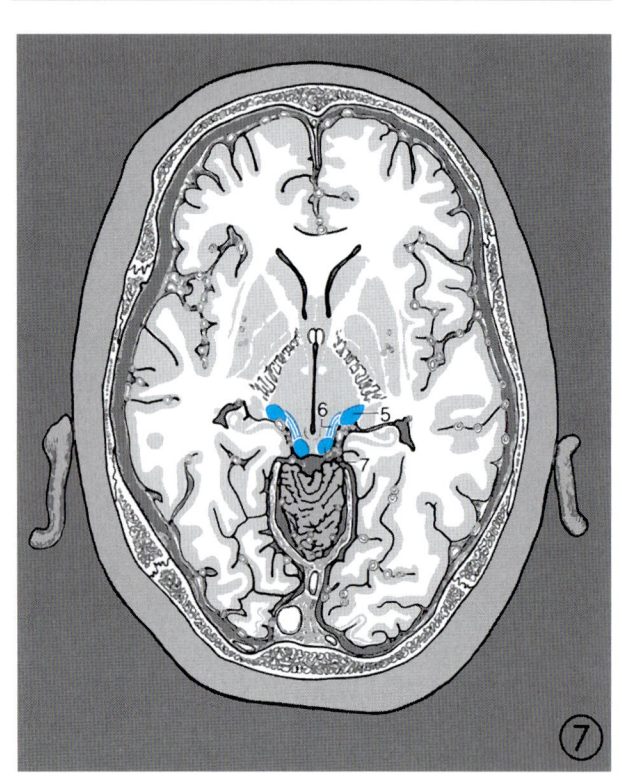

Fig. 125 Canthomeatally oriented serial illustrations of the auditory system. The encircled number indicates the number of the respective slice (Figs. 44, 45a,b, 46).

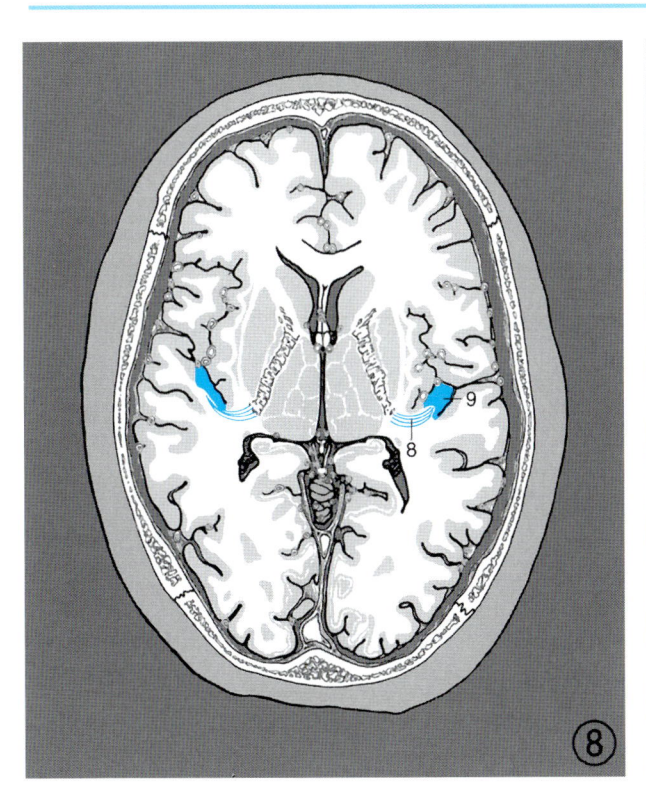

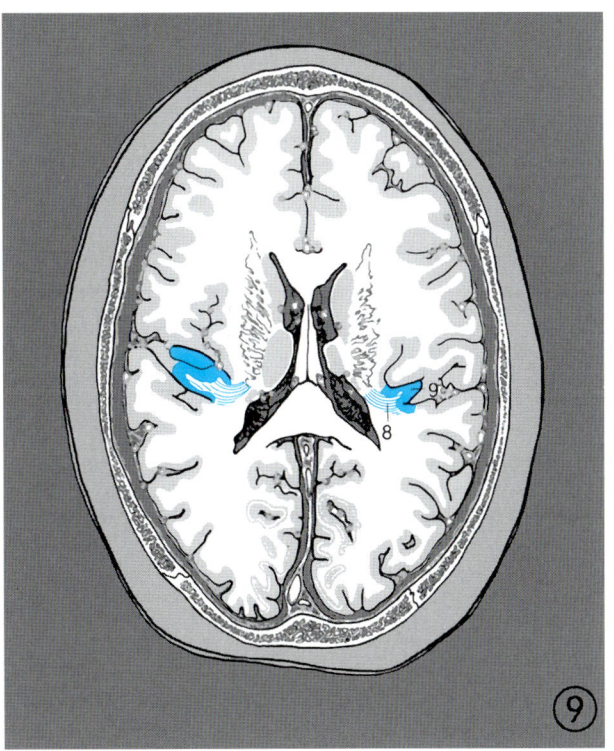

8 Acoustic radiation
9 Transverse temporal gyrus (of Heschl)

6.6 Visual System
(Figs. 126–129)

The photoreceptors of the visual system are located in the **retina**. Optical signals emitted from the rods and cones are transmitted through bipolar nerve cells to large multipolar ganglion cells. The axons of these ganglion cells extend along the inner layer of the retina and converge at the optic disc. These axons pass through the lamina cribrosa of the sclera and form the optic nerve. Within the orbit, the **optic nerve** measures 3 cm in length and pursues a slightly curved course to allow for free eye movements. The optic nerve crosses the canthomeatal plane at an acute angle and can, therefore, be seen in three of the 1-cm-thick slices (Fig. 129.2). Within the orbit, the optic nerve is sheathed by the pia, arachnoid, and dura mater with a narrow subarachnoid space. Whenever the eye rotates laterally, the optic nerve is repositioned somewhat medially in the orbit (396). The optic nerve proceeds through the **optic canal** a bony channel approximately 5 mm in length, to reach the **optic chiasm** (Fig. 129.3).

Inferior to the optic chiasm lie the sphenoidal sinus and the sella turcica containing the pituitary gland (hypophysis). The optic chiasm is located in front of the hypothalamus and medial to the internal carotid arteries. Fibers from the nasal half of the retina only (temporal visual field) cross in the optic chiasm, while fibers from the temporal half of the retina (nasal visual field) remain on the same side.

The **crossed and uncrossed fibers** form the **optic tract**, which is approximately 4 cm long. This arches along the border between the diencephalon and telencephalon to the lateral geniculate body where most of the fibers terminate (Figs. 127.7, 128.8, 129.5).

The **lateral geniculate body** is situated inferior to the pulvinar of the thalamus and immediately lateral to the medial geniculate body. The largest axial cut area of the lateral geniculate body resembles the shape of a hat, with a diameter of approximately 8 to 9 mm. Microscopically, the body is made up of six cell layers separated by thin white zones (fibers of the optic tract). Most fibers of the optic tract terminate in the lateral geniculate body. The crossed optic nerve fibers terminate in layers 1, 4, and 6, the uncrossed fibers in layers 2, 3, and 5. Layers 1 and 2 are made up of magnocellular nerve cells; these cells serve movement detection. The other layers 3 to 6 are parvocellular nerve cells; these cells serve recongnition of visual details and colors (127, 221).

About 10% of the optic tract fibers extend to the superior colliculi and pretectal areas. The reflexes of the intrinsic and extraocular muscles are modulated via this portion of the optic nerve. A third group of fibers forms the extrageniculate pathway leading to the cerebral cortex (see below).

The visual pathway leaves the lateral geniculate body as the **optic radiation** (geniculocalcarine tract) and loops over the temporal horn of the lateral ventricle before turning medially toward the visual cortex around the calcarine sulcus (82, 83, 203, 475). Nerve cells from the medial half of the lateral geniculate body project mainly into the superior lip of the primary visual cortex and those from its lateral half to the inferior lip of the primary visual cortex. In MR images and in histologic sections of brains of infants age 3 to 12 months, the optic radiation can be identified

(298, 361) in the area lateral to the temporal and occipital horns of the lateral ventricle in an approximately sagittal plane (Fig. 128.12). It appears hook-shaped in the coronal slices with the open part of the hook directed medially (Fig. 127.8). The upper layer of fibers in the optic radiation contains extramacular fibers which run to the anterior part of the upper lip of the primary visual cortex. The middle portion of the optic radiation contains the fibers that conduct the signals from the macula lutea of the retina to the occipital region of the primary visual cortex. The lower layer of fibers of the optic radiation runs through the loop (genu of optic radiation, Meyer's loop) at the anterior rim of the temporal horn of the lateral ventricle, passes underneath the lateral ventricle, then continues to the anterior part of the inferior lip of the primary visual cortex. If this portion only is damaged, perception in the peripheral (extramacular) part of the upper quadrant of the visual field is affected (179).

The **genu of optic radiation** (Meyer's loop) begins as a curved form sweeping forward into the temporal lobe (Figs. 127.6). It is not clearly demarcated in the histological specimens of juvenile and adult brains since this part is combined with other fibers and appears matted in the histological sections. The optic radiation can be stained and its course accurately determined only in the infants' brains (postnatal age 2 to 6 months) since these fibers develop initially in the white matter of the temporal and occipital lobes. When transferring these findings to the brains of adults it must be taken into account that the volume of the infants' brains doubles in size during the process of growth. We are only able to present a probable reconstruction of the temporal genu of the optic radiation. More in-depth research is required to clarify this point. The further course of the optic radiation in the external sagittal stratum is beside the temporal and occipital horns (Fig. 129.6) of the lateral ventricle.

The **primary visual cortex** (striate area or area 17 according to Brodmann), is positioned mainly in the medial part of the occipital lobe surrounding the entire length of the calcarine sulcus and extending about 1 cm onto the occipital pole. More than half of the primary visual cortex is positioned on the inner surface of the **calcarine sulcus** (Figs. 15b.6, 15d.6, 16b.6, 16d.6, 17b.5, 17d.5) that cuts deep into the occipital lobe. At the calcarine spur the white matter beneath the primary visual cortex borders the occipital horn of the lateral ventricle. Below the calcarine sulcus the visual cortex extends in an anterior direction before reaching the junction of the parieto-occipital sulcus. The shape of the primary visual cortex of the right and left hemispheres is asymmetrical and is individually variable (442). Its main course is similar to that of the bicommissural plane (453). Within the calcarine sulcus there are variable arches and depressions of the cortex (399). The primary visual cortex is histologically classified as granular. A macroscopically and microscopically visible fiber layer, known as the **occipital stripe** of Gennari, is formed by fibers of the optic radiation seeking neurons in the fourth layer of the primary visual cortex.

Clinical experience with temporal corticectomy showed no impairment of the visual field if the excision was more than 1 cm anterior to the verticofrontal plane of the posterior commissure (454). This plane runs through the posterior commissure and is vertical to the median plane and the bicommissural plane of Talairach. These findings suggest that the optic radiation is likely to run closer to the anterior end of the temporal horn of the lateral ventricle, and does not extend as far frontally as has been described (Meyer's loop) (203, 221). Furthermore, partial temporal lobectomy may result in small, large, or no visual defects (18). There may well be significant variability in the size of Meyer's loop.

In MR scans the **calcarine sulcus** is easily identified in the paramedian slices (Figs. 32b.17, 32d.17, 33b.12, 33d.12). The calcarine sulcus unites anteriorly with the parieto-occipital sulcus and both sulci enclose a wedge-shaped portion of the occipital lobe, the cuneus. In axial slices the superior and inferior lips of the visual cortex are not easy to differentiate as the calcarine sulcus takes a wavy course, almost parallel to the canthomeatal plane. In horizontal anatomic sections discernment of its superior and inferior lips can be difficult, whereas in the coronal slices the lips are obvious. The echo planar technique of fMRI is helpful in determining the ocular dominance columns of the primary visual cortex (96, 221).

Retinotopic Map

The lens of the eye ensures that objects in the field of vision are projected in reversed, inverted, and reduced format onto the photoreceptors of the retina in both eyes. The **spatial configuration** generated by the photoreceptors is retained from the retina to the primary visual cortex and is known as retinotopic map. The retinotopic localization has been confirmed with the aid of fMRI (96).

The following spatial arrangement exists between the photoreceptors of the retina and the ocular dominance columns of the primary visual cortex:

- As a result of the **partial crossing** of the optic nerve fibers in the optic chiasm, the optic signals arising from the right halves of both retinae (the left halves of the visual fields) reach the right primary visual cortex.
- The lower homonymous quadrants of the retina (the upper homonymous quadrants of the visual field) project into the portion of the visual cortex located below the calcarine sulcus (the lower lip of the primary visual cortex). The upper retinal quadrants project to the cortex above the calcarine sulcus.
- The macula lutea of the retina, the region with the most acute sight, has the largest field of projection

6.6 Visual System 363

1 Corresponding (homonymous) halves of visual field
2 Eyeball
3 Optic nerve
4 Optic chiasm
5 Optic tract
6 Temporal genu of optic radiation
7 Temporal (inferior) horn of lateral ventricle
8 Temporal lobe of cerebrum
9 Optic radiation
10 Lateral geniculate body
11 Pulvinar of thalamus
12 Superior colliculus
13 Central part (body) of lateral ventricle
14 Splenium of corpus callosum
15 Occipital (posterior) horn of lateral ventricle
16 Primary visual cortex
17 Calcarine sulcus

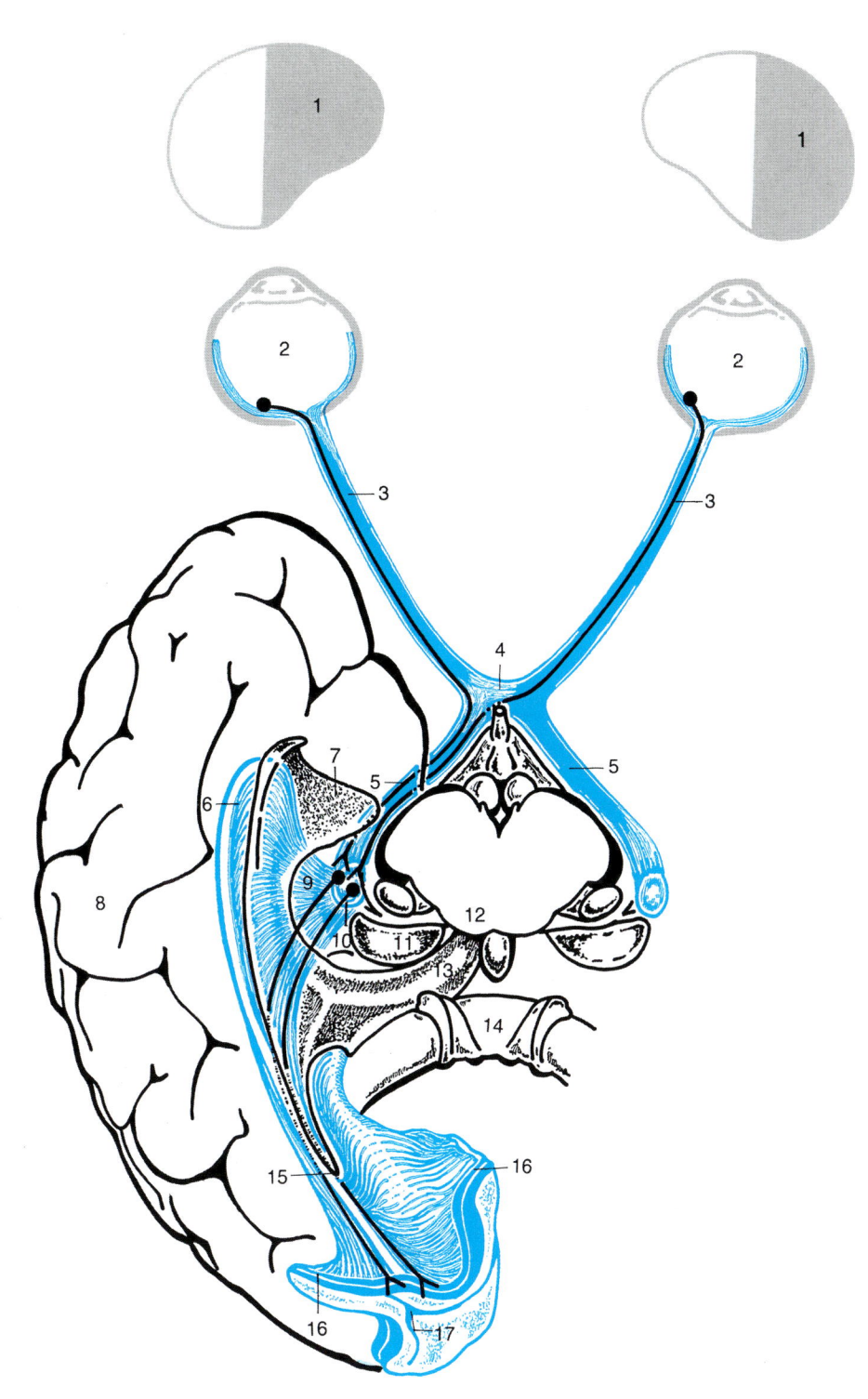

Fig. 126 The visual system (inferior view). The basal parts of the diencephalon and midbrain are located between the optic tracts. The temporal and occipital lobes are the only portions shown of the right telencephalon. Two homonymous halves of the visual field are portrayed in gray. The path of the neurons from one half of the retina to the respective visual cortex is shown. According to (332).

onto the primary visual cortex and is closest to the occipital pole. The visual cortex of the peripheral binocular visual field lies anterior to the occipital pole, and that of the peripheral monocular visual field is situated close to the parieto-occipital sulcus.

In addition to this major pathway of the optic nerve, there is also a small **extrageniculate supplementary pathway** that could partially compensate for deficits of the major pathway. This extrageniculate projection bypasses the lateral geniculate body and reaches the superior colliculi and the pulvinar of the thalamus. From the pulvinar, optic signals are transmitted to the primary and secondary visual cortical areas (357, 369, 430).

1 Optic disc
2 Retina
3 Optic nerve

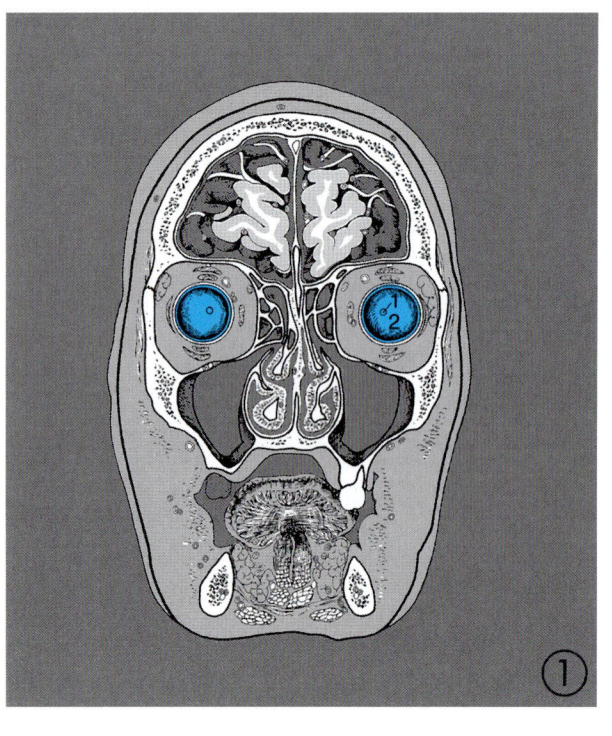

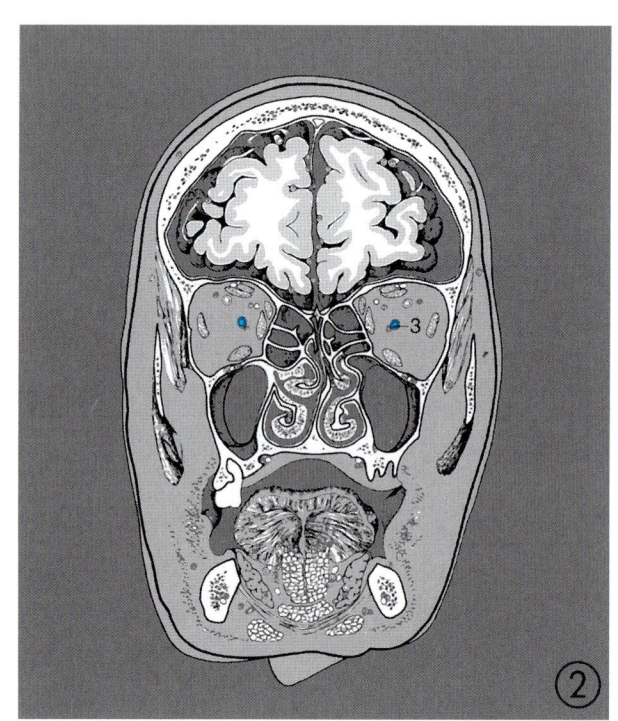

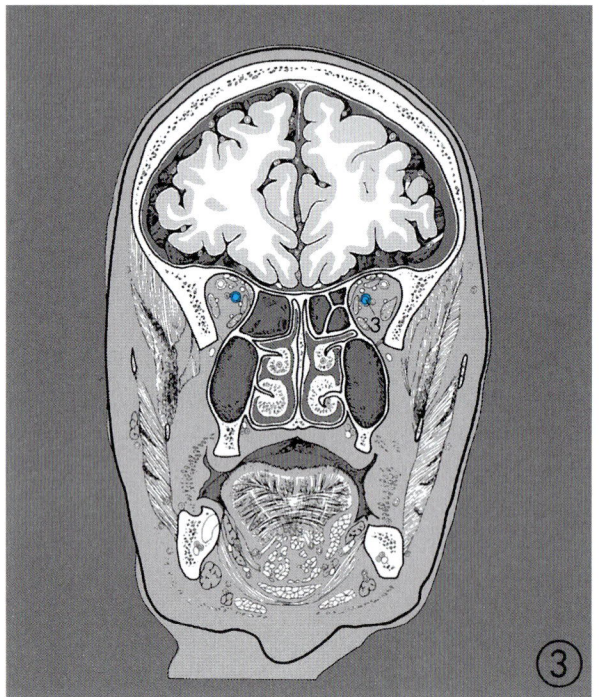

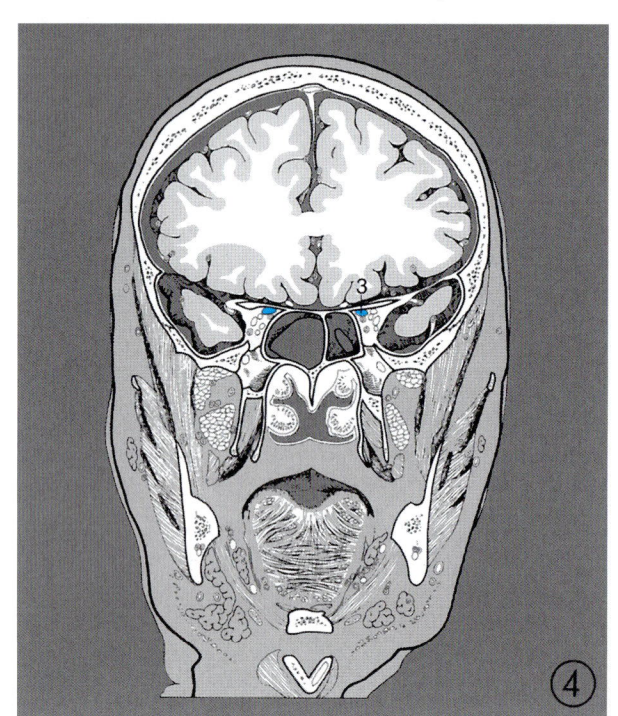

Fig. **127** Coronal serial illustrations of the visual system. The optic radiation (Meyer's loop) is included according to (454). The encircled numbers (1–8) indicate the number of the respective slice (Figs. 1, 2a,b, 3).

6.6 Visual System   365

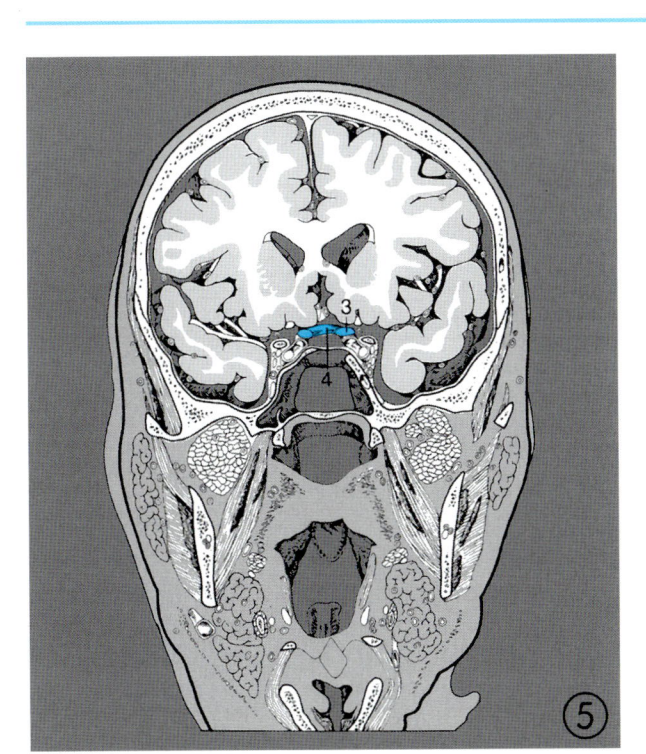

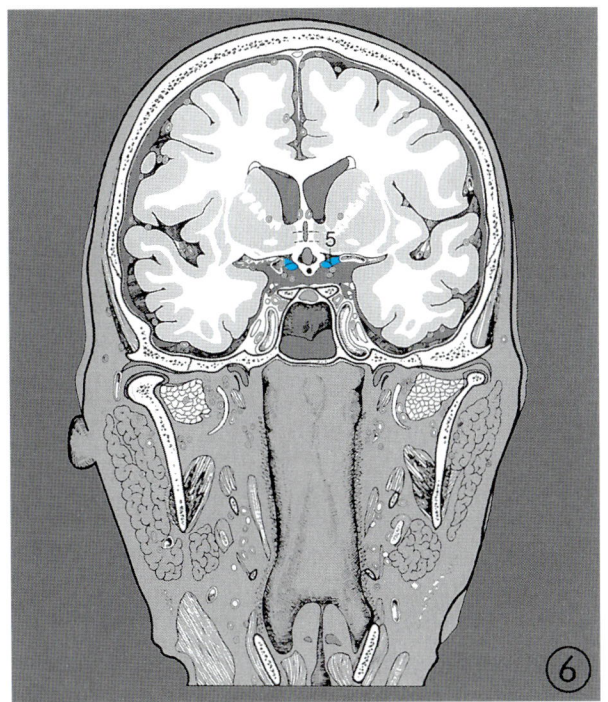

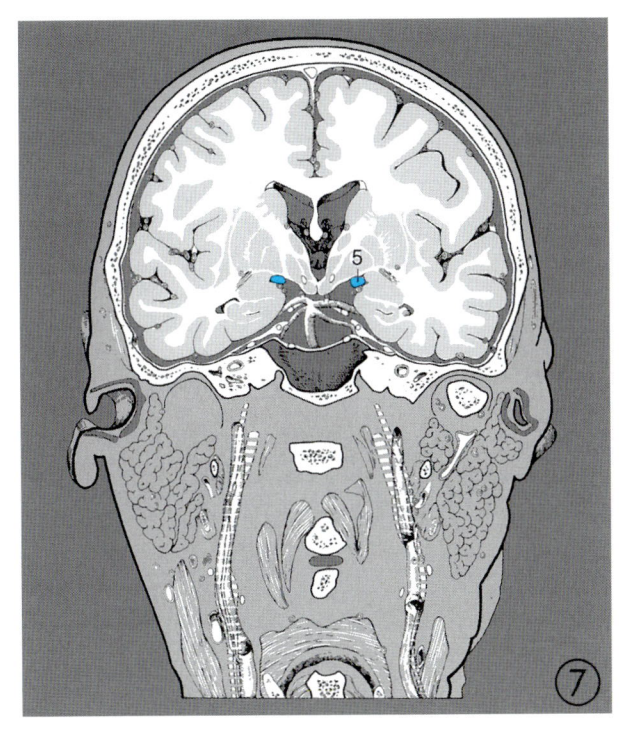

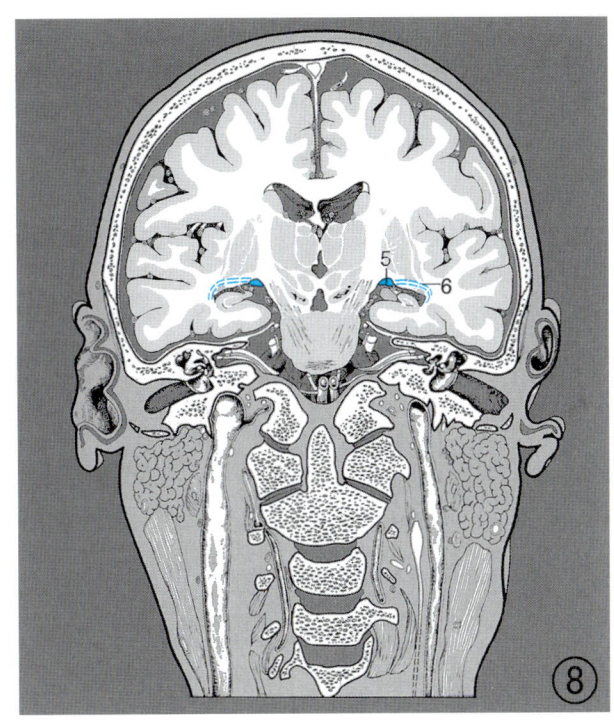

3 Optic nerve
4 Optic chiasm
5 Optic tract
6 Optic radiation, Meyer's loop

366   6 Neurofunctional Systems

7 Lateral geniculate body
8 Optic radiation
9 Primary visual cortex, inferior lip

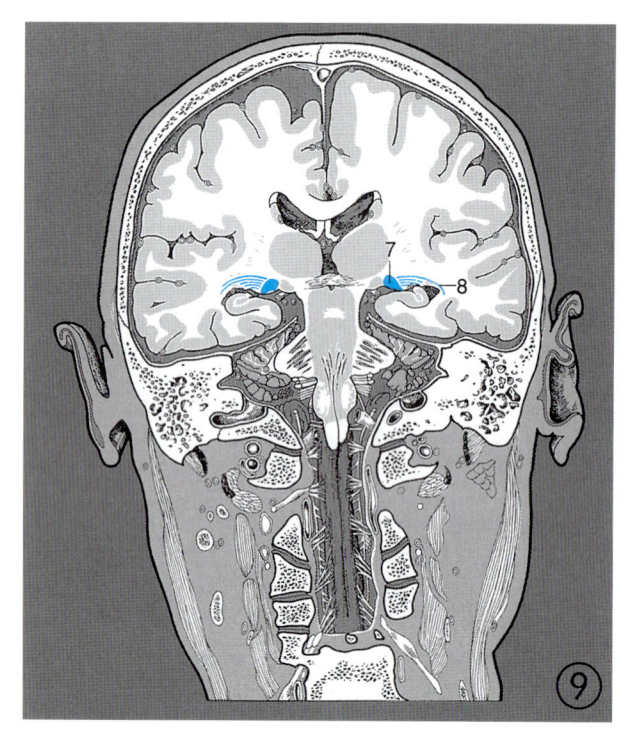

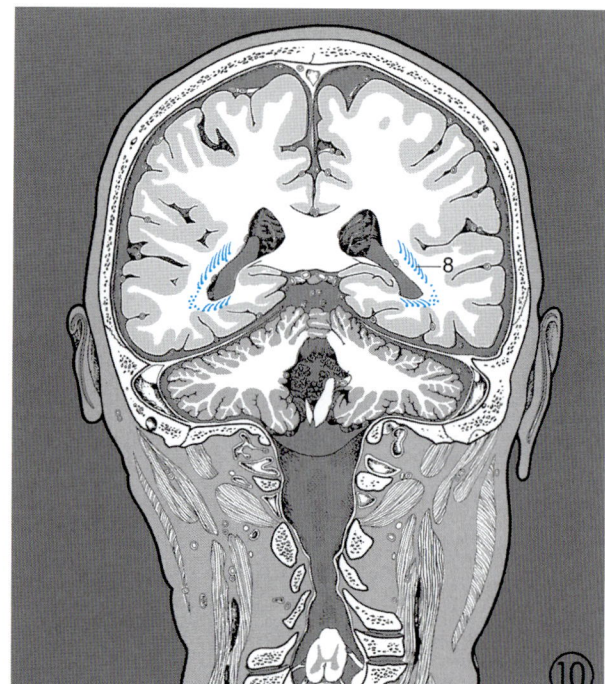

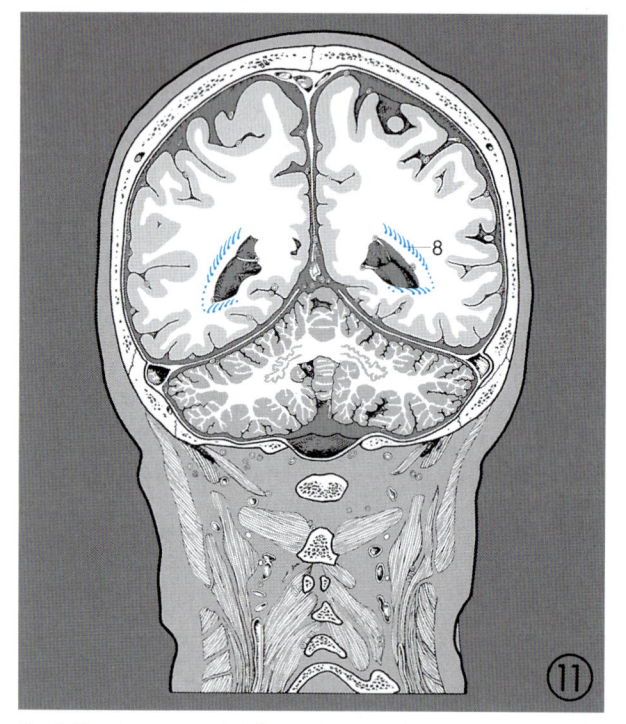

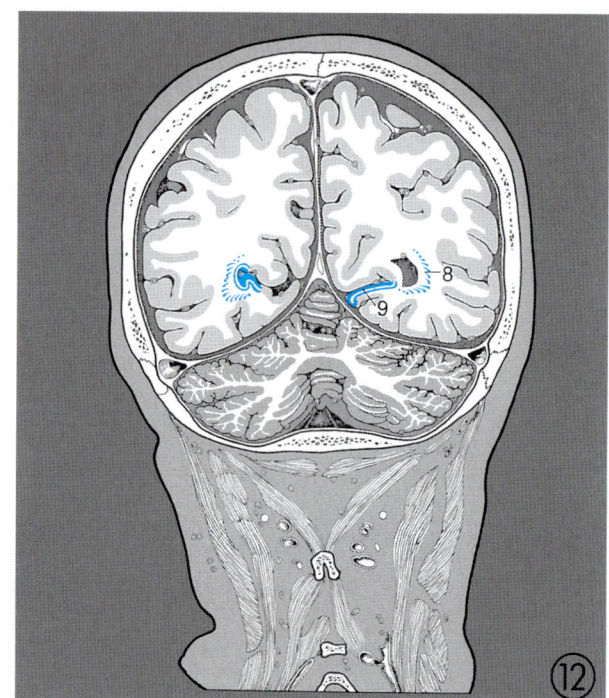

Fig. **127** Coronal serial illustrations of the visual system. The optic radiation is included according to (454). The encircled numbers (9–14) indicate the number of the respective slice (Figs. 1, 2a,b, 3).

6.6 Visual System

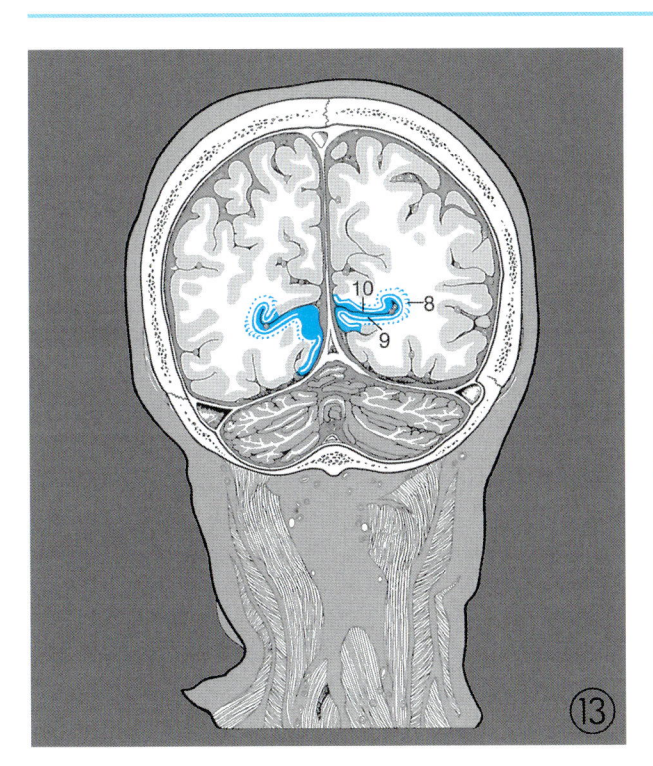

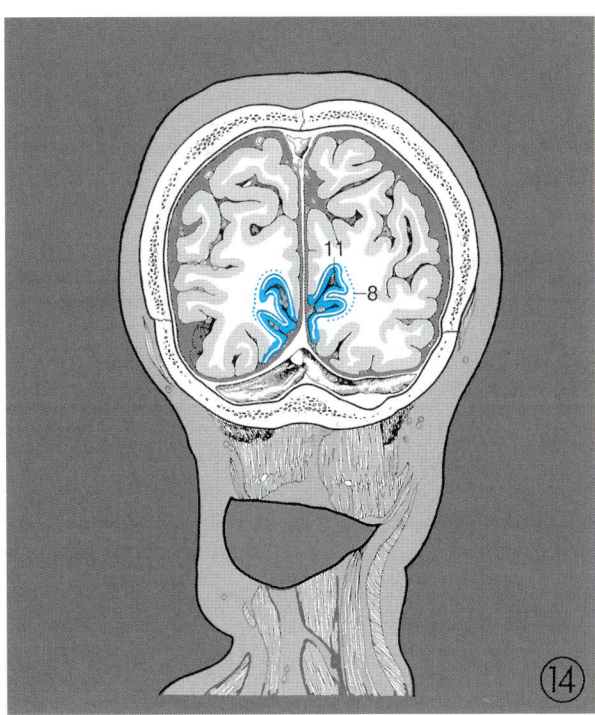

8 Optic radiation
9 Primary visual cortex, inferior lip
10 Primary visual cortex, superior lip
11 Primary visual cortex

368   6   Neurofunctional Systems

1 Optic nerve
2 Optic chiasm
3 Optic tract (within the slice)
4 Primary visual cortex, superior lip
5 Primary visual cortex, inferior lip
6 Optic nerve (within the slice)
7 Optic tract
8 Lateral geniculate body (within the slice)
9 Optic radiation
10 Primary visual cortex
11 Retina
12 Optic radiation (within the slice)

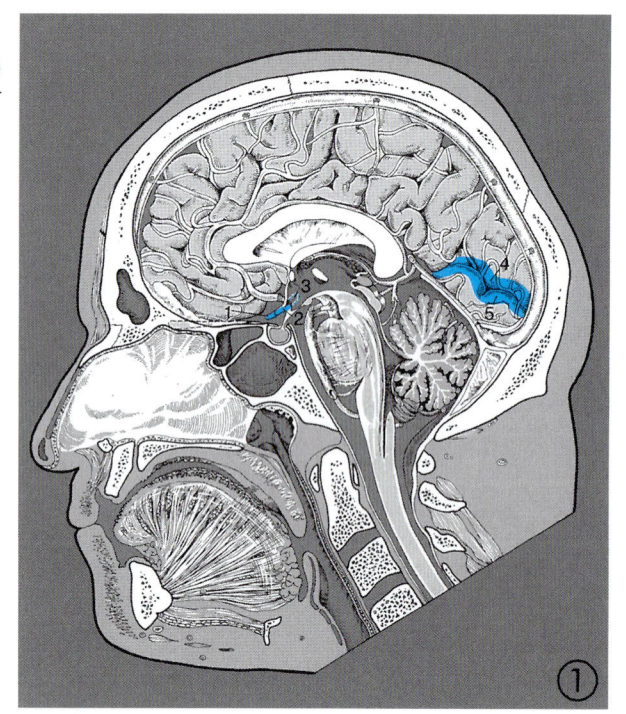

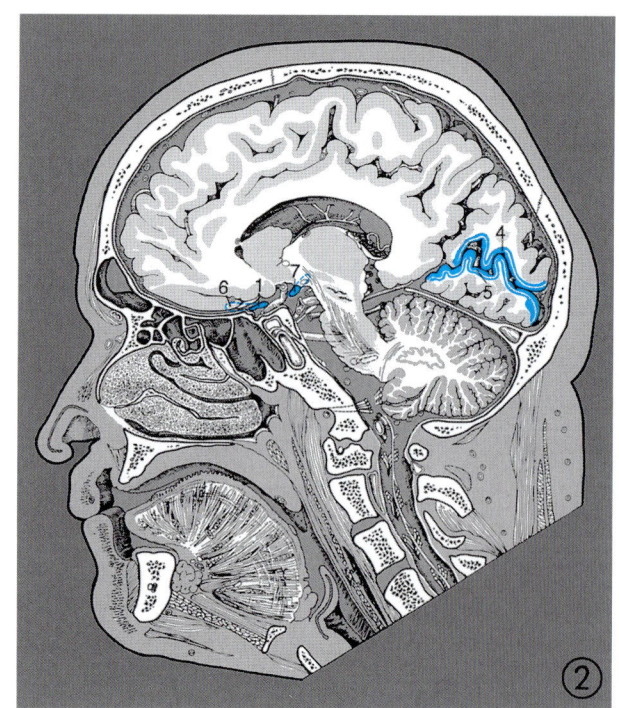

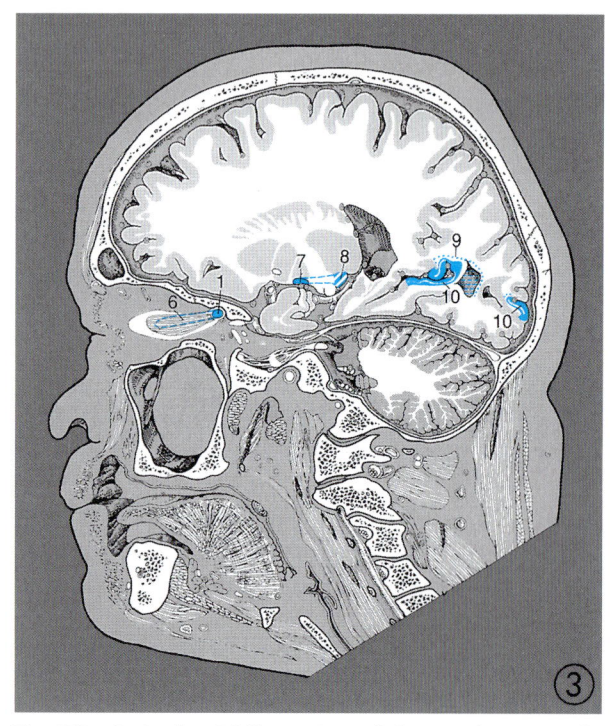

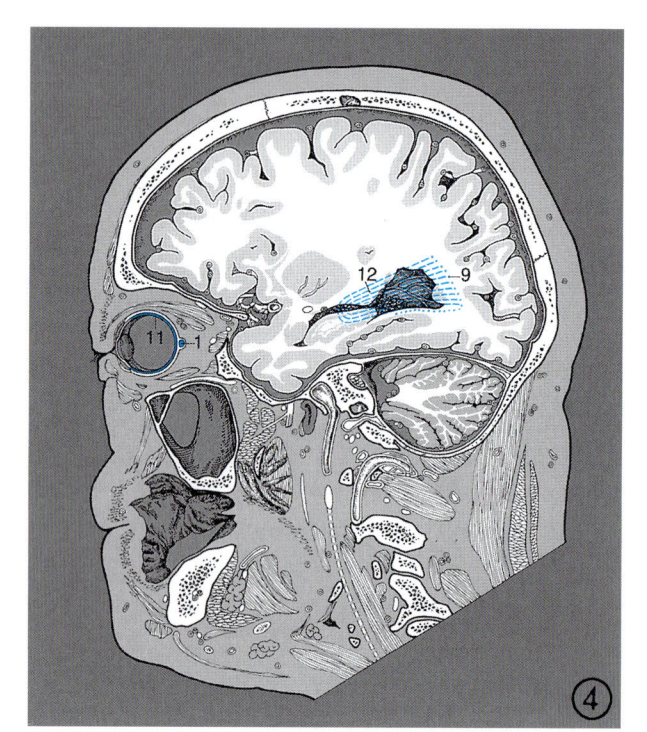

Fig. **128** Sagittal serial illustrations of the visual system. The optic radiation is included according to (454). The encircled number indicates the number of the respective slice (Figs. 29, 30a,b, 31).

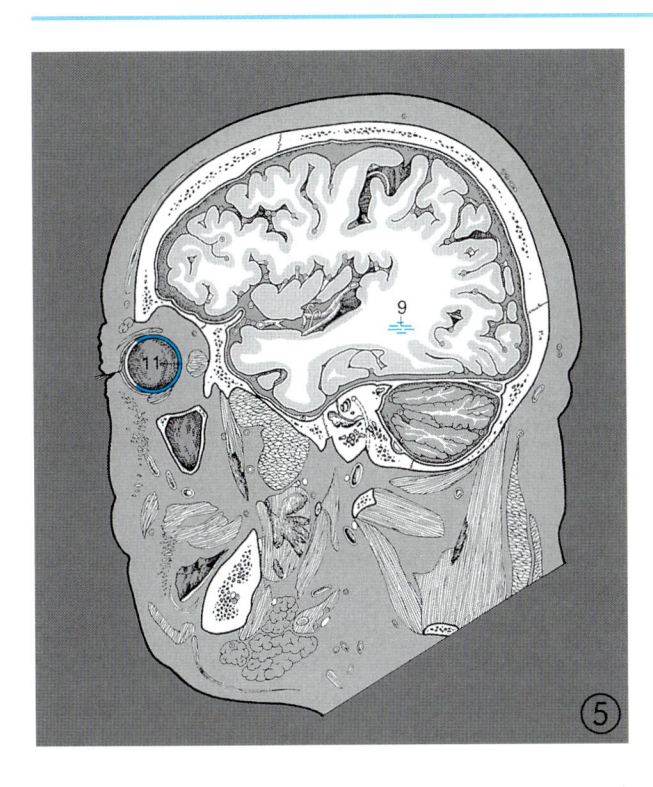

9 Optic radiation
11 Retina

Clinical Notes

Although the retina can be well evaluated with the ophthalmoscope, supplementary imaging procedures may be necessary, especially to identify lesions involving the anterior parts of the retina that cannot be seen with the ophthalmoscope. Supplementary imaging procedures can be helpful for identifying intraocular tumors and clouding of the refractive media, and for evaluating the **retrobulbar space** of the orbit. Clinical signs of a retrobulbar disorder may include monocular visual disturbances, pain upon movement of the eye, exophthalmos (forward displacement of the eyeball), and edema of the eyelids. Pathologic changes and functional disorders of the **optic nerve** as well as processes in the retrobulbar space are indications for the use of sonography, MRI, and CT. The reclining position of the head (preferred for this CT examination) sets the sectioning plane at 10° to the canthomeatal plane. This corresponds approximately to the infraorbitomeatal plane (321, 373). The optic nerve, the rectus, and the maximal circumference of the eyeball are clearly imaged and constantly reproducible in this plane. MR and CT images show alterations of the optic nerve and pathologic densities in the retrobulbar space. The diameter of the optic nerve can be determined exactly by choosing coronal as the sectioning plane (373). In cases involving minimal functional disorders of the optic nerve, especially in cases of postoptic nerve neuritis, elicitation of the visual evoked potentials (VEP) is a sensitive diagnostic-procedure (288). MRI is also able to detect foci of multiple sclerosis in the optic nerves.

Disorders in the region of the **optic chiasm** may result in bitemporal and, less frequently, in binasal hemianopia. Enlargement of the sella turcica caused by an adenoma of the pituitary gland or, more rarely, destruction of the sella turcica may appear in lateral radiographs of the skull. Further neuroimaging is required for premonitory symptoms, also in the case of hormonal defects or expansion of the sella turcica that might appear on X-rays of the skull. CT scans establish pathologic density patterns in the region of the optic chiasm and may occasionally identify bony destructions in the region of the sella turcica. Lesions in the optic tract or lateral geniculate body may result in a contralateral homonymous hemianopia. The greater sensitivity, the multiplanar imaging technique, and the absence of CT bony artifacts in the region of the skull base explain the preferential use of MRI versus CT when lesions of the optic nerve and the optic chiasm are suspected.

Homonymous quadrantanopia and homonymous hemianopia are clinical symptoms indicating a pathologic process in the region of the **optic radiation** or **primary visual cortex**. Symptoms of irritation such as **photopsy** and amaurosis fugax may be seen. Bilateral vascular or traumatic injuries affecting the visual cortex may result in cortical blindness.

370   6 Neurofunctional Systems

1 Retina
2 Optic nerve
3 Optic chiasm

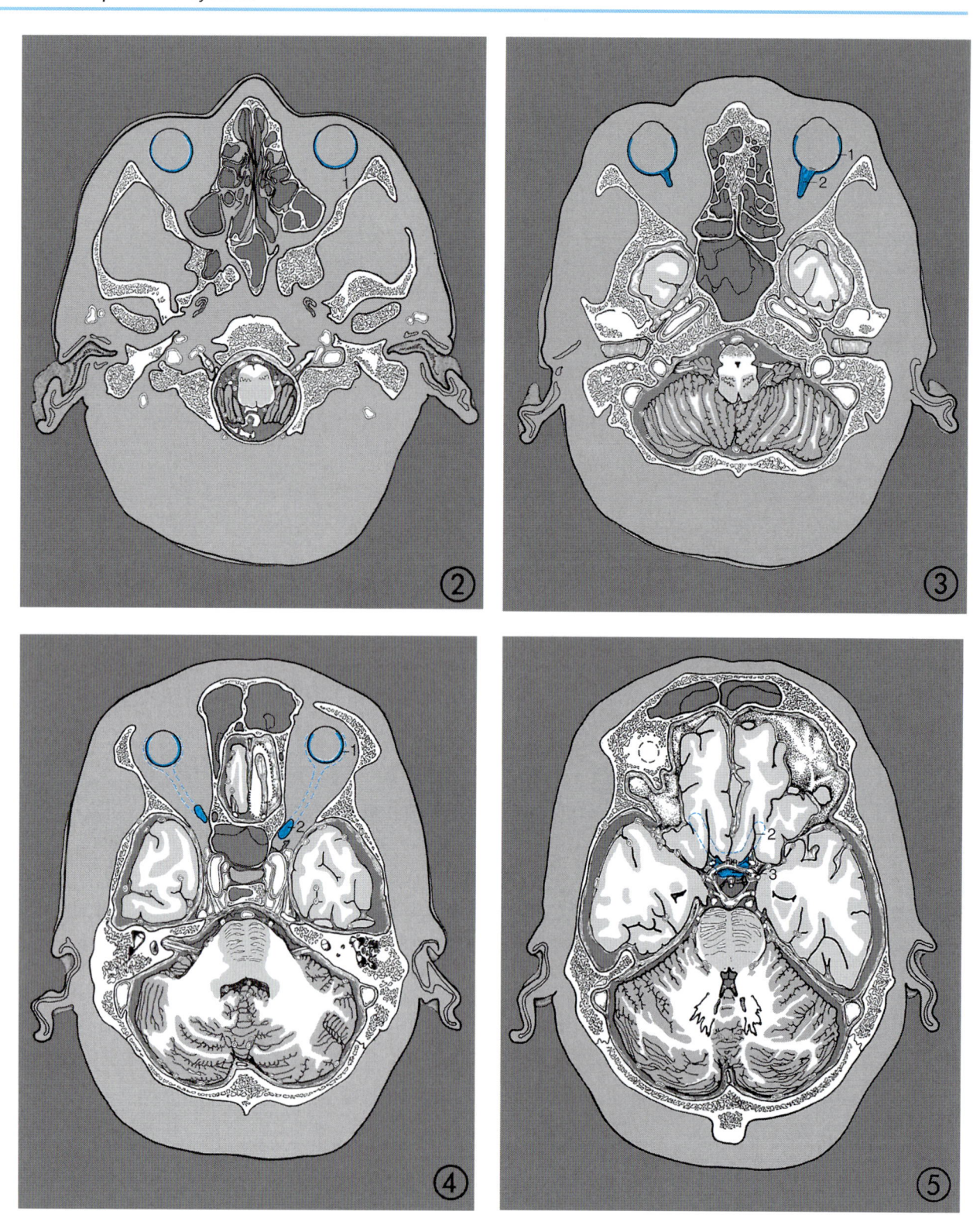

Fig. **129** Canthomeatally oriented serial illustrations of the visual system. The encircled number indicates the number of the respective slice (Figs. 44, 45a,b, 46).

6.6 *Visual System* 371

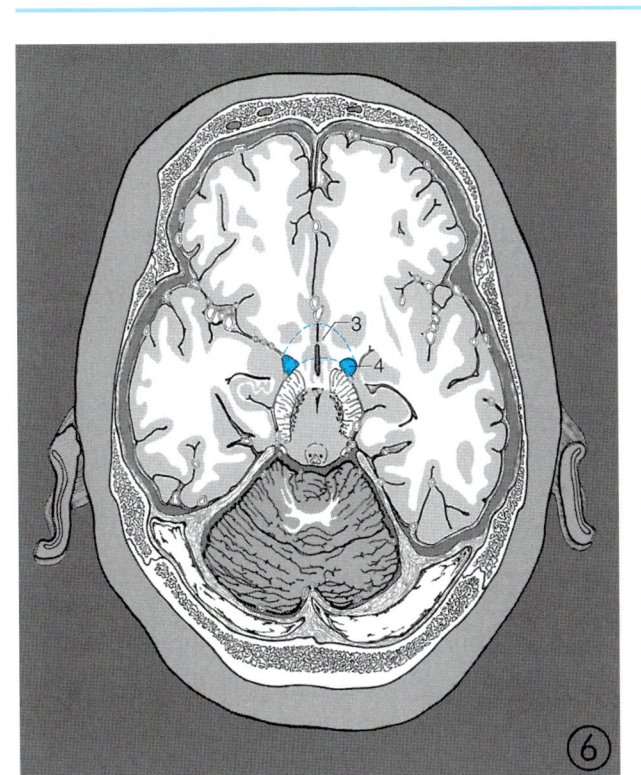

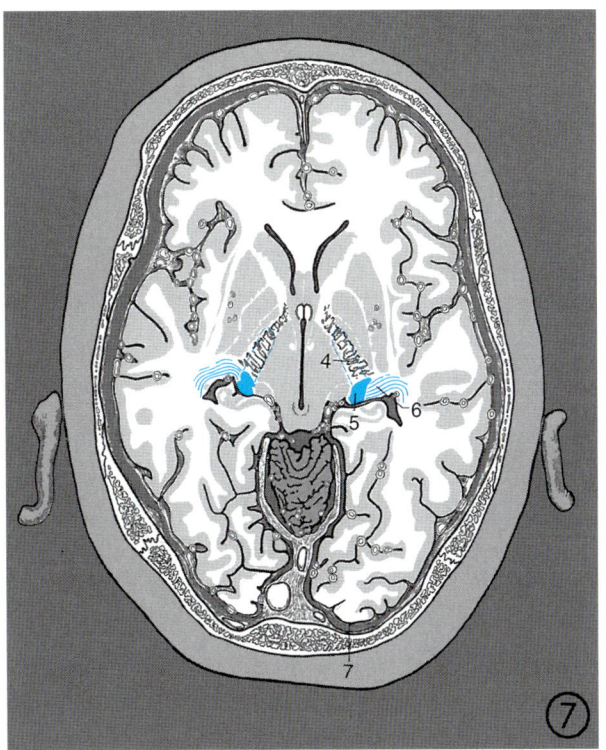

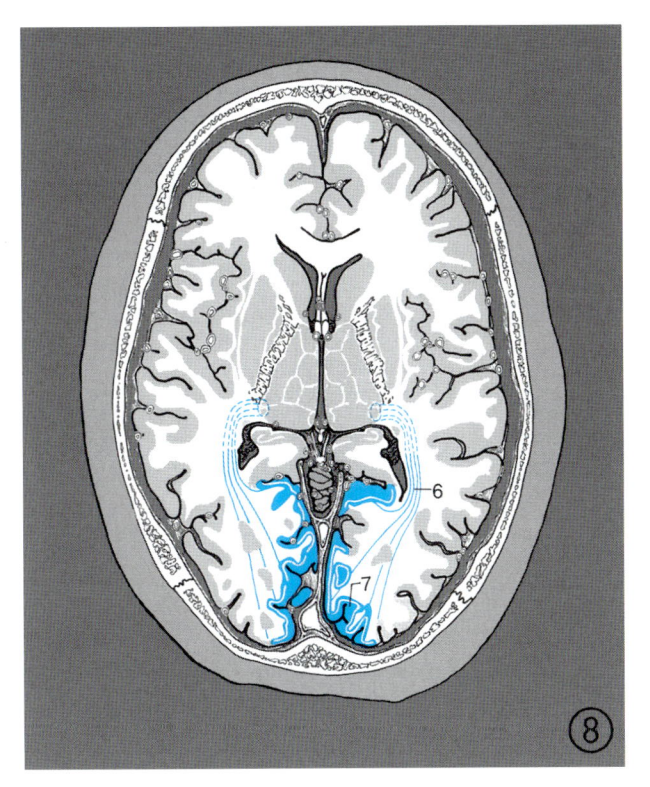

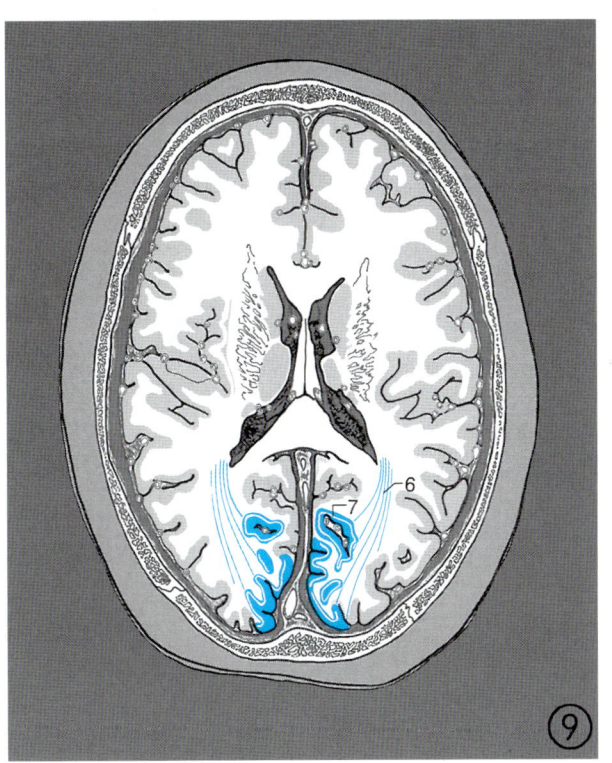

3 Optic chiasm
4 Optic tract
5 Lateral geniculate body
6 Optic radiation
7 Primary visual cortex

6.7 Olfactory System
(Figs. 147, 130, 131)

The **olfactory epithelium** lies in the upper and posterior part of the nasal cavity just below the cribriform plate of the ethmoid. This area of 2 cm² contains the olfactory receptor cells. Approximately 20 olfactory fila arise as the **olfactory nerve** in each side from the olfactory neurosensory cells of the nose and extend through the cribriform plate. The first-order neurons terminate in the olfactory bulb, forming several synaptic brushlike terminals, or the olfactory glomeruli. The synaptic glomeruli establish contact with the mitral cells. On average, the human olfactory bulb is 10 mm long, 4.5 mm wide, and horizontally flattened (416). It is considerably smaller than that of apes (444).

The axons of the mitral cells form the **olfactory tract**. This extends into small cortical areas at the base of the ipsilateral telencephalon (paleocortex) and is divided into medial and lateral olfactory striae. The medial olfactory stria extends towards the olfactory trigone below the genu of the corpus callosum (corresponding to the olfactory tubercle of macrosmatic animals). Olfactory projections passing through the lateral olfactory stria bend sharply around the edge of the insula and project into the **prepiriform cortex** and **periamygdaloid cortex** of the gyrus semilunaris (443) (Fig. 52a.15). These small cortical areas lie hidden in the angular space between the frontal lobe, the temporal lobe, and the neighboring edge of the insula. The periamygdaloid cortex is an area on the medial surface of the amygdaloid body. The olfactory pathway runs directly to the ipsilateral olfactory cortex. The left and right olfactory centers are connected by the anterior commissure.

Clinical Notes
Loss of the sense of smell (anosmia) results in a subjective impairment of the sense of taste. This is probably accounted for by the common cortical processing of olfactory and gustatory signals. Disturbances of olfaction arise as a result of injury to the olfactory epithelium or damage to the olfactory nerves and/or bulbs caused by a fracture or meningioma of the olfactory groove. Unilateral impairment is seldom noticed spontaneously by the patient. Olfactory hallucinations can arise due to lesions in the region of the olfactory tract and as a symptom of temporal lobe epilepsy (uncinate seizure).

1 Olfactory bulb
2 Olfactory tract

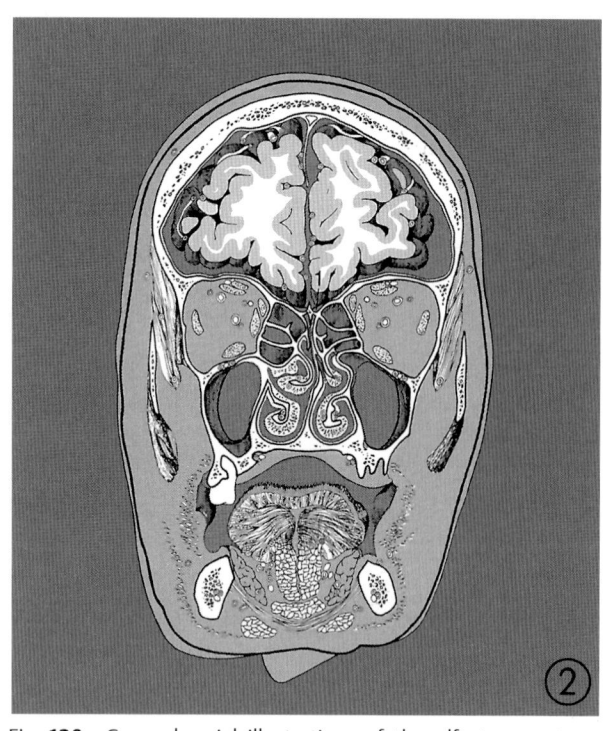

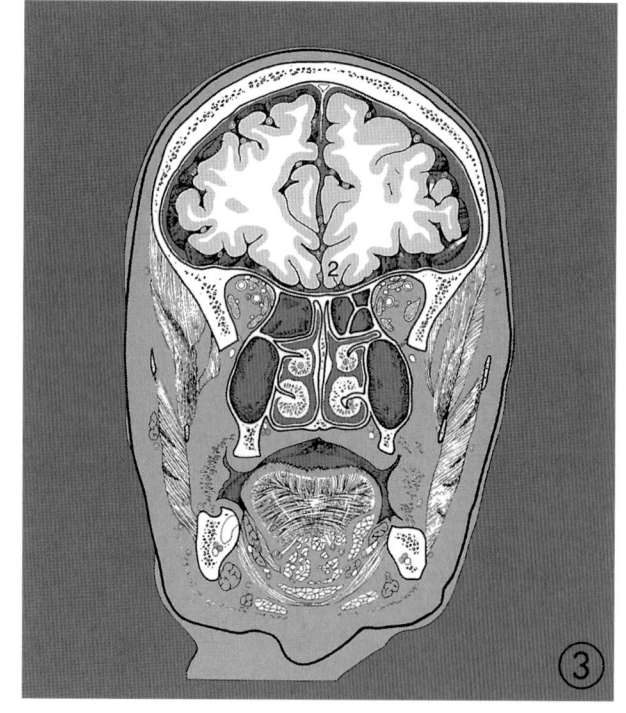

Fig. **130** Coronal serial illustrations of the olfactory system. The encircled numbers (2–3) indicate the number of the respective slice (Figs. 1, 2a,b, 3).

6.7 Olfactory System

2 Olfactory tract
3 Lateral olfactory stria
4 Prepiriform and periamygdaloid cortical areas
5 Periamygdaloid cortex

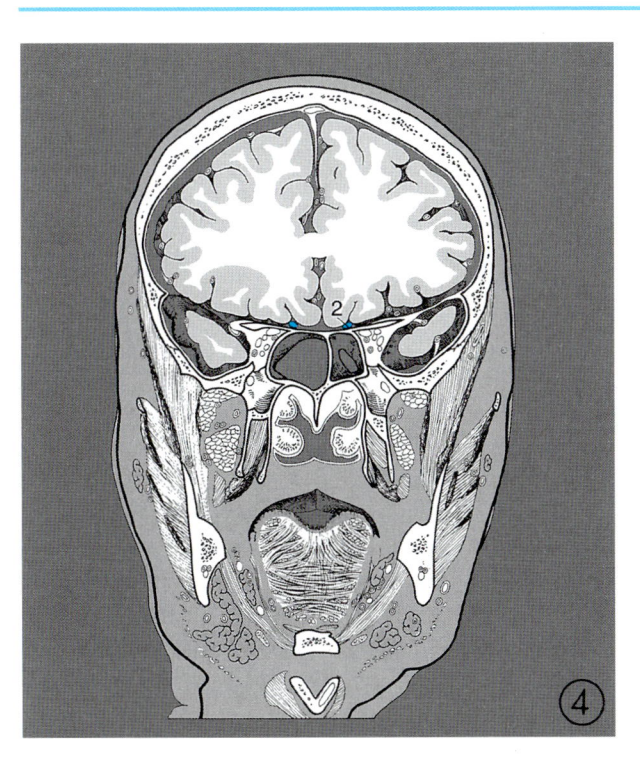

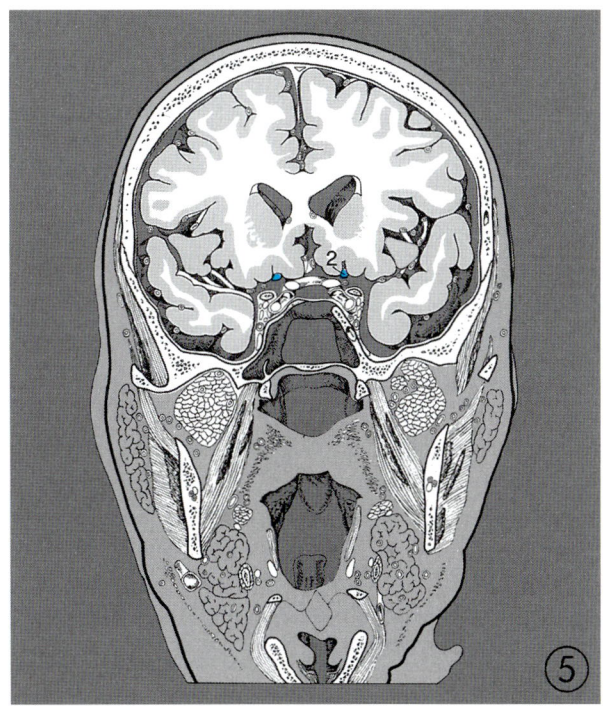

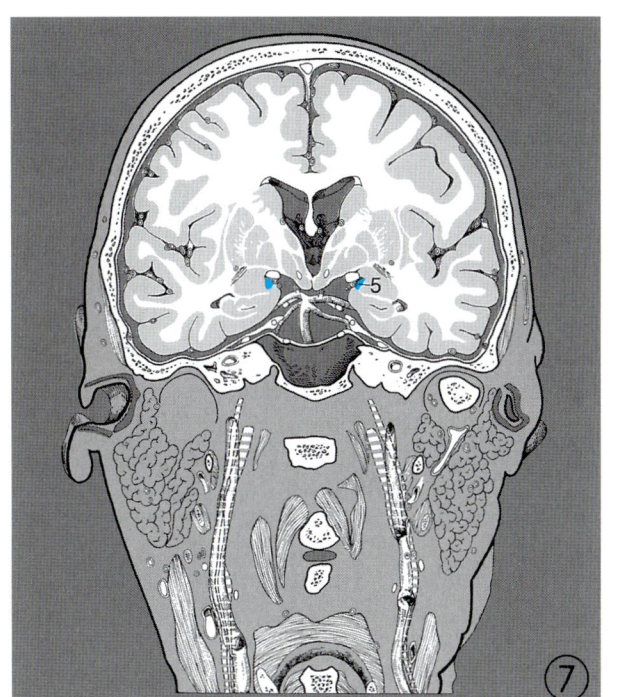

Fig. **130** Coronal serial illustrations of the olfactory system. The encircled numbers (4–7) indicate the number of the respective slice (Figs. 1, 2a,b, 3).

1 Olfactory bulb
2 Olfactory tract
3 Olfactory trigone (within the slice)
4 Prepiriform and periamygdaloid cortical areas (partially within the slice)

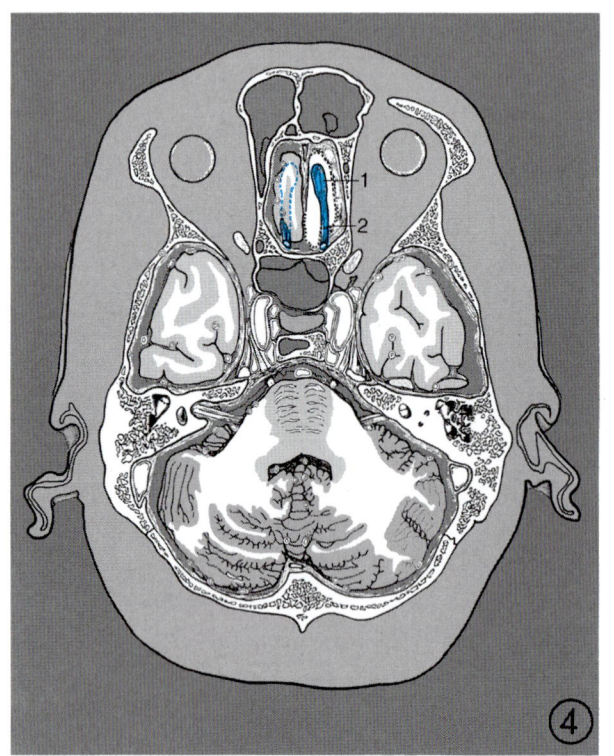

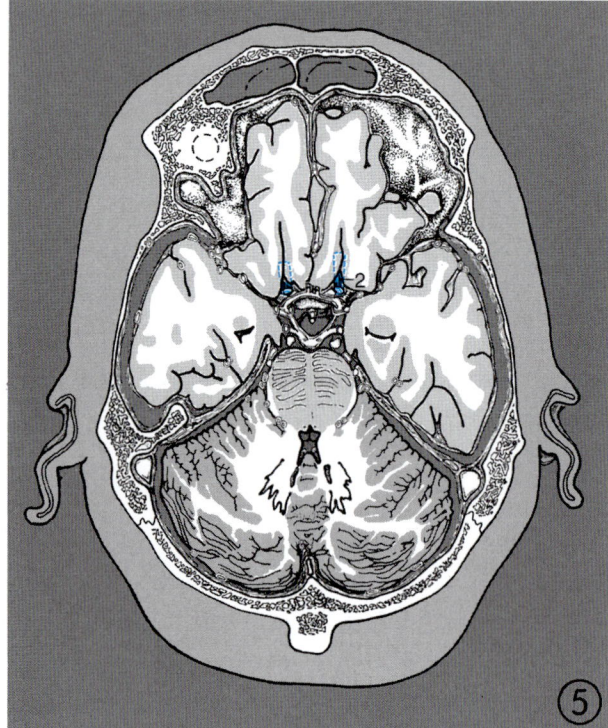

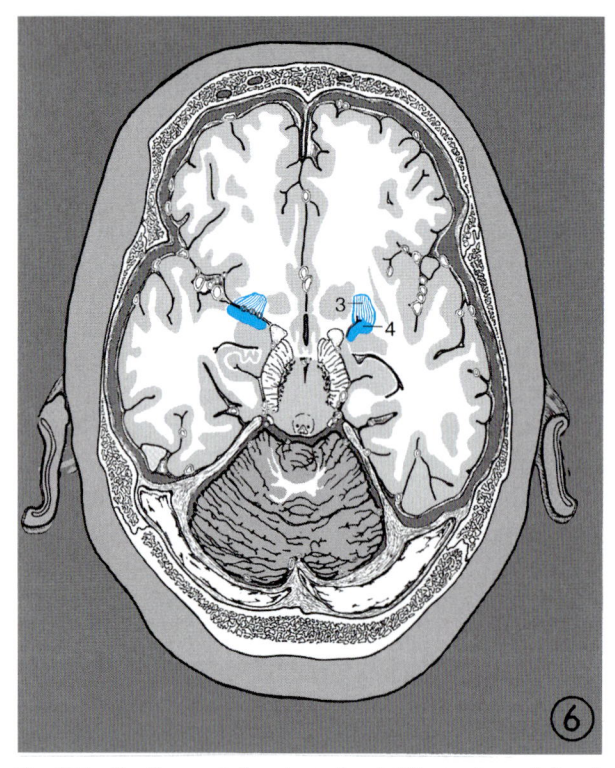

Fig. 131 Canthomeatally oriented serial illustrations of the olfactory system. The encircled number indicates the number of the respective slice (Figs. 44, 45a,b, 46).

6.8 Motor Systems

Cortical and subcortical neurons are joined by synapses with the motor neurons of the midbrain, pons, medulla oblongata, and spinal cord (221, 256, 257, 258, 374a, 465). Anatomic and physiologic research over the past few decades has shown that the cortical and subcortical nerve cells are closely linked by numerous control loops. This research has led to a revision of the classical concept of two separate motor systems, namely the pyramidal (voluntary) system and the extrapyramidal (involuntary) system. Commonplace activities, such as swinging the arms while walking or running, illustrate the connection between voluntary and automatic movements. Voluntary movement, therefore, is a combination of voluntary and involuntary action. Accordingly, the pyramidal pathway is also an important output route for individual basal ganglia, such as the striatothalamic main circuits.

Clinical Notes
Neuropathologic investigations and clinical examinations usually correlate neurologic symptoms with the pyramidal system or with specific systems of the basal ganglia. The Babinski reflex, for instance, may be seen as a result of a disorder in the pyramidal pathway or hypokinesia due to a lesion in the substantia nigra. For this reason, we will maintain the notion of a pyramidal system. The individual motor systems of the basal ganglia, however, will be treated separately.

Detection of disorders in the motor systems is of primary importance in clinical diagnosis. In many cases involving unconscious or only partially cooperative patients, an adequate examination of motor function is still possible. Motor disorders may be so obvious that a simple neurologic examination is sufficient for an approximate localization of the lesion. Therefore, more urgent diagnostic or therapeutic measures can be undertaken before a subtle neurologic examination of the patient is accomplished.

Damage to the so-called "**upper motor neurons**" is characterized by paralysis, loss of polysynaptic reflexes (e.g., superficial abdominal reflexes), and the appearance of pathologic **reflexes of the Babinski group**. An increase in the tonus (**spasticity**) of the paralyzed extremities and hyperreflexia develop at a variable rate. Finally, a typical clinical picture can be described, whereby a distally accentuated paralysis and a typical posture appear. Characteristic symptoms of a hemiplegic patient are the circumduction of the paralyzed leg and the adduction and flexion of the paralyzed arm (Wernicke-Mann's syndrome).

6.8.1 Pyramidal System
(Figs. 132–135)

The pyramidal system originates in pyramidal cells of the cerebral cortex. These cells are located anterior and posterior to the central sulcus in and around the precentral and postcentral gyri. Cytoarchitectonically, this primarily includes areas 4 and 6, also areas 3, 1, 2, and 5, in which regions like the primary motor and premotor areas, the supplementary motor area, and the somatic sensory areas are located (102, 132a, 270). In monkeys the retrograde tracing with horseradish techniques has ascertained the origin of the corticospinal fibers from these cortical areas.

The **primary motor cortex** (area 4) exhibits a fine somatotopic organization. Located on the medial surface of the hemisphere are the upper motor neurons that supply the spinal motor neurons of the leg muscles. Cortical regions responsible for innervation of the trunk, arm, facial, masticatory, lingual, and laryngeal muscles extend from the superior margin toward the lateral sulcus (Sylvian fissure). The lower motor neurons receive their input contralaterally. Ipsilateral innervation is also received by the lower motor neurons of the muscles of mastication, larynx, and upper face (occipitofrontalis and orbicularis oculi).

Three cerebral regions participate in initiating voluntary movements:
- Supplementary motor area (part of area 6)
- Premotor cortex (part of area 6)
- Upper parietal cortex (area 5).

The **supplementary motor area** (46, 356) lies on the medial surface of the hemisphere in the medial (not middle) frontal gyrus anterior to the paracentral lobule. A basic somatotopic organization is recognizable. Movements are planned in the supplementary motor area (103a, 130, 384, 465).

The **premotor cortex** occupies on the lateral surface of the hemisphere area 6, which lies anterior to area 4 in the frontal lobes. Complex and mainly learned movements are released from the premotor cortex (132, 351, 496).

The **upper parietal cortex** (area 5) lies posterior to the postcentral gyrus and sends out spatial information for the motor system.

The **primary motor cortex** (area 4) receives signals from the supplementary motor area, the premotor cortex, the upper parietal cortex, and the cerebellum. The pyramidal cells of the primary motor cortex analyze these signals and give out command signals to the motor neurons of the spinal cord (via the corticospinal fibers) and the brainstem (via the corticonuclear fibers).

The main origin of the **corticospinal system** is the motor cortex in the upper part of the precentral gyrus (Fig. 132.3)) on the lateral side and in the neighboring middle part of the paracentral lobule on the medial side of the hemisphere. Around 80% of the corticospi-

1 Postcentral gyrus and somatic sensory cortex
2 Central sulcus
3 Precentral gyrus
4 Primary motor cortex (area 4)
5 Premotor cortex (area 6)
6 Tail of caudate nucleus
7 Corticospinal tract
8 Head of caudate nucleus
9 Putamen
10 Substantia nigra
11 Cerebellum
12 Pons
13 Medulla oblongata
14 Pyramidal decussation

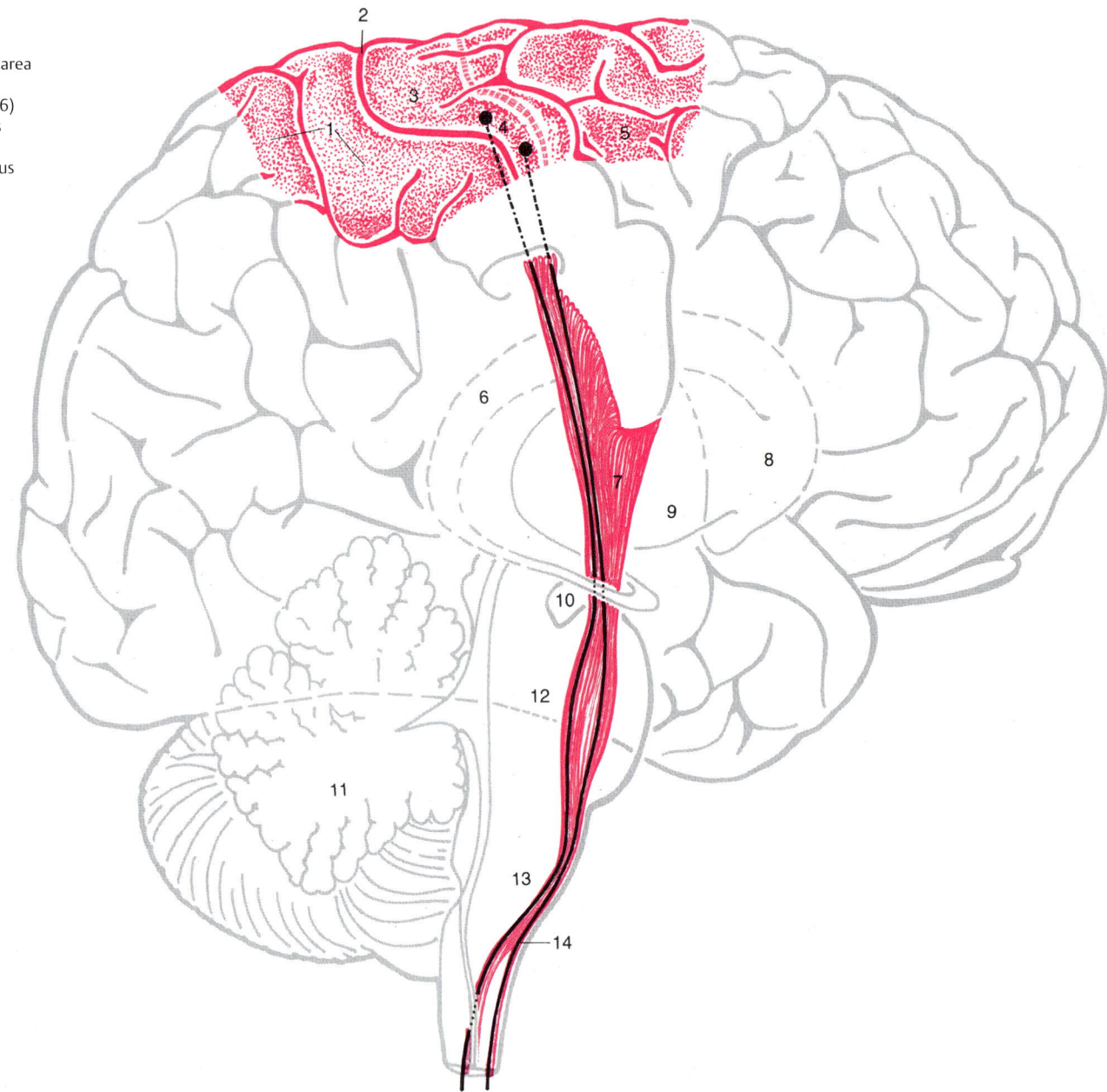

Fig. **132** Lateral view of the pyramidal (corticospinal) tract. The origin of the pyramidal tract in the cerebral cortex and the long corticofugal system are shown transparently. The brainstem and cerebellum are dissected in the median plane. The right half of both structures has been removed with the exception of the pyramidal tract and the substantia nigra. According to (332).

nal fibers stem from the precentral gyrus (127); fibers from the somatic sensory areas 3, 1, 2 end synaptically at the afferent nerve cells of the spinal posterior gray horns, thereby influencing the afferent signals (299). The primary motor cortex occupies both the precentral gyrus and the paracentral lobule. In close proximity to the superior margin of hemisphere, area 4 covers the width of the precentral gyrus and remains inferior as a tiny strip at its posterior lip (56). This corresponds with recent pigmentarchitectonic studies showing evidence that area 4 in the precentral gyrus lies close to the central sulcus, mainly in the area of its anterior wall. Area 4 covers approximately the middle third of the paracentral lobule (46).

The **corticospinal fibers** (pyramidal pathway) transmit motor impulses to the contralateral spinal motor neurons (64, 65, 490). Originating in the somatotopically organized regions of the cerebral cortex, the axons of the large and small pyramidal cells extend through the internal capsule, the cerebral crus, the anterior portion of the pons, and the medulla oblongata. The posterior limb of the **internal capsule** can be demarcated in axial slices between the thalamus and lentiform nucleus by means of an approximate rectangle (64). This narrow rectangle is divided into three parts in an anterior–posterior direction and the position of the corticospinal tract localized by specification of the anterior, middle, and

6.8.1 Pyramidal System 377

1 Superior frontal gyrus
2 Middle frontal gyrus
3 Corticospinal tract
4 Corticospinal tract in cerebral crus (within the slice)
5 Supplementary motor area
6 Precentral gyrus
7 Corticospinal tract in posterior limb of internal capsule (within the slice)
8 Precentral gyrus
9 Postcentral gyrus
10 Corticospinal tract in pyramid
11 Pyramidal decussation
12 Anterior corticospinal tract in anterior funiculus (within the slice)
13 Lateral corticospinal tract in lateral funiculus (within the slice)

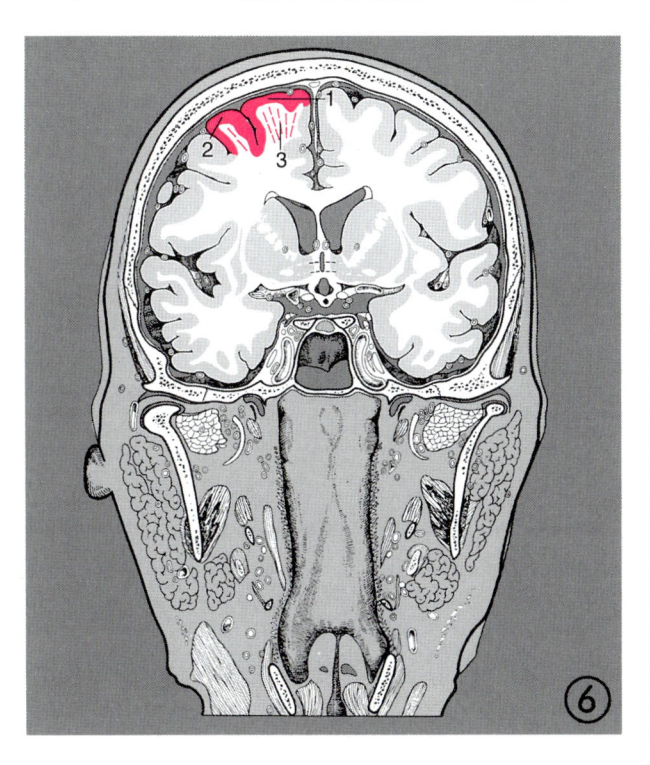

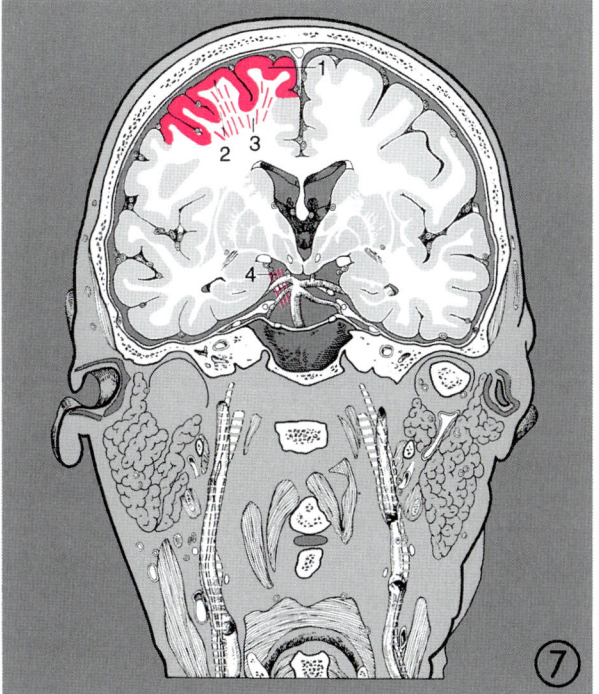

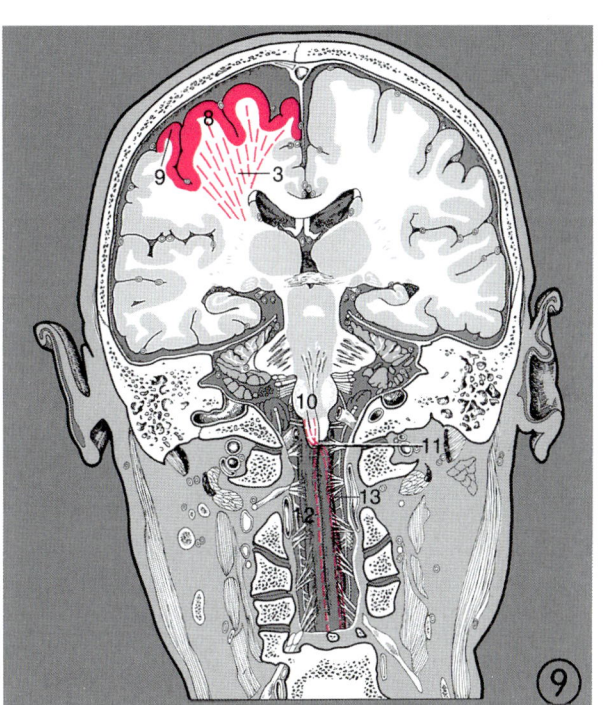

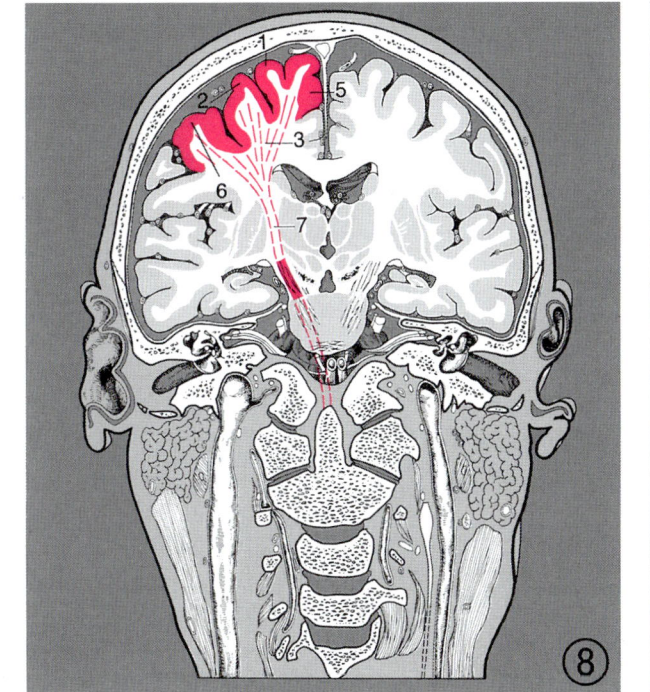

Fig. 133 Coronal serial illustrations of the pyramidal tract and its areas of origin. The encircled numbers (6–9) indicate the number of the respective slice (Figs. 1, 2a,b, 3).

posterior third. In the upper part of the diencephalon the corticospinal tract is located approximately in the middle third and in the lower part of the diencephalon approximaltey in the posterior third, with the exception of the most posterior region.

In the midbrain the corticospinal tract is located in the middle third of the **cerebral crus**. In the anterior part of the **pons** the pontine nuclei are found between the fibers of the corticospinal tract. Therefore its external circumference is larger compared to its compact fiber bundle in the cerebral crus. The pyramidal pathways form bilateral, cordlike protrusions on the anterior surface of the **medulla oblongata**—the **pyramids**—hence the name. Immediately above the spinal cord, 75–90% of the fibers cross at the **pyramidal decussation** and form the lateral corticospinal tract. This tract descends the entire length of the lateral funiculus. The smaller uncrossed portion of the pyramidal pathway, located in the anterior funiculus, descends as the anterior corticospinal tract to the middle of the thoracic spinal cord. It crosses at the level of the corresponding spinal segment. The interneurons, which act as relays between the pyramidal pathway and the spinal motor neurons, usually connect with numerous motor neurons or form parts of inhibitory feedback loops.

378   6 Neurofunctional Systems

3 Corticospinal tract
9 Postcentral gyrus
14 Precentral gyrus (muscles of the lower extremity)
15 Precentral gyrus (muscles of the foot)

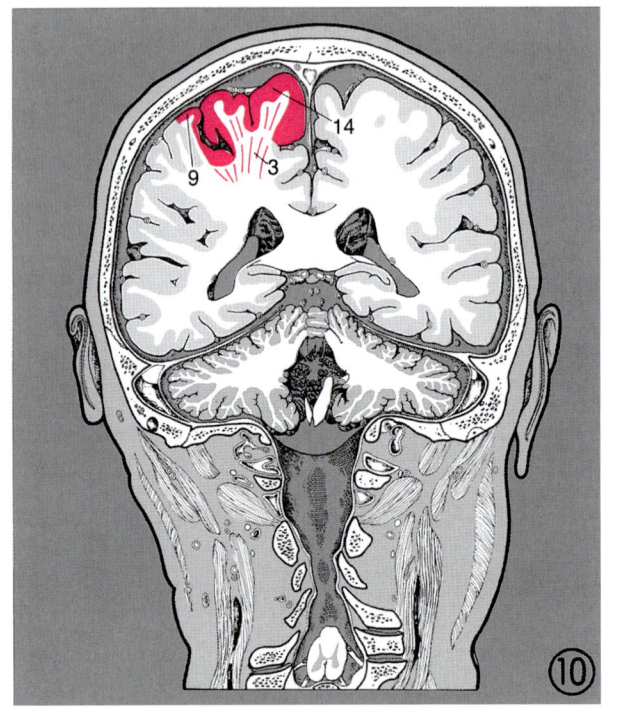

Fig. 133 Coronal serial illustrations of the pyramidal tract and its areas of origin. The encircled numbers (10–11) indicate the number of the respective slice (Figs. 1, 2a,b, 3).

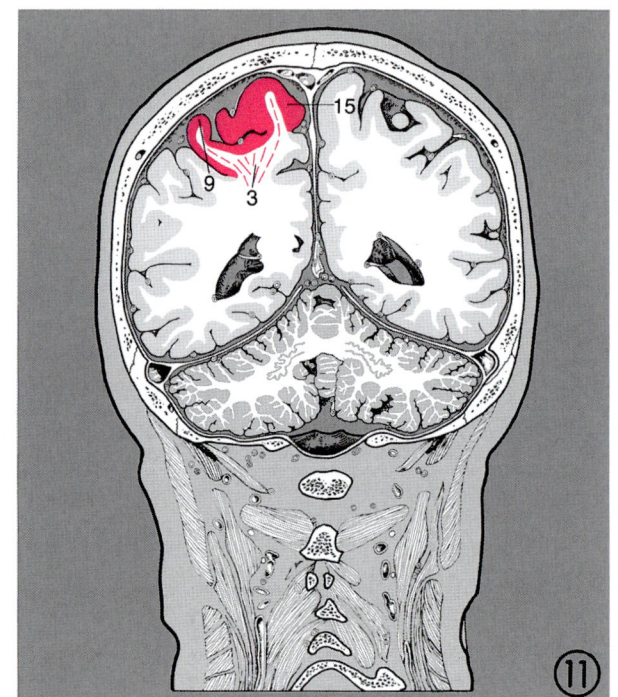

1 Supplementary motor area
2 Paracentral lobule
3 Corticospinal tract in cerebral crus (within the slice)
4 Corticospinal tract in pons (within the slice)
5 Corticospinal tract in pyramid
6 Pyramidal decussation
7 Anterior corticospinal tract (contralateral origin)
8 Precentral gyrus (muscles of the lower extremity)
9 Postcentral gyrus
10 Corticospinal tract
11 Corticospinal tract (within the slice)
12 Corticospinal tract in pons

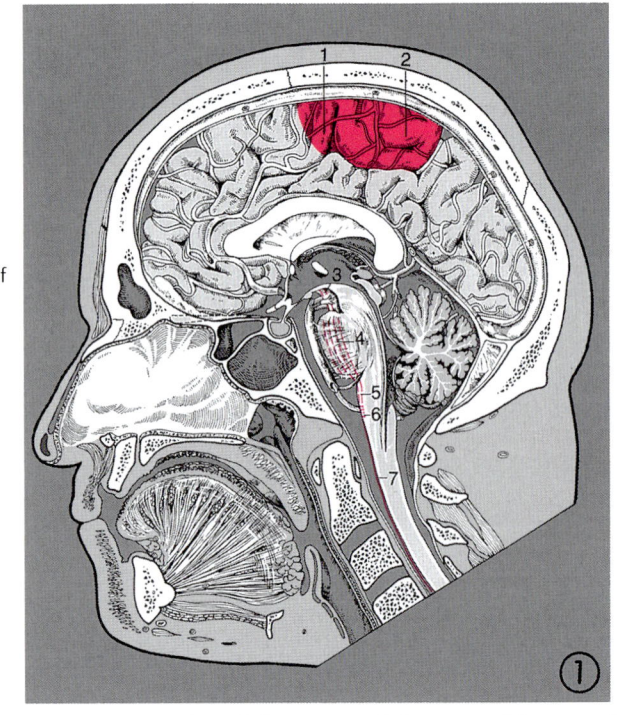

Fig. 134 Sagittal serial illustrations of the pyramidal tract and its areas of origin. The encircled numbers (1–2) indicate the number of the respective slice (Figs. 29, 30a,b, 31).

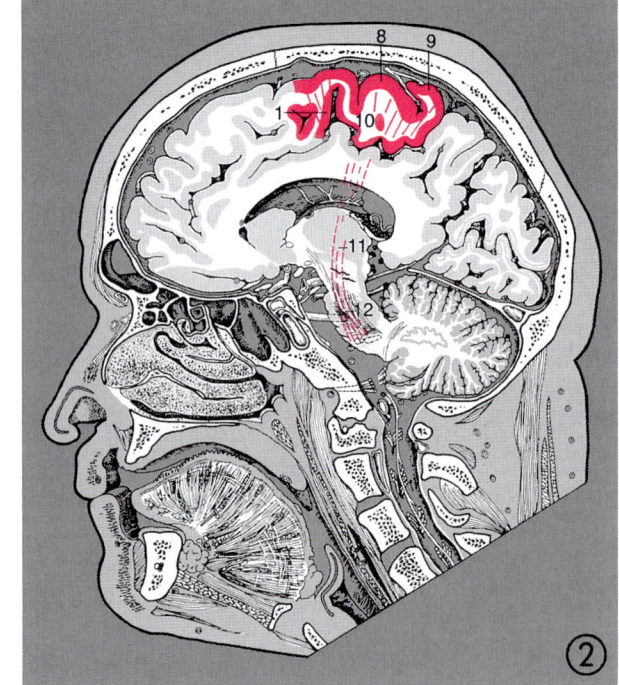

An increase in blood circulation can be seen with PET in the contralateral and ipsilateral motor cortex with movements of the individual muscles of one side. Furthermore, on one-sided magnetic stimulation of the motor cortex, a bilateral effect has been observed in the axial trunk muscles. From these observations, it may be deduced that there is both **contralateral** and **ipsilateral innervation** of the spinal motor neurons for the musculature of the axial trunk and the proximal extremities.

The **corticonuclear fibers** originate in the pyramidal cells of the inferior third of the precentral gyrus, the neighboring premotor cortex, the neighboring somatic sensory areas 3, 1, 2, and area 5. The corticonuclear fibers descend through the internal capsule, pass through the cerebral crus and reach the

6.8.1 Pyramidal System   379

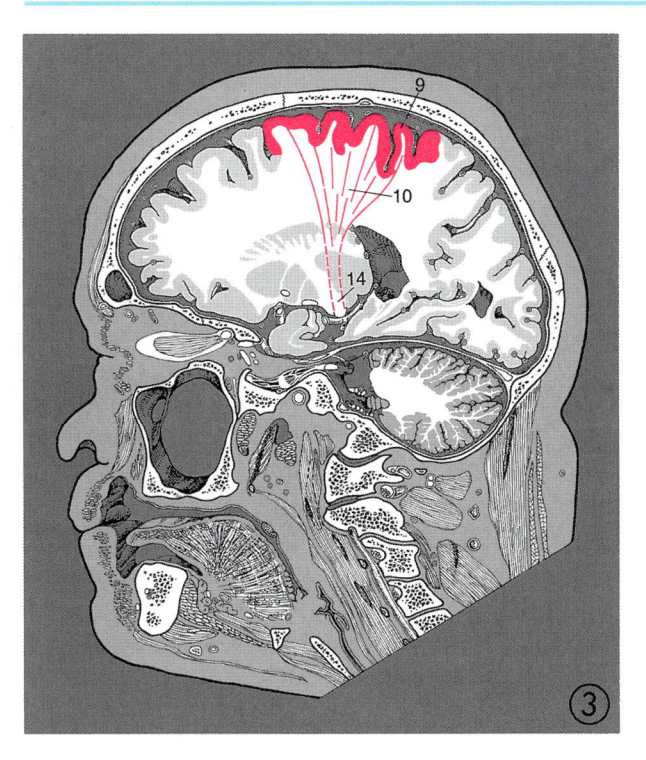

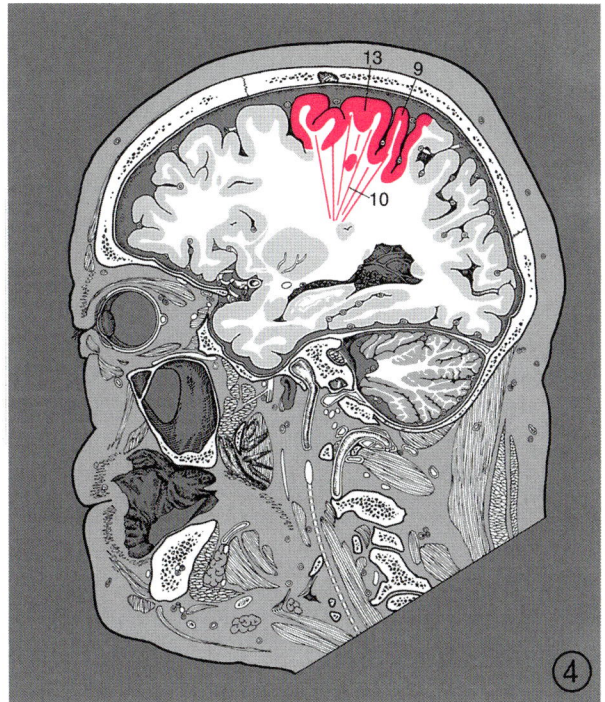

9 Postcentral gyrus
10 Corticospinal tract
13 Precentral gyrus
14 Corticospinal tract in posterior limb of internal capsule

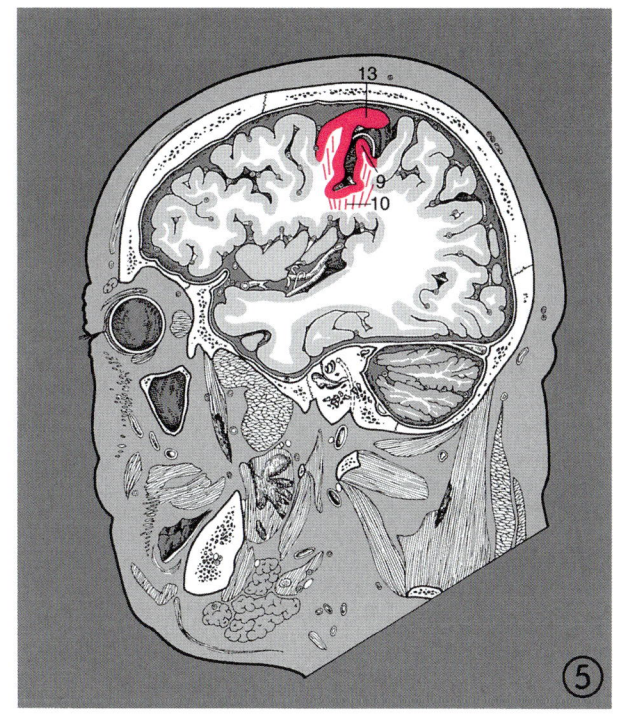

Fig. **134** Sagittal serial illustrations of the pyramidal tract and its areas of origin. The encircled numbers (3–5) indicate the number of the respective slice (Figs. 29, 30a,b, 31).

motor nuclei of **cranial nerves V, VII, IX, X, XII, and partially XI** on the contralateral side in the tegmentum of the pons and the medulla oblongata. The motor nuclei of cranial nerves V, IX, and X receive additional input from the ipsilateral motor cortex and, therefore, are bilaterally innervated. The motor nuclei of cranial nerves XI and XII receive their input from the contralateral cerebral cortex alone. The facial nucleus has two differently innervated regions. The motor neurons of the occipitofrontalis and the orbicularis oculi receive inputs via both ipsilateral and contralateral connections. The remaining facial muscles are innervated contralaterally only.

Clinical notes
When distinguishing between central and peripheral **facial paralysis** it is necessary to have some knowledge of both contralateral and ipsilateral innervation and of contralateral innervation alone for the motor nucleus of the facial nerve. A lesion of the corticonuclear fibers in the internal capsule of one side caused by a stroke, for example, results in a contralateral paralysis of all facial muscles except the occipitofrontalis and the orbicularis oculi. The patient is able to wrinkle the forehead on the side contralateral to the lesion, but the cheek and oral muscles of the face are paretic (central paralysis). Injury to the facial nucleus or nerve on one side results in a paralysis of all the facial muscles on that side (peripheral paralysis, Bell's palsy).
The somatotopic organization of the motor cortex with its relatively wide divergence of the corticospinal and corticonuclear fibers explains the frequent occurrence of partial paralyses or of **monopareses** in patients with lesions in and around the motor cortex. Irritative processes in the motor cortex may lead to focal epileptic seizures.
However, the tight bundling of all motor fibers of one hemisphere in the internal capsule accounts for extensive contralateral **hemiplegia** as a result of a lesion in the internal capsule. The topographic proximity of the motor pathway to the terminal part of the sensory pathway in the posterior portion of the internal capsule accounts for simultaneous hemisensory disorders in cases of hemiplegia. Lesions of the posterior and the retrolentiform part of the internal capsule may include the optic pathway and result in a homonymous hemianopia on the opposite side.

1 Lateral corticospinal tract
2 Anterior corticospinal tract
3 Corticospinal tract

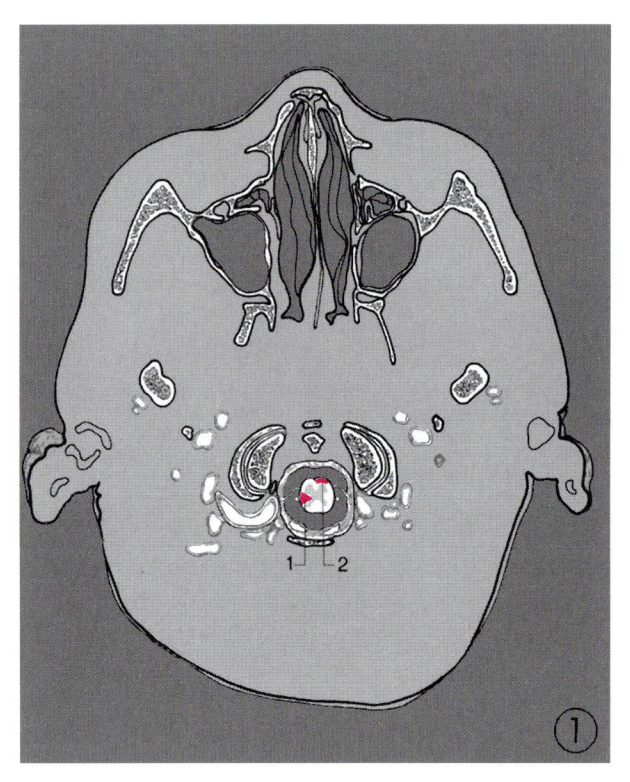

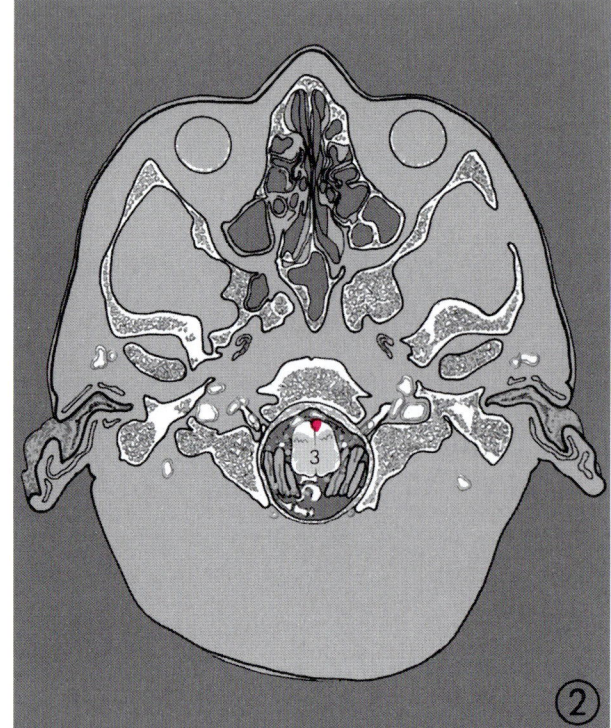

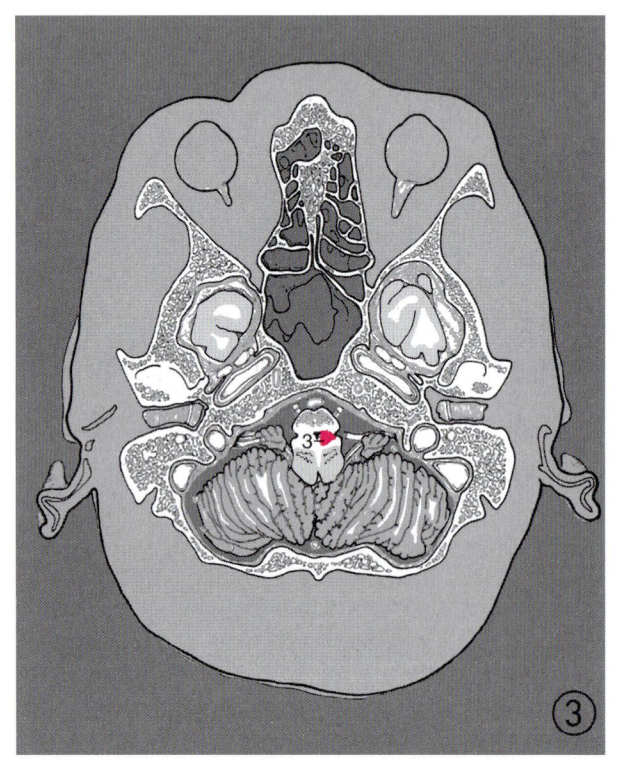

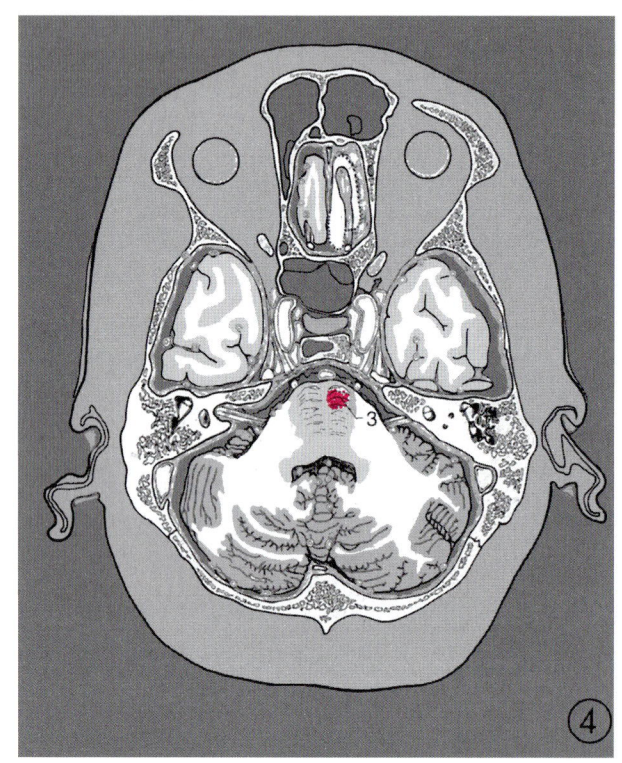

Fig. 135 Canthomeatally oriented serial illustrations of the pyramidal tract and its areas of origin. The encircled numbers (1–8) indicate the number of the respective slice (Figs. 44, 45a,b, 46).

Transcranial magnetic stimulation allows assessment of the functions of the motor pathways by determination of the central conduction time. This noninvasive measurement is carried out by generating a strong magnetic field in a electric coil, which is placed over the vertex, then measuring the motor response of the contralateral extremity. A lesion of the corticospinal fibers results in the loss of the response potential if the tract is completely disrupted, and in a reduction of amplitude if only a partial disruption exists (80a, 84, 167a, 288, 374a, 446).

A hemiplegia with eye muscle disorders and central facial paralysis indicates a lesion in the midbrain and/or the pons. Injuries affecting pons and medulla oblongata are a cause of ipsilateral cranial nerve disorders accompanied by swallowing and speech impairment (cranial nerves IX, X, and XII) and contralateral hemiparesis.

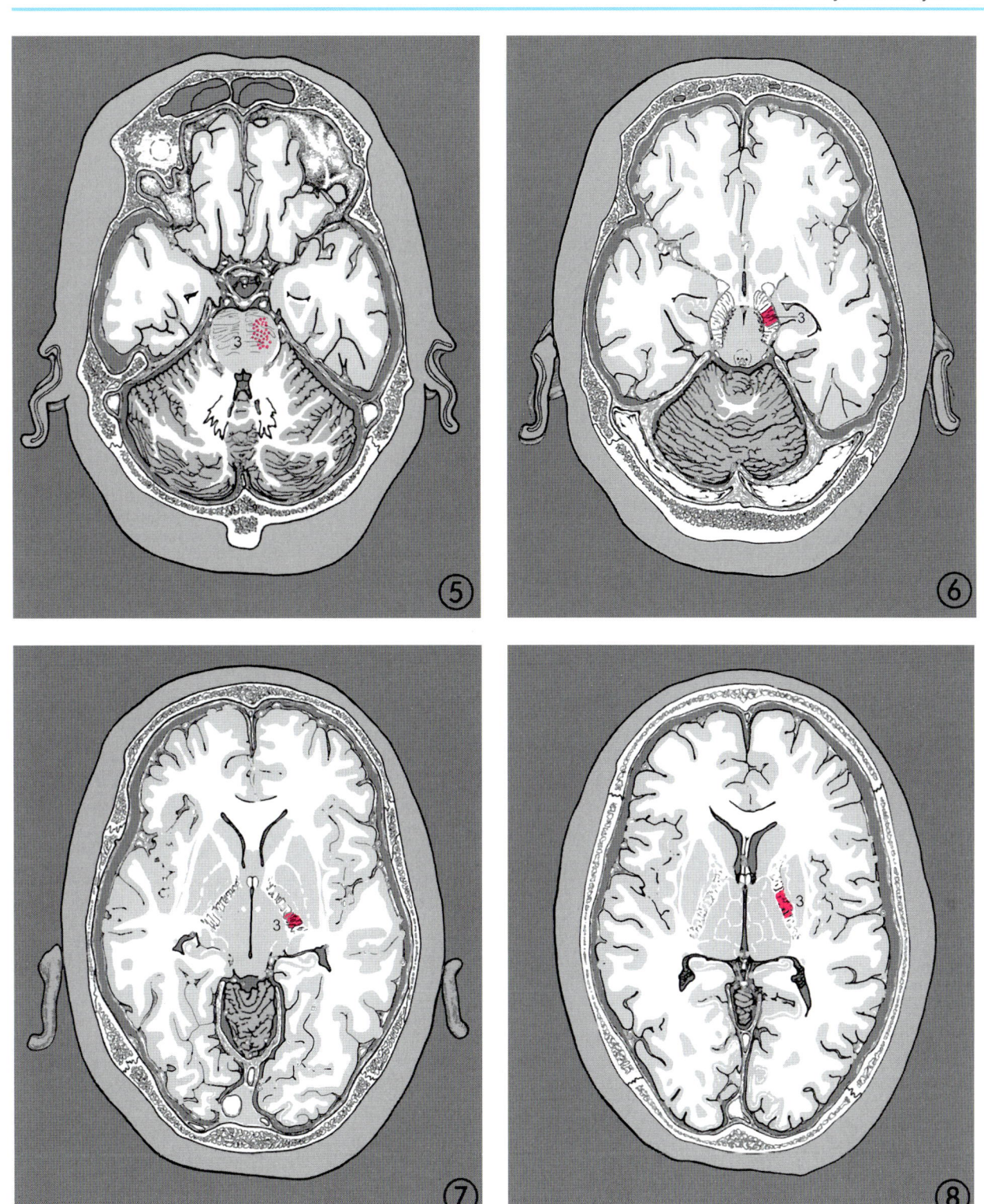

6.8.1 *Pyramidal System* 381

3   Corticospinal tract

382   6 Neurofunctional Systems

3 Corticospinal tract
4 Precentral gyrus
5 Premotor cortex
6 Somatic sensory cortex
7 Paracentral lobule

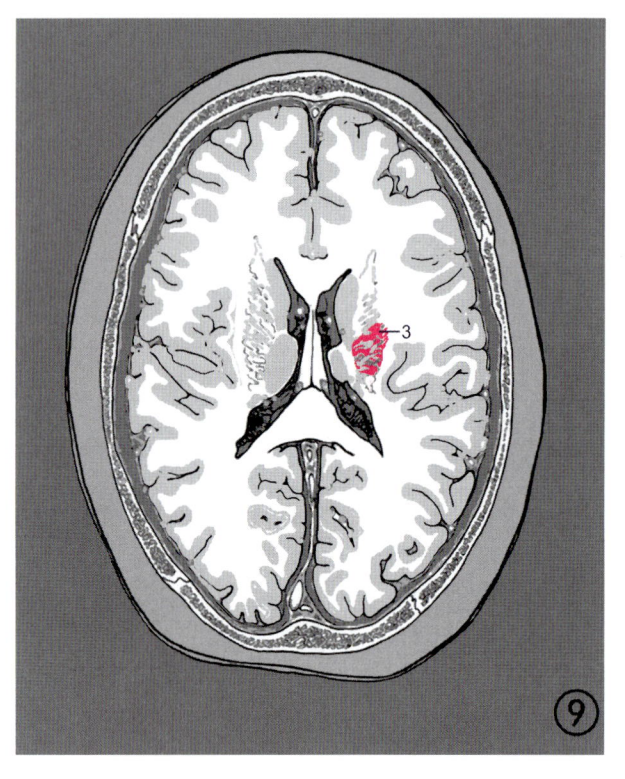

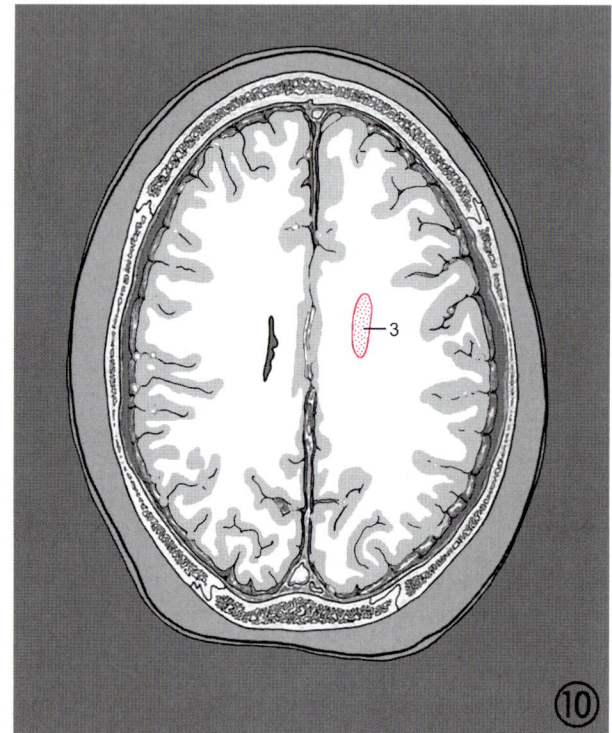

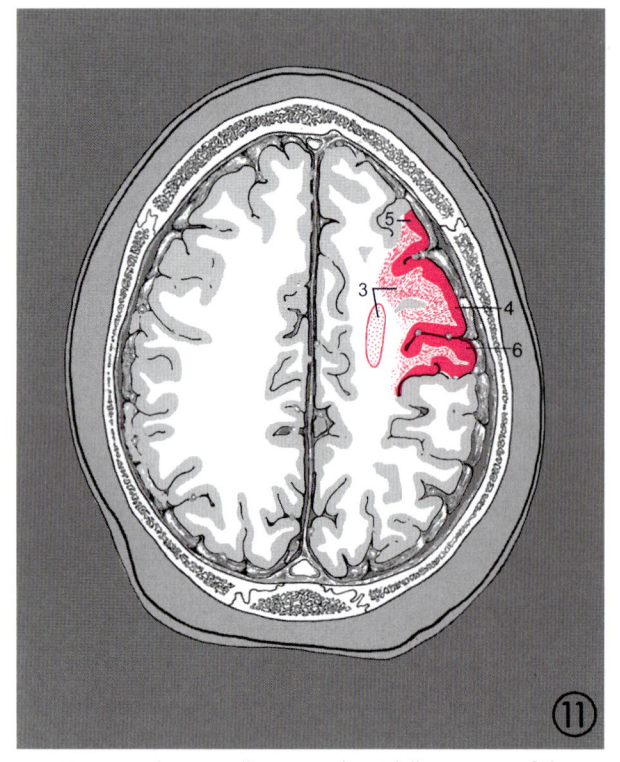

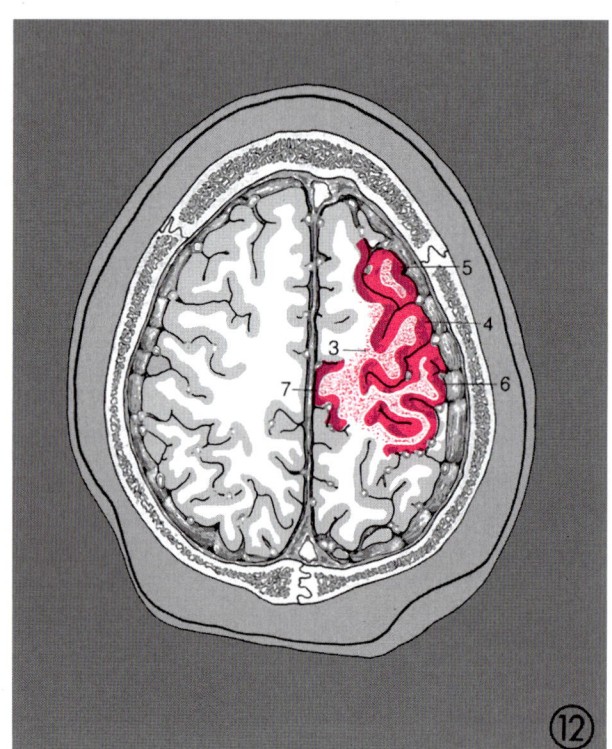

Fig. 135 Canthomeatally oriented serial illustrations of the pyramidal tract and its areas of origin. The encircled numbers (9–14) indicate the number of the respective slice (Figs. 44, 45a,b, 46).

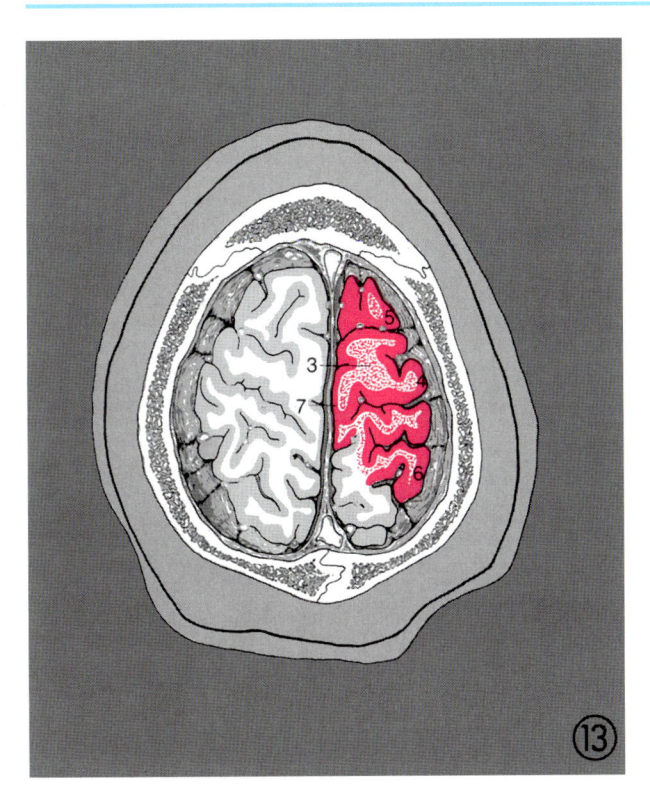

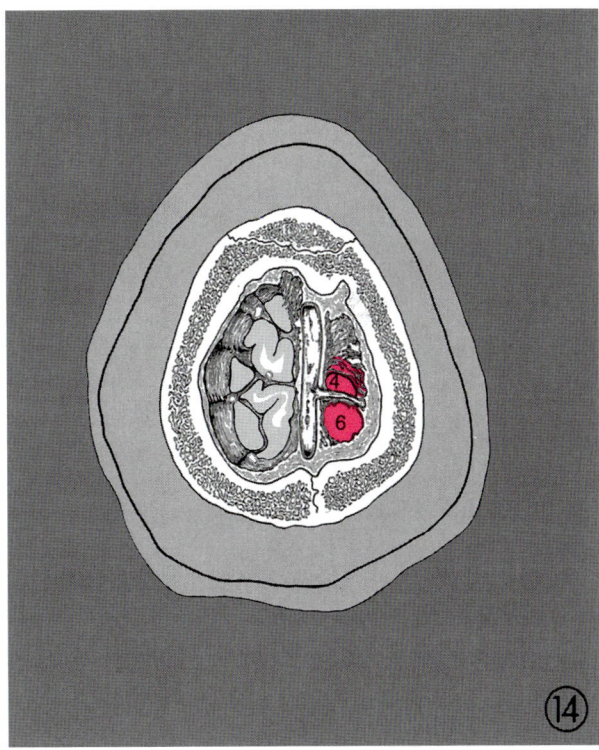

3 Corticospinal tract
4 Precentral gyrus
5 Premotor cortex
6 Somatic sensory cortex
7 Paracentral lobule

6.8.2 Motor Systems of the Basal Ganglia
(Figs. 136–138)

The motor systems of the basal ganglia are composed of subcortical groups of nuclei. These nuclei have extensive connections with the motor cortex and form several loops or circuits among themselves. In accordance with these neuronal loops, it appears that the neurons of the basal ganglia form several **control circuits**. The neurons receive their incoming signals (input) from cortical regions and from the reticular formation, vestibular system, and cerebellum. The outgoing signals (output) leave primarily via the pyramidal pathway; some, however, leave via the descending multisynaptic brainstem pathways including the reticulospinal and vestibulospinal pathways.

The main structures comprising the motor systems of the **basal ganglia** are the striatum (putamen, caudate nucleus, and nucleus accumbens), globus pallidus, subthalamic nucleus, substantia nigra, red nucleus, and lateral vestibular nucleus. Stereotactic operations have shown that small nuclei of the lateral thalamic nucleus, namely the ventral anterior and ventral lateral nuclei, can significantly influence rigidity and tremor. For this reason, these smaller nuclei may also be considered part of the basal ganglia.

Important **afferent signals** reaching the basal ganglia arrive in the striatum from the reticular formation via small thalamic nuclei, such as the intralaminar nuclei. Pathways project from the dentate nucleus in the cerebellum, via the ventral lateral nucleus of the thalamus, to the pallidum and the motor cortex. The mesostriatal serotoninergic system, the cell bodies of which lie in the posterior raphe nucleus of the midbrain, terminates in the striatum.

The **main control circuit** of the basal ganglia projects from the neocortex to the striatum, and is relayed via the globus pallidus into the ventral anterior and ventral lateral nuclei of the thalamus. These nuclei project to the motor and premotor cortex (areas 4 and 6). Apparently, this loop "collects" information from the entire neocortex and processes it for the motor and premotor cortex. In addition, three accessory circuits connect the previously mentioned nuclei of the basal ganglia. In these circuits, the striatum assumes a central role.

The **first accessory loop** extends from the striatum to the globus pallidus, from there to the centromedian nucleus of the thalamus, with a return to the striatum. The **second accessory loop** projects from the globus pallidus to the subthalamic nucleus and back. The **third accessory loop** (striatum–substantia nigra–striatum) uses two different neurotransmitters: GABA and dopamine. The striatonigral fibers use GABA, the nigrostriatal fibers are dopaminergic.

The corticonuclear and corticospinal fibers are important efferent pathways of the basal ganglia. These fibers originate in the motor and premotor cortex and receive an input from the first striatal loop. There is uncertainty, however, about the number of motor signals that are transmitted downward parallel to the pyramidal pathways. Parallel projections, originating in the basal ganglia, extend via the substantia nigra to the tectum and the reticular formation. The tectospinal and reticulospinal tracts descend from here into the spinal cord. Some descending fibers of the lateral vestibular nucleus, such as the lateral vestibulospinal tract, also belong to the output system of the basal ganglia as well.

384   6 *Neurofunctional Systems*

1 Head of caudate nucleus (in the posterior part of the slice)
2 Head of caudate nucleus
3 Putamen
4 Claustrum
5 Body of caudate nucleus
6 Ventral lateral nucleus of thalamus (within the slice)
7 Globus pallidus

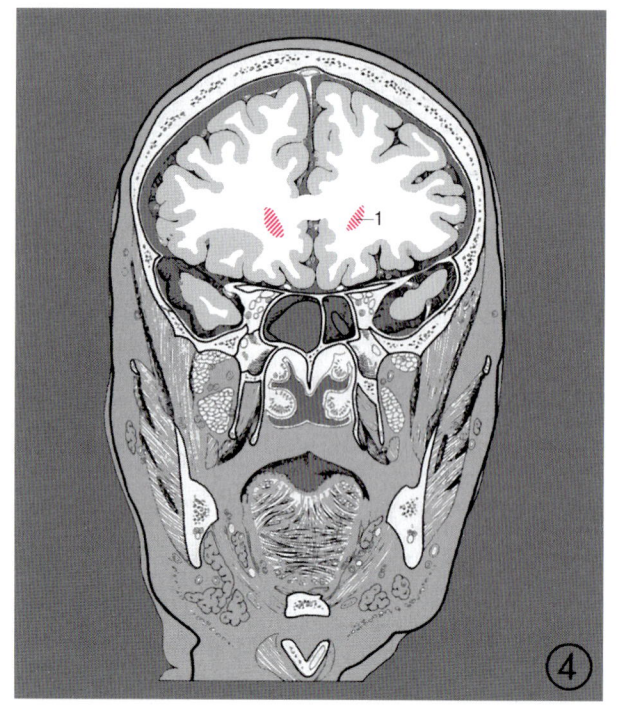

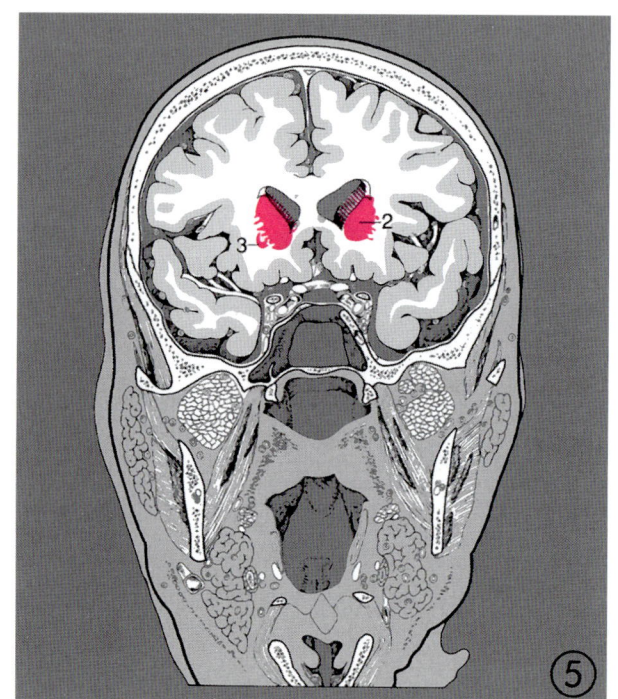

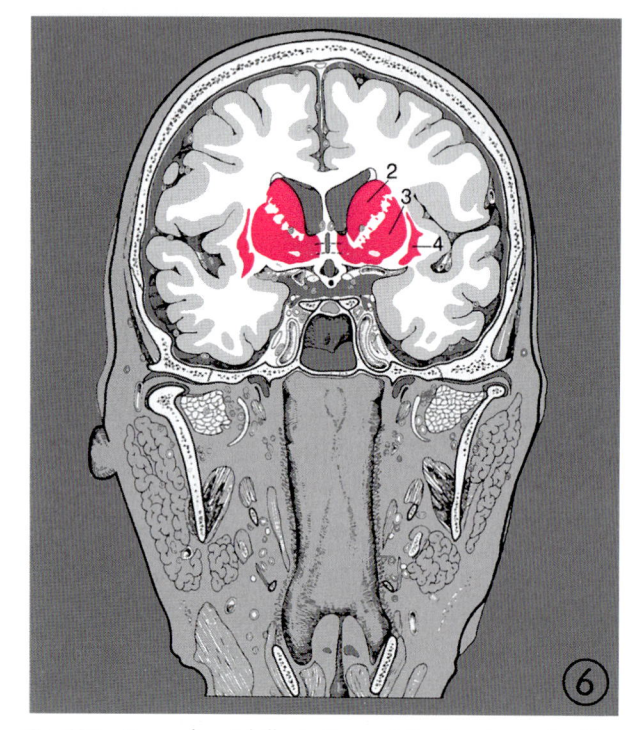

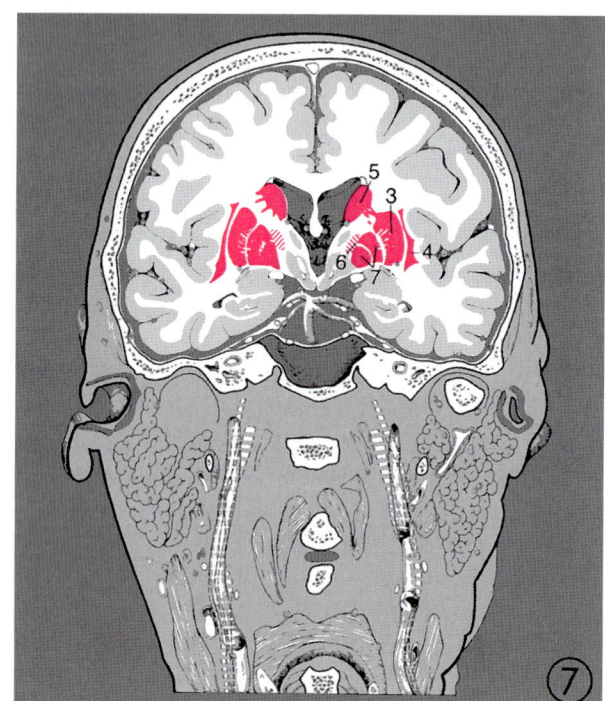

Fig. **136** Coronal serial illustrations of the basal ganglia. The encircled number indicates the number of the respective slice (Figs. 1, 2a,b, 3).

6.8.2 Motor Systems of the Basal Ganglia

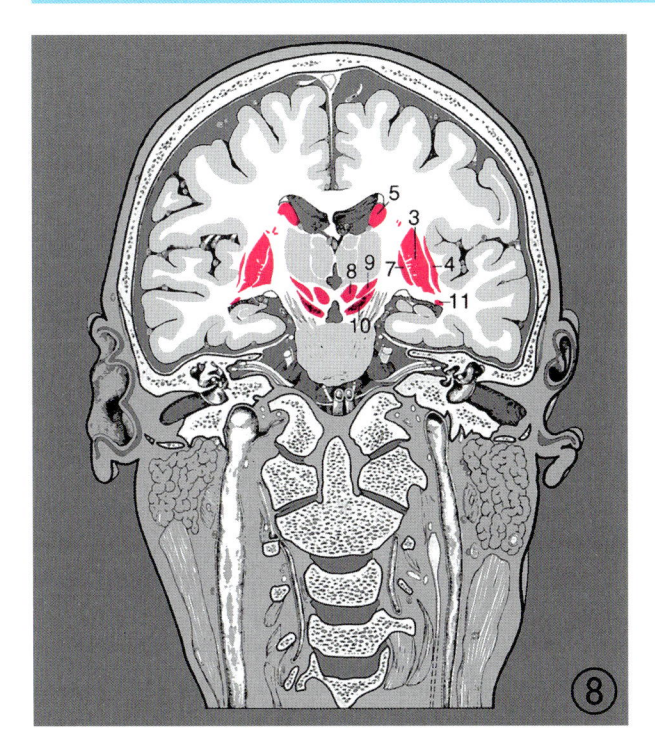

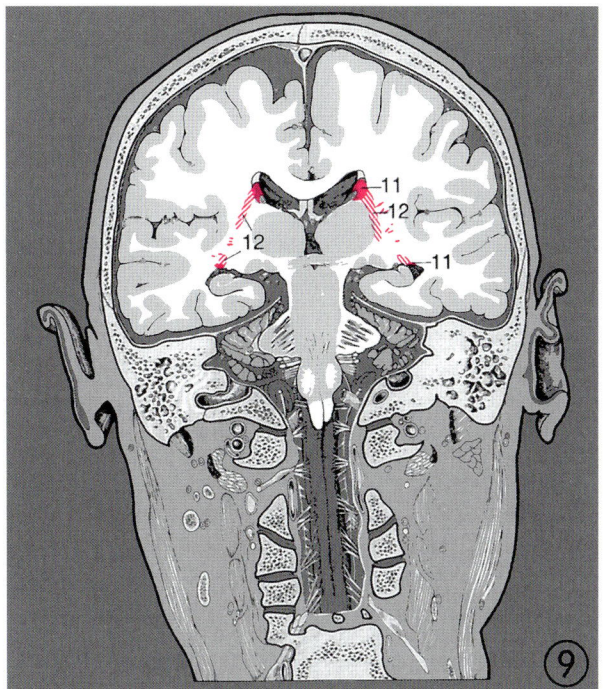

3 Putamen
4 Claustrum
5 Body of caudate nucleus
7 Globus pallidus
8 Red nucleus
9 Subthalamic nucleus
10 Substantia nigra
11 Tail of caudate nucleus
12 Tail of caudate nucleus (within the slice)

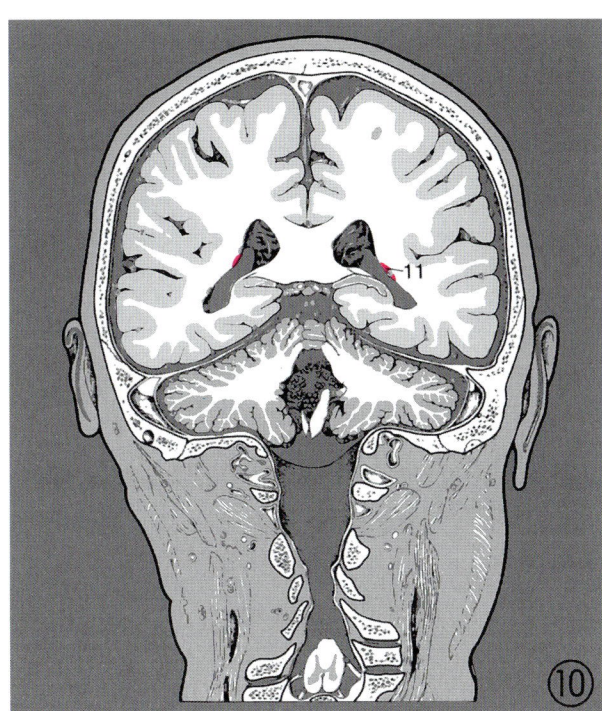

Fiber bundles connect the basal ganglia **with the limbic system**. The pallidohabenular fibers connect the medial segment of the pallidum with a portion of the limbic system (lateral habenular nucleus).

Clinical Notes

Disorders of the basal ganglia cause characteristic changes in motor functions, including speech. Such changes may be obvious, as in spontaneous hyperkinesia, tonus changes (especially rigidity), hypokinesia, tremor, and characteristic postural disorders. In hereditary **Huntington's disease** the severity of the clinical symptoms, hyperkinesia and dementia, often correlates with a widening of the ventricles as seen in CT and MR scans, which demonstrate typical atrophy of the caudate nucleus and putamen and also a diffuse, subcortically accentuated brain atrophy (374a, 447). With PET, reduction of the metabolism in the basal ganglia can be demonstrated even before the appearance of clinical symptoms, and before manifestation of brain atrophy (66, 489). In cases of **Parkinson's syndrome**, CT scans provide few consistent pathologic findings. In addition to rare abnormal findings, dilatation of the ventricles and/or subarachnoid spaces are common. Parkinson's syndrome is generally recognized as being primarily a disorder of the nigrostriatal dopaminergic system (Chap. 7.1.1). PET and SPECT can be used for differential diagnosis of Parkinson's disease and other similar motor impairments (32a, 32b, 66).

Athetosis arises as a result of anatomic lesions that vary from case to case. CT and MR findings, therefore, also vary considerably. **Hemiballism** (uncontrollable flailing movements of one or both limbs on the contralateral side) is often associated with a cerebrovascular lesion involving the subthalamic nucleus or its connections (471b).

386   6 Neurofunctional Systems

1. Subthalamic nucleus (within the slice)
2. Red nucleus (within the slice)
3. Substantia nigra (within the slice)
4. Body of caudate nucleus (within the slice)
5. Head of caudate nucleus
6. Ventral lateral nucleus of thalamus
7. Subthalamic nucleus
8. Substantia nigra
9. Body of caudate nucleus
10. Tail of caudate nucleus
11. Putamen
12. Lateral part of globus pallidus
13. Medial part of globus pallidus

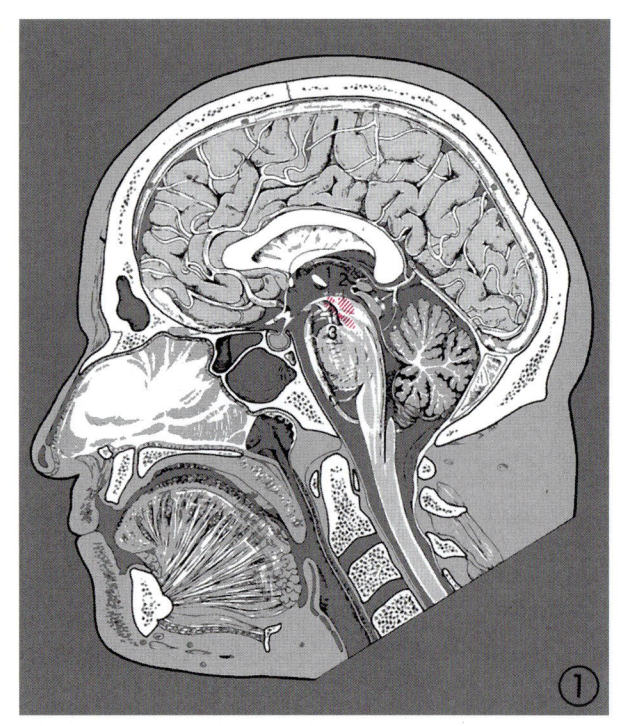

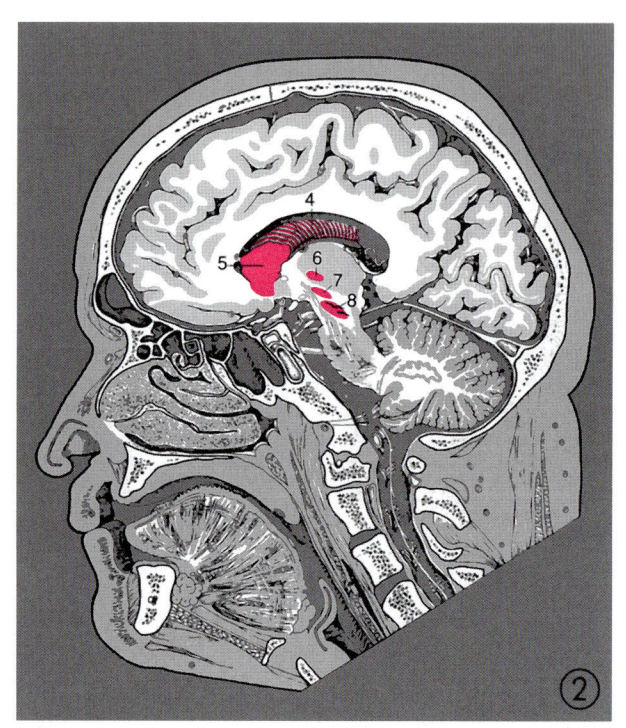

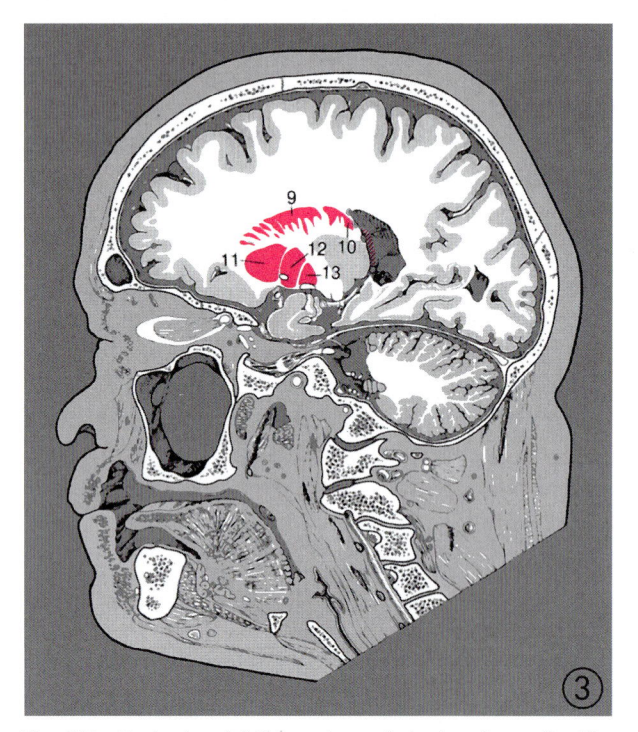

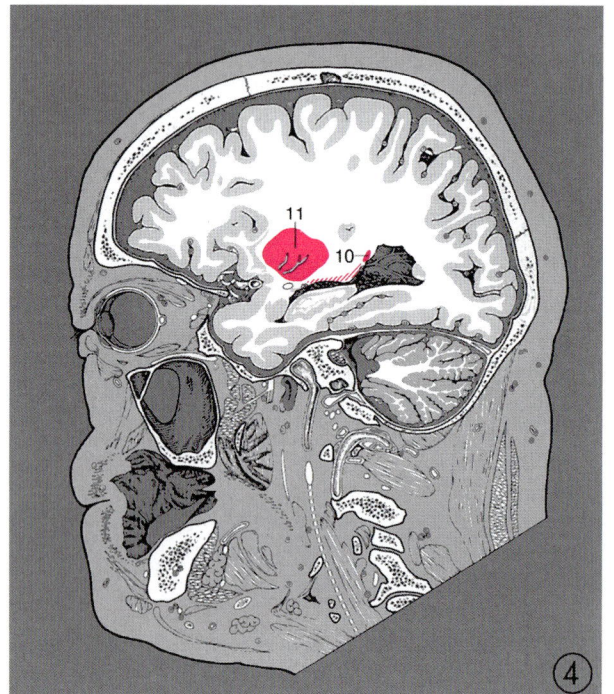

Fig. **137** Sagittal serial illustrations of the basal ganglia. The encircled number (1–4) indicates the number of the respective slice (Figs. 29, 30a,b, 31).

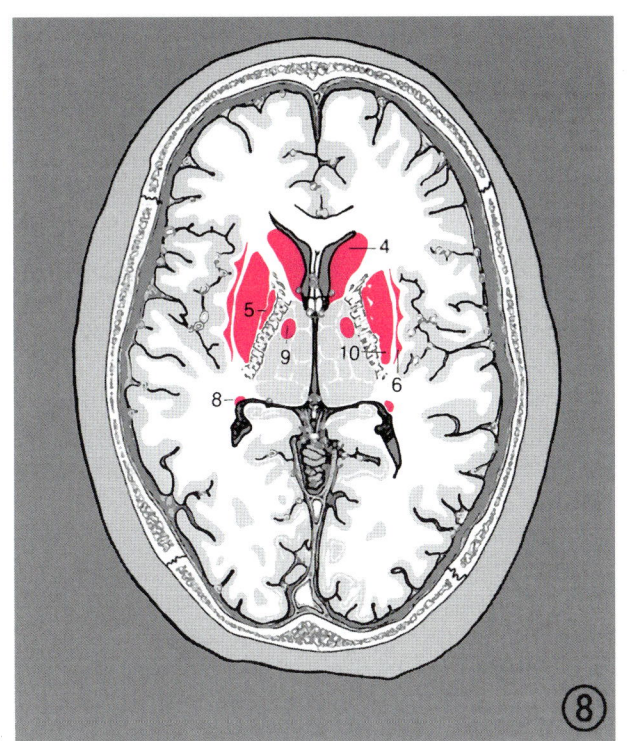

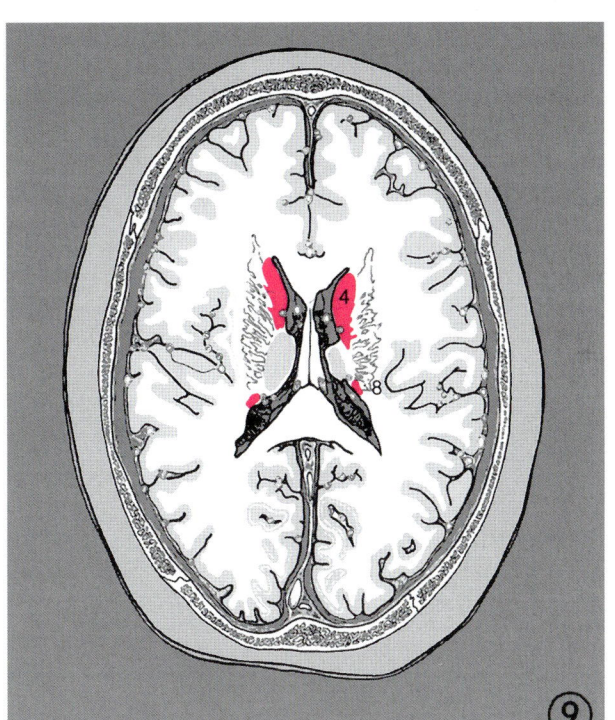

6.8.2 Motor Systems of the Basal Ganglia   387

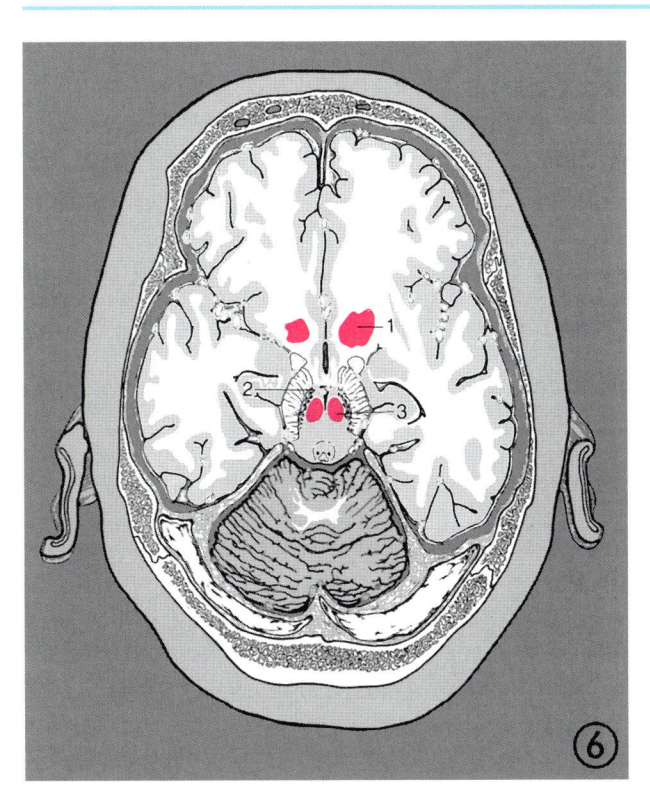

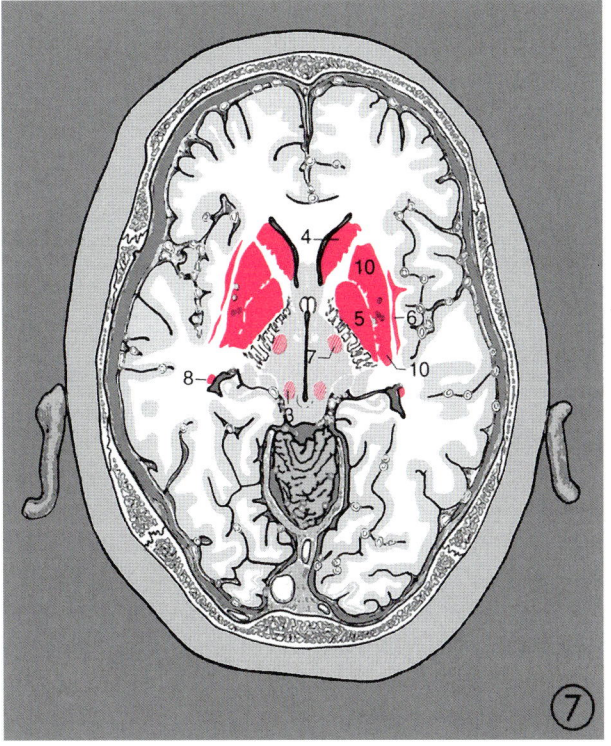

1 Floor of striatum, nucleus accumbens
2 Substantia nigra
3 Red nucleus (partially within the slice)
4 Head of caudate nucleus
5 Globus pallidus
6 Claustrum
7 Subthalamic nucleus (within the slice)
8 Tail of caudate nucleus
9 Ventral lateral nucleus of thalamus
10 Putamen

Fig. 138 Canthomeatally oriented serial illustrations of the basal ganglia. The encircled number (6–9) indicates the number of the respective slice (Figs. 44, 45a,b, 46).

6.8.3 Oculomotor Systems

(Figs. 139–141)

The oculomotor systems control the movements of the extraocular muscles via the third, fourth, and sixth cranial nerves. Disturbances of ocular movements are clinically important. Paralysis of gaze, impaired pupillary reactions, paralysis of vergence movements, nystagmus, and paralysis of the third, fourth, and sixth cranial nerves are obvious symptoms. Often the localization of a peripheral or central lesion can be achieved through a neurologic examination of eye movements alone (203, 276, 461, 471b).

One can divide eye movements into several types, such as saccades (rapid eye movements), smooth pursuit eye movements, vestibulo-ocular reflexes, and convergence movements, which are controlled by independent neuronal connections. These neuronal networks converge at the level of the motor neurons of the third, fourth, and sixth cranial nerves. The motor nuclei of the third and fourth cranial nerves are in the floor of the aqueduct in the tegmentum of the midbrain (Figs. 68.10, 68.11, 78b.20, 77b.27). The abducens nucleus (of the sixth cranial nerve) is in the pontine gray substance in the floor of the fourth ventricle (Figs. 68.14, 74b.28). In the last decade animal experiments, particularly in primates, have produced valuable information about these oculomotor connections (70, 196, 197, 203).

Saccades

Saccades are **fast conjugate movements** of the eyes, that lead both eyes from one fixation point to another (70). The fovea centralis of the retina of both eyes is centered on a specific object of view. These saccadic movements can be controlled voluntarily by various areas of the cerebral cortex or by the vestibular system as fast phases of nystagmus (Chap. 6.4). The frontal eye fields and the superior colliculus are both involved. Animal experiments have revealed that lesions in both these regions lead to permanent impairment of saccadic eye movements. These saccades are controlled by a **neuronal network of parietal and frontal cerebral areas** (Fig. 139). The posterior parietal cortex (Figs. 139.1, 140.14, 141.17) receives information from the primary visual cortex and transmits on to the frontal eye field (Figs. 139.3, 140.1, 141.16). The frontal eye field is also connected with a supplementary eye field and the dorsolateral prefrontal cortex (Fig. 139.4). The frontal eye field is localized with PET studies in the middle region of the precentral sulcus and at the border of the precentral gyrus (235, 359). The corticofugal paths of the frontal eye field extend through the internal capsule to reach the superior colliculus, the supranuclear center of fixation in the mesodiencephal junction, the pons, also the basal ganglia and the thalamus. The rostral interstitial nucleus of the medial longitudinal fasciculus (Figs. 139.6, 140.4, 141.3) and the interstitial nucleus of Cajal can be found in the mesodiencephal junction. The nerve cells of the rostal interstitial nucleus of the medial longitudinal fasciculus generate vertical and torsional saccades. The neurons of the interstitial nucleus of Cajal stabilize the vertical gaze holding (196, 197).

The horizontal saccades are triggered by the paramedian pontine reticular formation (PPRF) (Figs. 139.10, 140.9, 141.7). It projects into the ipsilateral abducens nucleus that contains motor neurons and internuclear neurons. The abducens internuclear neurons have strong synaptic connections via the medial longitudinal fasciculus with the motor neurons of the contralateral medial rectus in the oculomotor nucleus. This circuit is the basis for horizontal conjugate eye movements, because the two synergists of horizontal conjugate eye movements, lateral rectus and medial rectus, receive their commands from motor neurons and internuclear neurons within the same nuclear area, i. e. the abducens nucleus. A similar connection through internuclear neurons in the interstitiial nucleus of Cajal is suspected for vertical conjugate eye movements (70).

Smooth Pursuit Eye Movements

The smooth pursuit eye movements guide both eyes so that small moving objects are continuously portrayed on the fovea of the retina. Pursuit eye movements require motivation and attention and cannot be performed without a moving object. This system controls the eye muscles in such a way that the speed of the rotation angle of the eyes corresponds to the speed of the object. The visual signals reach the visual cortex via the retina, the optic nerve, and the lateral geniculate body. In experiments carried out on rhesus monkeys, lesions were made in the parieto-occipital cortex in an area that resulted in an impairment of smooth pursuit eye movements. The homologue of this parieto-occipital cortex in the human cerebrum is positioned approximately in the areas 19 and 39 according to Brodmann (460). Fiber connections are found from here to the frontal eye fields. Both the **parieto-occipital cortex** and the **frontal eye fields** have corticofugal paths leading to the posterolateral (dorsolateral) pontine nuclei. From the pons, neuronal pathways for smooth pursuit eye movements course via the middle cerebellar peduncle to the cerebellar flocculus (H X), the declive (VI), and the folium of vermis (VII A), project onto the vestibular nuclei, and finally to the eye muscle nuclei (235, 276). Cerebellectomized monkeys loose smooth pursuit eye movements completely (483).

Vestibulo-ocular Reflexes

The vestibulo-ocular reflexes compensate for movements of the head in space with eye movements that stabilize the visual image on the retina. If, for example, the head is turned left, both eyes turn right so that the fovea of the retina receives the same image of

6.8.3 Oculomotor Systems

1 Posterior parietal cortex
2 Supplementary eye field (on the medial side of the hemisphere)
3 Frontal eye field
4 Dorsolateral prefrontal cortex
5 Corticofugal fibers
6 Rostral interstitial nucleus of the medial longitudinal fasciculus
7 Superior colliculus
8 Oculomotor nucleus
9 Trochlear nucleus
10 Paramedian pontine reticular formation (PPRF)
11 Abducens nucleus

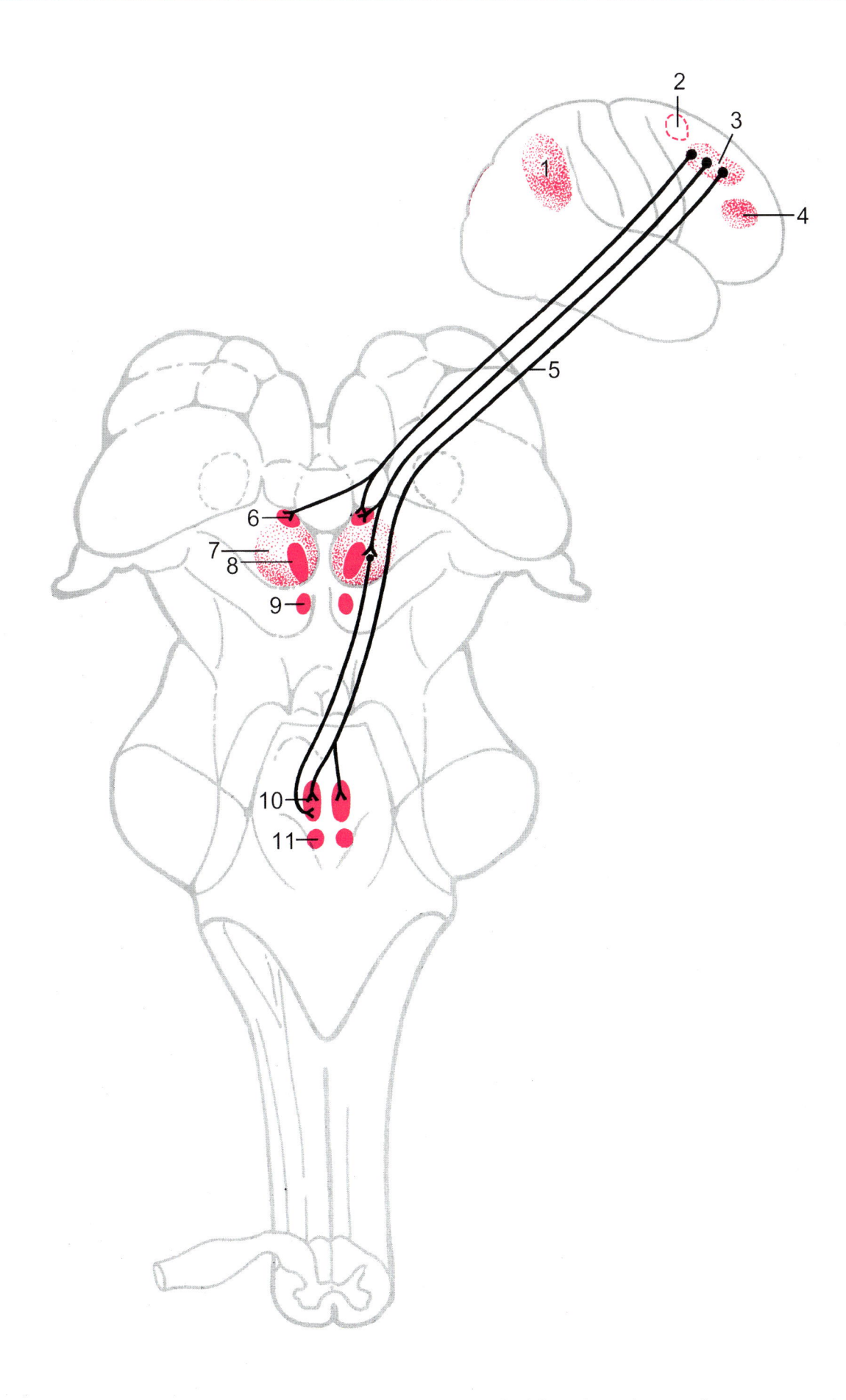

Fig. 139 Cortical and corticofugal parts of one oculomotor system controlling fast conjugate movements of the eyes (saccades). The neuronal pathway of the saccades to the supranuclear centers is demonstrated (rostral interstitial nucleus of medial longitudinal fasciculus and paramedian pontine reticular formation) in lateral view of the cerebrum and posterior view of the brainstem and diencephalon. According to (70, 196, 197, 235).

1 Frontal eye field
2 Corticofugal fibers
3 Supplementary eye field
4 Rostral interstitial nucleus of the medial longitudinal fasciculus
5 Dorsolateral pontine nuclei (within the slice)
6 Superior colliculus (in the posterior part of the slice)
7 Oculomotor nucleus (within the slice)
8 Trochlear nucleus (within the slice)
9 Paramedian pontine reticular formation (PPRF) (within the slice)
10 Vestibular nuclei
11 Abducens nucleus (within the slice)
12 Prepositus nucleus (within the slice)
13 Flocculus (H X)

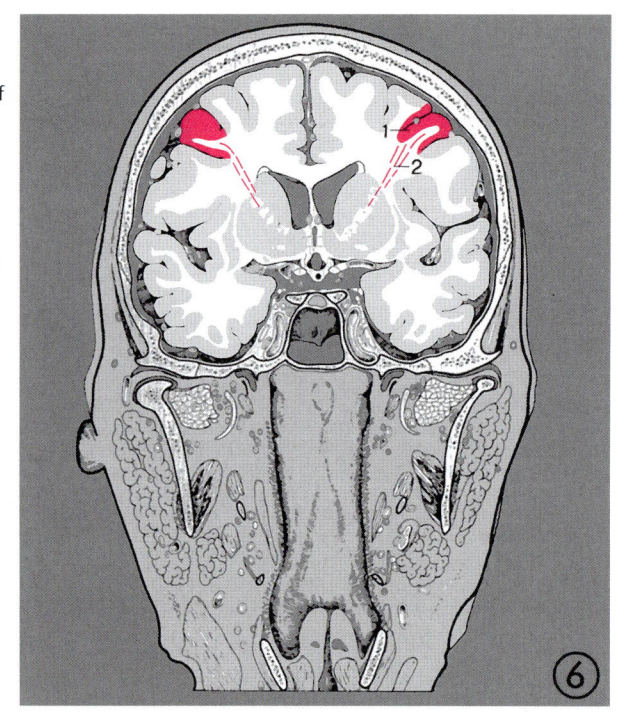

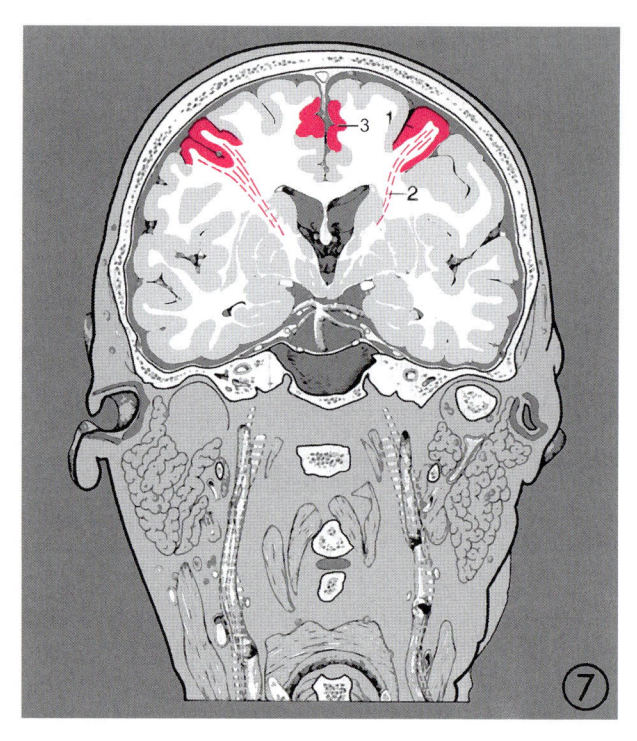

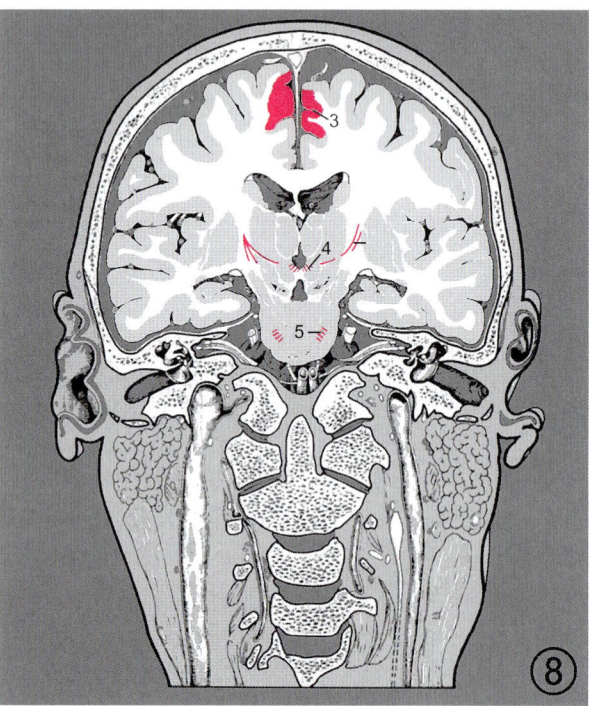

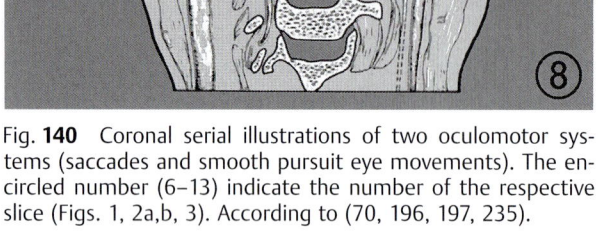

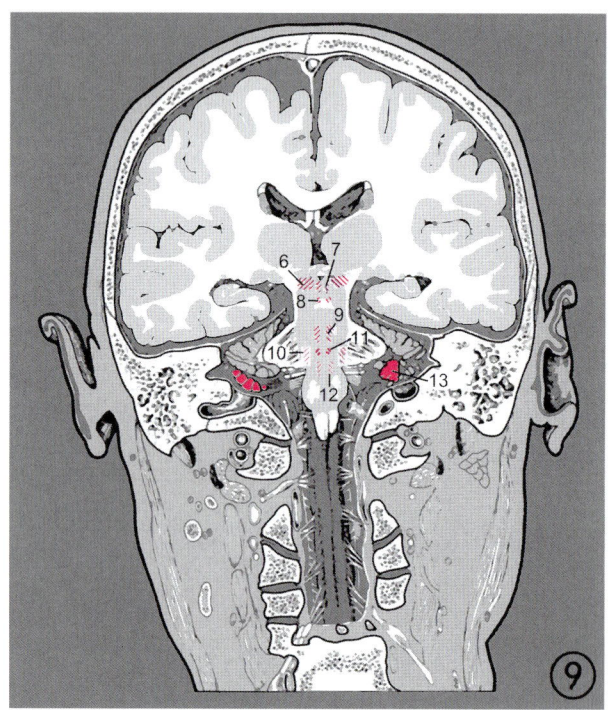

Fig. **140** Coronal serial illustrations of two oculomotor systems (saccades and smooth pursuit eye movements). The encircled number (6–13) indicate the number of the respective slice (Figs. 1, 2a,b, 3). According to (70, 196, 197, 235).

the outside world. The **vestibulo-ocular reflex** can be demonstrated even in unconscious patients. The network of this reflex consists basically of three sets of neurons concerning angular rotation: the first set is located in the vestibular ganglion; it receives its signals from the semicircular ducts and transmits them to the vestibular nuclei (second set). Signals of linear acceleration (i. e. gravity) are generated by the sensory cells of the utricle and saccule, called the otolithic organs and transmitted via the vestibular ganglion to the vestibular nuclei (Chap. 6.4). The neurons of the motor nuclei of the eye muscles form the third and effector set of neurons. The vestibulo-ocular reflex generates eye movements with a very short latency. This reflex pathway is depicted with the vestibular system (Fig. 119).

Vergence Movements

The convergence of both eyes serves the binocular fixation of near objects. Their premotor neurons lie in the mesodiencephal junction (196). The prepositus nucleus shown in Figure 141.9 (formerly nucleus

6.8.3 Oculomotor Systems   391

14 Posterior parietal cortex
15 Parieto-occipital cortex
16 Primary visual cortex
17 Declive (VI)
18 Folium of vermis (VII A)

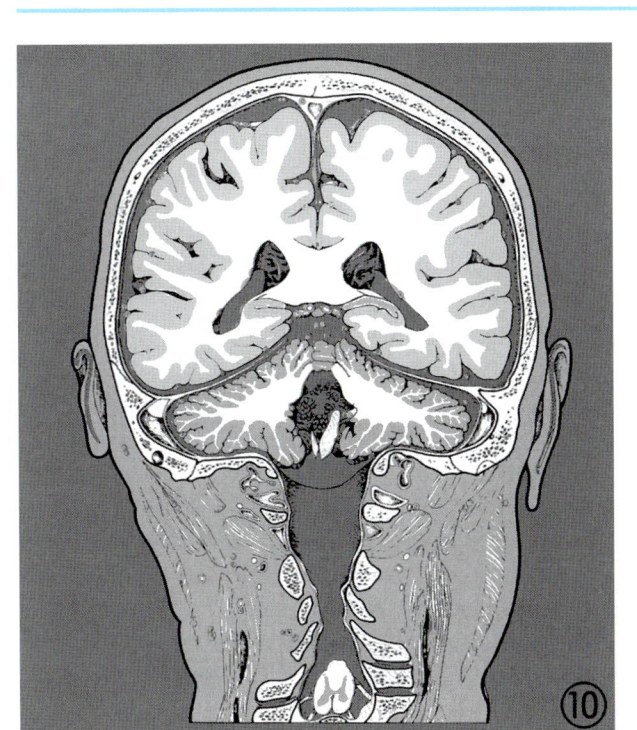

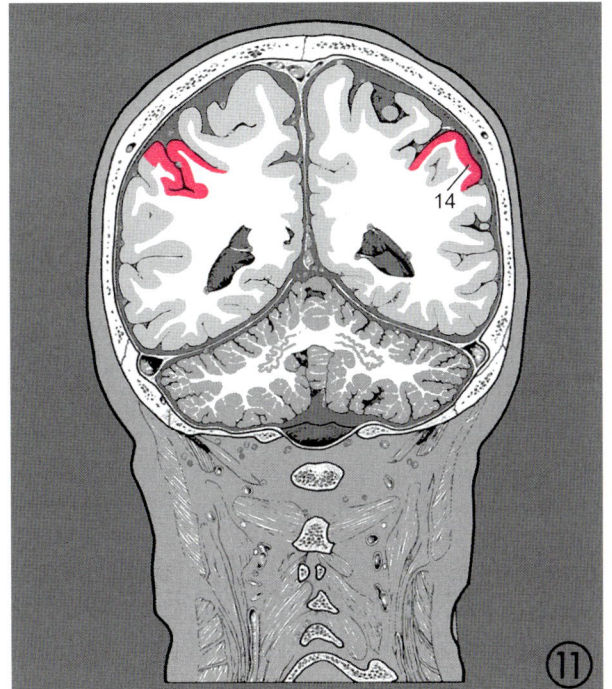

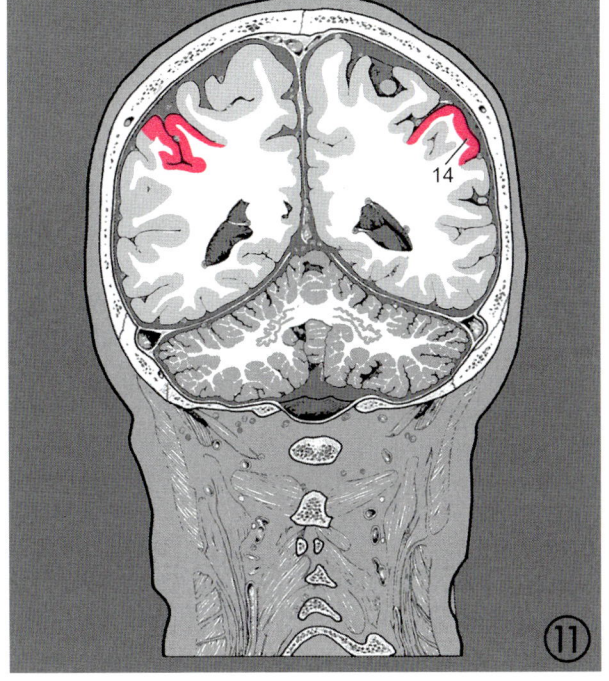

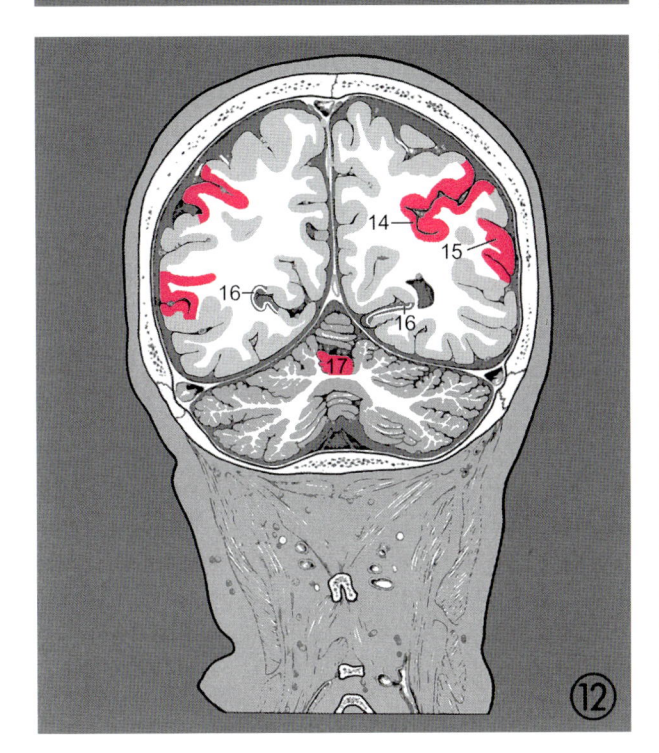

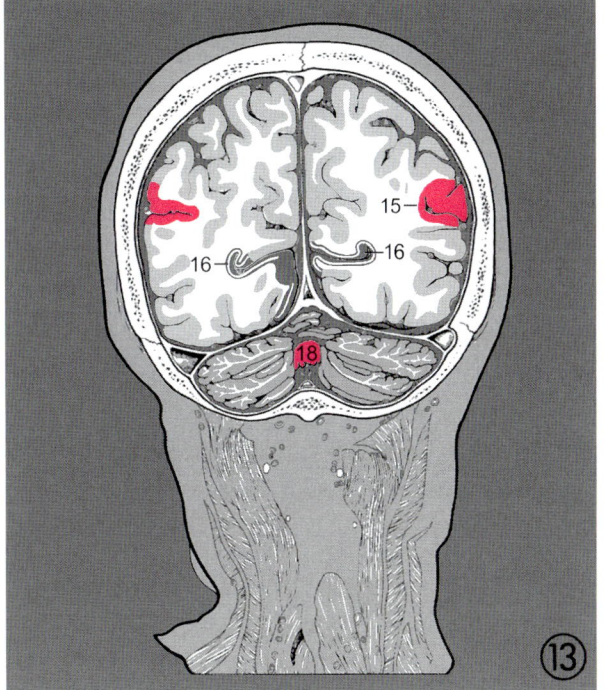

prepositus hypoglossi) has neuronal connections to and from most oculomotor areas, including the vestibular nuclei and parts of the cerebellum. Therefore, it may be supposed that the prepositus nucleus receives efference copies of the oculomotoricity and thus stabilizes the direction of fixation.

Clinical Notes
In **gaze palsies**, conjugate movements of the eyes are restricted or absent in the horizontal or vertical direction. Gaze palsies are predominantly supranuclear in origin. Hence the vestibulo-ocular reflexes and sometimes the smooth pursuit eye movements remain intact. As a rule there is no diplopia (3).

With a lesion of the abducens nucleus, not only are motor neurons destroyed, there is also a loss of the internuclear neurons, already mentioned above, that supply the contralateral medial rectus. Hence a gaze palsy to the ipsilateral side develops (internuclear ophthalmoplegia) (70). Therefore, an isolated lesion of the lateral rectus cannot be the result of an abducens nuclear lesion.

The horizontal gaze palsy to the contralateral side resulting from a unilateral lesion of the frontal lobe with the interruption of the corticopontine fibers is usually transient. It is accompanied by a conjugate deviation of both eyes. This **conjugate deviation** is directed toward the lesion and is

16 Primary visual cortex

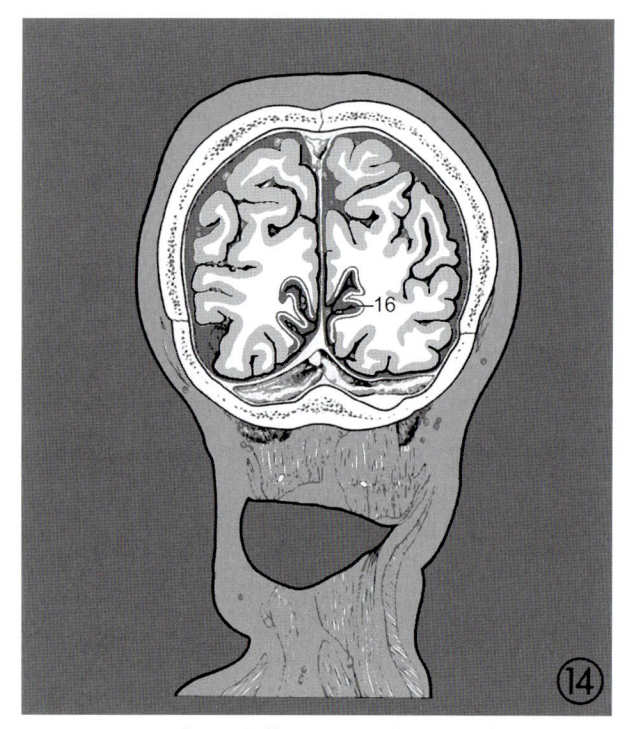

Fig. 140 Coronal serial illustrations of two oculomotor systems (saccades and smooth pursuit eye movements). The encircled number (14) indicates the number of the slice (Figs. 1, 2a,b, 3). According to (70, 196, 197, 235).

especially marked in unconscious patients. With cerebral irritation, such as epilepsy, a paroxysmal deviation of gaze occurs to the side contralateral to the lesion; its origin is unclear. Pontine lesions can cause a paralysis of gaze toward the side of the lesion with conjugate deviation to the opposite side. A **paralysis of vertical gaze** occurs only with bilateral lesions in the rostral interstitial nucleus of the medial longitudinal fasciculus, a paralysis of upward gaze being much more frequent. In combination with paralysis of convergence it is called **Parinaud's syndrome**.

After a lesion of the medial longitudinal fasciculus with interruption of the connections between the abducens and oculomotor nuclei, an **internuclear ophthalmoplegia** results. This includes an impairment of adduction of one or both eyes, as well as a gaze-evoked nystagmus during abduction. When looking straight ahead there is no diplopia. These disorders may be the result of multiple sclerosis or vascular lesions (235, 276).

Lesions of the oculomotor, trochlear, and abducens nerve cause **diplopia**. The clinical distinction between myogenic and neurogenic paresis can be difficult if there is no other neurologic symptom. With neurogenic lesions infranuclear and nuclear damages are to be considered. For the diagnosis, the history and **associated symptoms** are decisive.

Likewise, infranuclear paralyses of the ocular muscles and involvement of the first division of the trigeminal nerve occur as the "syndrome of the

1 Supplementary eye field
2 Primary visual cortex
3 Rostral interstitial nucleus of the medial longitudinal fasciculus
4 Superior colliculus
5 Oculomotor nucleus
6 Trochlear nucleus
7 Paramedian pontine reticular formation (PPRF)
8 Abducens nucleus
9 Prepositus nucleus
10 Declive (VI)
11 Folium of vermis (VII A)
12 Tuber of vermis (VII B)
13 Dorsolateral pontine nuclei

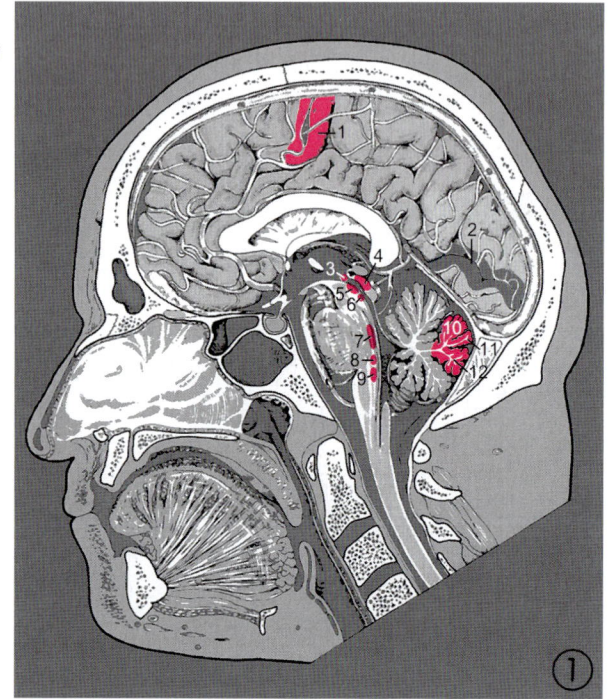

Fig. 141 Sagittal serial illustrations of two oculomotor systems (saccades and smooth pursuit eye movements). The encircled numbers (1–2) indicate the number of the respective slice (Figs. 29, 30a,b, 31). According to (70, 196, 197, 235).

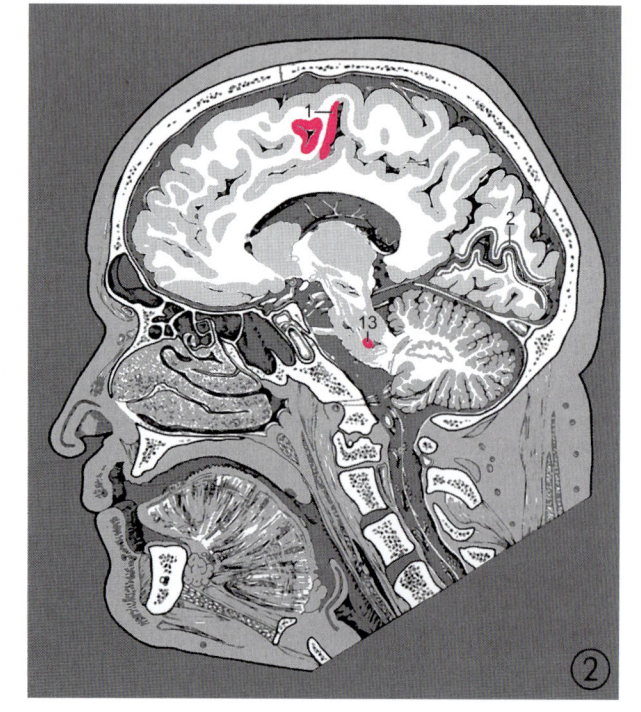

6.8.3 Oculomotor Systems

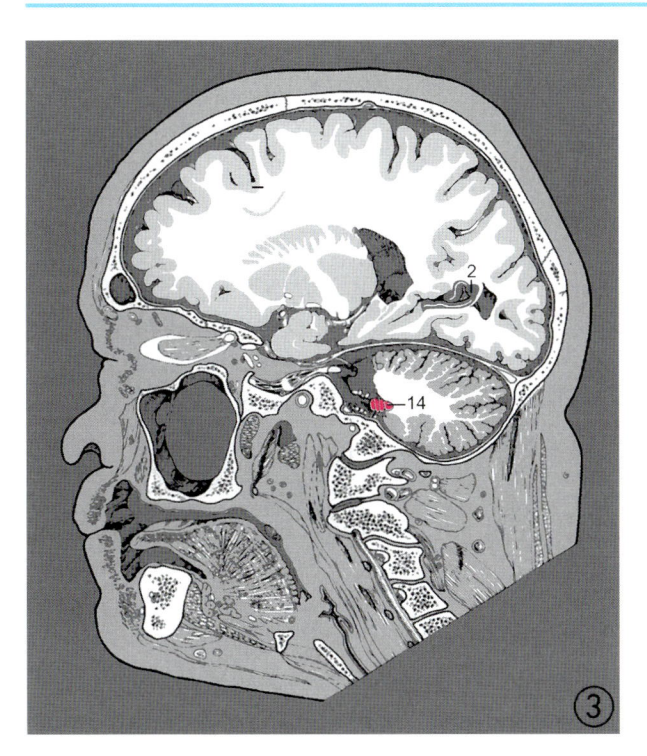

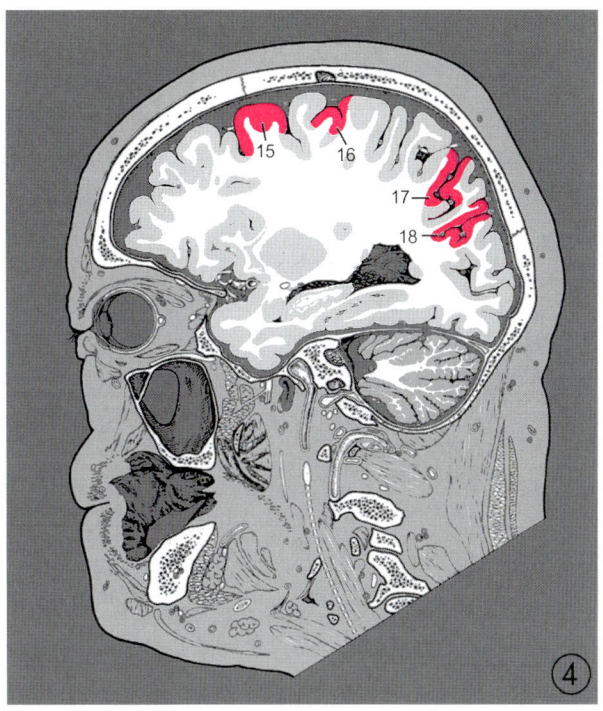

2 Primary visual cortex
14 Flocculus (H X)
15 Dorsolateral prefrontal cortex
16 Frontal eye field
17 Posterior parietal cortex
18 Parieto-occipital cortex

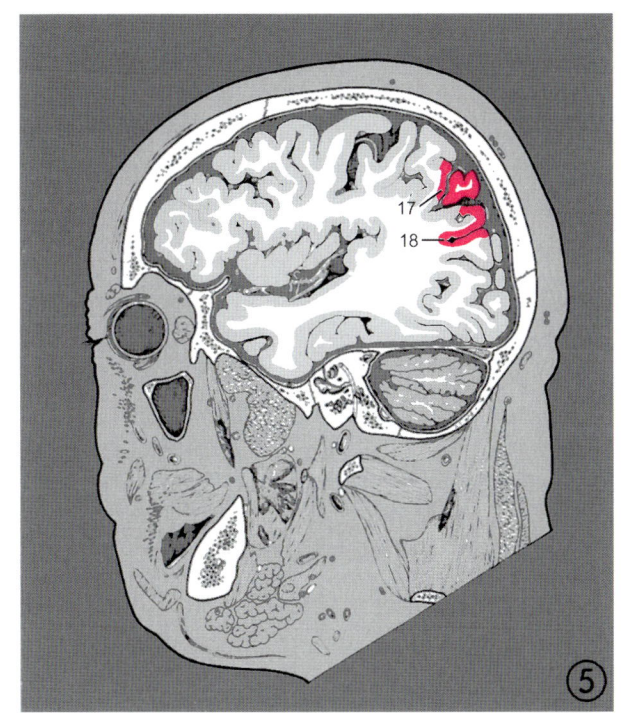

Fig. 141 Sagittal serial illustrations of two oculomotor systems (saccades and smooth pursuit eye movements). The encircled numbers (3–5) indicate the number of the respective slice (Figs. 29, 30a,b, 31). According to (70, 196, 197, 235).

superior orbital fissure." The orbital apex syndrome can be regarded as an advanced syndrome of the superior orbital fissure. Here disorders of the optic nerve, the ophthalmic artery, and the orbital veins accompany the defects already mentioned.

Pupillary anomalies play an important role in clinical diagnosis. Abnormal bilateral dilatation of the pupils is found with midbrain lesions. Abnormally small pupils indicate lesions in the pons. Pupils of unequal size may be the result of a unilateral mydriasis as seen in oculomotor paresis—frequently with ptosis and impaired motility of the eyes—or of a unilateral miosis (**Horner's syndrome**, a combination of miosis with ptosis and enophthalmos on the same side). Abnormal pupillary reactions may be caused by optic nerve lesions (amaurotic iridoplegia), an oculomotor nerve disorder, or, frequently, by lesions of the eyeball.

6.9 Cerebellar Systems

(Figs. 142–144a,b)

The cerebellum receives afferent connections from virtually all receptors in the human body. These include proprioceptive, exteroceptive, vestibular, auditory, visual, and other sensory receptors (55, 221, 374a). The neocortex projects via the pontine nuclei and through pontocerebellar tracts into the contralateral cerebellum. The corticopontocerebellar pathway extends through the massive middle cerebellar peduncle. Most of the efferent pathways originate in the cerebellar nuclei and leave the cerebellum mainly via the superior cerebellar peduncles. The ratio of afferent to efferent fibers in the cerebellum is 40:1 (180). This input : output ratio underlies the **coordinative role** of the cerebellum for all motor functions from standing and walking to speaking and writing.

The cerebellum receives information from the vestibular nuclei concerning the position of the head. The vestibulocerebellar tract forwards signals from the vestibular system mainly to the nodule of vermis (X). In the past the flocculonodular lobe was thought to be the recipient of these signals. More recent animal experiments have shown that the flocculus (H X) receives mainly visceromotor afferents (266). Proprioceptive signals from the musculoskeletal system of the extremities and the trunk are received by the cerebellum via the anterior and posterior spinocerebellar tracts (Figs. 144a.8, 144a.19) and via the cuneocerebellar tract ending in the anterior lobe, the pyramids of vermis (VIII), and the gracile lobe of the cerebellum (H VII B). Further afferent connections to the cerebellum include the auditory and visual systems. The olivocerebellar tract of the inferior olivary nucleus extends to all areas of the cerebellum (350). The fibers of noradrenergic and serotoninergic neurons of the brainstem reach also all areas of the cerebellar cortex. Under experimental conditions these seem to stimulate the excitatory transmissions to the mossy and climbing fibers. The afferent systems end mostly in the cerebellar cortex, afferent collaterals also reach the cerebellar nuclei. The axons of the inhibitory Purkinje cells link the cerebellar cortex with the cerebellar nuclei.

There are numerous connections between the neocortex and the cerebellar cortex in the lateral zone of the cerebellar hemisphere. The corticopontine tract extends from the cerebral cortex through the internal capsule to reach the pontine nuclei. The neurons of the pontine nuclei send their axons to the contralateral cerebellar cortex in the lateral zone of the cerebellar hemispheres after sending collaterals to the cerebellar nuclei. With this corticopontocerebellar connection the cerebellar cortex receives information on the intended motor activity from the neocortex.

The cerebellar cortex is divided functionally into **longitudinal zones** according to its efferent pathways. These zones are oriented perpendicular to the interlobular sulci. There are three corticonuclear zones described for each half of the cerebellum from medial to lateral:
- Vermis
- Narrow, intermediate zone at the transition of the vermis and hemisphere
- Large, lateral zone of the cerebellar hemisphere.

1 Culmen (IV, V)
2 Primary fissure
3 Declive (VI)
4 Folium of vermis (VII A)
5 Tuber of vermis (VII B)
6 Pyramis of vermis (VIII)
7 Uvula of vermis (IX)
8 Nodule of vermis (X)
9 Tonsil of cerebellum (H IX)
10 Dentate nucleus

- Anterior lobe
- Flocculonodular lobe
- Posterior lobe

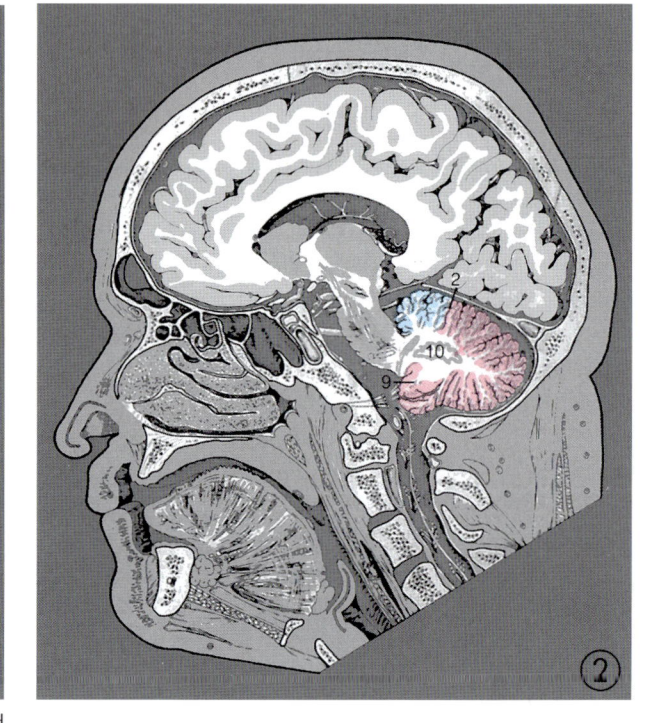

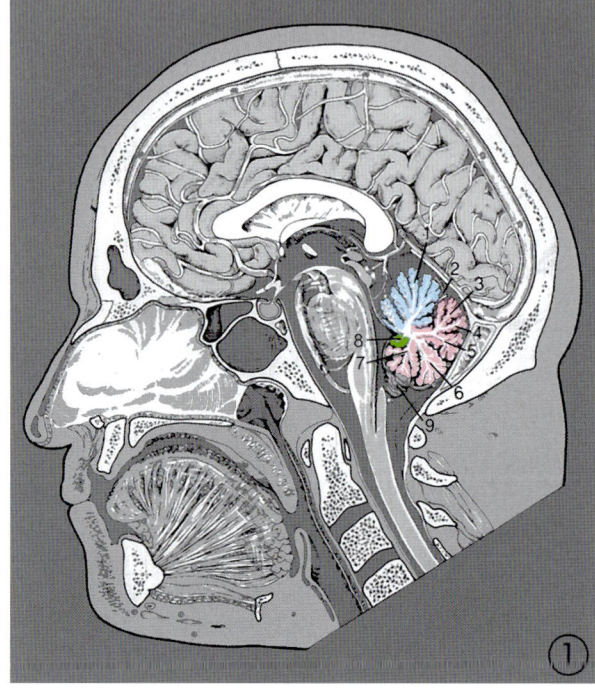

Fig. 142 Sagittal serial illustrations of the cerebellar lobes and lobules (Table 1, p. ■■). The encircled number (1–6) indicates the number of the respective slice (Figs. 29, 30a,b, 31).

6.9 Cerebellar Systems

2 Primary fissure
11 Flocculus (H X)

- Anterior lobe
- Flocculonodular lobe
- Posterior lobe

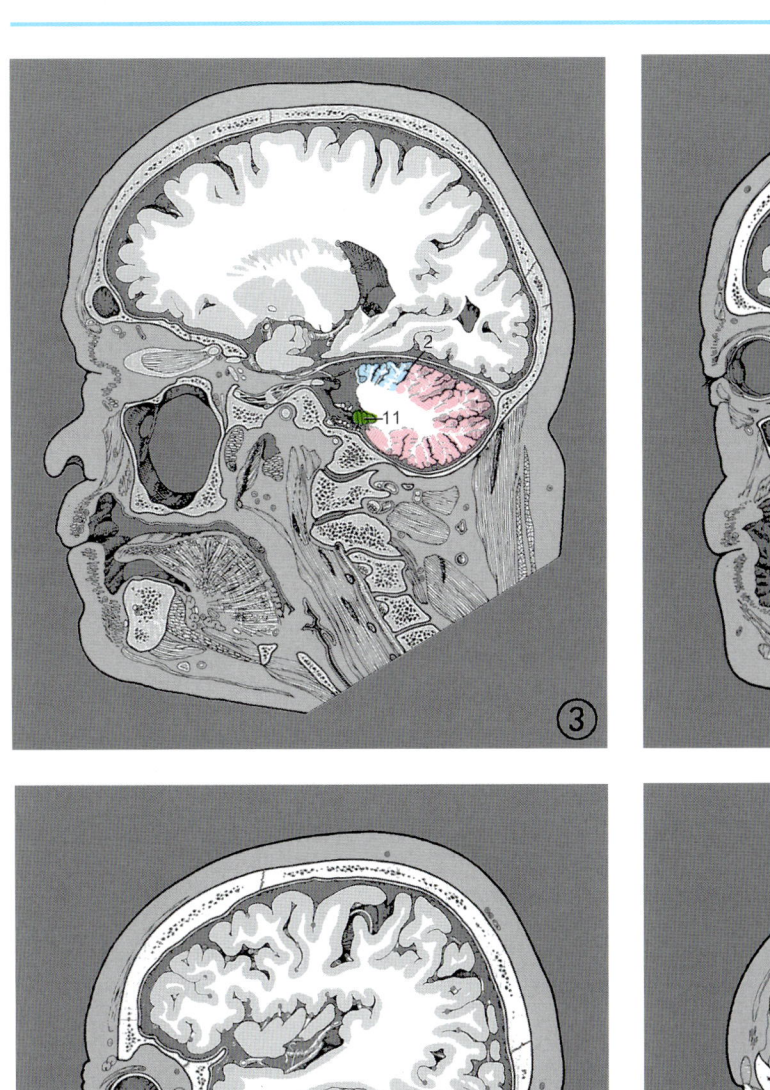

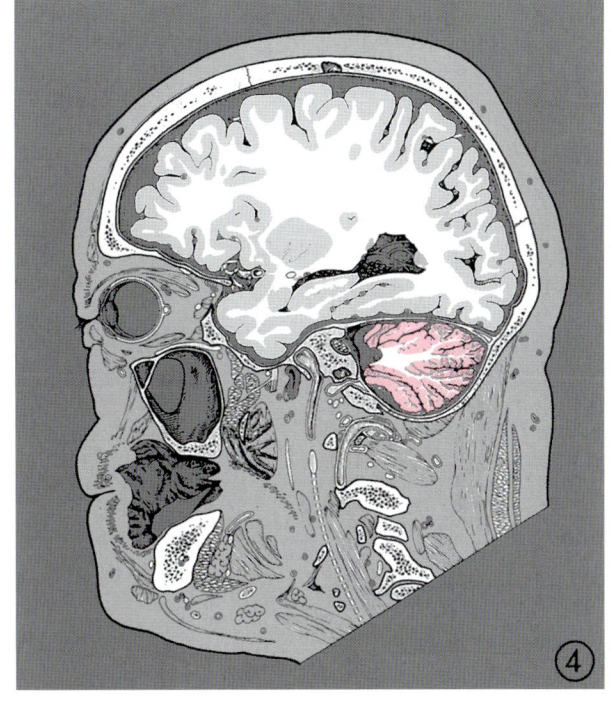

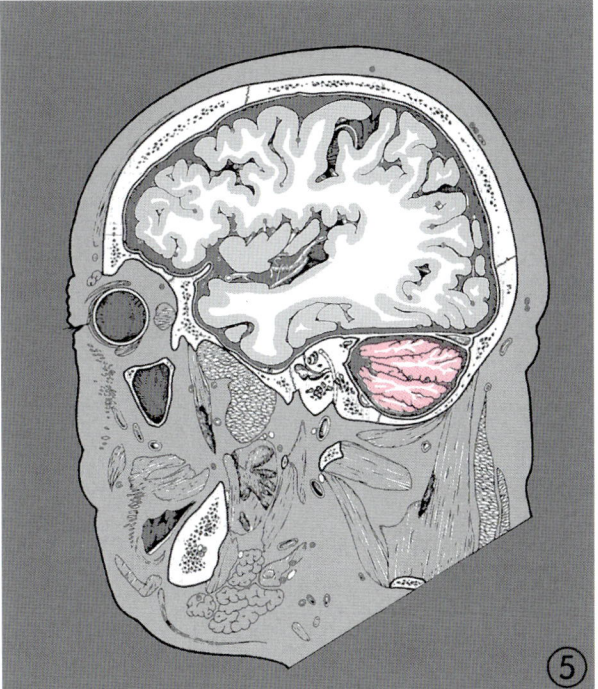

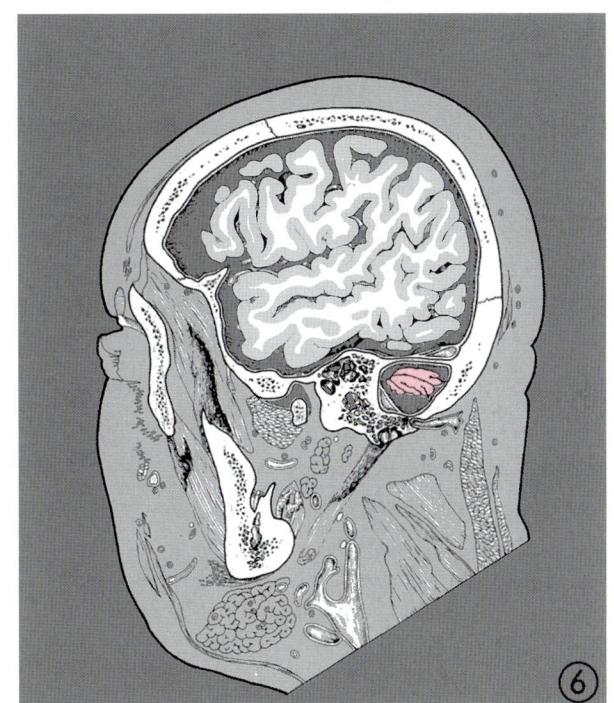

The transitions between the three zones are continuous and not separated by a visible macroscopic border.

The Purkinje cells of these projection zones are connected with the ipsilateral nuclei. The Purkinje cells of the vermis project to the fastigial nucleus and vestibular nuclei. The Purkinje cells of the intermediate zone project to the interpositus nuclei (globose and emboliform nuclei). The Purkinje cells of the lateral zone are connected with the dentate nucleus.

The axons of the interpositus and dentate nuclei extend through the superior cerebellar peduncle (Fig. 144b.6), cross in the lower midbrain, and end in the red nucleus (Fig. 144b.5) and in the ventral lateral nuclei of the thalamus (Fig. 144b.3). The red nucleus receives signals from the motor cortex via collaterals of the motor pathways. Therefore one could interpret the red nucleus as a synaptic station that is able to transfer the learning process of movement to the corticospinal pathways and automatic movements to the rubrospinal tract. The cerebellum can exert influence on the motor cortex in the frontal lobes via the ventral lateral nuclei. The Purkinje cells of the cerebellar cortex receive time signals via the afferents signaling the state of play of the musculoskeletal system and information about intended movements via the corticopontocerebellar pathways. Comparison of these signals allows harmonious functioning of the motor

1 Tonsil of cerebellum (H IX)
2 Flocculus (H X)
3 Uvula of vermis (IX)
4 Pyramis of vermis (VIII)
5 Nodule of vermis (X)

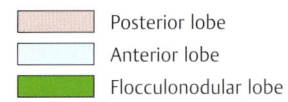

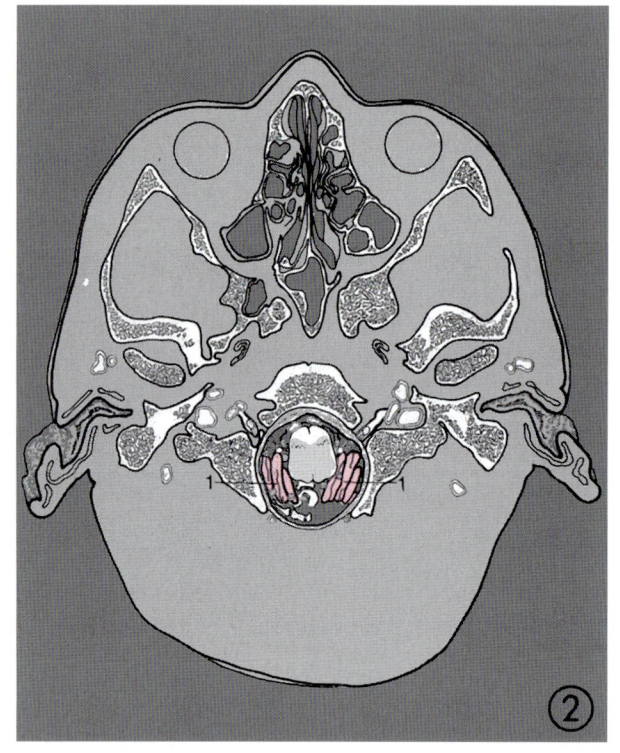

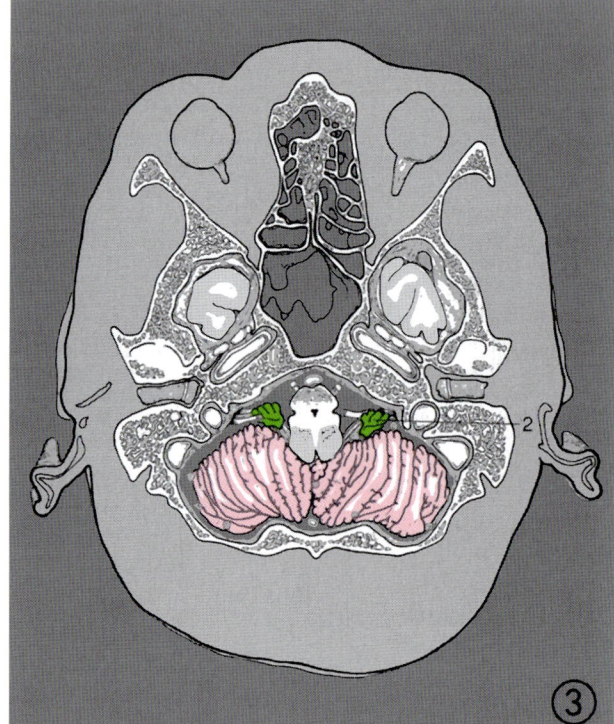

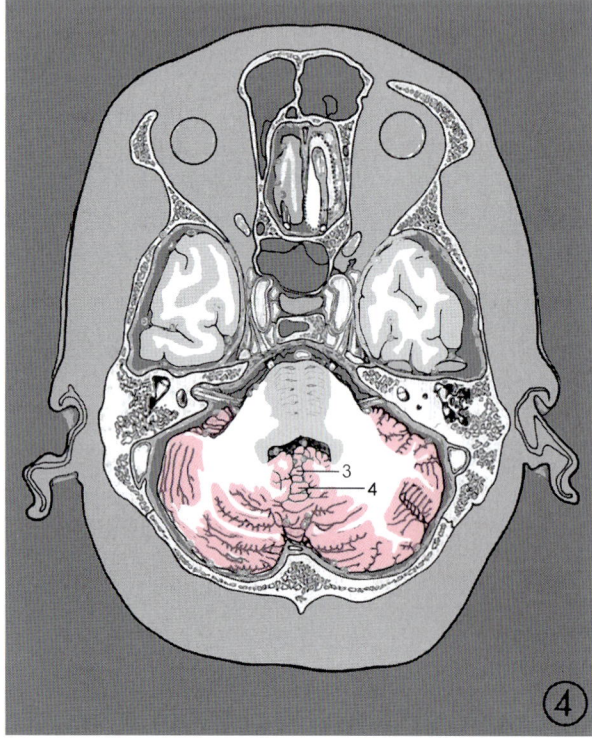

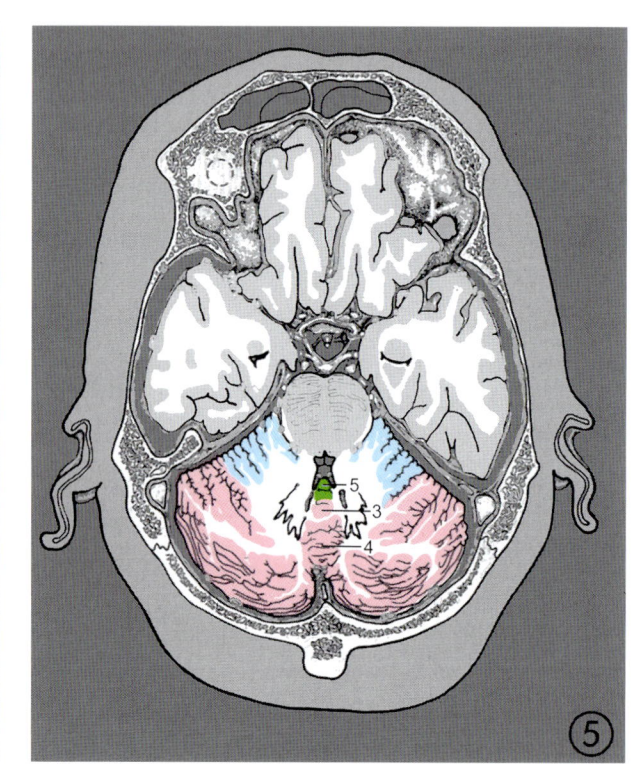

- Posterior lobe
- Anterior lobe
- Flocculonodular lobe

Fig. **143** Canthomeatally oriented serial illustrations of the cerebellar lobes and lobules (Table 1, p. 304). The encircled number (2–8) indicates the number of the respective slice (Figs. 44, 45a,b, 46).

6.9 Cerebellar Systems

Posterior lobe
Anterior lobe

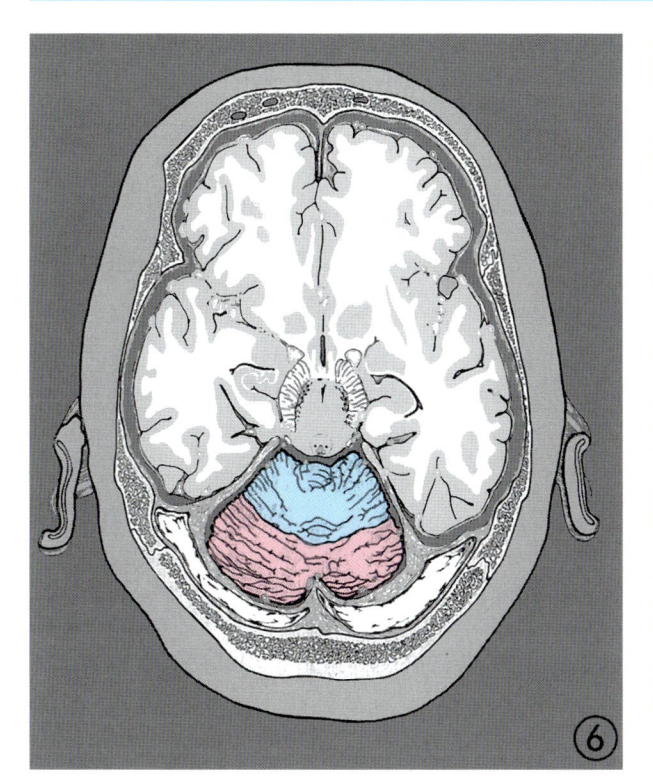

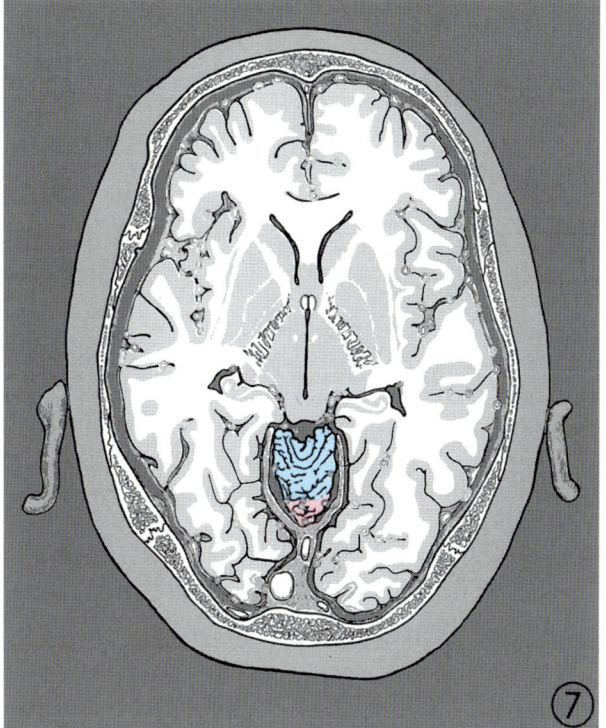

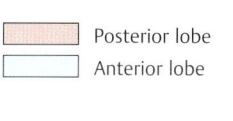

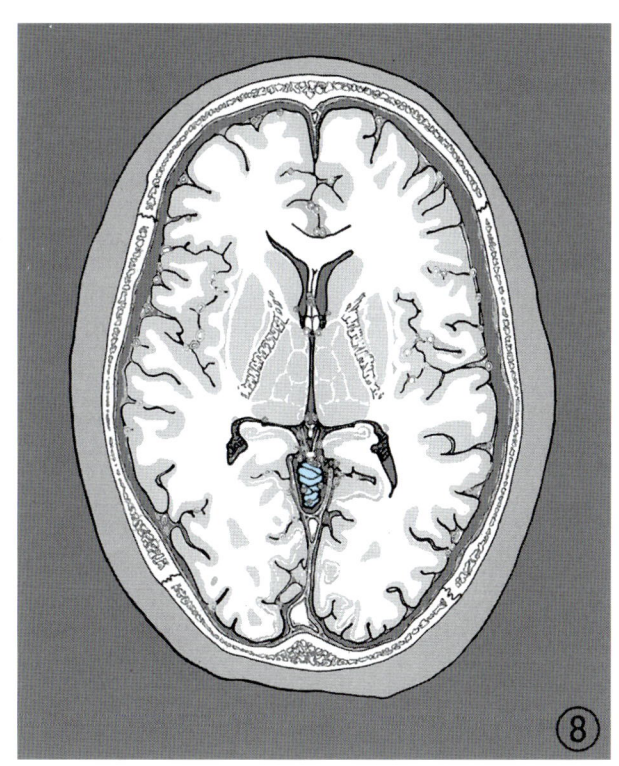

system. Impairment of the cerebellum therefore does not cause paralysis of the motor system, but rather an incoordination of movements in strength and accuracy.

Due to the **decussation** of the efferent cerebellar pathways in the midbrain, and to the **redecussation** of the rubrospinal tract and of the pyramidal pathways, each cerebellar hemisphere is connected with the ipsilateral spinal cord. Unilateral cerebellar lesions, therefore, lead to **ipsilateral dysfunctions**.

Clinical Notes
The vermis is primarily interconnected with the vestibular system. **Lesions of the vermis** result in truncal ataxia where the patient is unable to maintain an upright stance without further cerebellar symptoms (26, 127, 367).
The intermediate zone, notably in the anterior lobe, is the main target of the posterior spinocerebellar fibers from the lower limb. Accordingly, **lesions of the intermediate zone** are typically associated with a staggering ("drunken") gait.
Lesions of the lateral zone of the cerebellar hemisphere are characterized by impaired motor coordination. In cases of cerebellar ataxia, the muscles fail to work in harmony, even when the patient uses visual control. In finger-to-nose testing, intention tremor (action tremor) will appear even with the eyes open. Rapid repetition of movements is not possible (adiadochokinesis). Goal-oriented movement is incorrectly performed (dysmetria). Speech is often slow and words are broken up into syllables (the typical disorder being scanning dysarthria). Muscle tonus may be decreased (hypotonia of the musculature). A nystagmus is often observed.

398   6   Neurofunctional Systems

1 Thalamus
2 Corticopontine tract
3 Red nucleus
4 Tectum of midbrain
5 Decussation of superior cerebellar peduncles
6 Superior cerebellar peduncle
7 Vermis of anterior lobe of cerebellum
8 Anterior spinocerebellar tract
9 Primary fissure
10 Pons
11 Trigeminal nerve
12 Pontocerebellar tract
13 Inferior cerebellar peduncle
14 Middle cerebellar peduncle
15 Inferior olivary nucleus
16 Olivocerebellar tract
17 Hemisphere of posterior lobe
18 External arcuate fibers
19 Posterior spinocerebellar tract

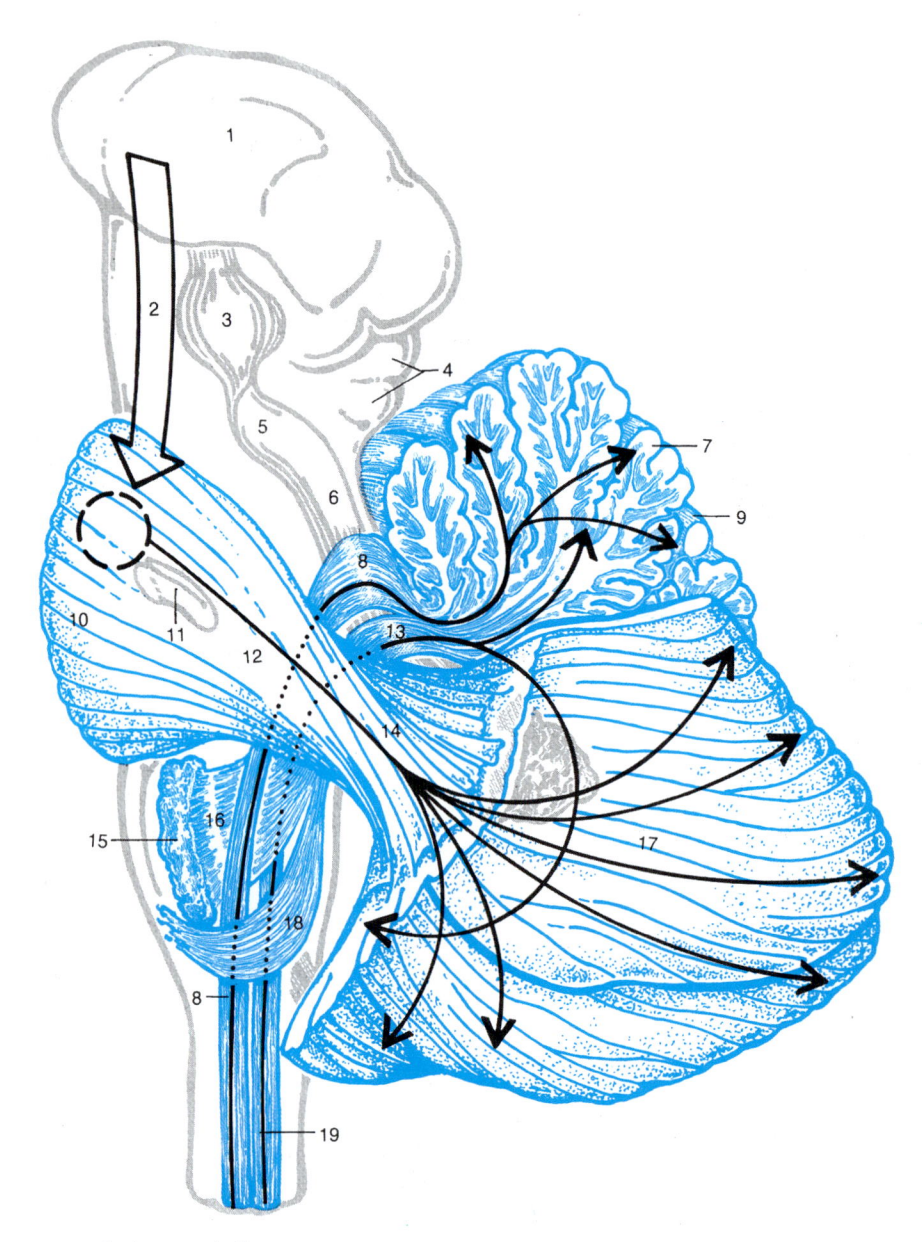

Fig. **144a** The afferent systems of the cerebellar cortex (lateral view). The left half of the anterior lobe of the cerebellum was removed. The flocculonodular lobe was separated and a part of the posterior lobe removed laterally and inferiorly from the middle cerebellar peduncle. According to (332).

6.9 Cerebellar Systems   399

1 Primary motor and premotor cortex (areas 4 and 6)
2 Pyramidal tract
3 Ventral lateral nucleus of thalamus
4 Ventral anterior nucleus of thalamus
5 Red nucleus
6 Superior cerebellar peduncle
7 Purkinje cells
8 Dentate nucleus
9 Fastigial nucleus
10 Vestibular nuclei

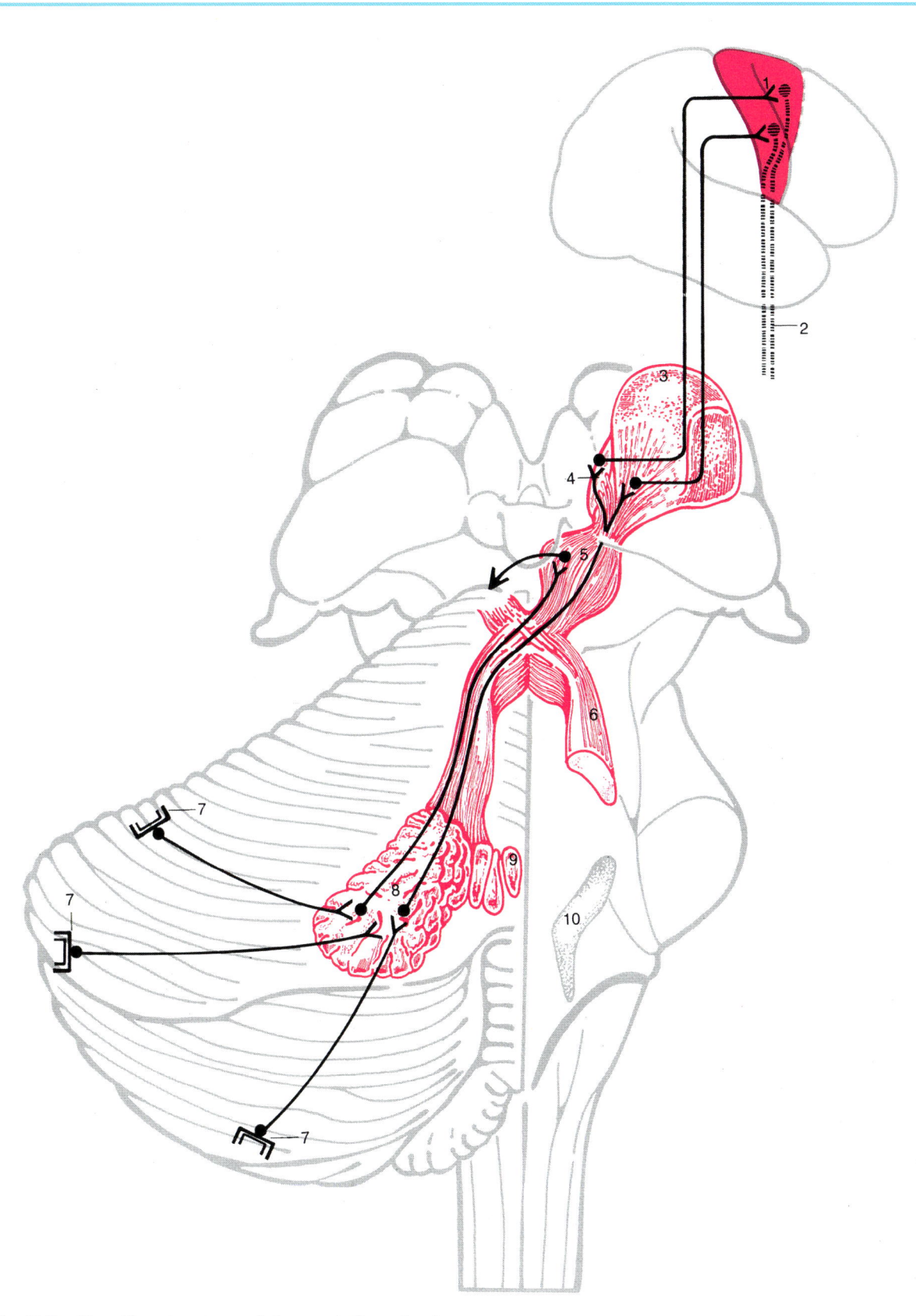

Fig. **144b** The efferent systems of the cerebellum showing the location of the pathways and the nuclei (posterior view). The cerebellum was dissected in the median plane and the right half was removed with the exception of the superior cerebellar peduncle. According to (332).

6.10 Language Areas
(Figs. 145, 146)

Language areas were first described by Broca in 1861 and Wernicke in 1874. Disorders affecting language processing after perisylvian lesions have been described in all the studied languages. The perisylvian association cortex comprises Wernicke's area, the supramarginal gyrus, the angular gyrus and Broca's area in the dominant hemisphere. The left hemisphere is dominant in more than 95% of right-handed individuals. Approximately 60–65% of the non-right-handed individuals are left hemisphere dominant, about 15–20% are right hemisphere dominant. The remainder appears to use both hemispheres for language processing. The localization of the language function in one hemisphere is not completely lateralized. The nondominant hemisphere is involved in many language operations (374a). In the past the topography of the language areas was determined by clinical and pathological findings. Language disorders are usually the result of vascular occlusion or cerebral bleeding (147, 173a, 174, 277, 374a). Therefore, the pathologic lesion may be larger than the actual main language area. The lack of neurohistologic characteristics for the language areas prevents pinpointing the exact extent of the language areas. Consequently different topical descriptions have been published. In Figures 145 and 146, the boundaries of the language areas are drawn according to the smallest sizes of the areas as given in lesion studies (147, 174, 277). Additional data are available thanks to PET investigations, with estimation of glucose metabolism, local oxygen utilization, and regional cerebral circulation and fMRI (2, 155a, 304, 327, 374a).

Wernicke's area lies in the superior temporal gyrus lateral from the primary auditory cortex. Wernicke's area is supplied by the posterior temporal artery that arises from the middle cerebral artery (174).

The **visual auditory conversion language area** is located in the angular gyrus (147) (Figs. 145.4, 146.3). The angular gyrus seems to contain a neural lexicon of words and other symbols that can be retrieved by visual signals (127).

Broca's area lies in the frontal lobe, anterior to the primary motor and premotor cortex. Broca's area occupies the opercular and triangular parts of the inferior frontal gyrus. Based on cytoarchitectonic criteria, this area corresponds to Brodmann's area 44 and 45 (110). An occlusion of the artery of the precentral sulcus (174, 367) affects Broca's area and, according to the analysis of CT scans, the neighboring insular region as well (40).

The superior longitudinal fasciculus (Fig. 145.1) lies on the posterolateral border of the putamen between the projection pathways of the external and internal capsules. These fibers of the superior longitudinal fasciculus (arcuate fasciculus) run between the temporal, parietal, and frontal lobes and join together Wernicke's area, the visual auditory conversion language area, and Broca's area. Further language areas have been identified in the supplementary motor area and head of the caudate nucleus (90).

1 Superior longitudinal (arcuate) fasciculus
2 Broca's area

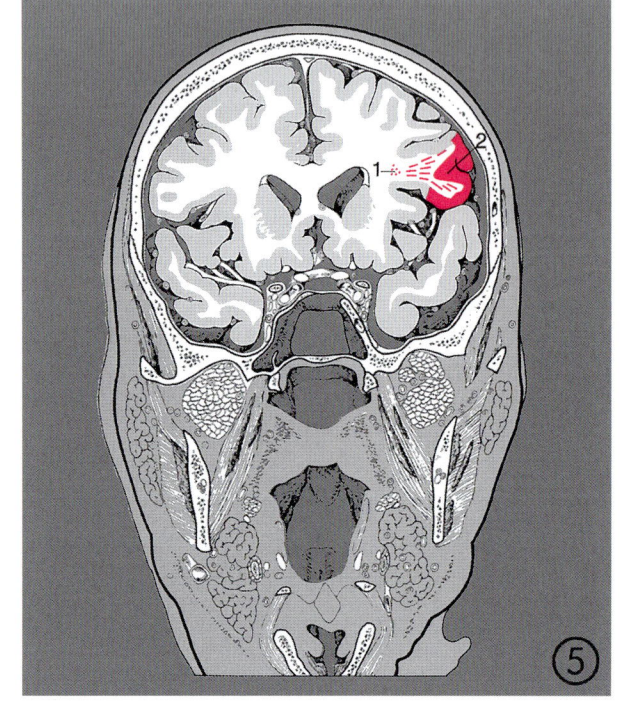

Fig. **145** Coronal serial illustrations of the language areas viewed from the front. The encircled numbers (5–10) indicate the number of the respective slice (Figs. 1, 2a,b, 3).

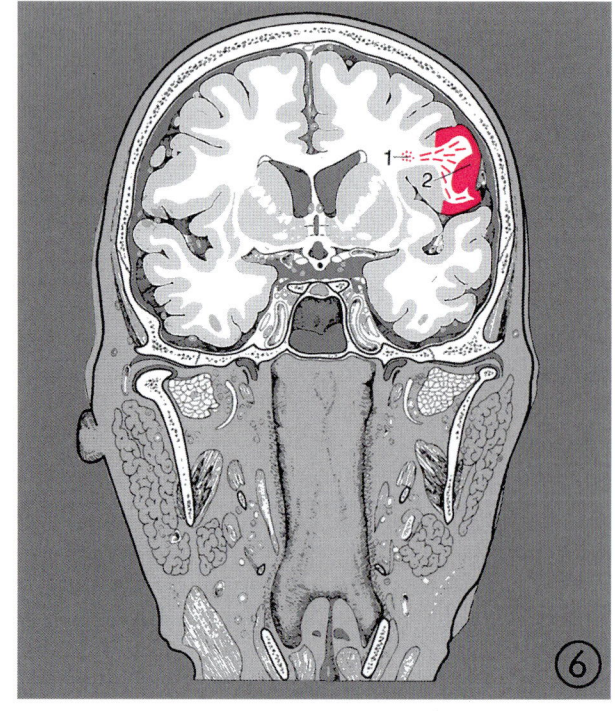

6.10 *Language Areas* 401

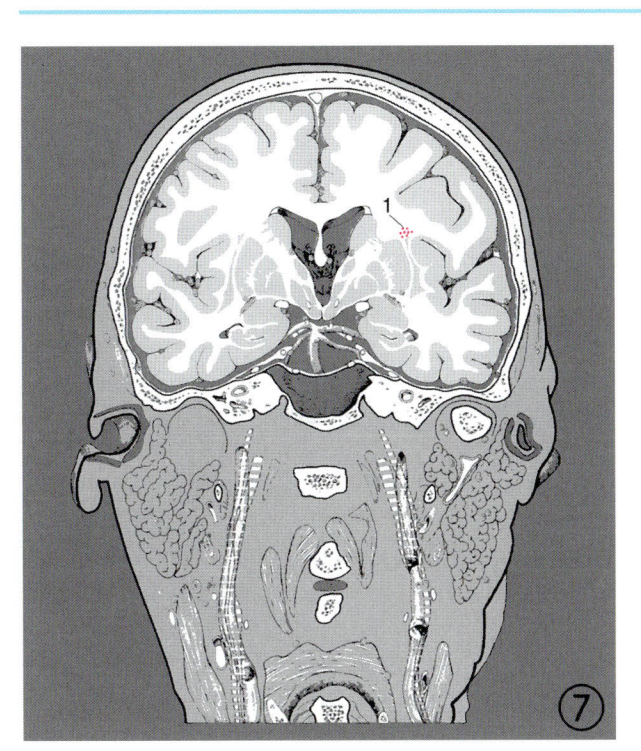

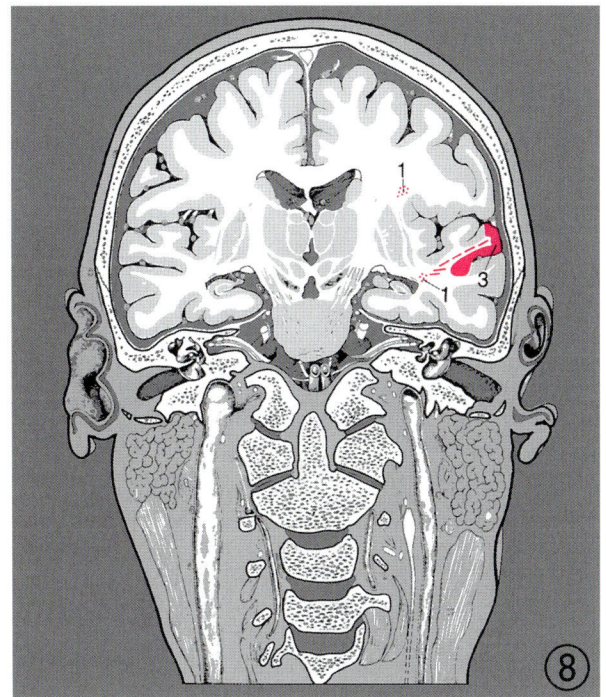

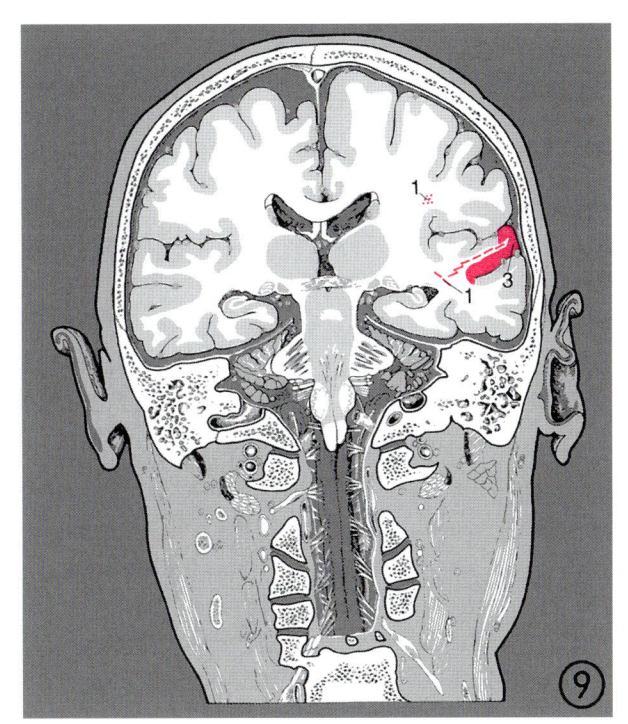

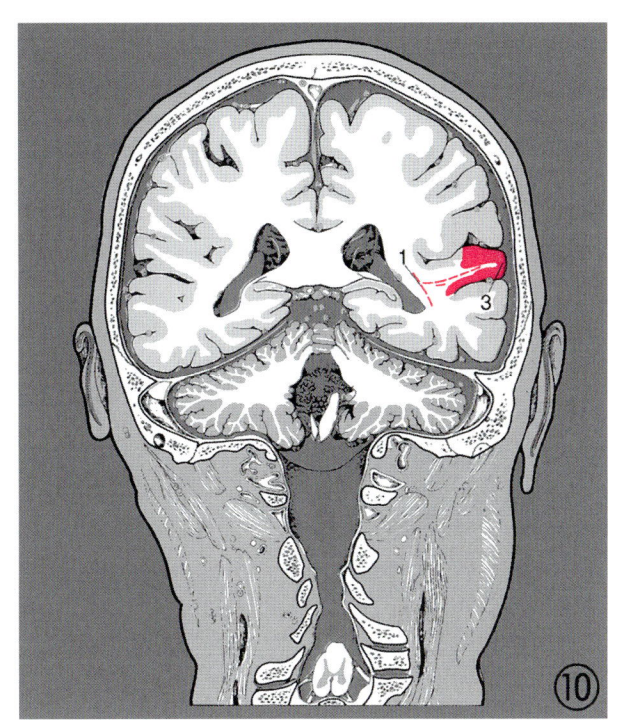

1 Superior longitudinal (arcuate) fasciculus
3 Wernicke's area

402   6   Neurofunctional Systems

1 Superior longitudinal (arcuate) fasciculus
4 Angular gyrus

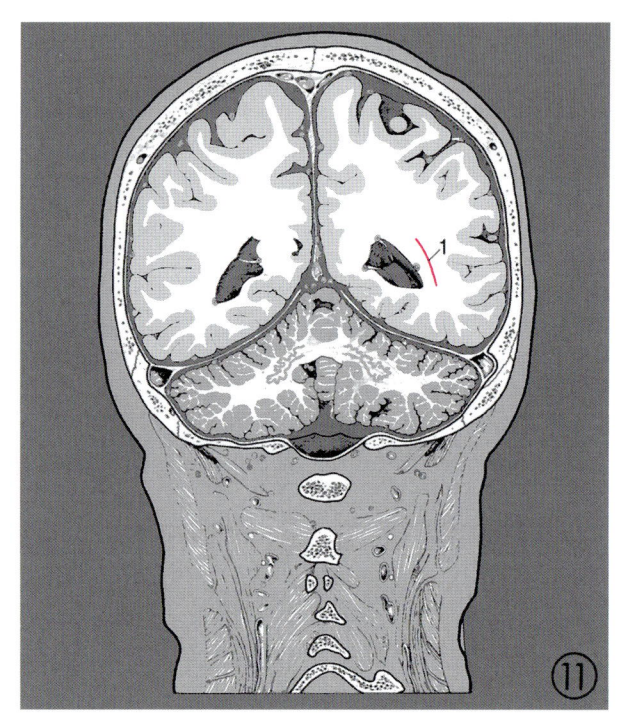

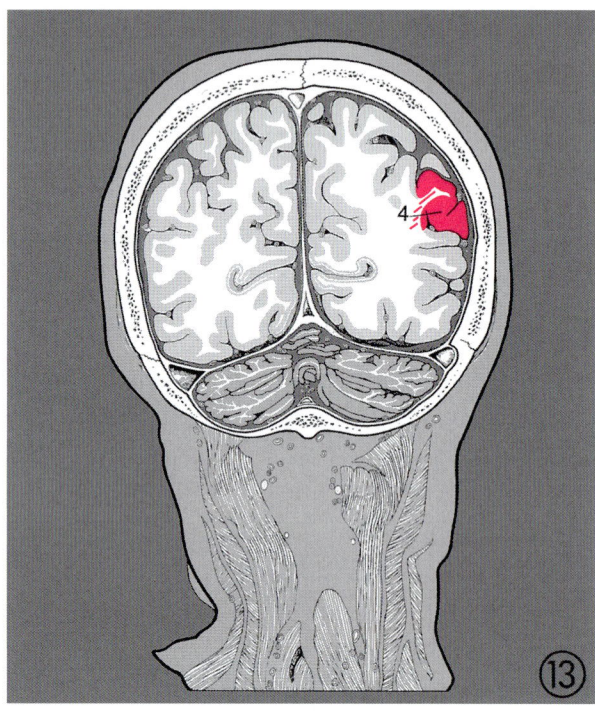

Fig. 145 Coronal serial illustrations of the language areas viewed from the front. The encircled numbers (11–13) indicate the number of the respective slice (Figs. 1, 2a,b, 3).

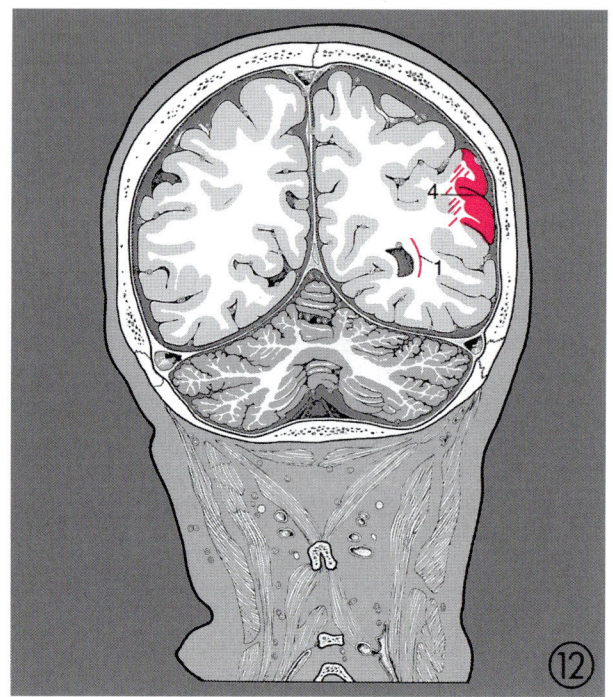

Clinical Notes
With **Wernicke's aphasia** a loss of understanding of language predominates. The flow of language is preserved. Phonetic and semantic paraphasias occur. Synonyms are sensory, receptive or syntactic aphasia.

Broca's aphasia usually arises from a lesion of Broca's area with agrammatism. The flow of language is slowed down. In addition articulation can be impaired if the neighboring premotor and motor cortex is affected. Synonyms are motor or expressive aphasia.

Descriptive divisions into fluent and nonfluent aphasia are also customary. Fluent aphasia is caused by a lesion located behind the central sulcus, whereas nonfluent aphasia is caused by a lesion located in front of the central sulcus (31). Apart from cortical lesions, aphasic disturbances can also be caused by subcortical brain lesions. For this the term striatocapsular aphasia is used. Recently special attention has been paid to aphasia in lesions of the left thalamus (6, 60, 339, 379). Clinically it is distinguished from striatocapsular aphasia by the fact that speech repetition is unaffected.

Infarcts of the supplementary motor area (Figs. 133.5, 134.1) of the dominant hemisphere initially cause a disturbance of mutistic language and later a slowing down of language. Most of these patients show a generalized akinesia. Lesions of the head of the caudate nucleus (Figs. 9a.10), and those of the anterior putamen and the anterior limb of the internal capsule of the dominant hemisphere, cause atypical disturbances of language. These lesions are typically caused by infarcts in the vascular territory of the central anterolateral arteries (lateral lenticulostriate) (Figs. 93, 94, 96)

6.10 Language Areas 403

1 Broca's area
2 Wernicke's area
3 Angular gyrus

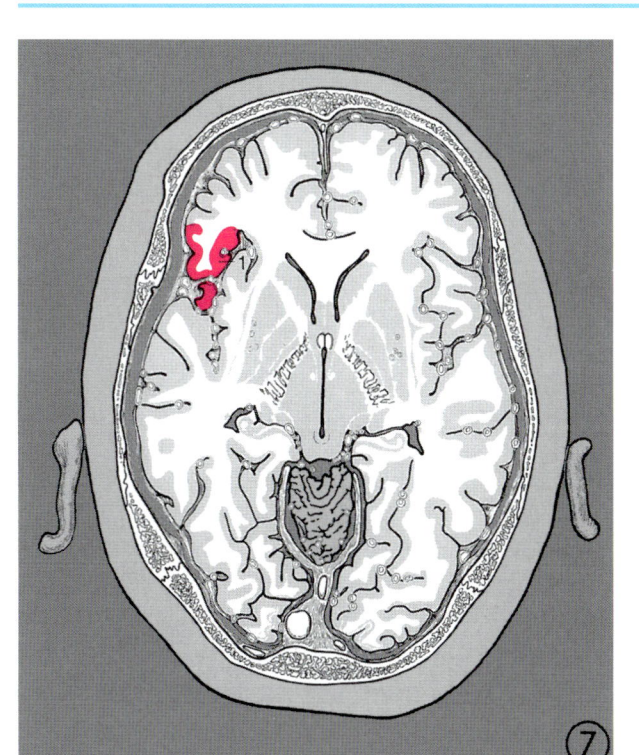

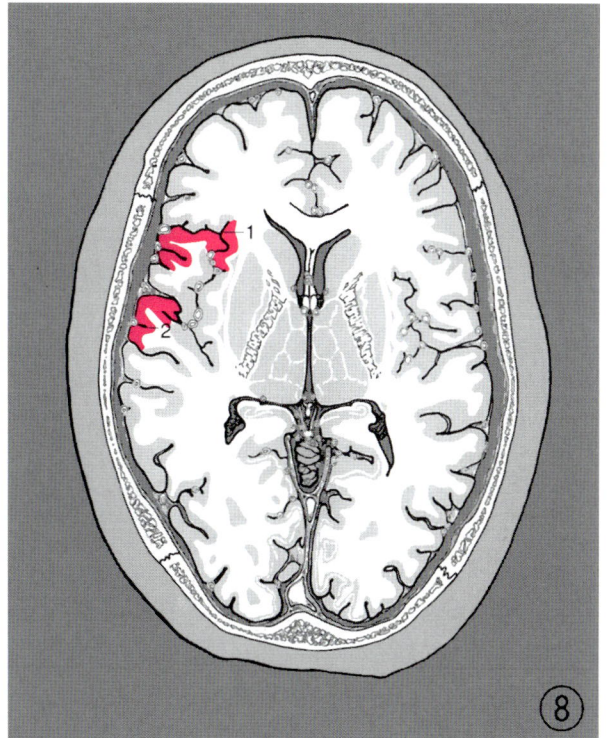

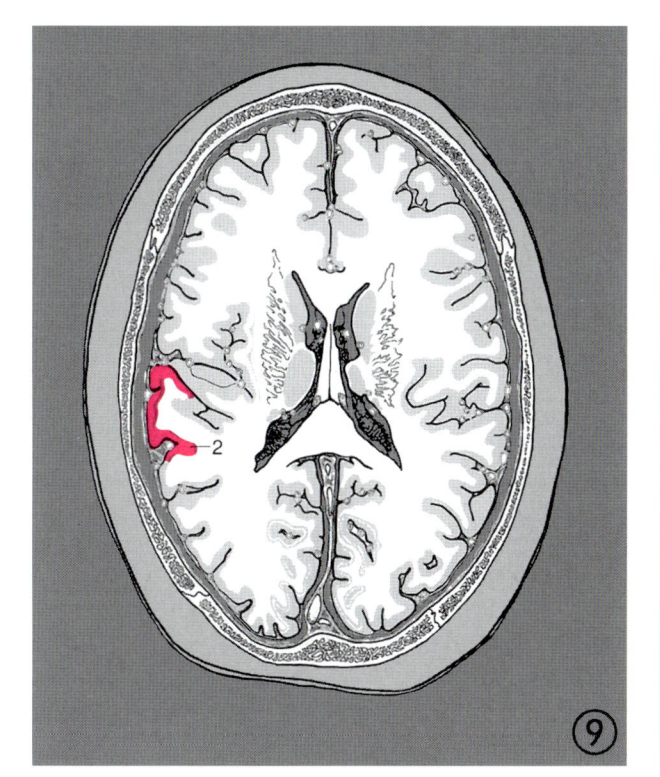

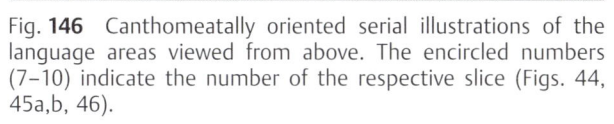

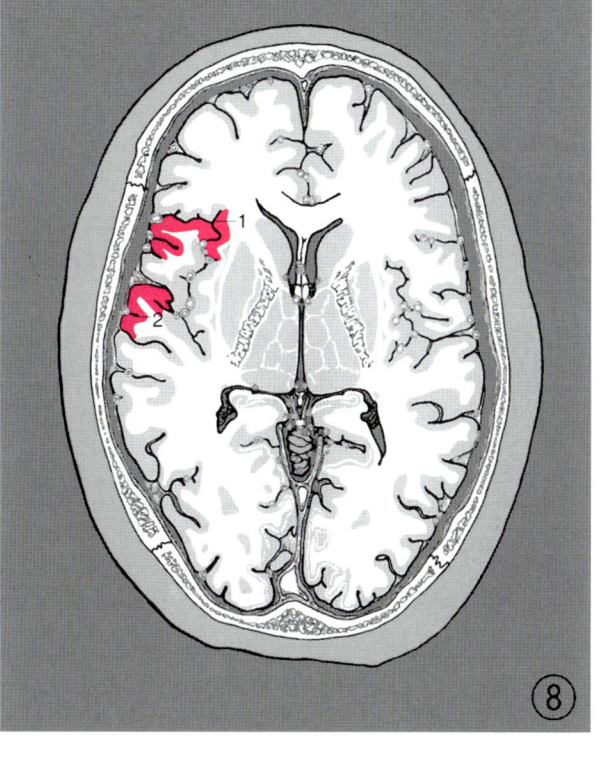

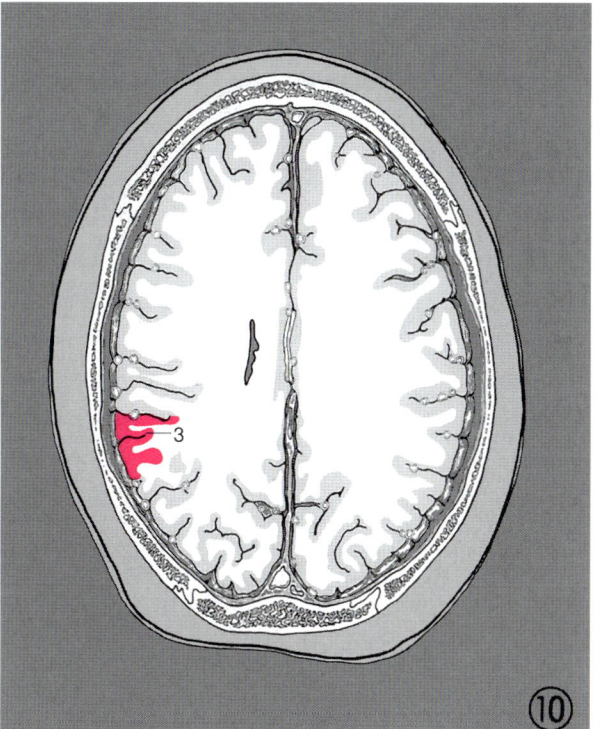

Fig. 146 Canthomeatally oriented serial illustrations of the language areas viewed from above. The encircled numbers (7–10) indicate the number of the respective slice (Figs. 44, 45a,b, 46).

3 Angular gyrus

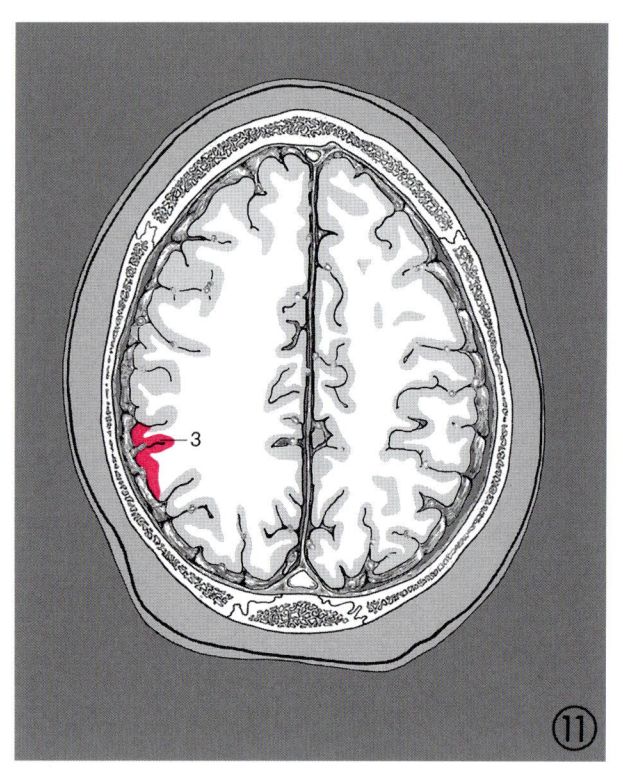

Fig. 146 Canthomeatally oriented serial illustrations of the language areas viewed from above. The encircled number (11) indicates the number of the slice (Figs. 44, 45a,b, 46).

(90). In these patients only some symptoms of Broca's and Wernicke's aphasias are seen. In summary, a large number of brain regions are involved in representing and processing language. The most important of these regions is the dominant perisylvian cortex (374a).

As an alternative to the invasive Wada-test, the noninvasive fMRI can be used for determination of the language-dominant hemisphere (291a, 437).

6.11 Limbic System
(Figs. 147–150)

The limbic system comprises cortical and subcortical portions. The cortical portions develop from the phylogenetically old archicortex and periarchicortex, and are pushed during evolution against the medial and inferior sides of both cerebral hemispheres by the development of the neocortex. These cortical parts form a margin around the corpus callosum and are named, therefore, "limbic" (rim). The archicortex and periarchicortex lie in front, above, and behind the corpus callosum and are divided into three corresponding subunits: the pre-, supra-, and retrocommissural cortical areas. The archicortical portions form the inner edge of the margin, and the periarchicortical portions the outer edge. The precommissural portion of the archicortex includes the inner part of the subcallosal area; the supracommissural portion includes the supracallosal indusium griseum; and the retrocommissural portion includes the hippocampal formation. The outer ring around the corpus callosum is formed by the outer part of the subcallosal area, the part of the cingulate gyrus close to the corpus callosum and the parahippocampal gyrus (443). Electrophysiologic stimulations of these regions lead to emotional reactions such as anger, fear, desire, sexual aggression, with corresponding effects on the autonomic nervous system. Such observations led MacLean to name the limbic system the "visceral brain."

The **cortical limbic regions** maintain afferent and efferent connections with certain subcortical structures. These subcortical structures—septal nuclei, preoptic area, mammillary body and other hypothalamic subnuclei, anterior nuclei of the thalamus, and limbic midbrain nuclei—are accordingly considered to be parts of the limbic system.

The subcallosal area and indusium griseum are relatively poorly developed in humans. However, the hippocampal formation is larger in man than in apes (239, 443). It is located in the medial portion of the temporal lobe and consists of three parts: the hippocampus, dentate gyrus, and subiculum. During ontogenesis, the hippocampal formation is folded inward and comes to lie medial to the temporal horn of the lateral ventricle. It encloses the hippocampal sulcus in a C-shaped structure with two curved lips. The **dentate gyrus** lies in the upper limb of this structure. The term dentate refers to the toothed appearance of the surface of the gyrus. The curved portion of the **hippocampus proper** (Ammon's horn) extends into the lateral ventricle. The lower limb of the C is formed mainly by the subiculum (113).

The hippocampal formation has afferent connections with the septal nuclei, hypothalamic subnuclei, parahippocampal gyrus, and the dopaminergic and serotoninergic centers of the brainstem (Chaps. 7.1.1 and 7.2). The fibers of the **fornix** form a partially afferent pathway that carries mainly efferent axons from the hippocampal formation. The initial segments of the fornical fibers make up the alveus, a thin white layer lining the ventricular surface of the hippocampus proper. The fibers proceed as the fimbria of hippocampus and arch beneath the corpus callosum as the posterior pillar (crus) of the fornix. Under the splenium of the corpus callosum, where the right crus of the fornix meets the left crus, some fibers cross in the fornical commissure. Beneath the trunk of the corpus callosum the fornix descends toward the interventricular foramen (of Monro). Here, the pathways separate into the two anterior pillars of fornix. These pillars skirt the interventricular foramen and continue in an inferior direction toward the hypothalamus. Directly above the anterior commissure, precommissural fibers extend to the **septal nuclei**, straight gyrus, and frontal cortex. Below the anterior commissure, fiber bundles reach the nuclei of the stria terminalis and the anterior nuclei of the thalamus.

                                                                    6.11 Limbic System   405

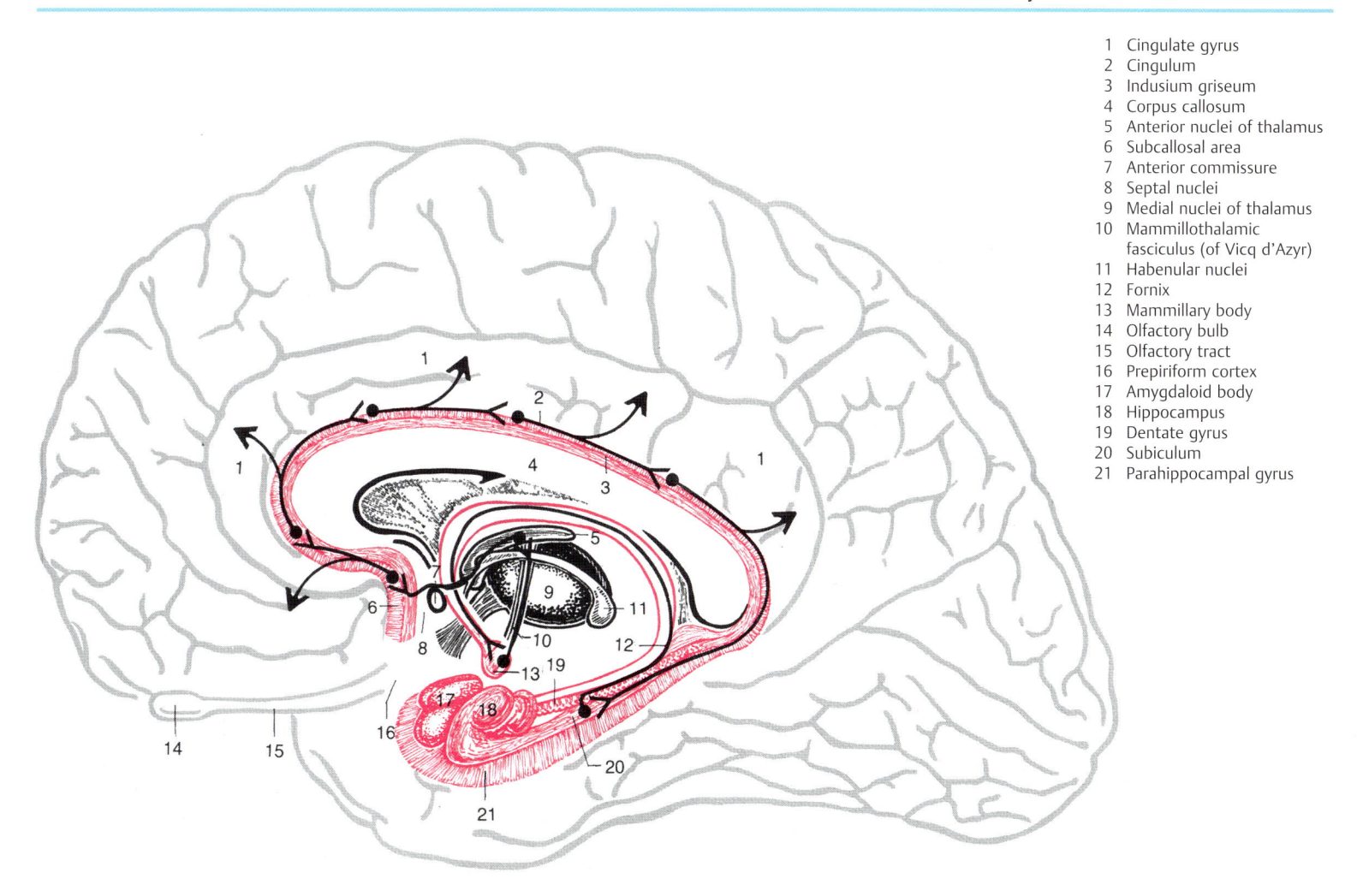

1 Cingulate gyrus
2 Cingulum
3 Indusium griseum
4 Corpus callosum
5 Anterior nuclei of thalamus
6 Subcallosal area
7 Anterior commissure
8 Septal nuclei
9 Medial nuclei of thalamus
10 Mammillothalamic
   fasciculus (of Vicq d'Azyr)
11 Habenular nuclei
12 Fornix
13 Mammillary body
14 Olfactory bulb
15 Olfactory tract
16 Prepiriform cortex
17 Amygdaloid body
18 Hippocampus
19 Dentate gyrus
20 Subiculum
21 Parahippocampal gyrus

Fig. 147 Medial view of the limbic and olfactory systems. The wall of the third ventricle is omitted revealing the Papez circuit, mammillothalamic fasciculus, and anterior nuclei of the thalamus. According to (332, 444).

The main bundle of the fornix projects into the **hypothalamus**, especially into the mammillary body.

The mammillothalamic fasciculus (Vicq d'Azyr's bundle) projects from the **mammillary body** to the **anterior nuclei of the thalamus**. Fiber pathways return via the cingulum to the hippocampal formation. This circuit (hippocampal formation – mammillary body – anterior nucleus of the thalamus – cingulate gyrus and cingulum – hippocampal formation) is known as the **Papez circuit**. Connections radiate from here into the frontal cortex, cingulate gyrus, and parahippocampal gyrus. These neuronal connections are likely to be damaged when a bilateral lesion of the hippocampal formation, the fornices, or the mammillary bodies causes a dramatic loss of recent memory (208, 387).

The **amygdaloid body** is a complex of several nuclei and a cortical area. It is located in a medial position at the tip of the temporal horn of the lateral ventricle and belongs partly to the olfactory centers (Chap. 6.7) and partly to the limbic system. The amygdaloid body has afferent connections with the olfactory bulb, hypothalamic nuclei, brainstem, and cortical regions of the telencephalon. The main efferent pathways are the stria terminalis and the ventral amygdalofugal fibers. The stria terminalis arches between the caudate nucleus and the thalamus and projects into the septal nuclei, hypothalamic nuclei, reticular formation, and into isolated telencephalic regions.

The **septal nuclei** (formerly septum verum or precommissural septum) plays a central role among the **subcortical nuclear areas** of the limbic system mentioned earlier. The medial forebrain bundle connects the septal nuclei with other centers in the hypothalamus and midbrain. This connection is twofold, namely septomesencephalic and mesencephaloseptal. These centers are the preoptic regions of the hypothalamus, lateral and medial hypothalamic nuclei, and limbic nuclear areas of the midbrain. The latter include an anterior region of the mesencephalic tegmentum, the interpeduncular nucleus, as well as the posterior raphe nucleus, the superior central nucleus, and the posterior tegmental

406   6 Neurofunctional Systems

1 Periarchicortex in cingulate gyrus (within the slice)
2 Periarchicortex in cingulate gyrus
3 Subcallosal area (partially within the slice)
4 Septal nuclei (within the slice)
5 Fornix (within the slice)

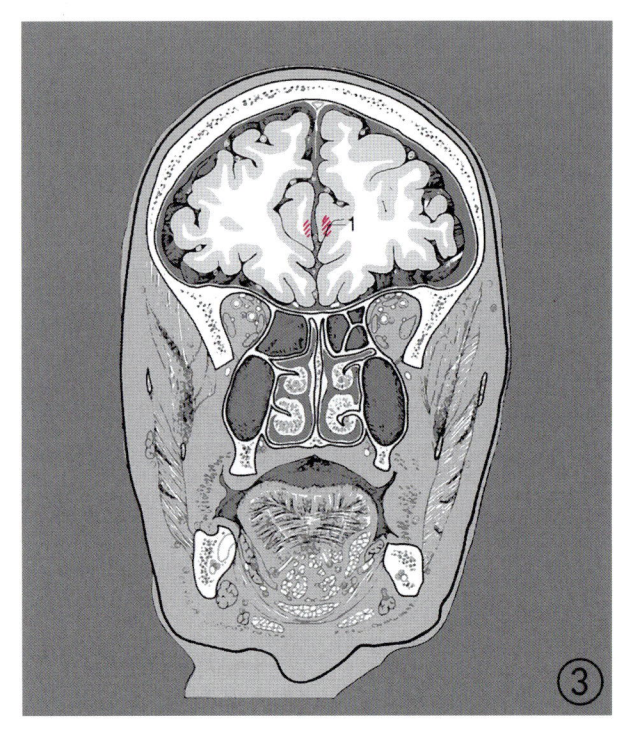

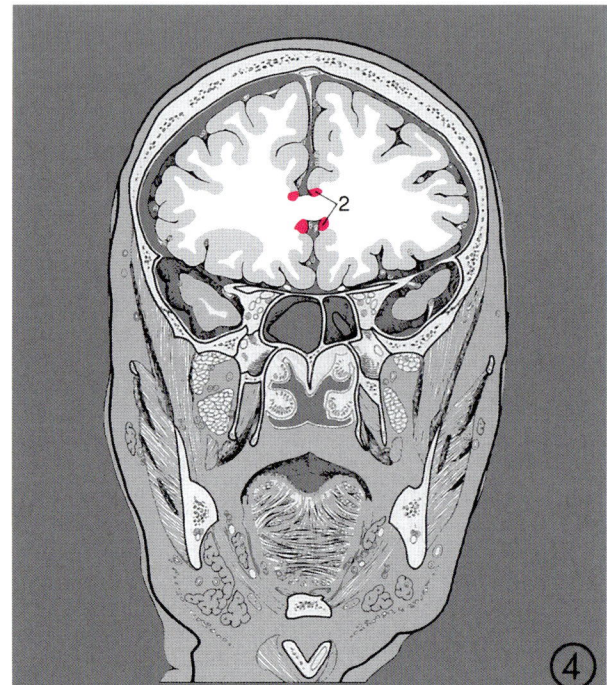

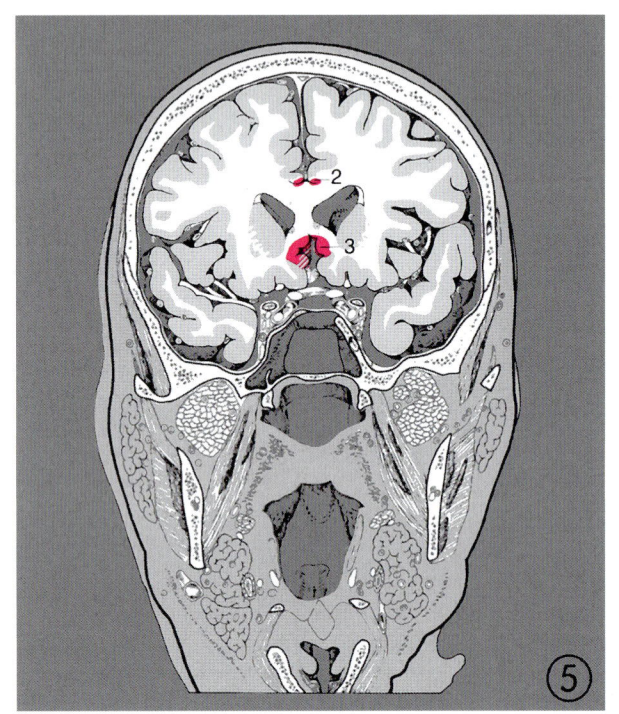

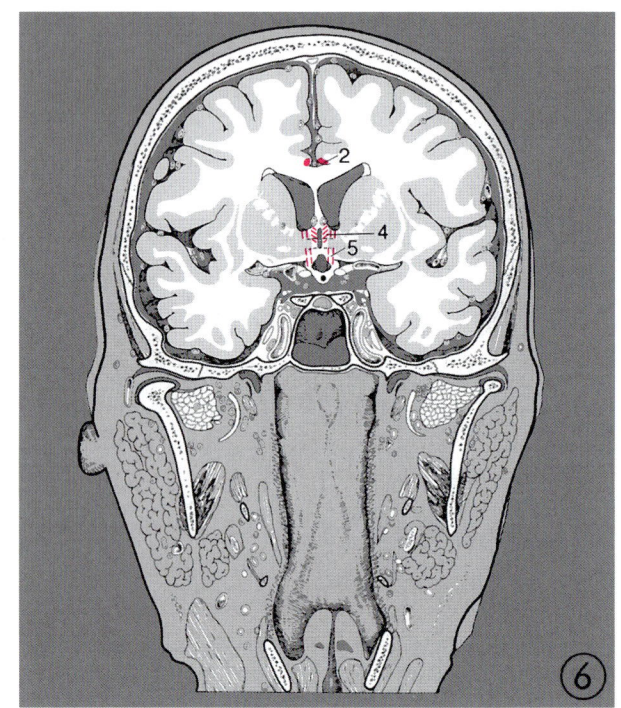

Fig. **148** Coronal serial illustrations of the cortical areas and important nuclear regions of the limbic system including the fornix and the mammillary body. The encircled numbers (3–10) indicate the number of the slice (Figs. 1, 2a,b, 3).

6.11 Limbic System

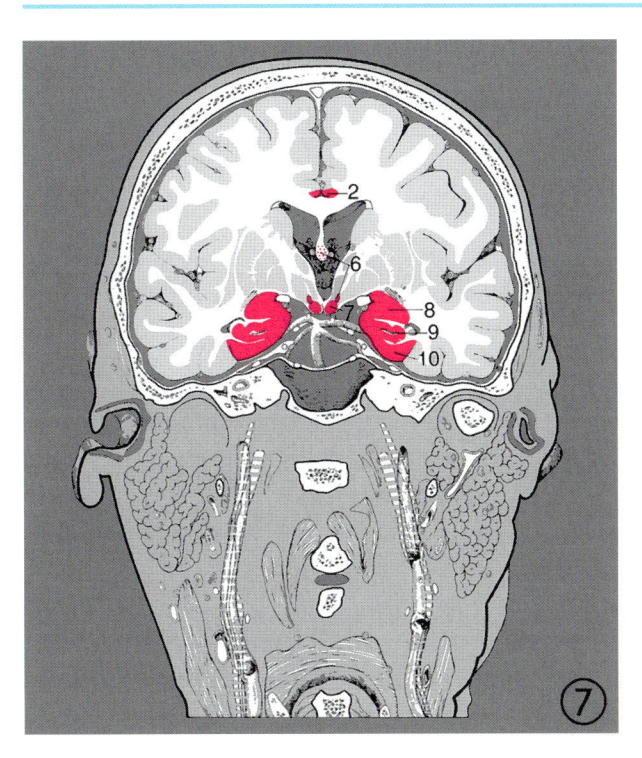

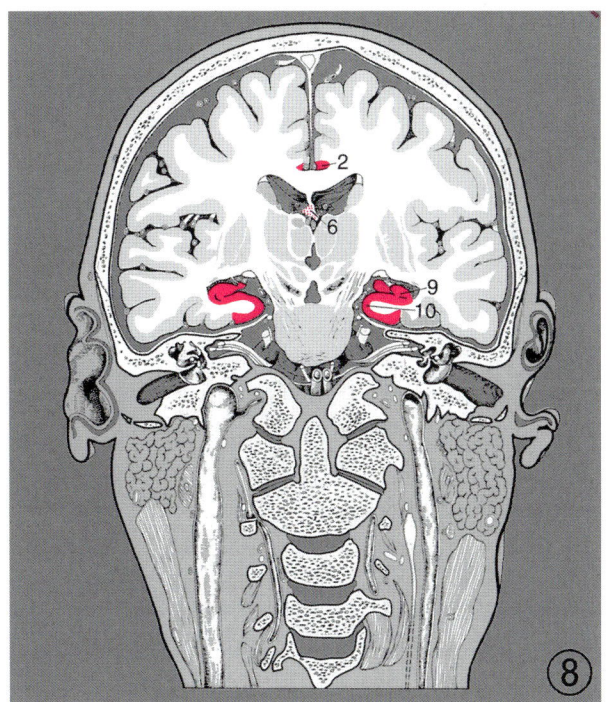

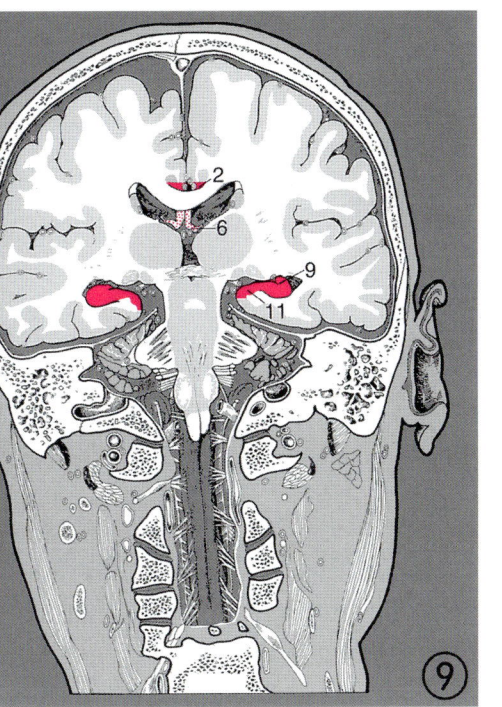

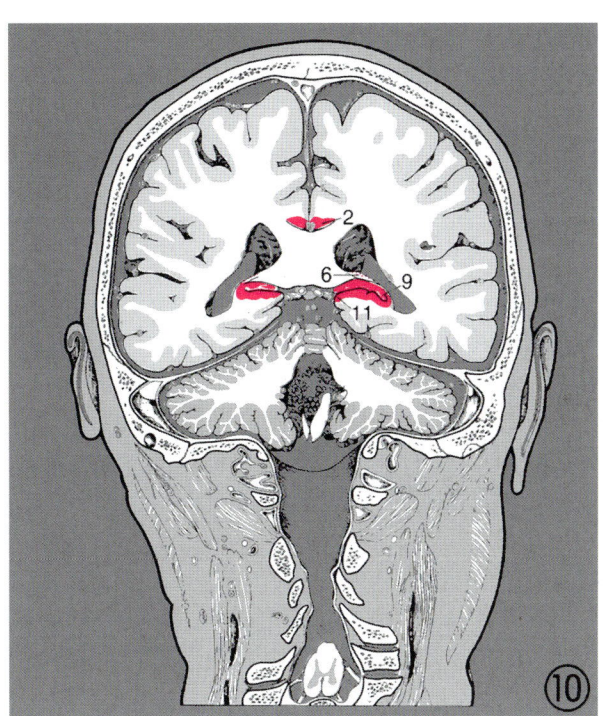

2 Periarchicortex in cingulate gyrus
6 Fornix
7 Mammillary body
8 Amygdaloid body (partially limbic)
9 Hippocampal formation
10 Parahippocampal gyrus
11 Periarchicortex

2 Periarchicortex in cingulate gyrus

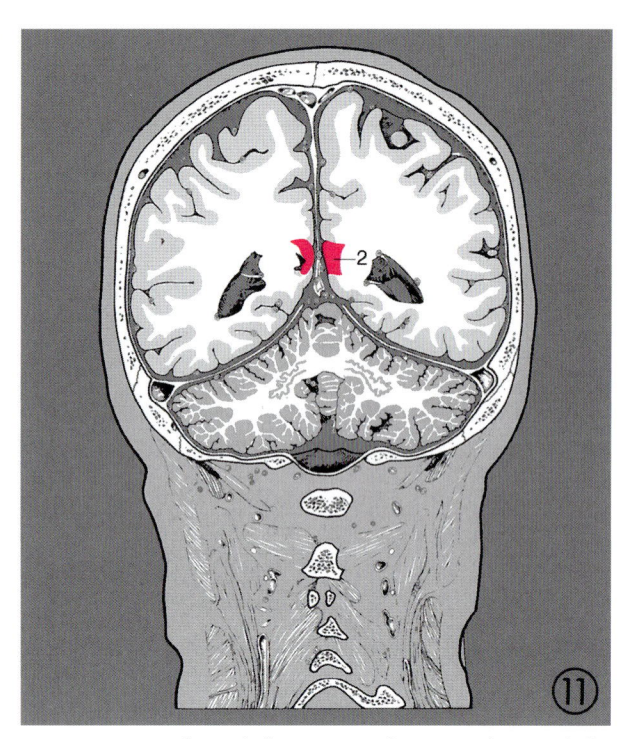

Fig. **148** Coronal serial illustrations of a cortical area of the limbic system. The encircled number (11) indicates the number of the respective slice (Figs. 1, 2a,b, 3).

6.11 Limbic System

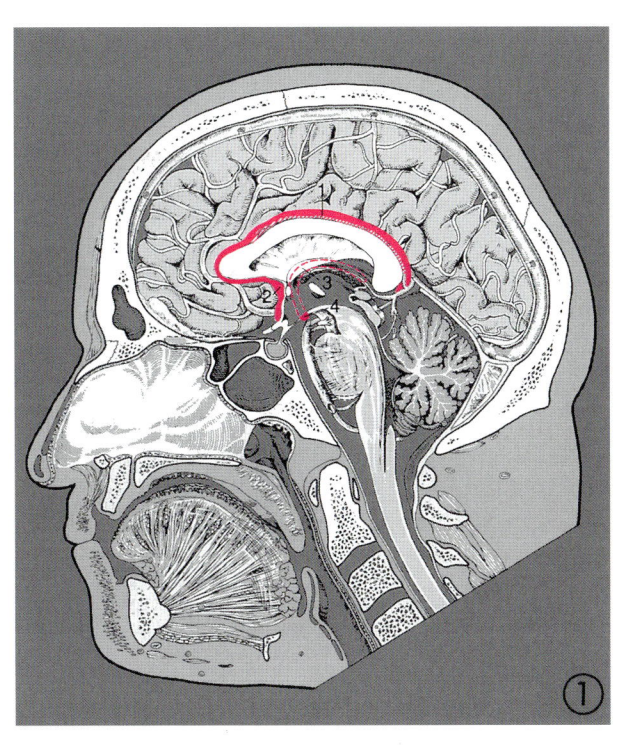

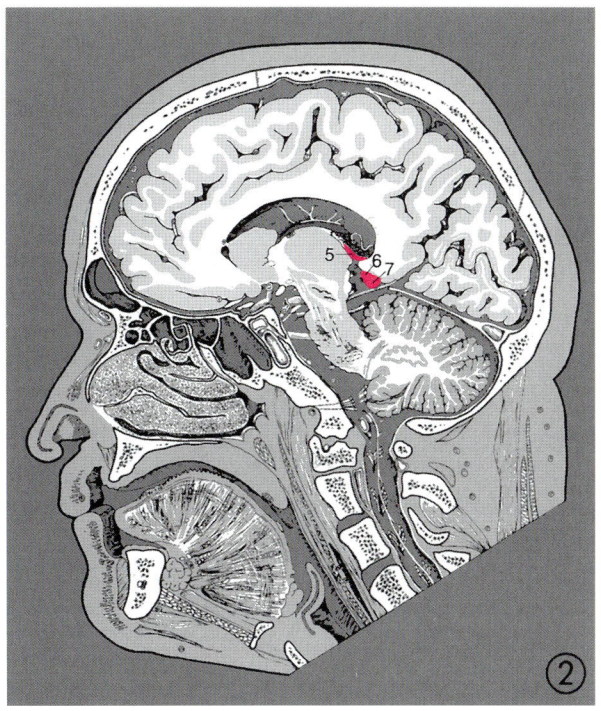

1 Periarchicortex in cingulate gyrus (partially within the slice)
2 Subcallosal area
3 Fornix (within the slice)
4 Mammillary body
5 Fornix
6 Fasciolar gyrus
7 Isthmus of cingulate gyrus
8 Amygdaloid body (partially limbic)
9 Uncus of parahippocampal gyrus
10 Hippocampal formation (in the lateral part of the slice)
11 Hippocampal formation
12 Parahippocampal gyrus

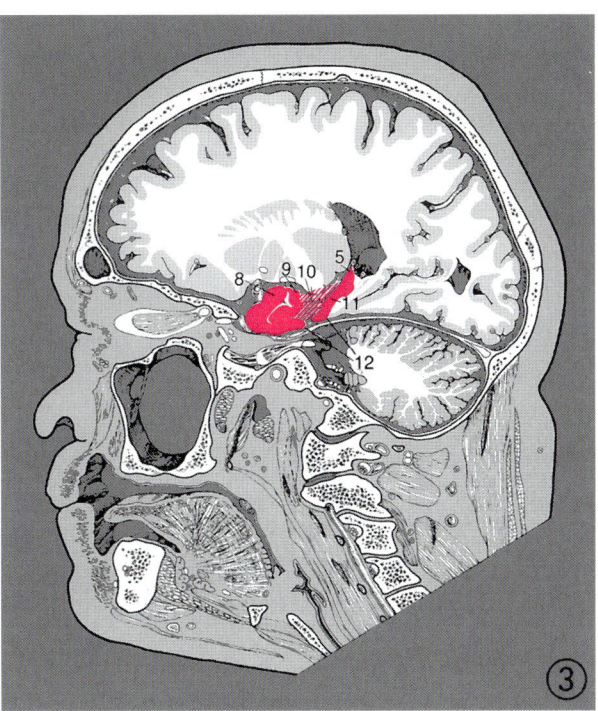

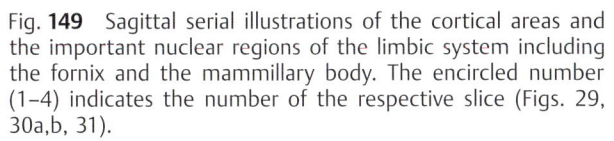

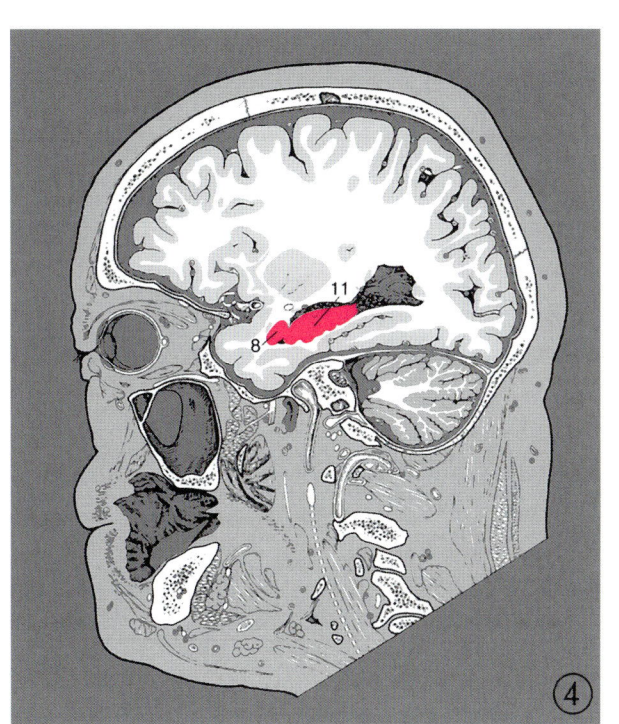

Fig. 149 Sagittal serial illustrations of the cortical areas and the important nuclear regions of the limbic system including the fornix and the mammillary body. The encircled number (1–4) indicates the number of the respective slice (Figs. 29, 30a,b, 31).

410   6 Neurofunctional Systems

1 Periarchicortex (retrocommissural part)
2 Amygdaloid body (partially limbic)
3 Hippocampal formation
4 Subcallosal area
5 Mammillary body (within the slice)
6 Uncus of parahippocampal gyrus
7 Parahippocampal gyrus
8 Periarchicortex in cingulate gyrus
9 Septal nuclei
10 Fornix

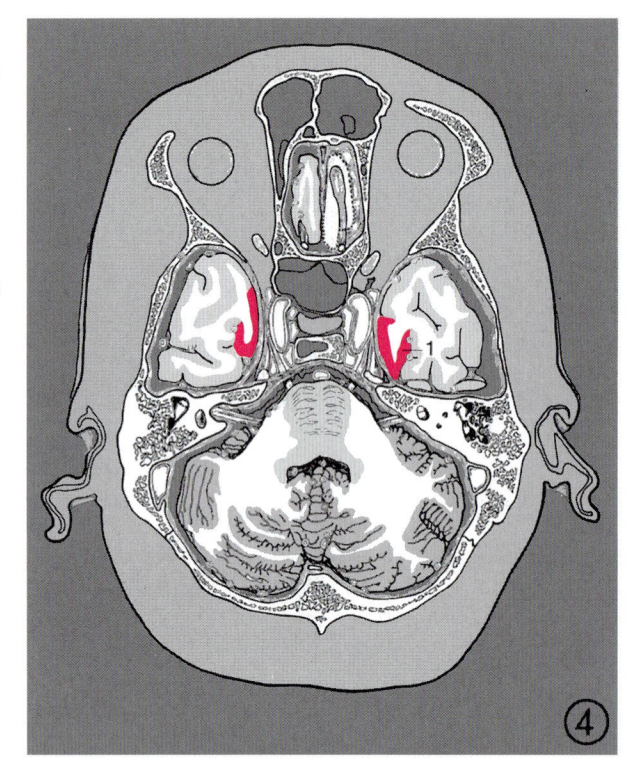

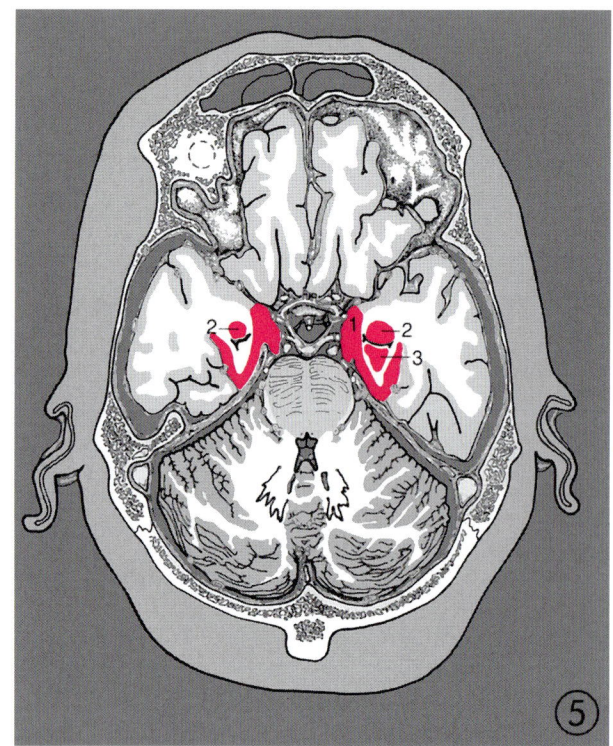

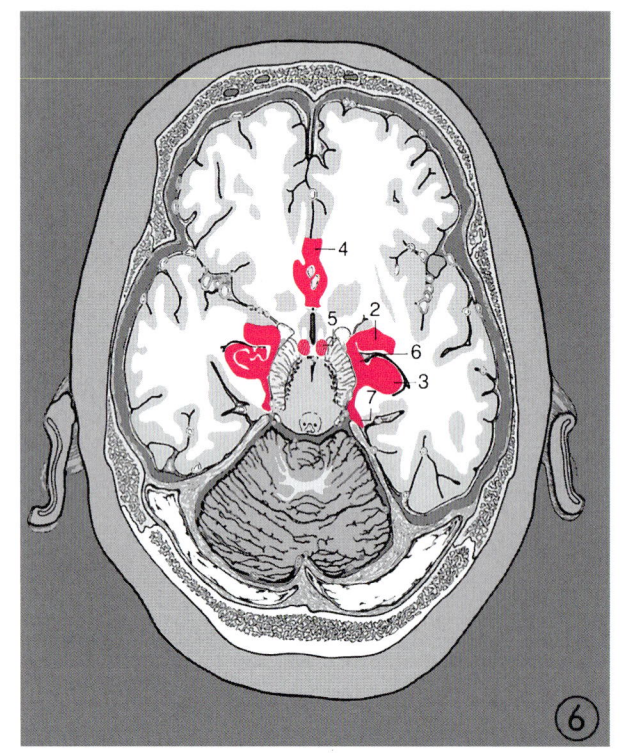

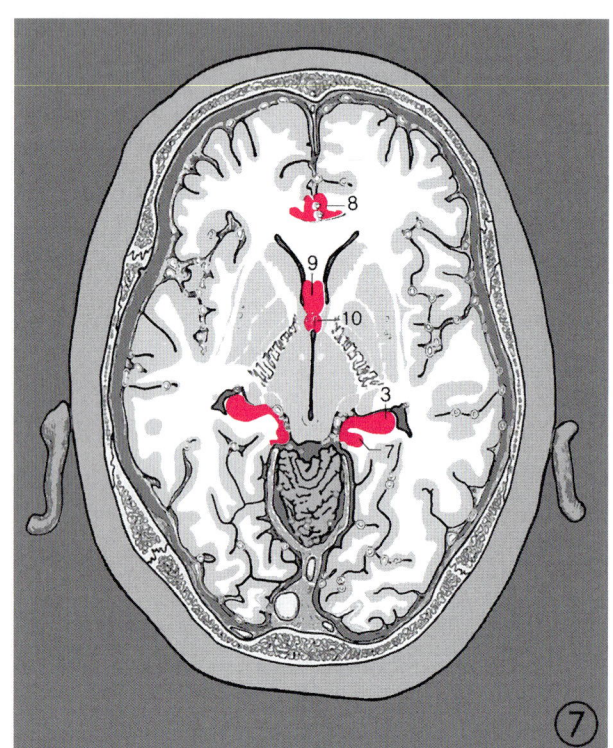

Fig. 150 Canthomeatally oriented serial illustrations of the cortical areas and the most important nuclear regions of the limbic system including the fornix and the mammillary body. The encircled number (4–10) indicates the number of the respective slice (Figs. 44, 45a,b, 46).

6.11 Limbic System

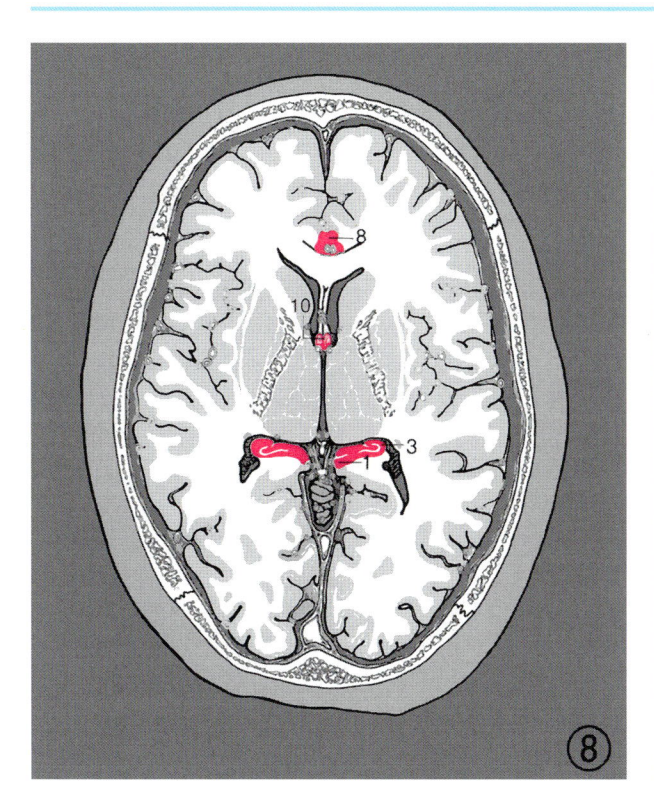

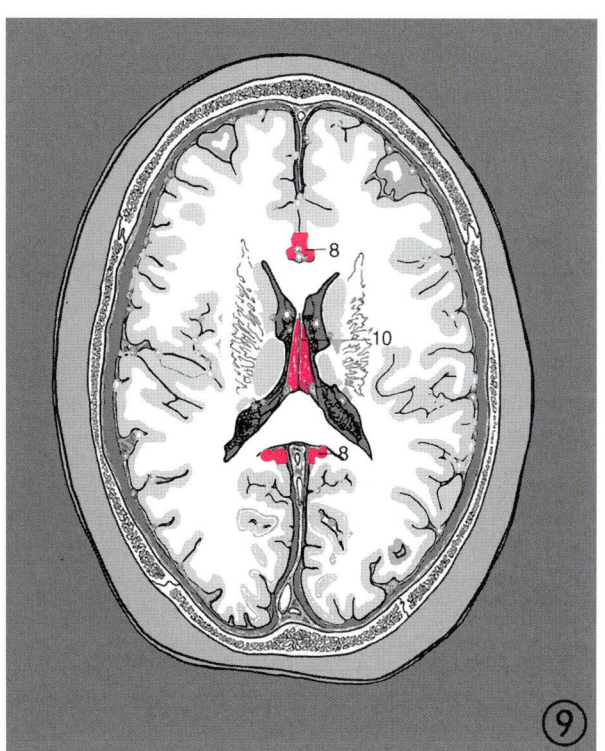

1 Periarchicortex (retrocommissural part)
3 Hippocampal formation
8 Periarchicortex in cingulate gyrus
10 Fornix

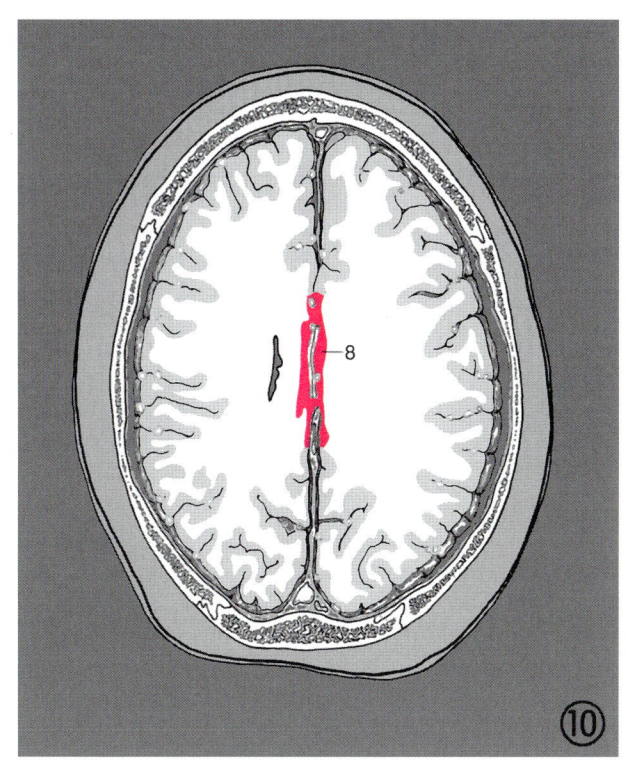

nucleus (of Gudden). The mammillotegmental fasciculus connects the mammillary body with the tegmentum of the midbrain. A further connection exists between the hypothalamic centers and the medulla oblongata via the **posterior longitudinal fasciculus** (of Schütz). The striae medullares of thalamus project from the septal nuclei to the habenular nuclei. The habenulo-interpeduncular tract continues from the habenular nuclei to the interpeduncular nucleus.

6.12 Autonomic Nervous System
(Fig. 151)

The autonomic nervous system of the head innervates the smooth muscle of the eye and the orbit, the lacrimal and salivary glands, the blood vessels and the sweat glands of the scalp, and the erectile smooth muscle of hairs on the scalp. This efferent innervation is, according to classical theory, bineuronal. The cell bodies of the primary neurons are located in the central nervous system (CNS), and those of the secondary neurons in the ganglia outside the CNS. The preganglionic fibers leave the CNS and are connected through a synapse with the secondary neurons. The postganglionic fibers run to the targets or end organs. As in other parts of the body these efferent autonomic fibers are divided into a parasympathetic part and a sympathetic part. The **parasympathetic part** assumes trophotropic functions of digestion and energy synthesis (anabolism); the **sympathetic part** assumes ergotropic functions of physical activity, in the sense of "fight or flight" and the associated output of energy. The classic concept of the autonomic nervous system has been broadened through the discovery of the synaptic effects of neuropeptides (Chap. 7.7) (127, 333). **Neuropeptides** are able to modulate the effects of the transmitter substances of the parasympathetic and sympathetic systems.

Parasympathetic Nervous System of the Head

The cell bodies of the primary parasympathetic neurons of the head are found in the midbrain, pons, and in the medulla oblongata. The preganglionic fibers leave the brain with the oculomotor, facial, and glossopharyngeal nerves. The parasympathetic (ciliary, pterygopalatine, submandibular, and otic) ganglia are close to their target organs. Therefore, the postganglionic course of the parasympathetic fibers is relatively short.

The parasympathetic **accessory nucleus of oculomotor nerve** (of Edinger–Westphal) is located in the tegmentum of the midbrain just anterolateral to the aqueduct. The preganglionic fibers join the oculomotor nerve and run through the superior orbital fissure into the orbit to the ciliary ganglion (Fig. 151.9). This is situated about 18 mm behind the eyeball, lateral to the optic nerve. The postganglionic fibers of the nerve cells in the ciliary ganglion reach the sphincter pupillae (pupillary constriction) and the ciliary muscle (accommodation of the eye). The bineuronal pathway from the accessory nucleus of oculomotor nerve (of Edinger–Westphal) to the sphincter pupillae is also the efferent pathway for the **pupillary reflex**.

1 Oculomotor nerve
2 Accessory nucleus of oculomotor nerve (of Edinger–Westphal)
3 Superior salivatory nucleus
4 Inferior salivatory nucleus
5 Sympathetic fibers in the wall of vertebral artery
6 Sympathetic fibers in the wall of internal carotid artery
7 Intermediate nerve
8 Glossopharyngeal nerve

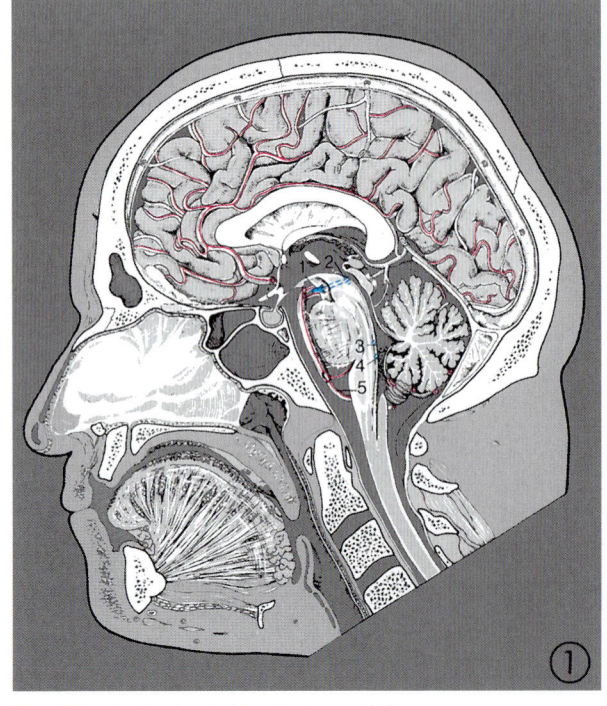

Fig. **151** Sagittal serial illustrations of the autonomic nervous system of the head: parasympathetic system (blue) and sympathetic system (red). The encircled number (1–6) indicates the number of the respective slice (Figs. 29, 30a,b, 31).

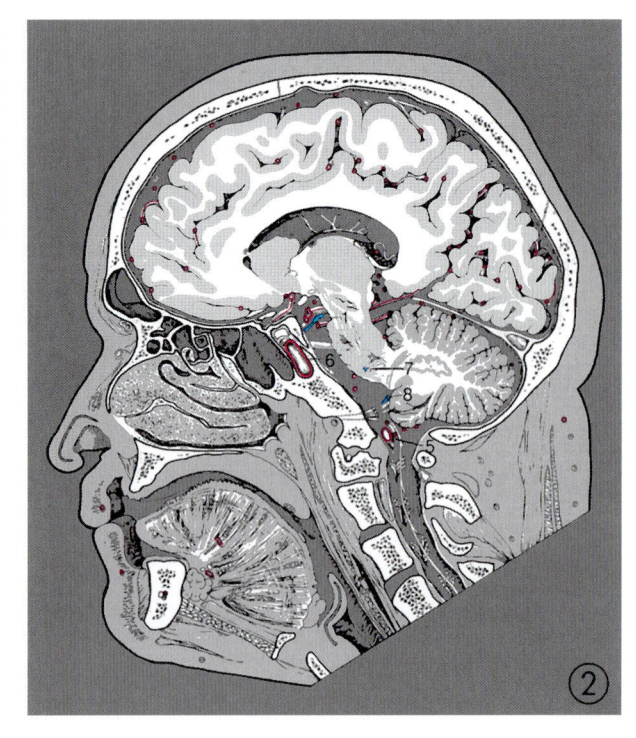

6.12 Autonomic Nervous System

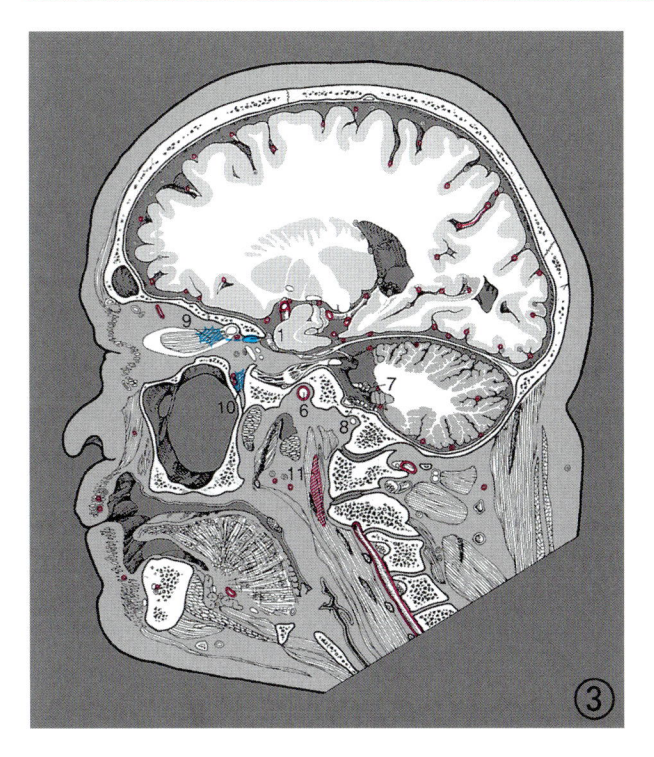

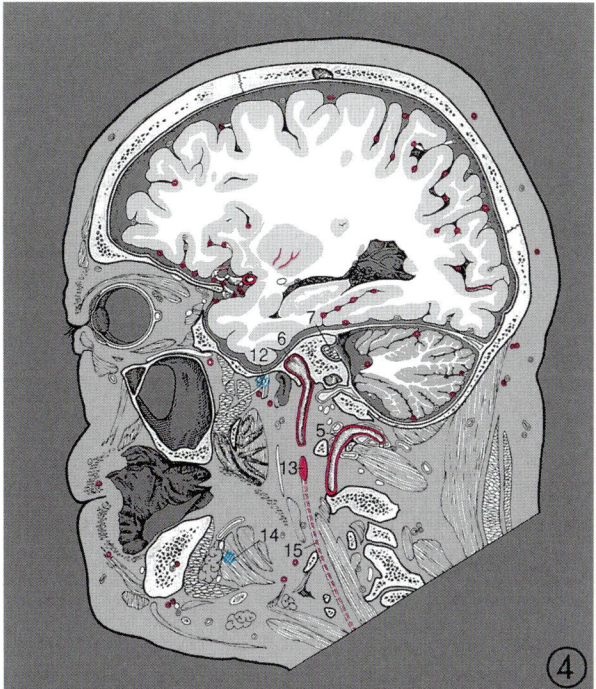

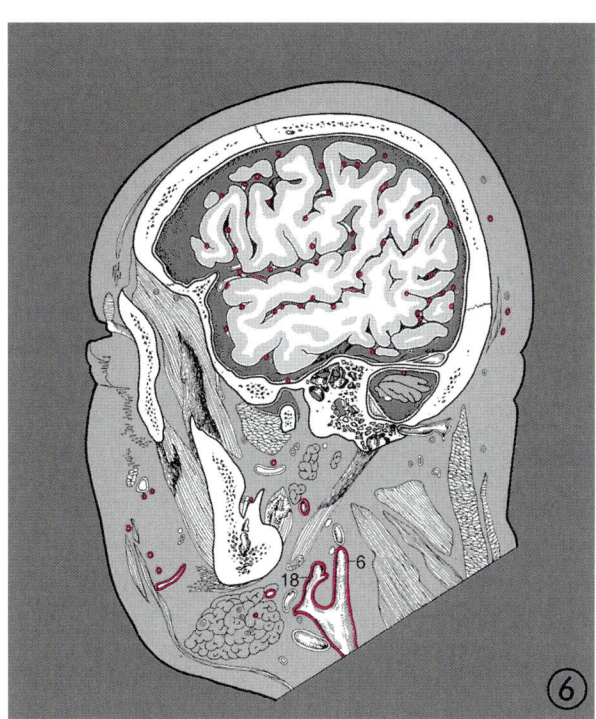

1 Oculomotor nerve
5 Sympathetic fibers in the wall of vertebral artery
6 Sympathetic fibers in the wall of internal carotid artery
7 Intermediate nerve
8 Glossopharyngeal nerve
9 Ciliary ganglion (in the lateral part of the slice)
10 Pterygopalatine ganglion (within the slice)
11 Superior cervical ganglion (in the lateral part of the slice)
12 Otic ganglion
13 Superior cervical ganglion
14 Submandibular ganglion (in the lateral part of the slice)
15 Sympathetic trunk
16 Greater petrosal nerve
17 Chorda tympani
18 Sympathetic fibers in the wall of external carotid artery

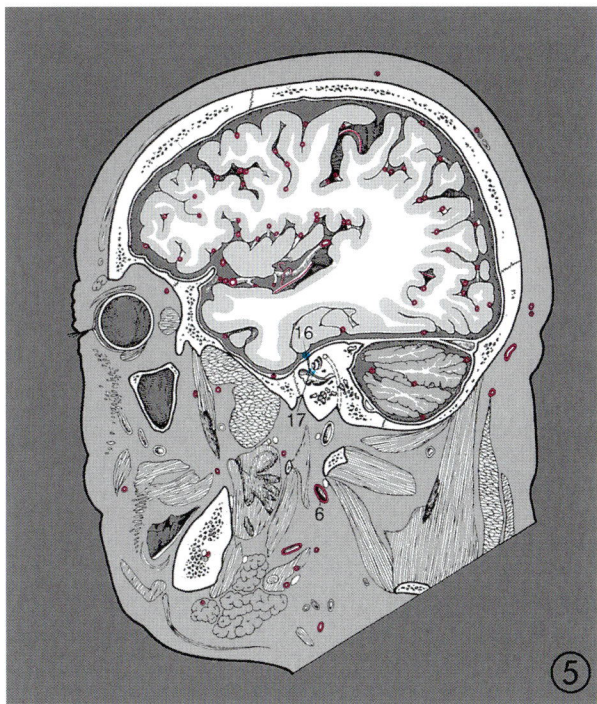

The cell bodies of the primary **parasympathetic neurons** of the facial nerve are found in the **superior salivatory nucleus** just underneath the floor of the rhomboid fossa, in the inferior part of the pons. The preganglionic fibers run in the intermediate nerve of the facial nerve to the internal acoustic meatus in the petrous bone. At the entrance of the facial canal the fibers leave the intermediate nerve as the greater petrosal nerve. This nerve leaves the petrous bone, runs underneath the dura of the middle cranial fossa, and, after running through a small bony canal, it reaches the **pterygopalatine ganglion**. This ganglion is located in the pterygopalatine fossa (Fig. 151.10). The postganglionic fibers run with the zygomatic nerve to the lacrimal gland and through the nasal nerves and the palatine nerves to the glands of the nasal cavity and of the palate. At the end of the facial canal, just above the stylomastoid foramen, the **chorda tympani** branches off the intermediate nerve. It runs underneath the mucous membrane of the tympanic cavity, passes through a fine bony canal and reaches the infratemporal fossa at the base of the skull, posteromedial to the temporomandibular joint (Chap. 3.6). Here the chorda tympani joins the lingual nerve. The preganglionic fibers reach the submandibular ganglion (Fig. 151.14) in the submandibular triangle at the posterior border of the mylohyoid. The postganglionic fibers run to the submandibular and sublingual glands and the glands of the tongue.

The cell bodies of the primary parasympathetic neurons of the glossopharyngeal nerve are located in the **inferior salivatory nucleus** close to the floor of the rhomboid fossa in the superior portion of the medulla oblongata. Its preganglionic fibers first run in the glossopharyngeal nerve through the jugular foramen and enter the petrous bone. The small, lesser petrosal nerve arises from a nerve plexus. It leaves the petrous bone, runs underneath the dura mater in the middle cranial fossa and after passing through a fine bony canal reaches the **otic ganglion** (Fig. 151.12). This ganglion lies close below the foramen ovale, on the medial aspect of the mandibular nerve. The postganglionic fibers join the auriculotemporal nerve and innervate the parotid gland.

The **vagus nerve** with its parasympathetic fibers leaves the lateral part of the medulla oblongata (Figs. 68.X, 71b.18, 71c.7, 71d.7) and runs through the jugular foramen (Figs. 70a.15). In the neck the vagus nerve runs in the neurovascular bundle between the internal carotid artery and the internal jugular vein (Fig. 11c.37). The parasympathetic innervation of the vagus nerve reaches the heart, lungs, and gastrointestinal tract. For this reason the vagus nerve is not depicted in Figure 151.

Sympathetic Nervous System of the Head

The cell bodies of the primary sympathetic neurons of the head are located in the **lateral gray horns of the spinal cord** in the segments C8, T1–T3 (333). The preganglionic fibers leave the spinal canal with the corresponding spinal nerves and ascend with the spinal sympathetic trunk mainly to reach the **superior cervical ganglion** where the second set of neurons is found. The superior cervical ganglion (Figs. 10a.41, 34a.36, 35a.34) is a spindle-shaped swelling, which is, on average, 28 mm long (260). This ganglion lies behind the internal carotid artery at the level of the first and second cervical vertebrae and is enclosed by the deep cervical fascia. The postganglionic fibers form periarterial plexuses around the cranial arteries and innervate the smooth muscle fibers of the dilator pupillae (pupillary dilatation) and the tarsal muscles (widening of the palpebral fissure), the smooth muscles of the arteries, the sweat glands of the scalp (excitatory), and the lacrimal and salivary glands (inhibitory).

Clinical Notes
In a unilateral lesion of the cervical sympathetic an ipsilateral **Horner's syndrome** is observed: the pupil is constricted due to the paralysis of the dilator pupillae (miosis). The upper lid droops because the tarsal muscle has lost its nerve supply (ptosis). Through the paralysis of the orbitalis (Figs. 6c.20, 35c.22) or a reduction of blood flow in the retrobulbar fat, an enophthalmos develops (471b). In addition a vasodilatation of the conjunctiva occurs. The secretion of sweat by the face is decreased or lost, and the secretion of tears is also decreased ipsilaterally.

7 Neurotransmitters and Neuromodulators

Neurotransmitters convey signals at the synapses between neurons or between neurons and effector organs (muscle cells, glandular cells). Neuromodulators **presynaptically** influence the amount of neurotransmitter being liberated or its reuptake into the nerve cells. Furthermore, the **neuromodulators** regulate the sensitivity of the transmitter receptors **postsynaptically**. A transmitter receptor is a protein in the cell membrane of a nerve cell or glia cell; one end of the receptor reaches the extracellular space and the other the intracellular space. The neuromodulators are thus able to regulate the level of excitability at the synapses and to alter the effect of the neurotransmitters. Hence, neuronal information processing in the synapses through different regulatory mechanisms is more complex than was previously assumed. Neurotransmitters and neuromodulators are grouped together as neuroactive substances.

Research on the neuroactive substances has developed remarkably during the last 40 years and is still ongoing. The significance of the neuroactive substances is considerable, particularly for neuropharmacology (221, 381a, 481). In addition, positron emission tomography (PET) and single photon emission computed tomography (SPECT) allow the in vivo study of regional distribution and concentration of neuroactive substances at macroscopic level (measurements of receptor binding potential, reuptake sites, transporter function, enzyme activity [e.g. MAO], transmitter synthesis [F-Dopa], transmitter [dopamine] release [amphetamine]) (66, 97a, 193, 206, 209). Therefore, an overview of the localization of neurotransmitters and neuromodulators in the brain will be given, although most of the data to date have been obtained from rat brains and to a lesser extent from primate brains. Their extrapolation to the human brain involves many uncertainties.

For a better understanding of neuroactive substances, we will briefly review the history of their discovery. Forty years ago neuronal theory was based on the following assumptions: each neuron provided only one and the same neurotransmitter to its synapses, each transmitter being either excitatory or inhibitory. The advances of electronmicroscopy and the use of microelectrodes made possible an intensive investigation of synaptology. In the textbooks of 1960 only six neurotransmitters were mentioned: acetylcholine, noradrenaline (norepinephrine), dopamine, adrenaline (epinephrine), histamine, and serotonin. By 1970 about ten were mentioned. In the last three decades more than 30 transmitter/modulator peptides have been discovered in the nervous system.

In the light of the new information the **neuronal theory** now acknowledges that many neurons contain more than one neuroactive substance (192, 291). Nerve cells that contain more than one neurotransmitter release only one transmitter when stimulated. One neurotransmitter, for example acetylcholine, can have an excitatory or an inhibitory effect. This depends on the transmitter receptors of the postsynaptic neurons. For dopamine it has been reported that it can function either as a neurotransmitter or a neuromodulator (333). These varying effects of the transmitters indicate their manifold functions in the central nervous system (CNS). Several neuroactive substances are usually involved within a neurofunctional system. One neuroactive substance generally influences several neurofunctional systems. This will be demonstrated, for example for the different sites of action of the dopaminergic groups of nerve cells. The nigrostriatal neurons are found in the motor system of the basal ganglia (Chap. 6.8.2), the mesolimbic neurons in the limbic system (Chap. 6.11), the tuberoinfundibular neurons in the hypothalamo-hypophysial system, and a small group (A 15) in the olfactory system. These dopaminergic neurons are only parts of different neurofunctional systems. This knowledge is important for interpretation of pharmacologic actions and side effects.

Nieuwenhuys (333) has provided a very good overview of our present knowledge of the chemoarchitecture of the brain. He suggested three new terms that describe the topical arrangement of some of the groups of neurons referred to in the following chapters:
- Core
- Median paracore
- Lateral paracore.

The **core** is a periventricular area in the brainstem and forebrain, the nerve cells of which are rich in neuromodulators. These nerve cells release their neuromodulators, usually paracrine, through the intercellular space to their adjoining cells (not through synapses). Most likely a functional connection exists with the circumventricular organs that have no blood–brain barrier and, therefore, seem to be particulary well-suited for neuroendocrine regulation. The following areas belong to the core: posterior (dorsal) nucleus of the vagus nerve (Figs. 68.18, 70b.25), the superficial zone of the spinal nucleus of the trigeminal nerve (Figs. 68.5, 69b.28, 70b.31), the parabrachial nuclei, periaqueductal gray substance (Fig. 12a.24), small periventricular nuclei of the hypothalamus, septal nuclei (Fig. 148.4), as well as parts of the limbic system (Chap. 6.11).

The **median paracore** is adjacent to the core in the median area of the tegmentum of the brainstem and consists of a series of raphe nuclei that contain, among others, serotoninergic nerve cells (Chap. 7.2).

The **lateral paracore** adjoins the core in the anterolateral part of the tegmentum of the brainstem. It contains catecholaminergic and some cholinergic neurons (Chaps. 7.1, 7.4).

7.1 Catecholaminergic Neurons

The catecholaminergic neurons contain in their perikarya and cell processes the transmitter substances dopamine, noradrenaline (norepinephrine), or adrenaline (epinephrine). These molecules are derived from the amino acid tyrosine. During the biosynthesis of these transmitters, dihydroxybenzol is produced as the basic framework, which is typical of the catecholamine compounds with a side-chain and an amino group. Dopamine, noradrenaline, and adrenaline are relatively small molecules. Consequently they diffuse out of neurons soon after death. Therefore, conventional histologic techniques cannot be used reliably to map the sites of production and storage of these compounds.

The discovery of dopaminergic, noradrenergic, and adrenergic neurons 40 years ago depended on the technical possibility of freezing living cells and drying them prior to processing them for fluorescence microscopy. In 1962 histologic techniques were successful in demonstrating a green fluorescence of dopamine and noradrenaline (120). Today, the more sensitive immunofluorescent methods enable a more accurate detection of catecholaminergic neurons. The noradrenergic and dopaminergic nerve cells were labelled A1 to A15 and the adrenergic nerve cells C1 to C3. The sequence of numbers was chosen in ascending order in the brainstem, i.e. from inferior to superior.

The localization of catecholaminergic neurons is still under investigation. Data obtained from rats and lower primate brains must be extrapolated to the human brain. The dopaminergic, noradrenergic, and adrenergic cell groups, however, correspond closely in the adult human brain with the neuromelanin-containing neurons (42, 401). Therefore, these neuromelanin-containing nerve cells provide the first line of information about catecholamines in neuropathologic specimens. The nigrostriatal dopaminergic system is of interest in Parkinson's disease and its therapy. Probably some catecholaminergic neurons and transmitter receptors are the site of action of antidepressive and neuroleptic drugs (303).

7.1.1 Dopaminergic Neurons

Dopamine-synthesizing nerve cells (A8–A15) are found in the midbrain, diencephalon, and telencephalon (221, 374a). The largest and most striking group of dopaminergic nerve cells is the **pars compacta of the substantia nigra** (A9) (Figs. 11a.28, 33a.20, 52a.29, 77b.21, 78b.15, 132.10, 138.2). Their axons form an ascending pathway that runs through the lateral part of the hypothalamus and traverses the internal capsule. The **nigrostriatal fibers** then run to the caudate nucleus (Figs. 8a.9, 10a.9, 12a.20, 33a.7, 34a.5, 35a.11, 53a.16, 54a.34) and putamen (Figs. 9a.14, 11a.16, 34a.7, 35a.10, 53a.13, 54a.17). Together with a small group of nerve cells A8 from the reticular formation of the midbrain, the nerve cell group A9 forms the nigrostriatal system. In accordance with its synaptic connections, the substantia nigra belongs to the basal ganglia (Chap. 6.8.2).

A second dopaminergic nerve cell group runs from the mesencephalic cell group A10 to parts of the **limbic system**. It is, therefore, called **mesolimbic**. Drugs affecting this system are believed to produce psychic effects (303). The A10 group forms a ventral cap on the interpeduncular nucleus in the tegmentum of the midbrain. The axons run in the medial forebrain bundle to the following structures of the limbic structures (Fig. 147): inner nucleus of the stria terminalis, olfactory tubercle, nucleus accumbens, septal nuclei, and several parts of the frontal, cingulate, and entorhinal cortex. Certain substances such as opiates, cocaine, and alcohol can stimulate the mesolimbic system and release the reward mechanism. Therefore this mechanism may be regarded as one neurobiologic basis for drug addiction.

A third dopaminergic system, called **tuberoinfundibular**, is found in the diencephalon. Cell group A12 is located in the tuber cinereum and projects to the infundibulum (Figs. 2b.28, 32a.25, 45b.30, 51a.9, 67.19, 76b.4). This system is thought to have a neuroendocrine function. The other diencephalic nerve cell groups A11, A13, and A14 and their target cells are also located in the hypothalamus.

A small group A15 is scattered throughout the olfactory bulb (Figs. 2b.24, 5a.10, 45b.27, 50a.3, 76a.6) and is the only telencephalic dopaminergic group of neurons.

The clinical significance of a deficiency in dopamine, particularly in the substantia nigra, provides us today with the possibility of substitution therapy in the management of Parkinson's syndrome (Chap. 6.8.2). Dopamine and the dopamine agonist bromocriptine function as an adenohypophysiotropic prolactin-inhibiting factor. This explains the clinical use of bromocriptine for the conservative treatment of prolactinomas, as well as its use in the treatment of Parkinson's disease.

7.1.2 Noradrenergic Neurons

The noradrenergic nerve cells are found only in a narrow anterolateral zone of the tegmentum of the medulla oblongata and pons. Although the cell groups A1 to A7 have been described originally in rats (86, 87), similar localizations were found in primates (123, 144, 201, 202, 303, 336). The fibers leaving these groups of nerve cells either ascend toward the midbrain or descend toward the spinal region. Furthermore, the noradrenergic cells are connected with the cerebellum. The noradrenergic fibers branch more widely than the dopaminergic ones. The proximity of the noradrenergic fibers to the cerebral arterioles and capillaries is striking and they have thus been thought to play a role in the regulation of cerebral blood flow (175, 374).

The largest noradrenergic cell group A6 is located in the **cerulean nucleus**. It contains almost half of all noradrenergic cells (449). In adults the cerulean nucleus holds neuromelanin-containing nerve cells that form a dark-blue, 1-cm-long strip in the cerulean nucleus (Figs. 51a.20, 52a.34, 75b.22, 76b.23, 77b.28), in the upper pontine region on the floor of the fourth ventricle. It extends upward to just below the inferior colliculi (Fig. 77b.34). The posterior noradrenergic bundle originates from the A6 group. It runs through the tegmentum of the midbrain anterolateral to the periaqueductal gray substance, enters the hypothalamus, runs to the septal nuclei and then into the cingulum. The posterior noradrenergic bundle is connected with the following structures:

- In the **midbrain** the posterior raphe nucleus and the inferior and superior colliculi (Figs. 2b.21, 2b.31, 32a.18, 32a.19, 78b.31, 77b.34).
- In the **diencephalon** the anterior nuclei of thalamus and the medial and lateral geniculate bodies (Figs. 12a.18, 12a.19, 34a.15, 53a.31, 53a.32).
- In the **telencephalon** the amygdaloid body (Figs. 10a.27, 35a.21, 51a.12, 52a.21), the hippocampal formation (Figs. 10a.30, 11a.31, 13a.15, 52a.24, 53a.36, 54a.37), the cingulate, retrosplenial, and entorhinal cortex, as well as the entire neocortex.

Additional fibers from the cell group A6 run to the cerebellum through the superior cerebellar peduncle (Figs. 51a.22, 75b.25, 76b.21, 144b.6). Descending fibers from the cerulean nucleus are joined by fibers from the neighboring cell group A7. They provide the posterior (dorsal) nucleus of the vagus nerve (Figs. 68.18, 70b.25, 71b.26), the inferior olivary nucleus (Figs. 12a.38, 70b.16, 71b.14, 72b.14), and the spinal cord. The anterolateral ceruleospinal tract gives off noradrenergic fibers to the ventral and dorsal gray horn in the spinal cord (338). As a whole, the few noradrenergic cells of the cerulean nucleus have a huge field of projection, reaching into separate regions of the forebrain, the brainstem, the cerebellum, and the spinal cord.

The nerve cell groups A1 and A2 are located in the medulla oblongata. Together with the pontine cell groups A5 and A7 they form the anterior ascending noradrenergic neurons. In the midbrain they project into the periaqueductal gray substance (Fig. 12a.24) and into the reticular formation, in the diencephalon into the whole hypothalamus (Figs. 52a.17, 53a.22, 67.11, 77b.9, 78b.5), and in the telencephalon into the olfactory bulb. From these cell groups (A1, A2, A5, A7) bulbospinal fibers also run into the spinal cord.

7.1.3 Adrenergic Neurons

The adrenaline (epinephrine)-synthesizing nerve cells are found only in the medulla oblongata in a narrow anterolateral area (lateral paracore [333]). The largest cell group C1 lies posterior to the inferior olivary nucleus (Figs. 12a.38, 70b.16, 71b.14, 72b.14), the middle cell group C2 in the neighborhood of the solitary nucleus (Figs. 68.8, 70b.23, 71b.23), and the cell group C3 close underneath the periventricular gray. The C1–C3 efferents run to the posterior (dorsal) nucleus of the vagus nerve, the solitary nucleus, cerulean nucleus, the periventricular gray of the pons, the periaqueductal gray substance of the midbrain, the hypothalamus, and the paraventricular nucleus. Physiologic experiments (91, 154) have shown that cell group C1 is a very sensitive vasopressor center.

7.2 Serotoninergic Neurons

The serotoninergic nerve cells were discovered by fluorescence microscopy 40 years ago, at the same time as the catecholaminergic nerve cells. The serotoninergic nerve cells show a yellow fluorescence (120). Serotonin is derived from the amino acid tryptophan.

The serotoninergic nerve cells B1 to B9 are found in the medulla oblongata, pons, and midbrain according to the nomenclature (86, 87). The majority of these cell groups are located in the median zone of the brainstem (fusion zone = raphe) and, therefore, are called the nuclei of the raphe. The raphe neurons B1 (pallidal raphe nucleus) and B2 (obscurus raphe nucleus) are located in the medulla oblongata, B3 (magnus raphe nucleus) in the border area between the medulla oblongata and pons, B5 (pontine raphe nucleus) in the pons, and B7 (posterior raphe nucleus) in the midbrain. The raphe neurons B6 and B8 (superior central nucleus) are found in the tegmentum of the pons and midbrain. In the raphe nuclei there are also nerve cells that contain other neurotransmitters such as dopamine, noradrenaline, GABA, enkephalin, and substance P (333). For this reason the raphe nuclei are also called **multiple transmitter centers**.

The projections of the serotoninergic nerve cells ascend and descend just like the noradrenergic fibers.

The main serotoninergic projection is directed toward the **limbic system** and also into the reticular formation and the spinal cord. A close association exists with the cerulean nucleus, the largest center of noradrenergic nerve cells.

The large anterior ascending tract arises from the cell groups B6, B7, and B8. It runs anteriorly through the tegmentum of the midbrain and laterally through the hypothalamus, then branches into the pathways of the fornix and the cingulum. Along this route the cell groups B6, B7, and B8 are synaptically connected with the:

- Interpeduncular nucleus and substantia nigra (Figs. 11a.28, 33a.20, 52a.29, 77b.21, 78b.15) in the **midbrain**
- Habenular nuclei (Figs. 54a.27, 147.11), subnuclei of the thalamus, and nuclei of the hypothalamus in the **diencephalon**.
- Septal nuclei (Fig. 148.4) and the olfactory bulb (Figs. 2b.24, 5a.10, 45b.27, 50a.3, 76a.6) in the **telencephalon.**

Numerous projections to other limbic areas, including the hippocampus (Figs. 10a.30, 11a.31, 13a.15, 52a.24, 53a.36, 54a.37), subiculum, cingulate, and entorhinal cortex also exist. In addition, there are connections to the striatum and the frontal neocortex. The shorter posterior ascending tract connects the cell groups B3, B5, and B7 through the posterior longitudinal fasciculus (of Schütz) with the periaqueductal gray substance and the posterior hypothalamic area. Furthermore, serotoninergic projections into the cerebellum (from B6 and B7) and into the spinal cord (from B1 to B3) exist. There are numerous fiber connections to the reticular formation.

Ascending serotoninergic fibers are possibly involved in the regulation of sleep. An inhibitory effect of the descending serotoninergic fibers to the first sympathetic neuron in the spinal cord has been demonstrated physiologically. The raphe neurons in the medulla oblongata are thought to control the conduction of pain in the anterolateral system (221, 333).

7.3 Histaminergic Neurons

The histaminergic nerve cells are located in the inferior part of the hypothalamus close to the infundibulum. Histamine is metabolized by the enzyme histidine decarboxylase from the amino acid histidine. Neurochemical, neurophysiologic, and neuropharmacologic findings have identified histamine as a neurotransmitter. The histaminergic nerve cells have been located with antibodies against histidine decarboxylase.

Short and long branching fibers from the histaminergic nerve cells in the inferior portion of the hypothalamus run to the:

- **Brainstem**, within the posterior and periventricular zone. Histaminergic fibers reach the periaqueductal gray substance, posterior raphe nucleus, medial vestibular nucleus, solitary nucleus (Figs. 68.8, 70b.23, 71b.23), posterior nucleus of vagus nerve (Figs. 68.18, 70b.25, 71b.26), facial nucleus (Figs. 68.15, 73b.21, 74b.23), anterior and posterior cochlear nuclei (Figs. 68.7, 72b.26), lateral lemniscus (Figs. 74b.20, 75b.18, 76b.18, 77b.30), and the inferior colliculus (Figs. 2b.31, 32a.19, 77b.34). These results were obtained with rat brains (478).
- **Diencephalon**, to the posterior, lateral, and anterior part of the hypothalamus. The mammillary body (Figs. 2b.22, 10a.25, 32a.15, 45b.22, 67.18, 77b.10) is rich in histaminergic fibers. In the thalamus histaminergic fibers branch into the periventricular nuclei and the lateral geniculate body (221).
- **Telencephalon**, to the diagonal band of Broca, the nucleus accumbens, amygdaloid body (Figs. 10a.27, 35a.21, 51a.12, 52a.21), and the cerebral cortex

7.4 Cholinergic Neurons

Acetylcholine has been known as a neurotransmitter since 1914. The first evidence of cholinergic perikarya was obtained with the help of acetylcholinesterase, but the results were not reliable. Only during the last 15 years has it been possible to accurately identify cholinergic nerve cells by using antibodies against choline acetyltransferase.

The alpha (α) and gamma (γ)-motor neurons of the oculomotor, trochlear, trigeminal, abducens, facial, glossopharyngeal, vagus, accessory, and hypoglossal nerves (Fig. 68) and of the spinal nerves are cholinergic (221). Acetylcholine influences the contraction of skeletal muscles (513). The preganglionic neurons of the autonomic system are cholinergic and stimulate the postganglionic neurons of the autonomic system (513). Other cholinergic nerve cells have been given an alphanumerical designation in a superior–inferior direction (in contrast to the catecholaminergic and the serotoninergic neurons). The cholinergic neurons Ch1 form about 10% of the cells of the medial septal nucleus, Ch2 neurons 70% of the cells of the vertical limb of the diagonal band (of Broca), and Ch3 neurons 1% of the cells of the horizontal limb of the diagonal band of Broca. All three groups of neurons project downward into the medial habenular nucleus and the interpeduncular nucleus. The neurons Ch1 are connected through ascending fibers via the fornix with the hippocampus (Chap. 6.11). The cell group Ch3 synapses with nerve cells of the olfactory bulb (Figs. 2b.24, 5a.10, 45b.27, 50a.3, 76a.6).

The cell group Ch4 is relatively large in the human brain and corresponds to the **basal nucleus** (of

Meynert) (Fig. 10a.23). It is located in the innominate substance below the globus pallidus (Fig. 10a.15). In the basal nucleus (of Meynert) 90% of all cells are cholinergic. This nucleus receives afferent input from the subcortical diencephalic-telencephalic regions and from the limbic-paralimbic cerebral cortex. The anterior cells of the basal nucleus project to the frontal and parietal neocortex and the posterior cells to the occipital and temporal neocortex. The basal nucleus is, therefore, a relay station between the limbic-paralimbic regions and the neocortex. These findings are of interest since in Alzheimer's disease the choline acetyltransferase is reduced in the basal nuclei, and the neurons show overt degeneration (485, 486). However, it has not been demonstrated whether this is a primary degeneration or a secondary following the loss of neocortical nerve cells (307). In younger patients suffering from Alzheimer's disease an even greater loss of cells in the cerulean nucleus (A6) has been observed than in the basal nucleus (296).

The two small cholinergic cell groups Ch5 and Ch6 are located in the pons and are regarded as part of the ascending reticular system (333).

A small group of cells (**periolivary nucleus**) that consists partly of cholinergic cells can be found on the edge of the trapezoid body in the lower part of the pons. Its efferent fibers run to the receptor cells of the auditory system (Chap. 6.5). This cholinergic system influences the transfer of auditory signals.

7.5 GABAergic Neurons

The GABAergic neurons contain the neurotransmitter amino acid gamma (γ)-aminobutyric acid (GABA). It is derived biochemically from glutamic acid by the action of the enzyme glutamic acid decarboxylase. GABA can be detected immunohistochemically with antibodies against this enzyme. In the CNS GABA is the most important **inhibitory neurotransmitter** (221, 513).

GABA is found in the spinal cord in interneurons that inhibit afferent systems presynaptically and postsynaptically. Individual hypothalamocortical connections are GABAergic. Intracortically connected GABAergic nerve cells are found in the olfactory system and in the limbic system (basket cells of the hippocampus). In the motor system of the the basal ganglia the following efferents contain γ-aminobutyric acid, namely striatonigral, pallidonigral, and subthalamopallidal tracts.

In the cerebellum the Purkinje cells contain GABA (Fig. 144b.7); their efferents end in the cerebellar nuclei and in the lateral vestibular nucleus. In the cerebellar cortex the Golgi cells, stellate cells, and basket cells are intracortical GABAergic nerve cells.

7.6 Glutamatergic and Aspartatergic Neurons

The two similar amino acids, glutamate (GLU) and aspartate (ASP), have been classified electrophysiologically as **excitatory neurotransmitters**. Immunohistochemically and autoradiographically they are usually not discriminated. For this reason they are also grouped together in this overview. Nerve cells with GLU- and/or ASP-transmitters have been identified in the auditory system. Probably these neurons are the first-order neurons of the auditory system (Fig. 122). In the olfactory system neurons with GLU/ASP-transmitters are the nerve cells that unite the olfactory bulb with the prepiriform cortex. In the limbic system the axons of the GLU/ASP-containing pyramidal cells of the hippocampus run to the septal nuclei. In the neocortex the pyramidal cells contain glutamate. Glutamate has also been detected in the following tracts that arise from the pyramidal cells: corticostriatal, corticothalamic, corticotectal, corticopontine, and corticospinal tracts (221, 333).

7.7 Peptidergic Neurons

Peptidergic neurons include:
- Hypothalamoneurohypophysial nerve cells with the peptides oxytocin and vasopressin (Chap. 5.7.4)
- Nerve cells with hypophysiotropic peptides such as somatostatin, corticoliberin, thyroliberin, luliberin (Chap. 5.7.4)
- Nerve cells with "gut-brain" peptides, such as substance P, vasoactive intestinal polypeptide (VIP), and cholecystokinin
- Nerve cells, the peptides of which are derivates of pro-opiomelanocortin, such as corticotropin and β-endorphin
- Enkephalinergic nerve cells.

The neurotransmitter and/or neuromodulator function of many peptides is still disputed (333). Therefore, only a few substances will be discussed.

7.7.1 SP-Containing Neurons

About 25 years ago the chemical structure of substance P (SP) was found to be an 11-amino-acid peptide. Soon after its discovery the slow onset and the long-lasting excitatory effects of SP on neurons were noticed.

About one-fifth of nerve cells in the **spinal ganglia** and the **trigeminal** (Gasserian) **ganglion** (Figs. 9a.31, 34a.28, 73b.3, 114.4) are SP-containing nerve cells. These cells are small and have no or thin myelin sheaths. They probably conduct pain signals. In the olfactory system the brush cells in the **olfactory bulb** contain SP. In the brainstem, particularly in the periventricular gray substance, there are numerous nerve cells containing SP. Efferent connections run into the spinal cord from three centers: magnus raphe nucleus; periaqueductal gray substance (Fig. 12a.24); accessory oculomotor nucleus (of Edinger–Westphal) (Figs. 68.9, 151.2).

SP-containing neurons of the habenular nuclei run from the diencephalon to the interpeduncular nucleus. The striatum has SP-containing nigrostriatal fibers that are assumed to be part of the motor system of the basal ganglia. Furthermore, substance P has been detected in certain parts of the baboon's neocortex in small cells, predominantly in layers V and VI.

7.7.2 VIP-Containing Neurons

The vasoactive intestinal polypeptide (VIP) is a 28-amino-acid peptide. In the gastrointestinal tract it dilates the blood vessels and stimulates the transformation of glycogen into glucose. In the nervous system vasoactive intestinal polypeptide is thought to be an excitatory neurotransmitter and/or a neuromodulator (333). In the brainstem, VIP-containing nerve cells are located in the solitary nucleus (Figs. 68.8, 70b.23, 71b.23) and are locally interconnected in this nuclear area. The **periaqueductal gray substance** (Fig. 12a.24) contains VIP-containing neurons that ascend to the hypothalamus, the bed nucleus of the stria terminalis, and the amygdaloid body (Figs. 10a.27, 35a.21, 51a.12, 52a.21), and are connected with the limbic system. In the suprachiasmatic nucleus there are many VIP-containing nerve cells that are connected with nuclei of the hypothalamus. Probably these are involved in regulating circadian rhythms. The highest concentration of VIP is found in the **neocortex**, mostly in bipolar cells that are interconnected intracortically. Possibly the VIP regulates the energy metabolism of the neocortex.

7.7.3 β-Endorphin-Containing Neurons

Beta (β)-endorphin is a 31-amino-acid peptide. It functions as an inhibitory neuromodulator in the brain. Endorphinergic cells are found in the mediobasal hypothalamus and in the inferior part of the solitary nucleus in the medulla oblongata (Figs. 68.8, 70b.23). Ascending efferents of the hypothalamic endorphinergic nerve cells run to the paraventricular nucleus, the preoptic area, the septal nuclei (Fig. 148.4), and parts of the amygdaloid body (Figs. 10a.27, 35a.21, 51a.12, 76b.5). Descending efferents run to the periaqueductal gray substance of the midbrain (Fig. 12a.24), to the cerulean nucleus (Figs. 51a.20, 75b.22, 76b.23), and to the reticular formation of the pons and the medulla oblongata. Intraventricular administration of β-endorphin or injection of this substance into the periaqueductal gray substance of the midbrain produces analgesia. Therefore, a role in the **central regulation of stress-induced analgesia** has been attributed to the endorphinergic nerve cells (221). Furthermore, it has been demonstrated that the endorphinergic nerve cells stimulate release of the growth hormone, prolactin, and vasopressin.

7.7.4 Enkephalinergic Neurons

Enkephalin is a 5-amino-acid peptide. It has been identified electrophysiologically as an inhibitory neurotransmitter. Enkephalin has been identified by immunohistochemistry in interneurons with short processes and in neurons with long projection fibers. Enkephalin functions as an endogenous **ligand for opiate receptors** (221).

The superficial dorsal layer of the dorsal gray horn of the spinal cord and the spinal nucleus of trigeminal nerve contain a dense plexus of enkephalinergic fibers and are rich in opiate receptors. In addition, numerous small enkephalinergic neurons are located in this layer. Probably they presynaptically inhibit the release of SP from the synaptic endings of the primary neurons in the pain-conducting systems. Enkephalin-containing nerve cells are also found in the periolivary nucleus (auditory system) and in the olfactory bulb (Figs. 2b.24, 5a.10, 45b.27, 50a.3, 76a.6) (olfactory system). Furthermore, there are abundant enkephalin-containing nerve cells in the raphe nuclei, particularly in the magnus raphe and posterior raphe nuclei. The periaqueductal gray substance (Fig. 12a.24) has the highest concentration of opiate receptors. Analgesia can be produced through an electric stimulus or a microinjection of an opiate in this area. Enkephalinergic nerve cells act on the hypothalamo-hypophysial regulation of oxytocin and vasopressin, as well as on the regulation of several liberins and statins. The substantia innominata is the area most rich in enkephalin. The striatum holds enkephalin-containing nerve cells that project to the pallidum. Enkephalin-containing nerve cells are located in the neocortex and allocortex and are connected intracortically.

8 Material and Methods

Using the neuroanatomic collection from the Hannover Medical School the authors have been able to gain valuable information about the sectional anatomy of the head and variability of neuroanatomic structures. The collection includes 35 brains, that have been fixed intracranially, from bodies donated to the Hannover Medical School for research and study as the result of bequests. In addition, the collection contains neurohistologic serial sections from 34 brains, that had been fixed after removal.

All **illustrations in this atlas** have been depicted with the help of original sections. The material was taken from 4 individuals whose age, sex, height, head measurements, and cause of death are given in Table 2. Maximum width of the head was measured above the external acoustic meatus. The length of the head was measured between the glabella (landmark between the two superciliary arches) and opisthion (midpoint of the posterior border of the foramen magnum). The facial height was measured between the nasion (median point in sutures between the intersection of frontal and nasal bones) and gnathion (lowest point on the midline of the mandible), and the greatest interzygomatic distance was measured between the most lateral points of the zygomatic bones.

The anatomic examination of the four heads revealed some unusual features. In the head of the **coronal series** S 63/86 the squamous suture and the anterior part of the sagittal suture was partially ossified. The brain belongs to the occipitopetal type (Chap. 1.2). The neck muscles were poorly developed.

In the head of the **sagittal series** S 58/86 the alveolar processes of the toothless upper and lower jaws were reduced in size. The submandibular gland was very large. There was a moderate exophthalmos. The frontal sinuses were asymmetrical (Fig. 30a.3). The arteries were partly sclerotic and elongated with increased tortuosity.

In the head of the **canthomeatal series** H 22/77 the paranasal sinuses were extremely large, particularly the sphenoidal sinus (Figs. 49c.7, 50c.8). The pineal gland was unusually small (Fig. 54c.18). As death was caused by strangulation (suicide by hanging), the veins were dilated. There was only a slight edema of the brain, the ventricles were very narrow. The brain is of the frontopetal type (Chap. 1.2).

In the head of the **brainstem series** S 66/87 the jugular vein, the sigmoid sinus, and the jugular foramen were hypoplastic on the left side (Fig. 70a.16). There was also a deviation of the nasal septum (Fig. 70a.3). These morphologic features can be clearly seen in the illustrations.

Cerebrospinal fluid (CSF) was withdrawn by suboccipital and lumbar puncture from the subarachnoid space of the cadavers and was replaced by an equal amount of 37% formalin solution (Merck) which was slowly injected into the subarachnoid space. Perfusion was carried out through the femoral artery with a fixative consisting of 86 parts of 96% alcohol, eight parts of 37% formalin, three parts of glycerine DAB 7, and three parts of saturated phenol DAB 8 solution. Lateral and posteroanterior teleradiographs of the head were then taken.

CT and MR images were taken of the heads of the coronal, sagittal, and brainstem series. With the head of the canthomeatal series only CT scans were performed. The sectioning planes were determined according to stereotactic principles. The coordinates of these planes for the coronally, sagittally, and canthomeatally oriented coordinate systems are described in Chapter 1.2. The description of Meynert's plane, which is used for the coordinate system of the brainstem series, is given in the same chapter.

The corresponding **coordinate planes** must be visible on the individual head slices in order that the slices can be spatially oriented in the coordinate system. Therefore, the corresponding coordinate planes,

Table 2 Material

	Protocol number	Age in years	Sex	Height of the body (cm)	Width of the head (cm)	Length of the head (cm)	Width–length index (%)	Facial height (cm)	Interzygomatic distance (cm)	Face index (%)	Cause of death
Coronal series	S 63/86	65	Female	163	15.5	18.9	82	11.0	13.7	80	Gastric cancer
Sagittal series	S 58/86	70	Male	175	17.0	20.2	84	12.6	16.6	76	Myocardial infarct
Canthomeatal series	H 22/77	43	Male	176	17.1	23.4	73	12.5	16.6	75	Suicide by hanging
Brainstem series	S 66/87	62	Male	170	16.0	19.8	81	13.4	15.0	89	Gastric cancer

namely the median, Reid's base line, meatovertical, canthomeatal, and Meynert's planes were marked by deep incisions into the skin. These skin incisions later assisted in the orientation of the individual slices, by enabling correct alignment of the slices within the coordinate framework.

The heads were then stored at –26°C for six days, sectioned using a band-saw KS 400 (Reich, Nürtingen, Germany) and finally cut into 1 cm slices using a special adjustment. For the brainstem series S 66/87, the slices were cut at intervals of 5 mm. Due to the cutting width of the band-saw blade, the thickness of each slice was reduced by 1 mm.

The **sectioning surfaces of the slices** were photographed and reproduced on a scale of 1 : 1. The illustrations were traced in permanent ink on transparent plastic overlays directly from the photographs. To ensure accuracy, the illustrations were compared with the original slices throughout the process. The individual structures were identified using a Zeiss stereomicroscope with an improved light source (Volpi halogen cold mercury lamp Intralux 150 H). With these visual aids, the Gennari's band in the visual cortex, the corona radiata, and the alveus of the hippocampus could be easily recognized in the alcohol–formalin-fixed brain slices. Small arteries were differentiated histologically from veins of similar size. The slices were compared with neurohistologic sections from the above-mentioned collection at the Hannover Medical School. In addition one of the authors (K) was able to study the brains of the Yakovlev Collection at the Armed Forces Institute of Pathology of Walter Reed Hospital in Washington D.C. with the financial help of a grant from the German Research Society (Kr 289/15).

The individual **gyri and sulci** of the cerebral hemispheres could only be identified with certainty after 1 : 1 brain models or plexiglass reconstructions were prepared and compared with a series of macroscopic sections from other brains and heads.

Towards the final phase of our examination, all the head sections were assembled together in order to ensure accurate localization of the sectioning planes in the radiographs. To compensate for the 1 mm loss in thickness of the slices due to the width of the blade (14 cuts account for 14 mm), the radiographs were cut into strips corresponding to the slices and remounted with a 1-mm space between the individual slices. Figures 2a, 30a, 45a were obtained in this way. The medial and lateral (anterior and superior respectively) views of the brain (Figs. 2b, 3, 30b, 31, 45b, 46) were obtained after a midline cut through the slices of the brain, and the freed halves were assembled into a complete hemisphere or brain. These were photographed, and corrections were made for the corresponding 1-mm intervals as described above. The lateral view of the ventricular system (Figs. 83b, 86b) was graphically reconstructed from the slices by computer (program by Dr. B. Sauer), and topographically superimposed on the radiographic image of the heads (Figs. 2a, 45a).

The small **cerebral arteries** that run in the sulci of the cerebrum are often very tortuous and have many branches. Exact reconstruction of the course of all these fine arteries within the 1-cm-thick slices was not possible in all regions. Therefore, when referring to these branches of the anterior cerebral artery we only speak of the precuneal artery (Figs. 57c.13, 58c.8, 59c.8) and do not attempt to differentiate between the superior and inferior precuneal arteries. In the same way the branches of the temporal and parietal arteries are not differentiated further (Figs. 55c.17, 56c.11, 57c.12, 51c.8, 52c.8, 53c.10). Small arteries running entirely within a slice, parallel to the sectioning plane, are not cut and, therefore, are not shown in the illustrations.

For printing, the **graphic illustrations in the atlas** were reduced in size; the coronal series (Figs. 4–17) to 82%, the sagittal series (Figs. 32–37) to 71%, the canthomeatal series (Figs. 47–60) to 78%, and the overall view of the brainstem series (Figs. 69a–78a) to 79%. The scale, in centimeters, can be read from the corresponding coordinate frame in the atlas illustrations of the coronal, sagittal, and brainstem series.

The technique of illustration of the canthomeatal series in the first edition of this book was geared toward computed tomography (CT) of the brain. For this reason the soft tissues of the facial skeleton and the craniocervical junction were not depicted and not described. The graphic illustrations in the second edition will do justice to the advances that have been made in cranial imaging techniques. Therefore, the three series depict in accurate detail the extracranial soft-tissue structures such as the muscles, glandular tissues, peripheral nerves, and blood vessels. In the third edition the contrast between the gray and white matter in the anatomic atlas illustrations and serial images was intensified for optimal comparison with the MR and CT images.

The MR and CT images were acquired so as to correspond as closely as possible to the anatomic atlas illustrations. Great care was given to aligning the cutting planes of digital neuroimaging to correspond to the anatomic serial sections. The images corresponding most favorably were selected from a series of several MR and CT images and positioned alongside the atlas illustration. The **MR images** were taken from a 38-year-old female. The MR investigations were carried out over a period of several days using a Magnetom Sonata 1.5 T (Tesla) magnetic resonance tomograph (Siemens, Erlangen). Four series were obtained (coronal, sagittal, canthomeatal, and brainstem series) in T1 and T2 evaluation. The measuring parameters of the MR images were selected for the processing and description of the anatomy of the brain. The reader will be able to determine the morphology of the individual structures from the spacial relation toward the anatomically neighboring struc-

Parameters	Notes
tir1_11 180	turbo inversion recovery, 1 Echo, Turbofactor 11, Refocusing angle 180°
TI 150 ms	Time of Inversion
TR 6500 ms	Time of Repetition
TE 60 ms	Time of Echo
TA 6–11 min	Time of Acquisition
AC 1–3	Acquisition
FoV 201*230 mm	Field of View
Ma 220*256	Matrix
SL 3 mm	Slice
gaps 3 mm	

Table 3 Parameters for T1-weighted MR images

Coronal and sagittal series	Brainstem series	Notes
tseva 160	ts1_15 180	tseva = Turbospinecho Volume Acquisition, turbofactor = 160, flip angle = variable, ts = Turbospinecho, 1 Echo, turbofactor = 15, refocusing angle 180°, 1SAT
1 SAT		transverse saturation
TR 2750 ms	TR 4600 ms	Time of Repetition
TE 328/1 ms	TE 120/1 ms	Time of Echo
TA 09:58 min/s	TA 3:59 min/s	Time of Acquisition
AC 1	AC3	Acquisition
FoV 160*256 mm	FoV 201*230 mm	Field of View
Ma 160*256	Ma 255*512	Matrix
SL 1.0 mm	SL 3 mm	Slice
no gap	gaps 0.9 mm	

Table 4 Parameters for T2-weighted MR images of the coronal, sagittal series, and brainstem series

tures in the same slice and also in the bordering slices.

For the choice of investigation sequence and window positioning it was our intention to present the best possible neuroanatomic structures with a clear differentiation between gray and white matter. Bones, muscle, tendons, and fat were suppressed in MR images.

All T1-weighted MR images were obtained using a Turbo-Inversion-Recovery-Sequence in real part reconstruction. The choice of inversion time T1 = 150 ms was made with regard to fat suppression, thus reducing the risk of artifacts and increasing the number of sections for the representation of the whole brain within a reasonable examination time. The parameters listed in Table 3 were generally used.

The **T1-weighted MR images** were obtained with a Turbo-Inversion-Recovery-Sequence with some minor optimization of the following parameters:

The following parameters were chosen for the **T2-weighted MR images** (316):

Some minor deviations between the T1- and T2-weighted MR images occurred due to new positioning. Additional MR images were obtained from the above-mentioned female in a 3D-block using the T1-weighted MPRAGE sequence (Magnetization Prepared Rapid Gradient Echo). The workstation 3D Virtuoso from Siemens, Erlangen enabled determination of anatomic structures, even when individual structures were difficult to locate on any specific level. This workstation allowed for high degree of accuracy in determining the structures in all three layers.

For the canthomeatal series, **CT images** were chosen to replace the T2-weighted MR images. The CT images were taken from a 70-year-old female. The investigation was undertaken with a Somatom Volume Zoom computed tomograph (Siemens, Erlangen) in

In the infratentorial space	In the supratentorial space	Notes
kV 140	kV 140	**k**ilo**V**olt
mAs 380	mAs 300	**M**illi**a**mpere **s**econds
TI 1.0 s	TI 1.0 s	rotation time in spiral mode
GT–4.5	GT–4.5	**G**antry **T**ilt
SL 1.25 mm	SL 5.0 mm	**Sl**ice, estimated layer thickness
1.0 mm	2–5 mm	collimated layer thickness
3.5 mm	8.8 mm	advancement by rotation

Table 5 Parameter for the **CT images**

four parallel slices (multislice technique) using the spiral procedure (helical technique). The infratentorial space was evaluated using 1.25 mm slices and the supratentorial space using 5 mm slices.

The best correlated CT images were presented together with the anatomic atlas images. The investigation parameters are shown in Table 5.

It should be pointed out to the reader that the **specimens for the anatomic atlas images** for the four series were taken from four different individuals (Table 2).

All **MR images** in the book were taken from one individual and the **CT images** from another individual. These interindividual differences in the anatomic structures correspond with findings in routine clinical practice. Considerable anatomic variants and pathologic intracranial mass displacements were disregarded in order to present a book featuring "normal" neuroanatomy as a prerequisite for the recognition of pathologic changes.

9 References

1. Ackermann, H., Mathiak, K.: Symptomatologie, pathologisch-anatomische Grundlagen und Pathomechanismus zentraler Hörstörungen (reine Worttaubheit, auditive Agnosie, Rindentaubheit). Fortschr. Neurol. Psychiat. 67 (1999) 509–523
2. Ackermann, H., Wildgruber, D., Grood, W.: Neuroradiologische Aktivierungsstudien zur zerebralen Organisation sprachlicher Leistungen. Fortschr. Neurol. Psychiat. 65 (1997) 182 – 194
3. Adams, R.D., Victor, M., Ropper, A.H.: Principles of neurology. New York: McGraw Hill 1997
4. Afshar, F., Watkins, E.S., Yap, J.C.: Stereotaxic atlas of the human brainstem and cerebellar nuclei. A variability study. New York: Raven Press 1978
5. Alexander, K., Daniel, W.G., Diener, H.C., Freund, M. et al.: Thiemes Innere Medizin TIM. Stuttgart, New York: Thieme 1999
6. Alexander, M.P., LoVerme, S.R.: Aphasia after left hemispheric intracerebral hemorrhage. Neurology 30 (1980) 1193–1202
7. Allon, N., Yeshurun, Y., Wollberg, Z.: Responses of single cells in the medial geniculate body of awake squirrel monkeys. Exp. Brain Res. 41 (1981) 222–232
8. Alpers, B.J., Berry, R.G.: Circle of Willis in cerebral vascular disorders. Arch. Neurol. 8 (1963) 398–402
9. Ambrose, J.: Computerized transverse axial scanning (tomography). Part 2: Clinical application. Brit. J. Radiol. 46 (1973) 1023–1047
10. Amunts, K., Zilles, K.: Advances in cytoarchitectonic mapping of the human cerebral cortex. Neuroimaging Clinics of North America 11 (2001) 151 – 169
11. Andrew, J., Watkins, E.S. A stereotaxic atlas of the human thalamus and adjacent structures. Baltimore: Williams and Wilkins 1969
12. Angevine, J.B. (Jr.), Mancall, E.L., Yakovlev, P.I.: The human cerebellum. An atlas of cross topography in serial sections. Boston: Little and Brown 1961
13. Arlart, I.P., Bongartz, G.M., Marchal, G. (Eds.): Magnetic resonance angiography. Berlin, Heidelberg, New York: Springer 2003
14. Armington, W.G., Harnsberger, H.R., Smoker, W.R.K., Osborn, A.G.: Normal and diseased acoustic pathway: evaluation with MR imaging. Radiology 167 (1988) 509–515
15. Arning, C.: Farbkodierte Duplexsonographie der hirnversorgenden Arterien. Stuttgart, New York: Thieme 2002
16. Atlas, S.W.: Pocket atlas of cranial magnetic resonance imaging. Philadelphia: Lippincott, Williams and Wilkins 2001
17. Atlas, S.W.: Magnetic resonance imaging of the brain and spine. Philadelphia, Baltimore: Lippincott Williams and Wilkins Vol. 1, 2 2002
18. Babb, T.L., Wilson, C.L., Crandall, P.H.: Asymmetry and ventral course of the human geniculostriate pathway as determined by hippocampal visual evoked potentials and subsequent visual field defects after temporal lobectomy. Exp. Brain Res. 47 (1982) 317–328
19. Baloh, R.W., Furman, J.M., Yee, R.D.: Dorsal midbrain syndrome: Clinical and oculographic findings. Neurology 35 (1985) 54–60
20. Bancaud, J., Talairach, J.: Organisation fonctionelle de l'aire motrice supplémentaire (einseignements apportés par la S.E.E.G.). Neurochirurgie 3 (1967) 343–356
21. Barkovich, A. J.: MR of the normal neonatal brain: assessment of deep structures. Amer. J. Neuroradiol. 19 (1998) 1397–1403
22. Barkovich, A. J.: Pediatric Neuroimaging New York: Raven 1997
23. Bauer, A., Langen-Müller, U.de, Glindemann, R., Schlenck, C., Schlenck, K.-J., Huber, W.: Qualitätskriterien und Standards für die Therapie von Patienten mit erworbenen neurogenen Störungen der Sprache (Aphasie) und des Sprechens (Dysarthrie). Akt. Neurol. 29 (2002) 63 – 75
24. Bauer, B.L., Hellwig, D.: Minimal invasive endoskopische Neurochirurgie (MIEN). Dtsch. Ärztbl. 92 (1995) A 2816–2835
25. Bauer, R., Flierdt, v. de E., Mörike, K.: MR Tomography of the central nervous system. Stuttgart, New York: Urban und Fischer 1993
26. Baumgartner, G.: Funktion und Symptomatik einzelner Hirnregionen. 1.77–1.112 In: Hopf, H.C., Poeck, K., Schliack, H. II. (Eds.): Neurologie in Praxis und Klinik. Band 1. Stuttgart: Thieme 1983
27. Bear, M.F., Connors, B.W., Paradiso, M.A.: Neuroscience: Exploring the brain. Baltimore, Philadelphia: Williams and Wilkins 1996
27a. Becker, G., Berg, D.: Neuroimaging in basal ganglia disorders: perspectives for transcranial ultrasound. Movement Disorders 16 (2001) 23 – 32
27b. Becker, G., Naumann, M., Schenbeck, M., Hofmann, E., Deimling, M., Lindner, A., Gahn, G., Reiners, C., Toyka, K., Reiners, K.: Comparison of transcranial sonography, magnetic resonance imaging and single photon emission computed tomography findings in idiopathic spasmodic torticollis. Movement Disorders 12 (1997) 79 – 88
28. Becker, H., Vonofakos, D.: Diagnostische Bedeutung von Hirntumorverkalkungen im Computertomogramm. Radiologe 23 (1983) 459–462
29. Beevor, C.E.: On the distribution of the different arteries supplying the human brain. Phil. Trans. B 200 (1909) 1–55
30. Benjamin, R.M., Burton, H.: Projection of taste nerve afferents to anterior opercular-insular cortex in squirrel monkey (Saimiri sciureus). Brain Res.7 (1968) 221–231
31. Benson, D.F.: Neurological correlates of aphasia and apraxia. 163–175. In: Matthews, W.B., Glaser, G.H. (Eds.): Recent advances in clinical neurology. Edinburgh, London, New York: Churchill Livingstone 1981
32. Bentivoglio, M.: The anatomical organization of corticospinal connections. 1–22 In: Non-invasive stimulation of brain and spinal cord: Fundamentals and clinical applications. New York: Liss 1988
32a. Berding, G., Brücke, T., Odin, P., Brooks, D.J., Kolbe, H., Gielow, P., Harke, H., Knoop, B.O., Dengler, R., Knapp, W.H.: [123 I] â – CIT SPECT imaging of dopamine and serotonin transporters in Parkinson's disease and multiple system atrophy. Nuklearmedizin 42 (2003) 31–38
32b. Berding, G., Schrader, C.H., Peschel, T., van den Hoff, J., Kolbe, H., Meyer, G.J., Dengler, R., Knapp, W.H.: [N-methyl 11C] meta-Hydroxyephedrine positron emission tomography in Parkinson's disease and multiple system atrophy. Eur. J. Nucl. Med. 30 (2003) 127–131
33. Bergstrand, G., Bergström, M., Nordell, B., Stählberg, F., Ericsson, A., Hemmingsson, A., Sperber, G. Thuomas, K.-A., Jung, B.: Cardiac gated MR imaging of cerebrospinal fluid flow. J. Comput. assist. Tomogr. 9 (1985) 1003–1006
34. Berlit, P. (Ed.): Klinische Neurologie. Berlin, Heidelberg, New York: Springer 1999
35. Berman, S.A., Hayman, L.A., Hinck, V.C.: Correlation of CT cerebral vascular territories with function: 1. Anterior cerebral artery. Amer. J. Roentgenol. 135 (1980) 253–257
36. Berman, S.A., Hayman, L.A., Hinck, V.C.: Correlation of CT cerebral vascular territories with function: 3. Middle cerebral artery. Amer. J. Roentgenol. 142 (1984) 1035–1040
37. Berns, T.F., Daniels, D.L., Williams, A.L., Haughton, V.M.: Mesencephalic anatomy: Demonstration by computed tomography. Amer. J. Neuroradiol. 2 (1981) 65–67
38. Bierny, J.-P., Komar, N.N.: The sylvian cistern on computed tomography scanning. J. Comput. assist. Tomogr. 1 (1977) 227–230
39. Binder, J.R., Frost, J.A., Hammeke, T.A., Cox, R.W., Rao, S.M., Prieto, T.: Human brain language areas identified by functional magnetic resonance imaging. J. Neurosci. 17 (1997) 353 – 362
39a. Binder, J.R.: Functional MRI of the language system. In: Moonen, C.T.W., Bandettini, P.A. (Eds.) Functional MRI. Berlin, Heidelberg, New York: Springer 2000 407–419

39b Binnie, C.D., Cooper, R., Fowler, C.F., Mauguière, F., Prior, P.F., Osselton, J.W.: Clinical neurophysiology EMG, nerve conduction and evoked potentials. Oxford: Butterworth (in press)
39c Blank, S.C., Scott, S.K., Murphy, K., Warburton, E., Wise, J.S.: Speech production: Wernicke, Broca and beyond. Brain 125 (2002) 1829–1838
40 Blunk, R., Bleser, R. de, Willmes, K., Zeumèr, H.: A refined method to relate morphological and functional aspects of aphasia. Europ. Neurol. 20 (1981) 69–79
41 Bo, W.J., Wolfman, N.: Basic atlas of sectional anatomy with correlated imaging. Philadelphia, London, Toronto: Saunders 1998
42 Bogerts, B.: A brainstem atlas of catecholaminergic neurons in man, using melanin as a natural marker. J. comp. Neurol. 197 (1981) 63–80
43 Bonneville, J.-F., Cattin, F., Dietemann, J.-L.: Computed tomography of the pituitary gland. Berlin, Heidelberg, New York: Springer 1986
44 Bosch, D.A.: Stereotactic techniques in clinical neurosurgery. Wien, New York: Springer 1986
45 Bowsher, D.: Diencephalic projections from the midbrain reticular formation. Brain Res. 95 (1975) 211–220
46 Braak, H.: Architectonics of the human telencephalic cortex. Berlin, Heidelberg, New York: Springer 1980
47 Braak, H.: The pigment architecture of the human temporal lobe. Anat. Embryol. 154 (1978) 213–240
48 Braak, H.: Über die Kerngebiete des menschlichen Hirnstammes. I. Oliva inferior, Nucleus conterminalis und Nucleus vermiformis corporis restiformis. Z. Zellforsch. 105 (1970) 442–456
49 Braak, H.: Über die Kerngebiete des menschlichen Hirnstammes. II. Die Raphekerne. Z. Zellforsch. 107 (1970) 123–141
50 Bradley, W.G.: MR of the brain stem: a practical approach. Radiology 179 (1991) 319–332
51 Brandt, T., Dichgans, J., Diener, H.C. (Eds.): Therapie und Verlauf neurologischer Erkrankungen. Stuttgart, Berlin, Köln: Kohlmeyer 2000
52 Brassow, F., Baumann, K.: Volume of brain ventricles in man determined by computer tomography. Neuroradiology 16 (1978) 187–189
53 Bredberg, G.: Innervation of the auditory system. Scandinavian Audiology 13 Suppl. (1981) 1–10
54 Broca, P.: Anatomie comparée circonvolutions cerebrales. Le grande lobe limbique et la scissure limbique dans la serie des mammiferes. Rev. Anthropol. 1 (1878) 384–498
55 Brodal, A.: Neurological anatomy in relation to clinical medicine. New York, Oxford: Oxford University Press 1981
56 Brodmann, K.: Vergleichende Lokalisationslehre der Großhirnrinde – in ihren Prinzipien dargestellt auf Grund des Zellenbaues. Leipzig: Barth 1909
57 Bron, A.J., Tripathi, R.C., Tripathi, B.J.: Wolff's anatomy of the eye and orbit. London: Chapman and Hall 1997
57a Brücke, T., Djamshidian, S., Benecsits, G., Pirker, W., Asenbaum, S., Podreka, I.: SPECT and PET imaging of the dopaminergic system in Parkinson's disease. J. Neurol. 247 Suppl. 4 (2000) IV/2 – IV/7
58 Bruhn, H.: Untersuchungen physiologischer und pathophysiologischer Stoffwechselzustände und Hirnfunktionen des Menschen mit Hilfe neuer methodischer Entwicklungen zur ortsaufgelösten Magnetresonanzspektroskopie und funktionellen Magnetresonanztomographie. Habilitationsschrift der Medizinischen Fakultät der Humboldt-Universität Berlin 2001
59 Brust, J.C.M.: Stroke. Diagnostic, anatomical, and physiological considerations. 853–861 In: Kandel, E.R., Schwartz, J.H. (Eds.): Principles of neural science. New York: Elsevier Science Publishing 1985
60 Bruyn, R.P.M.: Thalamic aphasia. A conceptional critique. J. Neurol. 236 (1989) 21–25
61 Bucher, O., Wartenberg, H.: Cytologie, Histologie und mikroskopische Anatomie des Menschen. Bern, Stuttgart, Toronto: Huber 1997
62 Buchner, H., Adams, L., Müller, A., Ludwig, I., Knepper, A., Thron, A., Niemann, K., Scherg, M.: Somatotopy of human hand somatosensory cortex revealed by dipole source analysis of early somatosensory evoked potentials and 3D-NMR tomography. Electroencephalogr. Clin. Neurophysiol. 96 (1995) 121–134
63 Büdingen, H.-J. von, Kaps, M., Reutern, G.-M. von: Ultraschalldiagnostik der hirnversorgenden Arterien. Stuttgart, New York: Thieme 2000
64 Buhmann, C., Kretschmann, H.-J.: Computer-assisted three-dimensional reconstruction of the corticospinal system as a reference for CT and MRI. Neuroradiology 40 (1998) 549–557
65 Buhmann, C.: Computergestützte 3D-Rekonstruktion des corticospinalen Systems als Referenz für die bildgebenden Verfahren CT, MRT und PET. Med. Dissertation, Med. Hochschule Hannover 1994
66 Büll, U., Schicha, H., Biersack, H.-J., Knapp, W.H., Reiners, C., Schober, O. (Eds.): Nuklearmedizin. Stuttgart, New York: Thieme 1999
66a Burgener, F.A., Meyers, S.P., Tan, R.K., Zaunbauer, W.: Differenzialdiagnostik in der MRT. Stuttgart, New York: Thieme 2003
67 Burton, H., Benjamin, R.M.: Central projections of the gustatory system. 148–164 In: Autrum, H., Jung, R., Loewenstein, W.R., Mackay, D.M., Teuber, H.L. (Eds.): Handbook of sensory physiology. Vol. 4: Chemical senses, part 2. Berlin, Heidelberg, New York: Springer 1971
68 Butler, P. (Ed.): Imaging of the nervous system. Berlin, Heidelberg, New York: Springer 1990
69 Butler, P., Mitchel, A.W.M., Ellis, H.: (Eds.): Applied Radiological Anatomy. Cambridge: Cambridge University Press 1999
70 Büttner-Ennever, J.A. (Ed.): Neuroanatomy of the oculomotor system. In: Robinson, D.A., Collewijn, H. (Eds.): Reviews of oculomotor research. Vol. 2. Amsterdam, New York, Oxford: Elsevier 1988
71 Büttner-Ennever, J.A., Büttner, U., Cohen, B., Baumgartner, G.: Vertical gaze paralysis and the rostral interstitial nucleus of the medial longitudinal fasciculus. Brain 105 (1982) 125–149
72 Büttner-Ennever, J.A.: A review of otolith pathways to the brainstem and cerebellum. Ann. N.Y. Acad. Sci. 871 (1999) 51 – 64.
73 Büttner-Ennever, J.A.: Overview of the vestibular system: Anatomy. 3 – 24 In Anderson, J.H. and Beitz, A.J. (Eds.) Neurochemistry of the Vestibular System. Boca Raton, London, New York: CRC Press 2000
74 Carpenter, M.B.: Anatomy and physiology of the basal ganglia. 233–268 In: Schaltenbrand, G., Walker, A.E. (Eds.): Stereotaxy of the human brain. 2nd ed. Stuttgart, New York: Thieme 1982
75 Carpenter, M.B.: Core text of neuroanatomy. Baltimore, London, Sydney: Williams and Wilkins 1991
76 Carson, R.E., Herscovitch, P., Daube-Witherspoon, M.: Quantitative functional brain imaging with positron emission tomography. San Diego, London, Boston: Academic Press 1998
77 Casselman, J.W., Francke, J.-P., Dehaene, I.: Imaging of the upper cranial nerves. CD-ROM Nycomed Amersham Buchler GmbH Fraunhoferstr. 7 D 85737 Ismaning b. München 1999
78 Celesia, G.G.: Organization of auditory cortical areas in man. Brain 99 (1976) 403–414
79 Chaheres, D.W., Schmalbrock, P.: Fundamentals of Magnetic Resonance Imaging. Baltimore, Hong Kong, London, Munich, Philadelphia, Tokyo: Williams and Wilkins 1992
80 Chee, M.W.L., Tan, E.W.L., Thiel, T.: Mandarin and English single word procressing studied with functional magnetic resonance imaging. J. Neurosci. 19 (1999) 3050 – 3056
80a Chiappa, K.H.: Evoked potentials in clinical medicine. Philadelphia: Lipincott-Raven 1997
81 Chollet, F.: Pharmacologic modulation of human cerebral activity: contribution of functional neuroimaging. Neuroimaging Clinics of North America 11 (2001) 375 – 380
82 Citrin, C.M., Alper, M.G.: Computed tomography of the visual pathways. Comput. Tomogr. 3 (1979) 305–331
83 Citrin, C.M., Alper, M.G.: Computed tomography of the visual pathways. Int. Ophthalmol. Clin. 22 (1982) 155–180
84 Claus, D.: Die transkranielle motorische Stimulation. Stuttgart, New York: Fischer 1989
85 Crosby, E.C., Humphrey, T., Lauer, E.W.: Correlative anatomy of the nervous system. New York: Macmillan 1962
85a Crossman, A.R.: Functional anatomy of movement disorders. J. Anat. 196 (2000) 519–525
86 Dahlström, A., Fuxe, K.: Evidence for the existence of monoamine neurons in the central nervous system. II. Experimentally induced changes in the intraneuronal amine levels of bulbospinal neuron systems. Acta physiol. scand. 64, Suppl. 247 (1965) 1–36
87 Dahlström, A., Fuxe, K.: Evidence for the existence of monoamine-containing neurons in the central nervous system. I. Demonstration of monoamines in the cell bodies of brainstem neurons. Acta physiol. scand. 62, Suppl. 232 (1964) 1–55
88 Dallel, R., Raboisson, P., Auray, P., Woda, A.: The rostral part of the trigeminal sensory complex is involved in orofacial nociception. Brain Res. 448 (1988) 7–19
89 Damasio, H.: A computed tomographic guide to the identification of cerebral vascular territories. Arch. Neurol. 40 (1983) 138–142

90 Damasio, H.: Neuroimaging contributions to the understanding of aphasia. In: Boller, F., Grafman, J. (Eds.) Handbook of neuropsychology, vol. 2. Amsterdam: Elsevier Science Publ. 1989
91 Dampney, R.A.L., Moon, E.A.: Role of ventrolateral medulla in vasomotor response to cerebral ischemia. Amer. J. Physiol. 239 (1980) H349-H358
92 Dani, S.U., Hori, A., Walter, G.F.: Principles of neural aging. Amsterdam, Lausanne, New York: Elsevier 1997
93 Danielsen, E.R., Ross, B.: Magnetic resonance spectroscopy diagnosis of neurological diseases. New York, Basel: Marcel Dekker 1999
94 Davidoff, R.: The pyramidal tract. Neurology 40 (1990) 332–339
95 De Armond, S.J., Fusco, M.M., Dewey, M.M.: Structure of the human brain. A photographic atlas. New York: Oxford Press 1989
96 Dechent, P., Frahm, J.: Direct mapping of ocular dominance columns in human primary visual cortex. Neuro Report 11 (2000) 3247 – 3249
97 DeCoene, B., Hajnal, J.V., Pennock, J.M., Bydder, G.M.: MRI of the brain stem using fluid attenuated inversion recovery pulse sequences. Neuroradiology 35 (1993) 327–331
97a DeDeyn, P.P., Dierckx, R.A., Alavi, A., Pickut, B.A. (Eds.): A textbook of SPECT in neurology and psychiatry. London: J. Libbey 1997
98 Deeg, K.-H., Peters, H., Schumacher, R., Weitzel, D.: Die Ultraschalluntersuchung des Kindes. Berlin, Heidelberg, New York: Springer 1997
99 Dejerine, J.: Anatomie des centres nerveux. Tome 1,2. Paris: Masson 1980
100 Delank, H.-W., Gehlen, W.: Neurologie. Stuttgart: Enke 1999
101 Demaerel, Ph.: Recent advances in diagnostic neuroradiology. Berlin, Heidelberg, New York: Springer 2001
102 Denny-Brown, D.: Relations and functions of the pyramidal tract. 131–139 In: Schaltenbrand, G., Walker, A.E. (Eds.): Stereotaxy of the human brain, 2nd ed. Stuttgart, New York: Thieme 1982
103 Deschauer, M., Georgiadis, D., Lindner, A.: Hörverlust als Leitsymptom von Arteria cerebelli inferior anterior Infarkten. Forschr. Neurol. Psychiat. 66 (1998) 109–112
103a Dettmers, C., Fink, G., Rijntjes, M., Stephan, K., Weiller, C.: Kortikale Kontrolle der Willkürmotorik: Funktionelle Bildgebung der motorischen Exekutive des ZNS. Neurol. Rehabil. 1 (1997) 15 – 27
104 Diehl, R.R., Berlit, P.: Funktionelle Dopplersonographie in der Neurologie. Berlin, Heidelberg, New York: Springer 1996
105 Dieterich, M., Brandt, T.: Vestibular system: anatomy and functional magnetic resonance imaging. Neuroimaging Clinics of North America 11 (2001) 263 – 273
106 Dieterich, M.: Ocular motor system: anatomy and functional magnetic resonance imaging. Neuroimaging Clinics of North America 11 (2001) 251 – 261
107 Donaghy, M. (Ed.): Brain's diseases of the nervous system. Oxford, New York: Oxford University Press 2001.
108 Drenckhahn, D., Zenker, W. (Eds.): Benninghoff: Makroskopische Anatomie, Embryologie und Histologie des Menschen. Band 2: Niere, Reproduktionsorgane, Nervensystem, Sinnesorgane, Haut. München, Wien, Baltimore: Urban und Schwarzenberg 1994
109 Dudel, J., Menzel, R., Schmidt, R.F.: Neurowissenschaft. Vom Mokekül zur Kognition. Berlin, Heidelberg, New York: Springer 2001
110 Duus, P.: Topical diagnosis in neurology. Stuttgart, New York: Thieme 1998
111 Duvernoy, H.M.: Human brain stem vessels. Berlin, Heidelberg, New York: Springer 1999
112 Duvernoy, H.M.: The human brain stem and cerebellum. Wien, New York: Springer 1995
113 Duvernoy, H.M.: The human hippocampus. Berlin, Heidelberg, New York: Springer 1998
114 Ebeling, U., Huber, P., Reulen, H.J.: Localization of the precentral gyrus in the computed tomogram and its clinical application. J. Neurol. 233 (1986) 73–76
115 Ebeling, U., Reulen, H.J.: Subcortical topography and proportions of the pyramidal tract. Acta Neurochir. (Wien) 118 (1992) 164–171
116 Economo, C. von, Koskinas, G.N.: Die Cytoarchitektonik der Hirnrinde des erwachsenen Menschen. Textband und Atlas. Wien, Berlin: Springer 1925
117 Edelman, R.R., Hesselink, J.R., Zlatkin, M.B.: Clinical magnetic resonance imaging. Philadelphia, London, Toronto: Saunders 1996
118 Englander, R.N., Netsky, M.G., Adelman, L.S.: Location of human pyramidal tract in the internal capsule: Anatomic evidence. Neurology 25 (1975) 823–826
119 Faerber, E.N.: Cranial computed tomography in infants and children. Clinics in development medicine no. 93. Spastics international medical publications (SIMP). Oxford: Blackwell Scientific 1991
120 Falck, B., Hillarp, N.-A., Thieme, G., Torp, A.: Fluorescence of catecholamines and related compounds condensed with formaldehyde. J. Histochem. Cytochem. 10 (1962) 348–354
121 Farruggia, S., Babcock, D.S.: The cavum septi pellucidi: Its appearance and incidence with cranial ultrasonography in infancy. Radiology 139 (1981) 147–150
122 Federative Committee on Anatomical Terminology (FCAT): Terminologia anatomica. International anatomical terminology. Stuttgart, New York: Thieme 1998
123 Felten, D.L., Laties, A.M., Carpenter, M.B.: Monoaminecontaining cell bodies in the squirrel monkey brain. Amer. J. Anat. 139 (1974) 153–166
124 Feneis, H.: Pocket atlas of human anatomy. Stuttgart, New York: Thieme 2000
125 Fischer, M.: Doppler-Sonographie und Doppler-Frequenzspektrumanalyse extrakranieller Hirngefäße. München, Wien, Baltimore: Urban und Schwarzenberg 1990
126 Fishman, E.K., Jeffrey, B.R.: Spiral-CT. Stuttgart, New York: Thieme 2000
127 FitzGerald, M.J.T, Folan-Curan, J.: Clinical Neuroanatomy and related neuroscience. Edinburgh, London: Saunders 2002.
128 Flechsig, P.: Zur Anatomie und Entwicklungsgeschichte der Leitungsbahnen im Grosshirn des Menschen. Arch. Anat. Entwicklungsgesch., Anat. Abt. (1881) 12–75
129 Foerster, O.: Motorische Felder und Bahnen. Sensible corticale Felder. In: Bumke, O., Foerster, O. (Eds.): Handbuch der Neurologie. Band 6. Berlin: Springer 1936 1–488
129a Fossett, D.T., Caputy, A.J.: Operative neurosurgical anatomy. New York, Stuttgart: Thieme 2002
130 Fox, P.T., Fox, J.M., Raichle, M.E., Burde, R.M.: The role of cerebral cortex in the generation of voluntary saccades: a positron emission tomographic study. J. Neurophysiol. 54 (1985) 348–369
131 Frackowiak, R., Friston, K.J., Frith, C.D., Dolan, R., Mazziotta, J.C.: Human brain function. San Diego, London, Boston: Academic Press 1997
132 Freund, H.J.: Premotor area and preparation of movement. Rev. Neurol. (Paris) 146 (1990) 543–547
132a Freund, H.J.: Motorische Störungen bei kortikalen Läsionen. Klin.Neurophysiol. 30 (1999) 113–119
133 Frick, H., Leonhardt, H., Starck, D.: Spezielle Anatomie, Band 2 Eingeweide, Nervensystem, Systematik der Muskeln und Leitungsbahnen. Stuttgart, New York: Thieme 1992
134 Fritsch, R., Hitzig, E.: Über die elektrische Erregbarkeit des Großhirns. Arch. Anat. Physiol. u. wissenschaftl. Med. 37 (1870) 300–332
135 Fritz, P., Lenarz, T., Haels, J., Fehrentz, D.: Feinstrukturanalyse des Felsenbeines mittels hochauflösender Dünnschicht-Computertomographie. Teil 1: Sensitivität der Strukturdarstellung bei einer standardisierten Untersuchungstechnik. Fortschr. Röntgenstr. 147 (1987) 266–271
136 Froriep, A.: Die Lagebeziehungen zwischen Großhirn und Schädeldach. Leipzig: Veit 1897
137 Gaa, J., Lehmann, K.-J., Georgi, M. (Eds.): MR-Angiographie und Elektronenstrahl-CT-Angiographie. Stuttgart, New York: Thieme 2000
138 Galaburda, A., Sanides, F.: Cytoarchitectonic organisation of the human auditory cortex. J. comp. Neurol. 190 (1980) 597–610
139 Galaburda, A.M., LeMay, M., Kemper, T.L., Geschwind, N.: Right-left asymmetries in the brain. Science 199 (1978) 852–856
140 Galaburda, A.M., Sanides, F., Geschwind, N.: Human brain. Cytoarchitectonic left-right asymmetries in the temporal speech region. Arch. Neurol. 35 (1978) 812–817
141 Galanski, M., Dickob, M., Wittkowski, W.: CT-Zisternographie der basalen Zisternen. Fortschr. Röntgenstr. 145 (1986) 149–157
142 Gallen, C.C., Sobel, D.F., Waltz, T., Aung, M., Copeland, B., Schwartz, B.J., Hirschkoff, E.C., Bloom, F.E.: Noninvasive presurgical neuromagnetic mapping of somatosensory cortex. Neurosurgery 33 (1993) 260–268
143 Garnett, E.S., Nahmias, C., Firnau, G.: Central dopaminergic pathways in hemiparkinsonism examined by positron emission tomography. Can. J. Neurol. Sci. 11 (1984) 174–179

144 Garver, D.L., Sladek, J.R. (Jr.): Monoamine distribution in primate brain. 1. Catecholamine-containing perikarya in the brain stem of Macaca speciosa. J. comp. Neurol. 159 (1975) 289–304
145 George, B., Laurian, C.: The vertebral artery. Wien, New York: Springer 1987
146 Gerke, M.: Computerunterstützte dreidimensionale Rekonstruktion des limbischen Systems als Referenz für die bildgebenden Verfahren (Computertomographie, Magnetische Resonanztomographie und Positronen-Emissionstomographie). Med. Dissertation, Med. Hochschule Hannover 1988
147 Geschwind, N.: Specializations of the human brain. A photographic guide. Scientific American 241 (1979) 180–199
148 Gillilan, L.A.: The correlations of the blood supply of the human brain stem with clinical brain stem lesions. J. Neuropath. Exp. Neurol. 23 (1964) 78–108
149 Gloger, A., Gloger, S.: Dreidimensionale Computerrekonstruktion der terminalen Äste der drei Großhirnarterien des Menschen als Referenz für die Magnetresonanztomographie (MRT), die Computertomographie (CT) und die Positronen-Emissionstomographie (PET). Med. Dissertation, Med. Hochschule Hannover 1993
150 Gloger, S., Gloger, A., Vogt, H., Kretschmann, H.-J.: Computer-assisted 3D reconstruction of the terminal branches of the cerebral arteries. 1. Anterior cerebral artery. Neuroradiology 36 (1994) 173–180
151 Gloger, S., Gloger, A., Vogt, H., Kretschmann, H.-J.: Computer-assisted 3D reconstruction of the terminal branches of the cerebral arteries. 2. Middle cerebral artery. Neuroradiology 36 (1994) 181–187
152 Gloger, S., Gloger, A., Vogt, H., Kretschmann, H.-J.: Computer-assisted 3D reconstruction of the terminal branches of the cerebral arteries. 3. Posterior cerebral artery and circle of Willis. Neuroradiology 36 (1994) 251–257
153 Gobel S., Binck J.M.: Degenerative changes in primary trigeminal axons in neurons in nucleus caudalis following tooth pulp extirpation in the cat. Brain Res. 132 (1977) 347–354
154 Goodchild, A.K., Moon, E.A., Dampney, R.A.L., Howe, P.R.C.: Evidence that adrenaline neurons in the rostral ventrolateral medulla have a vasopressor function. Neurosci. Lett. 45 (1984) 267–272
155 Gouaze, A., Salamon, G. (Eds.): Brain anatomy and magnetic resonance imaging. Berlin, Heidelberg, New York, London, Paris, Tokyo: Springer 1988
155a Grabowski, T.J., Damasio, A.R.: Investigating language with functional neuroimaging. In: Toga, A.W., Mazziotta, J.G. (Eds.): Brain mapping. The systems. San Diego, San Francisco, New York: Academic Press 2000
156 Graham, D.I., Lantos, P.L. (Eds.): Greenfield's Neuropathology. London: Arnold Publishers 2002
157 Grand, W., Hopkins, L.N.: Vasculature of the brain and cranial base. New York, Stuttgart: Thieme 1999
158 Greenberg, J.O.: Neuroimaging. New York, St. Louis, San Francisco: McGraw-Hill 1995
158a Greenberg, M.S.: Handbook of neurosurgery. New York: Thieme Medical Publishers 2001
159 Grehl, H., Reinhardt, F.: Checkliste Neurologie. Stuttgart, New York: Thieme 2002
160 Groot, J. de: Correlative neuroanatomy of computed tomography and magnetic resonance imaging. Philadelphia: Lea and Febiger 1991
161 Haaga, J.R., Alfidi, R.J. (Eds.): Computed tomography and magnetic resonance imaging of the whole body. St. Louis, Toronto, Princeton: Mosby 1994
162 Habel, U., Posse, S., Schneider, F.: Funktionelle Kernspintomographie in der klinischen Psychologie und Psychiatrie. Fortschr. Neurol. Psychiat. 70 (2002) 61–70
163 Hacke, W., Hennerici, M., Gelmers, H.J., Krämer, G.: Cerebral ischemia. Berlin, Heidelberg, New York: Springer 1991
164 Hacker, H., Kühner, G.: Die Brückenvenen. Radiologe 12 (1972) 45–48
165 Haddad, J., Christmann, D., Messer, J. (Eds.): Imaging techniques of the CNS of the Neonates. Berlin, Heidelberg: Springer 1991
166 Hagens, G. von, Whalley, A., Machke, R., Kriz, W.: Schnittanatomie des menschlichen Gehirns. Darmstadt: Steinkopff 1990
167 Haller, J.O.: Textbook of neonatal ultrasound. New York: Parthenon Publishing 1998
167a Halliday, A.M.: Evoked potentials in clinical testing. Livingstone: Churchill 1993
168 Hanaway, J.: The brain atlas a visual guide to the human central nervous system. Bethesda, MD: Fitzgerald 1998
169 Hanaway, J., Woolsey, T.A., Gado, M.H.: The brain atlas. Bethesda, Maryland: Fitzgerald Science Press 1998
170 Hanaway, J., Young, R., Netsky, M., Adelman, L.: Localization of the pyramidal tract in the internal capsule. Neurology 31 (1981) 365–367
171 Hanaway, J., Young, R.R.: Localization of the pyramidal tract in the internal capsule of man. J. Neurol. Sci. 34 (1977) 63–70
172 Hardy, T.L., Bertrand, G., Thompson, C.J.: The position and organization of motor fibers in the internal capsule found during stereotactic surgery. Appl. Neurophysiol. 42 (1979) 160–170
173 Harrison, J.M., Howe, M.E.: Anatomy of the afferent auditory nervous system of mammals. 283–336 In: Autrum, H., Jung, R., Loewenstein, W.R., Mackay, D.W., Teuber, H.L. (Eds.): Handbook of sensory physiology. Vol. 5: Auditory system, part 1. Berlin, Heidelberg, New York: Springer 1974
173a Hart jr, J., Selnes, O.A.: Acquired disorders of language. In Asbury, A.K., Mc Khann, G.M., Mc Donald, W.I., Goadsby, P.J., Mc Arthur, J.C.: Diseases of the nervous system. Cambridge University Press Vol I 2002 317–330
174 Hartje, W., Poeck, K.: Klinische Neuropsychologie. Stuttgart, New York: Thieme 2002
175 Hartman, B.K.: The innervation of cerebral blood vessels by central noradrenergic neurons. 91–96 In: Usdin, E., Snyder, S.H. (Eds.): Frontiers in catecholamine research. Oxford: Pergamon Press 1973
176 Hassler, R.: Architectonic organization of the thalamic nuclei. 140–180 In: Schaltenbrand, G., Walker, A.E. (Eds.): Stereotaxy of the human brain, 2nd ed. Stuttgart, New York: Thieme 1982
177 Haug, H.: The significance of quantitative stereologic experimental procedures in pathology. Path. Res. Pract. 166 (1980) 144–164
178 Haverling, M.: The tortuous basilar artery. Acta radiol. Diagn. 15 (1974) 241–249
179 Hayman, L.A., Berman, S.A., Hinck, V.C.: Correlation of CT cerebral vascular territories with function. II. Posterior cerebral artery. Amer. J. Radiol. 137 (1981) 13–19
180 Heidary, A., Tomasch, J.: Neuron numbers and perikaryon areas in the human cerebellar nuclei. Acta anat. (Basel) 74 (1969) 290–296
181 Heimer, L., Robards, M.J. (Eds.): Neuroanatomical tract-tracing methods. New York: Plenum 1989
182 Heimer, L.: The human brain and spinal cord. Functional neuroanatomy and dissection guide. New York, Berlin, Heidelberg, Tokyo: Springer 1995
183 Heindel, W., Kugel, H., Lackner, K. (Eds.): Rationelle MR-Untersuchungstechniken. Stuttgart, New York: Thieme 1997
183a Hennerici, M.G., Neuerburg-Heusler, D.: Vascular diagnosis with ultrasound. Stuttgart, New York: Thieme 1998
184 Henry, J.M.: Anatomy of the brainstem. 37–59 In: Schaltenbrand, G., Walker, A.E. (Eds.): Stereotaxy of the human brain, 2nd ed. Stuttgart, New York: Thieme 1982
185 Hentschel, F., Heuck, F., Vogt, K., Bast, B.: Schädel-Gehirn Wirbelsäule-Rückenmark. Stuttgart, New York: Thieme 1999
186 Heym, C. (Ed.): Histochemistry and cell biology of autonomic neurons and paraganglia. Berlin, Heidelberg, New York, Tokyo: Springer 1987
187 Hirayama, K., Tsubaki, T., Toyokura, Y., Okinaka, S.: The representation of the pyramidal tract in the internal capsule and basis pedunculi. Neurology 12 (1962) 337–342
188 Hobson, J.A., Brazier, M.A.B. (Eds.): The reticular formation revisited. Specifying function for a nonspecific system. New York: Raven 1980
189 Hofer, M.: CT-Kursbuch. Düsseldorf: Hofer Verlag Didamed 2000
190 Hofer, M.: Sono-Grundkurs. Stuttgart, New York: Thieme 1999
191 Hökfelt, T., Fuxe, K., Goldstein, M., Johansson, O.: Immunohistochemical evidence for the existence of adrenaline neurons in the rat brain. Brain Res. 66 (1974) 235–251
192 Hökfelt, T., Johansson, O., Ljungdahl, A., Lundberg, J.M., Schultzberg, M.: Peptidergic neurones. Nature 284 (1980) 515–521
193 Holman, B.L., Hill, T.C., Magistretti, P.L.: Brain imaging with emission computed tomography and radiolabeled amines. Invest. Radiol. 17 (1982) 206–215
194 Honda, H., Watanabe, K., Kusumoto, S., Hoshi, H., Nishikawa, K., Kakitsubata, Y., Jinnouchi, S., Kodama, T., Nakayama, S., Ono, S.: Optimal positioning for CT examinations of the skull base. Europ. J. Radiol. 7 (1987) 225–228

195 Hopf, H.C., Deuschl, G., Diener, H.C., Reichmann, H. (Hrsg.): Neurologie in Praxis und Klinik. Band 1 und 2. Stuttgart, New York: Thieme 1999

196 Horn, A., Büttner-Ennever, J.A.: Neuroanatomie der okulomotorischen Kerne, Hirnstammzentren und -bahnen. 34–47 In Huber, A. and Kömpf, A. (Eds.) Klinische Neuroroophthalmologie. Stuttgart, New York: Thieme 1998.

197 Horn, A., Büttner-Ennever, J.A.: Premotor neurons for vertical eye movements in the rostral mesencephalon of monkey and human: histologic identification by parvalbumin immunostainig. J. comp. Neurology 392 (1998) 413 – 427

198 Hosten, N., Liebig, T.: CT of the head and spine. Stuttgart, New York: Thieme 2001

199 Hounsfield, G.N.: Computerized transverse axial scanning (tomography). Part 1: Description of system. Brit. J. Radiol. 46 (1973) 1016–1022

200 Howe, P.R.C., Costa, M., Furness, J.B., Chalmers, J.P.: Simultaneous demonstration of phenylethanolamine N-methyltransferase immunofluorescent and catecholamine fluorescent nerve cell bodies in the rat medulla oblongata. Neuroscience 5 (1980) 2229–2238

201 Hubbard, J.E., Carlo, V. di: Fluorescence histochemistry of monoamine-containing cell bodies in the brain stem of the squirrel monkey (Saimiri sciureus). III: Serotonin- containing groups. J. comp. Neurol. 153 (1974) 385–398

202 Hubbard, J.E., Carlo, V.di: Fluorescence histochemistry of monoamine-containing cell bodies in the brain stem of the squirrel monkey (Saimiri sciureus). II: Catecholamine- containing groups. J. comp. Neurol. 153 (1974) 369–384

203 Huber, A., Kömpf, D.: Klinische Neuroophthalmologie. Stuttgart, New York: Thieme 1998

204 Hufschmidt, A., Lücking, C.H.: Neurologie compact. Stuttgart, New York: Thieme 1999

205 Huk, W.J., Gademann, G., Friedmann, G.: Magnetic resonance imaging of central nervous system diseases. Berlin, Heidelberg, New York, London, Paris, Tokyo, Hong Kong: Springer 1990

206 Hundeshagen, H. (Ed.): Handbuch der medizinischen Radiologie. Band 15, Teil 1 B. Fitschen, J., Helus, F., Jordan, K., Junker, D., Meyer, G.-J., Schober, O., Stöcklin, G.: Emissions-Computertomographie mit kurzlebigen zyklotron-produzierten Radiopharmaka. Berlin, Heidelberg, New York, London, Paris, Tokyo, Hong Kong: Springer 1988

207 Isaacson, R.L.: The limbic system. New York, London: Plenum 1982

208 Iversen, S.D.: Do hippocampal lesions produce amnesia in animals? Int. Rev. Neurobiol. 19 (1976) 1–49

209 Jamieson, D., Alavi, A., Jolles, P., Chawluk, J., Reivich, M.: Positron emission tomography in the investigation of central nervous system disorders. Radiologic Clinics of North America 26 (1988) 1075–1088

210 Jannetta, P.J., Bennett, M.H.: The pathophysiology of trigeminal neuralgia. 312–315 In: Samii, M., Jannetta, P.J. (Eds.): The cranial nerves. Berlin, Heidelberg, New York: Springer 1981

211 Jannetta, P.J.: Hemifacial spasm. In: Samii, M., Jannetta, P.J. (Eds.): The cranial nerves. Berlin, Heidelberg, New York: Springer 1981 484–493

212 Jannetta, P.J.: Observations on the etiology of trigeminal neuralgia, hemifacial spasm, acoustic nerve dysfunction and glossopharyngeal neuralgia. Definitive microsurgical treatment and results in 117 patients. Neurochirurgia 20 (1977) 145–154

212 a Jansen, O., Schellinger, P.D., Fiebach, J.B., Sartor, K., Hacke, W.: Magnetresonanztomographie beim akuten Schlaganfall. Deutsches Ärzteblatt 99 (2002) 1065–1070

212 b Jansen, O., Ulmer, S., Alfke, K., Straube, T.: Advances in brain tumor imaging. Klin. Neuroradiol. 13 (2003) 15–19

213 Jelgersma, G.: Atlas anatomicum cerebri humani. Amsterdam: Scheltema and Holkema N.V. 1931

214 Jinkins, J.R.: Atlas of neuroradiologic embryology, anatomy, and variants. Philadelphia, Baltimore: Lippincott, Williams & Wilkins 2000

215 Jolesz, F.A., Kikinis, R.: Intraoperative imaging revolutionizes therapy. Diagnostic imaging 150 (1995) 62–68

216 Jones, E.G.: The thalamus. New York: Plenum 1985

217 Joseph, J.-P.: Communications: Le rôle fonctionnel du cortex auditif: comparaison homme–animal. Revue de Laryngologie 101 (1980) 327–334

218 Jueptner, M., Krukenberg, M.: Motor system: cortex, basal ganglia, and cerebellum. Neuroimaging Clinics of North America 11 (2001) 203 – 219

219 Kahle, W., Frotscher, M.: Color atlas and textbook of human anatomy Vol. 3. Stuttgart: Thieme 2002

220 Kalender, W. A., K. Wedding, A. Polacin, M. Prokop, C. Schaefer-Prokop, M. Galanski: Grundlagen der Gefäßdarstellung mit Spiral-CT. Akt. Radiol. 4 (1994) 287–297

221 Kandel, E.R., Schwartz, J.H., Jessel, T.M. (Eds.): Principles of neural science. New York: McGraw Hill, Health Professions 2000

222 Kanski, J.J., Spitznas, M.: Lehrbuch der klinischen Ophthalmologie. Stuttgart, New York: Thieme 1996

223 Kassenärztliche Bundesvereinigung: Richtlinien über Kriterien zur Qualitätsbeurteilung der Kernspintomographie. Deutsches Ärzteblatt 98 (2001) 634–643

224 Kelter, S.: Aphasien. Hirnorganisch bedingte Sprachstörungen und kognitive Wissenschaft. Psychiatrie, Neurologie, Klinische Psychologie. Grundlagen – Methoden – Ergebnisse. In: Baumgartner, G., Cohen, R., Grüsser, O.-J., Helmchen, H., Schmidt, L.R. (Eds.) Stuttgart, Berlin, Köln: Kohlhammer 1990

225 Keyserlingk, D. Graf von, Niemann, K., Wasel, J.: A quantitative approach to spatial variation of human cerebral sulci. Acta anat. 131 (1988) 127–131

226 Kido, D.K., LeMay, M., Levinson, A.W., Benson, W.E.: Computed tomographic localization of the precentral gyrus. Radiology 135 (1980) 373–377

227 Kim, J.S., Lee, J.H., Choi, C.G.: Patterns of lateral medullary infarction. Vascular lesion – magnetic resonance imaging correlation of 34 cases. Stroke 29 (1998) 645–652

228 Kim, K.H.S., Reikin, N.R., Lee, K., Hirsch, J.: Distinct cortical areas associated with native and second languages. Nature 388 (1997) 171 – 174

229 Kleinschmidt, A., Nitschke, M.F., Frahm, J.: Somatotopy in the human motor cortex hand area. A high-resolution functional MRI study. Europ. J. Neuroscience 9 (1997) 2178–2186

230 Klingler, J.: Die makroskopische Anatomie der Ammonsformation. Denkschriften der Schweizerischen Naturforschenden Gesellschaft. Band 78, Teil 1. Zürich: Fretz 1948

231 Klötzsch, C., Mäurer, M., Seidel, G. Sliwka, U.: Stellenwert der transkraniellen Farbduplex-Sonographie. Deutsches Ärzteblatt 98 (2001) 548 – 552

232 Knaap, M.S. van der, Valk, J.: Magnetic resonance of myelin, myelination and myelin disorders. Berlin, Heidelberg, New York: Springer 1995

232 a Knecht, S., Deppe, M., Drager, B., Bobe, L., Ringelstein, E.-B., Henningsen, H.: Language lateralization in healthy righthanders. Brain 123 (2000) 74–81

232 b Knecht, S., Ringelstein, E.-B.: Neuronale Plastizität am Beispiel des somatosensorischen Systems. Nervenarzt 70 (1999) 889 – 898

233 Knudsen, P.A.: Ventriklernes storrelseforhold i anatomisk normale hjerner fra voksne mennesker. Odense: Andelsbogtrykkeriet 1958

234 Koenig, M., E. Klotz, B. Luka, D. J. Venderink, J. F. Spittler, L. Heuser: Perfusion CT of the brain: diagnostic approach for early detection of ischemic stroke. Radiology 209 (1998) 85–93

235 Kömpf, D., Heide, W.: Zentralnervöse Strukturen – two goals, two modes, six systems. 48–57 In Huber, A. and Kömpf, D. (Eds.) Klinische Neuroroophthalmologie. Stuttgart, New York: Thieme 1998

236 Konitzer, M.: Pathologie und Klinik des posterioren Thalamus. Nervenarzt 58 (1987) 413–423

237 Köster, O.: Computertomographie des Felsenbeines. Stuttgart, New York: Thieme 1999

238 Krayenbühl, H., Yasargil, M.G.: Cerebral angiography. Stuttgart, New York: Thieme 1982

239 Kretschmann, H.-J., Kammradt, G., Krauthausen, I., Sauer, B., Wingert, F.: Growth of the hippocampal formation in man. Bibliotheca anatomica. Basel: Karger Band 28 (1986) 27–52

240 Kretschmann, H.-J., Schleicher, A., Grottschreiber, J.-F.,Kullmann, W.: The Yakovlev Collection. A pilot study of its suitability for the morphometric documentation of the human brain. J. neurol. Sci. 43 (1979) 111–126

241 Kretschmann, H.-J., Tafesse, U., Herrmann, A.: Different volume changes of cerebral cortex and white matter during histological preparation. Microscopica Acta 86 (1982) 13–24

242 Kretschmann, H.-J., Weinrich, W. Gerke, M., Wesemann, M., Fresen, T.: Dreidimensionale Computergraphik neurofunktioneller Systeme. Stuttgart, New York: Thieme CD-ROM 1998

243 Kretschmann, H.-J., Weinrich, W. Gerke, M., Wesemann, M., Fresen, T.: Neurofunctional systems. Stuttgart, New York: Thieme CD-ROM 1999

244 Kretschmann, H.-J., Weinrich, W., Fiekert, W., Gerke, M., Vogt, H., Weirich, D., Wesemann, M.: Neurofunctional systems. Stuttgart, New York: Thieme 1998

245 Kretschmann, H.-J.: Localization of the corticospinal fibres in the internal capsule in man. J. Anat. 160 (1988) 219-225
246 Krieg, W.J.S.: Architectonics of human cerebral fiber systems. Evanston/Ill.: Brain Books 1973
247 Krieg, W.J.S.: Functional neuroanatomy. Bloomington/Ill.: Pantagraph Printing 1966
248 Krings, T., Coenen, V.A., Axer, H., Möller-Hartmann, W., Mayfrank, L., Weidemann, J., Kränzlein, H., Gilsbach, J.M., Thron, A.: Three-dimensional visualization of motor cortex and pyramidal tracts employing functional and diffusion weighted MRI. Klin. Neuroradiol. 11 (2001) 105-121
249 Krönauer, A.: Computerunterstützte dreidimensionale Rekonstruktion der Basalganglien als Referenz für die bildgebenden Verfahren (Computertomographie, Magnetische Resonanztomographie und Positronen-Emissionstomographie). Med. Dissertation, Med. Hochschule Hannover 1987
250 Kuhn, M.J.: Atlas der Neuroradiologie. Weinheim: Chapman & Hall 1994
251 Kummer, R. von, Bozzao, L., Manelfe, C.: Early CT diagnosis of hemispheric infarction. Berlin, Heidelberg, New York: Springer 1995
252 Kuni, C.C., DuCret, R.P.: Manual of nuclear medicine imaging. Stuttgart, New York: Thieme 1997
253 Kunze, K. (Ed.): Praxis der Neurologie. Stuttgart, New York: Thieme 1999
254 Kunze, K., Zangemeister, W.H., Arlt, A. (Eds.): Clinical problems of brainstem disorders. Stuttgart, New York: Thieme 1986
255 Künzle, H., Akert, K.: Efferent connections of cortical area 8 (frontal eye field) in Macaca fascicularis. A reinvestigation using the autoradiographic technique. J. comp. Neurol. 173 (1977) 147-164
256 Kuypers, H.G.J.M.: Anatomy of the descending pathways. 597-666 In: Brooks, V.B. (Ed.): Handbook of physiology. Sec. 1: The nervous system, vol. 2: Motor Control, part 2. (American physiological society. ser.) Baltimore: Williams and Wilkins 1981
257 Kuypers, H.G.J.M.: Central cortical projections to motor and somatosensory cell groups. Brain 83 (1960) 161-184
258 Kuypers, H.G.J.M.: Corticobulbar connexions to the pons and lower brain-stem in man. Brain 81 (1958) 364-388
259 Lanferann, H., Herminghaus, S., Pilatus, U., Raab, P., Wagner, S., Zanella, F.E.: Grundlagen der 1H-MR-Spektroskopie intrakranieller Tumoren. Klinische Neuroradiologie, 12 (2002) 1-17
260 Lang, J., Jensen, H.-P., Schröder, F.: Praktische Anatomie. In: Lanz, T. von, Wachsmuth W. (Eds.) Band 1, Teil 1 Kopf, Teil A Übergeordnete Systeme. Berlin, Heidelberg, New York, Tokyo: Springer 1985
261 Lang, J., Reiter, U.: Über die intrazisternale Länge der Hirnnerven VII-XII. Neurochirurgia 28 (1985) 153-157
262 Lang, J., Stefanec, P., Breitenbach, W.: Über Form und Maße des Ventriculus tertius, von Sehbahnteilen und des N. oculomotorius. Neurochirurgia 26 (1983) 1-5
263 Lang, J.: Klinische Anatomie der Nase, Nasenhöhle und Nebenhöhlen. Stuttgart, New York: Thieme 1988
264 Lang, J.: Clinical anatomy of the head. Berlin, Heidelberg, New York: Springer 1983
265 Lang, J.: Kopf Gehirn- und Augenschädel. In: Lanz, T. von, Wachsmuth, W. (Eds.): Praktische Anatomie, Band 1, Teil 1B. Berlin, Heidelberg, New York: Springer 1979
266 Langer, T., Fuchs, A.F., Scudder C.A., Chubb, M.C.: Afferents to the flocculus of the cerebellum in the rhesus macaque as revealed by retrograde transport of horseradish peroxidase. J. Comp Neurol 235 (1985) 1 - 25
267 Lanz, T. von, Wachsmuth, W: Praktische Anatomie. Band 1, Teil 2: Hals. Berlin, Göttingen, Heidelberg: Springer 1955
268 Larsell, O.: The comparative anatomy and histology of the cerebellum. Minneapolis: University of Minnesota Press 1970
269 Lasjaunias, P., Berenstein, A., ter Brugge, K.G.: Surgical neuroangiography. Berlin, Heidelberg, New York: Springer 2001
270 Lassek, A.M.: The pyramidal tract. Springfield/Ill.: Thomas 1954
271 Last, R.J., Tompsett, D.H.: Casts of the cerebral ventricles. Brit. J. Surg. 40 (1953) 525-543
272 Laubenberger, Th., Laubenberger, J.: Technik der medizinischen Radiologie. Köln: Deutscher Ärzteverlag 1999
273 Leblanc, A.: Encephalo-peripheral nervous system. Berlin, Heidelberg, New York, London, Paris, Tokyo: Springer 2001
274 Leblanc, A.: The cranial nerves. Anatomy, imaging, vascularisation. Berlin, Heidelberg, New York: Springer 1995
275 Lee, S. H., Rao, K.C.V.G., Zimmerman, R.A.: Cranial MRI and CT. New York, St. Louis: McGraw-Hill 1999
276 Leigh, R.J., Zee, D.S.: The neurology of eye movements. Philadelphia: Davis 1999
277 Leischner, A.: Aphasien und Sprachentwicklungsstörungen. Klinik und Behandlung. Stuttgart: Thieme 1987
278 LeMay, M.: Asymmetries of the skull and handedness. J. neurol. Sci. 32 (1977) 243-253
279 Lemke, B.: Validierung eines Matching-Verfahrens zur Projektion anatomischer 3D-Modelle von zentralen Gehirnstrukturen auf MR-Bilder. Medizin. Dissertation der Medizinischen Hochschule Hannover 1996
280 Leonard, C.M., Martinez, P., Weintraub, B.D., Hauser, P.: Magnetic resonance imaging of cerebral anomalies in subjects with resistance to thyroid hormone. Am. J. Med. Genet. 60 (1995) 238-243
281 Leonhardt, H.: Ependym und circumventriculäre Organe. 177-666 In: Möllendorff, W. von, Bargmann, W., Oksche, A., Vollrath, L. (Eds.): Handbuch der mikroskopischen Anatomie des Menschen. Band 4: Nervensystem, Teil 10. Berlin, Heidelberg, New York: Springer 1980
282 Levin, D.N., Pelizzari, C.A., Chen, G.T.Y., Chen, C.-T., Cooper, M.D.: Retrospective geometric correlation of MR, CT, and PET images. Radiology 169 (1988) 817-823
283 Liegeois-Chauvel, C., Musolino, A., Chauvel, P.: Localization of the primary auditory area in man. Brain 114 (1991) 139-153
283 a Liepert, J., Bauder, H., Miltner, W.H.R., Taub, E., Weiller, C.: Therapie-induzierte kortikale Reorganisation bei Schlaganfallpatienten. Neurol. Rehabil. 6 (2000) 177-183
284 Lindenberg, R.: Die Gefäßversorgung und ihre Bedeutung für Art und Ort von kreislaufbedingten Gewebsschäden und Gefäßprozessen. 1071-1164 In: Lubarsch, O., Henke, F., Rössle, R., Uehlinger, E. (Eds.): Handbuch der speziellen pathologischen Anatomie und Histologie. Band 13: Nervensystem, Teil 1/B. Berlin, Heidelberg, New York: Springer 1957
285 Lippert, H.: Lehrbuch Anatomie. München, Wien, Baltimore: Urban und Schwarzenberg 2000
286 Lissner, J., Seiderer, M. (Eds.): Klinische Kernspintomographie. Stuttgart: Enke 1990
287 Lloyd, G.A.S.: Diagnostic imaging of the nose and paranasal sinuses. London, Berlin, Heidelberg, New York, Paris, Tokyo: Springer 1988
288 Lowitzsch, K., Hopf, H.C., Buchner, H., Claus, D., Jörg, J., Rappelsberger, P., Tackmann, W.: Das EP-Buch. Stuttgart, New York: Thieme 2000
289 Lübke, W.T.: Computerunterstützte dreidimensionale Rekonstruktion des Kleinhirns als Referenz für die bildgebenden Verfahren (Computertomographie, Magnetische Resonanztomographie und Positronen-Emissionstomographie). Med. Dissertation, Med. Hochschule Hannover 1994
290 Ludwig, E., Klingler, J.: Atlas cerebri humani. Basel: Karger 1956
291 Lundberg, J.M., Hökfelt, T.: Coexistence of peptides and classical neurotransmitters. Trends Neuro. Sci. 6 (1983) 325-333
291 a Lurito, J.T., Dzemidzic, M.: Determination of cerebral hemisphere language dominance with functional magnetic resonance imaging. Neuroimaging Clinics of North America 11 (2001) 355 - 363
292 Mai, J.K., Assheuer, J.K., Paxinos, G.: Atlas of the human brain. San Diego, London, Boston: Academic Press 1997
293 Mai, J.K., Stephens, P.H., Hopf, A., Cuello, A.C.: Substance P in the human brain. Neuroscience 17 (1986) 709-739
294 Mai, J.K., Triepel, J., Metz, J.: Neurotensin in the human brain. Neuroscience 22 (1987) 499-524
295 Maiden-Tilsen, M.: Computergestützte 3D-Rekonstruktion des 3. Neurons des intrakraniellen somatosensorischen Trigeminussystems als Referenz für die bildgebenden Verfahren (not published)
296 Mann, D.M.A., Yates, P.O., Marcyniuk, B.: A comparison of changes in the nucleus basalis and locus caeruleus in Alzheimers disease. J. Neurol. Neurosurg. Psychiatry 47 (1984) 201-203
297 Marino, R., Rasmussen, T.: Visual field changes after temporal lobectomy in man. Neurology 18 (1968) 825-835
298 Martin, E., Kikinis, R., Zuerrer, M., Boesch, C., Briner, J., Kewitz, G., Kaelin, P.: Developmental stages of human brain: An MR study. J. Comput. assist. Tomography 12 (1988) 917-922
299 Martin, J.H.: Neuroanatomy. Text and atlas. New York: Mc Graw-Hill 2003
300 Martin, W.R.W., Beckman, J.H., Calne, D.B., Adam, M.J., Harrop, R., Rogers, J.G., Ruth, T.J., Sayre, C.I., Pate, B.D.: Cerebral glucose metabolism in Parkinson's disease. Can. J. Neurol. Sci. 11 (1984) 169-173
301 Maurer, J.: Neurootologie. Stuttgart, New York: Thieme 1999
302 Mawad, M.E., Silver, A.J., Hilal, S.K., Ganti, S.R.: Computed tomography of the brain stem with intrathecal metrizamide.

Part I: The normal brain stem. Amer. J. Roentgenol. 140 (1983) 553-563
303 McGeer, P.L., Eccles, J.C., McGeer, E.G.: Molecular neurobiology of the mammalian brain. New York, London: Plenum 1987
304 McGraw, P., Mathews, V.P., Wang Y., Phillips, M.D.: Approach to functional magnetic resonance imaging of language based on models of language organization. Neuroimaging Clinics of North America 11 (2001) 343 – 353
305 Meese, W., Kluge, W., Grumme, T., Hopfenmüller, W.: CT evaluation of the CSF spaces of healthy persons. Neuroradiology 19 (1980) 131-136
306 Meisenzahl, E.M., Schlösser, R.: Functional magnetic resonance imaging research in psychiatry. Neuroimaging Clinics of North America 11 (2001) 365 – 374
307 Mesulam, M.-M., Mufson, E.J., Levey, A.L., Wainer, B.H.: Cholinergic innervation of cortex by the basal forebrain: Cytochemistry and cortical connections of the septal area, diagonal band nuclei, nucleus basalis (substantia innominata), and hypothalamus in the rhesus monkey. J. comp. Neurol. 214 (1983) 170-197
308 Miller, D.H., Kesselring, J., McDonald, W.I., Paty, D.W., Thompson, A.J.: Magnetresonanz bei Multipler Sklerose. Stuttgart, Berlin, Köln: Kohlhammer 1998
309 Möller, T.B., Reif, E.: Taschenatlas der Schnittbildanatomie. Bd 1 Computertomographie, Kernspintomographie Kopf, Hals, Wirbelsäule, Gelenke. Stuttgart, New York: Thieme 1997
310 Möller, T.B., Reif, E.: MRI parameters and positioning. Stuttgart, New York: Thieme 2002
311 Moonen, C.T.W., Bandettini, P.A. (Eds.): Functional MRI. Berlin, Heidelberg, New York: Springer 2000
312 Moore, J.K., Karapas, F., Moore, R.Y.: Projections of the inferior colliculus in insectivores and primates. Brain Behav. Evol. 14 (1977) 301-327
313 Moore, R.Y., Bloom, F.E.: Central catecholamine neuron systems: Anatomy and physiology of the dopamine systems. Ann. Rev. Neurosci. 1 (1978) 129-169
314 Moore, R.Y., Bloom, F.E.: Central catecholamine neuron systems: Anatomy and physiology of the norepinephrine and epinephrine systems. Ann. Rev. Neurosci. 2 (1979) 113-168
315 Mori, K.: Anomalies of the central nervous system. In: Nadjmi, M., Harwood-Nash, D.E. (Eds.). Stuttgart, New York: Thieme 1985
316 Mugler III, J.P., Kiefer, B., Brookeman, J.R.: Three-dimensional T2-weighted imaging of the brain using very long spin-echo trains. Proceedings of the International Society for Magnetic Resonance in medicine 2000 Eighth meeting, Denver, Abstract 687
317 Müller, D.: (not published) 1996
317a Müller-Forell, W.: Bildgebende Diagnostik von Orbitaerkrankungen. Klin.Neuroradiol. 12 (2002) 101-126
318 Mumenthaler, M., Mattle, H.: Neurologie. Stuttgart, New York: Thieme 2002
319 Mumenthaler, M.: Neurologic differential diagnosis. Stuttgart: Thieme 1992
320 Muramoto, O., Kuru, Y., Sugishita, M., Toyokura, Y.: Pure memory loss with hippocampal lesions. A pneumoencephalographic study. Arch. Neurol. 36 (1979) 54-56
321 Nadjmi, M., Piepgras, U., Vogelsang, H.: Kranielle Computertomographie. Stuttgart, New York: Thieme 1981
322 Naidich, P., Valavanis, G., Kubik, S.: Anatomic relationships along the low-middle convexity: Part I. Normal specimens and magnetic resonance imaging. Neurosurgery 36 (1995) 517 – 531
323 Naidich, T., Brightbill, T.C.: Systems for localizing frontoparietal gyri and sulci on axial CT and MRI. Int. J. Neuroradiol. 4 (1996) 313 – 338
324 Naidich, T.P., Daniels, D.L., Haughton, V.M., Pech, P., Williams, A., Pojunas, K., Palacios, E.: Hippocampal formation and related structures of the limbic lobe: Anatomic-MR correlation. Part 2. Sagittal sections. Radiology 162 (1987) 755-761
325 Naidich, T.P., Daniels, D.L., Haughton, V.M., Williams, A., Pojunas, K., Palacios, E.: Hippocampal formation and related structures of the limbic lobe: Anatomic-MR correlation. Part 1. Surface features and coronal sections. Radiology 162 (1987) 747-754
326 Naidich, T.P., Daniels, D.L., Pech, P., Haughton, V.M., Williams, A., Pojunas, K.: Anterior commissure: Anatomic-MR correlation and use as a landmark in three orthogonal planes. Radiology 158 (1986) 421-429
327 Naidich, T.P., Hof, P.R., Gannon, P.J., Yousry, T.A., Yousry, I.: Anatomic substrates of language: emphasizing speech. Neuroimaging Clinics of North America 11 (2001) 305 – 341
328 Naidich, T.P., Hof, P.R., Yousry, T.A., Yousry, I.: The motor cortex: anatomic substrates of function. Neuroimaging Clinics of North America 11 (2001) 171 – 193
329 Naidich, T.P., Leeds, N.E., Kricheff, I.I., Pudlowski, R.M., Naidich, J.B., Zimmerman, R.D.: The tentorium in axial section. Radiology 123 (1977) 631-648
330 Neuerburg-Heusler, D., Hennerici, M.G.: Gefäßdiagnostik mit Ultraschall. Stuttgart, New York: Thieme 1999
331 Nieuwenhuys, R., Voogd, J., Huijzen, C. van: Das Zentralnervensystem des Menschen. Ein Atlas mit Begleittext. Berlin, Heidelberg, New York: Springer 1980
332 Nieuwenhuys, R., Voogd, J., Huijzen, C. van: The human central nervous system. Berlin, Heidelberg, New York, London, Paris, Tokyo: Springer 1988
333 Nieuwehuys, R.: Chemoarchitecture of the brain. Berlin, Heidelberg, New York: Springer 1985
334 Nitschke, M.F., Kleinschmidt, A., Wessel, K., and Frahm, J.: Somatotopic motor representation in the human anterior cerebellum. Brain 119 (1996) 1023 – 1029
335 Noback, C. R., Strominger, N.J., Demarest, R.J.: The human nervous system. Baltimore: Williams and Wilkins 1996
336 Nobin, A., Björklund, A.: Topography of the monoamine neuron systems in the human brain as revealed in fetuses. Acta physiol. scand., Suppl. 388 (1973) 1-40
337 Novelline, R.A., Rhea, J.T., Rao, P.M., Stuk, J.L.: Helical CT in emergency radiology. Radiology 213 (1999) 321 – 339
337a Nowinski, W.L. Thirunavuukarasuu, A., Bryan, R.N.: The cerefy ® atlas of brain anatomy. Stuttgart, New York: Thieme 2002
337b Nowinski, W.L. Thirunavuukarasuu, A., Kennedy, D.N.: Brain atlas of functional imaging. Stuttgart, New York: Thieme 2001
338 Nygrèn, L.-G., Olson, L.: A new major projection from locus coeruleus: The main source of noradrenergic nerve terminals in the ventral and dorsal columns of the spinal cord. Brain Res. 132 (1977) 85-93
339 Ojemann, G.A.: The intrahemispheric organization of human language, derived with electrical stimulation techniques. Trends in Neuroscience 6 (1983) 184-189
340 Oldendorf, W.H.: Isolated flying spot detection of radiodensity discontinuities-displaying the internal structural pattern of a complex object. IRE Trans. biomed. electr. (N.Y.) 8 (1961) 68-72
341 Olszewski, J., Baxter, D.: Cytoarchitecture of the human brain stem. Basel, New York: Karger 1982
342 Ono, M., Kubik, S., Abernathey, C.D.: Atlas of the cerebral sulci. Stuttgart: Thieme 1990
343 Osborn, A.G.: Diagnostic cerebral angiography. Philadelphia, Baltimore, New York: Lippincott Williams and Wilkins 1999
344 Osborn, A.G.: Diagnostic neuroradiology. St. Louis, Baltimore, Boston: Mosby 1994
345 Osborn, A.G.: The medial tentorium and incisura: normal and pathological anatomy. Neuroradiology 13 (1977) 109-113
346 Palacios, E., Fine, M., Haughton, V.M.: Multiplanar anatomy of the head and neck for computed tomography. New York: Wiley 1980
347 Palay, .L., Chan-Palay, V.: Cerebellar cortex. Cytology and organization. Berlin, Heidelberg, New York: Springer 1974
348 Panofsky, W., Staemmler, M.: Untersuchungen über Hirngewicht und Schädelkapazität nach der Reichardtschen Methode. Frankfurt. Z. Path. 26 (1922) 519-549
349 Papeschi, R.: Dopamine, extrapyramidal system, and psychomotor function. Psychiat. Neurol. Neurochir. (Amst.) 75 (1972) 13-48
350 Parent, A.: Carpenter's human neuroanatomy. Baltimore: Williams and Wilkins 1996
351 Passingham, R.E.: Premotor cortex and preparation for movement. Exp. Brain Res. 70 (1988) 590-596
352 Patten, J.P.: Neurological differential diagnosis. Berlin, New York: Springer 1996
352a Paulesu, E., Frackowiak, R.S.J., Bottini,G. Maps of somatosensory systems. In: Frackowiack, R.S.J., Friston, K.J., Frith, C.D., Mazziota, J.C. (Eds.) Human brain function p. 218-231 San Diego: Academic Press 1997
353 Paxinos, G. (Ed.): The human nervous system. New York, London: Academic Press 1990
354 Paxinos, G., Huang, X.-F.: Atlas of the human brainstem. San Diego, New York, Boston : Academic Press 1995
355 Penfield, W., Rasmussen, T.: The cerebral cortex of man. A clinical study of localization of function. New York: Hafner 1968
356 Penfield, W., Welch, K.: The supplementary motor area of the cerebral cortex. A clinical and experimental study. Arch. Neurol. Psychiat. (Chic.) 66 (1951) 289-317

357 Perenin, M.T., Jeannerod, M.: Subcortical vision in man. Trends in Neuroscience 2 (1979) 204–207

358 Peters, A., Palay, S.L., Webster, H.F. de: The fine structure of the nervous system: The neurons and supporting cells. Philadelphia, London, Toronto: Saunders 1991

359 Petit, L., Clark, V.P., Ingeholm, J., Haxby, J.V.: Dissociation of saccade-related and pursuit-related activation in human frontal eye fields as revealed by fMRI. J. Neurophysiol. 77(1997) 3386–3390

360 Pfeifer, R.A.: Myelogenetisch-anatomische Untersuchungen über das kortikale Ende der Hörleitung. Leipzig: Teubner 1920

361 Pfeifer, R.A.: Myelogenetisch-anatomische Untersuchungen über den zentralen Abschnitt der Sehleitung. Berlin: Springer 1925

362 Pfeifer, R.A.: Myelogenetisch-anatomische Untersuchungen über den zentralen Abschnitt der Taststrahlung, der Pyramidenbahn, der Hirnnerven und zusätzlicher motorischer Bahnen. Nova Acta Leopoldina (Neue Folge) 1 (1934) 341–473

363 Phillips, D.P.: Introduction to anatomy and physiology of the central auditory nervous system. 407–427 In: Jahn, A.F., Santos-Sacchi, J. (Eds.): Physiology of the ear. New York: Raven Press 1988

364 Piepgras, U.: Neuroradiologie. Stuttgart, New York: Thieme 1977

365 Platzer, W. (Ed.): Pernkopf: Atlas der topographischen und angewandten Anatomie des Menschen. Stuttgart, New York: Thieme 1994

366 Platzer, W.: Atlas of topographical anatomy. Stuttgart: Thieme 1985

367 Poeck, K., Hacke, W.: Neurologie. Berlin, Heidelberg, New York: Springer 2001

368 Pompeiano, O.: Reticular formation. 381–488 In: Autrum, H., Jung, R., Loewenstein, W.R., Teuber, H. (Eds.): Handbook of sensory physiology. Vol. 2: Somatosensory system. Berlin, Heidelberg, New York: Springer 1973

369 Pöppel, E., Held, R., Dowling, J.E.: Neuronal mechanisms in visual perception. Neurosci. Res. Program Bull. 15 (1977) 313–319, 323–353

369a Price, C.J.: The anatomy of language: contributions from functional anatomy. J. Anat. 197 (2000) 335–359

370 Putz, R., Pabst, R.: Sobotta Atlas of human anatomy Vol.1. Head, neck, upper limb. Munic, Jena: Urban und Fischer 2001

371 Quaknine, G.E.: Microsurgical anatomy of the arterial loops in the ponto-cerebellar angle and the internal acoustic meatus. 378–390 In: Samii, M., Jannetta, P.J. (Eds.): The cranial nerves. Berlin, Heidelberg, New York: Springer 1981

372 Raab, P., Pilatus, U., Lanfermann, H., Zanella, F.E.: Grundlagen und klinische Anwendung der MR-Spektroskopie des Gehirns. Akt. Neurol. 29 (2002) 53 – 62

373 Radü, E.W., Kendall, B.E., Moseley, I.F.: Computertomographie des Kopfes. Stuttgart, New York: Thieme 1994

374 Raichle, M.E., Hartman, B.K., Eichling, J.O., Sharpe, L.G.: Central noradrenergic regulation of cerebral blood flow and vascular permeability. Proc. nat. Acad. Sci. (Wash.) 72 (1975) 3726–3730

374a Ramachandran, V.S.: Encyclopedia of the human brain. Amsterdam, Boston: Academic Press 2002

375 Ramsey, R.: Neuroradiology. Philadelphia: Saunders 1994

376 Ramsey, R.: Teaching atlas of spine imaging. Stuttgart, New York: Thieme 1999

376a Reither, M.: Magnetresonanztomographie in der Pädiatrie. Berlin, Heidelberg, New York: Springer 2000

377 Rennie, J.M.: Neonatal cerebral ultrasound. Cambridge: Cambridge Univ. Press 1997

378 Retzius, G.: Das Menschenhirn. Studien in der makroskopischen Morphologie. Band 1. Stockholm: Norstedt 1896

379 Reynolds, A.F., Harris, A.B., Ojemann, G.A., Turner, P.T.: Aphasia and left thalamic hemorrhage. J. Neurosurg.48 (1978) 570–574

380 Riley, H.A.: An atlas of the basal ganglia, brain stem, and spinal cord. New York: Hafner 1960

381 Ring, A., Waddington, M.M.: Roentgenographic anatomy of the pericallosal arteries. Amer. J. Roentgenol. 104 (1968) 109–118

381a Rockstroh, S.: Einführung in die Neuropsychopharmakologie. Bern: H. Huber 2001

382 Rohen, J.W., Yokochi, C.: Color atlas of anatomy: photographic study of the human body. Baltimore: Schattauer 1998

383 Rohkamm, R.: Taschenatlas Neurologie. Stuttgart, New York: Thieme 2003

384 Roland, P.E., Skinhoj, E., Lassen, N.A.: Different cortical areas in man in organisation of voluntary movements in extrapersonal space. J. Neurophysiol. 43 (1980) 137–150

385 Roland, P.E.: Cortical organization of voluntary behavior in man. Human Neurobiol. 4 (1985) 155–167

386 Roland, P.E.: Metabolic measurement of the working frontal cortex in man. Trends in neurosciences 7 (1984) 430–435

387 Rosene, D.L., Hoesen, G.W. van: Hippocampal efferents reach widespread areas of cerebral cortex and amygdala in the rhesus monkey. Science 198 (1977) 315–317

388 Ross, E.D.: Localization of the pyramidal tract in the internal capsule by whole brain dissection. Neurology 30 (1980) 59–64

389 Röther, J., Gass, A., Busch, E.: Diffusions- und perfusionsgewichtete Magnetresonanztomographie bei der zerebralen Ischämie. Akt. Neurologie 26 (1999) 300 – 308

390 Röthig, W.: Korrelationen zwischen Gesamthirn- und Kleinhirngewicht des Menschen im Laufe der Ontogenese. J. Hirnforsch. 15 (1974) 203–209

391 Rubin, G.D., Shiau, M.C., Schmidt, A.J., Fleischmann, D., Logan, L., Leung, A.N., Jeffrey, R.B., Napel, S.: Computed tomographic angiography: historical perspective and new state-of-the-art using multi detector-row helical computed tomography. J. computer assisted tomography 23 (1999) 83 90

392 Rumeau, C., Tzourio, N., Murayama, N., Peretti-Viton, P., Levrier, O., Joliot, M., Mazoyer, B., Salamon, G.: Location of hand function in the sensimotor cortex: MR and functional correlation. Am. J. Neuroradiol. 15 (1994) 567–572

393 Rutherford, M. (Ed.): MRI of the neonatal brain. Londen, Edinburgh, New York: Saunders 2002

394 Sabattini, L.: Evaluation and measurement of the normal ventricular and subarachnoid spaces by CT. Neuroradiology 23 (1982) 1–5

395 Sadler, T.W.: Medizinische Embryologie. Stuttgart, New York: Thieme 2003

396 Salvolini, U., Cabanis, E.A., Rodallec, A., Menichelli, F., Pasquini, U., Iba-Zizen, M.T.: Computed tomography of the optic nerve. Part 1: Normal results. J. Comput. assist. Tomogr. 2 (1978) 141–149

397 Samii, M., Draf, W.: Surgery of the skull base. Berlin, Heidelberg, New York, London, Paris, Tokyo: Springer 1989

398 Samii, M., Jannetta, P.J. (Eds.): The cranial nerves. Berlin, Heidelberg, New York: Springer 1981

399 Sanides, F., Vitzthum, H.: Zur Architektonik der menschlichen Sehrinde und dem Prinzip ihrer Entwicklung. Dtsch. Z. Nervenheilkd. 187 (1965) 680–707

400 Sanides, F.: Representation in the cerebral cortex and its areal lamination patterns. In: Bourne, G.H. (Ed.): The structure and function of nervous tissue. New York, London: Academic Press 1972 329–453

401 Saper, C.B., Petito, C.K.: Correspondence of melanin-pigmented neurons in human brain with A1-A14 catecholamine cell groups. Brain 105 (1982) 87–101

402 Sarkisoff, S.A., Filimonoff, I.N.: Atlas du cerveau de l'homme et des animaux. Moscou: Institut du Cerveau de C.C.E. de-LURSS 1937

403 Sartor, K. (Ed.): Diagnostic and interventional neuroradiology. Stuttgart, New York: Thieme 2002

404 Sartor, K.: MR Imaging of the skull and brain. Berlin, Heidelberg, New York: Springer 1992

405 Savoiardo, M., Bracchi, M., Passerini, A., Visciani, A.: The vascular territories of the cerebellum and brainstem: CT and MR study. Am. J. Neuroradiol. 8 (1987) 199–209

406 Schaltenbrand, G., Walker, A.E. (Eds.): Stereotaxy of the human brain. Anatomical, physiological and clinical applications. Stuttgart: Thieme 1982

407 Schering: Lexikon der Radiologie. Bearbeitet von der Lexikonredaktion des Verlages. Berlin, Wien: Blackwell Wissenschaftsverlag 1996

408 Schiebler, T.H., Schmidt, W., Zilles, K. (Eds.): Anatomie. Berlin, Heidelberg, New York: Springer 1999

409 Schirmer, M.: Neurochirurgie. München: Urban und Schwarzenberg 1998

410 Schlegel, U., Westphal, M.: Neuroonkologie. Stuttgart, New York: Thieme 1998

411 Schliack, H., Hopf, H.C. (Eds.): Diagnostik in der Neurologie. Stuttgart, New York: Thieme 1988

412 Schmahmann, J.D.: Cerebellum and brainstem p. 207 – 259 in Toga, A.W., Mazziotta, J.C.: Brain Mapping. San Diego, San Francisco: Academic Press 2000

413 Schmahmann, J.D., Doyon, J., McDonald, D., Holmes, C., Lavoie, K., Hurwitz, A.S., Kabani, N., Toga, A., Evans, A., and Petrides, M.: Three-dimensional MRI atlas of the human

cerebellum in proportion stereotaxic space. NeuroImage. (1999) Vol. 10 issue 3 233–260
414 Schmahmann, J.D., Loeber, R.T., Marjani, J., and Hurwitz, A.S.: Topographic organization of cognitive functions in the human cerebellum. A meta-analysis of functional imaging studies. NeuroImage 7 (1998) 5721
414a Schmahmann, J.D., Sherman, J.C.: The cerebellar cognitive affective syndrome. Brain 121 (1998) 561–579
415 Schmalstieg, H., Becker, H.: 3D-CT der Schädelbasis. Klinische Neuroradiologie 5 (1995) 71–81
416 Schmid, H.-M.: Über Größe, Form und Lage von Bulbus und Tractus olfactorius des Menschen. Gegenbaurs morph. Jb. (Lpzg.) 119 (1973) 227–237
416a Schmidek, H.H., Sweet, W.H.: Operative neurosurgical techniques. Philadelphia: Saunders 2000
417 Schmidt, A. M.: Computergestützte 3D-Rekonstuktion des trigeminalen Systems – vom Hirnstamm bis zum Eintritt in den Thalamus – als Referenz für die bildgebenden Verfahren CT, MRT und PET. Dissertation der Medizinischen Hochschule Hannover 2002
418 Schmidt, A.M., Weber, B.P., Becker, H.: Functional magnetic resonance imaging of the auditory cortex as diagnostic tool in cochlear implant candidates. Neuroimaging Clinics of North America 11 (2001) 297 – 304
419 Schmidt, D., Malin, J.-P. (Eds.): Erkrankungen der Hirnnerven. Stuttgart, New York: Thieme 1995
420 Schmidt, R.F., Schaible, H.-G. (Eds.): Neuro- und Sinnesphysiologie. Berlin, Heidelberg, New York: Springer 2001
421 Schneider, J.S, Lidsky, T.L. (Eds.): Basal ganglia and behavior: Sensory aspects of motor functioning. Toronto, Lewiston, New York, Stuttgart: Huber 1987
422 Schnitzlein, H.N., Murtagh, F.R.: Imaging anatomy of the head and spine. Baltimore, Munich: Urban und Schwarzenberg 1990
423 Schnyder, H., Reisine, H., Hepp, K., Henn, V.: Frontal eye field projection to the paramedian pontine reticular formation traced with wheat germ agglutinin in the monkey. Brain Res. 329 (1985) 151–160
424 Schultze, W.H.: Über Messungen und Untersuchungen des Liquor cerebrospinalis an der Leiche. In: Schmidt, M.B., Berblinger, W. (Eds.): Centralblatt für allgemeine Pathologie und pathologische Anatomie. Ergänzungsheft zum Band 33. Jena: Fischer 1923 291–296
425 Schwartz, A., Kischka, U., Rihs, F.: Funktionelle bildgebende Verfahren 295 – 318 In Kischka, U., Wallesch, C.-W., Wolf, G. (Eds.) Methoden der Hirnforschung. Heidelberg, Berlin: Spektrum Akademischer Verlag 1997
426 Seeger, W.: Atlas of topographical anatomy of the brain and surrounding structures for neurosurgeons, neuroradiologists, and neuropathologists. Wien, New York: Springer 1985
427 Seifritz, E., Salle, F. Di, Bilecen, D., Radü, E.W., Scheffler, K.: Auditory System: functional magnetic resonance imaging. Neuroimaging Clinics of North America 11 (2001) 275–296
428 Silverman, S.G., Collick, B.D., Figuera, M.R., Khorasani, R., Adams, D.F., Newman, R.W., Topulos, G.P., Jolesz, F.A.: Interactive MR-guided biopsy in an open-configuration MR imaging system. Radiology 197 (1995) 175–181
429 Singer, M., Yakovlev, P.I.: The human brain in sagittal section. Springfield/Ill.: Thomas 1964
430 Singer, W.: Control of thalamic transmission by corticofugal and ascending reticular pathways in the visual system. Physiol. Rev. 57 (1977) 386–420
431 Skalej, M., Schiefer, U., Nägele, T., Grodd, W., Voigt, K.: Funktionelle Bildgebung des visuellen Kortex mit der MRT. Klin. Neuroradiol. 5 (1995) 176–183
432 Slegte, R.G.M. de, Valk, J., Lohman, A.H.M., Zonneveld, F.W.: Cisternographic anatomy of the posterior cranial fossa. Assen/Maastricht, Wolfeboro, New Hampshire: Van Gorcum 1986
433 Smith, C.G., Richardson, W.F.G.: The course and distribution of the arteries supplying the visual (striate) cortex. Amer. J. Ophthal. 61 (1966) 1391–1396
434 Smith, R.L.: Axonal projections and connections of the principal sensory trigeminal nucleus in the monkey. J. comp. Neurol. 163 (1975) 347–376
435 Snyder, E.Y.: Neural stem-like cells: developmental lessons with therapeutic potential. The Neuroscientist 4 (1998) 408–425
436 Soininen, H.S., Partanen, K., Pitkanen, A., Vainio, P., Hanninen, T., Hallikainen, M., Koivisto, K., Riekkinen, P.J.: Volumetric MRI analysis of the amygdala and the hippocampus in subjects with age-associated memory impairment: correlation to visual and verbal memory. Neurology 44 (1994) 1660–1668
437 Spreer, J., Ziyeh, S., Wohlfahrt, R., Hammen, A., Schreiber, A., Hubbe, U., Schmider, K., Schumacher, M.: Vergleich verschiedener Paradigmen für die fMRT zur Bestimmung der Hemisphärendominanz für sprachliche Funktionen. Klinische Neuroradiologie 8 (1998) 173 – 181
438 Starck, D.: Die Evolution des Säugetier-Gehirns. Wiesbaden: Steiner 1962
439 Starck, D.: Vergleichende Anatomie der Wirbeltiere. Band 3. Berlin, Heidelberg, New York: Springer 1982
440 Stark, .D., Bradley, W.G.: Magnetic resonance imaging. St. Louis, Baltimore, Boston: Mosby 1999
441 Steinmetz, H., Furst, G., Freund, H.J.: Cerebral cortical localization: application and validation of the proportional grid system in MR imaging. J. Comput. Assist. Tomogr. 13 (1989) 10–19
442 Stensaas, S.S., Eddington, D.K., Dobelle, W.H.: The topography and variability of the primary visual cortex in man. J. Neurosurg. 40 (1974) 747–755
443 Stephan, H., Andy, O.J.: Anatomy of the limbic system. 269–292 In: Schaltenbrand, G., Walker, A.E. (Eds.): Stereotaxy of the human brain. Stuttgart, New York: Thieme 1982
444 Stephan, H.: Allocortex. In: Möllendorff, W. von, Bargmann, W., Oksche, A., Vollrath, L. (Eds.): Handbuch der mikroskopischen Anatomie des Menschen. Band 4: Nervensystem, Teil 9. Berlin, Heidelberg, New York: Springer 1975
445 Stoeter, P., Schumacher, M., Huk, W., Zanella, F., Grodd, W., Thron, A., Mödder, U.: Magnetresonanztomographie in der Neuroradiologie. Leitlinien herausgegeben von der Deutschen Gesellschaft für Neuroradiologie. Klin. Neuroradiol. 11 (2001) 1–5
446 Stöhr, M., Dichgans, J., Diener, H.C., Buettner, U.W.: Evozierte Potentiale SEP – VEP – AEP – EKP – MEP. Berlin, Heidelberg, New York, London, Paris, Tokyo, Hong Kong: Springer 1996
447 Stoppe, G., Hentschel, F., Munz, D.L. (Eds.): Bildgebende Verfahren in der Psychiatrie. Stuttgart, New York: Thieme 2000
448 Sunaert, S., Yousry, T.A.: Clinical application of functional magnetic resonance imaging. Neuroimaging Clinics of North America 11 (2001) 221 – 236
449 Swanson, L.W.: The locus coeruleus: a cytoarchitectonic, Golgi, and immunohistochemical study in the albino rat. Brain Res. 110 (1976) 39–56
450 Swartz, J.D., Harnsberger, H.R.: Imaging of the temporal bone. Stuttgart, New York: Thieme 1998
451 Swobodnik, W., Herrmann, M., Altwein, J.E. (Eds.): Atlas of ultrasound anatomy. Stuttgart, New York: Thieme 1999
452 Takahashi, S. (Ed.): Illustrated computer tomography. Berlin, Heidelberg, New York: Springer 1983
453 Talairach, J., Szikla, G., Tournoux, P., Prossalentis, A., Bordas-Ferrer, M., Covello, L., Jacob, M., Mempel, E.: Atlas d'anatomie stéréotaxique du télencéphale. Paris: Masson 1967
454 Talairach, J., Tournoux, P.: Co-planar stereotaxic atlas of the human brain. Stuttgart, New York: Thieme 1988
455 Tamraz, J.C., Comair, Y.G.: Atlas of regional anatomy of the brain using MRI. Berlin, Heidelberg, New York: Springer 2000
456 Tatu, L., Moulin, T., Bogousslavsky, J., Duvernoy, H.: Arterial territories of the human brainstem and cerebellum. Neurology 47 (1996) 1125–1135
457 Taveras, J.M. (Ed.): Radiology. Vol. 3. Philadelphia: Lippincott – Raven 1996
458 Tei, H.: Monoparesis of the right hand following a localised infarct in the left »precentral knob„. Neuroradiology 41 (1999) 269 – 270
459 Terr, L.I., Edgerton, B.J.: Surface topography of the cochlear nuclei in humans: Two- and three-dimensional analysis. Hearing Research 17 (1985) 51–59
460 Thier, P.: Das System der langsamen Augenfolgebewegungen. 65–74 In Huber, A. and Kömpf, D. (Eds.) Klinische Neuroophthalmologie. Stuttgart, New York: Thieme 1998
461 Thömke, F.:Augenbewegungsstörungen. Stuttgart, New York : Thieme 2001
462 Thurn, P., Bücheler, E.: Einführung in die radiologische Diagnostik. Stuttgart, New York: Thieme 1998
463 Tiedemann, K.: Anatomy of the head and neck: a multiplanar atlas for radiologists and surgeons. Weinheim, Basel, Cambridge: VCH 1993
464 Timmann, D., Kolb, F.P., Diener, H.C.: Klinische Pathophysiologie der Ataxie. Klin. Neurophysiol. 30 (1999) 128 – 144
465 Toga, A.W., Mazziotta, J.C. (Eds.): Brain mapping. The systems. San Diego, San Francisco, New York: Academic Press 2000
466 Toole, J.F.: Cerebrovascular disorders. Philadelphia: Lippincott, Williams and Wilkins 1999
467 Truwit, C.: High resolution atlas of cranial neuroanatomy. Philadelphia: Lippincott, Williams and Wilkens 1994

468 Uhlenbrock, D.: MRT und MRA des Kopfes. Stuttgart, New York: Thieme 1996
469 Unterharnscheidt, F., Jachnik, D., Gött, H.: Der Balkenmangel. Berlin, Heidelberg, New York: Springer 1968
470 Valvassori, G.E., Mafee, M.F., Carter, B.L.: Imaging of the head and neck. Stuttgart, New York: Thieme 1995
471 Vanier, M., Lecours, A.R., Ethier, R., Habib, M., Poncet, M., Milette, P.C., Salamon, G.: Proportional localization system for anatomical interpretation of cerebral computed tomograms. J. Comp. assist. Tomogr. 9 (1985) 715–724
471a Verhoeff, N.P.L.G.: Radiotracer imaging of dopaminergic transmission in neuropsychiatric disorders. Psychopharmacology 147 (1999) 217–249
471b Victor, M., Ropper, A.H.: Adams and Victor's principles of neurology. New York: Mc Graw-Hill 2001
472 Vogt, H.: Ein Algorithmus zur Oberflächenrekonstrukton von Großhirnarterien. Dissertation der Medizinischen Hochschule Hannover 1997
473 Voogd, J.: The cerebellum of the cat. Assen: Van Gorcum 1964
474 Waddington, M.M.: Atlas of cerebral angiography with anatomic correlations. Boston: Little and Brown 1974
475 Wahler-Lück, M., Schütz, T., Kretschmann, H.-J.: A new anatomical representation of the human visual pathways. Graefe's Arch. Clin. Exp. Ophthalmol. 229 (1991) 201–205
476 Walker, A.E.: Normal and pathological physiology of the thalamus. In: Schaltenbrand, G., Walker, A.E. (Eds.): Stereotaxy of the human brain, 2nd ed. Stuttgart, New York: Thieme 1982 181–217
477 Warabi, T., Miyasaka, K., Inoue, K., Nakamura, N.: Computed tomographic studies of the basis pedunculi in chronic hemiplegic patients: Topographic correlation between cerebral lesion and midbrain shrinkage. Neuroradiology 29 (1987) 409–415
478 Watanabe, T., Taguchi, Y., Shiosaka, S., Tanaka, J., Kubota, H., Terano, Y., Tohyama, M., Wada, H.: Distribution of the histaminergic neuron system in the central nervous system of rats: A fluorescent immunohistochemical analysis with histidine decarboxylase as a marker. Brain Res. 295 (1984) 13–25
479 Weirich, D.: Computergestützte 3D-Rekonstruktion des medialen Lemniscussystems als Referenz für die bildgebenden Verfahren CT, MRT und PET. Med. Dissertation der Med. Hochschule Hannover 1994
480 Weismann, M., Yousry, I., Heuberger, E., Nolte, A., Ilmberger, J., Kobal, G., Yousry, T.A., Kettenmann, B., Naidich, T.P.: Functional magnetic resonance imaging of human olfaction. Neuroimaging Clinics of North America 11 (2001) 237–250
481 Wellhöner, H.-H.: Allgemeine und systematische Pharmakologie und Toxikologie. Berlin, Heidelberg, New York: Springer 1997
482 Wessely, W.: Biometrische Analyse der Frischvolumina des Rhombencephalon, des Cerebellum und der Ventrikel von 31 adulten menschlichen Gehirnen. J. Hirnforsch. 12 (1970) 11–28
483 Westheimer, G., Blair, S.M.: Oculomotor defects in cerebellectomized monkeys. Invest. Ophtalmol. 12 (1973) 618–621
484 Westrum, L.E., Canfield, R.C., Black, R.G.: Transganglionic degeneration in the spinal trigeminal nucleus following removal of tooth pulps in adult cats. Brain Res. 101 (1976) 137–140
485 Whitehouse, P.J., Price, D.L., Clark, A.W., Coyle, J.T., DeLong, M.R.: Alzheimer disease: Evidence for selective loss of cholinergic neurons in the nucleus basalis. Ann. Neurol. 10 (1981) 122–126
486 Whitehouse, P.J., Price, D.L., Struble, R.G., Clark, A.W., Coyle, J.T., DeLong, M.R.: Alzheimer's disease and senile dementia: Loss of neurons in the basal forebrain. Science 215 (1982) 1237–1239
487 Wicke, L.: Atlas der Röntgenanatomie. München, Jena: Urban und Fischer 2001
488 Widder, B.: Doppler- und Duplexsonographie der hirnversorgenden Arterien. Berlin, Heidelberg, New York: Springer 1988
489 Wienhard, K., Wagner, R., Heiss, W.-D.: PET Grundlagen und Anwendungen der Positronen-Emissions-Tomographie. Berlin, Heidelberg, New York, London, Paris, Tokyo: Springer 1989
490 Wiesendanger, M.: The pyramidal tract recent investigations on its morphology and function. Ergebn. Physiol. 61 (1969) 72–136
491 Wilkins, R.H., Rengachary, S.S. (Eds.): Neurosurgery. New York, St. Louis, San Francisco: McGraw-Hill 1995
492 Williams, P.L., Bannister, L.H.: Gray's anatomy. New York: Livingstone 1995
493 Williams, T.H., Gluhbegovic, N., Jew, J.Y.: The human brain [electronic resource]. Iowa City, Iowa: University of Iowa 2000
494 Willis, W.D. (Jr.): The pain system. Basel: Karger 1985
495 Winkler, P.: Localization of the motor hand area to a knob on the precentral gyrus. A new landmark. Brain 120 (1997) 141–157
495a Winn, H.R., Youmans, J.R.: Youmans neurological surgery. Philadelphia: Saunders 2003
496 Wise, S.P.: Frontal cortex activity and motor set. In: Ito, M. (Ed.): Neural programming. Basel: Karger 1989 25–38
497 Wolf, G.: Epiphysen- und Plexusverkalkungen in der Computertomographie. Med. Dissertation Medizinische Hochschule Hannover 1980
498 Wolf, K.-J., Fobbe, F.: Color duplex sonography. Stuttgart, New York: Thieme 1995
498a Woogd, J., Glickstein, M.: The anatomy of the cerebellum. Trends Neurosci. 21 (1998) 370–375
499 Woolsey, C.N., Erickson, T.C., Gilson, W.E.: Localization in somatic sensory and motor areas of human cerebral cortex as determined by direct recording of evoked potentials and electrical stimulation. J. Neurosurg. 51 (1979) 476–506
499a Woolsey, T.A., Hanaway, J., Gado, M.H.: The brain atlas. Hoboken, New Jersey: Wiley and Sons 2003
500 Yagishita, A., Nakano, I., Oda, M., Hirano, A.: Location of the corticospinal tract in the internal capsule at MR imaging. Radiology 191 (1994) 455–460
501 Yasargil, M.G.. Smith, R.D., Young, P.H., Teddy, P.J.: Microneurosurgery. Vol. 1. Stuttgart, New York: Thieme-Stratton 1984
502 Youmans, J.R.: Neurological surgery. A comprehensive reference guide to the diagnosis and management of neurosurgical problems. Philadelphia, London, Toronto: Saunders 1996
503 Yousry, I., Naidich, T.P., Yousry, T.A.: Functional magnetic resonance imaging: factors modulating the cortical activation pattern of the motor system. Neuroimaging Clinics of North America 11 (2001) 195–202
504 Yousry, T., Schmidt, D., Alkadhi, H., Winkler, P., Schmid, U. Peraud, A.: New anatomic landmark for the identification of the precentral gyrus: validation and characterization. Radiology 197 (1995) 373
505 Yousry, T.A., Fesl, G., Büttner, A., Noachter, S., Schmid, U.D.: Heschl's gyrus: anatomic description and methods of identification in MRI. Int. J. Neurorad. 3 (1997) 2–12
506 Yousry, T.A., Schmid U.D., Schmidt, D., Hagen, T., Jassoy, A., Reiser, M.F.: The central sulcal vein: a landmark for identification of the central sulcus using functional magnetic resonance imaging. J. Neurosurg. 85 (1996) 608–617
507 Yousry, T.A., Schmid, U.D., Alkadhi, H., Schmidt, D., Peraud, A., Buettner, A., Yousry, T.A., Schmidt, D., Alkadhi, H. et al.: Localization of the motor hand area to a knob on the precentral gyrus. A new landmark. Brain 120 (1997) 141–157
508 Yousry, T.A., Yousry, I., Naidich, T.P.: Progress in neuroanatomy. in: Demaerel, P. Recent advances in diagnostic neuroradiology. Berlin, Heidelberg, New York: Springer 2001
509 Zanella, F.E.: Bildgebung. In Schlegel, U., Westphal, M. (Hrsg.) Neuroonkologie. Stuttgart, New York: Thieme 1998
510 Zeumer, H., Hacke, W., Hartwich, P.: A quantitative approach to measuring the cerebrospinal fluid space with CT. Neuroradiology 22 (1982) 193–197
511 Zihl, J.: Zerebrale Sehstörungen. Akt. Neurologie 27 (2000) 13–21
512 Zihl, J., Cramon, D. von: Zerebrale Sehstörungen. Baumgartner, G., Cohen, R. Grüsser, O.-J., Helmchen, H., Schmidt, L.R. (Eds.): Psychiatrie, Neurologie, Klinische Psychologie. Grundlagen-Methoden-Ergebnisse. Stuttgart, Berlin, Köln, Mainz: Kohlhammer 1986
513 Zilles, K., Rehkämper, G.: Funktionelle Neuroanatomie. Berlin, Heidelberg, New York: Thieme 1998
514 Zilles, K.: The cortex. In: Paxinos, G. (Ed.): The human nervous system. 757–802 San Diego Academic Press 1990
515 Zimmerman, R.A., Gibby, W.A., Carmody, R.F.: Neuroimaging. Clinical and physical principles. Berlin, Heidelberg, New York: Springer 2000

10 Index for Text and Illustrations

Plain numbers refer to pages. Numbers preceded by the letter F refer to figures. On the inside front cover the reader will find a list giving the page numbers of each illustration.

Example: The venous angle F97a.8 can be found on page 284 in Figure 97a and is indicated by number 8.

A

A1-A7 (Noradrenergic neurons) 297, 417
A8-A15 (Dopaminergic neurons) 416
A-Amplitude 17
Abbreviations 11, 12
Abducens nerve 220, 226, 287, F3.32, F6a.15, F7a.18, F8a.22, F9a.30, F10a.34, F11a.41, F30b.18, F32a.35, F33a.31, F34a.24, F35a.19, F49a.5, F50a.9, F72b.8, F72b.10, F73b.7, F73b.13, F74b.6, F74b.17, F81, F82
– – near opening of dura mater F50a.11, F74b.9
– nuclear lesion 391
– nucleus 294, 388, F68.14, F74b.28, F119.9, F139.11, F140.11, F141.8
Accessory nerve 231, 233, 286, F3.37, F11a.45, F12a.39, F30b.26, F34a.31, F35a.32, F36a.25, F37a.20, F46.34, F49a.10, F81, F82
– – cranial and spinal roots 286
– – – near opening of dura mater F70a.17
– – nucleus of oculomotor nerve (of Edinger–Westphal) 298, 412, F68.9, F151.2
Accommodation of eyes 412
Acervulus 306
Acetylcholin 418
Acoustic radiation 355, F122.9, F123.2, F124.10, F124.13, F124.15, F125.8
– schwannoma 359
– window 2
ACTH 11, 307
Action tremor 397
Adenohypophysis 307, F75b.2
ADH 11, 305
Adiadochokinesis 397
Adrenaline-synthesizing nerve cells 417
Adrenergic neurons 297, 416, 417
Adrenocorticotropic hormone 11, 307
Advances in neuroradiology 1
Advantage of graphic illustrations 2
AEP 11, 359
AICA 11, 254, 263, F32c.29, F34c.24, F49c.15, F50c.18, F73b.28, F88.5, F89a.4
A-image 17
Air-filled cavities 18
Akinetic mutism 303
Alexia 278, 324
Allocating level of slices 12
Allocortex 322
Alpha-motor neurons 418
Alphanumeric abbreviations for cerebellum according to Larsell 304

Alveolar process of maxilla F5c.23, F38.33, F39.24
Alveus 253, 404, F52a.23, F53a.35
Alzheimer's disease 419
Amaurosis fugax 369
Amaurotic iridoplegia 393
Ambient cistern 238, 242, 298, F52b.18, F52d.18, F77a.16, F77c.13, F77d.13, F78b.30, F78c.11, F78d.11, F83a.6, F84.13, F85.27, F86a.8, F87.15
Ammon's horn 404
Ampulloglomerular organ 254
Amygdala 253, 309
Amygdaloid body 253, 308, 309, 372, 405, 417, 418, 420, F9b.20, F9d.20, F10a.27, F35a.21, F51a.12, F51b.11, F52a.21, F76b.5, F147.17, F148.8, F149.8, F150.2
Analgesia 420
Anastomoses 256
– between internal and external carotid arteries 220
– of cerebral arteries 271
Aneurysm 253
Angiogram 283
Angiography 1, 14
Angioma 253
Angle of mandible F2a.35
Angular artery 270, F12c.9, F13c.7, F14c.6, F15c.8, F16c.7, F17c.4, F35c.8, F36c.8, F37c.8, F55c.19, F56c.15, F57c.14, F91a,b.11
– gyrus 315, 400, F3.11, F15a.5, F16a.4, F31.14, F35a.4, F36a.9, F37a.8, F46.11, F56a.15, F57a.10, F145.4, F146.3
Anosmia 324, 372
Anterior arch of atlas 232, F2a.28, F10c.26, F23.15, F24.12, F32c.35, F38.29, F45a.27, F47a.14, F47b.8, F61.10
– auditory pathway 355
– basal cistern 239, 242, F83a.9, F84.2, F85.26 F86a.9, F87.3
– belly of digastric F4c.38, F5c.39, F6c.37, F33c.44, F34c.45
– cerebral artery 266, F7b.10, F7c.5, F7d.10, F8b.14, F8c.10, F8d.14, F32b.11, F32c.20, F32d.11, F33c.14, F51c.10, F52b.3, F52c.6, F53c.5, F54c.7, F77b.1, F78b.1, F78c.2, F78d.2, F90a,b.3, F91a,b.3, F91d.2
– – – artery A1- A2- segment 266
– – – cortical arteries 267
– – – postcommunicating part 267
– – – precommunicating part 266
– – – terminal arteries 267
– – vein 284
– choroidal artery 266, F9c.10, F10c.10, F33c.15, F92a, F93, F94, F95a, F96

– clinoid process 236, F2a.5, F8c.12, F22.2, F40.10, F45a.8, F65.7
– cochlear nucleus 354, 355, 418, F68.7, F72b.26, F122.20, F123.12, F124.9
– commissure 252, 305, 309, 323, 372, F2b.14, F9a.20, F9a.21, F9b.15, F32a.8, F32b.12, F33a.14, F34a.12, F35a.13, F45b.14, F53b.12, F67.5, F147.7
– communicating artery 267, F32c.18, F51c.9, F91c.13, F91d.3
– corticospinal tract 377, F133.12, F134.7, F135.2
– cranial fossa 239, F18.3, F19.3, F20.2, F38.8, F39.7, F40.6, F51c.4, F65.4
– ethmoidal artery 218, 220
– – foramen 218, 219
– horn of lateral ventricle 252, F7b.9, F7d.9, F8a.8, F8b.7, F8d.7, F9a.9, F9b.7, F9d.7, F10a.8, F10b.8, F10d.8, F53a.7, F53b.6, F53c.11, F53d.6, F54a.8, F54b.5, F54c.10, F54d.5, F55a.10, F55b.6, F55d.6, F83b.1, F84.4, F85.25, F86b.1, F91c.2, F91d.29
– inferior cerebellar artery 11, 254, 263, F32c.29, F34c.24, F49c.15, F50c.18, F73b.28, F88.5, F89a.4
– – temporal artery of posterior cerebral artery F91d.24
– intercavernous sinus F97b.2
– interpositus nucleus 304
– limb of internal capsule 323, F9a.12, F9b.6, F9d.6, F53a.17, F54a.7, F54b.6, F54d.6, F55b.9, F55d.9
– lobe of cerebellum 303, 304, 394, F12a.31, F13a.21, F14a.10, F15a.13, F33b.20, F33d.20, F51b.16, F74a.16, F74c.9, F74d.9, F75a.17, F75c.11, F75d.11, F76a.19, F76c.10, F76d.10, F77a.18, F78a.11, F142, F143
– – – pituitary gland 307
– median fissure of medulla oblongata 297, F12a.46, F47a.19, F48a.2, F69b.20, F70b.11, F71b.9
– nasal aperture F30a.14
– – spine F2a.27, F38.24, F45a.25
– nuclei of thalamus 306, 404, 405, 417, F10a.14, F54a.23, F147.5
– parietal artery 270, F12c.5, F13c.6, F14c.3, F15c.2, F91a,b.9
– part of muscle cone 233
– – – pons 294
– petroclinoidal fold F10a.33
– quadrangular lobule (H IV, H V) 304
– ramus of lateral sulcus (Sylvian fissure) 313, F3.15, F46.19, F108b.19
– root of fifth cervical spinal nerve F12a.47

10 Index for Text and Illustrations

Anterior root of first cervical spinal nerve F3.38, F12a.42, F30b.28, F33a.39, F34a.34, F47a.20
– – – of second cervical spinal nerve F12a.44, F33a.40
– – – of third cervical spinal nerve and ganglion F34a.38
– semicircular canal 237, F11b.24, F11d.24, F50b.18, F50c.17, F65.12, F74a.14, F74b.13
– spinal artery 254
– spinocerebellar tract 394, F69b.23, F70b.21, F71b.21, F144a.8
– spinothalamic tract 326, F109.7, F110.1
– temporal artery of middle cerebral artery F91a,b.15
– transverse temporal gyrus (of Heschl) 316, 322, 355, 357, F12a.11, F36a.11, F37a.11, F123.1, F124.14
– trigeminothalamic tract 338, 342, F114.11
– vein of septum pellucidum 283, F54c.11, F97a.6
Anterolateral central arteries 275, F52c.9, F52c.10, F53c.12, F77b.5
– system 326
– territory of medulla oblongata 257
– – – midbrain 263
– – – pons 263
Anteromedial central arteries 266, 275, F52c.10, F77b.4
– frontal artery F4c.3, F5c.2, F6c.5, F32c.11, F33c.7, F34c.5, F53c.4, F54c.4, F90a,b.7, F91d.8
– territory of medulla oblongata 257
– – – midbrain 263
– – – pons 263
Antidiuretic hormone 11
Anvil 237, F50c.14
Apex of petrous part of temporal bone F64.10
Aphasia 325
Aplasia of corpus callosum 325
Apraxia 324
Aqueduct of midbrain 252, 298, F2b.30, F12a.23, F32b.22, F45b.24, F52d.17, F53a.34, F53c.17, F67.16, F77a.17, F77b.32, F77c.12, F77d.12, F78a.10, F78b.27, F78c.10, F78d.10, F83b.11, F84.22, F85.15, F86b.11, F87.18
Arachnoid mater 239
Arch of axis F12c.29, F13c.28, F26.12, F27.10
– – fifth cervical vertebra F13c.31, F14c.25, F26.16, F27.13, F28.8
– – fourth cervical vertebra F12c.31, F13c.30, F26.15, F27.12
– – sixth cervical vertebra F14c.26, F28.9
– – third cervical vertebra F12c.30, F13c.29, F26.14, F27.11
Archicortex 322, 404
Arcuate eminence 237, F25.3, F42.6, F74a.18
– fasciculus 400, F145.1
– fibers 323
Area 4 375, 376, F132.4, F144b.1
– 5 375, 378
– 6 375, F132.5, F144b.1
– 19 388
– 39 388
– 41 355, 357
– 42 357
– 44 400
– on edge of insula 345

Areas (3, 1, 2) 375, 378
Arnold–Chiari malformation 234
Arterial territories 256–264, 271–282
– – in infratentorial space 3
– – – supratentorial space 3
– – of brainstem 256–263, F89b
– – – cerebellum 263, 264, F89b
– – – forebrain 271–278
– – – medulla oblongata 257, 263, F89b
– – – midbrain 263, F89b
– – – pons 263, F89b
Arteries in head and neck 234, 235
– – lateral facial region 229
– of brain 253–256, 264–271
– – oral cavity 228
– – orbit 220
– – pharyngeal wall 231
Artery of central sulcus 270, F10c.7, F11c.7, F12c.3, F13c.3, F35c.6, F36c.4, F37c.4, F55c.14, F56c.9, F57c.9, F91a,b.8
– – precentral sulcus 270, F9c.6, F10c.5, F11c.4, F35c.2, F36c.3, F37c.5, F54c.8, F55c.9, F56c.8, F57c.8, F91a,b.7
Articular disc of temporomandibular joint 228, F9c.22, F37c.18, F70a.11, F71a.11
– process of axis F12c.29, F26.12
– – – fifth cervical vertebra F26.16
– – – fourth cervical vertebra F12c.31, F26.15
– – – third cervical vertebra F12c.30, F26.14
– tubercle 228, F2a.17, F37c.16
Ascending pharyngeal artery 228, 231
– ramus of lateral sulcus (Sylvian fissure) 313 F3.14, F46.15, F53a.24, F108b.13
– reticular system 348
ASP 11, 419
Aspartate 11, 419
Aspartatergic neurons 419
Association areas 322
– fibers 323
Ataxia 303, 304, 325
Athetosis 385
Atlanto-occipital joint 232, F11c.29, F12c.24, F25.15, F26.10, F34c.30, F39.18, F40.23
– membrane 233, 254
Atlas 232, F30a.20, F33c.31, F67.42
– assimilation 234
– pictures 12
Atrium of lateral ventricle 253, F13a.9, F13b.10, F54b.26, F55c.16, F83b.6, F84.25, F85.34, F86b.6
Auditory evoked potentials 11, 358, 359
– pathway 355
– system 354–359
Auricle 229, F10c.25, F11c.19, F12c.17, F13c.18, F47a.18, F48c.19, F49c.21, F50.21, F51c.21, F52c.16, F53c.20, F61.16, F62.16, F69a.23, F70a.23, F71a.22, F72a.17, F73a.19, F74a.19, F75a.20
Autonomic nervous system 412, 414
Axial planes 4
Axis 232, 238, F2a.34, F10c.31, F11c.33, F24.16, F25.20, F33c.37, F34c.41, F35c.43, F39.25, F40.28, F41.20

B

B 11
B1–B9 (Serotoninergic neurons) 297, 417
Babinski reflex 375
– sign 324
Background of neuroimaging 1–4
BAEP 359
Basal ganglia of telencephalon 375, 383, 385, F99, F101, F103
– nucleus (of Meynert) 418, 419, F10a.23
– vein (of Rosenthal) 284, F8c.11, F9c.11, F10c.12, F11c.14, F12c.14, F13c.11, F51c.15, F52c.15, F53c.19, F78b.32, F97a.12
Base of frontal lobe F51d.4
– – middle cranial fossa F49d.5
– – occipital lobe F73a.27, F74a.27, F74c.12, F74d.12
– – temporal lobe F46.31, F49a.3, F49b.6, F73a.13, F73c.2, F73d.2
Basilar artery 254, 271, F10c.17, F32b.25, F32c.25, F32d.25, F49c.11, F50b.12, F50c.12, F50d.12, F51b.12, F51c.14, F51d.12, F72b.5, F73b.6, F73c.5, F73d.5, F74b.10, F74c.4, F74d.4, F75b.8, F75c.7, F75d.7, F76b.9, F76c.8, F76d.8, F88.4, F89a.3
– impression 234
– part of occipital bone F48c.11, F48d.6, F62.10
– plexus F97b.5
– sulcus F50a.12
Basion F45a.23, F62.11
Basket cells 419
Bed nucleus of stria terminalis 420
Bell's palsy 379
BERA 11, 359
Beta-emitting nuclide 17
Beta-endorphin 419
Beta-endorphin-containing neurons 420
Bicommissural line 5, 11, 19
– – defined by midpoints 5
– – Talairach 4, 5
– – (B) F32a
Bilateral lesion of hippocampal formation 405
B-image 17
Binasal hemianopia 369
Bineuronal pathway 412
Bipolar nerve cells in spiral ganglion F122.18
Bitemporal hemianopia 369
Biventral lobule (H VIII) 304
Blood vessels guideline structures 20
– – in head and neck 234, 235
– – of craniocervical junction 233
Blood–brain barrier 415
Blow-out fracture 218
Bochdalek's bouquet 239
Body of axis F23.18
– – caudate nucleus F10a.9, F10b.9, F10d.9, F34a.5, F136.5, F137.4, F137.9
– – corpus callosum F2b.5, F9a.7, F10a.6, F10b.6, F10d.6, F11a.6, F11b.6, F11d.6, F12a.8, F12b.7, F12d.7, F33b.7, F33d.7, F45b.5, F55a.8
– – fourth cervical vertebra F2a.40
– – hyoid bone F21.22
– – lateral ventricle 252, F11a.8, F11b.7, F11d.7, F12a.7, F12b.8, F12d.8, F55c.13, F56a.12, F56c.12, F56d.9, F83b.2, F84.19, F85.24, F86b.2, F91c.4, F91d.31, F126.13

– – mandible 211, F2a.37, F4c.33, F5c.31, F6c.29, F18.20, F19.18, F30a.25, F32c.44, F33c.39, F34c.44, F38.37, F39.27, F40.30
– – sphenoid 236
– – third cervical vertebra F2a.38, F11c.38
Bones of craniocervical junction 231, F79, F80
Bony artifacts in CT scans 237, 304
Border zone infarct 278
Brachiocephalic vein 233, 235
Brachium of inferior colliculus 355, F122.11, F123.8, F124.5, F125.6
Bracket sign 313
Brain volume 11
Brainstem 288
– acoustic evoked potential 359
– electric response audiometry 11, 359
– series 3, 421, 422
– syndrome 297
– tumors 298
Branch of lateral occipital artery F53c.22
– – middle meningeal artery F52c.4
Branches of middle cerebral artery F90a,b.2
– – ophthalmic artery 220
Bregma F38.1, F45a.1, F60c.2
Bridging vein 283, F8c.4, F11c.2, F32b.1, F32c.2, F53c.3
Brightness 17
Broad window 14
Broca's aphasia 277, 402
– area 313, 322, 400, F145.2, F146.1
Brodmann's areas (3, 1, 2) 322
Bromocriptine 416
Buccal fat pad (of Bichat) F5c.22
– nerve 229
Buccinator F4c.29, F5c.28, F6c.28
Bulb of internal jugular vein F69b.15, F70a.19
Bulbar palsy 298

C

C1–C3 (Adrenergic neurons) 417
Calcarine artery 256, F15c.11, F16c.8, F17c.5, F32a.15, F33c.12, F34c.11, F54c.22, F55c.23, F89a.11, F91d.19
– spur 253, 362
– sulcus 253, 315, 322, 362, F2b.23, F15a.12, F15b.6, F15d.6, F16a.9, F16b.6, F16d.6, F17a.8, F17b.5, F17d.5, F32b.17, F32d.17, F33a.16, F33b.12, F33d.12, F45b.20, F54a.44, F67.23, F77a.25, F78a.18, F78c.15, F78d.15, F108b.26, F126.17
Calcifications 21
Callosomarginal artery 267, F54c.5, F55c.6, F56c.7, F57c.7, F90a.5, F91d.5
Canthomeatal plane 2, 4
– series 421, 422
Carotid canal 237, 265, F23.10, F39.11, F40.16, F41.14, F63.14
– sulcus F22.4
– syphon F33b.18, F33d.18, F50b.10
Cartilage of pharyngotympanic tube F9c.24, F35c.29, F48c.9, F69b.5, F70b.2
Catecholaminergic neurons 416
Caudal part of spinal nucleus of trigeminal nerve 338, F69b.28, F70b.31
Caudate nucleus 306, 308, 323, 383, 385, 416, F9b.8, F9d.8, F11a.9, F12a.9, F33a.7, F34b.5, F34d.5

Cave of septum pellucidum F54a.9, F54b.8
Cavernous sinus 220, 235, 283, 287, F8c.15, F9c.13, F33c.21, F50c.9, F74b.2, F75b.4, F97a.4, F97b.3
– – syndrome 288
Central arterial territories of forebrain 271–278
Central artery of retina 220
– canal 288, F32a.43, F69b.26, F69c.9, F70b.30, F85.21
– dysregulation of body temperature 306
– lobule (II, III) 304
– nervous system 11
– part of lateral ventricle 252, 253, 306, F11a.8, F11b.7, F11d.7, F12a.7, F12b.8, F12d.8, F55c.13, F56a.12, F56c.12, F56d.9, F83b.2, F84.19, F85.24, F86b.2, F91c.4, F91d.31, F126.13
– sulcus 309, F3.4, F11a.4, F12a.4, F12b.4, F12d.4, F13a.3, F13b.3, F13d.3, F31.9, F33b.1, F33d.1, F34b.1, F34d.1, F35b.1, F35d.1, F36a.4, F36b.3, F36d.3, F37a.3, F37b.1, F37d.1, F46.2, F54a.29, F55a.11, F56a.7, F56b.7, F56d.7, F57a.4, F57b.8, F57d.8, F58a.5, F58b.9, F58d.9, F59a.4, F59b.9, F59d.9, F60a.2, F60b.3, F60d.3, F108b.2, F132.2
Centromedian nucleus of thalamus 383, F12a.16
Cerebellar ataxia 397
– cortex 394
– hypoplasia 325
– nuclei 394, 419
– peduncles 288, 394
– systems 394–397
Cerebellopontine angle 359
– – syndrome 288
– cistern 239, 304, F50d.13, F73b.16, F73c.9, F73d.9, F74b.12, F75b.12, F84.18, F85.33, F87.6
Cerebellum 303, 304, 394, 417, F3.35, F12b.26, F12d.26, F34b.13, F34d.13, F35b.15, F35d.15, F45b.33, F46.29, F98, F99, F100, F101, F102, F103, F119.6, F132.11
Cerebral angiography 253
– arteries 422
– cortex 308, 317, 418
– crus 298, 303, 378, F52a.28, F52b.12, F52d.12, F77a.14, F77c.10, F77d.10, F78b.9, F78c.8, F78d.8
– edema 238
– ischemia 253
– lobes 309
– peduncle of midbrain 293, 298, 303
Cerebrospinal fluid 11
Cerebrospinal-fluid-containing spaces 239–253
Cerulean nucleus 297, 417–419, F51a.20, F52a.34, F75b.22, F76b.23, F77b.28
Cervical spinal nerves 233, F81, F82
Ch 11
Ch1–Ch6 (Cholinergic neurons) 418
Chance of errors 16
Chemoarchitecture 415
Chiari malformation 234, 304
Chiasmatic cistern 242, F83a.10, F84.7, F85.13, F86a.10
Choanae 211, 236
Cholinergic 11
– neurons 297, 418
Chorda tympani 228, 229, 414, F118.2, F151.17

Choreoathetoid movements 307
Choroid 226
Choroid plexus F10a.11, F72b.13
– – in atrium of lateral ventricle F54c.20, F54d.25
– – of central part of lateral ventricle 253
– – – fourth ventricle 242, F13a.24, F74b.31, F85.19
– – – inferior horn of lateral ventricle F35a.14
– – – lateral ventricle F11a.10, F13d.9, F33a.9, F53d.22, F55c.16, F85.29
– – – temporal horn of lateral ventricle F35a.14
– – – third ventricle 252, F85.4
Ciliary body 226
– ganglion 226, 412, F151.9
– muscle 226, 287, 412
Cingulate cortex 416, 418
– gyrus 316, 322, 323, 326, 404, F2b.3, F6a.5, F6b.4, F6d.4, F7a.5, F7b.6, F7d.6, F8a.5, F8b.3, F8d.3, F9a.5, F9b.4, F9d.4, F10a.4, F10b.4, F10d.4, F11a.5, F11b.4, F11d.4, F12a.5, F12b.6, F12d.6, F13a.6, F13b.6, F13d.6, F32b.2, F32d.2, F33a.5, F45b.4, F52a.6, F53a.4, F54a.5, F55a.5, F55b.4, F55d.4, F56a.8, F56b.10, F57a.6, F147.1
– sulcus F2b.2, F6a.4, F7a.3, F8a.4, F9a.4, F32a.1, F33b.6, F33d.6, F45b.3, F55a.4, F56a.4, F56b.4, F56d.4, F57a.5, F57d.5, F108b.23
Cingulum 323, 405, 417, 418, F56a.9, F56b.11, F147.2
Circadian rhythms 420
Circle of Willis 271, 307
Circled number of slices 12
Circular sulcus of insula F52a.9, F53a.8, F54a.33
Circumventricular organs 415
Cistern of great cerebral vein 242, F52b.20, F52d.20, F53b.21, F53d.21, F83a.7, F84.26, F85.8, F86a.5, F87.19
– – lamina terminalis 242, F83a.3, F84.6, F85.9, F86a.4, F87.12
– – lateral cerebral fossa 242, F11b.11, F11d.11, F36b.9, F36d.9, F52b.4, F52d.4, F53b.16, F53d.16, F54b.17, F54d.17, F55b.14, F55d.14, F84.5, F85.36, F87.13
– – Sylvian fissure 242, F11b.11, F11d.11, F36b.9, F36d.9, F52b.4, F52d.4, F53b.16, F53d.16, F54b.17, F54d.17, F55b.14, F55d.14, F84.5, F85.36, F87.13
– – transverse cerebral fissure 242, F83a.2, F84.20, F85.5, F86a.2
– – vallecula cerebri 242, F51d.8, F78c.3, F78d.3, F84.10, F85.30, F87.8
Cisterna magna 239, F13b.27, F13b.22, F13d.22, F14a.19, F15a.21, F32b.36, F32d.36, F48b.16, F48d.16, F67.41, F69a.24, F69b.34, F69c.12, F69d.12, F70a.25, F83a.13, F84.28, F85.22, F86a.13, F87.2
Cisternal puncture 234, 239
Cisterns 239
– guideline structures 19, 20
Claustrum 308, 309, 323, F9a.16, F10a.22, F10b.17, F35a.9, F52a.13, F53a.11, F54a.15, F55a.13, F136.4, F138.6
Clinical significance of craniocervical junction 233
– value of new imaging techniques 21

Clivus 236, F2a.13, F32c.28, F38.18, F45a.17, F49b.7, F49c.10, F49d.7, F63.12, F67.27, F70a.13, F70c.4, F70d.4, F71b.4, F71c.2, F71d.2, F72a.11, F72c.2, F72d.2, F73c.3, F73d.3
Closed portion of medulla oblongata 288, F69c.8, F69d.8
CNS 11
Cochlea F24.6, F36c.19, F49b.11, F64.11, F73b.5
Cochlear nerve 354, F122.19, F123.6, F124.8, F124.12, F125.1
– nuclei 294, F125.2
Collateral circulation 253
– sulcus F52a.36, F53a.43
– trigone 253
Collaterals 256
Collicular artery 256
Column of fornix 309, F53a.21, F53b.11, F54b.12
Commissural fibers 323
Commissure of inferior colliculus F122.13
Common carotid artery 234, F10c.38, F37c.44
– pathway 325
– tendinous ring 219, 220
Computed tomographs with spiral technique 2
– tomography 1, 11, 14, 18
– – angiography 11, 15
Computergraphic representation of neurofunctional systems 3
Condylar process 211, F43.11
Cones 226, 361
Confluence of sinuses 233, 236, 284, F17c.8, F32b.29, F32c.26, F32d.29, F53c.25, F74a.26, F74c.11, F74d.11, F97a.14, F97b.14
Congenital malformations 234
Conjugate deviation 391
Conjunctiva 219
Constrictor of pharynx 230, 231, F9c.33, F10c.36, F33c.35
Contralateral hemiplegia 379
– innervation of spinal motor neurons 378
– paresis 297
Contrast medium 15, 16, 359
Control circuits 383
– of autonomic activities 305
Conventional neuroradiologic procedures 18
Coordinate crosses 10
– frames 10
– framework 422
– planes 421
– system 3, 10
Coordinative role of cerebellum 394
Core 415
Cornea 226
Corneoscleral junction 219
Corona radiata F55a.16
Coronal planes 5
– series 421, 422
– suture 5, 238, F32c.1, F33c.1, F34c.1, F35c.1, F36c.1, F37c.1, F38.1, F39.1, F40.1, F41.1, F42.1, F43.1, F53c.7, F54c.6, F55c.7, F56c.6, F57c.6, F58c.5, F59c.3, F60c.3
Coronoid process 211, 228, F2a.21, F6c.25, F7c.23, F20.14, F37c.22, F43.10, F69a.7
Corpus callosum 93, 307, 323, 324, F8b.5, F8d.5, F9b.5, F9d.5, F54a.6, F55b.5, F55d.5, F67.1, F108b.24, F147.4

Corresponding (homonymous) halves of visual field F126.1
Cortex of frontal lobe F105, F106, F108a
– – insula F35a.6, F36a.10
– – occipital lobe F105, F106, F108a
– – parietal lobe F105, F106, F108a
– – telencephalon F98, F99, F100, F101, F102, F103
– – temporal lobe F105, F106, F108a
Cortical blindness 324, 369
– deafness 324
Corticectomy 362
Corticofugal fibers F139.5, F140.2
Corticoliberin 419
Corticonuclear fibers 375, 378, 383
– tract 303, F77b.16, F78b.11
Corticopontine fibers 294
– tract 394, 419, F144a.2
Corticospinal fibers 375, 376, 380, 383
– – of cerebral crus 377
– – – internal capsule 376
– – – medulla oblongata 377
– – – pons 377
– system 375
– tract 303, 419, F69b.21, F70b.12, F71b.10, F72b.9, F73b.11, F74b.11, F75b.9, F76b.13, F77b.17, F78b.12, F132.7, F133.3, F134.10, F134.11, F135.3
– – in cerebral crus F133.4, F134.3
– – in pons F134.4, F134.12
– – in posterior limb of internal capsule F133.7, F134.14
– – in pyramid F133.10, F134.5
Corticostriatal tract 419
Corticotectal tract 419
Corticothalamic tract 419
Corticotropic cells 307
Cranial cavity 238, 239
– fossae 239
– nerves 286–288
– roots of accessory nerve F70b.22
Craniocervical junction 231
Cribriform plate of ethmoid 210, 238, 239, 287, 317, 372, F5c.13, F19.4, F38.12
Cricoid cartilage F10c.37, F23.21
Crista galli 210, 238, 239, F4c.7, F18.2, F30a.4, F32c.16, F38.7, F50c.3, F51d.2, F64.3, F77a.4, F78a.2
Crossed impairment 342
– paralysis 264
Crossing of auditory pathway 355
– – optic nerves 218
CSF 11, 239
– spaces 18, 19, 239–253
CT 11, 18
– angiography 253
– bony artifacts 369
– images 422–424
– investigation 211
CTA 11, 15, 253, 278
CT-Angio 11
Culmen (IV, V) 303, 304, F2b.32, F32a.20, F32b.23, F32d.23, F67.13, F142.1
Cuneate fasciculus 331, F111.8, F112.11, F113.1
– nucleus (of Burdach) 293, 331, F69b.29, F70b.27, F71b.22, F111.6, F112.8, F113.4
– tubercle F48a.8, F49a.15
Cuneocerebellar tract 394
Cuneus 315, 362, F2b.16, F15a.9, F16a.7, F17a.6, F45b.12, F55a.26, F56a.20, F57a.15, F91d.33

D

Damage to upper motor neurons 375
Dandy-Walker malformation 234
Declive (VI) 303, 304, 388, F2b.35, F32a.29, F32b.27, F32d.27, F67.26, F140.17, F141.10, F142.3
Decussation of efferent cerebellar pathways 397
– – superior cerebellar peduncles F77b.22, F144a.5
– – trochlear nerves F77b.33
Deep cerebral vein of anterior perforated substance 284
– lateral facial region 229
– veins of brain 283
Dementia 385
Dens of axis 232, 238, F2a.29, F11b.26, F11c.30, F11d.26, F24.13, F25.16, F30a.18, F32c.36, F38.31, F45a.28, F47a.15, F47b.11, F61.12
Dentate gyrus 322, 404, F78b.24, F147.19
– – nucleus 304, 383, 395, F14a.17, F33a.27, F51a.24, F73a.21, F73b.32, F74a.21, F74b.34, F142.10, F144b.8
Dermatome 331
Descending palatine artery F6c.24
– – vein F6c.24
Detailed recognition of anatomic structures 18
Deutsche Horizontale 4, 11
DH 4, 11
Diabetes insipidus 305
Diagonal band (of Broca) 418
– sulcus F108b.21
Diaphragma sellae 307
Diencephalon 305–307, F98, F99, F101, F102, F103
Digastric 227
– tendon F7c.34, F8c.37, F35c.47
Digital subtraction angiography 11, 14
Dilator pupillae 226, 414
Diploic veins 235
Diplopia 392
Disadvantages of MRI and CT 1
Discrepancy between clinical findings and neuroimaging 3
Dislocations of craniocervical junction 233
Disorders of basal ganglia 385
Dissociated nystagmus 349
– sensory disorder 342
Distal medial striate artery 266, 275
Disturbances of equilibrium 304, 349
– of olfaction 372
– – speech 304
Dopamine 383
– agonist 416
Dopaminergic neurons 303, 404, 416
Doppler sonography 17, 19, 20, 235
Dorsal cochlear nucleus F68.7, F72b.26, F122.23, F123.12, F124.9
– column–lemniscal pathway 331, 332
– funiculus F47a.22
– gray horn of spinal cord 420
– nucleus of vagus nerve 294, 415, 417, F68.18, F70b.25, F71b.26
– root of second cervical spinal nerve F33a.40
– – – spinal nerve F109.9, F111.10
– – – third cervical spinal nerve and ganglion F34a.38
Dorsolateral pontine nuclei 388, F140.5, F141.13
– prefrontal cortex 388, F139.4, F141.15

Dorsum sellae 236, F38.11, F45a.9, F50c.11, F65.11, F75b.6, F76b.6
Drunken gait 397
DSA 11, 14
Duplex scan 17
– sonography 19
Dura mater 239, F4a.5, F5a.4, F6a.6, F7a.8, F15a.7, F16a.11, F17a.9, F36a.1, F37a.1, F48a.10, F49a.19, F50a.21, F51a.27, F52a.43, F53a.46, F56a.18, F57a.13, F58a.13, F59a.8, F60a.4, F69b.13
Dural pouch 287
– structures guideline structures 20, 21
Dynamic CT 15
Dysarthria 397
Dysbasia 324
Dysdiadochokinesia 304
Dysmetria 397
Dyssynergia 304

E

Eardrum 229
Edema of eyelids 369
Edge of insula 322
Edinger–Westphal nucleus 298, 412, F68.9, F151.2
EEG 11
Efferent pathways of amygdaloid body 405
Eighth cranial nerve 286
Electroencephalogram 11
Eleventh cranial nerve 286
Emboliform nucleus 304, 395
Emissary vein 233, 283, F37c.25
Emission computed tomography 1, 16–18, 278
Enhanced contrast 20
Enhancement 16
Enkephalinergic neurons 419, 420
Enophthalmos 393, 414
Entorhinal cortex 322, 416–418
EP 11
Epiglottis F8c.34, F32c.42, F33c.41
Epilepsy 392
Epileptic seizures 379
Epinephrine-synthesizing nerve cells 417
Epithalamus 252, 306
Erector spinae 232
Ethmoid 210, 238, F5c.13, F49c.3, F63.4
Ethmoidal bulla F4a.10, F74a.6
– cells 210, F2a.9, F4a.7, F5a.12, F6a.14, F6b.16, F6d.16, F18.7, F19.6, F20.6, F30a.9, F33a.22, F33b.17, F33d.17, F39.9, F45a.11, F48c.4, F49b.2, F49c.1, F49d.2, F50b.2, F50d.2, F62.3, F63.1, F64.5, F67.21, F74a.7, F75a.6, F75c.2, F75d.2
Eustachian tube 230, 237
Evoked potentials 11
Evolution of human brain 2
Excitatory neurotransmitters 419
Exophthalmos 369
Expressive aphasia 402
External acoustic meatus 229, 237, 354, F10c.22, F11c.24, F24.8, F37c.20, F43.8, F45a.18, F48d.9, F49b.16, F49c.14, F49d.16, F63.15, F67.34, F70a.14, F71a.12
– – opening F2a.16
– arcuate fibers F144a.18
– capsule 309, 323, F9a.15, F10a.20, F35a.8, F53a.12, F54a.16

– carotid artery 228, 229, 234, F10c.27, F10c.33, F37c.33
– jugular vein 233
– occipital protuberance 231, 232, 236, F32c.30, F38.19, F45a.20, F51c.26, F65.19
– sagittal stratum 362
Extracranial fixation of brains 11
Extrageniculate supplementary pathway 363
Extraocular muscles 218, 219
Extrapyramidal system 375
Extreme capsule 309, F9a.17, F10a.21, F35a.5, F53a.10, F54a.14
Eye muscle nuclei 388
Eyeball 218, 226, F4a.11, F4b.6, F4d.6, F5b.8, F5d.8, F35a.17, F35b.10, F35d.10, F36a.14, F36b.10, F36d.10, F48a.1, F49a.1, F49b.1, F49d.1, F50a.1, F50b.1, F50d.1, F74a.4, F75a.4, F75c.1, F75d.1, F76a.3, F76c.2, F76d.2, F126.2
Eyelids 219

F

Facial artery 220, 228, 234, F6c.30, F8c.33, F9c.36, F36c.44, F37c.40
– canal 237, F25.7, F36a.22, F36c.28, F42.11, F49c.18, F63.17
– nerve 227, 229, 286, 345, F3.28, F11a.39, F11a.44, F11b.23, F11d.23, F12a.34, F30b.17, F33a.29, F34a.29, F35a.27, F35b.14, F35d.14, F36a.22, F37a.18, F49a.13, F50a.14, F50d.14, F69a.15, F70a.20, F71a.15, F73b.12, F73b.14, F73c.8, F73d.8, F81, F82, F114.VII, F117.VII, F118.2
– nucleus 294, 379, 418, F68.15, F73b.21, F74b.23
– paralysis 379
– skeleton 210, 211
– – guideline structures 18
– vein 220, 235, 283, F6c.30
Falx cerebelli 239, F51a.26
– cerebri 238, 307, F4a.3, F4b.3, F5a.2, F5b.3, F6a.1, F7a.1, F7b.3, F8a.2, F9a.2, F10a.3, F11a.2, F13a.2, F13b.5, F14a.4, F15a.3, F15b.3, F15c.6, F16a.5, F16b.2, F16c.5, F17a.4, F17b.2, F51a.1, F52a.3, F53a.3, F53d.3, F54a.3, F54d.2, F55a.3, F55d.3, F56a.3, F56d.3, F57a.14, F57b.4, F57d.4, F58a.10, F58b.3, F58d.3, F59a.7, F59b.3, F59d.3, F60b.5, F76a.25, F77a.24, F78a.17
Fascial sheath 219
Fasciolar gyrus F149.6
Fast conjugate movements of eyes 388
– imaging with steady precession 11, 15
– low angle shot 11, 15
Fastigial nucleus 304, 395, F51a.23, F144b.9
Fastigium of fourth ventricle F67.28
Fat pad of Bichat 229
Fifth cervical vertebra F11c.41, F12c.33, F25.23
– cranial nerve 287
Fimbria of hippocampus 324, 404, F54a.36
Finger-to-nose testing 397
First accessory loop of basal ganglia 383
– cranial nerve 287
– molar tooth F4c.27, F18.19
First-order neurons 326
FISP 11, 15
Fixation nystagmus 349

Flaccid hemiplegia 324
FLAIR sequences 286
FLASH 11, 15
Flocculonodular lobe 304, 349, 394, F142, F143
Flocculus (H X) 293, 304, 388, 394, F3.31, F12a.37, F30b.21, F46.32, F49a.12, F49b.18, F72a.14, F72b.12, F72c.5, F72d.5, F73b.23, F140.13, F141.14, F142.11, F143.2
Floor of anterior cranial fossa F2a.4, F41.4, F45a.6
– – external acoustic meatus F48c.14
– – frontal sinus F64.2
– – middle cranial fossa F2a.14, F45a.16, F63.7, F72a.9
– – mouth 227
– – orbit F4c.22, F5c.20, F18.9, F19.8, F30a.11, F34c.20, F35c.27, F40.14, F41.11
– – posterior cranial fossa F2a.25, F45a.21, F63.19
– – rhomboid fossa F13a.26, F71a.19, F71c.8, F71d.8, F72b.23, F72c.7, F72d.7
– – striatum F52a.12, F138.1
Flow phenomenon 253
– void 20
Fluent aphasia 402
Fluorescence microscopy 416
fMRI 12, 16
– signal output 16
Folium of vermis (VII A) 304, 388, F2b.40, F16a.15, F32a.30, F32b.28, F32d.28, F67.30, F140.18, F141.11, F142.4
Follicular stimulating hormone 12, 307
Follow-up examinations 21
Foramen cecum 297, F45b.38, F49a.7
– lacerum F63.10
– magnum 231, 236, 238, 286, F2a.26, F14c.13, F25.11, F26.9, F27.8, F38.23, F48c.20, F62.15, F67.39
– ovale 229, 236, 239, 287, F41.12, F63.8
– rotundum 236, 239, 287, F21.10, F40.12, F63.5
– spinosum 236, 239, F62.8, F63.11
– transversarium 238, F61.13
Forebrain 288
Forel's axis 2, 288
– fields 306
Fornical commissure 404
Fornix 324, 404, 418, F2b.10, F9d.10, F10a.10, F10a.25, F10b.10, F10d.10, F11a.12, F11b.8, F11d.8, F12a.12, F12b.11, F12d.11, F13a.13, F32a.5, F32b.7, F34a.16, F45b.10, F52a.19, F54a.21, F55a.19, F55b.12, F55d.12, F67.2, F78b.7, F147.12, F148.5, F148.6, F149.3, F149.5, F150.10
Four walls of orbit 218
Fourth cervical vertebra F11c.40, F24.18, F25.22, F38.38, F39.29, F40.32, F41.24
– cranial nerve 287
– ventricle 242, 288, F2b.38, F13b.19, F13d.19, F32a.32, F32b.32, F32d.32, F45b.32, F49b.19, F49d.19, F50a.16, F50b.20, F50d.20, F51a.21, F51b.15, F51d.15, F71a.20, F72b.23, F73b.29, F73c.10, F73d.10, F74c.10, F74d.10, F75b.23, F75c.10, F75d.10, F76b.22, F83b.12, F85.18, F86b.12, F87.7
Fovea centralis of retina 226, 388, F4a.9
Fractures of craniocervical junction 233
Frankfurt line 4

Frontal bone 237, F2a.1, F4c.4, F5c.3, F6c.2, F18.1, F19.1, F20.1, F30a.1, F32c.4, F33c.5, F35c.3, F36c.2, F37c.2, F38.3, F39.3, F40.3, F41.3, F42.3, F43.3, F45a.3, F50c.1, F51c.1, F52b.1, F52c.1, F52d.1, F53c.1, F53d.1, F54c.1, F55c.1, F55d.1, F56c.1, F56d.1, F57c.1, F57d.1, F58c.1, F58d.1, F59c.1, F59d.1, F60c.1, F64.1, F65.1, F66.1, F77a.1, F78a.3
- branch of middle meningeal artery F49c.6, F50c.7, F51c.7
- cortex 404, 416
- eye field 388, F139.3, F140.1, F141.16
- forceps 323, F55a.6
- horn of lateral ventricle 252, 253, F7b.9, F7d.9, F8a.8, F8b.7, F8d.7, F9a.9, F9b.7, F9d.7, F10a.8, F10b.8, F10d.8, F53a.7, F53b.6, F53c.11, F53d.6, F54a.8, F54b.5, F54c.10, F54d.5, F55a.10, F55b.6, F55d.6, F83b.1, F84.4, F85.25, F86b.1, F91c.2, F91d.29
- lobe 313, F91c.1, F104a, F104b, F107a, F107b, F108b.9
- – syndrome 288
- neocortex 418
- nerve 226, F6a.12, F35a.12, F115.7
- operculum 313, 317
- pole F2b.8, F3.17, F31.1, F45b.7, F46.16, F52a.2
- sinus 217, F2a.3, F4b.5, F4d.5, F5b.7, F5d.7, F30a.3, F32a.13, F33a.13, F34a.11, F38.6, F39.6, F40.5, F45a.4, F50c.2, F51b.1, F51c.2, F51d.1, F52c.2, F65.2, F66.2, F67.10, F77a.2, F78a.1
Frontopetal type of telencephalon 10, 313
Frontopontine tract 303, F77b.15, F78b.10
Frontozygomatic suture F18.5, F30a.5, F43.4
FSH 12, 307
functional magnetic resonance imaging 12, 16

G

GABA 12, 383, 419
GABAergic neurons 419
Gadolinium-Diamid 16
Gadolinium-DTPA 16
Gamma-aminobutyric acid 12, 419
Gamma-motor neurons 418
Garcin's syndrome 287
Gaze palsies 391
Gaze-dependent nystagmus 349
Gaze-evoked nystagmus 392
Geniculate body lesion 369
- ganglion 345
Geniculocalcarine tract 361
Genioglossus F4c.30, F5c.32, F6c.33, F32c.41
Geniohyoid 227, F4c.34, F5c.37, F6c.38, F32c.45, F33c.42, F34c.47
Genu of corpus callosum 323, F2b.9, F7a.6, F7b.8, F7d.8, F8a.7, F32a.3, F32b.5, F32d.5, F45b.8, F53a.6, F53d.5, F54b.4, F54d.4
- – facial nerve 237, 294, F68.13, F74b.27
- – internal capsule 323, F10a.12, F53a.18, F54a.19
- – optic radiation 362
GH 12, 307
Glabella 421
Glands of tongue 414

Global aphasia 277
Globose nucleus 304, 395
Globus pallidus 305, 306, 309, 323, 383, F9b.11, F9d.11, F10a.15, F10b.12, F10d.12, F11a.23, F34a.8, F34b.11, F34d.11, F53b.13, F53d.13, F54a.18, F54b.14, F136.7, F138.5
Glossopharyngeal nerve 228, 231, 286, 345, 414, F3.33, F9a.37, F11a.42, F12a.36, F30b.22, F33a.34, F34a.31, F35a.31, F46.34, F49a.9, F69b.10, F70b.4, F71b.11, F81, F82, F114.IX, F117.IX, F118.1, F151.8
- neuralgia 287
GLU 12, 419
Glutamate 12, 419
Glutamatergic neurons 419
Gnathion 421
Golgi cells 419
Gonadotropic cells 307
Gracile fasciculus 331, F111.9, F112.10, F113.2
- lobe of cerebellum (H VII B) 304, 394
- nucleus (of Goll) 293, 331, F69b.30, F70b.28, F111.7, F112.9, F113.5
- tubercle F48a.7, F48b.13, F49a.16, F69c.10, F69d.10
Gradenigo's syndrome 288
Graphic illustrations in the atlas 422
Gray matter of telencephalon 308
Great cerebral vein (of Galen) 283, 285, F32b.9, F32c.13, F32d.9, F54c.19, F55c.20, F97a.10
Greater cornu of hyoid bone F8c.38, F9c.42, F22.12, F23.19
- occipital nerve 233, F13a.29, F14a.20, F15a.22, F16a.17, F17a.12
- palatine artery F5c.26
- – canal F39.16
- – nerve F5a.22, F115.5
- – vein F5c.26
- petrosal nerve 414, F73b.8, F151.16
- wing of sphenoid 236, F6c.14, F20.5, F45a.5
Green fluorescence of dopamine and noradrenaline 416
Groove for sigmoid sinus F27.3
Growth hormone 12, 307, 420
Guideline structures 18–21
Gustatory cortical area near insula F117.2
- fibers in posterior (dorsal) trigeminothalamic tract F117.4, F118.4
- system 345
Gut-brain peptides 419
Gyri of cerebral hemispheres 422
Gyrus semilunaris 372, F52a.15

H

H1 and H2 306
Habenular commissure 252
- nuclei 306, 412, 418, 420, F54a.27, F147.11
Habenulo-interpeduncular tract 412
Hammer 237, F50c.13, F73a.14
Hand area 309
Hard palate 211, 227, F2a.30, F4c.25, F5c.24, F6c.23, F18.16, F19.15, F20.15, F33c.28, F38.27, F39.20
Head and neck region guideline structures 19
- joints 232
- of caudate nucleus 308, F8a.9, F8b.8, F8d.8, F9a.10, F33d.10, F53a.16, F53b.7, F53d.7, F54a.10, F54b.9, F54d.9,

F55a.12, F55b.8, F55d.8, F132.8, F136.1, F136.2, F137.5, F138.4
- – mandible 228, F2a.20, F9c.23, F10c.24, F23.12, F30a.13, F37c.19, F45a.19, F63.13, F67.36, F69a.13, F70a.12, F71c.3, F71d.3
Helical CT 2
- CT technique 14
Hemianopia 325
Hemiataxia 307
Hemiballism 307, 385
Hemifacial spasm 287
Hemiplegia with eye muscle disorders and central facial paralysis 380
Hemisphere of anterior lobe of cerebellum F52a.39
- – cerebellum (H II – H X) 303, 304, F48b.15, F48d.15, F51d.20, F71c.10, F71d.10, F72c.10, F72d.10
- – posterior lobe of cerebellum F16b.14, F16d.14, F49a.18, F49b.21, F49d.21, F50a.20, F50b.24, F50d.24, F52a.42, F69c.13, F69d.13, F144a.17
Hemorrhage 253, 298
Heubner's recurrent artery 266, 275
High sensitivity for pathologic lesions 16
High-resolution technique 19, 211, 288
Hippocampal formation 324, 404, 417, F148.9, F149.10, F149.11, F150.3
- sulcus 404, F52a.26
Hippocampus 253, 316, 322, 418, F10a.30, F10b.22, F10d.22, F11a.31, F11b.18, F11d.18, F12b.17, F12d.17, F13a.15, F13b.13, F13d.13, F34b.12, F35a.22, F35b.9, F35d.9, F51a.14, F51b.13, F52a.24, F52b.16, F53a.36, F53b.24, F54a.37, F76b.11, F77b.19, F78b.25, F147.18
- proper 404
Histaminergic neurons 418
Histologic preparation of brains 11
Hodology 2
Homonymous hemianopia 278, 307, 324, 369, 379
- quadrantanopia 369
- quadrants of visual field 362
Horizontal gaze palsy 391
Horner's syndrome 264, 298, 393, 414
Hounsfield units 12, 14, 18
HR-CT 19
HU 12, 14, 18
Huntington's disease 385
Hydrocephalus 253
Hyoid bone F2a.39, F7c.35, F32c.47, F33c.46, F38.39, F39.30, F40.34
Hyperacusis 359
Hyperkinesia 385
Hyperreflexia 375
Hypoglossal canal 231, 236, 239, 286, F33a.36, F39.15, F48c.16, F48d.10, F62.13, F69b.16, F69b.16
- nerve 227, 231, 286, F3.34, F4a.23, F5a.26, F6a.31, F7a.29, F8a.31, F9a.38, F10a.44, F11a.43, F12a.40, F30b.27, F33a.36, F33a.47, F34a.33, F35a.33, F36a.29, F46.33, F48a.5, F69b.17, F70b.9, F70b.15, F71a.14, F71b.7, F71b.15, F81, F82
- nucleus 294, F68.19, F70b.24, F71b.25
Hypokinesia 375, 385
Hypopharynx 230
Hypophysial fossa 236, 307, F2a.7, F22.3, F38.13, F45a.10, F65.8
- portal system 305

Hypophysiotropic peptides 419
Hypophysis 307, 361
Hypothalamic nuclei 405
- subnuclei 404
- sulcus 305
Hypothalamo-hypophysial system 415
Hypothalamoneurohypophysial nerve cells 419
Hypothalamus 252, 305, 361, 405, 416–418, 420, F52a.17, F53a.22, F67.11, F77b.9, F78a.7, F78b.5
Hypothetical fibers from thalamus to parietal cortical area F120.4, F121.8
– – – – – parietal operculum F118.7
Hypotonia of musculature 397

I

i. v. 12
IF 12, 305
Illustration technique 2
Illustrations in this atlas 421
Image pathology 1
Immunofluorescent methods 416
Impaired motor coordination 397
- pupillary reactions 388
Incisive canal of maxilla 227, F32c.34, F38.32
Incus 237, F50c.14
Indusium griseum 404, F147.3
Infarct 275
Inferior alveolar artery F4c.35, F5c.34, F6c.31, F8c.27, F36c.43
– – – in mandibular canal F7c.28
– – – – foramen F37c.31
– – nerve 229, F4a.24, F5a.27, F6a.30, F7a.28, F8a.27, F33a.46, F34a.39, F35a.37, F36a.24, F37a.19, F115.3
– – vein F4c.35, F5c.34, F6c.31, F8c.27, F36c.43
– – – in mandibular canal F7c.28
– – – – foramen F37c.31
- branch of oculomotor nerve F6a.17
- central veins 284
- cerebellar peduncle 304, 355, F71b.28, F72b.25, F73b.27, F144a.13
- cerebral veins 283
- colliculus 298, 354, 355, 359, 418, F2b.31, F32a.19, F45b.25, F52d.19, F53a.39, F67.17, F77b.34, F77c.14, F77d.14, F122.12, F123.9, F124.1, F125.7
- frontal gyrus 313, F3.13, F5a.6, F6a.7, F6b.5, F6d.5, F7a.7, F7b.11, F7d.11, F8a.6, F8b.9, F8d.9, F9a.8, F9b.9, F9d.9, F30b.6, F31.5, F36a.7, F36b.5, F36d.5, F37a.7, F37b.6, F37d.6, F46.13, F52a.5, F53a.5, F54a.4, F55a.7
- – sulcus F3.12, F30b.5, F31.6, F46.14
- ganglion of vagus nerve 345
- genu of central sulcus F108b.8
- horn of lateral ventricle 252, F9b.21, F9d.21, F10a.29, F10b.21, F10d.21, F11a.24, F11b.19, F11d.19, F12a.21, F12b.18, F12d.18, F35b.8, F35d.8, F51a.13, F51b.10, F52a.31, F52b.13, F76b.8, F76c.7, F76d.7, F77b.20, F78b.26, F78c.13, F78d.13, F83b.10, F84.14, F85.35, F86b.10, F91c.11, F91d.37, F126.7
- hypophysial arteries 307
- lip of primary visual cortex 361
- medullary velum 242
- nasal concha 210, F4a.20, F4b.8, F4d.8, F5a.20, F5b.10, F5d.10, F6a.23, F6b.19, F6d.19, F7a.24, F7b.16, F7d.16, F18.15, F19.14, F20.13, F33a.35, F33b.26, F33d.26, F47b.2, F69a.2, F69c.2, F69d.2, F70a.2
– – meatus 217, F4a.18, F5a.21, F6a.25
- oblique 220, F4c.21, F35c.20, F36c.18, F73a.4
- olivary nucleus 293, 295, 394, 417, F12a.38, F48a.4, F49a.8, F70b.16, F71b.14, F71c.6, F71d.6, F72b.14, F144a.15
- olive 288, F30b.19, F70c.8, F70d.8, F71a.17
- ophthalmic vein 220
- orbital fissure 218, F7c.11
- petrosal sinus F34c.25, F71a.13, F74b.5, F97a.5, F97b.8
- portion of medulla oblongata 288
– – – pons 293, F73c.7, F73d.7
- precuneal artery F90a,b.13, F91d.13
- rectus 220, F4c.20, F5c.18, F6b.15, F6c.19, F6d.15, F35c.21, F73a.7, F74a.9, F75d.3
- sagittal sinus 283, F56c.14, F97a.11
- salivatory nucleus 294, 414, F68.16, F151.4
- semilunar lobules (H VII A) 304
- tarsal muscle 219
- temporal gyrus 315, F3.26, F9a.32, F9b.23, F9d.23, F10a.39, F11a.35, F11b.20, F11d.20, F12a.28, F12b.23, F12d.23, F13a.20, F13b.18, F13d.18, F14a.14, F14b.11, F14d.11, F15a.16, F35a.26, F35b.12, F35d.12, F36a.19, F36b.13, F36d.13, F37a.16, F46.26, F50a.8, F50b.9, F51a.17, F52a.32
– – sulcus 315, F3.25, F9a.33, F46.22
- thyroid artery 231
- vestibular nucleus 349, F119.11
Infranuclear paralyses of ocular muscles 392
Infraorbital artery F4c.23, F5c.19,
- canal 219, F18.10, F19.10, F47a.6, F61.4
- nerve 226, F4a.15, F5a.14, F6a.20, F35a.25, F115.2
- vein F4c.23, F5c.19
Infratemporal fossa 227, 229
Infratentorial space 10, 238
Infundibular recess 252, 305, F9a.26, F77b.8, F83b.9, F84.9, F85.11, F86b.9
- stalk 307
Infundibulum 242, 305, 307, 416, F2b.28, F32a.25, F45b.30; F51a.9, F67.19, F76b.4, F76c.6, F76d.6, F77c.6, F77d.6
Inhibiting factor 12, 305
Inhibitory neurotransmitter 419
Inion 236, F32c.30, F38.19, F45a.20, F51c.26, F65.19
Injury of lateral geniculate body 307
Insula 308, 317, F8a.10, F8b.11, F8d.11, F9a.18, F9b.13, F9d.13, F10a.17, F10b.14, F10d.14, F11a.17, F11b.10, F11d.10, F36b.7, F36d.7, F52a.14, F52b.8, F52d.8, F53a.9, F53b.9, F53d.9, F54a.13, F54b.11, F54d.11, F55a.14, F55b.11, F55d.11
Insular arteries 270, F8c.9, F9c.8, F10c.9, F11c.11, F35c.9, F36b.6, F36c.9, F36d.6, F52c.7, F53c.6, F54c.9, F55c.10, F78b.2, F78a.6, F91a,b.5
- cortex 322, 349
Intention tremor 397
Interhemispheric cistern 238, 242, F4d.2, F5d.2, F7d.2, F16d.4, F17d.3, F76d.11, F78c.1, F78d.1, F84.1, F85.1, F87.11
- disconnection effect 324
- fibers 323
- fissure 307, F4a.1, F7a.9, F15a.2, F16a.2, F17a.2, F30b.1, F31.2, F77a.22, F78a.4
Intermediate mass 252, 306
- nerve 286, 414, F3.28, F11a.39, F12a.34, F30b.17, F33a.29, F34a.29, F35a.27, F50a.14, F73b.12, F151.7
– – parasympathetic fibers 286
- zone of cerebellar cortex 394
Intermediomedial frontal artery F4c.2, F5c.4, F6c.3, F7c.2, F8c.5, F32c.8, F33c.9, F34c.4, F55c.4, F56c.4, F57c.4, F90a,b.8, F91d.9
Internal acoustic meatus 237, 239, 286, 349, 354, F11b.23, F11c.20, F11d.23, F25.4, F35b.14, F35c.23, F35d.14, F41.9, F49b.14, F50b.15, F50d.15, F64.12, F73a.15, F73b.9, F73c.6, F73d.6
– – opening F50c.15
- arcuate fibers 331, F111.5, F112.7, F113.3
- capsule 323, 342, 378, 388, F8b.6, F8d.6, F34b.6, F34d.6
- carotid artery 220, 231, 234, 235, 265, 271, 307, 361, 414, F8b.18, F8c.13, F8d.18, F9b.22, F9c.17, F9d.22, F10b.24, F10c.23, F10d.24, F33c.17, F34b.14, F34c.23, F34d.14, F35b.13, F35c.35, F35d.13, F36c.38, F37b.12, F37c.41, F37d.12, F47a.11, F48b.5, F48c.12, F49b.8, F49c.9, F49d.8, F50c.10, F51b.6, F51d.6, F69a.14, F69b.14, F69c.5, F69d.5, F70b.3, F70d.5, F71b.5, F72b.4, F73b.2, F73c.4, F73d.4, F74b.3, F74c.2, F74d.2, F75b F75c.6, F75d.6, F76b.2, F76c.5, F76d.5, F88.9, F89a.15, F90a,b.1, F91a,b.1
– – – C1–C5 segment 265
- cerebral vein 283, F11c.10, F11b.8, F11d.8, F12b.12, F12c.10, F12d.12, F13b.12, F13c.10, F13d.12, F32b.10, F32c.12, F32d.10, F54c.12, F55b.19, F97a.9
- jugular vein 228, 231, 235, 283, F11c.37, F35c.30, F36c.32, F37c.38, F47a.13, F48c.13, F49c.17, F69b.11, F70a.16, F70b.6, F97a.17, F97b.9
- occipital protuberance 236, F2a.18, F32c.27, F38.15, F45a.15, F51c.24, F65.17, F73a.28
- vertebral venous plexus 283
Interneurons 377, 419
Internuclear neurons 388
Internuclear ophthalmoplegia 391, 392
Interpeduncular cistern 242, 298, F11a.30, F11b.17, F11d.17, F52b.11, F52d.11, F77a.13, F77c.9, F77d.9, F83a.5, F84.17, F85.14, F86a.7
- fossa 298, F30b.12, F77b.14
- nucleus 405, 412, 416, 418, 420
Interpolar part of spinal nucleus of trigeminal nerve 338, F71b.27
Interpositus nuclei 395
Interstitial nucleus (of Cajal) 388
Interthalamic adhesion 252, 306, F2b.13, F32a.9, F32b.13, F45b.15, F67.4
Interventional neuroradiology 1
Interventricular foramen (of Monro) 252, 253, 306, 323, F2b.11, F10a.13, F10b.11, F10d.11, F45b.13, F54a.22, F54b.13, F54d.13, F83b.3, F84.12, F85.3, F86b.3
Intervertebral disc F11c.36, F32c.40

Intracerebral coordinates 5
Intracranial fixation of brains 11
Intrahemispheric fibers 323
Intralaminar nuclei of thalamus 306, 326, 348, 383, F109.4
Intraparietal sulcus 322, 349, F108b.6
intravenous 12
Intravital neuroanatomy 10, 11
Investigation sequence of MRI 423
Ipsilateral auditory pathway 355
- dysfunctions of unilateral cerebellar lesions 397
- innervation of spinal motor neurons 378
- strabismus 287
Iris 226
Ischemic brain infarction 256
Isocortex 322
Isthmus of cingulate gyrus F149.7
- of fauces 227, F8a.30

J

Jacksonian motor seizure 324
Jugular foramen 231, 235, 239, 286, F25.6, F49c.16, F62.12, F63.16, F69a.17, F70a.15
- – syndrome 287

K

Knob 309

L

Labyrinth 237
Lacrimal apparatus 219
- bone 211
- gland 219, 414, F4c.14, F36c.12, F76a.4
- – innervation 219
- nerve 226
Lambdoid suture 231, 238, F32c.10, F33c.8, F34c.7, F35c.11, F36c.11, F37c.12, F38.4, F39.4, F40.4, F41.5, F42.4, F43.5, F50c.22, F51c.22, F52c.18, F53c.24, F54c.25, F55c.24, F56c.17, F57c.17, F64.16, F65.16, F66.4, F74a.25, F75a.25, F76a.26, F77a.26, F78a.19
Lamina affixa 253, 306
- cribrosa of sclera 226, 361
- terminalis 252, 305, F2b.17, F32a.14, F45b.21, F52a.16, F67.9, F78b.3
Language areas 277, 400, 402, 404
Laryngopharynx 230
Lateral aperture (of Luschka) of fourth ventricle 239, 242, F72a.15, F72b.21, F72c.6
- atlantoaxial joint 232, F11c.34, F24.15, F25.19, F34c.40, F40.27
- branches of pontine arteries 254
- corticospinal tract 377, F133.13 F135.1
- dorsal nucleus of thalamus F11a.11
- facial region 228
- frontobasal artery 270, F6c.6, F7c.6, F35c.10, F36c.10, F91a,b.4
- geniculate body 306, 361, 388, 417, 418, F12a.19, F53a.32, F78b.17, F126.10, F127.7, F128.8, F129.5
- gray horns of spinal cord 414
- habenular nucleus 385
- lemniscus 303, 354, 355, 418, F74b.20, F75b.18, F76b.18, F77b.30, F122.15, F123.10, F124.2, F124.6, F125.4
- lenticulostriate arteries 275
- mass(-es) of atlas 232, F11c.31, F12c.28, F25.17, F26.11, F34c.35, F39.23, F40.26, F47a.17, F47b.9, F61.14
- occipital artery 256, F12c.15, F13c.14, F14c.10, F15c.13, F16c.12, F17c.7, F34c.15, F52c.13, F53c.18, F89a.12, F91d.21
- occipitotemporal gyrus 315, 316, F9a.35, F10a.38, F11a.34, F12a.27, F12b.22, F12d.22, F13a.19, F13b.17, F13d.17, F14a.13, F14b.9, F14d.9, F15a.15, F15b.9, F15d.9, F16a.13, F16b.10, F16d.10, F17a.11, F36a.18, F52a.37, F53a.42
- olfactory stria 322, 372, F130.3
- paracore 416, 417
- part of globus pallidus F53a.14, F137.12
- pharyngeal space 231
- posterior nucleus of thalamus F54a.26
- pterygoid 228, 229, F7c.18, F8c.22, F9c.27, F35c.32, F36c.25, F37c.23, F69a.11, F69c.4, F69d.4, F70a.10, F71a.8
- – plate 228, F7c.17, F21.17, F35c.33, F41.18, F47b.5, F47a.9, F61.8, F69b.2
- rectus 220, F5c.15, F6b.13, F6c.17, F6d.13, F35c.18, F36c.15, F50b.6, F50d.6, F75a.10, F76a.9, F76c.4, F76d.4
- semicircular canal F50b.17
- spinothalamic tract 326, F109.7, F110.1
- sulcus 313, F8a.11, F9a.13, F9b.14, F9d.14, F10a.18, F10b.15, F10d.15, F11a.19, F11b.12, F11d.12, F12b.10, F12d.10, F13a.8, F13b.7, F13d.7, F30b.7, F36a.8, F37a.9, F37b.8, F37d.8, F46.18, F52a.7, F53b.8, F53d.8, F108b.17
- territory of medulla oblongata 263
- – – midbrain 263
- – – pons 263
- trigeminothalamic tract 338, 342, F114.14, F115.21, F116.3, F116.4
- ventricle 252, F32b.6, F32d.6, F33b.8, F33d.8, F34b.7, F34d.7, F35b.6, F35d.6, F53b.23, F55b.18, F55d.18, F84.16, F85.28, F87.10, F122.7
- vestibular nucleus (of Deiters) 349, 383, 419, F119.13, F120.6, F121.5
- vestibulospinal tract 349, 383, F119.14, F120.8, F120.10, F121.2
- zone of cerebellar hemisphere 394
- – – reticular formation 295
Lateralization of language areas 400
Lens 226, F4b.6, F4d.6, F35a.16, F35c.16, F49b.1, F49d.1, F75a.2, F76a.2, F76c.1, F76d.1
Lentiform nucleus 309, 323
Leptomeningeal anastomoses 271
Lesion in postcentral gyrus 324
- of abducens nucleus 391
- – medial geniculate body 307
Lesions of intermediate zone of cerebellar cortex 397
- – lateral zone of cerebellar hemisphere 397
- – vermis 397
Lesser cornu of hyoid bone F21.21
- petrosal nerve 414
- wing of sphenoid 236, F7c.8, F21.4, F41.6
Levator palpebrae superioris 219, F4c.10, F5c.8, F6b.7, F6c.10, F6d.7, F35c.13, F36c.13, F76a.11, F77a.7
- scapulae 233, F37c.39
- veli palatini 227, 230, F9c.26, F33c.29, F34c.29

LH 12, 307
Liberins 305
Ligamentum nuchae F16c.19, F17c.14
Limbic lobe 317
- midbrain nuclei 404
- system 316, 322, 385, 404, 405, 412, 416, 418
Limbus corneae 219
Lingua 227
Lingual artery 228, 231, F8c.36, F9c.41, F36c.45
- nerve 228, 229, F5a.25, F6a.29, F7a.27, F8a.29, F33a.44, F34a.40, F35a.38, F36a.26, F115.6
Lingula (I) 304
Lobules of the cerebellum 304
Localization of direction of a sound source 355
Long central artery 266, 275
Longissimus capitis 232, F37c.34
Longitudinal axis of brainstem 2, 288
- – – forebrain 2, 288
- cerebral fissure 307, F4a.1, F7a.9, F15a.2, F16a.2, F17a.2, F30b.1, F31.2, F77a.22, F78a.4
- zones of cerebellar cortex 394
Longus capitis 233, F33c.30, F69b.8
Lower eyelid F35a.24, F74a.2
- jaw 211
Luliberin 419
Luteinizing hormone 12, 307

M

M 12
MA 12
Macrophotography 2
Macula lutea of retina 362
Magnetencephalogram 12
Magnetic field 15
- resonance 12
- – angiography 12, 15
- – imaging 1, 12, 15, 16, 18
- – spectroscopy 16
- stimulation of motor cortex 378
Magnocellular nerve cells 361
Magnus raphe nucleus 417
Main control circuit of basal ganglia 383
- sensory nucleus of the trigeminal nerve 338
Major forceps 253, 323, F55a.24
Malleus 237, F50c.13, F73a.14
Mammillary body 242, 305, 404, 405, 418, F2b.22, F10a.25, F32a.15, F32b.19, F32d.19, F45b.22, F52b.9, F67.18, F77a.12, F77b.10, F77c.7, F78c.7, F78d.7, F147.13, F148.7, F149.4, F150.5
Mammillotegmental fasciculus 412
Mammillothalamic fasciculus (of Vicq d'Azyr) 405, F53a.23, F78b.8, F147.10
Mammotropic cells 307
Mandible 211, F36c.42, F41.21, F45a.30, F47a.10, F47b.7, F48b.4, F48c.10, F48d.4, F61.9, F62.9
Mandibular canal 211, F18.21, F19.19, F20.18, F21.20, F22.10, F39.28, F40.31, F41.23, F42.17
- foramen 211, 229, F43.15
- fossa 228, 237, F9c.21, F23.8, F37c.17, F43.7
- nerve 227, 229, 287, F9a.36, F35a.29, F49a.4, F71a.9, F71b.1, F72b.2, F115.12, F116.V/3
Marginal branch of cingulate sulcus 313, 332, F33b.5, F33d.5, F57b.12, F108b.22

Mass of orbital fat 19
Masseter 228, F5c.25, F6c.27, F7c.26, F8c.28, F9c.37, F37c.29, F69a.9
– reflex 342
Masticatory apparatus 228
Mastoid cells 237, F25.10, F43.13, F48d.12, F49c.20, F49d.20, F69a.18
– process 231, 237, F2a.23, F12c.23, F25.12, F26.8, F30a.19, F37c.24, F43.14, F45a.24, F48c.17, F62.14, F63.18, F69a.20
Material 421
Maxilla 211, F4c.24, F6c.22, F18.17, F19.16, F20.12, F33c.27, F34c.33, F35c.40, F36c.22, F39.21, F40.24, F41.17, F42.10, F47a.3, F61.2, F69a.1, F70a.1, F71a.1
Maxillary artery 218, 228, 229, 234, F7c.16, F8c.21, F9c.28, F36c.24, F37c.26, F69b.6
– nerve 218, 228, 287, F7a.20, F8a.24, F34a.27, F49a.4, F73a.10, F115.10, F116.V/2
– sinus 211, 229, F2a.24, F4a.19, F5a.19, F6a.22, F6b.18, F6d.18, F18.14, F19.13, F20.10, F30a.15, F34a.32, F34b.15, F34d.15, F35b.16, F35d.16, F36a.21, F40.20, F41.16, F45a.22, F47a.7, F47b.3, F48b.2, F48c.6, F48d.2, F61.6, F62.6, F67.40, F69a.3, F69c.1, F69d.1, F70a.4, F70c.2, F70d.2, F71a.3, F72a.4
ME 12
Measuring sequences 15
Meatovertical line (MV) 12, F32a
Meckel's cave 287
Medial branches of pontine arteries 254
– forebrain bundle 405
– frontal gyrus F91d.25
– frontobasal artery 267, F4c.8, F5c.7, F6c.8, F32c.19, F33c.13, F51c.5, F90a,b.4, F91d.6
– geniculate body 306, 355, 417, F12a.18, F34a.15, F53a.31, F78b.18, F122.10, F123.4, F123.7, F124.11, F125.5
– lemniscus 303, 331, F70b.14, F71b.13, F72b.11, F73b.17, F74b.18, F75b.16, F76b.16, F77b.23, F78b.22, F111.4, F112.3, F112.6, F113.6
– – system 331, 332
– lenticulostriate arteries 266, 275
– longitudinal fasciculus 349, F69b.22, F70b.19, F71b.20, F72b.16, F73b.25, F74b.26, F75b.21, F76b.20, F77b.26, F78b.21, F119.7
– nuclei of thalamus 306, F11a.13, F33a.8, F54a.24, F147.9
– occipital artery 256, F12c.13, F13c.12, F14c.9, F33c.16, F34c.10, F52c.12, F53c.15, F54c.21, F89a.9, F91d.17
– occipitotemporal gyrus 315, 316, F13a.18, F13b.15, F13d.15, F14a.11, F14b.8, F14d.8, F15a.14, F15b.8, F15d.8, F16a.12, F16b.9, F16d.9, F17a.10, F34a.19, F35a.23, F53a.44
– olfactory stria 372
– orbital part of frontal lobe F91d.36
– part of globus pallidus F53a.15, F137.13
– pterygoid 228, 229, F7c.19, F8c.26, F9c.31, F35c.34, F36c.36, F37c.32
– – plate F7c.20, F21.18, F39.19, F69b.1
– rectus 220, F4c.15, F5c.14, F6b.14, F6c.15, F6d.14, F34c.16, F50b.4, F50d.4, F75a.8, F76a.7
– reticular nucleus 326, F109.6
– vestibular nucleus 349, 418, F119.12

– vestibulospinal tract F119.15, F120.9, F120.10, F121.1
– zone of reticular formation 295
Median aperture (of Magendie) 242
– atlantoaxial joint 232, F38.28
– paracore 416
– plane (M) 4, 12, F4c, F69a
– sulcus 293, F71b.24
– zone of reticular formation 294
Medulla oblongata 288–293, 342, 348, 412, 414, F2b.44, F12b.27, F12d.27, F32a.36, F32b.34, F32d.34, F45b.39, F46.35, F48b.11, F48d.11, F49a.14, F49b.17, F49d.17, F67.35, F69a.19, F69c.8, F70a.18, F71a.16, F72a.13, F98, F99, F100, F101, F102, F103, F122.25, F132.13
Medullary laminae of thalamus 306
– striae of fourth ventricle 354, F124.4
– – – thalamus 252
MEG 12
Mental foramen 229
MEP 12
Mesencephalic dysfunctions 303
– nucleus of trigeminal nerve 294, 298, 342, F68.2, F74b.29, F75b.24, F76b.24, F77b.31, F78b.28, F114.6, F116.10
– tract of trigeminal nerve F68.1
Mesencephalon 298
Mesocortex 322
Mesodiencephal junction 388
Mesolimbic system 416
Metathalamus 305, 306, 323
Methods 421–424
Meyer's loop 362, F127.6
Meynert's axis (MA) 2, 10, 12, 288, F67
– plane (ME) 12, F69a
Midbrain 298–303, 348, 412, F12b.20, F12d.20, F33b.14, F33d.14, F45b.23, F91c.15, F98, F99, F100, F101, F102, F103
– syndrome 238
Middle cerebellar peduncle 304, 388, F12a.32, F12b.25, F12d.25, F50a.17, F50b.21, F73b.24, F73c.12, F73d.12, F74b.15, F74c.8, F74d.8, F144a.14
– cerebral artery 267–271, F8b.13, F8d.13, F9c.9, F34c.13, F35b.7, F35c.14, F35d.7, F51c.11, F51d.7, F77b.7, F77c.5, F77d.5, F78c.4, F78d.4, F91a,b.2
– – – bifurcation 270
– – – insular part 270
– – – M1- M2-segment 270
– – – sphenoid part 270
– cranial fossa 239, F21.7, F22.5, F23.4, F40.13, F41.8, F42.7, F64.9, F65.9
– ear deafness 359
– frontal gyrus 313, F3.8, F4a.4, F5a.3, F5b.5, F5d.5, F6a.3, F6b.3, F6d.3, F7a.4, F7b.5, F7d.5, F8a.3, F8b.4, F8d.4, F9a.3, F9b.3, F9d.3, F10a.2, F10b.3, F10d.3, F30b.3, F31.4, F35a.1, F35b.3, F35d.3, F36b.1, F36d.1, F37b.2, F37d.2, F46.10, F52a.4, F53a.2, F53b.4, F53d.4, F54a.2, F54b.3, F54d.3, F55a.2, F56a.2, F57a.2, F58a.2, F58b.6, F58d.6, F133.2
– inferior temporal artery of posterior cerebral artery F91d.23
– meningeal artery 220, 236, F10c.19, F36c.26, F71b.3, F72a.10, F72b.3, F73a.12, F74a.11, F76a.15
– nasal concha 210, F4a.14, F5a.16, F6a.18, F6b.17, F6d.17, F7a.22, F18.12, F19.9, F20.8, F33a.32, F33b.25, F33d.25, F72a.6, F73a.3
– – meatus 217, F4a.13, F5a.15, F6a.19

– portion of pons 293
– temporal artery of middle cerebral artery F91a,b.14
– – gyrus 315, F3.23, F8a.20, F8b.16, F8d.16, F9a.25, F9b.18, F9d.18, F10a.28, F10b.20, F10d.20, F11a.27, F11b.16, F11d.16, F12a.22, F12b.19, F12d.19, F13a.16, F13b.14, F13d.14, F14a.9, F14b.10, F14d.10, F15a.11, F30b.10, F35a.20, F35b.11, F35d.11, F36a.16, F36b.11, F36d.11, F37a.15, F37b.9, F37d.9, F46.25, F51a.6, F52a.22, F52b.10, F52d.10, F53a.38, F53b.19, F53d.19, F54a.38, F54b.23, F54d.23
Minor forceps 323, F55a.6
Miosis 393, 414
Mitral cells 372
Mobility of equipment 17
Monocular visual field 363
Monopareses 379
Motor aphasia 402
– cortex 379
– disorders 375
– evoked potentials 12
– language area 313
– neurons 375
– – of eye movements 388
– – – third, fourth, and sixth cranial nerves 388
– nucleus of cranial nerve V, VII, IX, X, XII, and partially XI 379
– – – trigeminal nerve 294, F68.12, F74b.24
– root of trigeminal nerve F68.Vm, F74b.21, F81, F82
– systems 375–393
– – of basal ganglia 383, 385
Mouth 227
– proper 227
MR 12
– angiography 253
– images 422
MRA 12, 15, 253, 278
MRI 12, 15, 18
– signal 16, 253
MRS 16
Multiplanar imaging technique 369
– sections 2
Multiple sclerosis 1, 298, 369, 392
– transmitter centers 417
Muscle cone of craniocervical junction 232
Muscles of craniocervical junction F79, F80
– – floor of mouth 287
– – mastication 228, 287
– – neck 232
Musculotubal canal 237
Mutism 324
MV 12
Mydriasis 393
Myelography 1, 14
Mylohyoid 227, F4c.37, F5c.38, F6c.39, F7c.30, F32c.46, F33c.43, F34c.46, F35c.46
Myogenic paresis 392

N

Names for arteries 253
Narrow window 14
Nasal bone 211, F2a.11, F32c.24, F38.14, F45a.12, F47a.1, F48c.1, F61.1, F62.1

Nasal cavity 211–217, F4a.16, F5a.18, F6a.24, F7a.23, F69a.5, F70a.6, F71a.5, F72a.1, F73a.1, F79, F80
– septum 211, F4a.17, F4b.7, F4d.7, F5a.17, F5b.9, F5d.9, F6a.21, F7a.21, F18.13, F19.11, F20.11, F21.15, F30a.12, F32a.34, F38.21, F47a.2, F47b.1, F48b.1, F48c.2, F48d.1, F61.3, F62.2, F69a.6, F70a.3, F70c.1, F70d.1, F71a.6, F71c.1, F71d.1, F72a.3, F72c.1, F72d.1, F73a.6, F74a.1, F75a.5
– skeleton 210
– vestibule 211, F33a.37
Nasion 421
Nasociliary nerve 218, 226, F5a.9, F6a.13, F115.4
Nasolacrimal canal 219
– duct 217, 219, F71a.2, F72a.2
Nasopharynx 230, F8a.25, F8b.20, F8c.23, F8d.20, F32a.42, F47b.6, F69a.10, F69b.4, F69c.3, F69d.3, F70a.9, F70b.1, F70c.3, F70d.3
Neck of mandible 211, F2a.22, F23.14
Neencephalic projection fibers 323
Neocortex 322, 404, 417, 419, 420
Nerves of craniocervical junction 233
– – lateral facial region 229
– – nasal cavity 218
– – oral cavity 228
– – orbit 226
– – pharyngeal wall 231
Neuroactive substances 415
Neuroanatomic collection from Hannover medical school 421
Neurocranium 236–238
– guideline structures 19
Neurofunctional systems 2, 3, 256, 325–414
Neurogenic paresis 392
Neurohypophysis 305, 307, F75b.5
Neuroimaging 1, 14–21
Neuroleptic drugs 416
Neuromodulators 415–420
Neuronal network of parietal and frontal cerebral areas 388
– theory 415
Neuropeptide-containing cells 297
Neuropeptides 412
Neuropharmacology 415
Neurotransmitters 415–420
New orientation of cerebral anatomy 2
Nigrostriatal dopaminergic system 385
– fibers 416
Ninth cranial nerve 286
Nodule of vermis (X) 293 ,304, 394, F2b.39, F13b.20, F13d.20, F32a.33, F32b.33, F32d.33, F45b.34, F67.29, F73b.30, F73c.11, F73d.11, F74b.32, F142.8, F143.5
Nondominant hemisphere 400
Nonfluent aphasia 402
Nonspecific nuclei of thalamus 306
Noradrenergic neurons 297 416, 417
Notes for reader 11–13
Nuclear resonance signals 15
Nuclei of hypothalamus 418
– of lateral lemniscus 355, F122.14
– – trapezoid body 355, 359, F122.22
Nucleus accumbens 308, 309, 383, 416, 418, F52a.12, F138.1
– ambiguus 294, F68.17, F70b.20, F71b.16, F72b.17
– ovalis 345, F117.5
– prepositus hypoglossi 390, 391
– proprius of dorsal gray horn 326
Nystagmus 304, 349, 388, 397

O

Obex of medulla oblongata 242, 288, F32a.40, F32b.35, F32d.35, F67.37, F70b.29, F70c.9, F70d.9
Objectives of neuroimaging 1–4
Obliquus capitis inferior 233, F13c.26, F14c.20, F34c.42, F35c.41, F36c.35
– – superior 233, F13c.22, F14c.16
Obscurus raphe nucleus 417
Occipital artery 233, 234, F10c.28, F11c.35, F12c.25, F13c.25, F14c.18, F15c.18, F16c.16, F17c.11
– bone 231, 236, F2a.8, F12c.22, F13c.19, F14c.14, F15c.17, F16c.15, F17c.10, F24.10, F26.6, F27.7, F28.3, F33c.23, F35c.26, F36c.17, F37c.15, F38.9, F39.12, F40.18, F41.10, F42.5, F43.9, F45a.7, F49c.23, F49d.23, F50b.25, F50c.24, F50d.25, F51c.25, F52c.20, F52d.22, F53c.26, F53d.29, F54c.26, F55c.25, F55d.25, F56c.18, F56d.18, F57c.16, F57d.15, F63.19, F64.17, F65.18, F66.5, F69a.26, F70a.26, F71a.26, F72a.21, F73a.29, F74a.29, F75a.27, F76a.28, F77a.28, F78a.21
– condyle 231, 236, F11c.26, F25.13, F30a.16, F34c.27, F39.17, F40.22, F47a.16, F47b.12
– forceps 253, 323, F55a.24
– gyri 315, F3.18, F16a.8, F17a.5, F17b.4, F17d.4, F31.17, F33a.12, F34a.6, F35a.7, F36a.17, F36b.12, F36d.12, F46.17, F53a.45, F53b.28, F53d.28, F54a.42, F54b.30, F54d.30, F55a.27, F55b.23, F55d.23, F56a.19, F56b.16, F56d.16
– horn of lateral ventricle 252, 253, F14a.6, F14b.6, F14d.6, F15a.10, F15b.7, F15d.7, F16b.7, F16d.7, F55b.22, F78a.12, F83b.8, F84.29, F85.31, F86b.7, F91c.5, F91d.34, F126.15
– lobe 315, F91c.16, F91d.35, F104a, F104b, F107a, F107b, F108b.16
– pole 363, F2b.34, F3.21, F31.18, F45b.26, F46.21, F54a.45, F74a.28
– protuberance 231
– sinus F49b.22, F49c.22, F50c.23, F51c.23, F97b.12
– stripe (of Gennari) 322, 362
Occipitofrontalis 375, 379, F34c.8
Occipitomastoid suture F26.7, F27.6
Occipitopetal type of telencephalon 10, 313
Occipitopontine tract 303, F77b.18, F78b.13
Occlusion of cerebellar artery 254
Occlusions of major brain arteries 253
Ocular dominance columns 322, 362
Oculomotor nerve 220, 226, 287, F2b.29, F7a.15, F8a.18, F9a.27, F10a.31, F10c.14, F30b.13, F32a.16, F33a.23, F34a.21, F51a.11, F76b.7, F77b.13, F77d.8, F78b.14, F81, F82, F151.1
– nerve parasympathetic fibers 287
– nucleus F68.10, F78b.20, F119.3, F139.8, F140.7, F141.5
– systems 388–393
Olfactory bulb 239, 242, 308, 317, 372, 405, 416–418, 420, F2b.24, F3.22, F5a.10, F6b.12, F6d.12, F30b.11, F32a.22, F45b.27, F46.27, F50a.3, F76a.6, F130.1, F131.1, F147.14
– cortex 322
– epithelium 218, 372
– glomeruli 372

– groove syndrome 288
– nerve 218 ,287, 372
– pathway 372
– sulcus 315, F51a.5
– system 372
– tract 308, 317, 322, 372, F32a.22, F2b.25, F3.24, F6a.11, F7a.12, F8a.15, F33a.17, F45b.28, F46.28, F50a.4, F51a.7, F76a.12, F130.2, F131.2, F147.15
– trigone 372, F131.3
– tubercle 372, 416
Olivocerebellar tract 394, F144a.16
Olivocochlear tract (of Rasmussen) 359
Omega form of transverse temporal gyrus (of Heschl) 316
Open portion of medulla oblongata 288
Opened orbit F51c.3
Opening for internal carotid artery 231
– of trigeminal cistern F74b.7
Openings of orbital cavity 218
Opercular part of inferior frontal gyrus 400
Ophthalmic artery 218, 220, 393, F5c.12, F6c.16, F7c.9, F76a.8
– nerve 218, 226, 287, F7a.17, F8a.21, F34a.23, F115.9
– vein 283
Ophthalmoscope 369
Opiate receptors 420
Opisthion 421
Optic canal 217, 218, 226, 236, 239, 361, F21.3, F65.6, F76a.13
– chiasm 218, 242, 305, 361, 362, 369, F2b.20, F8a.16, F8b.15, F8d.15, F32a.24, F32b.18, F32d.18, F45b.29, F51a.8, F67.14, F77b.3, F77c.4, F77d.4, F122.1, F126.4, F127.4, F128.2, F129.3
– disc 226, F4a.8, F127.1
– nerve 217, 218, 226, 287, 361, 369, 393, F2b.26, F5a.11, F6a.16, F6b.10, F6d.10, F7a.13, F7b.14, F7d.14, F8a.17, F32a.23, F33a.18, F34a.20, F35a.18, F49a.2, F50a.5, F50b.5, F50d.5, F75a.9, F76a.14, F76b.1, F77b.2, F77c.1, F77d.1, F126.3, F127.3, F128.1, F128.6, F129.2
– pathway 379
– radiation 361, 362, F126.9, F127.6, F127.8, F128.9, F128.12, F129.6
– – lesion 369
– tract 242, 361, F9a.24, F9b.19, F9d.19, F10a.26, F10b.19, F10d.19, F11a.26, F33a.19, F33b.13, F33d.13, F34a.13, F52a.20, F52b.7, F77b.6, F78b.6, F78c.5, F78d.5, F126.5, F127.5, F128.3, F128.7, F129.4
– – lesion 369
Oral cavity 227, 228, F4a.21, F5a.23, F6a.27, F7a.25, F32a.44, F33a.41, F34a.35, F35a.35, F79, F80
– – proper 227
– part of spinal nucleus of trigeminal nerve 338, F72b.19, F73b.22
– vestibule 227, F36a.28
Orbicularis oculi 219, 375, 379, F4c.19
– oris F33c.34, F34c.32
Orbit 218–226, F18.8, F19.7, F20.3, F30a.6, F40.11, F41.7, F47a.4, F48c.5, F49c.4, F50c.4, F62.4, F63.2, F64.4, F79, F80
Orbital apex syndrome 288, 393
– floor 218
– gyrus(-i) 315, F5a.5, F6a.8, F6b.6, F6d.6, F7a.11, F7b.12, F7d.12, F46.24, F51a.2
– plate 210, F4c.16, F5c.17, F18.6, F19.5, F75a.3

- roof 218
- vein 393
Orbitalis 414, F6c.20, F35c.22
Orbitomeatal plane 4
Oropharynx 230, F32a.48, F33a.45
Otic ganglion 229, 412, 414, F35a.29, F151.12
Otolithic organs 390
Otoliths 349
Oxytocin 305, 419, 420

P

Pain perception disorder 326
Pain-conducting system 420
Palatine bone 211, F47a.8, F61.7
- nerves 414, F6a.26, F34a.26, F115.8
- tonsil 227, F8a.28, F33a.42
Palatoglossal arch 227
Palatoglossus 227, F33c.36, F34c.43
Palatopharyngeal arch 227, 230
Palatopharyngeus 227
Paleocortex 322
Pallidal raphe nucleus 417
Pallidohabenular fibers 385
Pallidonigral tract 419
Papez circuit 323, 405
Paracavernous sinus 283
Paracentral artery F8c.7, F9c.4, F10c.3, F11c.3, F12c.2, F13c.2, F32c.6, F33c.3, F34c.2, F57c.10, F58c.7, F59c.7, F90a,b.11, F91d.11
- lobule 313, 331, 332, 376, F2b.1, F13a.4, F14a.3, F45b.1, F58a.8, F59a.6, F91d.26, F134.2, F135.7
Parahippocampal gyrus 316, 404, F9a.29, F10a.36, F10b.23, F10d.23, F11a.32, F11b.21, F11d.21, F12a.26, F12b.21, F12d.21, F51a.15, F52a.27, F53a.37, F147.21, F148.10, F149.12, F150.7
Paralysis of gaze 388
- - third, fourth, and sixth cranial nerves 388
- - vergence movements 388
- - vertical gaze 392
Paramagnetic substances 16
Paramedian pontine reticular formation 12, 295, 388, F75b.15, F76b.19, F139.10, F140.9, F141.7
- zone of reticular formation 294
Parameters for CT images 424
- - T1-weighted MR images 423
- - T2-weighted MR images 423
Paranasal sinus(-es) 211, 217, 218, F79, F80
Parapharyngeal space 230, 231, F79, F80
Paraplegia 234
Parasympathetic innervation of parotid gland 286
- nervous system of head 412
- part of autonomic nervous system 412
Paraterminal gyrus 322, F32a.7
Paraventricular nucleus 420
Parietal artery F35c.7, F36c.7, F37c.6, F55c.17, F56c.11, F57c.12
- bone 238, F2a.2, F8c.2, F9c.3, F10c.4, F11c.5, F12c.6, F13c.4, F14c.4, F15c.3, F16c.4, F17c.3, F21.1, F22.1, F23.1, F24.1, F25.1, F26.1, F27.1, F28.1, F32c.3, F33c.4, F35c.5, F36c.5, F37c.3, F38.2, F39.2, F40.2, F41.2, F42.2, F43.2, F45a.2, F53c.8, F54c.14, F54d.16, F55c.18, F55d.16, F56c.13, F56d.14, F57c.11, F57d.13, F58c.6, F58d.12, F59c.6, F59d.13, F60c.6, F60d.4, F75a.23, F76a.24, F77a.21, F78a.16
- cortical area 349, F119.1, F120.11, F121.9
- lobe 313, 315, F91c.12, F104a, F104b, F107a, F107b, F108b.7
- operculum 317, 322, 345, F109.2, F117.1, F118.6
Parietoinsular cortex 349
Parieto-occipital artery 256, F15c.7, F16c.6, F17c.2, F32c.14, F33c.10, F34c.6, F55c.21, F56c.16, F57c.15, F89a.10, F91d.18
- cortex 388, F140.15, F141.18
- sulcus 313, 315, 362, F2b.6, F15a.6, F15b.4, F15d.4, F16a.6, F16b.5, F16d.5, F17a.3, F31.16, F32a.2, F32b.4, F33a.6, F33b.9, F33d.9, F34a.4, F34d.8, F45b.6, F54a.39, F55a.25, F55b.21, F56.17, F56b.15, F56d.15, F57a.12, F57d.14, F58a.12, F67.3, F91d.32, F108b.12
Parinaud's syndrome 392
Parkinson's syndrome 385, 416
Parotid duct 229, F6c.26, F7c.24
- gland 229, 414, F8c.24, F9c.34, F10c.30, F37c.28
Pars compacta of substantia nigra 416
- gustatoria of solitary nucleus F117.6
Partial crossing of optic nerve fibers 362
- volume effect 15
Parvocellular nerve cells 361
Pecommissural septum 405
Penetrating arteries 275
- branches of anterior cerebral artery F93, F94, F96
- - - middle cerebral artery F93, F94, F96
- - - posterior cerebral artery F93, F94, F96
- - - - communicating artery F93, F94, F96
Pentagonal cistern 242
Peptidergic neurons 419
Perception of pain and vibration 324
Periamygdaloid cortex 322, 372, F130.4, F130.5, F131.4
Periaqueductal gray substance 416–418, 420, F12a.24
Periarchicortex 322, 404, F148.11, F150.1
- in cingulate gyrus F148.1, F148.2, F149.1, F150.8
Pericallosal artery 267, F7b.7, F7c.4, F7d.7, F8c.8, F9c.5, F10c.6, F11c.8, F12c.7, F32b.3, F32c.9, F55c.8, F56c.10, F90a,b.9, F91d.4
- cistern 238, 242, F83a.1, F84.3, F85.2, F86a.1, F87.17
Periolivary nucleus 419, 420
Peripaleocortex 322
Peripheral paresis of hypoglossal nerve 227
Perisylvian lesions 400
Periventricular gray substance 420
- nuclei of hypothalamus 416
Perpendicular plate 210
PET 12, 17, 378, 415
Petro-occipital synchondrosis F25.9
Petrosal vein 285
Petrous part of temporal bone 237, F49d.10, F50b.19, F50.19, F64.13
Pharyngeal opening of pharyngo-tympanic tube F33c.24, F69b.3
- tonsil 230, 32a.39
- tubercle 231, F23.13, F32c.32, F38.22
Pharyngotympanic tube 230, 237, F34c.26, F69a.12, F71b.2
Pharynx 230, F79, F80
Photopsy 324, 369
Physiologic acoustic window 17
Pia mater 239
PICA 12, 254, 257, 263, F11c.21, F12c.20, F13c.17, F14c.12, F15c.16, F16c.14, F32c.33, F33c.25, F34c.28, F35c.38, F36c.31, F48c.18, F70b.13, F88.2, F88.3, F89a.2
Picture element 14
Pineal gland 252, 306, F2b.19, F12b.16, F12d.16, F13a.14, F32a.12, F32b.16, F32d.16, F45b.17, F54b.22, F54c.18, F54d.22, F67.7, F83a.4, F85.7, F86a.3, F122.6
- recess 252
Pinna 229, F10c.25, F11c.19, F12c.17, F13c.18, F47a.18, F48c.19, F49c.21, F50c.21, F51c.21, F52c.16, F53c.20, F61.16, F62.16, F69a.23, F70a.23, F71a.22, F72a.17, F73a.19, F74a.19, F75a.20
Pituitary gland 307, 361, F2b.27, F8b.17, F8d.17, F9c.14, F32a.27, F32b.24, F32d.24, F45b.30, F50a.7, F50b.11, F67.22, F75a.13, F75c.5, F75d.5
Pixel 2, 14
Plane of fastigium 10
- - orbital roof 4
Plasticity 325
Platysma F5c.36, F6c.40, F7c.33, F8c.39, F9c.43, F33c.45, F37c.42
Ploughshare 210
Pneumoencephalography 1, 14
Polar frontal artery 267, F4c.5, F5c.5, F6c.7, F32c.17, F33c.11, F34c.9, F52c.3, F90a,b.6, F91d.7
- temporal artery of middle cerebral artery F7c.7, F91a,b.16
Pole of frontal lobe F91d.28
- - occipital lobe F75c.12, F75d.12
- - temporal lobe F7a.16, F7b.15, F7d.15, F30b.14, F75c.4, F75d.4
Polysynaptic reflexes 375
Pons 293–298, 348, 412, 414, F2b.37, F3.29, F10a.35, F11a.37, F11b.22, F11d.22, F12a.30, F12b.24, F12d.24, F30b.15, F32a.28, F32b.31, F32d.31, F33a.24, F33b.19, F33d.19, F45b.31, F46.30, F49a.6, F49b.15, F50a.13, F50b.16, F50d.16, F51a.18, F51b.14, F51d.14, F67.25, F73a.16, F74a.15, F74c.6, F74d.6, F75a.16, F75c.8, F75d.8, F76a.18, F76c.9, F76d.9, F98, F99, F100, F101, F102, F103, F122.16, F132.12, F144a.10
Pontine arteries 254
- cistern 239, F74c.5, F74d.5, F83a.11, F84.15, F85.17, F86a.11, F87.4
- nuclei 294, 394, F73b.10, F74b.14, F75b.10, F76b.12
- raphe nucleus 417
Pontocerebellar tract F144a.12
Portal circulation of pituitary gland 307
Portio major of trigeminal nerve 338
Position of slices 210
Positions of neurofunctional systems 325
Positron emission tomography 12, 17, 415

Postcentral gyrus 312, 315, 322, 326, 331, 332, 338, 342, 349, 375, F3.3, F11a.7, F11b.5, F11d.5, F12a.3, F12b.5, F12d.5, F13a.5, F13b.4, F13d.4, F14a.2, F31.12, F33a.2, F33b.3, F33d.3, F34a.3, F34b.4, F34d.4, F35a.3, F35b.4, F35d.4, F36a.5, F36b.4, F36d.4, F37a.4, F37b.4, F37d.4, F46.7, F54a.30, F55a.15, F56a.10, F56b.8, F56d.8, F57a.7, F57b.9, F57d.9, F58a.6, F58b.11, F58d.11, F59a.5, F59b.10, F59d.10, F60a.3, F60b.6, F109.1, F110.4, F111.1, F112.4, F112.12, F113.9, F114.1, F115.14, F115.16, F116.13, F132.1, F133.9, F134.9
– sulcus 313, F3.5, F31.13, F46.1, F56a.11, F57b.10, F57d.10, F58b.13, F59b.11, F59d.11, F108b.4
Posterior acoustic stria F122.24
– arch of atlas 232, F2a.32, F13c.24, F14c.17, F27.9, F28.4, F32c.38, F38.30, F45a.29, F47a.26, F61.17
– ascending ramus of lateral sulcus (Sylvian fissure) F108b.10
– basal cistern 239, F83a.12, F84.23, F85.20, F86a.12, F87.1
– belly of digastric F9c.39, F10c.32, F11c.32, F12c.26, F36c.46, F37c.37
– cerebellomedullary cistern 239, F13a.27, F13b.22, F13d.22, F14a.19, F15a.21, F32b.36, F32d.36, F48b.16, F48d.16, F67.41, F69a.24, F69b.34, F69c.12, F69d.12, F70a.25, F83a.13, F84.28, F85.22, F86a.13, F87.2
– cerebral artery 256, F10c.13, F11c.15, F32c.21, F33b.15, F33c.19, F33d.15, F34c.14, F51c.13, F52b.15, F77b.11, F78b.23, F88.7, F89a.6, F91d.16
– – – fetal type 256
– – – postcommunicating part 256
– – – precommunicating part 256
– choroidal artery F11c.13, F12c.12
– clinoid process 236, F2a.6, F9c.12, F23.3, F33c.18, F39.8, F45a.9, F51a.10, F65.10
– cochlear nucleus 354, 355, 418, F68.7, F72c.26, F122.23, F123.12, F124.9
– commissure 252, 306, 323, F2b.18, F12a.17, F32a.11, F32b.15, F45b.18, F67.8
– communicating artery 265, F10c.11, F51c.12, F76b.3, F88.8, F89a.14, F91c.9, F91d.14
– – – fetal type 265
– cranial fossa 239, F25.5, F26.3, F27.4, F28.2, F38.20, F39.14, F40.19, F41.15, F42.9, F64.15, F65.15
– descending ramus of lateral sulcus (Sylvian fissure) F108b.15
– ethmoidal foramen 219
– funiculus F47a.22
– horn of lateral ventricle 252, F14a.6, F14b.6, F14d.6, F15a.10, F15b.7, F15d.7, F16b.7, F16d.7, F55b.22, F78a.12, F83b.8, F84.29, F85.31, F86b.7, F91c.5, F91d.34, F126.15
– inferior cerebellar artery 12, 254, 263, F11c.21, F12c.20, F13c.17, F14c.12, F15c.16, F16c.14, F32c.33, F33c.25, F34c.28, F35c.38, F36c.31, F48c.18, F70b.13, F88.2, F88.3, F89a.2
– – – artery caudal localization 254
– – temporal artery of posterior cerebral artery F91d.22
– intercavernous sinus F97b.4
– interpositus nucleus 304

– lateral choroidal arteries 256, F52c.14, F53c.16, F54c.16, F55c.15, F78b.33 F89a.8
– limb of internal capsule 306, 323, F11a.15, F34a.14, F53a.19, F53d.17, F54a.20, F54d.20
– lobe of cerebellum 303, 304, F13a.25, F13b.21, F13d.21, F14a.18, F14b.15, F14d.15, F15a.19, F15b.13, F15d.13, F16a.16, F33b.24, F33d.24, F36a.23, F36b.14, F36d.14, F37a.17, F37b.11, F37d.11, F69a.25, F70a.24, F70c.11, F70d.11, F71a.24, F72a.20, F73a.24, F74a.23, F75a.21, F76a.21, F142, F143
– – – pituitary gland 305, 307
– longitudinal fasciculus (of Schütz) 412, 418
– medial choroidal arteries 256, F52c.14, F53c.16, F54c.17, F89a.8
– nasal spine F2a.31, F38.25, F45a.26
– nucleus of vagus nerve 294, 415, 417, 418, F68.18, F70b.25, F71b.26
– parietal artery 270, F14c.5, F15c.5, F16c.3, F91a,b.10
– – cortex F139.1, F140.14, F141.17
– part of auditory pathway 354
– – – pons 294
– pericallosal artery F91d.20
– pharyngeal wall of nasopharynx F9c.29
– – – – oropharynx F9c.35
– quadrangular lobule (H VI) 304
– ramus of lateral sulcus (Sylvian fissure) F3.16, F46.12, F53a.25, F54a.12, F55a.17, F108b.14
– – – sulcus 315
– raphe nucleus 383, 405, 417, 418
– recess of fourth ventricle 293, F73b.31, F73c.13, F73d.13, F74b.33
– root of second cervical spinal nerve F33a.40
– – – spinal nerve F109.9, F111.10
– – – third cervical spinal nerve and ganglion F34a.38
– semicircular canal F49b.13, F65.13, F73a.17
– spinal artery 263
– spinocerebellar tract 394, F69b.27, F70b.26, F144a.19
– tegmental nucleus (of Gudden) 405, 412
– temporal artery of middle cerebral artery F91a,b.13
– territory of medulla oblongata 263
– – – midbrain 263
– – – pons 263
– transverse temporal gyrus 357, F12a.10, F36a.12, F37a.12
– trigeminothalamic tract 338, F114.8, F116.8
– wall of sphenoidal sinus F10a.40
Posterolateral central arteries 256, 275, F89a.7
– fissure 304
– pontine nuclei 388
Posteromedial central arteries 256, 275, F77b.12, F89a.7
– frontal artery F8c.3, F9c.2, F10c.2, F32c.5, F33c.2, F34c.3, F58c.3, F59c.4, F90a,b.10, F91d.10
Postmortem MR images 10
– neuroanatomy 10
Postsynaptical neuromodulators 415
PPRF 12, 295, 388, F75b.15, F76b.19, F139.10, F140.9, F141.7
Precentral artery F11b.3, F11d.3

– gyrus 312, 313, 322, 375, 376, F3.10, F10a.5, F10b.5, F10d.5, F11a.3, F12a.2, F12b.3, F12d.3, F13a.1, F13b.2, F13d.2, F14a.1, F31.10, F33a.1, F33b.2, F33d.2, F34a.2, F34b.3, F34d.3, F35a.2, F35b.2, F35d.2, F36a.3, F36b.2, F36d.2, F37a.2, F37b.3, F37d.3, F46.3, F54a.11, F55a.9, F56a.6, F56b.6, F56d.6, F57a.3, F57b.7, F57d.7, F58a.4, F58b.8, F58d.8, F59a.3, F59b.8, F59d.7, F59d.8, F60a.1, F60b.2, F132.3, F133.6, F133.8, F133.14, F133.15, F134.8, F134.13, F135.4
Precentral sulcus 313, F3.7, F31.8, F36a.2, F37a.5, F46.4, F56a.5, F56b.5, F56d.5, F57b.6, F57d.6, F58a.3, F58d.7, F59a.2, F59b.6, F59d.6, F108b.1
Precommissural septum 309
Precommunicating part of anterior cerebral artery F91c.8
– – – posterior cerebral artery F91c.14
Precuneal artery F11c.6, F12c.4, F13c.5, F14c.2, F15c.4, F16c.2, F32c.7, F33c.6, F57c.13, F58c.8, F59c.8
Precuneus 315, F2b.4, F15a.4, F16a.3, F17a.1, F33a.4, F45b.2, F56a.16, F57a.11, F58a.11, F59a.10, F91d.27
Prefrontal artery 270, F6c.4, F7c.3, F8c.6, F35c.4, F36c.6, F37c.7, F55c.5, F56c.5, F57c.5 F91a,b.6
– cortex 326
Preganglionic neurons of autonomic system 418
Premotor cortex 375, 378, 383, F132.5, F135.5, F144b.1
Preoccipital notch F3.27
Preoptic area 404, 420
Prepiriform cortex 322, 372, 419, F130.4, F131.4, F147.16
Prepositus nucleus 390, F72b.22, F140.12, F141.9
Prerolandic artery 270
Pressure cone 238
Presynaptical neuromodulators 415
Pretectal areas 361
Primary auditory cortex 355, 357
– – – in transverse temporal gyrus (of Heschl) F122.4
– cortical areas 322
– fissure of cerebellum 303, 304, F2b.33, F12a.33, F13a.22, F14a.15, F15a.18, F32a.26, F32b.26, F32d.26, F33b.21, F33d.21, F52a.41, F67.20, F74a.17, F74b.16, F75a.18, F75b.20, F76a.20, F142.2, F144a.9
– intermediate sulcus F108b.11
– motor cortex 322, 375, F132.4, F144b.1
– somatic sensory cortex 332
– – – in paracentral lobule F110.5, F112.12, F113.10
– technical diagnostic tools 1
– visual cortex 315, 362, 388, F15a.8, F16a.10, F17a.7, F33a.11, F34a.18, F54a.43, F55a.28, F77a.23, F78a.15, F126.16, F127.11, F128.10, F129.7, F140.16, F141.2
– – – lesion 369
– – – inferior lip F127.9, F128.5
– – – superior lip F127.10, F128.4
Principal sensory nucleus of trigeminal nerve 294, 338, F68.3, F74b.25, F114.9, F115.19, F116.6
PRL 12, 307
Projection fibers of cerebral cortex 323
– – – hippocampal formation 324
Prolactin 12, 307, 420

Prolactinomas 416
Protons 15
Psychomotor epilepsy 324
Pterygoid canal 236, F21.12
– fossa 236, F21.16
– hamulus 236, F7c.25, F20.16, F34c.34, F39.22, F40.25
– process 236, F40.21, F70a.8
– venous plexus 218, 220, 229, 235, 283, F9c.25, F37c.27, F69b.7
Pterygopalatine fossa 236, F7c.13, F20.7, F21.13, F34c.21, F40.15
– ganglion 218, 412, 414, F151.10
Ptosis 393, 414
Pulley 220
Pulvinar of thalamus 306, 363, F12a.13, F12b.13, F12d.13, F33a.10, F34a.10, F54a.28, F126.11
Pupillary anomalies 393
– constriction 412
– dilatation 414
– reflex 412
Purkinje cells 394, 419, F144b.7
Putamen 308, 309, 323, 383, 385, 416, F8a.12, F8b.10, F8d.10, F9a.14, F9b.12, F9d.12, F10a.16, F10b.13, F10d.13, F11a.16, F34a.7, F34b.10, F34d.10, F35a.10, F35b.5, F35d.5, F53a.13, F53b.10, F53d.10, F54a.17, F54b.10, F54d.10, F55b.10, F132.9, F136.3, F137.11, F138.10
Pyramid of medulla oblongata 288, 377, F30b.24, F48a.3, F48b.8, F69b.19, F69c.7, F69d.7, F70b.10, F70c.7, F70d.7, F71b.8, F71c.5, F71d.5, F72b.7, F72c.4
Pyramidal cells of cerebral cortex 375
– – – hippocampus 419
– – – neocortex 419
– decussation 377, F12a.41, F132.14, F133.11, F134.6
– pathway 375–380, 383
– system 303, 375–380
– tract F144b.2
Pyramis of vermis (VIII) 304, 394, F2b.43, F15a.20, F32a.38, F32b.39, F32d.39, F45b.37, F67.33, F71a.25, F71c.11, F71d.11, F72a.19, F72c.9, F72d.9, F73a.23, F142.6, F143.4

Q

Quadrantanopia 324
Quadrigeminal cistern 242, 298, F52b.20, F52d.20, F53b.21, F53d.21, F83a.7, F84.26, F85.8, F86a.5, F87.19
– plate 298
Quinsy 230

R

Radiofrequency 15
Ramus of mandible 211, 229, F2a.33, F7c.27, F8c.31, F9b.25, F9c.30, F9d.25, F20.17, F21.19, F22.9, F23.16, F30a.22, F37c.30, F42.16, F43.16
Raphe nuclei 416, 420
Rapid eye movements 388
– gradient-echo sequence 15
Recent memory 405
Receptive aphasia 402
Rectus capitis anterior 233, F69b.9
– – posterior major 233, F15c.20
– – – minor 233, F14c.15, F15c.19

Red nucleus 298, 383, 395, F11a.25, F78b.16, F136.8, F137.2, F138.3, F144a.3, F144b.5
Redecussation of pyramidal pathway 397
– – rubrospinal tract 397
References to anatomic structures 13
Reflexes of Babinski group 375
Regulation of sleep 418
Reid's base line (DH) 4, 10, 11, 239, F1a, F2a, F29, F32a, F44, F83b
Release of SP 420
Releasing factor 12, 305
Repetition time 15
Reticular formation 294, 348, 359, 383, 405, 418, 420, F69b.25, F70b.18, F71b.19, F72b.15, F73b.20, F74b.22, F75b.14, F76b.15, F77b.25, F78b.19
– nucleus of thalamus F53a.29
Reticulospinal tract 383
Retina 226, 361, 369, 388, F36a.15, F127.2, F128.11, F129.1
Retinotopic map 362
Retrobulbar space of orbit 369, F49b.3, F49d.3, F50d.3, F76c.3, F76d.3
Retrocochlear hearing impairment 354, 359
Retrolentiform part of acoustic radiation 357
Retromandibular vein 235
Retrosplenial cortex 417
Reversal of direction of blood flow 271
Reward mechanism 416
RF 12, 15, 305
Rhinal sulcus F108b.27
Rhomboid fossa 242, 288
Right-handed individuals 400
Rigidity 383
Rods 226, 361
Rolandic artery 270
Roof of fourth ventricle F13a.23, F84.27
– – midbrain 298
– – mouth 227
– – orbit 237, F4c.9, F5c.6, F18.4, F19.2, F30a.2, F34c.12, F35c.12, F40.7, F41.4, F65.3
Rostral interstitial nucleus of medial longitudinal fasciculus 388, 392, F139.6, F140.4, F141.3

S

Saccades 388
Saccule 348, 390
Sagittal planes 4
– series 421, 422
– slices 5, 93
– suture 238, F58c.9, F59c.9, F60c.7
Salivary glands 414
Salpingopharyngeus 231
Saw cut F38.5, F39.5
Scalp F58c.10, F60c.8
Scintigraphy 16
Sclera 219, 226
Scoutview 4
SE 15
Second accessory loop of basal ganglia 383
– cervical spinal ganglion F12a.45
– – – nerve F3.40, F30b.29
– cranial nerve 287
– molar tooth F4c.26, F5c.27, F18.18, F19.17
Secondary visual cortex 363

Sectioning surfaces of the slices 422
Sector (of Sommer) of the hippocampal formation 256
Sella turcica 236, 361, F45a.10, F65.8
Semicircular ducts 348, 390
Semilunar hiatus 210, 217, F4a.12, F5a.13, F33a.28, F73a.2, F74a.3
Semioval center 324, 342, F56a.14, F56b.12, F56d.12, F57a.8, F57b.11, F57d.11, F58a.7, F58b.10, F58d.10
Semispinalis capitis 232, F16c.17, F17c.12, F33c.32, F34c.37, F35c.39, F36c.39
Sensory aphasia 402
– root of trigeminal nerve 338, F114.5
SEP 12, 342
Septal nuclei 308, 309, 404, 405, 416–420, F53a.20, F147.8, F148.4, F150.9
Septum pellucidum 253, F2b.7, F9a.11, F10a.7, F10d.7, F32a.4, F45b.9, F54d.7, F55d.7
– verum 308, 309, 405
Serial illustrations 12
– slices of equal thickness 3
Serotoninergic neurons 297, 404, 417
Seventh cranial nerve 286
Short central arteries 266
Sigmoid sinus 233, 283, 285, F12c.19, F13c.16, F26.5, F35c.31, F36c.30, F37c.21, F49c.19, F50c.20, F50d.22, F51b.19, F51c.20, F69a.21, F69b.32, F70a.21, F71a.21, F72a.16, F73a.20, F97a.16, F97b.10
Signal intensity of MRI 15
SII 323
Single photon emission computed tomography 12, 17, 415
Sixth cranial nerve 287
Skin of the head F58c.11, F60c.9
Skull base 19, 238
Smooth pursuit eye movements 388, 391
Soft palate 227, F7c.21, F8c.25
Solitary nucleus 294, 345, 417, 418, 420, F68.8, F70b.23, F71b.23, F118.3
Somatic sensory cortex F135.6
– – – of postcentral gyrus F132.1
Somatosensory evoked potentials 12, 342
Somatostatin 419
Somatotopic organization 322, 326, 332
– – of motor cortex 379
Somatotropic cells 307
– hormone 12
Sonography 14, 17
SP 12, 419
Spasticity 324, 375
Spatial configuration of photoreceptors 362
– orientation of an image 18
SP-containing neurons 419
Special notes in atlas section 13
Specific nuclei of thalamus 306
SPECT 12, 17, 415
Speech impairment 380
Sphenoethmoidal recess 217
– suture 236
Sphenofrontal suture 238, F40.8
Sphenoid 236, F8c.19, F9c.18, F10c.21, F21.11, F22.8, F23.11, F24.7, F38.17, F39.13, F40.9, F49c.5, F50c.5, F51c.6, F63.7, F64.6, F65.5, F73a.8, F74a.8, F75a.7, F77a.8

Sphenoidal sinus 217, F2a.12, F7a.19, F8a.23, F8b.19, F8d.19, F9a.34, F9b.24, F9d.24, F10a.40, F20.6, F21.6, F22.7, F23.6, F32a.31, F32b.30, F32d.30, F33a.25, F33b.23, F33d.23, F38.16, F39.10, F45a.13, F48c.8, F49b.4, F49c.7, F49d.4, F50b.7, F50c.8, F50d.7, F63.6, F64.8, F67.24, F72b.1, F73a.11, F73b.1, F73c.1, F73d.1, F74a.10, F74b.1, F74c.1, F74d.1, F75a.12, F75b.1
Spheno-occipital synchondrosis F24.9
Sphenopalatine artery 227
Sphenoparietal sinus 283, F97b.1
– suture 238
Sphenosquamous suture F21.9, F23.7
Sphincter pupillae 226, 287, 412
Spinal cord 418, F2b.46, F3.41, F12a.43, F12b.28, F13a.31, F30b.30, F32a.45, F32b.40, F32d.40, F45a.41, F46.37, F47a.21, F47b.13, F67.43
– dura mater F47a.25
– ganglion 326, 331, 419, F109.10, F111.11
– motor neurons 376
– nucleus of accessory nerve F68.20
– – – trigeminal nerve 294, 338, 415, 420, F68.5, F114.12, F115.20, F116.2
– posterior gray horns 376
– root of accessory nerve F3.39, F33a.38, F46.38, F47a.23, F48a.6, F49a.11, F69b.31, F70b.22
– subarachnoid space F83a.14, F84.24, F85.23
– tract of trigeminal nerve F68.4, F114.13, F116.1
Spin-echo technique 15
Spinoreticular tract 326, F109.8
Spinothalamic tract F69b.24, F70b.17, F71b.17, F72b.18, F73b.18, F74b.19, F75b.17, F76b.17, F77b.29, F78b.29
Spinous process of axis F2a.36, F14c.21, F15c.22, F28.5, F32c.39, F38.34, F45a.31
– – – fifth cervical vertebra F15c.25
– – – fourth cervical vertebra F14c.24, F15c.24, F28.7
– – – third cervical vertebra F14c.23, F28.6, F38.35
Spiral ganglion 354, F122.18
– organ (of Corti) 354, 359
Splenium of corpus callosum 253, 323, F2b.12, F13a.10, F13b.8, F13d.8, F32a.6, F32b.8, F32d.8, F45b.11, F55a.23, F55b.17, F55d.17, F122.8, F126.14
Splenius capitis 232, F14c.19, F15c.21, F16c.18, F17c.13, F33c.38, F34c.38, F35c.44, F36c.40, F37c.35
Squamous part of temporal bone 237
– suture 238, F21.2, F23.2, F24.2, F25.2, F26.2, F27.2
Staggering gait 397
Stapedius 359
Stapes 237
Statins 305
Stellate cells 419
Sternocleidomastoid F9c.45, F10c.35, F11c.39, F12c.32, F13c.27
STH 12
Stirrup 237
Straight gyrus 315, 404, F5a.7, F5b.6, F5d.6, F6a.9, F6b.9, F6d.9, F7a.10, F7b.13, F7d.13, F8a.14, F50a.2, F51a.3, F51b.3, F77a.9, F77c.2, F77d.2
– sinus 236, 283, 284, F14b.4, F14c.7, F14d.4, F15b.5, F15c.9, F15d.5, F16b.8, F16c.10, F16d.8, F32c.23, F53b.26, F53c.23, F54b.28, F54c.24, F55b.20, F55c.22, F55d.20, F75a.24, F76a.23, F77a.20, F78a.14, F78c.14, F78d.14, F97a.13
Stratum subependymale F9a.6
Stria medullaris of thalamus 306, 412
– of Gennari 322
– terminalis 405, F55c.11
Striate area 362
Striatocapsular aphasia 402
Striatonigral tract 419
Striatum 308, 309, 383, 418, 420
Strongly myelinated hypothalamus 305
Styloglossus 231, F8c.30, F9c.32, F35c.42
Stylohyoid 231, F8c.37, F36c.37
– ligament F8c.35, F9c.38, F10c.29, F22.11, F23.17, F24.14
Styloid process 227, 237, F11c.27, F24.11, F25.14, F30a.17, F36c.33, F42.14, F47a.12, F47b.10, F61.11
Stylomastoid foramen 229, 237, F11c.28, F42.13
Stylopharyngeus 231, F9c.40
Subarachnoid space 239
Subcallosal area 316, 404, F52a.11, F147.6, F148.3, F149.2, F150.4
Subclavian vein 235
Subdivisions of brain 288–324
Subdural hematoma 283
Subiculum 322, 404, 418, F147.20
Sublingual artery F4c.31, F5c.33, F6c.34, F7c.29
– gland 414, F4c.32, F5c.29, F33c.40
– vein F4c.31
Submandibular duct F4c.28, F5c.30, F6c.32
– ganglion 229, 412, 414, F151.14
– gland 414, F6c.36, F7c.32, F8c.32, F36c.47, F37c.43
Submental artery 228 ,4c.36, F5c.35, F6c.35, F7c.31
– vein F4c.36, F5c.35, F6c.35, F7c.31
Subnuclei of thalamus 305, 418
Suboccipital nerve 233, F13a.28
– venous plexus 233, F13c.23, F14c.22, F15c.23
Substance P 12, 417, 419
Substantia innominata 420
– nigra 298, 375, 383, 418, F11a.28, F33a.20, F52a.29, F77b.21, F78b.15, F132.10, F136.10, F137.3, F137.8, F138.2
Subthalamic nucleus 305, 383, 385, F11a.22, F33a.15, F136.9, F137.1, F137.7, F138.7
Subthalamopallidal tract 419
Subthalamus 305
Sulci of cerebral hemispheres 422
Superficial abdominal reflexes 375
– lateral facial region 229
– middle cerebral vein 283, F52c.5, F53c.9, F97a.3
– temporal artery 220, 229, 235, F9c.20
– – – frontal branch F6c.13, F7c.12, F8c.17
– veins of brain 283
Superior bulb of internal jugular vein F70b.7, F71b.12
– central nucleus 405, 417
– cerebellar artery 255, 256, 264, F10c.18, F11c.17, F12c.16, F13c.13, F14c.8, F15c.12, F32c.22, F33b.16, F33c.20, F33d.16, F34c.18, F35c.24, F36c.21, F51c.16, F76b.10, F88.6, F89a.5
– cistern 239, F14b.5, F14d.5, F83a.8, F84.30, F85.16, F86a.6, F87.20
– peduncle 298, 304, 395, F51a.22, F51b.18, F75b.25, F76b.21, F144a.6, F144b.6
– cerebral vein 283, F54c.3, F55c.3, F56c.3, F57c.3, F58c.4, F59c.5, F60c.4, F97a.1
– cervical ganglion 414, F10a.41, F34a.36, F35a.34, F151.11, F151.13
– choroid vein 283, F55c.12
– colliculus 298, 359, 361, 388, 417, F2b.21, F32a.18, F45b.19, F53b.20, F67.12, F78b.31, F78c.12, F78d.12, F126.12, F139.7, F140.6, F141.4
– frontal gyrus 313, F3.1, F4a.2, F4b.4, F4d.4, F5a.1, F5b.4, F5d.4, F6a.2, F6b.2, F6d.2, F7a.2, F7b.4, F7d.4, F8a.1, F8b.2, F8d.2, F9a.1, F9b.2, F9d.2, F10a.1, F10b.2, F10d.2, F11a.1, F11b.2, F11d.2, F12a.1, F12b.2, F12d.2, F30b.4, F31.3, F33a.3, F33b.4, F33d.4, F34a.1, F34b.2, F34d.2, F46.6, F52a.1, F52b.2, F53a.1, F53b.2, F53d.2, F54a.1, F54b.1, F54d.1, F55a.1, F55b.2, F55d.2, F56a.1, F56b.2, F57a.1, F57b.3, F57d.3, F58a.1, F58b.5, F58d.5, F59a.1, F59b.4, F59d.4, F133.1
– – sulcus 313, F3.2, F30b.2, F31.7, F46.8, F58b.4, F58d.4, F59b.5, F59d.5, F108b.5
– ganglion of glossopharyngeal nerve 345
– genu of central sulcus F108b.3
– hypophysial arteries 307
– laryngeal nerve F10a.45
– lip of primary visual cortex 361
– longitudinal fasciculus 400, F145.1
– margin of cerebral hemisphere 307
– – – petrous part of temporal bone 237, F2a.10, F24.3, F30a.10, F45a.14
– medullary velum 242
– nasal concha 210
– – meatus 217
– oblique 220, F4c.12, F5c.9, F6b.11, F6c.12, F6d.11, F76a.5, F77a.5
– olivary nucleus 355, F73b.19, F122.17, F123.11, F124.7
– ophthalmic vein 220, F4c.11, F5c.11, F6c.9, F7c.10
– orbital fissure 218, 226, 239, 287, F20.4, F21.5, F30a.7, F34c.17, F50c.6, F64.7, F75a.11
– parietal lobule 315, F3.6, F14b.2, F14d.2, F15a.1, F15b.2, F15d.2, F16a.1, F16b.3, F16d.3, F31.15, F46.5, F58a.9, F58b.14, F58d.14, F59a.9, F59b.12, F59d.12
– petrosal sinus 283, F51c.19, F75b.7, F97b.7
– portion of medulla oblongata 288
– – – pons 293
– – – skull 238
– precuneal artery F90a,b.12, F91d.12
– rectus 219, F4c.13, F5c.10, F6b.8, F6c.11, F6d.8, F35c.17, F76a.10, F77a.6
– sagittal sinus 236, 283, 284, F4b.1, F4c.1, F5b.1, F5c.1, F6b.1, F6c.1, F7b.1, F7c.1, F7d.1, F8b.1, F8c.1, F8d.1, F9b.1, F9c.1, F9d.1, F10b.1, F10c.1, F10d.1, F11b.1, F11c.1, F11d.1, F12b.1, F12c.1, F12d.1, F13b.1, F13c.1, F13d.1, F14b.1, F14c.1, F14d.1, F15b.1, F15c.1, F15d.1, F16b.1, F16c.1, F16d.1, F17b.1, F17c.1, F17d.1, F32b.1, F32c.2, F32d.1, F53b.27,

F53c.2, F53d.27, F54b.29, F54c.2, F54d.29, F55b.24, F55c.2, F55d.24, F56b.17, F56c.2, F56d.17, F57b.2, F57c.2, F57d.2, F58b.2, F58c.2, F58d.2, F59b.2, F59c.2, F60b.1, F60c.5, F60d.1, F75a.26, F76a.27, F76c.12, F76d.12, F77a.27, F77c.16, F78a.20, F78c.16, F78d.16, F97a.2, F97b.13
– salivatory nucleus 294, 414, F68.16, F151.3
– semilunar lobules (H VII A) 304
– tarsal muscle 219
– temporal gyrus 315, 400, F3.19, F8a.13, F8b.12, F8d.12, F9a.19, F9b.16, F9d.16, F10a.19, F10b.16, F10d.16, F11a.20, F11b.15, F11d.15, F12a.15, F12b.15, F12d.15, F13a.12, F13b.11, F13d.11, F14a.8, F14b.7, F14d.7, F30b.8, F36a.13, F37a.10, F37b.7, F37d.7, F46.20, F51a.4, F51b.5, F52a.10, F52b.5, F52d.5, F53a.27, F53b.14, F53d.14, F54a.31, F54b.15, F55a.20
– – sulcus 315, F3.20, F9a.22, F14a.7, F30b.9, F37a.14, F46.23
– thalamostriate vein 283, F9c.7, F10c.8, F11c.9, F12c.8, F13c.8, F55c.11, F97a.7
– thyroid artery 231, 234, F9c.44
– vestibular nucleus 349, F74b.30, F119.8
Supplementary areas 323
– auditory area 323
– eye field 388, F139.2, F140.3, F141.1
– motor area 323, 375, 400, F133.5, F134.1
– somatic sensory area 323, 326
– visual area 323
Suprachiasmatic nucleus 420
Supramarginal gyrus 315, 400, F3.9, F12a.6, F12b.9, F12d.9, F13a.7, F14a.5, F14b.3, F14d.3, F31.11, F36a.6, F37a.6, F37b.5, F37d.5, F46.9, F56a.13, F56b.13, F57a.9
Supraoptic recess 252, F83b.7, F85.10, F86b.8
Supraorbital nerve 226, F4a.6, F5a.8, F115.1
Supraorbitomeatal plane 5
Suprapineal recess 252, F83b.5, F84.21, F85.6, F86b.5
Suprasellar cistern 242, F87.9
Supratentorial space 5, 238
Surgical intervention 1, 238
Swallowing impairment 380
Sylvian fissure 313, F8a.11, F9a.13, F9b.14, F9d.14, F10a.18, F10b.15, F10d.15, F11a.19, F11b.12, F11d.12, F12b.10, F12d.10, F13a.8, F13b.7, F13d.7, F30b.7, F36a.8, F37a.9, F37b.8, F37d.8, F46.18, F52a.7, F53b.8, F53d.8, F108b.17
Sympathetic fibers in the wall of external carotid artery F151.18
– – – – of internal carotid artery F151.6
– – – – of vertebral artery F151.5
– nervous system of head 414
– part of autonomic nervous system 412
– trunk 231, F10a.43, F11a.46, F35a.36, F151.15
Synapses 415
Syndrome of apex of petrous part of temporal bone 288
– – sphenoid wing 288
– – superior orbital fissure 288, 392, 393

Syndromes of cranial nerves 287
Syntactic aphasia 402

T

T1-weighted MR images 1, 15, 423
T2-weighted MR images 1, 15, 423
Table 1 304
– 2 421
– 3 423
– 4 423
– 5 424
Tail of caudate nucleus 253, 308, F11a.29, F12a.20, F13a.11, F35a.11, F53a.33, F54a.34, F54b.24, F55a.22, F132.6, F136.11, F136.12, F137.10, F138.8
Tarsal muscle 414
TE 12
Tectal plate 298, F32b.21, F32d.21
Tectospinal tract 383
Tectum of midbrain 298, F144a.4
Tegmen tympani 237
Tegmentum of medulla oblongata 417
– – midbrain 298, 355, 388, 412, 417, F32a.17, F32b.20, F32d.20, F52a.30, F52b.14, F52d.14, F67.15, F77a.15, F77c.11, F77d.11, F78a.9, F78c.9, F78d.9
– – pons 294, 417
Tela choroidea of third ventricle 252
Telencephalic nuclei 308
Telencephalon 307–324
Temperature perception disorder 326
Temporal artery of middle cerebral artery F8c.14, F9c.16, F10c.16, F11c.12, F12c.11, F13c.9, F36c.16, F37c.11, F51c.8, F52c.8, F53c.10
– – – posterior cerebral artery F11c.16, F35c.19, F89a.13
– bone 237, F8c.16, F9c.19, F10c.20, F11c.18, F12c.18, F13c.15, F21.8, F22.6, F23.5, F24.5, F25.8, F26.4, F27.5, F34c.22, F35c.28, F36c.29, F40.17, F41.13, F42.12, F43.12, F49c.8, F50c.19, F51c.18, F51d.17, F52c.11, F53c.14, F63.9, F64.14, F65.14, F66.3, F70a.22, F71a.18, F72a.12, F73a.18, F74a.20, F75a.19, F76a.17, F77a.11, F78a.8
– genu of optic radiation F126.6
– horn of lateral ventricle 252, 253, 361, F9b.21, F9d.21, F10a.29, F10b.21, F10d.21, F11a.24, F11b.19, F11d.19, F12a.21, F12b.18, F12d.18, F35b.8, F35d.8, F51a.13, F51b.10, F52a.31, F52b.13, F76b.8, F76c.7, F76d.7, F77b.20, F78b.26, F78c.13, F78d.13, F83b.10, F84.14, F85.35, F86b.10, F91c.11, F91d.37, F126.7
– lobe 313, 315, F2b.36, F45b.35, F50a.6, F50d.8, F51b.9, F51d.9, F52a.8, F53a.26, F74a.12, F74c.3, F74d.3, F91c.6, F91d.38, F104a, F104b, F107a, F107b, F108b.20, F122.2, F126.8
– – epilepsy 372
– operculum 317
– plane 316, 357, 358, F37a.13
Temporalis 228, F4c.6, F5c.16, F6c.18, F7c.15, F8c.18, F9c.15, F10c.15, F36c.23, F37c.10, F69a.8, F70a.7, F71a.7, F72a.8, F73a.9, F74a.13, F75a.14, F76a.16, F77a.10, F77d.3, F78a.5
Temporomandibular joint 228, F23.9, F71a.10
Temporo-occipital artery 270, F15c.10, F16c.9, F17c.6, F35c.15, F36c.14, F37c.9, F54c.15, F91a,b.12

Temporopontine tract 303, F77b.18, F78b.13
Tendon of lateral rectus F4c.18
Tensor tympani 287
– veli palatini 227, 237, F7c.22, F34c.31
Tenth cranial nerve 286
Tentorial incisura 20, 238
– notch 20, 238
Tentorium of cerebellum 236, 238, 315, F11a.36, F12a.29, F13a.17, F14a.12, F15a.17, F15c.14, F16a.14, F16c.11, F16d.11, F32a.21, F33a.21, F36a.20, F51a.19, F51c.17, F52a.40, F52c.17, F53a.40, F53c.21, F54a.40, F54c.23, F73a.25, F74a.24, F75a.22, F75b.19, F76a.22, F76b.25, F77a.19, F78a.13
Terminal branches of anterior cerebral artery F92a, F92b, F93, F94, F95a, F95b, F96
– – – middle cerebral artery F92a, F92b, F93, F94 F95a, F95b, F96
– – – posterior cerebral artery F92a, F92b, F93, F94, F95a, F95b, F96
– part of basilar artery F91c.7, F91d.15
– – – internal carotid artery F91c.10, F91d.1
– territories of anterior cerebral artery 277
– – – forebrain 271–278
– – – middle cerebral artery 277
– – – osterior cerebral artery 278
– vein 283, F9c.7, F10c.8, F11c.9, F12c.8, F13c.8, F97a.7
Terminologia Anatomica 11, 288
Terminology 11
Thalamic dysfunctions 307
Thalamoparietal fibers 331, 332, F109.3, F110.3, F111.2, F112.1, F112.5, F113.8, F114.2, F115.15, F116.12
Thalamus 252, 306, 323, F11b.9, F11d.9, F33b.11, F33d.11, F34b.9, F34d.9, F53b.18, F53d.18, F54b.19, F54d.19, F55a.18, F55b.13, F55d.13, F122.5, F144a.1
Therapy control 1
Third accessory loop of basal ganglia 383
– cervical vertebra F10c.34, F24.17, F25.21, F30a.24, F32c.43, F38.36, F39.26, F40.29, F41.22
– cranial nerve 287
– occipital nerve F13a.30, F14a.21, F15a.23, F16a.18
– ventricle 252, 305, F2b.15, F9a.23, F9b.17, F9d.17, F10a.24, F10b.18, F10d.18, F11a.21, F11b.14, F11d.14, F32a.10, F32b.14, F32d.14, F45b.16, F52a.18, F52b.6, F52d.6, F53a.28, F53b.15, F53c.13, F53d.15, F54a.35, F54b.18, F54c.13, F54d.18, F67.6, F78b.4, F78c.6, F78d.6, F83b.4, F84.8, F85.12, F86b.4, F87.14, F91c.3, F91d.30, F108b.25, F122.3
Three terraces of cranial fossae 239
Three-dimensional coordinate systems 4–10
– knowledge of anatomic structures 210
Thrombosis of cerebral veins 285
– – venous sinuses 285
Thyroid cartilage F7c.36, F8c.41, F9c.46, F10c.39, F22.13, F23.20, F40.33
Thyroliberin 419
Thyrotropic cells 307
– hormone 12, 307

Time of echo 12
- of repetition 12
Tongue 227, F4a.22, F5a.24, F6a.28, F6b.20, F7a.26, F7b.17, F32a.47, F33a.43, F34a.37
Tonsil of cerebellum (H IX) 304, F2b.45, F3.36, F30b.25, F32a.41, F32b.37, F32d.37, F33a.33, F45b.40, F46.36, F48a.9, F48b.14, F48d.14, F49a.17, F67.38, F69a.22, F69b.33, F69c.11, F69d.11, F70c.10, F70d.10, F142.9, F143.1
Tonsillar herniation 238
Topogram 4
Topographic pattern of fifth through twelfth cranial nerve nuclei 294
Topography of craniocervical junction 230–235
- – facial skeleton 210–229
- – neurocranium 236–238
- – neurofunctional systems 3
- – pharynx 230, 231
- – sensory disorders 342
TR 12, 15
Transcranial magnetic stimulation 380
Transition of aqueduct into fourth ventricle F52a.33, F87.16
Transmitter receptor 415
Transverse cerebral fissure 307, F16d.11
- ligament of atlas 232, 234, F32c.37
- occipital sulcus F108b.18
- process of atlas F25.18, F30a.21, F35c.36, F36c.34, F41.19, F42.15
- – – axis F30a.23
- sinus 236, 283, 285, F14b.13, F14c.11, F14d.13, F15b.11, F15c.15, F15d.11, F16b.12, F16c.13, F16d.12, F17b.6, F17c.9, F17d.6, F33b.22, F33c.22, F33d.22, F34c.19, F35c.25, F36c.20, F37b.10, F37c.14, F37d.10, F52c.19, F73a.26, F74a.22, F97a.15, F97b.11
- temporal gyrus (of Heschl) 315, 324, 357, F11a.18, F11b.13, F11d.13, F12a.14, F12b.14, F12d.14, F36b.8, F36d.8, F54a.32, F54d.21, F55a.21, F55b.15, F55.15, F123.3, F123.5, F125.9
- X-ray tomographic procedure 14
Trapezius 232, F16c.20, F17c.15, F33c.33, F34c.39, F35c.45, F36c.41, F37c.36
Trapezoid body 355, F122.21, F124.3, F125.3
Tremor 303, 383, 385
Triangle in paracentral lobule 332
Triangular area (of Wernicke) 331
- part of inferior frontal gyrus 313, 400
- – – trigeminal nerve F74b.8
Trigeminal (Gasserian) ganglion 242, 287, 338, 419, F9a.31, F34a.28, F73b.3, F114.4, F115.11, F116.5
- cistern 242, F84.11, F85.32, F87.5
- impression 237, F74b.4
- lemniscus 342, F114.7, F115.18, F116.9
- nerve 287, 293, 338, F10a.37, F11a.38, F30b.16, F33a.26, F34a.25, F50a.10, F73b.4, F74c.7, F74d.7, F75a.15, F75b.11, F75b.13, F75c.9, F75d.9, F114.V, F115.13, F116.V, F144a.11
- neuralgia 287
- system 338–342
Trigeminothalamic tract from principal sensory nucleus of trigeminal nerve F114.10, F116.7
Trochlea 220, F77a.3
Trochlear nerve 220, 226, 287, 298, F6a.10, F7a.14, F8a.19, F9a.28, F10a.32, F11a.33, F12a.25, F34a.22, F51a.16, F52a.35, F76b.14, F77b.24, F81
- nucleus 298, F68.11, F77b.27, F119.4, F139.9, F140.8, F141.6
Truncal ataxia 304, 397
Trunk of corpus callosum 323, F2b.5, F9a.7, F10a.6, F10b.6, F10d.6, F11a.6, F11b.6, F11d.6, F12a.8, F12b.7, F12d.7, F33b.7, F33d.7, F45b.5, F55a.8
TSH 12, 307
Tuber cinereum 305, 416
- of vermis (VII B) 304, F2b.42, F67.31, F141.12, F142.5
Tuberculum sellae 236, F38.10
Tuberoinfundibular dopaminergic system 305
- neurons 415
- system 416
Turkish saddle 236
Twelfth cranial nerve 286
Tympanic cavity 229, 237, F11c.22, F36c.27, F42.8, F49c.12, F50c.16
- membrane 229, F11c.23, F49c.13
- part of temporal bone 237

U

Ultrasound diagnosis 2
- examination of brain 17
- scanning 1
- techniques 17, 18
Uncinate seizure 372
Uncus of parahippocampal gyrus 316, F34a.17, F52a.25, F149.9, F150.6
Unilateral cerebellar lesions 397
Upper eyelid F35a.15, F75a.1, F76a.1
- jaw 211
- parietal cortex 375
Utricle 348, 390
Uvula of palate 227, 230, F8a.26, F8c.29, F32a.46
- – vermis (IX) 304, F2b.41, F14a.16, F32a.37, F32b.38, F32d.38, F45b.36, F50a.18, F67.32, F71a.23, F71c.9, F71d.9, F72a.18, F72b.27, F72c.8, F72d.8, F73a.22, F142.7, F143.3

V

Vagus nerve 228, 231, 286, 345, 414, F3.33, F10a.42, F11a.42, F12a.36, F30b.23, F33a.34, F34a.31, F35a.30, F36a.27, F37a.21, F46.34, F49a.9, F68.X, F69b.12, F70b.5, F71b.18, F71c.7, F71d.7, F81, F82, F114.X, F117.X, F118.1
- – parasympathetic nerve 286
Var. 12
Variability of arteries 253
Variant 12
Vasoactive intestinal polypeptide 12, 420
Vasopressin 305, 419, 420
Vasopressor center 417
Veins in head and neck 235
- of brain 283–285
- – orbit 220
Velum palatinum 227
Venous angle 283, F97a.8
- plexus of foramen ovale F97b.6
Ventral anterior nucleus of thalamus 383, F144b.4
- cochlear nucleus F68.7, F72b.26, F122.20, F123.12, F124.9
Ventral intermediate nucleus of thalamus 349, F119.2, F120.1, F121.7
- lateral nucleus of thalamus 306, 383, 395, F11a.14, F54a.25, F136.6, F137.6, F138.9, F144b.3
- posterolateral nucleus of thalamus 306, 326, 331, 349, F34a.9, F53a.30, F109.5, F110.2, F111.3, F112.2, F113.7
- posteromedial nucleus of thalamus 306, 338, 342, 345, F114.3, F115.17, F116.11, F117.3, F118.5
- root of fifth cervical spinal nerve F12a.47
- – – first cervical spinal nerve F3.38, F12a.42, F30b.28, F33a.39, F34a.34, F47a.20
- – – second cervical spinal nerve F12a.44, F33a.40
- – – third cervical spinal nerve and ganglion F34a.38
Ventricles 242
Ventricular system guideline structures 19, 20
Ventriculography 1, 14
VEP 12, 369
Vergence movements 388, 390
Vermis of anterior lobe of cerebellum F13b.16, F13d.16, F14b.12, F14d.12, F15b.10, F15d.10, F16b.13, F16d.13, F52a.38, F52b.21, F52d.21, F53a.41, F53b.25, F54a.41, F54b.27, F77c.15, F77d.15, F144a.7
- – cerebellum (I – X) 303, 304, 394, F14b.14, F14d.14, F15b.12, F15d.12, F50a.19, F50b.23, F50d.23, F51a.25, F51b.21, F51d.21
Vernet's syndrome 288
Vertebral artery 233, 254, F11b.25, F11c.25, F11d.25, F12b.29, F12c.21, F12d.29, F13c.21, F32c.31, F33c.26, F34c.36, F35c.37, F47b.14, F48b.7, F48c.15, F48d.7, F49b.9, F49d.9, F69b.18, F69c.6, F69d.6, F70b.8, F70c.6, F70d.6, F71b.6, F71c.4, F71d.4, F72b.6, F72c.3, F72d.3, F88.1, F89a.1
- – V3- V4- segment 254
- – V3 segment F47a.24
- canal F26.13, F38.26, F61.15
- vein 233, F12c.27, F13c.20
Vertigo 349
Vessels of nasal cavity 218
Vestibular fold F8c.40
- ganglion 349, 390
- nerve 349, F119.10, F120.3, F121.3
- nuclei 294, 388, 390, 394, 395, F68.6, F72b.24, F73b.26, F120.7, F121.4, F140.10, F144b.10
- reflexes 349
- system 348, 349
Vestibule F24.4, F49b.12
Vestibulocerebellar tract 394
Vestibulocochlear nerve 286, 355, F3.30, F11a.40, F11b.23, F11d.23, F12a.35, F30b.20, F33a.30, F34a.30, F35a.28, F35b.14, F35d.14, F50a.15, F50d.14, F72b.20, F73b.15, F73c.8, F73d.8
Vestibulo-ocular reflexes 349, 388, 391
Vestibulospinal pathways 383
Vestibulothalamic tract F119.5, F120.2, F120.5, F121.6
VIP 12, 420
VIP-containing neurons 420
Visceral brain 404
Visual auditory conversion language area 400
- axis 219
- cortex 388

- evoked potentials 12, 369
- system 361–369
Vocal fold F8c.42
Vomer 210
Voxel 1

W

Wada-test 404
Wall of eyeball 226
Wallenberg tract 338
Wallenberg's syndrome 264, 297, 298, 342
Weakly myelinated hypothalamus 305

Wernicke-Mann's syndrome 375
Wernicke's aphasia 277, 324, 402
- area 323, 400, F145.3, F146.2
Whiplash 233
White commissure of spinal cord F109.11
- matter of telencephalon 308, 323
Window level 14
- width 14
Wing of central lobule (H II, H III) 304

X

X-ray density 14

Z

Zona incerta 305, 306
Zygomatic arch 228, 237, F2a.15, F6c.21, F7c.14, F8c.20, F20.9, F21.14, F48c.7, F48d.3, F62.7, F72a.7
- bone 211, F2a.19, F4c.17, F5c.21, F18.11, F19.12, F30a.8, F37c.13, F43.6, F47a.5, F47b.4, F48c.3, F49c.2, F61.5, F62.5, F63.3, F69a.4, F70a.5, F71a.4, F72a.5, F73a.5, F74a.5